Audiology
Diagnosis

Audiology
Diagnosis

Edited by

Ross J. Roeser, Ph.D.
Professor and Director
Callier Center for Communication Disorders
School of Human Development
University of Texas at Dallas
Dallas, Texas

Michael Valente, Ph.D.
Professor of Clinical Otolaryngology
Division of Audiology
Department of Otolaryngology–Head and Neck Surgery
Washington University School of Medicine
St. Louis, Missouri

Holly Hosford-Dunn, Ph.D.
President
Tucson Audiology Institute, Inc.
Managing Member
Arizona Audiology Network, LLC
Tucson, Arizona

2000
Thieme
New York • Stuttgart

Thieme New York
333 Seventh Avenue
New York, NY 10001

Audiology: Diagnosis
Ross J. Roeser, Ph.D.
Michael Valente, Ph.D.
Holly Hosford-Dunn, Ph.D.

Senior Medical Editor: Andrea Seils
Editorial Director: Avé McCracken
Editorial Assistant: Thomas Soper
Director, Production and Manufacturing: Anne Vinnicombe
Senior Production Editor: Eric L. Gladstone
Marketing Director: Phyllis Gold
Sales Manager: Ross Lumpkin
Chief Financial Officer: Seth S. Fishman
President: Brian D. Scanlan
Cover Designer: Kevin Kall
Compositor: V&M Graphics, Inc.
Printer: Maple-Vail

Library of Congress Cataloging-in-Publication Data

Audiology : diagnosis / edited by Ross J. Roeser, Michael Valente, Holly Hosford-Dunn.
    p. ; cm.
   Companion volume to: Audiology : treatment, and Audiology : practice management.
   Includes bibliographical references and index.
   ISBN 0-86577-857-4 (TNY)—ISBN 313116431X (GTV)
   1. Hearing disorders—Diagnosis.   2. Audiometry.   I. Roeser, Ross J.   II. Valente, Michael.
III. Hosford-Dunn, Holly.
   [DNLM: 1. Hearing Disorders—diagnosis.   WV 270 A912 2000]
RF294 .A824 2000
617.8'075—dc21   99-052571

Important note: Medical knowledge is ever-changing. As new research and clinical experience broaden our knowledge, changes in treatment and drug therapy may be required. The authors and editors of the material herein have consulted sources believed to be reliable in their efforts to provide information that is complete and in accord with the standards accepted at the time of publication. However, in view of the possibility of human error by the authors, editors, or publisher of the work herein, or changes in medical knowledge, neither the authors, editors, publisher, nor any other party who has been involved in the preparation of this work, warrants that the information contained herein is in every respect accurate or complete, and they are not responsible for any errors or omissions or for the results obtained from use of such information. Readers are encouraged to confirm the information contained herein with other sources. For example, readers are advised to check the product information sheet included in the package of each drug they plan to administer to be certain that the information contained in this publication is accurate and that changes have not been made in the recommended dose or in the contraindications for administration. This recommendation is of particular importance in connection with new or infrequently used drugs.

Some of the product names, patents, and registered designs referred to in this book are in fact registered trademarks or proprietary names even though specific reference to this fact is not always made in the text. Therefore, the appearance of a name without designation as proprietary is not to be construed as a representation by the publisher that it is in the public domain.

Printed in the United States of America

5   4   3   2   1

TNY ISBN 0-86577-857-4

GTV ISBN 3-13-116431-X

Contents

Principles of Diagnostic Audiology

Applications in Diagnostic Audiology

Behavioral Applications

Physiologic Applications

Future Directions

Preface

This book is on the topic of diagnostic audiology, and is one in a series of three texts prepared to represent the breadth of knowledge covering the multi-faceted profession of audiology in a manner that has not been attempted before. The companion books to this volume are *Treatment* and *Practice Management.* In total, the three books provide a total of 73 chapters covering material on the range of subjects and current knowledge audiologists must have to practice effectively. Because many of the chapters in the three books relate to each other, our readers are encouraged to have all three of them in their libraries, so that the broad scope of the profession of audiology is made available to them.

A unique feature of all three books is the insertion of highlighted boxes (pearls, pitfalls, special considerations, and controversial points) in strategic locations. These boxes emphasize key points authors are making and expand important concepts that are presented.

The 26 chapters in this book cover all aspects of diagnostic audiology. In the first chapter, we review diagnostic procedures as they relate to the profession of audiology. Included in Chapter 1 is a review of the scope of practice in audiology, specifically as it relates to diagnostic procedures; a review of the classical diagnostic audiological tests; and a presentation on the effectiveness of classical diagnostic audiological tests. Two additional topics in Chapter 1 are whether audiologists have the prerogative to diagnose hearing loss and the issue of how we refer to those we serve, whether it be "patients" or "clients."

Chapters 2 through 10 present basic and advanced information on fundamental principles in diagnostic audiology including: anatomy and physiology of the auditory and vestibular systems, disorders of the auditory system, radiology and functional brain imaging, pharmacology, acoustics and psychoacoustics, and instrumentation and calibration. An example of the expanding scope of practice for the profession of audiology is that the topics of radiology, brain imaging, and pharmacology have never been included in an audiology textbook.

Diagnostic audiological procedures are reviewed in Chapters 11 through 24. The diverse topics covered in these chapters include: pure tone tests, clinical masking, speech audiometry, central auditory tests in children and adults, middle ear measures, clinical electrophysiology, otoacoustic emissions, neonatal hearing screening, intraoperative monitoring, and assessment of vestibular function.

In Chapter 25 a new dimension in diagnostic audiology, genetics, is reviewed. Finally, in Chapter 26 insights into the future of diagnostic audiological procedures are provided by several leading audiologists.

This book could not have been completed without the tireless efforts of Ms. Debbie Moncrieff and Dr. Jackie Clark. Ms. Moncrieff, a doctoral candidate at UTDallas/Callier Center, assisted as an editorial consultant in reading and editing chapters. Her suggestions added immensely to the quality of the material in the chapters. Dr. Clark co-authored a chapter and added many substantive comments to several chapters; her input was invaluable.

The three of us were brought together by Ms. Andrea Seils, Senior Medical Editor at Thieme Medical Publishers, Inc. During the birthing stage of the project Andrea encouraged us to think progressively—out of the box. She reminded us repeatedly to shed our traditional thinking and concentrate on the new developments that have taken place in audiology in recent years and that will occur in the next 5 to 10 years. With Andrea's encouragement and guidance, each of us set out what some would have considered to be the impossible—to develop a series of three cutting-edge books that would cover the entire profession of audiology *in a period of less than 2 years.* Not only did we accomplish our goal, but as evidenced by the comprehensive nature of the material covered in the three books, we exceeded our expectations! We thank Andrea for her support throughout this 2-year project.

The authors who were willing to contribute to this book series have provided outstanding material that will assist audiologists in-training and practicing audiologists in their quest for the most up-to-date information on the areas that are covered. We thank them for their diligence in following our guidelines for preparing their manuscripts and their promptness in following our demanding schedule.

The consideration of our families for their endurance and patience with us throughout the duration of the project must be recognized. Our spouses and children understood our mission when we were away at editorial meetings; they were patient when we stayed up late at night and awoke in the wee hours of the morning to eke out a few more paragraphs; they tolerated the countless hours we were away from them. Without their support and encouragement we would never have finished our books in the timeframe we did.

Finally, each of us thanks our readers for their support of this book series. We would welcome comments and suggestions on this book, as well as the other two books in the series. Our email addresses are below.

Ross J. Roeser—*roeser@callier.utdallas.edu*
Michael Valente—*valentem@msnotes.wustl.edu*
Holly Hosford-Dunn—*tucsonaud@aol.com*

Acknowledgments

The editors of this book series, Ross J. Roeser, Ph.D., Michael Valente, Ph.D., and Holly Hosford-Dunn, Ph.D., would like to extend their deepest gratitude to the following companies and manufacturers who, through the generosity of their financial support, helped defray the costs incurred by our hard-working authors in the development of their contributions.

Beltone Electronics
Oticon
Siemens
Sonus USA, Inc.
Starkey Labs
Widex Hearing Aid Company

Contributors

Kathryn A. Albright, M.S.
Hearing Health Institute
Fort Worth, TX

Prudence Allen, Ph.D.
Associate Professor
School of Communication Sciences and Disorders
National Centre for Audiology
University of Western Ontario
London, Ontario
Canada

Lynn S. Alvord, Ph.D.
Associate Professor
Department of Communication Disorders
University of Utah
Salt Lake City, UT

Sally A. Arnold, Ph.D.
Assistant Professor
Department of Speech-Language Pathology
Buffalo State College
Buffalo, NY

Bopanna Ballachanda, Ph.D.
University of New Mexico
Albuquerque, NM

Kristi A. Buckley, M.S.
Teaching Assistant
Callier Center for Communication Disorders
School of Human Development
University of Texas at Dallas
Dallas, TX

Robert B. Burr, Ph.D.
Assistant Professor
Department of Neurosurgery
University of Utah Medical Center
Salt Lake City, UT

Jackie L. Clark, Ph.D.
Faculty and Research Associate
Callier Center for Communication Disorders
University of Texas at Dallas
Dallas, TX

John A. Ferraro, Ph.D.
Professor and Chairman
Department of Hearing and Speech
University of Kansas Medical Center
Kansas City, KS

Terese Finitzo, Ph.D.
Director
Hearing Health Institute
Fort Worth, TX

Tom Frank, Ph.D.
Professor of Communication Disorders
Department of Communication Disorders
Pennsylvania State University
University Park, PA

Theodore J. Glattke, Ph.D.
Professor
Departments of Speech and Hearing Sciences and Surgery
University of Arizona
Tucson, AZ

Linda Gray, M.D.
Associate Professor of Neuroradiology
Department of Radiology
Duke University Medical Center
Durham, NC

Alison M. Grimes, M.A.
Director of Audiology
Providence Speech and Hearing Center
Orange, CA

Holly Hosford-Dunn, Ph.D.
President
Tucson Audiology Institute, Inc.
Managing Member
Arizona Audiology Network, LLC
Tucson, AZ

Lisa L. Hunter, Ph.D.
Associate Professor
Department of Otolaryngology
University of Minnesota
Minneapolis, MN

Gary P. Jacobson, Ph.D.
Director
Division of Audiology
Department of Otolaryngology–Head and Neck Surgery
Henry Ford Hospital
Detroit, MI

James F. Jerger, Ph.D.
Distinguished Scholar in Residence
School of Human Development
University of Texas at Dallas
Dallas, TX

Jennifer A. Jordan, M.D.
Clinical Faculty Member
Department of Otolaryngology
University of Texas Southwestern Medical Center–Dallas
Dallas, TX

Bronya J. B. Keats, Ph.D.
Professor of Genetics
Department of Biometry and Genetics
Louisiana State University Medical Center
New Orleans, LA

Robert W. Keith, Ph.D.
Professor and Director
Division of Audiology and Vestibular Testing
University of Cincinnati Medical Center
Cincinnati, OH

Thomas A. Littman, Ph.D.
Department of Audiology
Virginia Mason Medical Center
Seattle, WA

Robert H. Margolis, Ph.D.
Professor and Director of Audiology
Department of Otolaryngology
University of Minnesota
Minneapolis, MN

Cynthia A. McCormick, Ph.D.
Assistant Professor
Department of Communication Disorders
University of Utah
Salt Lake City, UT

Sandra L. McFadden, Ph.D.
Research Assistant Professor
Hearing Research Lab
University of Buffalo
Buffalo, NY

David L. McPherson, Ph.D.
Hearing and Speech Science Lab
Brigham Young University
Provo, UT

Aage R. Moller, Ph.D.
Professor and M.F. Jonsson Chair
Callier Center for Communication Disorders
University of Texas at Dallas
Dallas, TX

Deborah Moncrieff, Ph.D.
Assistant Professor
Department of Communication Sciences and Disorders
University of Florida
Gainesville, FL

Frank E. Musiek, Ph.D.
Professor of Otolaryngology and Neurology
Department of Surgery and Medicine
Dartmouth-Hitchcock Medical Center
Lebanon, NH

Joy O'Neal, M.F.A.
Director
Audiology Services
Texas Department of Health
Bureau of Children's Health
Austin, TX

Victoria B. Oxholm, M.A.
Department of Surgery and Medicine
Dartmouth-Hitchcock Medical Center
Lebanon, NH

Martin S. Robinette, Ph.D.
Professor of Audiology
Department of Otolaryngology–Head and Neck Surgery
Mayo Clinic Scottsdale
Scottsdale, AZ

Ross J. Roeser, Ph.D.
Professor and Director
Callier Center for Communication Disorders
School of Human Development
University of Texas at Dallas
Dallas, TX

Peter S. Roland, M.D.
Professor and Vice Chairman
Department of Otolaryngology–Head and Neck Surgery
University of Texas Southwestern Medical Center–Dallas
Dallas, TX

Richard J. Salvi, Ph.D.
Professor
Hearing Research Lab
University of Buffalo
Buffalo, NY

Nathan D. Schwade, Ph.D.
Assistant Professor
Department of Otolaryngology–Head and Neck Surgery
University of Texas Southwestern Medical Center–Dallas
Dallas, TX

Angela G. Shoup, Ph.D.
Director
Division of Communicative and Vestibular Disorders
Assistant Professor
Department of Otolaryngology–Head and Neck Surgery
University of Texas Southwestern Medical Center–Dallas
Dallas, TX

Brad A. Stach, Ph.D.
Professor of Audiology
Nova Scotia Hearing and Speech Clinic
Dalhousie University
Halifax, Nova Scotia
Canada

Ginger S. Stickney, M.S.
Teaching Assistant
Callier Center for Communication Disorders
School of Human Development
University of Texas at Dallas
Dallas, TX

Linda M. Thibodeau, Ph.D.
Associate Professor
Callier Center for Communication Disorders
School of Human Development
University of Texas at Dallas
Dallas, TX

Debara L. Tucci, M.D.
Assistant Professor of Otolaryngology
Department of Surgery
Duke University Medical Center
Durham, NC

Michael Valente, Ph.D.
Professor of Clinical Otolaryngology
Division of Audiology
Department of Otolaryngology–Head and Neck Surgery
Washington University School of Medicine
St. Louis, MO

Jian Wang, M.D.
Research Assistant Professor
Hearing Research Lab
University of Buffalo
Buffalo, NY

Charles G. Wright, Ph.D.
Associate Professor
Department of Otolaryngology–Head and Neck Surgery
University of Texas Southwestern Medical Center
Dallas, TX

M. Wende Yellin, Ph.D.
Assistant Professor
Department of Speech Pathology and Audiology
Northern Arizona University
Flagstaff, AZ

## Chapter 1

Diagnostic Procedures in the Profession of Audiology

Ross J. Roeser, Michael Valente, and Holly Hosford-Dunn

Outline

The word *audiology* literally means the science of hearing. Over the years, audiology has evolved into an autonomous profession, and today audiologists are the primary health-care professionals involved in the identification, prevention, and evaluation of auditory and related disorders. In addition, audiologists are the single most important resource for non-medical habilitation/rehabilitation services for individuals with hearing disorders through the application of hearing aids, associated rehabilitation devices (assistive listening devices and implantable devices), and (re) habilitation programs for children and adults. Audiologists are also involved in related research pertinent to the prevention, identification, and management of hearing loss and related disorders.

PEARL

Audiology is defined as the science of hearing, the art of hearing assessment, and the (re) habilitation of individuals with hearing impairment.

SCOPE OF PRACTICE IN AUDIOLOGY

The scope of practice for a profession is defined by professional organizations, government agencies, and licensing laws. Scope of practice information is used as a reference for issues on service delivery, third-party reimbursement, legislation, consumer education, regulatory action, state and professional licensure, legal intervention, and interprofessional relations. As expected, in the 50 years the profession of audiology has been in existence the scope of practice has grown. This metamorphosis has occurred gradually as a result of emerging clinical, technological, and scientific developments, which are now commonplace in our modern world. Whereas only 25 years ago audiologists were primarily performing behavioral tests of auditory function, today the typical audiologist has a wide range of electrophysiological assessment tools to select from, and audiology is the primary discipline involved in hearing rehabilitation with hearing aids, implantable hearing instruments, and assistive listening devices.

Two professional organizations have developed scope of practice statements for audiology: The American Speech-Language-Hearing Association (ASHA) and the American Academy of Audiology (AAA). Copies can be found in Appendix 2 of *Practice Management*. The activities listed range from the application of procedures for assessment, diagnosis, management, and interpretation of test results related to disorders of human hearing, balance, and other neural systems to participation in the development of professional and technical standards. The ASHA Scope of Practice document makes it clear that the list of activities is not intended to be exhaustive but reflects the current practice of the profession of audiology.

Scope of practice statements relate to what a profession does; they are also based on what a profession is. Traditionally, audiology is a profession that has been associated with hearing and disorders of hearing. Based on this, some have argued that audiologists should not be involved with procedures outside of assessment or rehabilitation of the auditory system. Their rationale is that to continue to be within the mainstream of the profession, audiology practice should focus exclusively on hearing and hearing disorders. However, it is clear that audiologists are practicing in related areas, such as intraoperative monitoring and balance assessment. Chapters 23 and 24 cover these topics respectively; they are reflected on in *Practice Management*.

The process for changing the scope of professional practice for any profession is either to change professional codes or

Audiology: Diagnosis. Edited by Roeser, Valente, and Hosford-Dunn. Thieme Medical Publishers, Inc., New York © 2000

state licensing laws that govern the profession or to simply extend the practice until challenged legally and have the courts adjudicate the issue. Modifying scope of practice by changing professional codes and state licensing laws is a time-consuming and expensive process. For example, before the mid-1970s the ASHA Code of Ethics prohibited audiologists from dispensing hearing aids. It took years to make the necessary amendments to allow audiologists to engage in this critical practice. In addition, definitions contained in codes and licensure must be broad, so it is not appropriate to specify all functions or procedures. Professional preparation and clinical experience are the important criteria that define the limits within which a profession can operate.

It is not uncommon for a profession to extend its practice until legally challenged. The courts are constantly challenging professional boundaries. For example, after extended litigation, optometrists are now able to prescribe antibiotics for conjunctivitis after extended litigation. When challenged, audiologists must be prepared to defend their practices with evidence of their qualifications and competencies through documentation of adequate academic preparation and experience. Because the scope of practice in audiology is expanding, the necessary academic preparation is undergoing critical review and the professional doctorate (Au.D.) has been accepted by ASHA and AAA as the minimum entry level for the profession.

The broad range of activities and services within the scope of practice for audiologists, as defined by the ASHA Task Force on Clinical Standards, is listed in Table 1–1. Most of the 23 procedures are broadly defined, requiring complex knowledge and years of experience for clinical competency. An important point made in this table, one that relates directly to this textbook, is that many of the activities listed in Table 1–1 include diagnostic procedures. Moreover, preferred practice patterns have been written for these and other diagnostic audiological procedures performed by audiologists and are available from ASHA (ASHA, 1995).

In the remaining portion of this chapter traditional and current diagnostic tests are reviewed, the effectiveness and use of diagnostic audiological tests is discussed, and the role of audiologists in diagnostic testing is covered.

DIAGNOSTIC AUDIOLOGICAL TESTS

Table 1–1 lists traditional and current diagnostic audiological tests that have been developed through the years. By reading the chapters in this book, it is clear that in recent years major advances have been made in diagnostic audiology. Today, audiologists are performing diagnostic procedures that not only rely on behavioral psychoacoustic tests with pure tones and speech but also on radiology, brain imaging, middle ear measures, auditory electrophysiology, earcanal emissions, and sophisticated tests of vestibular function. More and more, tests are being developed to assess central auditory function in children and adults. The importance of genetics is even becoming an important factor in diagnostic testing. These topics are covered in detail by the most prominent audiologists and audiology researchers in the country within the chapters of this text.

TABLE 1–1 Activities within the scope of practice for audiologists*

Hearing screening
Speech screening
Language screening
Follow-up procedures
Consultation
Prevention
Counseling
Aural rehabilitation assessment
Aural rehabilitation
Product dispensing
Product repair/modification
Basic audiological assessment[+]
Pediatric audiological assessment
Comprehensive audiological assessment[+]
Electrodiagnostic test procedures[+]
Auditory evoked potential assessment[+]
Neurophysiological intraoperative monitoring[+]
Balance system assessment[+]
Hearing aid assessment
Assistive listening system/device selection
Sensory aids assessment[+]
Hearing aid fitting/orientation
Occupational hearing conservation

*Preferred practice patterns are available from ASHA for each of these procedures
[+]Diagnostic procedures

In the remaining portion of this chapter the traditional diagnostic audiological tests are reviewed and their effectiveness is discussed. Some of these tests are still in use today, but many are not; they are presented primarily for historical purposes.

Tuning Fork Tests

The use of tuning forks provided the first diagnostic procedures for diagnosing the magnitude and type (conductive, sensorineural, or mixed) of hearing loss. With current sophisticated diagnostic equipment and procedures, tuning fork tests have limited application. However, because tuning forks are readily available, and it is even possible to use a standard bone conduction vibrator to perform audiometric tuning fork tests, physicians and audiologists will find some of the procedures useful for some patients in some situations. Chapter 11 reviews the procedures followed in tuning fork tests.

Air Conduction and Bone Conduction Comparison

The most basic diagnostic audiological information comes from comparison of air conduction (A/C) to bone conduction (B/C) thresholds. From this comparison the diagnosis of the magnitude and type of hearing loss can be made (normal- or abnormal-hearing, and conductive, sensorineural, and

TABLE 1–2 Summary of diagnostic audiological tests
(NOTE: Those tests marked with an asterisk are presented for historical purposes only)

Tuning fork tests
  Weber
  Schwabach
  Bing
Air conduction (A/C) and bone conduction (B/C)
  comparison
Loudness balancing
Bekesy (self-recording) Audiometry*
  Classical diagnostic Bekesy audiometry
  Reverse sweep Bekesy
  Bekesy comfort loudness (BCL)
Short Increment Sensitivity Index (SISI)*
Threshold Tone Decay Tests
  Classical (Carhart) Threshold Tone Decay Test
  Owens Threshold Tone Decay Test
Supra Threshold Adaptation Test (STAT)*
Speech audiometry
Immittance measures (tympanometry)
  Tympanogram
  Ipsilateral/contralateral comparison
  Acoustic reflex decay
Auditory evoked potentials
Otoacoustic emissions
Tests for pseudohypoacusis
Tests of central auditory function

mixed). Chapter 11 provides a comprehensive review of pure tone A/C and B/C procedures.

The configuration of the audiogram is an important factor when interpreting diagnostic tests. It is not always possible to determine the cause of a hearing loss by reviewing the type and configuration of the hearing loss, but many conditions have stereotypical findings. A few classical examples are the following.

- *Meniere's syndrome (endolymphatic hydrops)* is a condition in which increased pressure is in the endolymph in the inner ear, which first presents with fluctuating low-frequency rising sensorineural hearing loss. As the disease process continues, the loss changes to flat and then sloping in the latter stages. Accompanying the hearing loss are the symptoms of low-frequency (roaring) tinnitus, vertigo, and nausea.

- *Noise-induced hearing loss* occurs over time gradually when ears are exposed to high-intensity sounds. The stereotypical finding for hearing loss caused by noise exposure is a reduction of hearing in the 4000- to 6000-Hz region, with improvement of hearing at 8000 Hz. Over time, if the ear continues to be exposed to high-intensity sounds, the hearing loss in the 4000- to 6000-Hz region increases and gradually spreads to lower frequencies.

- *Presbyacusis* (or presbycusis) is hearing loss caused by advancing age, and begins in the fourth or fifth decades

of life. The loss is sensorineural and initially affects high frequencies only. As the loss progresses, it gradually invades the lower frequencies but continues to influence high frequencies the most.

- *Otosclerosis* is a condition in which a buildup of spongy material occurs in the bony capsule of the inner ear and on the footplate of the stapes, which results first in a conductive hearing loss. As the condition progresses, the loss becomes mixed and sloping with the classical "Carhart's notch"—an increased depression in bone conduction thresholds of 5 dB at 500 and 4000 Hz, 10 dB at 1000 Hz, and 15 dB at 2000 Hz. Bone conduction thresholds will improve by the amount of the Carhart's notch with successful surgery.

Loudness Balancing

Loudness balancing procedures were among the first diagnostic audiological tests to be developed. During loudness balancing tests, the loudness of stimuli presented to a patient's normal-hearing ear are compared with the loudness in the ear with hearing loss. Implicit in loudness balancing is the requirement that one ear have normal threshold sensitivity, at least at some frequencies.

Loudness balancing procedures are performed to determine whether recruitment is present or absent in an ear with hearing loss. Originally, the alternate binaural loudness balancing (ABLB) and the monaural loudness balancing (MLB) tests were developed. However, patient requirements used for the MLB were so difficult that the MLB procedure was not used clinically. The ABLB is performed by alternating a pure tone between the two ears, keeping the intensity in one ear (usually the ear with normal-hearing) fixed and varying the intensity in the other ear until the two tones are judged equally loud by the patient. The test begins at 20 dB SL in the fixed (normal) ear. After equal loudness is judged, the intensity is increased in 20 dB increments until either the patient's tolerance level or the maximum limits of the audiometer are reached.

Findings from the ABLB are plotted graphically with laddergrams, which are shown in Figure 1–1. No recruitment is indicated if the decibel difference between the two ears remains constant (Fig. 1–1A). However, if the loudness difference between the two ears decreases, with less intensity increase in the abnormal ear required for equal loudness in the normal ear, then either partial or complete recruitment is indicated. Partial recruitment is present when a decrease exists in the difference between the two ears but equal intensities are not established (Fig. 1–1B). Complete recruitment is present if equal loudness occurs at equal intensities (± 10 dB; Fig. 1–1C). In derecruitment an increase occurs in the intensity difference between the two ears to achieve equal loudness (Fig. 1–1D).

Recruitment was originally thought to be an abnormal finding, in that the loudness growth in the impaired ear appeared to be abnormally fast (see Fig. 1–1C). That is, in ears showing recruitment, even though a loss of threshold hearing sensitivity exists, at high intensities no difference in loudness is found when compared with the normal loudness function. On the basis of this, recruitment was first defined as an abnormal growth of loudness in an ear with sensorineural hearing loss. However, a number of clinical research studies have

---

PEARL

Recruitment is the rapid growth of loudness in an ear with sensorineural hearing loss. The presence of recruitment in an ear with sensorineural hearing loss suggests cochlear site of lesion. The absence of recruitment suggests a noncochlear (or retrocochlear) site of lesion.

---

changed this original concept, and it is now recognized that recruitment is not the abnormal finding but represents the impaired ear's ability to respond normally to loudness at high intensities (Sanders, 1979).

The abnormal finding from tests of recruitment, such as the ABLB, is the absence of recruitment, or derecruitment, which is an unusually slow growth of loudness in an ear with sensorineural hearing loss. The presence of recruitment has been and continues to be associated with cochlear site of lesion. In an ear with sensorineural hearing loss the absence of recruitment does not rule out pathological cochlear condition but is considered a possible retrocochlear sign. The most abnormal finding on loudness balancing tests is derecruitment, which is a highly positive sign for retrocochlear involvement.

Bekesy (Self-Recording) Audiometry

Bekesy (1947) described an audiometer that allows patients to track their own thresholds—a self-recording audiometer. Threshold testing is performed with the self-recording (Bekesy) audiometer by instructing the patient to activate a handheld switch when the test signals are just heard and release the switch immediately when the test signals become inaudible. As the patient is responding, the self-recording audiometer marks the responses on an audiogram form, and thresholds are calculated from the tracings. With this procedure, thresholds can be obtained for a variety of stimuli using

sweep frequency (for example 100 to 10,000 Hz) or fixed frequency recordings and continuous or pulsed tones.

PEARL

The term *retrocochlear* refers to areas in the auditory system beyond the cochlea, including the brain stem and higher levels. The term *central* refers to areas in the auditory system beyond the brain stem.

Classical Diagnostic Bekesy Audiometry

J. Jerger (1960) was among the first to use the Bekesy audiometer for diagnostic purposed. In the *classical Bekesy procedure* thresholds for a pulsing (p) pure tone are compared with those using a continuously (c) presented pure tone. The pulsing tone has a duration of 200 ms, a rise-fall time of 50 ms, and a 50% duty cycle. Originally, four patterns were described (types I to IV), but later Jerger and Herer (1961) added one more, type V. The five classical Bekesy patterns are shown in Figure 1–2. Results were consistent with the following:

- *Type I*—Normal-hearing, conductive hearing loss, and sensorineural hearing loss of unknown origin
- *Type II*—Sensorineural hearing loss caused by a cochlear site of lesion
- *Type III*—Retrocochlear site of lesion oftentimes caused by an acoustic neuroma or cerebellopontine angle tumor
- *Type IV*—Cochlear or retrocochlear site of lesion
- *Type V*—Pseudohypoacusis

On the basis of results from numerous clinical studies using the classical Bekesy procedure, a number of modifications were developed; the most were reverse-sweep Bekesy and Bekesy comfort level.

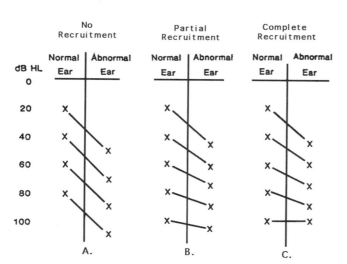

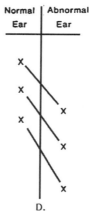

Figure 1–1 Laddergrams from the ABLB test. For each example, the normal ear has a 0 dB HL threshold and the abnormal ear a 30 dB HL threshold.

Continuous (Sweep) Frequency Bekesy Tracings

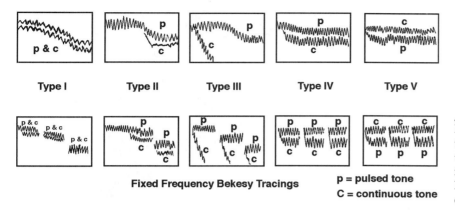

Type I Type II Type III Type IV Type V

Fixed Frequency Bekesy Tracings

p = pulsed tone
C = continuous tone

Figure 1–2 Classical Bekesy diagnostic patterns showing thresholds for pulsed (*p*) tones and continuous (*c*) tones. The top tracings are for sweep frequencies (100 to 10,000 Hz) and the bottom for the fixed frequencies of 250, 1000, and 4000 Hz.

Reverse-Sweep Bekesy

In the classical sweep frequency Bekesy procedure the pulsed and continuous tones are presented from low to high frequencies. In the reverse-sweep procedure the sweep of the continuous tones are from high to low frequencies and are compared with the pulsed tone tracings from low to high frequencies (Rose, 1962). This modification revealed more hearing loss for the continuous reverse sweep. The advantage of this modification is that patients with sensorineural hearing loss as a result of retrocochlear pathological condition in the region of the brain stem had more hearing loss with the reverse-sweep procedure. In addition, patients with pseudohypoacusis were also found to have abnormal reverse-sweep tracings.

Bekesy Comfort Level

In the Bekesy comfort level (BCL) procedure patients are instructed to respond to the stimuli at suprathreshold, rather than threshold, levels. The rationale for the BCL procedure is that because retrocochlear disorders initially appear at suprathreshold level, recordings above threshold would be more sensitive. Reports using this procedure revealed six types of recordings and suggest it was more sensitive than

the classical procedure in identifying retrocochlear disorders (Jerger & Jerger, 1974).

Short Increment Sensitivity Index (SISI)

The SISI test (Jerger et al, 1959) is based on the differential intensity function of the ear (see Chapter 9). That is, the test determines the ability of the patient to detect a 1 dB change of intensity in a pure tone stimulus when superimposed on a continuous tone presented at 20 dB SL. The classical SISI procedure is graphically illustrated in Figure 1–3. During the test, a pure tone is presented continuously at 20 dB SL (a 20 dB pedestal), and 25 to 28 presentations of 1- to 5-dB are superimposed on it. The increases in intensity are 300 ms in duration, have a 50 ms rise/fall time, and a 200 ms on time. One increment is presented every 5 seconds, and the patient is instructed to respond when the increments are detected. During the test, only the 1 dB increments are used to calculate the SISI score. The first five 5 dB increments are used for practice to see whether the patient can perform the task. During the 11th, 17th, and 23rd trials, the stimuli are changed. If the patient is not responding, 5 dB increments are presented to ensure that the patient is attending to the task. However, if a high rate of responding occurs for the 1 dB increments, they

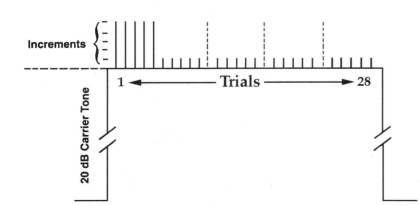

Figure 1–3 Diagram of the procedure used in the SISI test.

are removed during these trials to prevent rhythmic responding. The SISI score is calculated by multiplying the number of 1 dB increments that are correctly detected by 5, giving a percentage of correct responses. Scores between 0 and 70% are negative for cochlear pathological conditions. Scores of 75% and above are positive for cochlear pathological conditions. Modifications to the classical procedure included reducing the initial five 5 dB practice increments in 1 dB steps (that is, 4 dB, 3 dB, and 2 dB) to eliminate the sudden reduction of the signal to 1 dB and to reduce the number of 1 dB increments from 20 to 10.

Through the years the classical SISI test was shown to be an accurate predictor of a cochlear pathological condition. A tendency exists for the test to be more predictive of cochlear hearing loss at higher frequencies (2000 to 4000 Hz) than at low frequencies (250 to 500 Hz).

A high intensity modification of the classical procedure was introduced to detect retrocochlear pathological conditions. When the 20 dB SL pedestal is raised to 75 dB HL, patients with normal-hearing and cochlear hearing loss are able to detect the 1 dB increments, but patients with retrocochlear pathological conditions are not. As a result, patients with normal-hearing and sensorineural hearing loss of cochlear origin will have high SISI scores, but those with a retrocochlear pathological condition will have low scores.

Threshold Tone Decay Tests

Threshold tone decay tests quantify the amount of auditory fatigue present when stimuli are presented at or near threshold sensitivity for each patient. The general procedure is to quantify the ability of a patient to perceive and maintain a pure tone presented continuously. The classical procedure was described by Carhart (1957), and a modification was introduced by Owens (1964).

Classical (Carhart) Threshold Tone Decay Test

In the classical procedure the patient is instructed to respond when the tone is perceived by raising a finger and continue to respond as long as the tone is heard. The tone is initially presented below threshold and increased slowly in 5-dB steps until the patient first responds. As soon as the patient responds, timing begins, and if the tone is heard for a full minute, the test is terminated. If, however, the signal fades into inaudibility and the patient stops responding before the 1-minute period is over, the intensity is increased by 5 dB *without interruption* and timing begins again. This procedure continues until the patient is able to sustain the tone for 1 full minute or until the signal reaches 30 dB SL.

The classical procedure can be time-consuming, possibly requiring as much as 4 to 4½ minutes for each frequency tested. To shorten the test, Olsen and Noffsinger (1974) suggested that the initial stimulus be presented at 20 dB SL. This is not only a time-saving procedure that maintains the sensitivity but it also makes the test easier for patients because stimuli are easier to perceive at 20 dB SL.

The extent of the decay, both in the number of frequencies at which decay occurs and the intensity and rapidity of the decay, provides differential diagnostic information in the following areas: (1) slow tone decay is associated with cochlear pathological conditions but marked or rapid decay with retrocochlear pathological conditions; (2) tone decay in excess of 30 dB is very likely associated with retrocochlear pathological conditions, regardless of its rapidity; and (3) the greater the number of frequencies involved, the greater the likelihood of retrocochlear involvement.

Rosenberg Modification

The Carhart procedure can be time-consuming, possibly requiring as much as 4 to 4½ minutes for each frequency tested. To shorten the test, Rosenberg (1958) suggested measuring the decay only for a total of 60 seconds. In this procedure after the initial response, the tone is presented for 60 seconds, and the amount of tone decay occurring in the 60-second period is measured in decibels. Interpretation of results is similar to the Carhart procedure. Because Rosenberg modification reduces the sensitivity of the test, it is considered a screening procedure.

Owens Threshold Tone Decay Test

Owens (1964) described a modification of the classical tone decay test that incorporates a 20-second rest period between each stimulus presentation. In the Owens procedure, each tone presentation begins at 5 dB SL, and if the patient does not perceive the tone for 60 seconds, the stimulus is discontinued for 20 seconds before reintroduction at successive 5 dB increments. This procedure continues until the stimulus is perceived for 60 seconds or a level of 20 dB SL is reached.

It is possible to differentiate between decay occurring with cochlear versus retrocochlear site of lesion with the Owens procedure. Patients with retrocochlear lesions characteristically show decay at all frequencies, and the rapidity of the decay does not change as the intensity is increased. Patients with cochlear pathological conditions, on the other hand, show decay at one or two frequencies, and the decay is slower as the intensity of the test signal is increased. Table 1–3 shows the three types of decay found with the Owens procedure. Type I is associated with normal ears, type II with ears having cochlear pathological conditions, and type III with ears having retrocochlear pathological conditions.

Suprathreshold Adaptation Test (STAT)

Jerger and Jerger (1975) developed the STAT on the basis of the observation that abnormal adaptation (fatigue) associated with retrocochlear pathological conditions occurs first at high intensities. During the STAT procedure a continuous pure tone stimulus is presented at a level of 110 dB SPL (about 90- to 100-dB HL depending on the test frequency) for 60 seconds to determine whether it can be perceived for the full duration. Because of the intensity of the test signal and the distinct possibility of crossover (see Chapter 12), masking usually must be presented to the nontest ear. If the stimulus is perceived for less than 60 seconds, an interrupted pure tone (500 ms on/ 500 ms off) is presented at the 110 dB SPL level. Results are considered positive for retrocochlear pathological conditions when the continuous tone cannot be perceived for the 60 second duration only if the interrupted tone can be perceived for the 60 second duration. The STAT test is most effective in identifying retrocochlear pathological conditions when positive results are obtained below 2000 Hz.

TABLE 1–3 Threshold tone decay patterns from the Owens* test

Levels above threshold	Type I	A	B	C	D	E	Type III
60	60	27	8	12	13	6	15
		60	36	29	26	18	17
			60	45	31	21	13
				60	47	38	12

*Owens (1964)

A recent concern with the STAT has to do with the intensity at which the stimuli are presented. After it was developed, the procedure was in widespread use by audiologists for diagnostic applications without any significant consequences. However, isolated reports of patients having potential threshold shifts from using high-intensity procedures such as the STAT have dissuaded the use of this procedure.

Speech Audiometry

Pure tones are used in diagnostic audiology primarily because they are simple to generate and are capable of differentially assessing the specific effects of auditory system pathological conditions. However, pure tone measurements provide only limited information concerning the communication difficulty a patient may experience and/or diagnostic site of lesion information. Speech audiometry assesses the patient's ability to respond to standardized material for threshold assessment (speech recognition threshold—SRT) and speech perception ability with words (word recognition scores) and/or sentences (speech recognition scores). The topic of speech audiometry is covered in detail in Chapter 13.

Speech audiometry provides data to assess the validity of pure tone thresholds and obtain diagnostic information regarding site of lesion. Validation of pure tone data is accomplished by comparing thresholds for speech materials, the SRT, to thresholds for pure tones in the 500- to 2000-Hz range (pure tone average, or PTA). Such comparison should reveal close agreement (within ± 6- to 8-dB). Whenever a difference exists between the SRT and the PTA, the validity of the results are in question, and the equipment, the procedures used to obtain the data, and patient cooperation must be checked (see Chapters 11 and 14).

Diagnostic information from speech audiometry is obtained by comparing word and speech intelligibility scores at different intensities. The shape of the performance intensity (PI) function and the difference in the functions for words and sentences provides diagnostic information. Figure 1–4 provides classical results showing PI functions using words and sentences for different sites of lesions. The findings for this procedure were obtained with standard phonetically balanced (PB) word lists and sentences from the Synthetic Sentence Identification (SSI) test (Jerger & Hayes, 1977).

> **PEARL**
>
> **A PI function compares percent of correct responses for speech materials with words (word intelligibility scores) or sentences (speech intelligibility scores) at various levels of presentation.**

1. *Normal findings:* Patients have high speech recognition scores (between 90 and 100%) for both types of stimuli at low and high intensities (Fig. 1–4A).
2. *Cochlear site:* Patients with a cochlear site of lesion have PI functions that are predictable in the following ways:
   A. With flat audiometric configurations, identical or similar PI functions are obtained for words (PI-PB) and sentences (PI-SSI; Fig. 1–4B).
   B. With sloping high-frequency losses, the PI function for words (PI-PB) is reduced compared with the PI function for sentences (PI-SSI; Fig. 1–4C).
   C. With rising audiometric configurations, the PI function for words (PI-PB) is elevated compared with the PI function for sentences (PI-SSI; Fig. 1–4D).
3. *Eighth nerve site:* The direction and magnitude of the PI function is not predictable, but significant PI rollover occurs. Rollover is defined as a significant reduction in PI scores that occurs at high intensities. That is, scores reach a maximum in the mid-range intensities, and when the intensity is increased a sharp decrease in performance occurs (Fig. 1–4E).

> **PEARL**
>
> *Rollover* **is observed on the PI function obtained during word/speech recognition testing when a significant reduction in scores occurs as the intensity of the scores increases. Rollover is associated with retrocochlear involvement.**

4. *Central site:* The PI function for words (PI-PB) is typically elevated compared with the PI function for sentences (PI-SSI) similar to cochlear losses with rising configurations (Fig. 1–4D).

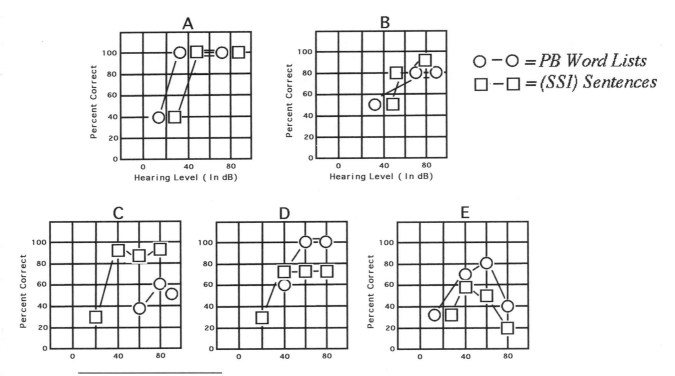

Figure 1–4 Examples of PI functions for words (PI-PB) and sentences (PI-SSI) for **(A)** normal-hearing, **(B-D)** cochlear hearing loss with different configurations, and **(E)** eighth nerve site. Patients with central site and presbyacusis have configurations similar to example **D**.

5. *Presbyacusis:* The PI functions for words (PI-PB) and sentences (PI-SSI) are below normal. Typically, the PI function for words (PI-PB) is elevated compared with the PI function for sentences (PI-SSI; Fig. 1–4D).

Immittance Measures

Immittance measures do not assess hearing. They provide objective information on the mechanical transfer function of sound in the outer and middle ear and, depending on the status of the outer and middle ear and cochlear function, provide data on the neural integrity of the auditory nerve function at the level of the brain stem. With the immittance test battery it is possible to obtain diagnostic information on the status of the outer and middle ear and cochlear function and the status of the eighth nerve and brain stem. Chapter 17 is a comprehensive review of basic and advanced middle ear measurement techniques.

Table 1–4 lists the procedures used in immittance measures including the tympanogram, tympanogram height, physical volume, and acoustic reflex. In this table a comparison is made between the measures obtained with the classical (descriptive) immittance method and the absolute (microprocessor-based) method. Although each test provides significant information by itself, immittance tests are not performed or interpreted in isolation. Diagnostic information from immittance measures is strengthened when results from all test procedures are interpreted together.

As shown in Table 1–4, the classical (descriptive) and the absolute (microprocessor-based) methods measure findings in different units and classify results differently, especially for the tympanogram.

Tympanogram

The tympanogram is a graphic display of tympanic membrane compliance as a function of pressure changes in the external earcanal. As shown in Figure 1–5 the classical (descriptive) method types normal and abnormal tympanogram shape into five categories (type A, As, Ad, B, and C). The absolute method provides objective measures of the tympanogram: tympanometric peak pressure (TPP), tympanometric width/gradient (TW or GR), and tympanogram height (static admittance-peak Y). Normal middle ear function is necessary before the acoustic reflex can be measured with the immittance procedure.

Acoustic Reflex

The acoustic reflex occurs when a small muscle in the middle ear, the stapedius muscle in humans, contracts as a result of acoustic stimulation at intensities between 70- and 90- or 100-dB HL; normally this reflex occurs in both ears (bilaterally). The fact that the acoustic reflex is bilateral means that a signal directed to one ear can elicit a reflex in both ears (the ipsilateral and contralateral ears) simultaneously.

When the stapedius muscle contracts in the normal ear, a resulting stiffening of the tympanic membrane occurs. The stiffening of the tympanic membrane during stapedial contraction changes the amount of reflected energy from the probe tone of the immittance instrument. It is important to realize that the immittance procedure does not measure middle ear muscle contraction directly but measures *the effect of middle ear muscle contraction on tympanic membrane stiffening.*

TABLE 1–4 Summary of immittance tests and comparison of classical and absolute (microprocessor-based) procedures

Procedure	Purpose	Classical Description	Units of Measurement	Absolute Description	Unit of Measurement
Tympanogram	Assess the pressure/ compliance function of the eardrum	Type A, B, C	Relative units	Tympanometric peak pressure (TPP) ------------------ Tympanometric width (TW) gradient (GR)	DaPa ---------------- DaPa
Tympanogram height	Classification of tympanogram	Static compliance	Cm^3/ml*	Static admittance (Peak Y)	Mmho or cm^3/ml*
Physical volume	Measures the equivalent volume of the space between the probe tip and the eardrum	Physical volume test	Cm^3/ml*	Equivalent earcanal volume (V^{ec})	cm^3/ml*
Acoustic reflex	Indirect measure of stapedial muscle contraction to intense sound	Acoustic reflex	Relative change in eardrum admittance (compliance)	Acoustic reflex (AR)	Relative change in eardrum admittance (compliance)

*Cubic centimeters (cm^3) and milliliters (ml) are identical volumes (1 cm^3 = 1 ml).

This has an important implication in interpreting the clinical value of acoustic reflex results because mechanical changes in the middle ear can obliterate recording the acoustic reflex when it occurs. That is, the middle ear muscles may contract, but the presence of middle ear pathological conditions will obliterate the effect of the contraction on the stiffness change necessary to record the contraction with the immittance instrument. Acoustic reflex measures provide a powerful diagnostic assessment of three areas: middle ear function, neurological functioning of the auditory system, and an index of auditory sensitivity. The acoustic reflex will be affected if any of these three functions is impaired.

Ipsilateral/Contralateral Comparison

Table 1–5 provides clinical interpretations for results from ipsilateral and contralateral acoustic reflexes. As shown, six patterns can be identified that provide data on middle ear involvement, and involvement at cochlear, eighth nerve, seventh nerve, or brain stem sites. Table 1–5 shows findings from left side involvement; if the right side was involved, the findings would be reversed. The acoustic reflex provides clinicians with a powerful differential diagnostic tool that is particularly helpful because of its ease in administration.

Acoustic Reflex Decay

If the acoustic reflex stimulus is presented continuously over an extended period (10 seconds or longer), in the normal ear the acoustic reflex will be sustained at maximum amplitude during stimulation. This function is evaluated during the acoustic reflex decay test. Acoustic reflex decay is tested with low-frequency stimuli (500 and 1000 Hz) because at higher frequencies abnormal results can occur in the absence of negative otologic histories and no clinical symptoms. The standard procedure is to present the stimulus at 10 dB SL (re: the threshold of the acoustic reflex), and the stimulus is presented for 10 seconds. The normal acoustic reflex function is graphically displayed in Figure 1–6. As shown, the amplitude is constant over the 10 second period. However, in patients with abnormal reflex decay an inability to maintain full amplitude for the duration of stimulation is present. As shown in Figure 1–6, the amplitude of the reflex decreases to less than half the maximum amplitude within 5 seconds.

Abnormal reflex decay can be observed in patients with either cochlear and eighth nerve pathological conditions. When the decay occurs within 5 seconds or at frequencies less than 1000 Hz, results are suggestive of an eighth nerve site. As pointed out later in this chapter, the test has a high degree of sensitivity to retrocochlear pathological conditions. As a result, because of its ease of administration, the acoustic reflex decay is considered a valuable diagnostic test. However, some concern exists about presenting acoustic stimuli for extended periods at high intensities. For this reason, the acoustic reflex decay test should be administered judiciously. When deemed necessary, it is best to administer the test at the end of the test session, especially after threshold testing. This way, thresholds will not be affected by the intense stimulation and, if they are, a record is available if concerns exist regarding threshold shifts caused by the intense stimulation.

Auditory Evoked Potentials

Auditory stimuli are capable of evoking responses in the electrical activity of the central nervous system and with the use of computer technology can be recorded from electrodes placed on the head. Figure 1–7 provides an example of the composite

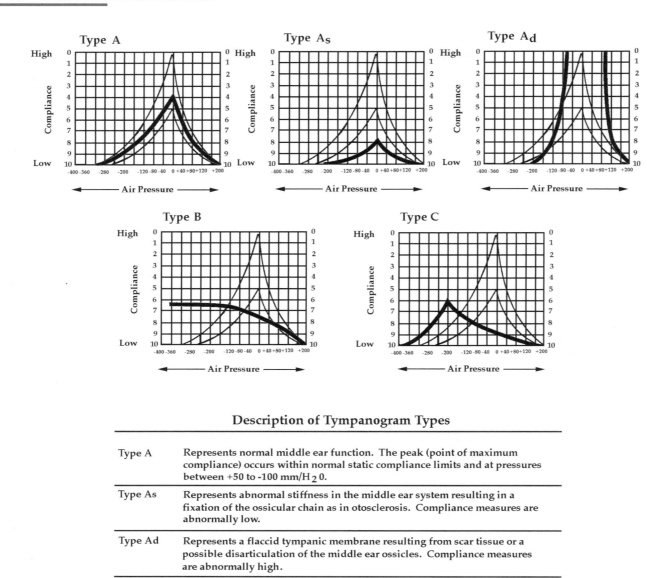

Description of Tympanogram Types

Type A	Represents normal middle ear function. The peak (point of maximum compliance) occurs within normal static compliance limits and at pressures between +50 to -100 mm/H_2O.
Type As	Represents abnormal stiffness in the middle ear system resulting in a fixation of the ossicular chain as in otosclerosis. Compliance measures are abnormally low.
Type Ad	Represents a flaccid tympanic membrane resulting from scar tissue or a possible disarticulation of the middle ear ossicles. Compliance measures are abnormally high.
Type B	Represents restricted tympanic membrane mobility and would indicate that some pathological condition exists in the middle ear. Static compliance measures are abnormally low.
Type C	Represents significant negative pressure in the middle ear cavity (considered significant for treatment when more negative than -200 mm/H_2O). This may indicate a precursory state of otitis media or the resolution of an ear infection. Compliance measures are usually within normal limits.

Figure 1–5 Tympanograms and their description using the classical (A, B, and C) system.

auditory evoked response, including the short latency (electrocochleographic) response (SLR), the middle latency response (MLR), and the long latency (LLR) response. Auditory evoked responses have been used in diagnostic audiology for more than 3 decades, and as more knowledge is being made available in this area, it is clear that auditory electrophysiological measures will become an even more prominent diagnostic tool in audiology in the future. Topics related to auditory evoked potentials in diagnostic audiology are covered in Chapters 18 to 20.

Otoacoustic Emissions

Otoacoustic emissions are recorded by introducing a brief acoustic signal into the earcanal and measuring the acoustic energy that is emitted. Otoacoustic emissions were discovered only within the past two decades, but their use in studying auditory physiology and diagnostic audiology has already made a significant difference in everyday clinical practice. Chapter 21 presents an excellent review on otoacoustic emissions and Chapter 22 discusses, among other issues, the application of otoacoustic emissions in neonatal hearing screening.

TABLE 1–5   Ipsilateral-contralateral, acoustic reflex pattern interpretation

Reflex Pattern Name	Visual (Probe Ear) Hz	R	L	Verbal	Clinical Interpretations
Normal	Crossed	□	□	Normal for both ears	1. Normal
	Uncrossed	□	□		
Vertical	Crossed	□	■	Abnormal whenever probe is in the affected ear	1. Mild middle ear disorder (in the left ear)
	Uncrossed	□	■		2. Seventh (facial) nerve disorder (on the left side)
Diagonal	Crossed	■	□	Abnormal with sound to affected ear	1. Right nerve disorder (on the left side)
	Uncrossed	□	■		2. Severe cochlear loss (in the left ear)
Inverted L-shape	Crossed	■	■	Abnormal on both ears to crossed stimulation, abnormal on affected ear to uncrossed stimulation	1. Unilateral middle ear disorder (in the left ear)
	Uncrossed	□	■		2. Intra-axial brain stem disorder eccentric to one side (left side)
					3. Combined seventh and eighth nerve disorder
Horizontal	Crossed	■	■	Abnormal to crossed stimulation on both ears	1. Extra-axial and/or intra-axial brain stem disorder
	Uncrossed	□	□		
Uni-box	Crossed	■	□	Abnormal with sound to affected ear on crossed stimulation only	1. Extra-axial and/or intra-axial brain stem disorder
	Uncrossed	□	□		

Adapted from Jerger and Jerger (1977, p.455). Reprinted by permission. □, Reflex present; ■, reflex absent.

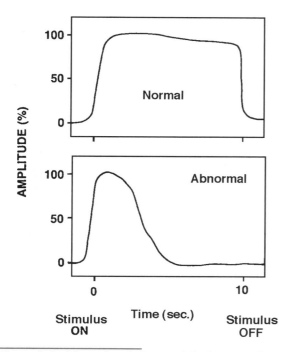

Figure 1–6   Normal and abnormal findings on the acoustic reflex decay test.

Tests for Pseudohypoacusis

Pseudohypoacusis literally means false (pseudo) reduced hearing (hypoacusis) and refers to patients who for some reason have exaggerated hearing loss. Some patients demonstrating pseudohypoacusis have no hearing loss, but for most hearing loss is present; the degree of impairment is exaggerated. Through the years, other terms, including nonorganic hearing loss, functional hearing loss, psychogenic hearing loss, hysterical deafness, and malingering have been used to describe patients whose hearing loss is questionable. Each of these terms has specific connotations, and for this reason they must be used carefully in describing these patients. The topic of pseudohypoacusis is covered in detail in Chapter 14.

Tests of Central Auditory Function

In Chapter 26, leading experts in audiology provide their views about the future direction of diagnostic audiology. From the discussion on this topic, it is clear that assessment of central auditory function is an area of significant importance in diagnostic audiology and will provide audiologists with the most significant advances in the future. Although some of the procedures will involve auditory electrophysiology and brain imaging, behavioral tests of central auditory function will also prove to be of significant value in the clinical setting. Chapters 15 and 16 cover the topics of central auditory function in children and adults, respectively.

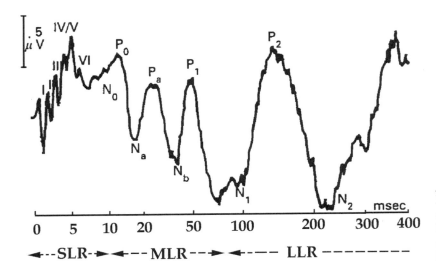

Figure 1–7 Example of the composite human auditory evoked response, including the short latency (electrocochleography) response (*SLR*), middle latency response (*MLR*), and long latency response (*LLR*).

THE EFFECTIVENESS OF DIAGNOSTIC AUDIOLOGICAL TESTS

All diagnostic procedures, whether for the auditory system or any other system, are designed to identify the presence of a disorder as early as possible. When indicated, diagnostic procedures can also help to identify the cause or nature of the disorder. The value of a diagnostic test depends on the ability to perform as intended. That is, the procedure must accurately identify those patients with the disorder while clearing those patients without the disorder. In diagnostic audiology a variety of procedures are available, so the question becomes which test(s) is most effective. In answering this question the primary criterion is based on the reliability and validity of the test.

PEARL

Reliability measures the intraexaminer and interexaminer consistency of a test. *Validity* is a measure of the ability of a test to detect the disorder for which it was designed.

Reliability deals with consistency; if the test is administered and then repeated (test-retest) at a different time by the same (intraexaminer) or a different (interexaminer) individual, to what extent will the test results be the same? Without a high degree of reliability, the test is not effective because the results of the test will vary either from session to session, from tester to tester, or possibly both. Test reliability can be controlled and maintained at a high level by standardizing test administration, ensuring proper equipment calibration, and controlling patient variables. Careful attention to these matters will help ensure a high level of reliability, but does not guarantee it.

It is easy to see how poor reliability has serious consequences for diagnostic procedures; the reliability of a test

must be high for it to be effective. However, just because a test is reliable, it still may not be an effective test if it fails to identify the problem for which it is being conducted. That is, the test must be a *valid* measure of the disorder for which it was designed.

Audiological test validity has been studied through the application of mathematical models, including clinical decision analysis (CDA) and information theory analysis (Jerger, 1983; Turner & Nielsen, 1983). CDA allows for decisions to be made about tests when uncertainty exists: uncertainty is always present with diagnostic procedures because they are not perfect. That is, certain predictable errors are associated with each test.

In applying CDA to audiological tests, assumptions must be made. Traditionally, one basic assumption has been made on the basis of whether tests are positive for retrocochlear disorder (a positive result) or negative for retrocochlear disorder (a negative result), with negative results for retrocochlear disorders being positive for cochlear disorder. By considering diagnostic procedures in this way, it is possible to model the outcomes in a matrix relating to the actual presence or absence of retrocochlear disorder.

Table 1–6 provides a model for analyzing diagnostic test data. As shown, the diagnostic test results can be grouped by the number of test outcomes suggesting positive (fail) and negative findings (pass) outcomes and by the number of patients with retrocochlear (condition present) or cochlear (condition absent) site of lesion. With these parameters, classification of the data into four cells is possible: correct identification of the abnormal condition (cell *A*—sensitivity), correct identification of the normal condition (cell *D*—specificity), false positive (cell *B*), and false negative (cell *C*).

These four possible outcomes allow one to evaluate the effectiveness of a diagnostic test by calculating its sensitivity, specificity, predictive values (of positive and negative results), and efficiency as described in the following (see Table 1–6).

1. *Sensitivity*: The sensitivity of a test is its accuracy in correctly identifying disordered subjects; in the case of site-of-

TABLE 1–6 Hypothetical data analyzing the effectiveness of a diagnostic audiological test

	Condition Present	Condition Absent	
Positive (Fail)	**A** Correct identification of abnormal condition (sensitivity) 21	**B** False positive 6	A + B = 27
Negative (Pass)	**C** False negative 3	**D** Correct identification of normal condition (specificity) 586	C + D = 589
	(A + C = 24)	(B + D = 592)	616

Sensitivity =	$\dfrac{A}{A + C} \times 100$	$\dfrac{21}{24} = 88\%$
False negative =	$\dfrac{C}{A + C} \times 100$	$\dfrac{3}{24} = 13\%$
Specificity =	$\dfrac{D}{B + D} \times 100$	$\dfrac{586}{592} = 99\%$
False positive =	$\dfrac{B}{B + D} \times 100$	$\dfrac{6}{592} = 1\%$
Predictive value (positive result) =	$\dfrac{A}{A + B} \times 100$	$\dfrac{21}{27} = 78\%$
Predictive value (negative results) =	$\dfrac{D}{C + D} \times 100$	$\dfrac{586}{589} = 99\%$
Efficiency =	$\dfrac{A + D}{A + B + C + D} \times 100$	$\dfrac{607}{616} = 99\%$

lesion tests, sensitivity is the ability to identify a retrocochlear disorder. Sensitivity is calculated by dividing the true positive results by the total number of patients with retrocochlear disorder.

2. *Specificity*: The specificity of a test is its accuracy in correctly rejecting patients without retrocochlear disorder. That is, these patients would be classified as having cochlear site-of-lesion. Specificity is calculated by dividing true negative results by the total number of patients with cochlear disorder. Sensitivity and specificity are generally related inversely; as one increases, the other decreases.

3. *Predictive value*: The predictive value (PV) of a test is related to the number of false negative results in patients with retrocochlear disorders and the number of false positive results in patients with cochlear disorders. PV is influenced by the prevalence of the disorder. However, the prevalence of retrocochlear disorders in patients with sensorineural hearing loss is unknown. Therefore to calculate the PV of audiological tests, an estimate must be made regarding prevalence. Using the estimate makes it possible to calculate the PV of the positive result (PV+) and the PV of the negative result (PV−). The PV+ is calculated by dividing the true positive findings by the total number of positive tests, whereas the PV− is calculated by dividing the true negative findings by the total number of negative tests.

4. *Efficiency*: Efficiency specifies a test's overall accuracy. When applied to site-of-lesion procedures, it is the ability to accurately identify both cochlear and retrocochlear disorders. Efficiency is calculated by dividing the true positive plus the true negative findings by the total number of patients.

In each case the results of all the above measures are multiplied by 100 to derive a percentage.

In addition to these four measures, the false negative rate (those with the disorder who are missed by the diagnostic test) and false positive rate (those without the disorder but who are identified as having the disorder) can be calculated. The ideal diagnostic audiological test is one that has high true positive (sensitivity) and true negative (specificity) rates and low false positive and false negative rates. The hypothetical data shown in Table 1–6 show sensitivity and specificity rates of 88 and 99%, and false negative and false positive rates of 13 and 1%, respectively. In addition, the predictive value of a positive and negative result is 78 and 99% respectively, and the efficiency is 99%.

Whether the results from the test being evaluated in Table 1–6 support routine clinical use depends on a variety factors, such as the possible use of other diagnostic tests, the consequences of incorrectly identifying or failing to identify the condition, and costs. Costs include not only the funding required to perform the tests but other factors such as time, inconvenience, and consequences if the test results are not accurate.

The preceding principles have been applied to diagnostic audiological test procedures by a number of investigators (Jerger, 1983; Turner & Nielsen, 1983). For example, Jerger and Jerger (1983) reported on the sensitivity, specificity, predictive value of positive and negative results, and efficiency of six diagnostic audiological tests from data reported by Jerger and Jerger (1983) and Musiek et al (1983). Results shown in Table 1–6 indicate that the sensitivity of the six tests ranged from 45 to 97%, with auditory brain stem response (ABR) audiometry being the most sensitive (97%) and Bekesy and STAT being the least sensitive (50 and 45%, respectively). Specificity ranged from 70 to 100%, with Bekesy and STAT having high specificity (90 to 100%) and acoustic reflexes and BCL the lowest specificity (70%). Although some variability exists, these results agree with reports of other investigators. The general inverse relationship between the sensitivity of a test and its specificity is demonstrated by Bekesy audiometry. This procedure had next to the lowest sensitivity but the highest specificity. An exception to this trade-off is ABR audiometry, which had unusually high sensitivity and specificity rates.

The derived predictive values were based on a prevalence rate of 50%. The predictive value for positive results ranged from 74 to 100%, whereas negative results ranged from 62 to 96%. As with sensitivity and specificity, generally a trade-off was present between the predictive values for positive and negative results. For example, Bekesy audiometry had the highest positive predictive value (100%), indicating that no false positive findings for any patient with cochlear disorder were present, but a low negative predictive value (67%) was present. Overall, positive predictive values were high for ABR, PI-PB, Bekesy, and STAT. Negative predictive values were high for ABR, acoustic reflex, and BCL.

Of the six procedures evaluated, efficiency ranged from 68 to 91%. ABR had the highest efficiency at 91% and STAT the lowest at 68%. The remaining four procedures varied only slightly from 75 to 78%.

These types of data help to quantify the overall usefulness of diagnostic audiological tests performed in isolation. However, when a test battery approach is used, additional factors must be considered, such as the complex interactions between the various test procedures and the interpretation when discrepancies exist between test outcomes.

Two factors that have had an impact on diagnostic audiological tests and the diagnostic audiological test battery, especially with respect to identifying retrocochlear disorders, are the advancement of radiographic techniques, specifically magnetic resonance imaging (MRI), and an increased sensitivity to financial costs and reimbursement through managed care. Studies have reported the sensitivity of enhanced MRI in detecting acoustic neuromas, even those considered small, to be near 100% (Wilson et al, 1997). Coupled with data that show the cost of diagnostic audiological testing can exceed an MRI screening procedure, it is easy to see why MRI has become the "gold standard" for detecting acoustic neuromas (Hirsch et al, 1996). These are the types of advances that have had a major impact on current diagnostic audiolological practice.

WHAT ARE AUDIOLOGISTS DOING?

In selecting a test battery, because of time and reimbursement constraints, that which is ideal may not be that which is real. The question arises as to which tests are preferred in clinical practice; the answer has to do with efficiency. Two types of efficiency are in play when audiologists construct a test battery for clinical use. Besides its definition as a measure of validity, as discussed in the previous section, efficiency can also refer to functionality and serviceability. In practical application some tests are easier for patients to manage and faster for audiologists to perform. Some tests lend themselves to quick interpretation and to modifications that reduce test time. Such tests have practical efficiency.

In the absence of published practice guidelines for audiology that are widely accepted in the profession,* two trends are at work to establish de facto test batteries. First, audiologists in busy practice settings tend to gravitate to test protocols that allow rapid testing, especially if clinic scheduling only allows 30 minutes for a "comprehensive" audiometric evaluation. Second, managed care organizations and other third-party payors allow reimbursement for only certain procedural codes, which effectively eliminates noncovered tests from the audiological batteries applied to patients under those plans (see Chapter 26).

As to what tests are "popular," two recent surveys of AAA members report on current audiological practices in the United States. Martin et al (1998) surveyed 218 audiologists on specific procedures they used most often. Chermak et al (1998) surveyed 185 audiologists, asking them to identify and

---

*At the time of writing (Spring, 1999), the Joint Audiology Committee, with representatives from the VA, AAA, and ASHA, has developed draft versions of statements and clinical algorithms for clinical practices in five areas, including comprehensive audiologic assessment.

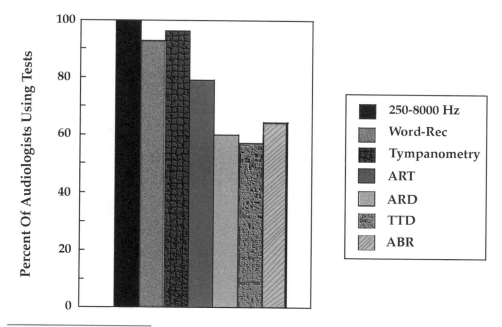

Figure 1–8 De facto audiometric test battery based on combined results from surveys of AAA members conducted by Chermak et al (1998) and Martin et al (1998). 250-8000 Hz: pure tone audiometric testing; Word-Rec, word recognition testing; ART, acoustic reflex test; ARD, acoustic reflex decay test; TTD, threshold tone decay; ABR, auditory brain stem response.

rank order the central auditory tests they used. Figures 1–8 through 1–10 combine and summarize portions of findings from these two surveys, yielding de facto test batteries that reflect the present standard of care for audiology in the United States.

Figure 1–8 shows that most practicing audiologists (>80%) currently apply a combination of pure tone audiometry, speech audiometry, acoustic immittance, and acoustic reflex testing in their daily routine. Acoustic reflex decay, threshold tone decay (TTD), and ABR also are used but by fewer audiologists (about 60% of respondents). This does not mean that every patient receives the de facto battery suggested by Figure 1–8 but that those tests are available in many practices and are used to evaluate patients. A few audiologists (<10%) eschew tympanometry and seem to get by with only pure tone and speech audiometry. Of the available site-of-lesion tests, only ABR and threshold tone decay appear to be used by more than 60% of audiologists (Fig. 1–8).

According to Martin et al (1998), it is not only the test armamentarium that is pared down in actual practice but also the test procedures. The following shortcuts and percentage of respondents surveyed were reported:

- Bone conduction testing performed only if acoustic immittance results are abnormal (6% of respondents)
- Use of monitored live voice presentation in SRT and word/speech recognition tests (94 and 91%, respectively)
- Elimination of familiarization component in SRT and word recognition tests (42 and 82%, respectively)
- Use of 5 dB step sizes for SRT determination (>90%)
- SRT criterion based on "two out of three correct" SRT criterion (60%)

- Use of half lists for word-recognition testing (56%)
- Set masking levels for speech, independent of speech presentation level

Not all trends suggested compromise. Martin et al (1998) also found that more audiologists are testing 3000-Hz and 6000-Hz thresholds than in the past. Also, 24% of the respondents reported the use of insert earphones in clinical evaluations.

Figure 1–9 details data for (electro)physiological tests, including ABR, electronystagmography (ENG), and otoacoustic emissions (OAE). Between 50 and 70% of the audiologists surveyed reported using ABR, ENG, or both 30 to 35% reported using OAEs, and 25 to 30% reported no use of the procedures. This situation is likely to change as ABR equipment ages, OAE equipment becomes more accessible, and the OAE procedures are recognized for reimbursement (see Chapter 26).

Figure 1–10 compares the percent of audiologists using site-of-lesion tests over time, from 1972 to 1997. As shown, a significant decline occurred in the general use of site-of-lesion testing. Compared with 75 to 80% of audiologists using Bekesy, SISI, and ABLB tests in 1972, only between 10 and 15% were using the same tests in 1997. The one exception is TTD testing, which appears to have remained constant at 55 to 60% of the respondents. Most of the audiologists who use TTD use a modified procedure that is faster to administer (Rosenberg or Olsen-Noffsinger).

Data from Chermak et al (1998) indicate that SCAN and SCAN-A are the most popular behavioral tests for central auditory function. All other central auditory tests (Willeford, competing sentences, SSI (ICM and CCM), speech in noise, SSW, filtered speech, and PIPB) showed uniform declines in use from 1972 to 1997, and no more than half of the audiologists reported using CAPD tests at all.

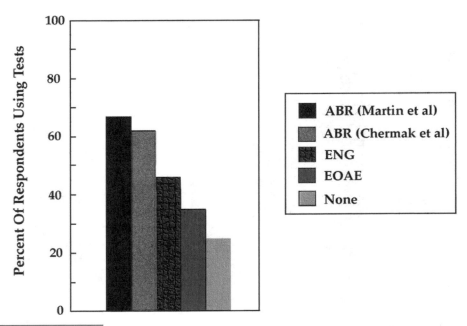

Figure 1–9 Popularity of electrophysiological and electroacoustic tests, based on percent of respondents to surveys by Chermak et al (1998) and Martin et al (1998).

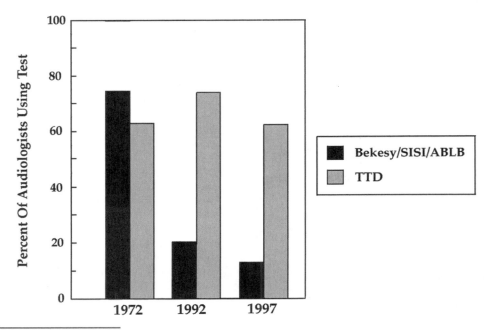

Figure 1–10 Comparison of use of behavioral site-of-lesion tests by audiologists in a 25-year period. Bekesy/SISI/ABLB percentages are averages of percent use reported for respondents for each of the three tests (data from Martin et al, 1998).

Overall, available data clearly show that the procedures used in diagnostic audiology have changed significantly in the past 25 years. The behavioral diagnostic test battery for retrocochlear lesions has all but been abandoned, save for the TTD test. Many of the subsequent chapters in this book refer to the emerging potential use of central auditory tests as a key to diagnostic audiology. In view of the low number of audiologists reporting their current use, if the optimism for their future application is to be realized, a major thrust must be made to develop and standardize procedures that can be put into widespread use.

CAN AUDIOLOGISTS DIAGNOSE HEARING LOSS?

A question posed at times, especially in matters dealing with litigation, is whether audiologists can "diagnose" hearing loss. In the courtroom or in a deposition during the qualifying period, it is not uncommon for the opposing attorney to challenge the legality of an audiologist rendering a "medical diagnosis" regarding the cause of hearing loss. Because the question posed includes the term "medical diagnosis," the opposing attorney will attempt to disqualify the audiologist because giving a medical diagnosis requires medical training and licensing. The implication is that audiologists, because they are not physicians, are not qualified to "diagnose" hearing loss. As a result, the opinions of the audiologist regarding hearing loss cannot be entered into the proceedings.

CONTROVERSIAL ISSUE

Some argue that audiologists cannot provide a diagnosis because they are not physicians, and only physicians have the credentials to give medical diagnoses.

One could go to several dictionaries and debate the meaning of the word "diagnose" and its use in various settings: in everyday language, in the clinic, in legal matters, and the like. For certain, to diagnose a condition a need to administer and interpret diagnostic tests exists. In the case of hearing loss diagnostic audiological tests would be administered and interpreted. This book testifies to the fact that many relatively simple and very complex diagnostic protocols are used by audiologists on a regular basis and that audiologists in various settings are the ones interpreting the results.

However, the real question is whether the training and experience that audiologists receive qualify them to give an opinion about the possible cause or causes of a patient's hearing loss and its impact on the patient's ability to communicate. A corollary to this is that if the audiologist is not the professional who can render an opinion regarding the cause of a patient's hearing loss and its impact on communication ability, who is?

Evidence suggests that audiologists are the primary professionals who are trained in hearing loss. As a result of the extensive training audiologists receive in the anatomy and physiology of the ear, pathophysiology of the auditory system, clinical experience, and professional skills, they are the most logical professionals to render an opinion regarding the effect of hearing loss on the communication function of patients. No other professional has the academic preparation. Otologists are the primary medical professionals who have expertise in diseases affecting the ear and auditory system. However, in most cases the otologist's expertise is limited to medical conditions of the ear, not hearing loss. In fact, in most medical schools audiologists are the faculty members who teach otology residents the curricula on hearing, hearing loss, and the impact of hearing loss on communication ability.

What about causation? Can audiologists render an opinion regarding causation? Certainly, by viewing audiometric results it is oftentimes possible to relate audiometric data to possible causation. For example, patients with conductive hearing loss cannot claim causation from continuous exposure to workplace noise of moderately high intensities. On the other hand, audiologists can confirm the causation of a patient's hearing loss with a history of noise exposure and the stereotypical 4000- to 6000-Hz sensorineural notch in the audiometric configuration to noise exposure. By examining other data, such as the intensity of workplace noise, the degree of threshold symmetry (or asymmetry), and social/medical history, including hobbies, sports, recreational activities, and medical conditions, an opinion can be given regarding the influence of each. These are clear examples of how the audiologist can, in fact, provide an opinion regarding the causation of hearing loss within the bounds of professional standards.

The Scope of Practice in Audiology by the American Speech-Language-Hearing Association states that, "Audiologists provide comprehensive *diagnostic* and rehabilitiative services for all areas of audiology, vestibular and related disorders" (ASHA, 1995). This statement gives audiologists national recognition that they can provide diagnostic testing and interpretation of results as they relate to hearing loss. However, care must be taken that audioligsts keep within their recognized bounds. Performing diagnostic audiological tests properly is one thing, interpreting them properly *and* reporting them within acceptable limits is another. For example, audiologists cannot, on the basis of their test results, "recommend" surgery for a patient. Instead, referral of surgical candidates for possible treatment to be determined by the otologic surgeon is appropriate. Moreover, audiologists should not state that test findings are indicative of a specific otologic disease but rather suggest that test results are consistent with an otologic condition to be determined by the physician. In the ideal situation audiologists will collaborate closely with physicians, preferably otologists, in developing diagnostic information for each patient served.

It is unlikely that any audiologist who is not a physician would want to be perceived as a physician. The fact that audiologists function in the healthcare profession sometimes confuses patients, and every effort should be made to make it clear that the audiologist is not a medical practitioner. A way to prevent any misunderstanding about using "medical diagnosis" is that "audiological diagnosis" is proposed as the terminology to be used to describe the contribution that audiologists make to the diagnostic process (Lipscomb, personal communication, 1999). That is, "audiological diagnoses" can be made by audiologists, which clearly implies that "medical diagnoses" are in the exclusive purview of medical practitioners.

PEARL

Physicians provide medical diagnoses; audioloigsts provide audiological diagnoses.

PATIENTS VERSUS CLIENTS

A question seldom posed formally, but having significant implications on how professionals perceive themselves and how they are perceived by others, is the terminology used to refer to those who are served. Put into a more specific framework, how should audiologists refer to those they serve? Are they "patients," "clients," or simply "customers?"

The noun "patient" is from the Latin "patiens," the present participle of pati, to suffer, and is used to denote an individual undergoing therapy; one with (or possibly with) an affliction, who is seeking therapy or a remedy. The word *patient* is associated with services provided by professions in healthcare (physicians, dentists, nurses, podiatrist, etc). The word *client*, on the other hand, is from the Latin "cliens," meaning dependent or follower, and refers to a customer or patron, one dependent on the patronage of another, or one for whom professional services are rendered. The word *client* is traditionally associated with professional services outside of healthcare, such as attorneys, accountants, and social workers.

In addressing the issue of what to call those served by audiologists, Harford (1995) asks the question, "Are audioloigists hearing healthcare professionals?" He indicates that within the professions of speech-language pathology and audiology organizations and segments within organizations promote the widespread use of the term *clients*, primarily because most of the members are providing services in the public schools where the use of the term *patients* would be questionable. He further states that audiologists are being influenced to use the term *clients* because of "lexical inbreeding," a process of exposing individuals to the use of terminology early in their careers as a result of the required exposure of audiologists-in-training to speech-language pathology instruction. Harford argues that many reasons exist why audiologists should use the term *patient*, including to be recognized as a viable part of the healthcare profession, to be recognized as the entry point into the healthcare system (the gatekeepers) for individuals with hearing impairment, to advance to a "doctoring profession," to be recognized by the health insurance industry, and to be favored in government healthcare regulations.

Practitioners will choose to call those they serve by whatever name they select. Audiologists working in the public schools are unlikely to talk to teachers about the students in the school as their "patients." However, audiologists working in health care facilities, clinical settings, or private practices, providing diagnostic audiological services and rehabilitative programs, should carefully consider the professional implications, both internal and external, of how they refer to those they serve.

The editors of all three volumes of this series have chosen to use the term *patients* when referring to those served by audiologists are in agreement with Harford that audiology is a healthcare profession. Using terminology identified with healthcare will enhance the ability of audioloigsts to serve those with hearing loss, as well as the profession, to become a recognized and viable component of healthcare programs.

REFERENCES

AMERICAN SPEECH-LANGUAGE-HEARING ASSOCIATION. (1995). *Scope of Practice in Audiology*. Rockville, MD: The Association.

BEKESY, G.V. (1947). A new audiometer. *Acta Otolaryngologica, (Stockholm), 35*; 411–422.

CARHART, R. (1957). Clinical determination of abnormal auditory adaptation. *Archives of Otolaryngology, 65*,32–39.

CHERMAK, G.D., TRAYNHAM, W.A., SEIKEL, J.A., & MUSIEK, F.E. (1998). Professional education and assessment practices in central auditory processing. *Journal of the American Academy of Audiology, 9*,452–465.

HARFORD, E. (1995) Are audiologists hearing healthcare professionals? *Audiology Today, 7*(3),10–11.

HIRSCH, B.E, DURRANT, J.D., YETISER, S., KAMERER, D.B., & MARTIN, W.H. (1996). Localizing retrocochlear hearing loss. *American Journal of Otology, 15*,537–546.

JERGER, J. (1960). Bekesy audiometry in analysis of auditory disorders. *Journal of Speech and Hearing Research, 3*, 275–287.

JERGER, S. (1983). Decision matrix and information theory analysis in the evaluation of neuroaudiologic tests. *Seminars in Hearing, 4*,121–132.

JERGER, J., & HAYES, D. (1977). Diagnostic speech audiometry. *Archives of Otolaryngology, 103*,216–222.

JERGER, J., & HERER, G. (1961). Unexpected dividend in Bekesy audiometry. *Journal of Speech and Hearing Disorders, 26*,390–391.

JERGER, J., & JERGER, S. (1975). A simplified tone decay test. *Archives of Otolaryngology, 101*,403–407.

JERGER, S., & JERGER, J. (1974). Diagnostic value of Bekesy comfort loudness tracings. *Archives of Otolaryngology, 99*,351–360.

JERGER, S., & JERGER, J. (1977). Diagnostic value of crossed vs. uncrossed acoustic reflexes. *Archives of Otolaryngology, 103*,455–466.

JERGER, S., & JERGER, J. (1983). The evaluation of diagnostic audiomteric tests. *Audiology, 22*, 144–161.

JERGER, J., SHEDD, J., & HARFORD, E. (1959). On the detection of extremely small changes in sound intensity. *Archives of Otolaryngology, 69*,200–211.

MARTIN, F.N., CHAMPLIN, C.A., & CHAMBERS, J.A. (1998). Seventh Survey of Audiometric Practices in the United States. *Journal of the American Academy of Audiology, 9*(2),95–104.

MUSIEK, F. E., MUELLER, R.J., KIBBE, K.S., & RACKLIFFE, L.S. (1983). Audiological test selection in the detection of eighth nerve disorders. *American Journal of Otolaryngology, 4*,281–287.

OLSEN, W. O., & NOFFSINGER, D. (1974). Comparison of one new and three old tests of auditory adaptation. *Archives of Otolaryngology, 99*,94–99.

OWENS, E. (1964). Tone decay in eighth nerve and cochlear lesions. *Journal of Speech and Hearing Disorders, 29*,14–22.

ROSE, D.E. (1962). Some effects and case histories of reversed frequency sweep in Bekesy audiometry. *Journal of Auditory Research, 2*,267–278.

ROSENBERG, P.E. (1958). *Rapid clinical measurement of tone decay*. Paper presented at the annual meeting of the American Speech and Hearing Association, New York.

SANDERS, J.W. (1979). Recruitment. In W.F. Rintelmann. (Ed.). *Hearing assessment*. Austin, TX: Pro-Ed.

TURNER, R.G., & NIELSEN, D.W. (1983). Application of clinical decision analysis to audiological tests. *Ear and Hearing, 5*,125–133.

WILSON, D.F., TALBOT, J.M., & LEIGH, M. (1997). A critical appraisal of the role of auditory brain stem response and magnetic resonance imaging in acoustic neuroma diagnosis. *American Journal of Otology, 18*,673–681.

## Chapter 2

Anatomy and Physiology of the Peripheral Auditory System

Richard J. Salvi, Sandra L. McFadden, and Jian Wang

Outline

The human auditory system is an extraordinary signal-processing device that enables a listener to extract critical information from a noisy acoustic environment. The system has an enormous dynamic range that allows a listener to detect extremely weak sounds that are close to the theoretical limits of detection and extremely high-level signals that are a million times more intense than sounds near the threshold of hearing. The system can also "tune in" and allow a listener to selectively attend to the speech sounds produced by a particular speaker in a noisy environment—a phenomenon referred to as the "cocktail party effect." Unfortunately, when the inner ear is damaged, the auditory system not only becomes less sensitive but also less selective. To appreciate how the auditory system operates in both normal-hearing and hearing-impaired individuals, it is necessary to understand some of the anatomical, biomechanical, and physiological characteristics of the inner ear or cochlea.

ANATOMY OF THE INNER EAR

The temporal bone, which lies medial to the external ear (i.e., the pinna and external earcanal or external auditory meatus), contains the cochlea, a fluid-filled bony structure shaped like a snail. The cochlea contains the sensory cells that are responsible for transforming acoustic information into neural activity. The human cochlea consists of a tube approximately 35-mm long, housed in a bony shell, and coiled around a bony central core known as the modiolus. The cochlea is coiled into roughly three turns that increase in diameter from the base to the apex (Fig. 2–1A). Acoustic information is transmitted to the cochlea along a path consisting of the external ear, the tympanic membrane, and the middle ear, an air-filled cavity that houses three ossicles known as the malleus, incus, and stapes. The footplate of the stapes inserts into the oval window, a kidney-shaped foramen near the base of the cochlea, and is held in place by the annular ligament. Motion of the stapes against the oval window initiates fluid motion in the cochlea.

The cochlea is subdivided into three longitudinal, fluid-filled canals known as the scala vestibuli, the scala tympani, and the scala media (Fig. 2–1B). A thin layer of cells known as Reissner's membrane separates the scala vestibuli from the scala media. The scala tympani is separated from the scala media by the basilar membrane. The basilar membrane extends from the osseous spiral lamina, a bony ledge on the modiolus, to the spiral ligament along the lateral wall of the cochlea. Although the scala vestibuli and the scala tympani are separate, parallel compartments, they share the same fluid content and communicate with one another through the helicotrema, a small opening at the apex of the cochlea. The scala tympani ends blindly at the base of the cochlea near the round window. Because the scala vestibuli and scala tympani are connected, inward motion of the stapes at the oval window will cause the fluids to move through the helicotrema and push the round window membrane outward into the air-filled middle ear space. The stria vascularis, a highly vascularized region containing numerous secretory cells, lies along the lateral wall of the scala media.

Endolymphatic and Perilymphatic Spaces

The scala vestibuli and scala tympani are filled with perilymph, a fluid similar to cerebrospinal fluid, that has a low

Audiology: Diagnosis. Edited by Roeser, Valente, and Hosford-Dunn. Thieme Medical Publishers, Inc., New York © 2000

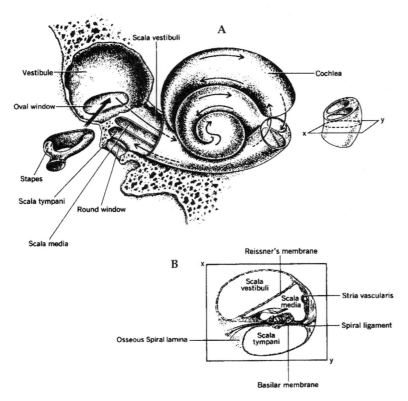

Figure 2–1   **(A)** Schematic drawing of the cochlea showing the relative positions of the scala vestibuli, scala media, and scala tympani. The stapes is attached to the oval window. The scala tympani ends blindly at the round window. The scala media is a membranous sac inside the bony labyrinth. The cochlea is shown cut away at its origin at the floor of the vestibule and again in its first turn. **(B)** Cross section of the cochlea at plane *xy*, showing the three scalae. The scala media is separated from the scala tympani by the basilar membrane and from the scala vestibuli by Reissner's membrane. The stria vascularis, adjacent to the spiral ligament along the lateral wall of the cochlea, forms the lateral boundary of the scala media. The organ of Corti sits on the basilar membrane in the scala media. (From Melloni [1957], with permission.)

concentration of potassium ions (K$^+$) and a high concentration of sodium ions (Na$^+$). The extracellular spaces surrounding the cells in the organ of Corti are also filled with perilymph. Most of scala media (i.e., the portion above the organ of Corti) contains endolymph, a fluid with a high concentration of K$^+$ and a low concentration of Na$^+$ and calcium ions (Ca^{2+}). The lower boundary of the endolymphatic space in the scala media is believed to be the reticular lamina on the upper surface of the organ of Corti (Fig. 2–2). The lateral boundary of the endolymphatic space is the stria vascularis, and the superior boundary is Reissner's membrane. Tight junctions between adjacent cells in the boundary tissues limit

diffusion of ions between the endolymphatic and perilymphatic compartments. The ionic composition of the endolymph in the scala media gives rise to an electrical potential called the endolymphatic or endocochlear potential (EP). As will be seen later, the EP is an electrochemical battery created by the stria vascularis that plays an essential role in cochlear transduction (Davis, 1965).

Organ of Corti

The organ of Corti rests on the basilar membrane in the scala media (Fig. 2–2). A prominent feature of the sensory

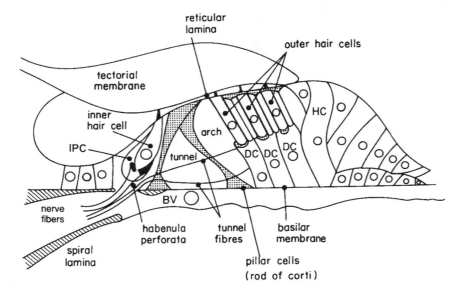

Figure 2–2   Detailed cross section of the organ of Corti. Outer hair cells are supported by Deiters' cells (DCs). Inner hair cells are closely surrounded by inner pillar cells (IPCs). The heads of the pillar cells forming the tunnel of Corti are joined at the reticular lamina. Peripheral processes of nerve fibers enter the organ of Corti through the habenula perforata. BV, basilar vessel. HC, Hensen cell. (From Bess & Humes [1990], with permission.)

epithelium is the tunnel of Corti formed by inner and outer pillar cells. The feet of the pillar cells rest on the basilar membrane and the heads of the pillar cells are joined at the reticular lamina at the apical surface of the organ of Corti. The organ of Corti contains two distinct types of sensory cells, inner hair cells (IHCs) and outer hair cells (OHCs). The flask-shaped IHCs are located medial to the inner pillar cells on the side closer to the modiolus. The human ear contains more than 3000 IHCs aligned in a single row that extends longitudinally from the base to the apex of the cochlea. The cylindrical-shaped OHCs are located lateral to the outer pillar cells on the side closer to the lateral wall. Approximately 12,000 OHCs are in the human cochlea; they are aligned in three parallel rows that extend from the base to the apex of the cochlea. The basal pole of each OHC rests in a cuplike process of a supporting cell, called a Deiters' cell, whereas its apical surface is coupled to the reticular lamina. The tectorial membrane, an acellular, gelatinous-like structure, is attached near the inner sulcus and projects out over the IHCs and OHCs.

Sensory Hair Cells

The apical pole of each hair cell is covered by a cuticular plate into which numerous rodlike stereocilia are embedded (Fig. 2–3). The stereocilia on the IHCs tend to be arranged in a gently curving arc (Fig. 2–3A), whereas those on the OHCs tend to be arranged in a W pattern (Fig. 2–3B). The stereocilia bundle contains several rows of stereocilia that increase in height in a stairstep fashion. The shortest row of stereocilia is located on the modiolar side of the hair cell, and the tallest row faces the lateral wall of the cochlea. The stereocilia are composed of polymerized actin filaments from which they derive their rigidity. Each individual stereocilium narrows at the point where its rootlet enters the cuticular plate, as shown schematically in Figure 2–4. The stereocilia pivot around the rootlet when the bundle is deflected. Side links along the side of the stereocilia tie the stereocilia together so that the entire bundle moves as a unit when deflected (Flock, 1977; Flock et al, 1977; Pickles et al, 1984).

Current theories assume that the mechanically gated transduction channels on hair cells are located near the tips of the stereocilia bundle (Fig. 2–4) (Corey & Hudspeth, 1979; Hudspeth & Corey, 1977; Pickles & Corey, 1992). Fine fibers called tip links connect the transduction channels at the tips of the shorter stereocilia to the sides of the taller stereocilia. Consequently, when the stereocilia bundle is deflected in the direction of the tallest stereocilia, tension on the fibers pulls the transduction channels open. This allows positively charged ions to flow in, which "depolarizes" the hair cell (i.e., the membrane potential becomes less negative). Deflection of the stereocilia bundle in the opposite direction closes transduction channels, decreasing ion flow into the hair cell and resulting in relative hyperpolarization. As shown in Figure 2–4, depolarization of the IHC increases the firing rate of primary auditory nerve (AN) fibers greater than their spontaneous rate, whereas hyperpolarization decreases the firing rate of spontaneously active AN fibers. Thus the back-and-forth movement of the IHC stereocilia produces cycles of excitation and suppression in cochlear output by way of AN.

Auditory Nerve

The auditory portion of the eighth cranial nerve contains the fibers that transmit neural activity from the cochlea to the central auditory system. The cell bodies of the AN fibers, called spiral ganglion cells or primary auditory neurons (Fig. 2–5), are located in the osseous spiral lamina. The peripheral processes of these bipolar neurons pass through narrow channels in the bony modiolus called the habenula perforata, enter the organ of Corti, and travel to the IHCs and OHCs. The central processes of the spiral ganglion neurons form the AN bundle that enters the cochlear nucleus (CN) in the brain stem. Approximately 50,000 fibers are in the AN of the cat. Approximately 90 to 95% of these are classified as type I fibers, and each of these synapses on a single IHC (Fig. 2–5). Each IHC is contacted by many (up to 20) type I fibers; thus type I AN fibers are more numerous than IHCs. The

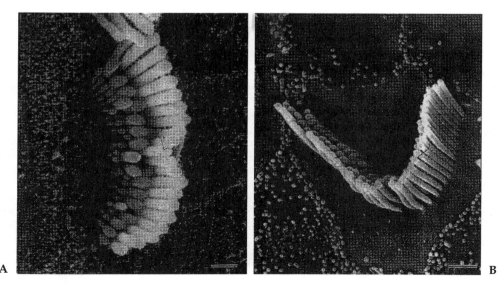

Figure 2–3   Stereocilia on an IHC (**A**) and an OHC (**B**) of chinchilla.

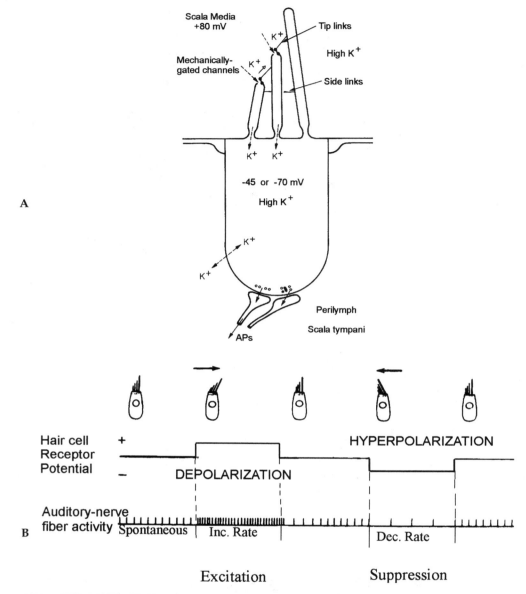

Figure 2–4 Schematic drawing of the transduction process, incorporating Davis' electromechanical model. **(A)** Transduction channels at the tips of the stereocilia are coupled to the next tallest stereocilia by a flexible transduction link. When open, the channels allow ions (primarily K^+ because this is the most abundant ion in endolymph) to flow into the cell, driven by the batteries of the EP +80 mV in the scala media) and the intracellular potential of the hair cell (−45 mV for IHC; −70 mV for OHC). Note that the stereocilia narrow at the point where they insert into the cuticular plate of the hair cell. **(B)** Current flow through the hair cell is modulated by deflection of the stereocilia. At rest, approximately 5 to 15% of transduction channels are open, resulting in a standing current through the hair cell. When the stereocilia bundle is deflected toward the tallest stereocilia, more transduction channels are opened, increasing ion flow and depolarizing the cell. Deflection of the bundle in the opposite direction closes channels and reduces K^+ current, leading to hyperpolarization of the cell. For IHCs, depolarization increases the rate of neurotransmitter release and increases the firing rate of AN fibers, whereas hyperpolarization decreases neurotransmitter release and decreases the firing rate of AN fibers. (Adapted from Pickles [1988], with permission, and Durrant & Lovrinic [1995].)

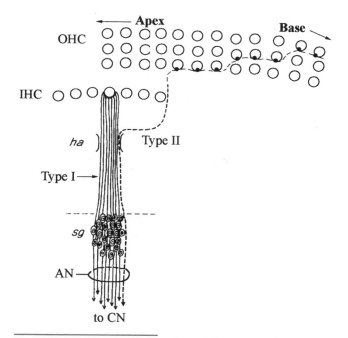

Figure 2–5   Afferent innervation of the organ of Corti. The peripheral processes of spiral ganglion (*sg*) neurons enter the cochlea through the habenula perforata (*ha*) and travel to the hair cells. Approximately 95% of the sg neurons are type I cells whose peripheral processes innervate IHCs. The remaining 5% of sg neurons are type II cells that innervate OHCs. The central processes of sg fibers form the auditory nerve (AN) that projects to the cochlear nucleus (CN) in the brain stem. (Adapted from Spoendlin [1978], with permission.)

remaining 5 to 10% of AN fibers are classified as type II fibers. As shown in Figure 2–5, the type II fibers travel to the OHCs. Unlike each type I fiber, which innervates a single IHC, each type II fiber branches profusely and innervates approximately 10 different OHCs (Spoendlin, 1972). The type II fibers cross the tunnel of Corti (see the "tunnel-crossing fibers" in Fig. 2–7) and spiral toward the base of the cochlea before making contact with the OHCs.

Efferent Innervation of the Cochlea

An intriguing aspect of cochlear anatomy is the presence of efferent nerve fibers that project to the cochlea from cell bodies in the superior olivary region of the brain stem. As illustrated in Figure 2–6, the efferent nerve fibers arise from two major cell groups, one located in the region of the medial superior olive (MSO) and the other located in the vicinity of the lateral superior olive (LSO). Collectively, the axons of these neurons are referred to as olivocochlear efferent fibers. Fibers arising from cells near the MSO are large, myelinated fibers called medial olivocochlear (MOC) efferents. Fibers arising from cells near the LSO are small, unmyelinated fibers referred to as lateral olivocochlear (LOC) efferents. LOC and MOC fibers can be further divided into crossed and uncrossed divisions, depending on whether their axons project to the

opposite or same ear. The crossed division consists of many more MOC efferents than LOC efferents, whereas the uncrossed division is dominated by LOC efferents.

MOC and LOC efferents gather together in the brain stem to form the olivocochlear bundle (OCB). As shown in Figure 2–6, the efferent fibers travel within the inferior vestibular nerve (IVN) to the vestibulocochlear anastomosis of Oort, which is the junction between the vestibular nerve and the AN in the periphery. Here, the efferent fibers cross over to the AN and enter the cochlea as the intraganglionic spiral bundle (Fig. 2–7). Within the organ of Corti, LOC efferents travel primarily within the inner spiral bundle, and terminate on the dendrites of type I afferent nerve fibers beneath the IHCs. MOC efferents travel primarily as upper tunnel radial fibers and terminate directly on the OHCs (Robertson et al, 1989; Warr & Guinan, 1979). In most species MOC efferents branch profusely, and a single MOC efferent can innervate as many as 100 OHCs (Emmerling & Sobkowicz, 1988; Liberman & Brown, 1986; Warr, 1975).

PEARL

Although most anatomical studies have been performed on animals, the main features of the efferent system are likely to be similar in humans.

Anatomical studies have shown that LOC neurons outnumber MOC neurons in a variety of species (Aschoff et al, 1988; Bishop & Henson, 1987; Warr, 1992; Warren & Liberman, 1989). LOC efferents comprise approximately 65% of the olivocochlear efferents in the cat and up to 100% in some types of bats. In all species LOC fibers project predominantly to the cochlea on the ipsilateral side, whereas MOC fibers project predominantly to the cochlea on the contralateral side. Because LOC fibers innervate type I afferent dendrites, whereas MOC fibers innervate OHCs, the two fiber systems influence cochlear functioning in much different ways.

Interestingly, although the anatomy of the OCB efferents has been well known since Rasmussen first described them in 1942 (see Fig. 2–6), the precise function of the OCB is still a mystery. Studies have suggested that the MOC efferents may be important for: (a) improving the ability to detect and discriminate signals in the presence of background noise (Buno, 1978; Dewson, 1967, 1968; Nieder & Nieder, 1970a,b; May & McQuone, 1995; Winslow & Sachs, 1987, 1988); (b) focusing (or unfocusing) attention on auditory stimuli (Desmedt, 1962; Giard et al, 1994; Igarashi et al, 1974; Pfalz, 1962); and (c) protecting the ear from damage caused by acoustic overstimulation (Cody & Johnstone, 1982; Handrock & Zeisberg, 1982; Rajan & Johnstone, 1983, 1988a,b, 1989; Zheng et al, 1997b,c). These effects are presumably mediated by the influence of the MOC fibers on OHC electromotility, which in turn affects the sensitivity of the cochlea. Extremely little is known about the functional significance of the LOC system. Recent studies suggest that LOC fibers play a role in the development and maintenance of normal cochlear function (Walsh et al, 1998; Zheng et al,

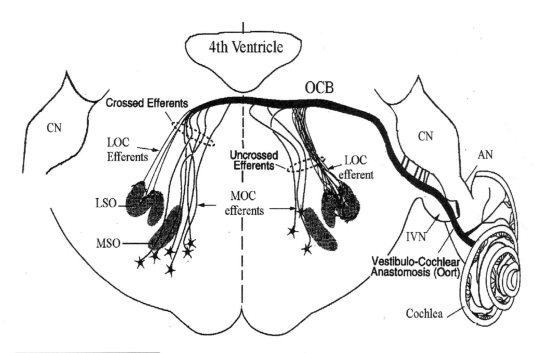

Figure 2–6 Sources of efferent fibers projecting to the cochlea from the superior olivary region of the brain stem. Cells in the region of the lateral superior olive (*LSO*) give rise to lateral olivo-cochlear (*LOC*) fibers that dominate an uncrossed efferent pathway. Cells in the region of the medial superior olive (*MSO*) give rise to medial olivocochlear (*MOC*) fibers that dominate a crossed efferent pathway. All fibers gather together beneath the floor of the fourth ventricle to form the olivocochlear bundle (*OCB*). The OCB travels with the inferior vestibular nerve (*IVN*) into the internal auditory meatus. At the junction between the vestibular nerve and the auditory nerve (*AN*), known as Oort's vestibulocochlear anastomosis, the efferent fibers cross over to the AN and enter the cochlea. (Adapted from Liberman [1990], with permission.)

Figure 2–7 Comparison of the pathways taken by the afferent (*hatched*) and efferent (*solid black*) nerve fibers within the organ of Corti, the position of the afferent type I and type II ganglion cells and the spiral efferents in the osseous spiral lamina, and the afferent processes running toward the cochlear nucleus in the modiolus. (From Slepecky [1996], with permission.)

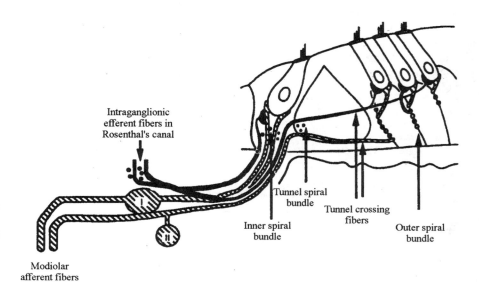

1999). Clearly, much more research is needed before we have a full understanding of the functional significance of the OCB, particularly the enigmatic LOC division.

COCHLEAR MECHANICS

Sound-induced motion of the stapes gives rise to pressure fluctuations in the cochlear fluids that cause the basilar membrane to vibrate. George von Békésy, who received the Nobel Prize for his pioneering work in hearing, provided the first comprehensive description of basilar membrane motion. With a microscope and stroboscopic illumination, von Békésy was able to observe the motion of the cochlear partition in cochleas extracted from human and animal cadavers (von Békésy, 1960). The inward and outward motion of the stapes is opposed by the inertia of the fluid mass, the stiffness of the tissue, and the frictional resistance generated by fluid motion within the scalae. Because the fluids in the inner ear are incompressible, the pressure fluctuations in the fluids occur almost instantaneously along the entire length of the cochlea. Nevertheless, the entire basilar membrane does not move in unison because the mechanical impedance of the cochlear partition varies from base to apex. The stiffness of the basilar membrane gradually decreases from base to apex, whereas its mass increases from base to apex. Because the base of the cochlea is stiffer and lighter than the apex, it responds sooner than the apex when pressure is applied to the basilar membrane. Because of the mass and stiffness gradient, the motion of the basilar membrane gradually shifts from the base toward the apex, giving the appearance of a "traveling wave" displacement pattern.

Figure 2–8 shows the traveling wave displacement pattern along the length of the cochlea during stimulation with a high-frequency tone (8 kHz), a mid-frequency tone (2 kHz), and a low-frequency tone (200 Hz). Each line represents a series of snapshot views of basilar membrane motion, showing how the peak response shifts from the base toward the apex of the cochlea. High-frequency sounds produce a traveling wave envelope that has a peak near the base of the cochlea, but no activity occurs in the middle or the apex of the cochlea. The peak for mid-frequency sounds is located near the middle of the cochlea. Low-frequency sounds produce a peak near the apex of the cochlea. However, low frequencies also activate the base and middle of the cochlea at high sound levels. The shift in the location of the peak results in a frequency to place transformation of sound. That is, the basilar membrane segregates different frequencies according to the position of maximal excitation along the cochlear partition.

The mass and stiffness gradient of the cochlear partition also influences its temporal response. Because the base of the cochlea is stiffer and lighter than the apex, it responds more quickly to stimulation. Thus although the pressure wave initiated by stapes motion is applied to the entire basilar membrane almost simultaneously, the basilar membrane near the base of the cochlea starts to move sooner than that in the apex. This results in a wave of motion that appears to move from base to apex over time. The time required for initiation of basilar membrane movement at any given point along the basilar membrane can be expressed in terms of phase angle or phase lag. The phase lag or phase angle can be referenced (compared) to

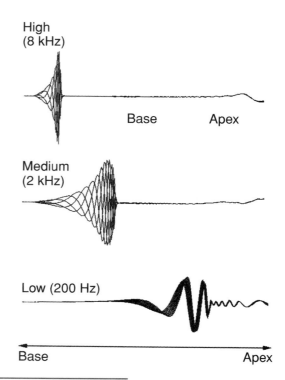

Figure 2–8 Traveling wave displacement patterns along the basilar membrane, for high-frequency tones (*top*), mid-frequency tones (*middle*), and low-frequency tones (*bottom*). The dashed lines show the envelope of the basilar membrane response.

the phase of the stimulus or the phase angle of another point on the basilar membrane. This is illustrated in Figure 2–9 which shows the phase angle (θ) at different points along the basilar membrane for four stimulus frequencies. (Note: $\theta = 2\pi ft$, where f = frequency and t = time. Because of this relationship, phase angle is proportional to the time required to move through a certain number of degrees of a stimulus cycle at a certain frequency.) Location along the basilar membrane is expressed in terms of distance from the stapes from base to apex. The phase angle for a point near the base of the cochlea is less than that near the apex for each frequency.

The traveling wave displacement envelope measured by von Békésy was extremely broad. Consequently, the results were difficult to reconcile with psychophysical measurements that suggested that the internal auditory filters were extremely narrow. The source of the discrepancy can be traced back to the fact that von Békésy's measurements were made on dead ears with abnormal mechanical properties. More recent measurements from intact animals with healthy cochleas have shown that the basilar membrane displacement patterns are extremely sharply tuned (Khanna & Leonard, 1982; Sellick et al, 1982). The most recent measurement techniques have used lasers to measure displacement or velocity of a given point on the basilar membrane as stimulus frequency and sound level are varied. The schematic diagram in Figure 2–10A shows a frequency-threshold-tuning curve for a point near the base of the cochlea. Threshold was defined as the minimum intensity required to elicit a just-

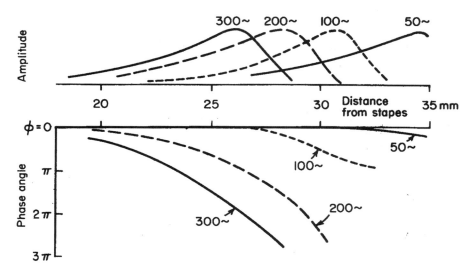

Figure 2–9 Von Békésy's classic data showing amplitude and phase measurements of the traveling wave at different points along the basilar membrane for four different frequencies (300, 200, 100, and 50 Hz). Top portion shows the relative amplitude of basilar membrane displacement for a constant stapes displacement. Bottom portion shows the corresponding phase angle (proportional to time delay) for each of the four frequencies. Measurements were made from the human cadaver cochlea. (From von Békésy [1960], with permission.)

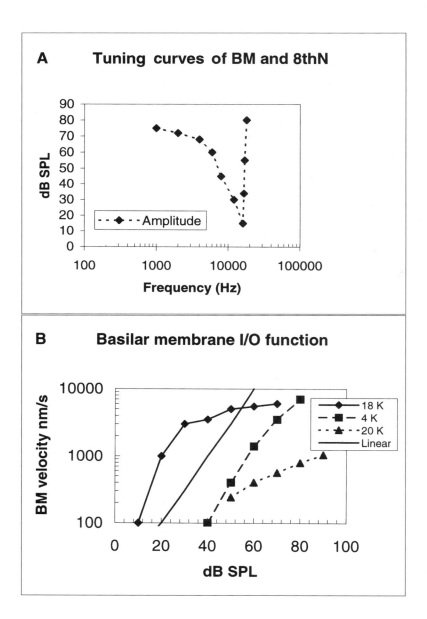

Figure 2–10 **(A)** Frequency tuning curve for the basilar membrane at a point near the base of the cochlea. **(B)** Basilar membrane velocity at the characteristic frequency (18 kHz) place on the basilar membrane using the Mossbauer technique. The solid line represents the response of a linear system, in which input level and output level are equivalent. Responses near the characteristic frequency are characterized by compressive nonlinearity.

detectable displacement of the basilar membrane. The frequency with the lowest threshold is referred to as the characteristic frequency (CF). Threshold increases significantly at frequencies greater than and less than CF. The tuning curve in a healthy ear consists of a low-threshold, narrowly tuned tip near CF and a high-threshold, broadly tuned tail less than CF. The high-frequency side of the tuning curve has an extremely steep slope because the basilar membrane displacement envelope shifts further toward the base of the cochlea as frequency increases (see Fig. 2–8).

The schematic diagram in Figure 2–10B shows basilar membrane displacement (proportional to velocity) as a function of sound level for three different frequencies, one at CF (18 kHz), a second frequency less than CF (4 kHz), and a third frequency greater than CF (20 kHz). For comparison, the solid line shows the response of a linear system in which the slope is 1 at all sound levels, indicating that the magnitude of the output is equivalent to the magnitude of the input. Because the basilar membrane is most sensitive to tones near CF, the input/output function at CF is located furthest to the left (lower intensities). The input/output functions greater than and less than CF are located further to the right (higher intensities) to reflect the decreased sensitivity to off-CF frequencies. For frequencies less than CF (represented by the 4 kHz input/output function in Fig. 2–10B), the slope of the input/output function is close to 1, indicating that the basilar membrane response is essentially linear, at least up to moderately high intensities. By contrast, the input/output function at CF and frequencies near CF show a compressive nonlinearity. That is, the input/output function rises rapidly at low intensities but begins to saturate at high intensities resulting in a slope that is less than 1 at high sound levels.

COCHLEAR ELECTROPHYSIOLOGY

Electrical activity is an integral part of the functioning of cells in the cochlea and the central auditory system. Several types of electrical potentials can be measured from electrodes placed in or near the cochlea that reflect the physiological state of the cochlea and the AN. The electrical potentials can be divided into two broad classes: resting potentials and stimulus-evoked potentials. Resting potentials are those that occur in the absence of acoustic stimulation and include the EP and the intracellular resting potentials of IHCs and OHCs. Stimulus-evoked potentials are those that occur in response to acoustic stimulation and include the cochlear microphonic (CM) potential, the summating potential (SP), and the compound action potential (CAP). The latter potentials arise when the activity of a group of cells becomes entrained to a specific stimulus, resulting in synchronous electrical activity.

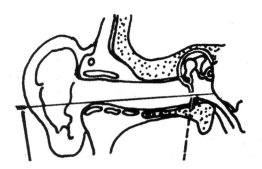

Silver electrode coated with vinyl chloride (Diamter: 0.2 mm, Length: 5 cm)

Perforation (Diameter: 0.5mm)

Figure 2–11 Transtympanic electrode used to record electrical potentials from the cochlea and auditory nerve. The electrode is inserted through the tympanic membrane and placed against the promontory of the cochlea that projects into the middle ear space. (From Tanahashi et al [1976], with permission.)

A second way of classifying electrical potentials is according to the type of electrode that is used to record them and, consequently, the size of the cellular population that contributes to the response. Cellular potentials, including the membrane and intracellular potentials of IHCs and OHCs and the action potentials of individual AN fibers, are recorded using fine-tipped, high-impedance metal microelectrodes or glass micropipettes. These potentials provide detailed information regarding the behavior of individual cells. Local field potentials (LFPs), reflecting the extracellular electrical activity arising from groups of cells, are recorded by means of low impedance (typically less than 100 kΩ) electrodes that are inserted directly into the cochlea or AN. The contribution of any given cell to the total LFP will depend on its proximity to the recording electrode and the size of its extracellular field potential. LFPs are typically quantified in terms of amplitude (total voltage) and provide information regarding the behavior of aggregates of cells. Finally, gross potentials are generated by large populations of cells and are recorded with relatively large, low-impedance electrodes, including transtympanic electrodes that are sometimes used to record the CM and CAP in humans (Fig. 2–11). Gross potentials such as the CAP can be used clinically to evaluate the functioning of the auditory periphery. Other potentials measured from the cochlea can provide insight into how the various elements and structures of the cochlea function in normal and impaired ears. Figure 2–12 shows a typical response recorded from a gross electrode placed near the round window. The response consists of three individual components that are evoked and recorded concurrently: the CM, the CAP (consisting of two negative peaks, labeled N1 and N2), and the SP. Special recording techniques can be used to isolate each of the components of the evoked response.

Resting Potentials of the Cochlea

Von Békésy first explored the electrical properties of the fluid spaces of the cochlea by recording changes in electrical potential as an electrode was advanced through the cochlea of a

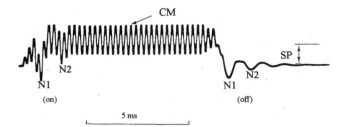

Figure 2–12 Diagram of the response to a tone burst, recorded with gross electrodes. The evoked response includes three components: the cochlear microphonic (*CM*), N1 and N2 phases of the CAP, and the summating potential (*SP*). The CM is an AC potential that mimics the stimulus waveform. The SP is a DC potential that shifts the CM from the baseline, in this example in the positive direction. The CAP occurs at both the beginning of the stimulus and at the end of the stimulus. (Reprinted from Pickles [1988], with permission.)

guinea pig. A hypothetical experiment similar to the one conducted by von Békésy is shown schematically in Figure 2–13. Potential differences are measured between a reference (ground) electrode that is inserted in the plasma and a micropipette recording electrode that is inserted into the cochlea through a small hole drilled in the bony labyrinthine wall. Changes in electrical potential relative to ground are observed on an oscilloscope as the recording electrode is advanced (a) into the scala tympani, (b) into the fluid surrounding the organ of Corti, (c) into a cochlear hair cell, (d) through the reticular lamina into the scala media, and (e) across Reissner's membrane into the scala vestibuli.

When the electrode enters the perilymph in the scala tympani, a small DC (unidirectional) potential of approximately +7 mV is recorded (Johnstone & Sellick, 1972). The potential changes very little as the electrode passes through the basilar membrane into the fluid surrounding the organ of Corti. Analysis of the fluid surrounding the organ of Corti indicates that its ionic content is essentially the same as perilymph (Anniko & Wroblewski, 1986; Ryan et al, 1980). As the electrode enters a cochlear hair cell, an abrupt change from a positive to a negative potential is observed. If the electrode has entered an OHC, the electrical potential will be approximately −70 mV. If the electrode has instead pierced an IHC, the potential will be close to −45 mV (Cody & Russell, 1987; Dallos et al, 1982). These intracellular potentials, recorded in the absence of acoustic stimulation, are the resting potentials of the hair cells. When the electrode crosses the reticular lamina and enters the endolymph of the scala media, an abrupt increase in electrical potential, to approximately +80 mV DC, occurs. The +80 mV EP can be recorded in the absence of any acoustic stimulation (Bosher & Warren, 1971; Peake et al, 1969). Finally, when the recording electrode is advanced through Reissner's membrane into the perilymph of the scala vestibuli, the potential drops abruptly to approximately +2 to 5 mV (Johnstone & Sellick, 1972).

The EP was originally thought to be a diffusion potential resulting from differences in ion concentration between endolymph and perilymph. However, studies have shown that decreasing the K^+ concentration gradient between endolymph and perilymph by injecting potassium chloride into the perilymph has little effect on the amplitude of the EP (Konishi & Kelsey, 1968; Tasaki et al, 1954). Thus the source of the EP is not simply the concentration gradient between the scala media and the perilymphatic spaces.

Several lines of evidence indicate that the stria vascularis is the source of endolymph and the EP and that generation of the EP is an active (energy-consuming) process. First, the EP decreases significantly when the stria is damaged surgically or with ototoxic drugs (Davis et al, 1958; Sewell, 1984). Second, Na^+/K^+-dependent ATPase activity is very high in stria vascularis (Kuijpers & Bonting, 1970). Ouabain, a drug that inhibits Na^+/K^+-ATPase activity, decreases the concentration of K^+ and increases the concentration of Na^+ in the scala media and reduces the EP (Konishi et al, 1978; Konishi & Mendelsohn, 1970). Third, positive electrical potentials can be recorded from the marginal cells of the stria vascularis even after Reissner's membrane is destroyed (Tasaki & Spyropoulos, 1959). Fourth, the EP declines rapidly during anoxia (Johnstone & Sellick, 1972). These results indicate that the EP is a metabolic potential, generated by energy-consuming activities of cells in the stria vascularis. Electrogenic pumps located in the basolateral walls of marginal cells in the stria vascularis actively take up K^+ and extrude Na^+ in order to maintain the ionic composition of the endolymph (Kuijpers & Bonting, 1970).

Davis Model of Transduction

Davis (1965) proposed a model of cochlear transduction that has served as a cornerstone in our understanding of cochlear electrophysiology. According to Davis' mechanoelectrical model, the EP and the intracellular potential of the hair cell act as batteries that drive the transduction process. Modern versions of the Davis model (Hudspeth, 1985b; Pickles, 1985) describe the transduction process in the following way. The transduction process begins with motion of the basilar membrane, which leads to stimulation of the hair cell stereocilia either by mechanical displacement of the tectorial membrane relative to the reticular lamina (OHCs) or by the motion of the fluid surrounding the stereocilia (IHCs). Measurements of the voltage gradients around the apical surface of hair cells indicate that the transduction channels are located near the tips of the stereocilia bundles (Corey & Hudspeth, 1979; Hudspeth, 1982; Hudspeth, 1985a). When the stereocilia are deflected, changes in electrical potential occur within a few microseconds. The time course of the electrical response suggests that the transduction channels are opened directly by mechanical tension.

A model of the transduction process was shown in Figure 2–4. The transduction channels near the tips of the stereocilia are coupled to the next tallest row of stereocilia by a flexible link (Pickles et al, 1984). These channels are nonselective cation channels, which means that they will allow virtually any type of positively charged ion to pass through them. However, because K^+ is the most abundant ion in endolymph, current through the channels is carried primarily by

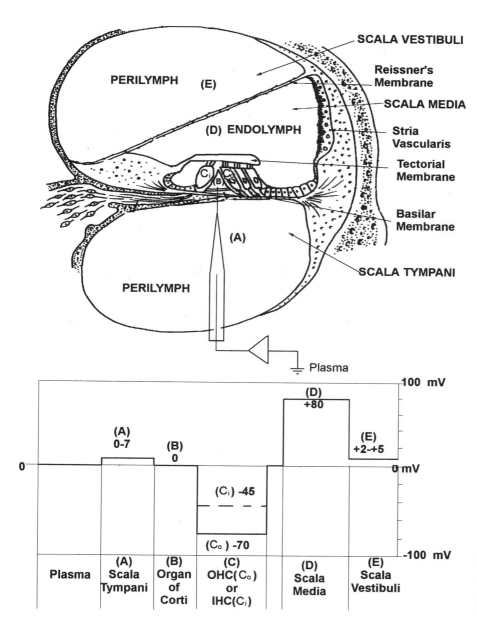

Figure 2–13 Potential differences recorded between a reference (ground) electrode located in the plasma and a micropipette recording electrode as it moves through the cochlea. DC potentials are recorded as the recording electrode moves through (A) the perilymph of the scala tympani; (B) through the basilar membrane into the fluid surrounding cells in the organ of Corti; (C) into an OHC (C_o) or an IHC (C_i); (D) through the reticular lamina into the endolymph of the scala media; and (E) through Reissner's membrane into the perilymph of the scala vestibuli. Top panel shows the position of the recording electrode. Bottom panel shows the amplitude and polarity of the DC potential.

K^+ ions. In the absence of stimulation approximately 5 to 15% of the ion channels are open at any given time, resulting in a "standing current" of K^+ through the hair cell (Crawford & Fettiplace, 1981; Hudspeth & Corey, 1977; Russell et al, 1986). The stria vascularis is primarily responsible for the standing current, because it secretes K^+ into the endolymph and generates the EP that drives K^+ current through the scala media.

When the basilar membrane moves toward the scala vestibuli, the stereocilia bundles on the hair cells are deflected toward the tallest stereocilia (see Fig. 2–4). This increases the tension in the transduction links, thereby increasing the proportion of nonselective cation channels that are open (Corey & Hudspeth, 1979; Hudspeth, 1982; Pickles et al, 1984). More K^+ current flows through the ion channels, resulting in depolarization of the hair cell. Conversely, movement of the basilar

membrane toward the scala tympani causes the hair cell stereocilia bundle to deflect toward the shortest stereocilia. This closes more channels, thereby decreasing current flow and hyperpolarizing the hair cell.

The K^+ current is driven across the apical surface of the hair cell by the combined effects of two batteries, one associated with the +80 mV EP in the scala media and the other associated with the negative intracellular potential of the hair cell (see Fig. 2–13). The EP battery and the intracellular battery are in series, so the total voltage available to drive K^+ current across the apical surface of the hair cell is approximately 125 mV for IHCs and 150 mV for OHCs. Increased movement of K^+ ions through the hair cell membrane depolarizes the cell, whereas decreased current leads to relative hyperpolarization (Fig. 2–4B). For IHCs, depolarization results in increased release of neurotransmitter from the base of the hair cell above the resting (spontaneous) level, which in turn increases the firing rate of the AN fibers synapsing on it. Conversely, hyperpolarization of the IHC decreases the rate of neurotransmitter release, thereby decreasing the discharge rates of AN fibers to less than their spontaneous rates. Depolarization and hyperpolarization of the OHC causes the cell to contract and elongate along its main axis. The voltage-induced change in OHC length (electromotility) is believed to modulate basilar membrane mechanics and thereby control the sensitivity of the cochlea to acoustic stimuli.

Stimulus-Evoked Potentials Measured from the Cochlea

Cochlear Microphonics

During acoustic stimulation, an AC (frequency-following) potential called the cochlear microphonic can be recorded from electrodes placed on or near the cochlea (see Fig. 2–12). The original recordings of the CM were made by Wever and Bray (1930), who observed that the cochlea acts like a microphone, transducing sound into analog changes in voltage. If the voltages are amplified and fed to a loudspeaker, as Wever and Bray did, the original stimulus will be reproduced with remarkable fidelity. For example, if the ear is stimulated with a 1 kHz pure tone of varying level, a 1 kHz electrical sine wave, with amplitude proportional to the stimulus level, will be produced by the cochlea.

Wever and Bray believed they were recording gross potentials from the AN. However, we now know that the CM is derived from currents flowing through the hair cells in response to acoustic stimulation. An experiment by Tasaki et al (1954) provided the first evidence that hair cells are the source of the CM. Tasaki et al measured the CM while advancing a recording electrode through the cochlea. The CM grew in amplitude as the electrode neared the reticular lamina, then reversed polarity as the electrode entered the scala media. These results indicated that the CM was generated by the hair cells or some other structure close to the reticular lamina. More recent studies have shown that large, sharply tuned CM potentials can be recorded from electrodes close to the hair cells (Goodman et al, 1982).

The extent to which IHCs contribute to the CM is unknown. Because OHCs are approximately three times as numerous as IHCs, the OHCs would be expected to be the main source of the CM. An experiment by Dallos (1973) provided support for the dominance of OHCs in CM production. When Dallos selectively destroyed OHCs with kanamycin, leaving IHCs intact, the CM was reduced to approximately 1/30 its normal size. Experiments with chinchillas that have selective basal IHC lesions associated with sectioning the AN show that basal IHC loss has no appreciable effect on the CM recorded from the round window (Zheng et al, 1997a). Other experiments that used a unique animal model in which the IHCs are selectively destroyed by carboplatin while OHCs remain intact provide further evidence that IHCs make little, if any, contribution to the CM (Takeno et al, 1994; Trautwein et al, 1996). Collectively, these results suggest that the CM is predominantly generated by the OHCs.

> ## PEARL
>
> **From a clinical standpoint, the CM recorded with electrocochleography or earcanal electrodes could be used to assess the integrity of the OHCs near the base of the cochlea.**

The CM appears to follow the waveform of the acoustic stimulus because it reflects the instantaneous displacement of the basilar membrane. It has no apparent threshold (Dallos, 1973) because the lowest level at which the CM can be recorded is limited by the noise floor of the recording apparatus and internal (biological) noise. Nevertheless, a threshold is often defined operationally (e.g., as the stimulus intensity at which CM amplitude exceeds some arbitrary voltage, such as 1 μV). The amplitude of the CM represents the vector sum of the potentials generated by a large number of individual hair cells (Whitfield & Ross, 1965). Interestingly, the CM shows little change in amplitude for long-duration stimuli, indicating that the sensory receptor does not adapt. This finding is consistent with recent intracellular measurements of the hair cell receptor potential (Cody & Russell, 1985). CM amplitude varies with stimulus sound pressure level (SPL), as shown by the input/output function (i.e., the function relating response magnitude to stimulus level) in Figure 2–14. At low to moderate sound levels, a linear relationship exists between CM amplitude and stimulus SPL, with CM increasing a little more than three times (10 dB) for every 10 dB increase in stimulus level. The amplitude of the CM eventually saturates and then rolls over slightly at the highest levels (Dallos, 1973; Tasaki et al, 1952). At very high stimulus levels, the CM may contain a considerable amount of harmonic distortion and bear little resemblance to the original signal (Dallos, 1973). The range of stimulus SPLs over which CM increases linearly and the maximum CM amplitude that is observed will depend on a combination of factors, including recording

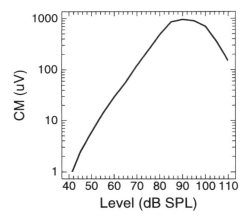

Figure 2–14 Input-output function of the CM recorded from a round window electrode in a chinchilla. At high stimulus levels, the CM saturates and rolls over.

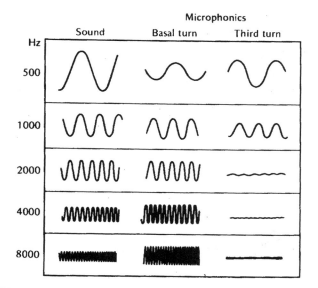

Figure 2–15 Spatial distribution of the CM recorded from the first and third turns of the guinea pig cochlea. The first column shows the waveform of the acoustic stimulus. The second column shows the CM recorded from an electrode in the basal turn. The third column shows the CM recorded from an electrode in the apical turn. Note that for a 500-Hz stimulus, the CM is larger in the apical turn than in the basal turn. The CM also shifts 180 degrees out of phase because of the time it takes for the traveling wave to reach the third turn. Low-frequency stimuli produce CM responses in both the apex and the base, whereas high-frequency stimuli produce responses in the base only. (From Yost [1994], with permission.)

technique, recording site, and the frequency and level of the sound stimulus.

Because the CM is initiated by basilar membrane displacement, it is spatially distributed along the cochlear partition according to both frequency and level (Tasaki et al, 1952). As shown in Figure 2–15, the pattern of the CM follows the pattern of the traveling wave that was originally observed by von Békésy. The CM recorded from an electrode placed in the first turn (base) is compared with the CM recorded from an electrode in the third turn (apex) of the cochlea. A low-frequency tone generates a CM that can be measured from both the base and the apex electrodes. However, the amplitude of the CM is greater in the apex than in the base, and a phase shift occurs between the two recording sites. In contrast, a high-frequency tone generates a CM only in the base of the cochlea. As stimulus level increases, the CM in response to a low-frequency tone will spread toward the base of the cochlea. The CM resulting from high-frequency tonal stimulation, on the other hand, will be primarily confined to the base of the cochlea at all stimulus levels. Thus the spatial distribution of the CM approximates the envelope of basilar membrane vibration.

Summating Potential

The SP appears as a steplike DC shift in potential that lasts as long as the stimulus, as shown in Figure 2–12. The SP can be

either positive or negative, depending on the stimulus parameters, recording site, and recording techniques (Dallos et al, 1970). SPs recorded from the scala tympani or the scala vestibuli can be either positive or negative, and they can reverse polarity, depending on the frequency, level, and duration of the stimulus. SPs recorded from the round window tend to be positive at low stimulus levels but negative at high stimulus levels (Margolis et al, 1992; Tilanus et al, 1992).

For some time, the SP has been thought to arise from distortion generated by the hair cell transduction process. Results obtained from animals treated with aminoglycoside antibiotics suggested that the OHCs may contribute significantly to the SP at low to moderate intensities, whereas IHCs may contribute to the SP at higher SPLs (Dallos, 1975). However, recent experiments with chinchillas with selective IHC loss (Zheng et al, 1997a) suggest that the IHCs are the major source of SPs recorded from the round window, particularly at low to moderate stimulus levels. Animals with a 40 to 50% loss of IHCs in the base of the cochlea showed a 60 to 80% decrease in SP amplitude at stimulus levels less than 80 dB SPL, despite having normal CM, normal distortion product otoacoustic emissions (DPOAEs), and a normal complement of OHCs. Similar results have been obtained from animals with selective carboplatin-induced IHC lesions (Durrant et al, 1998), in which lesions involving both IHCs and OHCs abolished the SP.

Compound Action Potential

The CAP is the extracellular field potential produced by the synchronous depolarization of a large number of AN fibers in response to a stimulus. Although not a true cochlear potential, it can be recorded from electrodes placed in or near the cochlea, and it provides information regarding the functional status of the cochlea. The CAP consists of two prominent negative peaks, referred to as N1 and N2 (Figs. 2–12 and 2–16). The N1 response occurs approximately 1.0 ms after the onset of the stimulus (approximately 0.7 ms after the onset of the CM), and N2 appears approximately 1 ms later. Like the CM, the CAP is a graded response that represents the summation of electrical activity from many cells (Antoli-Candel & Kiang, 1978), and its amplitude varies with stimulus level (Salvi et al,

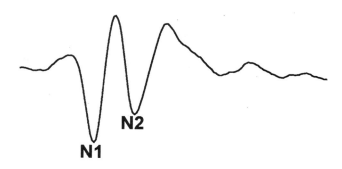

Figure 2–16 CAP recorded from a gross electrode, representing the massed activity of AN fibers. The CAP consists of two prominent negative peaks, N_1 and N_2. (From Durrant [1981], with permission.)

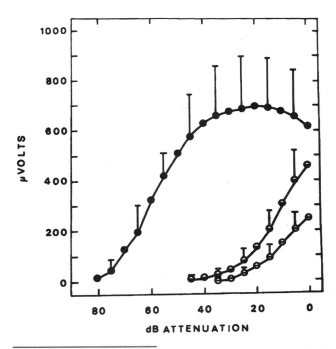

Figure 2–17 Amplitude of the CAP as a function of the intensity of a 0.1 ms click. Filled circles are from a chinchilla with normal hearing; open and half-filled circles are from animals with 40- to 50-dB hearing loss caused by noise exposure. (Reprinted from Salvi [1983a], with permission.)

1979). As stimulus level increases, CAP amplitude increases over a 40 dB to 50 dB range before saturating and then rolling over (Fig. 2–17). In addition, the latency of the CAP gradually decreases from approximately 2 ms at low stimulus levels to approximately 1 ms at high stimulus levels.

The lowest SPL at which the CAP can be detected defines its threshold. CAP thresholds for pure tones are generally 15 to 20 dB higher than behavioral thresholds. This probably occurs because behavioral thresholds are typically measured using long-duration (>200 ms) stimuli, whereas CAPs are elicited with brief-duration stimuli. Longer duration stimuli are more easily detected than short-duration stimuli because of temporal integration (Gerken et al, 1990). In addition, neural thresholds decrease by roughly 6- to 7-dB for each 10-fold increase in stimulus duration out to around 500 ms (Clock et al, 1993). Thus differences in stimulus duration probably account for the differences between CAP and behavioral thresholds.

In the clinic CAPs can be recorded from specially designed electrodes placed in the earcanal. In some cases a physician may insert an electrode through the tympanic membrane to touch the bony wall of the cochlea (Fig. 2–11). Measurement of the CAP provides information regarding the functional integrity of the AN. When tone bursts are used to elicit the CAP, the threshold can be determined over a range of frequencies, and the CAP audiogram can be measured. More commonly, however, clicks are used to elicit the CAP. The amplitude of the peaks can provide an estimate of the number of AN fibers contributing to the response, and the width of the CAP can provide an estimate of the synchrony of firing. A common finding in ears with sensorineural hearing loss is

a loss of sensitivity and decreased amplitude of the CAP (Fig. 2–17). The decrease in amplitude is a reflection of the reduced number of AN fibers contributing to the response. From a clinical perspective, an absence or greatly diminished CAP in the presence of a robust CM might be indicative of some type of neuropathy of the auditory nerve (Starr, 1996). This contrasts with a pure conductive hearing loss, in which the CAP input/output function would simply be shifted toward higher sound levels. That is, although higher stimulus levels would be required to evoke the CAP, the slope of the amplitude function would be minimally affected. The latency of the CAP can also be useful in differentiating between a conductive hearing loss, in which latency is prolonged, and a sensorineural hearing loss, in which latency is normal.

HAIR CELL PHYSIOLOGY

Potentials Measured from Individual Hair Cells

In the absence of acoustic stimulation, the resting potential of IHCs ranges from −35 to −45 mV. When a tone burst is presented, the IHC produces both an AC and a DC response (Sellick & Russell, 1978). In Figure 2–18, the upper trace of each pair represents the amplitude of the DC response and the lower trace represents the amplitude of the AC response. When low-intensity tone bursts are presented to the ear, the IHC generates low-amplitude AC and DC responses over a narrow range of frequencies. When tone bursts of high intensity are presented, the amplitudes of the AC and the DC responses increase near CF, and AC and DC responses occur over a broader range of frequencies. The tuning curve of an IHC is measured by increasing the SPL until it produces a just-detectable DC voltage (threshold response) over a range of test frequencies (Fig. 2–19) (Russell & Sellick, 1978). The frequency to which the hair cell is most sensitive (18-kHz in the example shown) is referred to as the CF. Threshold is lowest at the CF, but then increases rapidly as the frequency moves above or below CF. Thus the tuning curve of an IHC consists of a low-threshold, narrowly tuned tip and a high-threshold, broadly tuned tail that resembles the mechanical tuning curve of the basilar membrane (see Fig. 2–10A).

The broadening of the tuning curve that occurs at high sound levels is related to the nonlinear response of the IHC receptor potential. Fig. 2–20 shows DC amplitude-level functions at several frequencies (Russell & Sellick, 1978). The input/output function at the cell's CF is located furthest to the left (lower sound levels), whereas those associated with frequencies above or below CF are located further to the right (higher intensities). The input/output function at CF increases linearly at low intensities, but the slope of the

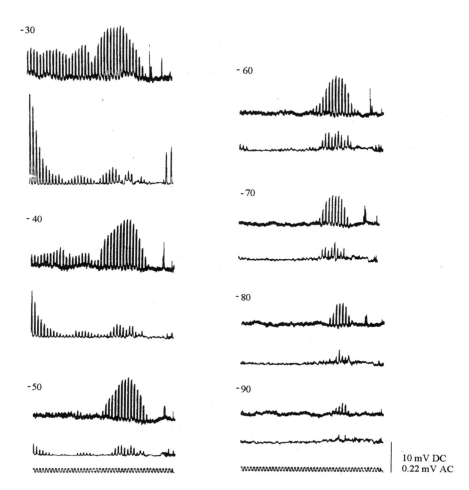

Figure 2–18 Intracellular responses from an IHC to 80-msec tone bursts presented from −40- to −90-dB of signal attenuation. The upper trace of each pair shows the amplitude of the DC response, and the lower trace shows the AC response. Notches in the tracings at −40- and −50-dB attenuation were caused by leakage through the electrical switch. (From Russell & Sellick [1978], with permission.)

function decreases at higher intensities. This behavior is similar to the compressive nonlinearity seen in the mechanical motion of the basilar membrane (Fig. 2–10B).

In response to toneburst stimulation, OHCs in the apex of the cochlea produce AC potentials similar to those of apical turn IHCs. However, resting potentials of apical OHCs (−53 mV) tend to be somewhat larger than those of apical IHCs (−32 mV) (Dallos, 1985; Dallos et al, 1982). IHCs and OHCs in the apex also produce DC receptor potentials to tone burst stimuli; those from IHCs are always depolarizing, whereas those from OHCs can be both hyperpolarizing and depolarizing (Dallos, 1985). OHCs in the base of the cochlea have large resting potentials (−71 mV) and produce AC receptor potentials of up to 15 mV in response to toneburst stimulation. However, their DC receptor potentials are quite small, particularly to tones near CF.

Outer Hair Cell Electromotility

Recent studies have shown that isolated OHCs can elongate and contract in response to DC or AC electrical stimulation (Brownell et al, 1985; Evans et al, 1986). AC stimulation results in a cycle-by-cycle change in cell length around some mean value. OHCs contract when their membrane is depolarized and elongate when hyperpolarized. Electrical partitioning experiments have shown that the change in OHC length is distributed along

the length of the cell between the nucleus and the cuticular plate region (Brownell et al, 1985; Dallos et al, 1991; Evans et al, 1986). Electromotile responses have been observed at frequencies as high as 8 kHz (Ashmore & Brownell, 1986). Static depolarization or hyperpolarization of OHCs by DC electrical stimulation or by application of chemicals results in a static change in cell length. These results indicate that the OHCs are capable of moving in response to a change in the cell's membrane potential. Because acoustic stimulation can depolarize and hyperpolarize the OHCs, the change in the cell's potential could induce AC or DC movements of the basilar membrane that could provide positive or negative feedback to the incoming sound vibration.

Figure 2–21 provides an anatomical framework for understanding how OHC movements could influence basilar membrane motion. In the intact organ of Corti, the OHCs are separated from one another by the spaces of Nuel, allowing the cells to slide freely by one another. The base of each OHC sits in a cuplike structure formed by the Deiters' cells. The Deiters' cell phalangeal process projects toward the cuticular plate where it contacts an adjacent OHC. When an OHC elongates or contracts along its main axis, the cell is able to exert an axial force that could cause the organ of Corti to move. Static DC movements could influence the stiffness of the cochlear partition and alter its vibration to sound. Because the OHCs are attached to the overlying tectorial membrane by their stereocilia, a change in the length of the OHC could

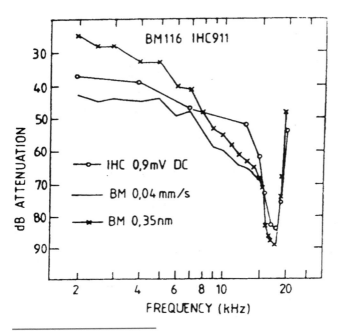

Figure 2–19 Frequency-intensity combinations necessary to produce a criterion DC receptor potential (0.9 mV) in an IHC *(open circle)*, a constant displacement (0.035 nm; *crosses*), or constant velocity (0.04 mm/sec; *solid line*) of the basilar membrane. (From Russell & Sellick [1978], with permission.)

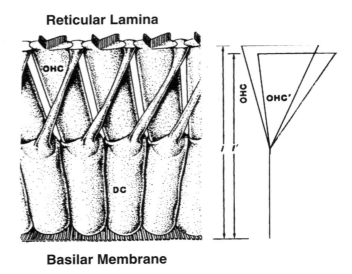

Figure 2–21 Diagram of a section of the organ of Corti *(left panel)* showing how the base of each OHC is cupped by a Deiters' cell *(DC)*. The phalangeal processes of the Deiters' cells project at an angle toward the reticular lamina and terminate between OHCs. The schematic drawing on the right illustrates an OHC at rest *(OHC)* and during contraction *(OHC')*. The distance between the basilar membrane and the reticular lamina is shown before (1) and during (1') contraction. (Reprinted from Brownell et al [1985], with permission.)

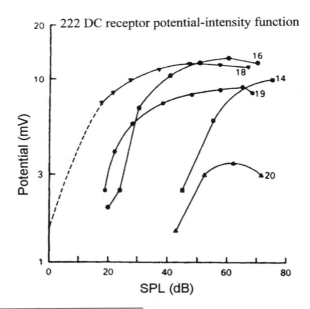

Figure 2–20 Input/output functions for the DC receptor potential of an IHC. The number above each curve indicates the stimulus frequency in kHz. The CF of the IHC shown is 18 kHz. (From Russell & Sellick [1978], with permission.)

deflect the stereocilia bundle or alter the position of the overlying tectorial membrane.

Recent experiments suggest that the electromotile response observed in vitro can influence the motion of the basilar membrane. When electrical stimulation is applied to an isolated segment of the organ of Corti (Mammano & Ashmore, 1993) or the intact cochlea, the basilar membrane moves at the same frequency as the electrical stimulus (Mountain et al, 1980; Nuttall et al, 1995; Nuttall and Ren, 1995; Xue et al, 1995a,b). The electrically induced motion of the basilar membrane results in the production of traveling waves that propagate in the reverse direction out of the cochlea and into the earcanal (Ren et al, 1996; Xue et al, 1995a). These electrically evoked sounds are referred to as electrically evoked otoacoustic emissions (EEOAEs).

Otoacoustic Emissons

The electromotile response of the OHCs provides a biological basis for understanding and interpreting a class of sounds that is generated in the inner ear and transmitted back through the ossicles of the middle ear and into the earcanal, where they can be recorded by a sensitive microphone and, in some cases, heard without the aid of amplification. Otoacoustic emissions are generated in healthy ears but are reduced in amplitude or absent in ears with certain types of damage, such as loss of OHCs. Consequently, otoacoustic emissions provide a way of assessing the functional integrity of the circuit composed of the OHCs and stria vascularis. Although several classes of otoacoustic emissions exist, the three types that are most frequently measured are spontaneous otoacoustic emissions (SOAEs), transient otoacoustic emissions (TOAEs), and DPOAEs.

Spontaneous Otoacoustic Emissions

Sounds are normally transmitted from the environment into the inner ear. However, the ear can act as a robust sound generator in the absence of acoustic stimulation, transmitting sounds (SOAEs) into the environment that, in some cases, are intense enough to be heard by individuals standing nearby (Glanville et al, 1971; Huizing & Spoor, 1973). Approximately one third of all human subjects with normal hearing have been reported to have SOAEs (Probst et al, 1991; Zurek, 1981, 1985). In most cases human SOAEs are less than 20 dB SPL, and they generally occur in narrow frequency bands less than 2 kHz. SOAEs generally remain stable within an ear, but the amplitude and spectrum of SOAEs vary from one ear to the next. One of the interesting features of SOAEs is that they can be suppressed by an external tone. The frequency-intensity combinations needed to suppress the SOAE by a fixed amount (e.g., by 3 dB) define the SOAE suppression contour.

Figure 2–22 shows the SOAE measured from a chinchilla In this animal the SOAE was so intense (>30 dB SPL) that it could be heard by people in a quiet room. The SOAE consisted of a narrow band signal at 4500 Hz. The emission, which was stable over time, could be temporarily abolished by sodium salicylate (Powers et al, 1995) and suppressed by external tones. The SOAE suppression contour consisted of a low SPL, narrowly tuned tip and a high SPL, broadly tuned, low-frequency tail. The narrowly tuned tip of the suppression contour was located slightly higher than the frequency of the SOAE. Interestingly, the shape of the SOAE suppression contour is similar to the shape of the tuning curve for the basilar membrane displacement pattern.

Transient Otoacoustic Emissions

TOAEs are elicited by presenting a short-duration acoustic impulse (click) or tone burst and then recording the subsequent acoustic activity in the earcanal with a sensitive microphone sealed in the earcanal. The amplitude of the signal recorded during the first 5 to 7 ms decays rapidly as the sound energy is absorbed by the external, middle and inner ear. This initial component of the waveform behaves linearly so that when the signal level increases 10 dB, the acoustic waveform recorded in the earcanal increases by the same amount. After the initial acoustic wave dies away, a second acoustic signal begins to emerge from the background noise in the earcanal. This second component, which is emitted from the cochlea, is the TOAE. The TOAE is considerably smaller than the initial acoustic signal by 25 dB or more (Fig. 2–23). The amplitude of the second component increases nonlinearly at high stimulus levels. Consequently, a 3 dB increase in the input signal may be required to produce a 1 dB

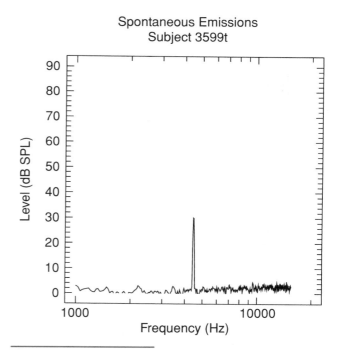

Figure 2–22   SOAE at 4400 Hz measured from a chinchilla. The emission was intense enough (34 dB SPL) to be heard by people in a quiet room.

increment in the level of the TOAE. The TOAE has a biological origin because conditions that damage that cochlea, such as acoustic trauma, metabolic inhibitors, or ototoxic drugs, reduce the amplitude of the TOAE (Kemp, 1978, 1982; Siegel & Kim, 1982).

One interesting property of the TOAE is that its short-term spectrum varies over time. The initial portion of the TOAE contains mainly high-frequency energy. Over time, the spectrum of the TOAE shifts to lower frequencies. The temporal dispersion of the TOAE appears to be related to the time delay imposed by the forward and reverse transmission of spectral components of the click to their respective transduction sites along the cochlear partition. If tone bursts are used to elicit the TOAEs, the spectrum of the TOAEs is similar to the eliciting stimulus; however, the time delay between stimulus onset and the emergence of the TOAE is inversely related to frequency. Consequently, low-frequency sounds take longer to emerge from the cochlea than high-frequency sounds. For reasons that are still not clear, the latency of the TOAE is somewhat longer than the time it would take for a particular frequency to travel to its characteristic place in the cochlea and then back into the earcanal.

Distortion Product Otoacoustic Emissions

Because the normal cochlea is a nonlinear system, its output includes distortion. Cochlear distortion can be demonstrated experimentally by presenting two primary tones, f_1 and f_2, and measuring the spectrum of the sound in the earcanal. If the

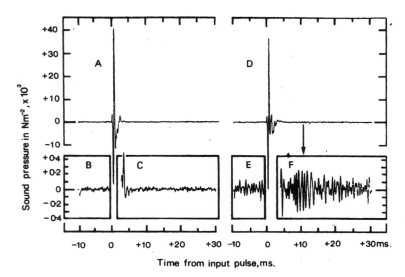

Figure 2–23 Click-evoked otoacoustic emissions measured in a test cavity (**A**) versus the human earcanal (**D**). Insets show highly amplified views of what is recorded before and after the click in the test cavity (**B, C**) and in the human earcanal (**E, F**). Only background noise is evident in the test cavity (**C**), whereas an otoacoustic emission is seen in the response from the earcanal (**F**). (Reprinted from Kemp, D [1978], with permission.)

cochlea were a linear system, only sounds corresponding to f_1 and f_2 would be detected in the earcanal. However, when two tones are presented to a healthy ear, additional frequency components can be detected in the earcanal at intermodulation frequencies, such as $2f_1-f_2$ and f_2-f_1. If, for example, primaries of 4000 Hz and 4800 Hz are presented to the ear, cubic ($2f_1-f_2$) and quadratic (f_2-f_1) distortion products would be produced at 3200 Hz and 800 Hz, respectively. In a healthy ear the largest distortion product, $2f_1-f_2$, is sometimes only 30- to 40-dB below the level of the primary tones. The amplitude of the distortion product increases as the level of the primary tones increases as illustrated in Figure 2–24 using data from a chinchilla. In this example the primary tones were of equal level, and the level increased from 0- to 80-dB SPL in 5 dB steps. At low intensi-

ties, the distortion product cannot be measured because its amplitude is less than the noise floor of the measurement system. However, as stimulus level increases, the cubic DPOAE amplitude rises above the noise floor at a rate of approximately 1 dB of DPOAE per 1 dB increase in signal level.

Selective destruction of all of the IHCs with the ototoxic drug, carboplatin, eliminates the CAP and causes a profound hearing loss in the chinchilla with no effect on the amplitude of the DPOAE (Trautwein et al, 1996; Wang et al, 1997). Although complete destruction of the IHCs does not alter the amplitude of the DPOAE, the amplitude of the DPOAE is reduced by OHC damage. In the chinchilla, DPOAE amplitude decreases at the rate of 2- to 4-dB for every 10% loss of OHCs (Hofstetter et al, 1997). The amplitude of the DPOAE is also altered by electrical or acoustic stimulation of the efferent neurons that synapse on the OHCs (Mott et al, 1989; Siegel & Kim, 1982). This suggests that DPOAEs are produced by OHCs in combination with the driving voltage produced by the endocochlear potential. From a clinical perspective, it is clear that DPOAEs primarily assess the functional integrity of the OHC system. They do not assess the functional integrity of the IHCs that transmit virtually all of the input to the central nervous system by way of the auditory nerve.

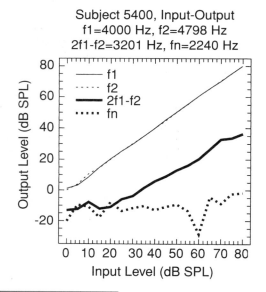

Figure 2–24 Cubic DPOAE input/output function from a chinchilla. Frequency of f_1, f_2, $2f_1-f_2$ and fn (noise floor) indicated; level of f_1 and f_2 were equal and were incremented from 0- to 80-dB SPL in 5 dB steps.

AUDITORY NERVE FIBER RESPONSES

Because each type I spiral ganglion neuron contacts only one IHC (see Fig. 2–5), the neural activity from each fiber reflects the output from a very small segment of the cochlea. With an extremely fine microelectrode, one can record the all-or-none spike discharges from individual nerve fibers that send their messages to the cochlear nucleus, the first auditory relay station in the brain. Most AN fibers discharge spontaneously in the absence of controlled acoustic stimulation and their spontaneous rates of discharge typically range from 0 to slightly more than 100 spikes/s (Fig. 2–25). A large proportion of fibers have spontaneous rates less than 18 spikes/s or more than 30 spikes/s, resulting in a bimodal distribution (Kiang et al, 1986; Liberman, 1978).

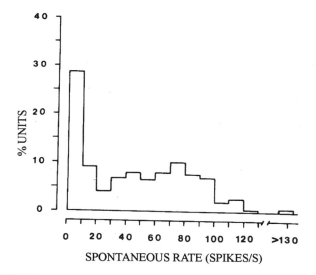

Figure 2–25 Histogram showing the bimodal distribution of spontaneous firing rates in a population of auditory nerve fibers in chinchilla. (From Salvi et al [1983b], with permission.)

When a tone burst with the appropriate frequency-intensity combination is presented to the ear, the discharge rate of the fiber will increase (Fig. 2–26). The stimulus intensity needed to produce a just-detectable increase in the discharge rate defines the neuron's threshold. The tuning curve represents the neuron's threshold over a broad range of frequencies (Fig. 2–27). The frequency at which a response can be elicited at the lowest stimulus intensity is the unit's CF. Threshold increases significantly greater than and less than CF, resulting in a narrow, low-threshold tip. Responses can be elicited to a broad range of frequencies less than CF, but only at high SPLs. Thus the neural tuning curves of AN fibers

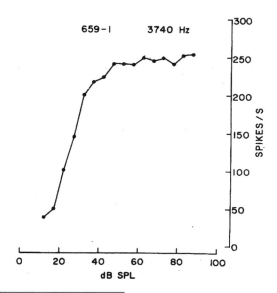

Figure 2–26 Input/output function from an AN fiber in response to stimulation with CF tone bursts. (From Salvi et al [1983b], with permission.)

closely parallel the shape of the basilar membrane iso-amplitude response curves.

The thresholds of neurons with similar CF can vary considerably (Fig. 2–27), even by as much as 50- to 60-dB. Neurons with low CF thresholds tend to have high spontaneous rates, whereas those with the highest CF thresholds have spontaneous rates near zero. By injecting a dye-tracer into a neuron, it has been possible to determine where the nerve fiber terminates in the organ of Corti. All the labeled neurons that respond to sound have been found to synapse on IHCs (Liberman, 1980, 1982; Robertson, 1984). Thus all the acoustic information transmitted to the central auditory system appears to be conveyed by the type I AN fibers that make up 90 to 95% of all AN fibers. No evidence exists that type II fibers, which contact OHCs, transmit spike activity to the central auditory system (Robertson, 1984).

AN fibers respond to sound by increasing their discharge rate over the time when the stimulus is present, but the amount of neural activity varies with stimulus level and the time since stimulus onset. The variation in discharge rate over the duration of the stimulus is illustrated by peristimulus or poststimulus time histograms to a series of tone burst stimuli presented at different sound levels (Fig. 2–28). For stimulus levels near threshold, the discharge rate is low and remains fairly constant over the duration of the stimulus. However, at suprathreshold intensities, the number of spikes increases. The discharge rate is high near stimulus onset and then rapidly decreases over the next 15 to 30 ms (Smith, 1980). The rapid decline in neural activity after stimulus onset presumably occurs because the pool of available neurotransmitter in the IHC is partially depleted (Furukawa & Matsuura, 1978). After the stimulus is turned off, the spontaneous discharge rate of the neuron is depressed, but gradually builds up to its normal rate as the pool of neurotransmitter is replenished. If the neuron is given sufficient time to recover from adaptation, it will again respond robustly at stimulus onset.

Figure 2–26 shows the discharge rate-intensity function for a typical AN fiber. As the stimulus rises above the neuron's threshold, the discharge rate increases monotonically over a range of 30- to 50-dB and then remains fairly constant at higher stimulus levels. Thus most neurons can only encode changes in sound level over a relatively narrow range of intensities, whereas normal listeners can detect changes in the loudness of a stimulus over a range of levels exceeding 100 dB. A solution to the discrepancy between human perception and single neuron performance can be found in the large range of CF thresholds at each CF (see Fig. 2–27). Low-threshold, medium-threshold, and high-threshold neurons can process changes in intensity over their respective dynamic ranges so that the total dynamic range from all the neurons at the same CF begins to approximate the human dynamic range for loudness (Viemeister, 1983).

Because the hair cells are depolarized by sounds that deflect the stereocilia toward the tallest stereocilia, increases in neurotransmitter release from IHCs occurs only during the excitatory half of every stimulus cycle (Kiang et al, 1965; see Fig. 2–4B). Therefore, when a low-frequency sound is presented, AN fibers discharge within a preferred 180 degree phase of each cycle as shown in Figure 2–29. This periodic firing to low-frequency sounds is referred to as phase locking.

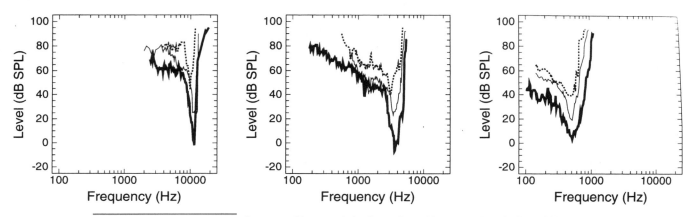

Figure 2–27 Tuning curves from AN fibers with high, mid, and low CF. Thresholds of fibers with similar CF can vary by as much as 50- to 60-dB. As a result, the proportion of fibers responding to a stimulus will increase as the stimulus level increases.

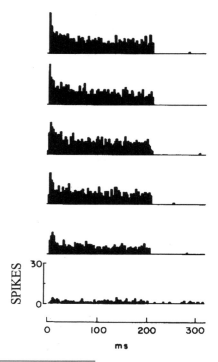

Figure 2–28 PST histograms from an AN fiber in response to CF tone bursts. Stimulus intensity was incremented in 10 dB steps. As stimulus intensity increases *(from bottom to top)*, the onset portion of the response becomes more prominent. (From Salvi et al [1983b], with permission.)

Neural phase locking is fairly robust at the low frequencies (<1500 Hz) where pitch perception is believed to be based on periodicity cues (Patterson, 1969; Schouten et al, 1962).

CONCLUSIONS

Many important aspects of hearing are determined by the biomechanical, anatomical, and physiological properties of the inner ear. The traveling wave displacement patterns provide a mechanism for segregating sounds of different frequencies into different locations along the basilar membrane. This provides a basis for place theories of pitch. From a clinical standpoint, damage to a specific place in the cochlea results in a hearing loss in a specific frequency region. The morphological polarization of the hair cell and the phase-locking behavior observed in AN fibers provide an anatomical and physiological basis for models of periodicity pitch. An understanding of cochlear physiology provides a basis for clinical diagnosis by use of electrocochleography (assessment of CAP and SP). The use of otoacoustic emissions for infant hearing screening requires a thorough understanding of cochlear mechanics and cochlear anatomy. Patients with sensorineural hearing loss are not only less sensitive to sound but many are also unable to extract specific features of an acoustic signal from its complex spectrum. The ability to resolve the spectral components of a complex sound depends on the ear's sharp mechanical and neural tuning, which depends on the functional integrity of the OHC. Because the CM and DPOAEs are generated by the OHCs, the clinician can use either or both of these measures to assess the functional condition of the OHC system in hearing-impaired patients. For example, DPOAEs could be used to monitor the ototoxic effects of aminoglycoside antibiotics and anticancer drugs such as cisplatin and carboplatin. The battery of physiological measures available to the clinician has proven useful in the diagnosis of subjects with auditory neuropathy (Starr, 1996). Patients with auditory neuropathy have normal DPOAEs and CM, suggesting that their OHCs are intact. However, the CAP is absent or of greatly diminished amplitude, suggesting that relatively little information is being transmitted to the central auditory system through the auditory nerve. Knowledge of the auditory periphery provides a scientific basis for understanding many facets of hearing and hearing loss.

ACKNOWLEDGMENT

Supported in part by NIH grant R01DCD01685 to RJS.

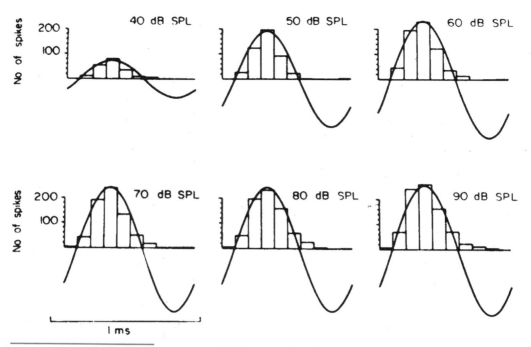

Figure 2–29   Period histograms of an AN fiber stimulated with a low-frequency tone (1100 Hz) of increasing intensity (40- to 90-dB SPL). The histograms have been fitted with a sinusoid of the best fitting amplitude but fixed phase. Note that spikes are evoked in only half of the stimulus cycle and that despite saturation of the firing rate at stimulus levels greater than 60 dB SPL, the histogram still follows the sinusoidal pattern of the stimulus. (From Rose et al [1971], with permission.)

REFERENCES

ANNIKO, M., & WROBLEWSKI, R. (1986). Ionic environment of cochlear hair cells. *Hearing Research, 22*;279–293.

ANTOLI-CANDEL, A., & KIANG, N. (1978). Unit activity underlying the N1 potential. In: R. Nauton, & C. Fernandez (Eds.), *Evoked electrical activity in the auditory nervous system*: New York: Academic Press.

ASCHOFF, A., MULLER, M., & OTT, H. (1988). Origin of cochlear efferents in some gerbil species. *Experimental Brain Research, 71*;252–262.

ASHMORE, J., & BROWNELL, W. (1986). Kilohertz movements induced by electrical stimulation in outer hair cells isolated from the guinea-pig cochlea. *Journal of Physiology, 376*;49.

BESS, F.H., & HUMES, L.E. (1990). *Audiology: The fundamentals.* Baltimore: Williams & Wilkins.

BISHOP, A.L., & HENSON O.W.J. (1987). The efferent cochlear projections of the superior olivary complex in the mustached bat. *Hearing Research, 31*;175–182.

BOSHER, S.K., & WARREN, R.L. (1971). A study of the electrochemistry and osmotic relationships of the cochlear fluids in the neonatal rat at the time of the development of the endocochlear potential. *Journal of Physiology (London), 212*;739–761.

BROWNELL, W.E., BADER, C.R., BERTRAND, D., & DE RIBAUPIERRE, Y. (1985). Evoked mechanical responses of isolated cochlear outer hair cells. *Science, 227*;194–196.

BUNO, JR., W. (1978). Auditory nerve fiber activity influenced by contralateral ear sound stimulation. *Experimental Neurology; 59*:62–74.

CLOCK, A.E., SALVI, R.J., SAUNDERS, S.S., & POWERS, N.L. (1993). Neural correlates of temporal integration in the cochlear nucleus of the chinchilla. *Hearing Research, 71*;37–50.

CODY, A.R., & JOHNSTONE, B.M. (1982). Acoustically evoked activity of single efferent neurons in the guinea pig cochlea. *Journal of the Acoustical Society of America, 72*;280–282.

CODY, A.R., & RUSSELL, I.J. (1985). Outer hair cells in the mammalian cochlea and noise-induced hearing loss. *Nature, 315*;662–665.

CODY, A.R., & RUSSELL, I.J. (1987). The response of hair cells in the basal turn of the guinea-pig cochlea to tones. *Journal of Physiology, 383*;551–569.

COREY, D.P., & HUDSPETH, A.J. (1979). Ionic basis of the receptor potential in a vertebrate hair cell. *Nature, 281*;675–677.

CRAWFORD, A., & FETTIPLACE, R. (1981). An electrical tuning mechanism in turtle cochlear hair cells. *Journal of Physiology (London), 315*;377–422.

DALLOS, P. (1973). *The auditory periphery: Biophysics and physiology.* New York: Academic Press.

DALLOS, P. (1975). Electrical correlates of mechanical events in the cochlea. *Audiology, 14*;408–418.

DALLOS, P. (1985). Response characteristics of mammalian cochlear hair cells. *Journal of Neuroscience, 5*;1591–1608.

DALLOS, P., EVANS, B.N., & HALLWORTH, R. (1991). Nature of the motor element in electrokinetic shape changes of cochlear outer hair cells. *Nature, 350*;155–157.

DALLOS, P., SANTOS-SACCHI, J., & FLOCK, A. (1982). Intracellular recordings from cochlear outer hair cells. *Science, 218*;582–584.

DALLOS, P., SCHOENY, Z.G., & CHEATHAM, M.A. (1970). Cochlear summating potentials: Composition. *Science, 170*;641–644.

DAVIS, H. (1965). A model for transducer action in the cochlea. *Cold Spring Harbor Symposia on Quantitative Biology, 30*;181–189.

DAVIS, H., DEATHERAGE, B.H., ROSENBLUT, B., FERNANDEZ, C., KIMURA, R., & SMITH, C.A. (1958). Modification of cochlear potentials by streptomycin poisoning and by extensive venous obstruction. *Laryngoscope, 68*;596–627.

DESMEDT, J.E. (1962). Auditory-evoked potentials from cochlea to cortex as influenced by activation of the efferent olivo-cochlear bundle. *Journal of the Acoustical Society of America, 34*;1478–1496.

DEWSON, III, J.H. (1967). Efferent olivocochlear bundle: Some relationships to noise masking and to stimulus attenuation. *Journal of Neurophysiol, 30*;817–831.

DEWSON, III, J.H. (1968). Efferent olivocochlear bundle: Some relationships to stimulus discrimination in noise. *Journal of Neurophysiology, 31*;122–130.

DURRANT, J., & LOVRINIC, J.H. (1995). *Bases of hearing science* (3rd ed.) (p. 144). Baltimore: Williams & Wilkins.

DURRANT, J., WANG, J., DING, D., & SALVI, R. (1998). Are inner or outer hair cells the source of summating potentials recorded from the round window? *Journal of the Acoustical Society of America, 104*;370–377.

DURRANT, J.D. (1981). Auditory physiology and an auditory physiologist's view of tinnitus. *Journal of Laryngology and Otology Supplement, 4*;21–28.

EMMERLING, M.R., & SOBKOWICZ, H.M. (1988). Differentiation and distribution of acetylcholinesterase molecular forms in the mouse cochlea. *Hearing Research, 32*;137–145.

EVANS, B., WARNER, R., & YONOVITZ, A. (1986). Measurements of in vitro outer hair cell motility in the mammalian cochlea. *Journal of the Acoustical Society of America, 79*;S49.

FLOCK, A. (1977). Physiological properties of sensory hairs in the ear. In: E. Evans, & J. Wilson (Eds.), *Psychophysical and physiology of hearing*. London: Academic Press.

FLOCK, A., FLOCK, B., & MURRAY, E. (1977). Studies on the sensory hairs of receptor cells in the inner ear. *Acta OtoLaryngologica, 83*;85–91.

FURUKAWA, T., & MATSUURA, S. (1978). Adaptive rundown of excitatory post-synaptic potentials at synapses between hair cells and eighth nerve fibres in the goldfish. *Journal of Physiology (London), 276*;193–209.

GERKEN, G.M., BHAT, V.K., & HUTCHISON-CLUTTER, M. (1990). Auditory temporal integration and the power function model. *Journal of the Acoustical Society of America, 88*;767–778.

GIARD, M.H., COLLET, L., BOUCHET, P., & PERNIER, J. (1994). Auditory selective attention in the human cochlea. *Brain Research, 633*;353–356.

GLANVILLE, J., COLES, R., & SULLIVAN, B. (1971). A family with high-tonal objective tinnitus. *Journal of Otolaryngology, 85*;1–10.

GOODMAN, D., SMITH, R., & CHAMBERLIN, S. (1982). Intracellular and extracellular responses in the organ of Corti of the gerbil. *Hearing Research, 7*;161–179.

HANDROCK, M., & ZEISBERG, J. (1982). The influence of the effect system on adaptation, temporary and permanent threshold shift. *Archives of Oto-Rhino-Laryngology, 234*;191–5.

HOFSTETTER, P., DING, D., POWERS, N., & SALVI, R.J. (1997). Quantitative relationship of carboplatin dose to magnitude of inner and outer hair cell loss and the reduction in distortion product otoacoustic emission amplitude in chinchillas. *Hearing Research, 112*;199–215.

HUDSPETH, A.J. (1982). Extracellular current flow and the site of transduction by vertebrate hair cells. *Journal of Neuroscience, 2*;1–10.

HUDSPETH, A.J. (1985a). The cellular basis of hearing: The biophysics of hair cells. *Sciences, 230*; 745–752.

HUDSPETH, A.J. (1985b). Models for mechanoelectrical transduction by hair cells. *Progress in Clinical and Biological Research, 176*;193–205.

HUDSPETH, A.J., & COREY, D.P. (1977). Sensitivity, polarity, and conductance change in the response of vertebrate hair cells to controlled mechanical stimuli. *Proceedings of the National Academy of Sciences USA, 74*;2407–2411.

HUIZING, E., & SPOOR, A. (1973). An unusual type of tinnitus. *Archives of Otolaryngology, 98*;134–136.

IGARASHI, M., ALFORD, B.R., GORDON, W.P., & NAKAI, Y. (1974). Behavioral auditory function after transection of crossed olivo-cochlear bundle in the cat. II. Conditioned visual performance with intense white noise. *Acta Otolaryngologies, 77*;311–317.

JOHNSTONE, B.M., & SELLICK, P.M. (1972). Dynamic changes in cochlear potentials and endolymph concentrations. *Journal of the Oto-Laryngological Society of Australia, 3*;317–319.

KEMP, D. (1978). Stimulated acoustic emissions from within the human audtiory system. *Journal of the Acoustical Society of America, 64*;1386–1391.

KEMP, D.T. (1982). Cochlear echoes: Implications for noise-induced hearing loss. In: R.P. Hamernik, D. Henderson, & R.J. Salvi (Eds.), *New perspectives on noise-induced hearing loss* (pp. 189–207). New York: Raven Press.

KHANNA, S.M., & LEONARD, D.G.B. (1982). Basilar membrane tuning in the cat cochlea. *Sciences, 215*;305–306.

KIANG, N.Y., LIBERMAN, M.C., SEWELL, W.F., & GUINAN, J.J. (1986). Single unit clues to cochlear mechanisms. *Hearing Research, 22*;171–182.

KIANG, N.Y.S., WATANABE, T., THOMAS, E.C., & CLARK, L.F. (1965). Discharge patterns of single fibers in the cat's auditory nerve (Research Mongr. No. 35).

KONISHI, T., HAMRICK, P., & WALSH, P. (1978). Ion transport in guinea pig cochlea. *Acta Otolaryngologica, 86*;22–34.

KONISHI, T., & KELSEY, E. (1968). Effect of sodium deficiency on cochlear potentials. *Journal of the Acoustical Society of America, 43*;462–470.

KONISHI, T., & MENDELSOHN, M. (1970). Effect of ouabain on cochlear potentials and endolymph composition in guinea pigs. *Acta Oto-laryngologica, 69*;192–199.

KUIJPERS, W., & BONTING, S.L. (1970). The cochlear potentials. II. The nature of the cochlear endolymphatic resting potential. *Pflügers Archives, 320*;359–372.

LIBERMAN, M.C. (1978). Auditory-nerve response from cats raised in a low-noise chamber. *Journal of the Acoustical Society of America, 63*;442–455.

LIBERMAN, M.C. (1980). Morphological differences among radial afferent fibers in the cat cochlea: An electron-microscopic study of serial sections. *Hearing Research, 3*;45–63.

LIBERMAN, M.C. (1982). The cochlear frequency map for the cat: Labeling auditory-nerve fibers of known characteristic frequency. *Journal of the Acoustical Society of America, 72*;1441–1449.

LIBERMAN, M.C. (1990). Effects of chronic cochlear de-efferentation on auditory-nerve response. *Hearing Research, 49*;209–224.

LIBERMAN, M.C., & BROWN, M.C. (1986). Physiology and anatomy of single olivocochlear neurons in the cat. *Hearing Research, 24*;17–36.

MAMMANO, F., & ASHMORE, J.F. (1993). Reverse transduction measured in the isolated cochlea by laser Michelson interferometry. *Nature, 365*;838–841.

MARGOLIS, R.H., et al. (1992). Tympanic electrocochleography: Normal and abnormal patterns of response. *Audiology, 31*;8–24.

MAY, B.J., & MCQUONE, S.J. (1995) Effects of bilateral olivocochlear lesions on pure-tone intensity discrimination in cats. *Audiology Neurosciences, 1*;385–400.

MELLONI, B.J. (1957). In *What's new*, No. 199. North Chicago: Abbott Laboratories.

MOTT, J.T., NORTON, S.J., & WARR, W.B. (1989). Changes in spontaneous otoacoustic emissions produced by acoustic stimulation of the contralateral ear. *Hearing Research, 38*;229–242.

MOUNTAIN, D.C., GEISLER, C.D., & HUBBARD, A.E. (1980). Stimulation of efferents alters the cochlear microphonic and the sound-induced resistance changes measured in scale media of the guinea pig. *Hearing Research, 3*;231–240.

NIEDER, P., & NIEDER, I. (1970a). Antimasking effect of crossed olivocochlear bundle stimulation with loud clicks in guinea pig. *Experimental Neurology, 28*;179–188.

NIEDER, P., & NIEDER, I. (1970b). Stimulation of efferent olivocochlear bundles causes release from low level masking. *Nature, 227*;184–185.

NUTTALL, A.L., KONG, W.J., REN, T.Y., DOLAN, D.F. (1995). Basilar membrane motion and position changes induced by direct current stimulation. In: A. Flock, D. Ottoson, & M. Ulfendahl (Eds.), *Active Hearing* (pp. 283–293). Oxford: Elsevier Science Ltd.

NUTTALL, A.L., & REN, T. (1995). Electromotile hearing: Evidence from basilar membrane motion and otoacoustic emissions. *Hearing Research, 92*;170–177.

PATTERSON, R.D. (1969). Noise masking of a change in residue pitch. *Journal of the Acoustical Society of America, 45*;1520–1524.

PEAKE, W., SOHMER, J., & WEISS, T. (1969). Microelectrode recordings of intracochlear potentials (pp. 293–304). M.I.T. Research Laboratory of Electronics: Quarterly Progress Report.

PFALZ, R.K.J. (1962). Centrifugal inhibition of afferent secondary neurons in the cochlear nucleus by sound. *Journal of the Acoustical Society of America, 34*;1472–1479.

PICKLES, J.O. (1985). Recent advances in cochlear physiology. *Progress in Neurobiology, 24*;1–42.

PICKLES, J.O. (1988). *An introduction to the physiology of hearing* (2nd ed). London: Academic Press.

PICKLES, J.O., COMIS, S.D., & OSBORNE, M.P. (1984). Cross-links between stereocilia in the guinea pig organ of Corti, and their possible relation to sensory transduction. *Hearing Research, 15*;103–112.

PICKLES, J.O, & COREY D.P. (1992). Mechanoelectrical transduction by hair cells. *Trends in Neuroscience, 15*;254–259.

POWERS, N.L., SALVI, R.J., WANG, J., SPONGR, V., & QIU, C.X. (1995). Elevation of auditory thresholds by spontaneous cochlear oscillations. *Nature, 375*;585–587.

PROBST, R., LONSBURY-MARTIN, B.L., & MARTIN, G.K. (1991). A review of otoacoustic emissions. *Journal of the Acoustical Society of America, 89*;2027–2067.

RAJAN, R., & JOHNSTONE, B.M. (1983). Efferent effects elicited by electrical stimulation at the round window of the guinea pig. *Hearing Research, 12*;405–417.

RAJAN, R., & JOHNSTONE, B.M. (1988a). Electrical stimulation of cochlear efferents at the round window reduces auditory desensitization in guinea pigs. I. Dependence on electrical stimulation parameters. *Hearing Research, 36*;53–74.

RAJAN, R., & JOHNSTONE, B.M. (1988b). Electrical stimulation of cochlear efferents at the round window reduces auditory desensitization in guinea pigs. II. Dependence on level of temporary threshold shifts. *Hearing Research, 36*;75–88.

REN, T., NUTTALL, A.L., & MILLER, J.M. (1996). Electrically evoked cubic distortion product otoacoustic emissions from gerbil cochlea. *Hearing Research, 102*;43–50.

ROBERTSON, D. (1984). Horseradish peroxidase injection of physiologically characterized afferent and efferent neurons in the guinea pig spiral ganglion. *Hearing Research, 15*;113–121.

ROBERTSON, D., HARVEY, A.R., & COLE, K.S. (1989). Postnatal development of the efferent innervation of the rat cochlea. *Developments in Brain Research, 47*;197–207.

ROSE, J.E., HIND, J.E., ANDERSON, D.J., & BRUGGE, J.F. (1971). Some effects of intensity on response of auditory nerve fibers in the squirrel monkey. *Journal of Neurophysiology, 34*;685–699.

RUSSELL, I.J., CODY, A.R., & RICHARDSON, G.P. (1986). The responses of inner and outer hair cells in the basal turn of the guinea-pig cochlea and in the mouse cochlea grown in vitro. *Hearing Research, 22*;199–216.

RUSSELL, I.J., & SELLICK, P.M. (1978). Intracellular studies of hair cells in the mammalian cochlea. *Journal of Physiology, 284*;261–290.

RYAN, A.F., WICKHAM, M.G., & BONE, R.C. (1980). Studies of ion distribution in the inner ear: Scanning electron microscopy and x-ray microanalysis of freeze-dried cochlear specimens. *Hearing Research, 2*;1–20.

SALVI, R., HENDERSON, D., & HAMERNIK, R.P. (1979). Single auditory nerve fiber and action potential latencies in normal and noise-treated chinchilla. *Hearing Research, 1*;237–251.

SALVI, R.J., HAMERNIK, R.P., & HENDERSON, D. (1983a). Response patterns of auditory nerve fibers during temporal threshold shift. *Hearing Research, 10*;37–67.

SALVI, R.J., HENDERSON, D., & HAMERNIK, R.P. (1983b). Physiological basis of sensorineural hearing loss. In: J.V. Tobias, & E.D. Schubert (Eds.), *Hearing research and theory* (Vol. 2). New York: Academic Press.

SCHOUTEN, J.F., RITSMA, R., & CARDOZO, B. (1962). Pitch of the residue. *Journal of the Acoustical Society of America, 34;* 1418–1424.

SELLICK, P.M., PATUZZI, R., & JOHNSTONE, B.M. (1982). Measurement of basilar membrane motion in the guinea pig using the Mossbauer technique. *Journal of the Acoustical Society of America, 72;*131–141.

SELLICK, P.M., & RUSSELL, I.J. (1978). Intracellular studies of cochlear hair cells: Filling the gap between basilar membrane mechanics and neural excitation. In: R.F Naunton, & C. Fernandez (Eds.), *Evoked electrical activity in the auditory nervous system* (pp. 113–139). New York: Academic Press.

SEWELL, W.F. (1984). The effects of furosemide on the endo-cochlear potential and auditory nerve fiber tuning curves in cats. *Hearing Research, 14;*305–314.

SIEGEL, J.H., & KIM, D.O. (1982). Efferent neural control of cochlear mechanics? Olivocochlear bundle stimulation affects biomechanical nonlinearity. *Hearing Research, 6;*245–248.

SLEPECKY, N.B. (1996). Structure of the mammalian cochlea. In: P. Dallos, A.N. Popper, & R.R. Fay (Eds.), *The cochlea.* New York: Springer.

SMITH, R. (1980). Adaptation, saturation, and physiological masking in single auditory nerve fibers. *Journal of the Acoustical Society of America, 65;*166–178.

SOHMER, H., & COHEN, D. (1976). Responses of the auditory pathway in several types of hearing loss. In: F.J. Ruben, C. Elberling, & G. Salomon (Eds.), *Electrocochleography* (p. 431–439). Baltimore: University Park Press.

SPOENDLIN, H. (1972). Innervation densities of the cochlea. *Acta Oto-laryngologica, 67;*235–248.

SPOENDLIN, H. (1978). The afferent innervation of the cochlea. In: R.F. Naunton, & C. Fernandez (Eds.), *Evoked electrical activity in the auditory nervous system* (p. 35). New York: Academic Press.

STARR, A., PICTON, T.W., SINNIGER, Y., HOOD, L.J., & BERLIN, C.I. (1996). Auditory neuropathy. *Brain, 119;*741–753.

TAKENO, S., HARRISON, R.V., IBRAHIM, D., WAKE, M., & MOUNT, R.J. (1994). Cochlear function after selective inner hair cell degeneration induced by carboplatin. *Hearing Research, 75;*93–102.

TANAHASHI, T., MATSUMURA, K., NIWA, H., & IWATA, H. (1976). Cochlear microphonics and eighth nerve action potentials: Clinical and experimental studies. In: F.J. Ruben, C. Elberling, & G. Salomon (Eds.), *Electrocochleography* (p. 480). Baltimore: University Park Press.

TASAKI, I., DAVIS, H., & ELDREDGE, D. (1954). Exploration of cochlear potentials with a microelectrode. *Journal of the Acoustical Society of America, 26;*765–773.

TASAKI, I., DAVIS, H., & LEGOUIX, J. (1952). The space-time pattern of the cochlear microphonics (guinea pig), as recorded by differential electrodes. *Journal of the Acoustical Society of America, 24;*502–519.

TASAKI, I., & SPYROPOULOS, C.S. (1959). Stria vascularis as source of endocochlear potential. *Journal of Neurophysiology, 22;*149–155.

TILANUS, C.C., KLIS, S.F., & SMOORENBURG, G.F. (1992). Effects of anoxia on the cochlear summating potential in the guinea pig. *European Archives of Oto-Rhino-Laryngology, 249;*12–15.

TRAUTWEIN, P., HOFSTETTER, P., WANG, J., SALVI, R., NOSTRANT, A. (1996). Selective inner hair cell loss does not alter distortion product otoacoustic emissions. *Hearing Research, 96;*71–82.

VIEMEISTER, N.F. (1983). Auditory intensity discrimination at high frequencies in the presence of noise. *Science, 221;*1206–1208.

VON BÉKÉSY, G.V. (1960). *Experiments in hearing.* New York: John Wiley & Sons.

WALSH, E.J., MCGEE, J., MCFADDEN, S.L., LIBERMAN, M.C. (1998). Long-term effects of sectioning the olivocochlear bundle in neonatal cats. *Journal of Neuroscience, 18;*3859–3869.

WANG, J., POWERS, N.L., HOFSTETTER, P., TRAUTWEIN, P., DING, D., SALVI, R. (1997). Effects of selective inner hair cell loss on auditory nerve fiber threshold, tuning and sponta-neous and driven discharge rate. *Hearing Research, 107;*67–82.

WARR, W. (1975). Olivocochlear and vestibular efferent neurons of the feline brain stem: Their location, morphology and number determined by retrograde axonal transport and acetylcholinesterase histochemistry. *Journal of Comparative Neurology, 161;*159–182.

WARR, W.B. (1992). Organization of olivocochlear efferent systems in mammals. In: R.R. Fay, & A.N. Popper (Eds.), *The mammalian auditory pathway: Neuroanatomy* (pp. 410–448). New York: Springer-Verlag.

WARR, W.B., & GUINAN, J.J. (1979). Efferent innervation of the organ of Corti: Two separate systems. *Brain Research, 173;*152–155.

WARREN, E.H., & LIBERMAN, M.C. (1989). Effects of contralateral sound on auditory-nerve responses. I. Contributions of cochlear efferents. *Hearing Research, 37;*80–104.

WEVER, E., & BRAY, C. (1930). Action currents in the auditory nerve in response to acoustic stimulation. *Proceedings of the National Academy of Sciences USA, 16;*34–350.

WHITFIELD, I., & ROSS, H. (1965). Cochlear microphonic and summating potentials and the outputs of individual hair cell generators. *Journal of the Acoustical Society of America, 38;*126–131.

WINSLOW, R.L., & SACHS, M.B. (1987). Effect of electrical stimulation of the crossed olivocochlear bundle on auditory nerve response to tones in noise. *Journal of Neurophysiology, 57;*1002–1021.

WINSLOW R.L., & SACHS, M.B. (1988). Single-tone intensity discrimination based on auditory-nerve rate responses in backgrounds of quiet, noise, and with stimulation of the crossed olivocochlear bundle. *Hearing Research, 35;*165–190.

XUE, S., MOUNTAIN, D.C., HUBBARD, A.E. (1995a). Acoustic enhancement of electrically evoked otoacoustic emissions reflects basilar membrane tuning: A model. *Hearing Research, 91;*93–100.

XUE, S., MOUNTAIN, D.C., HUBBARD, A.E. (1995b). Electrically evoked basilar membrane motion. *Journal of the Acoustical Society of America, 97;*3030–3041.

YOST, W.A. (1994). *Fundamentals of hearing: An introduction* (3rd ed). San Diego: Academic Press.

ZHENG, X.Y., DING, D.L., MCFADDEN, S.L., & HENDERSON, D. (1997a). Evidence that inner hair cells are the major source of cochlear summating potentials. *Hearing Research, 113;*76–88.

ZHENG, X.Y., HENDERSON, D., HU, B.H., DING, D.L., & MCFADDEN, S.L. (1997b). The influence of the cochlear efferent system on chronic acoustic trauma. *Hearing Research, 107;*147–159.

ZHENG, X.Y., HENDERSON, D., MCFADDEN, S.L., & HU, B.H. (1997c). The role of the cochlear efferent system in acquired resistance to noise-induced hearing loss. *Hearing Research, 104;*191–203.

ZHENG, X.Y., HENDERSON, D., MCFADDEN, S.L., DING. D.L., & SALVI, R.J. (1999). Auditory nerve fiber responses following chronic cochlear de-efferentation. *Journal of Comparative Neurology, 406;*72–86.

ZUREK, P. (1985). Acoustic emissions from the ear: A summary of results from humans and animals. *Journal of the Acoustical Society of America, 78;*340–344.

ZUREK, P.M. (1981). Spontaneous narrow-band acoustic signals emitted by human ears. *Journal of the Acoustical Society of America, 69;*514–523.

## Chapter 3

Anatomy and Physiology of the Central Auditory Nervous System: A Clinical Perspective

Frank E. Musiek and Victoria B. Oxholm

Outline

ANATOMY, PHYSIOLOGY, AND THE CLINICIAN

One might question the necessity of a chapter on anatomy and physiology (A&P) in a clinical handbook of audiology. Many clinicians may believe such a chapter would have little relevance to their daily duties. Also, many clinicians who know well the value of knowledge of the structure and function of the auditory system are hesitant to embrace such knowledge. Most of the introductory comments are aimed at these clinicians.

Certain areas of clinical audiology require more knowledge of A&P than do others. For example, it is difficult to imagine a good diagnostician who is not well versed in A&P. Conversely, clinicians who work essentially with hearing aids may not feel the need to know as much about the structure and function of the auditory system. However, although the demand for knowledge of A&P may vary across different areas of audiology, this knowledge is indeed relevant, necessary, and helpful to all aspects of clinical audiology. Following are the areas in which knowledge of A&P can help the clinician.

Communication

Communication with medical personnel about clinical topics is easier and more relevant if audiologists are knowledgeable about the structure and function of the auditory system. Long-lasting opinions about our profession are often formed by these medical personnel on the basis of our knowledge of A&P. Knowledge of A&P is also helpful during the frequent communications with hearing scientists and other audiologists.

Test Selection

Most audiological tests assess in some manner the function of the auditory system. Thus to select tests to evaluate different parts of the auditory system one should understand the relevant biology of a particular system. For example, because of A&P research it is known that certain tests are necessary to measure the integrity of interhemispheric transfer. Without this knowledge and the correct selection of tests, interhemispheric dysfunction may never be detected by the clinician.

Test Interpretation

Perhaps the most critical need for A&P is in the interpretation of audiological test results (especially diagnostic results). Test results combined with the patient's history can provide valuable information if interpreted with knowledge of A&P. For example, the acoustic reflex is of little value if one does not understand the anatomy of the reflex circuit. If one knows this circuit well, relevant clinical insight can be gained about the peripheral and part of the central auditory nervous system (CANS).

Radiology

Radiology is a medical specialty based on anatomy. The diagnostic audiologist must have at least a cursory knowledge of radiology to evaluate the audiological tests administered because imaging techniques are often the "gold standard" to which many diagnostic hearing test results are compared. In addition, radiologists look at brain images in a general sense and not for specifics as would an auditory anatomist. Therefore specific anatomical data on auditory structures often must be supplied by the clinician to optimize interpretation. These writers would suggest that fundamental information on radiology be included in courses of medical audiology, diagnostic audiology, and A&P.

Hearing Disorders

The understanding of various hearing disorders, both peripheral and central, depends on knowledge of A&P. Hearing disorders can relate to dysfunction at a certain locus or loci. For example, we now know that kernicterus primarily affects the cochlear nucleus (CN) in the brain stem, and even though high-frequency pure tone hearing loss is common, the cochlea is usually unaffected. This type of information is linked closely to A&P; without this information the clinician cannot fully understand the disorder and its consequences for hearing.

Patient Counseling

It is difficult to counsel patients if one does not have a good understanding of the condition's underlying A&P. For example, if a patient asks why two hearing aids are recommended instead of one, part of the appropriate answer relates to the physiology of binaural hearing and even plasticity of the brain. Patient questions can often be best answered with the help of an anatomical model because a visual aid gives the patient something tangible with which to work. The aforementioned are only a few of the many ways in which knowledge of A&P has an impact on the clinician.

At present in the field of audiology, many tests and clinical behaviors are associated with the CANS. Most auditory-evoked potentials have a profound interaction with the CANS, as do the various behavioral central auditory tests. The audiology-CANS relationships go beyond these obvious procedures. For example, maturational factors in children, auditory deprivation influences, and auditory training procedures all are closely related to the CANS. However, although modern audiology interacts increasingly with the CANS, the education and training of audiologists in the CANS have failed to keep pace. This is unfortunate, especially because current technology can help us learn more about the brain. The use of imaging techniques, such as positron emission

tomography (PET), magnetic resonance imaging (MRI), and functional MRI, allows knowledge of the human brain A&P to be acquired. Before the availability of these techniques, neuroanatomists and physiologists depended on cadaver specimens and animal studies to learn about the CANS.

It is difficult to use data from animal studies to generalize about the human A&P of the CANS (Moore, 1987). Fortunately, with the greater availability of imaging techniques relevant human data can be acquired. In this chapter we refer to human data as much as possible without compromising the critical knowledge gained from animal studies.

A Parallel and Sequential Processing System

In viewing the CANS (or the entire auditory system) overall, it is important to consider the concepts of sequential and parallel processing (Ehret & Romand, 1997). Sequential processing could be seen as consistent with a hierarchal organization of the auditory system. This means that information is transferred from one center to another in a progressive manner, moving from lower nuclei in the brain stem to the key structures in the cortex. As the information progresses from one auditory center to the next, the different structures along the pathway influence impulses. These actions alter or preserve the pattern of information in ways that make it usable to more central centers. The sequence of processing in the CANS implies that if certain sequences are skipped, optimal information flow is not achieved. This may be the case when nerves or nuclei are damaged and less-than-optimal auditory perception takes place. Parallel processing depends on having at least two separate channels for information as it progresses through the system. At the auditory nerve level, type I and type II fibers could be viewed as two channels representing parallel processing. Further up in the system much more parallel processing occurs as many channels come into play. Sequential and parallel processing are ways in which much information can be analyzed in abbreviated time periods, which is critical in the auditory system.

The auditory structures and their associated functions make up a system. Because it is a system, it is difficult to assign specific functions to each structure. Rather, the different structures interact to provide an end result of hearing. Although physiologically certain events appear to take place at a given structure, the manner in which a particular event contributes to overall hearing is uncertain.

CENTRAL AUDITORY NERVOUS SYSTEM: ANATOMICAL DEFINITION

We define the anatomical limits of the CANS as beginning at the CN and ending at the auditory cortex. However, the end point of the CANS is unclear because it might be someplace in the efferent system or possibly in a nonauditory area of the cerebrum. The end point of the CANS may also depend on the types of acoustic stimuli and the task to be completed. Thus it may be physiologically rather than anatomically determined (Fig. 3–1).

Brain Stem

Cochlear Nucleus

The CN is located in the cerebellopontine angle area, a lateral recess formed at the juncture of the pons, medulla, and cerebellum. It consists of three principal sections: the anterior ventral cochlear nucleus (AVCN), the posterior ventral cochlear nucleus (PVCN), and the dorsal CN. Auditory nerve fibers enter this complex at the junction of the AVCN and PVCN, where each fiber then divides and sends branches to the three individual nuclei (Schuknecht, 1974) (Figs. 3–1 and 3–2).

The CN is composed of multiple cell types. Among the most prominent of these are the pyramidal (fusiform), octopus, stellate, spherical (bushy), globular (bushy), and multipolar cells (Osen, 1969; Pfeiffer, 1966). The pyramidal cells in the cat are at the dorsal fringe of the dorsal CN, octopus cells are in the PVCN, and spherical cells are in the AVCN. Globular and multipolar cells are found between the AVCN and PVCN (Osen, 1969; Rouiller, 1997) (Figs. 3–3 and 3–4).

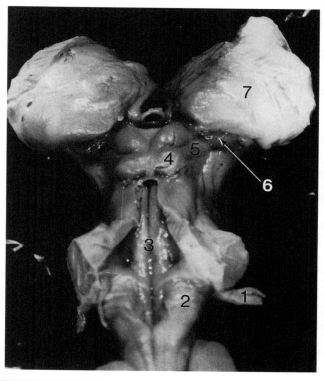

Figure 3–2 Posterior view of the human brain stem (cerebellum and vessels removed). 1, Eighth nerve (entering cochlear nucleus just below the cerebellar peduncle); 2, cochlear nucleus; 3, fourth ventricle; 4, inferior colliculus; 5, brachium of inferior colliculus; 6, medial geniculate body; 7, thalamus. (Courtesy of W. Mosenthal, & F. Musiek, Anatomy Laboratory, Dartmouth Medical School, Hanover, NH.)

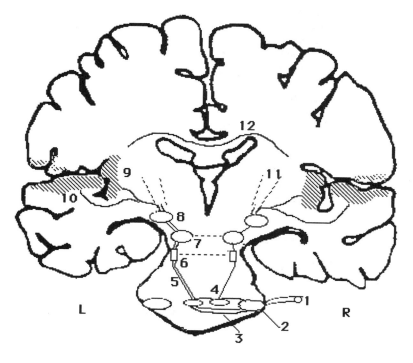

Figure 3–1 Coronal view of the brain with key auditory structures and areas defined. 1, Auditory nerve; 2, cochlear nucleus; 3, stria (dorsal, intermediate, ventral); 4, superior olivary complex; 5, lateral lemniscus; 6, nuclei of lateral lemniscus; 7, inferior colliculus; 8, medial geniculate bodies; 9, insula (shaded); 10, primary auditory region in temporal and parietal lobes (shaded); 11, internal capsule; 12, corpus callosum.

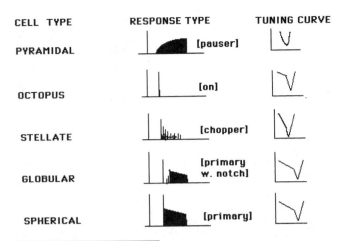

Figure 3–3 Examples of five cell types found in the cochlear nucleus with associated poststimulatory histogram types and tuning curve configurations.

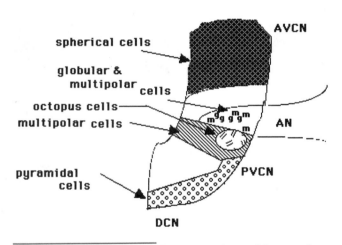

Figure 3–4 Location of cell types in the cochlear nucleus. AVCN, Anterior ventral cochlear nucleus; AN, auditory nerve; PVCN, posterior ventral cochlear nucleus; DCN, dorsal cochlear nucleus. (Based on Osen, K.K. [1969]. *Journal of Comparative Neurology, 136;453–484.*)

Incoming neural impulses can be modified by these cells in a characteristic manner that provides the basis for coding information by the type of neural activity within the CN. The average response of a particular neural unit over time to a series of short tones presented at the unit's characteristic frequency is shown in poststimulatory histograms (Rhode, 1985). The principal response patterns include the following: (1) primary-like, an initial spike proceeded by a steady response until the stimuli ceases; (2) the chopper poststimulatory response, an extremely rapid oscillatory neural response to the stimulus; (3) the onset response, a solitary initial spike at the onset of the stimulus; and (4) the pauser response, similar to the primary-like response but it ends soon after the initial spike and resumes a graded response (Kiang, 1975). An additional pattern, the "build-up" response, is when the cell fires increasingly throughout the stimulus

presentation (Kiang, 1975; Rhode, 1985). This correspondence between cell type and response pattern proposes a significant relationship between anatomy (structure) and physiology (function) of the cells within the CN. Poststimulatory histograms from the CN supply details regarding the complex processing of auditory information at the CN, such as precise timing needed for localization and distinguishing interaural time differences (Rhode, 1991). The various cell types also have associated tuning curves; the main difference among the cell types is the shape of their tails (Figs. 3–3 and 3–4).

The auditory nerve enters the brain stem on the lateral posterior aspect of the pontomedullary juncture and projects to the cochlear nuclear complex. Auditory nerve fibers entering each section of the CN are arranged in a systematic fashion that preserves the frequency organization from the cochlea (Sando, 1965; Webster, 1971). All three sections of the CN contain this tonotopic organization, with low frequencies represented ventrolaterally and high frequencies represented dorsomedially within each nucleus (Sando, 1965; Webster, 1971) (Fig. 3–5A). Some tuning curves derived from AVCN units using tone bursts have a similar shape to those of the auditory nerve (Rhode, 1991; Rose et al, 1959). However, some CN fibers produce wider tuning curves than do auditory nerve fibers (Moller, 1985). Frequency resolution of acoustic information coming from the auditory nerve may thus be maintained but not necessarily enhanced by CN units.

The tuberculoventral tract, a fiber pathway thought to be primarily inhibitory in nature, connects the dorsal and ventral portions of the CN (Ortel, personal communication, 1990). Three main neural tracts continue from the CN complex to the superior olivary complex (SOC) and higher levels of the CANS.

A large fiber tract called the dorsal acoustic stria emanates from the dorsal CN and continues contralaterally to the SOC, lateral lemniscus (LL) (Whitfield, 1967), and inferior colliculus (IC) (Kiang, 1975). The intermediate acoustic stria originates in the PVCN and communicates with the contralateral lemniscus (ventral nucleus) as well as the central nucleus of the contralateral IC (Kiang, 1975) (Fig. 3–5B). The ventral acoustic stria, the largest tract, arises from the AVCN and merges with the trapezoid body as it nears the midline of the brain stem (Whitfield, 1967). The ventral stria extends contralaterally along the LL to the SOC and other nuclear groups. Interestingly, in animal studies for simple detection tasks of tones or noise, performance was not affected by sectioning of the intermediate and dorsal acoustic stria. However, severe deficits were noted with sectioning of the ventral stria (Masterton & Granger, 1988).

In addition to these three primary tracts, other fibers project ipsilaterally from each division of the CN. Some of these fibers synapse at the SOC and nuclei of the LL within the pons. Other fibers synapse at the IC only and completely bypass the SOC and the nuclei of the LL. The contralateral pathways carry the largest number of fibers even though many neural tracts project both ipsilaterally and contralaterally from the CN (Noback, 1985).

The CN is a unique brain stem auditory structure in that its only afferent input is ipsilateral, coming from the cochlea by way of the auditory nerve. Consequently, damage to the CN can mimic auditory nerve dysfunction (Jerger & Jerger, 1974) because it may only produce ipsilateral pure tone deficits (Dublin, 1976, 1985; Matkin & Carhart, 1966). Extraaxial tumors, such as acoustic neuromas, often affect the CN

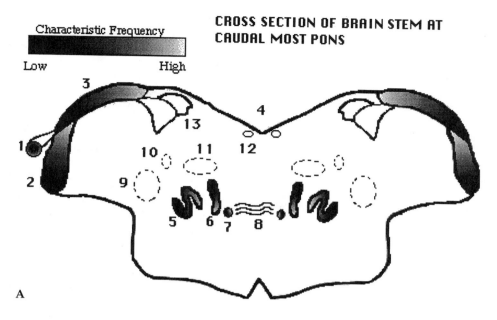

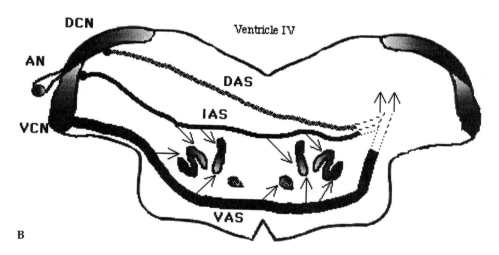

1. auditory nerve	5. lat. sup. olive	9. lateral lemniscus
2. ventral coch. nucleus	6. med. sup. olive	10. facial nuclei
3. dorsal coch. nucleus	7. trap. body med. nuclei	11. retic. form.
4. 4th ventricle	8. trap. body tract	12. MLF
		13. vestibular nuc.

Figure 3–5 **(A)** Cross section of the lower pons focusing on the cochlear nucleus, superior olivary complex, and associated structures in this region of the brain stem. **(B)** The same cross section as shown in Figure 3–5A, showing the three acoustic stria coursing from the left cochlear nucleus only. AN, Auditory nerve; VCN, ventral cochlear nucleus; DCN, dorsal cochlear nucleus; DAS, dorsal acoustic stria; IAS, intermediate acoustic stria; VAS, ventral acoustic stria (arrows indicate fibers ascending through the lateral lemnicus).

because of its posterolateral location on the brain stem surface (Dublin, 1976; Musiek & Kibbe-Michael, 1986; Nodar & Kinney, 1980).

Tumors situated in this cerebellopontine region can often affect the CN and may produce central auditory deficits. Nevertheless, the cerebellopontine angle is large enough in some cases to accommodate lesions of sizeable mass without

compromising neural function (Musiek & Gollegly, 1985; Musiek, et al, 1986).

Superior Olivary Complex

The SOC is positioned ventral and medial to the CN in the caudal portion of the pons (Noback, 1985) (Fig. 3–5A). The

SOC consists of numerous groups of nuclei, but this discussion will be limited to the following five: the lateral superior olivary complex (LSO), the medial superior olivary nucleus (MSO), the nucleus of the trapezoid body, and the lateral and medial preolivary nuclei. In humans evidence suggests that the MSO is the largest of these nuclei (Brugge & Geisler, 1978). In some animal species, however, the largest and most prominent nucleus is the S-shaped LSO (Moore, 1987).

Similar to that of the CN, tonotopic organization in the SOC seems to be preserved in all groups of nuclei. The LSO and MSO have been studied most extensively. In the LSO lower frequencies are represented laterally and the higher frequencies medially following the S-shaped contour of the nucleus, which gives it a unique tonotopic organization (Tsuchitani & Boudreau, 1966). The MSO has a primarily low-frequency representation, whereas the LSO responds to a broader range of frequencies (Noback, 1985). The nucleus of the trapezoid body has a tonotopic orientation, with the low frequencies represented laterally and the high frequencies medially.

The tuning curves for the trapezoid body, LSO, and MSO are mainly quite sharp, denoting good frequency selectivity (Rouiller, 1997). The trapezoid and MSO poststimulatory responses are primary-like with a notch, whereas the LSO has shown chopper and primary-like type responses (Keidel et al, 1983; Rouiller, 1997).

Within the SOC the LSO is innervated bilaterally (Strominger & Hurwitz, 1976) and receives ipsilateral input from the AVCN and contralateral innervation from both the AVCN and PVCN (Warr, 1966). Both ipsilateral and contralateral input from the AVCN are also received in the MSO (Strominger & Strominger, 1971). Afferent input to the trapezoid body is not understood fully, but a significant contribution seems to arise from the contralateral CN (Strominger & Hurwitz, 1976). Innervation of the lateral and the medial preolivary nuclei may come primarily from the ipsilateral AVCN, but this is also unclear and appears to differ among species (Strominger & Hurwitz, 1976).

The SOC is a complex relay station in the auditory pathway. It is the first, but not only, place where a variety of ipsilateral and contralateral inputs provide the system with the anatomical foundation for unique functions in binaural listening. Sound localization is determined mainly by interaural time (Masterson et al, 1975) and intensity (Boudreau & Tsuchitani, 1970) variations reflected in inputs to the SOC. The SOC has excitatory and inhibitory cells (and also some cells that are both excitatory and inhibitory) that are time (hence directionally) sensitive. These excitatory and inhibitory responses help clarify directional cues for the higher auditory system (Tsuchitani & Johnson, 1991). Tasks that necessitate the integration and interpretation of binaurally presented signals depend on the SOC and convergence of neural information from each ear. For example, audiological tests, such as rapidly alternating speech perception and the binaural fusion test (see Chapter 17), rely on binaural integration and the interaction of information in the SOC (Tobin, 1985). Abnormal results are often seen on these tests in cases with signal degradation before the SOC or SOC pathosis (Matzker, 1959). Binaural integration is also necessary for the measurement of masking levels differences (MLDs), which are a sensitive index of brain stem integrity (Lynn et al, 1981). Changing the phase of the stimulus (tones or speech) in the presence of noise results in a change in the ability to detect the signal, which makes temporal cueing at the SOC critical in MLDs. The importance of the SOC in the measurement of MLDs and the fusion of binaural signals is supported by several studies that show low brain stem lesions affect MLDs whereas lesions in the upper brain stem or auditory cortex do not (Cullen & Thompson, 1974; Lynn et al, 1981).

The SOC also appears to be an important relay station in the reflex arc of the acoustic stapedius muscle reflex (Borg, 1973). The reflex is thought to entail both direct and indirect neural pathways (Musiek & Baran, 1986), but the neurophysiology of the reflex arc is not entirely understood (Hall, 1985). The direct reflex arc appears to consist of a three-neuron or four-neuron chain that is activated when a sufficiently intense acoustic stimulus is presented to one or both ears. Neural impulses are conveyed through the auditory nerve to the AVCN and then proceed to the ipsilateral MSO and/or facial nerve nucleus. Transverse input seems to arise from the AVCN and travels to the contralateral MSO by way of the trapezoid body. Neurons originating in the MSO region eventuate in the motor nucleus of the facial nerve area, where motor fibers then descend to innervate the stapedius muscle. Consequently, unilateral acoustic stimulation results in bilateral stapedius muscle contractions (Borg, 1973).

The existence of an indirect pathway for the acoustic reflex has also been postulated. A slower polysynaptic pathway, possibly including the extrapyramidal system of the reticular formation, has been contemplated by Borg (1973) as this indirect reflex arc. Although all the pathways involved in the neural arc are not specified, significant clinical acoustic reflex data support the existence of this neural pathway (Hall, 1985).

Lateral Lemniscus

The LL is the primary auditory pathway in the brain stem and is composed of both ascending and descending fibers. The ascending portion extends bilaterally from the CN to the IC in the midbrain and contains both crossed and uncrossed fibers of the CN and SOC (Goldberg & Moore, 1967) (Fig. 3–1).

Within the LL are two main cell groups: the ventral and dorsal nuclei of the lateral lemniscus (NLL), and a minor cell group called the intermediate nucleus of the LL. These nuclei are located posterolaterally in the upper portion of the pons, near the lateral surface of the brain stem (Ferraro & Minckler, 1977). Afferent input to the NLL arises from the dorsal CN on the contralateral side and from the ventral CN from both sides of the brain stem (Jungert, 1958). Both the ipsilateral and contralateral SOC also provide input to the NLL (Noback, 1985). The dorsal NLL from either side of the brain stem are interconnected by a fiber tract called the commissure of Probst (Kudo, 1981). Lemniscal fibers may also cross from one side to the other through the pontine reticular formation (Ferraro & Minckler, 1977). Most neurons of the dorsal segment of the LL can be activated binaurally. However, most neurons from the ventral segment can be activated only by contralateral stimulation (Keidel et al, 1983). As with the CN and the SOC, definite tonotopic organization has been demonstrated for both the dorsal and ventral NLL (Brugge & Geisler, 1978). However, recent work has questioned the tonotopic arrangement of the LL and indicated a possible concentric organization (Merchan et al, 1994). Tuning curves are highly variable, and temporal resolution appears to be markedly decreased at the LL compared with more caudal auditory nuclei (Rouiller, 1997).

Inferior Colliculus

The IC is one of the largest and most identifiable auditory structures of the brain stem (Oliver & Morest, 1984). The IC is located on the dorsal surface of the midbrain, approximately 3 to 3.5 cm rostral to the pontomedullary junction (Fig. 3–2).

From the dorsal aspect of the midbrain, the IC is clearly visible as two spherical mounds (Musiek & Baran, 1986). Two additional rounded projections, the superior colliculi, can be seen on the dorsal surface of the midbrain, slightly rostral and lateral to the IC (Musiek & Baran, 1986).

Two major divisions exist within the IC: the central nucleus—or core—which is composed of purely auditory fibers, and the pericentral nucleus—or belt—which surrounds the central nucleus and consists mainly of somatosensory and auditory fibers (Keidel et al, 1983).

Most auditory fibers from the LL and the lower auditory centers synapse directly or indirectly at the IC (Barnes et al, 1943). Van Noort (1969) found that the IC receives input from the dorsal and ventral CN, lateral and medial superior olivary nuclei, dorsal and ventral nuclei of the LL, and contralateral IC. Other reports (Keidel et al, 1983; Pickles, 1988; Whitfield, 1967) suggest that the lower nuclei provide both contralateral and ipsilateral input to the IC. Many interneurons appear to exist in the IC, suggesting the presence of strong neuronal interconnections (Oliver & Morest, 1984). The superior colliculi, generally associated with the visual system, also receives input from the auditory system, which is integrated into the reflexes involving the position of the head and eyes (Gordon, 1972).

Many of the functional properties of the IC have been described. As with other brain stem auditory structures, the IC has a high degree of tonotopic organization (Merzenich & Reid, 1974). In the IC, the high frequencies are ventral and the low frequencies are dorsally positioned (Merzenich & Reid, 1974).

Moreover, the IC contains a large number of fibers that yield extremely sharp tuning curves, suggesting a high level of frequency resolution (Aitkin et al, 1975). The IC contains many time-sensitive and spatial-sensitive neurons (Knudson & Konishi, 1978; Pickles, 1982) and neurons sensitive to binaural stimulation (Benerento & Coleman, 1970). This suggests a role in sound localization (Musiek & Baran, 1986). Finally, in considering its neural connections and its position astride the auditory pathways, the IC has been referred to as the obligatory relay nuclear complex in transmitting auditory information to higher levels (Noback, 1985).

Similar to the LL, the IC has a commissure that permits neural communication between the left and right IC (Whitfield, 1967). A unique feature of the IC is its brachium, a large fiber tract that lies on the dorsolateral surface of the midbrain. This tract projects fibers ipsilaterally to the medial geniculate body (MGB), which is the principal auditory nucleus of the thalamus. Three cell types make up most neural elements in the IC. Disk-shaped cells represent 75 to 85% of the cells in the central nucleus. Simple and complex stellate cells also exist in the IC (Oliver & Shneiderman, 1991). In terms of response properties, the IC has two main types of responses: transient onset and sustained. The transient onset is an increase in response that grows only at the beginning of the stimulus; the sustained response gradually increases for the duration of the stimulus (Moore & Irvine, 1980). It is important to know that in the IC all the response types described at the CN are also present, although apparently to a lesser degree (Ehret & Merzenich, 1988). The temporal resolution of the IC, as with the LL, is less efficient than at the lower brain stem auditory structures (Rouiller, 1997). Interestingly, intensity coding at the IC reveals a large number of neurons with nonmonotonic functions (Ehret & Merzenich, 1988).

Medial Geniculate Body

The MGB is located on the inferior dorsolateral surface of the thalamus just anterior, lateral, and slightly rostral to the IC (Fig. 3–2). Although the MGB sits in the thalamus and the IC in the midbrain, these structures are located only approximately 1 cm apart. The MGB contains ventral, dorsal, and medial divisions (Morest, 1964). Cells in the ventral division respond primarily to acoustic stimuli, whereas the other divisions contain neurons that respond to both somatosensory and acoustic stimulation (Keidel et al, 1983; Pickles, 1988). The ventral division appears to be the portion of the MGB that transmits specific discrimination (speech) auditory information to the cerebral cortex (Winer, 1984, 1985). The dorsal division projects axons to association areas of the auditory cortex. This division may maintain and direct auditory attention (Winer, 1984). The medial division may function as a multisensory arousal system (Winer, 1984).

Afferent inputs to the MGB are primarily uncrossed, arriving from the IC by way of the branchium. It is possible, however, that some input may come from the contralateral IC and that some lower nuclei may input directly on the MGB (Pickles, 1982). In the cat crossed inputs from the IC connect to the medial division of the MGB (Morest, 1964; Winer, 1984).

Tonotopic organization has been reported in the ventral segment of the MGB, with low frequencies represented laterally and high frequencies represented medially (Aitkin & Webster, 1972). Tuning curves range from broad to sharp, but MGB fibers in general are not as sharply tuned as are those of the IC (Aitkin & Webster, 1972). As reviewed by Rouiller (1997), the MGB has neurons with response properties that include transient onset, sustained, offset, and inhibitory. The MGB also has sharp tuning curves that allow good frequency selectivity. Both monotonic and nonmonotonic neurons code the intensity. Temporal resolution varies across the three regions of the MGB, and the ventral division has the best fidelity (measured by phase locking or synchronization to individual clicks). In general, the temporal resolution of the ventral portion is similar to that of the IC and much poorer than that of the CN.

As with the IC, the MGB has many neurons sensitive to binaural stimulation and interaural intensity differences (Aitkin & Webster, 1972; Pickles, 1988).

Reticular Formation

The auditory system, like other sensory and motor systems, is intricately connected to the reticular formation. The reticular formation can be viewed as having two subsystems: the sensory or ascending reticular activating system (ARAS) and the motor activating system. Our remarks pertain to the ARAS.

The reticular formation, which forms the central core of the brain stem, is a diffusely organized area with intricately connected nuclei and tracts (Sheperd, 1994). The reticular formation is connected to the spinal cord by reticulospinal tracts and to the cerebrum by many (but poorly defined) tracts, such as the medial forebrain bundle, the mamillary peduncle, and the dorsal longitudinal fasciculus. The reticular formation also contains many brain stem nuclei. The reticular formation has both ascending and descending tracts on each side of the brain stem. These tracts extend from the caudal areas of the spinal cord through the medulla, pons, and midbrain, where diffuse tracts are sent throughout the cerebrum. Connections to the cerebellum also exist.

When the ARAS is stimulated, the cortex becomes more alert and aware. This increased alertness has been shown by changes in electroencephalogram patterns (French, 1957). Conversely, when the reticular formation is turned off, sleep or coma ensues (Mosenthal, personal communication, 1991). The ARAS is a general alarm that responds the same way to any sensory input. The ARAS responses prepare the entire brain to act appropriately to the incoming stimulus (Carpenter & Sutin, 1983). Evidence suggests that the ARAS can become sensitive to specific stimuli (French, 1957). For example, this system has a greater reaction to important stimuli than to unimportant stimuli. This may be one of the mechanisms underlying selective attention and could be related to the ability to hear in the presence of noise. General listening skills may also be affected by the state of awareness. The profuse connections of sensory structures to the reticular formation and their extensive interactions may make it unnatural to try to separate attention from sensory or cognitive processing of information.

Vascular Anatomy of the Brain Stem

Many auditory dysfunctions of the brain stem and periphery have a vascular basis. For example, vertebrobasilar disease, ministrokes, vascular spasms, aneurysms, and vascular loops have all been shown to affect the auditory system (Colclasure & Graham, 1981; Moller & Moller, 1985; Musiek & Gollegly, 1985).

The major blood supply of the brain stem is the basilar artery, which originates from the left and right vertebral arteries 1 to 2 mm below the pontomedullary junction on the ventral side of the brain stem (Fig. 3–6). At the low to midpons level, the anterior inferior cerebellar artery branches from the basilar artery to supply blood to the CN. The CN also may receive an indirect vascular supply from the posterior inferior cerebellar artery (Waddington, 1984). In many cases the anterior inferior cerebellar artery gives rise to the internal auditory artery, which supplies the VIII nerve, and then branches into three divisions to supply the cochlear and vestibular periphery. The internal auditory artery sometimes branches directly from the basilar artery (Portman et al, 1975).

At the midpons level small pontine branches of the basilar artery, perhaps with the circumferential arteries, indirectly supply the SOC and possibly the LL (Tsuchitani & Boudreau,

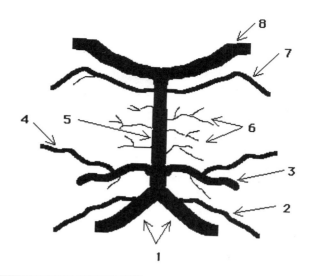

Figure 3–6 A drawing of the key vessels of the rostral medulla and pons segment of the brain stem. These vessels are located on the ventral side of the pons/medulla. 1, Vertebral arteries; 2, posterior inferior cerebellar artery (PICA); 3, anterior inferior cerebellar artery (AICA); 4, internal auditory artery; 5, basilar artery; 6, pontine arteries; 7, superior cerebellar artery; 8, posterior cerebral artery.

1966). In addition, a strong possibility exists that the paramedian branches of the artery supply the SOC and LL. The superior cerebellar arteries are located at the rostral pons or midbrain level. Their branches supply the IC and, in some cases, the NLL (Carpenter & Sutin, 1983). At the midbrain level, the basilar artery forms the posterior cerebral arteries. Each posterior cerebral artery has circumferential branches that supply the MGB ipsilaterally (Waddington, personal communication, 1985).

Significant variability has been shown in the vasculature of the brain stem (Waddington, 1974, 1984). Because vascular patterns vary among specimens, no one description can encapsulate all vascular patterns. Because most brain stem auditory structures are on the dorsal side of the brain stem, they may receive secondary and tertiary branches of the key arteries mentioned previously.

KEY CONCEPTS IN FUNCTION

The following segment introduces concepts about general auditory A&P and reviews them in reference to auditory brain stem structures.

Intensity Coding

As sound intensity increases, the firing rate of many of the auditory fibers in the brain stem increases; exceptions to this will be discussed later. Because the range between the threshold and saturation point of any given fiber is much smaller than the range of intensities audible to the human ear, large-intensity increases cannot be encoded by individual nerve fibers (Moller, 1983). Rather, at high intensities many neurons must interact to achieve accurate coding. The mechanisms of this interaction are poorly understood (Phillips, 1990; Pickles, 1988) because most information on intensity coding is gained on the basis of the study of individual neurons.

Neurons of various brain stem nuclei respond to stimulus intensity in three principal ways (Pickles, 1988; Whitfield, 1967). One type of response is monotonic, meaning that as the stimulus intensity increases the firing rate of the neuron(s) increases proportionally. The second type of intensity function is monotonic for low intensities, but as stimulus intensity increases, the firing rate levels off. The third type of intensity function is nonmonotonic. With this type of function the neuronal firing rate reaches a plateau at a relatively low intensity and sometimes actually decreases as intensity increases, resulting in a rollover phenomenon. For example, some neurons in the IC reach their maximum firing rate 5 dB above their threshold (Whitfield, 1967). These three types of intensity coding appear to be common throughout the auditory brain stem, although the extent of each type varies among nuclei groups. On the other hand, most fibers in the CN have monotonic intensity function. The CN fibers have a 30 dB to 40 dB dynamic range and in this regard are similar to the auditory nerve fibers (Rouiller, 1997).

One can hypothesize that a high-intensity signal would not be coded appropriately when damage to brain stem auditory neurons of the first type (monotonic) exists but not to the latter two types of neurons. This could result in higher intensities being coded incorrectly, which might result in what is known clinically as the rollover phenomenon (Jerger & Jerger, 1971).

Aspects of Temporal Coding

PEARL

The CANS is an elegant timekeeper. Physiological measures of latency, phase locking, phase difference, and synchronicity are common ways of detailing temporal processing. The latency of brain stem neuronal responses varies, depending on the type of auditory stimulus and the neuron or neuron group analyzed (Pickles, 1988; Whitfield, 1967). Some neurons react quickly to stimulation, whereas others have lengthy latency periods. Some neurons respond only on termination of the stimulus.

Phase locking is another phenomenon related to timing in the auditory system (Keidel et al, 1983; Moller, 1985). Many auditory neurons appear to lock onto the stimulus according to phase and fire only when the stimulus waveform reaches a certain point in its cycle. This is particularly evident with low-frequency sounds. Moreover, at lower frequencies certain neurons fire on every cycle, whereas at higher frequencies they fire only at every third or fifth cycle. This phase relationship is especially apparent in lower auditory brain stem

neurons and may have considerable relevance to the mechanisms underlying masking level differences (Jeffress & McFadden, 1971). Generally, the firing rates of brain stem auditory neurons are higher than those of cortical nerve fibers for steady-state signals or for periodic signals. The speed with which a neuron can respond to repeated stimuli depends on its refractory period. The refractory period is the time interval between two successive discharges (depolarization) of a nerve cell. The refractory period depends on the cell metabolism, and dysfunction of metabolic activity will lengthen the refractory period (Tasaki, 1954). Phase locking could be viewed as a form of synchronicity in that responses occur repeatedly in the same time domain. A good example of auditory synchronicity is the auditory brain stem response (ABR). In an ABR the waves represent synchronous electrical activity.

In reviewing timing of the auditory system it is necessary to discuss temporal processing. As Phillips (1995) conveys, this phrase may mean different things to different people. Clinicians often use the phrase temporal processing to indicate performance on an audiological test that requires some type of timing decision about the stimuli presented. Basic scientists look at various types of temporal processing and how these contribute to other auditory functions. Phillips (1995) provides several examples of how timing is key to certain auditory processes. Localization of a sound source requires relative timing of acoustic signal arriving at the two ears. The auditory system has a temporal sensitivity to phase differences (of the signal) that may help us hear in noise. Masking level difference is a good example of phase differential sensitivity. The pitch percept of complex sounds depends on timing (and related coding) of rapidly repeating acoustic events. In addition, sequencing of successive stimuli, masking of signals (existing close in time), discrimination of element duration and time intervals, integration of acoustic energy, and pitch changes can all be considered aspects of temporal processing. Even detection, recognition, and discrimination processes operate over critical time periods and thus may be considered as having a temporal element.

Frequency Coding

The three concepts relevant to our discussion of frequency coding include tonotopicity, frequency discrimination, and physiological tuning curves. The central auditory system is tonotopically arranged, and certain neurons respond best to certain frequencies. This arrangement provides a "spatial array" of various frequencies to which the system responds. The characteristic frequency is the frequency at which a neuron has its lowest threshold to a pure tone stimulus (the frequency that requires the least amount of intensity to raise a neuron's activity just above its spontaneous firing rate). A physiological tuning curve refers to a plot of the intensity level needed to reach the threshold of a nerve cell over a wide range of frequencies. This measure can convey much information about the frequency resolution of a neuron (or group of neurons). Frequency discrimination is the differential sensitivity to various frequencies. This differential measurement can be accomplished psychophysically and is often referred to as a difference limen, which is the smallest frequency difference that can be discerned between two acoustic stimuli. An electrophysiological correlate to the frequency difference limen can be accomplished using the evoked potential mismatched negativity (MMN). Differential sensitivity to intensity and duration of tones can be accomplished in the same way but is not used in physiological studies on audition as much as the frequency parameter is used.

The Auditory Brain Stem Response

In concluding this section on the auditory pathways of the brain stem it is important to discuss aspects of the ABR (see Chapter 21). The ABR has gained most of its popularity because of its clinical applications, but it has also been a valuable addition to basic science. The ABR has provided a physiological approach to the study of multiple neuron groups and the way they interact in the brain stem. This avenue of study is different from the single-neuron studies that have been common in auditory brain stem A&P.

The exact origins of some elements of the ABR are uncertain, but research on humans has helped clarify the subject (Moller, 1985; Wada & Starr, 1983). Moller (1985) indicated that wave I of the ABR is generated from the lateral aspect of the auditory nerve, whereas wave II originates from the medial aspect. Wave III likely has more than one generator, as do other subsequent waves of the ABR, but the CN is probably the principal source of wave III (Moller, 1985; Wada & Starr, 1983). In a study on patients with multiple sclerosis who underwent detailed MRIs and ABRs, observations indicated that waves I and II were generated peripheral to the rostral ventral acoustic stria (Levine et al, 1993). This same study indicated that wave III was generated by the AVCN and rostral ventral stria, with the IV/V complex generated rostrally to these structures. Clinical studies have shown that a midline lesion in the low pons that did not affect the cochlear nuclei preserved waves I, II, and III and delayed the IV/V wave complex. This lesion appeared to compromise the SOC (Musiek et al, 1994). Wave IV probably has multiple generator sites as well, but it arises predominantly from the SOC and has a contralateral influence that may be stronger than the ipsilateral contribution. According to Moller (1985) and Wada and Starr (1983), wave V is generated from the LL. Levine et al (1993) relate that the IV/V complex may be generated by the MSO system, perhaps where it projects contralaterally onto the LL or IC. In a simplified view of the ABR origins, it is plausible that the first five ABR waves may be generated entirely within the auditory nerve and pons. However, the IC may exert some influence on wave V, and this has been shown in detailed analyses of the ABR (Durrant et al, 1994).

The typical clinical findings of ABR abnormalities on the ear ipsilateral to a brain stem lesion (Chiappa, 1983; Musiek & Geurkink, 1982; Oh et al, 1981) seem to be inconsistent with known neuroanatomy, which shows most of the auditory fibers crossing to the contralateral side at the level of the SOC. It is unclear what these ABR findings mean in reference to brain stem pathways and associated physiology. However, it is important to consider these clinical findings in the framework of how the brain stem pathways may function in the pathological situation.

Animal studies by Wada and Starr (1983) and our own observations with humans show that the first five waves of the ABR are not affected by specific lesions of the IC, with the exceptions noted earlier. Unfortunately, the ABR may not be a useful tool in evaluating lesions at or above the IC. Powerful clinical tests such as the ABR, MLDs, and acoustic reflexes appear to be restricted to detecting lesions below the midbrain level. In cases in which lesions of the IC or the MGB (midbrain and thalamic levels) are suspected, other procedures are necessary to detect and define the abnormality.

THE CEREBRUM

Auditory Cortex and Subcortex

Neurons originating in the MGB and radiating outward to the auditory areas of the brain create the ascending auditory system that proceeds from the thalamic area to the cerebral cortex (Fig. 3–7).

The cerebral cortex, the gray matter overlay on the brain surface, consists of three principal types of cells: pyramidal, stellate, and fusiform. Six cell layers in the cortex can be distinguished by type, density, and arrangement of the nerve cells (Carpenter & Sutin, 1983). In the auditory region of the cortex, cells responsive to acoustic stimuli exist in all the layers, with the exception of layer one (Phillips & Irvine, 1981).

> ### CONTROVERSIAL POINT
>
> **Researchers disagree on which areas constitute the auditory cortex. This controversy results from adapting animal models to the human brain and from disagreement as to whether to include "association" areas as part of the auditory cortex (Musiek, 1986a). We believe these association areas are critical to understanding the system, although they also contain some fibers that are not sensitive to auditory stimuli.**

The principal auditory area of the cortex is considered to be Heschl's gyrus, sometimes referred to as the transverse gyrus (Fig. 3–8). This gyrus is located in the sylvian fissure, approximately two thirds posterior on the upper surface of the temporal lobe (supratemporal plane). It courses in a posterior and medial direction. Heschl's gyrus can be defined by the acoustic sulcus at its anterior and transverse sulcus at its posterior fringes. The temporal lobe must be displaced inferiorly or separated from the brain to expose the supratemporal plane to examine Heschl's gyrus.

Campain and Minckler (1976) analyzed numerous human brains and concluded that the configuration of Heschl's gyrus differed on the left side compared with the right. In some brains double gyri were present unilaterally, whereas in other brains double gyri were present on both sides. Musiek and Reeves (1990) studied 29 human brains and reported that a number of Heschl's gyri ranged from one to three per hemisphere, although no significant left-right asymmetry existed

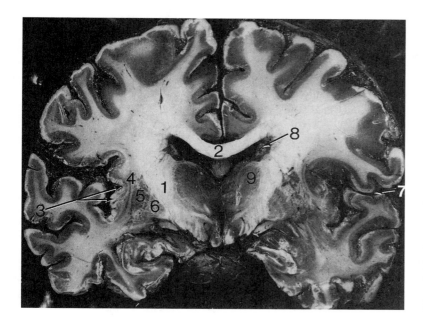

Figure 3–7 Coronal section through a human brain (gray matter stained), emphasizing the subcortical structures. 1, Internal capsule; 2, corpus callosum; 3, insula; 4, external capsule with the claustrum (gray matter strip); 5, putamen; 6, globis pallidus; 7, sylvian fissure; 8, caudate; 9, thalamus. (Courtesy of W. Mosenthal, & F. Musiek, Anatomy Laboratory, Dartmouth Medical School, Hanover, NH.)

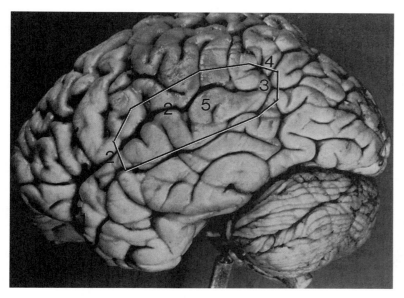

Figure 3–8 Lateral view of the left hemisphere of the brain with the auditory responsive area encircled. 1, temporal pole; 2, sylvian fissure; 3, supra marginal gyrus; 4, angular gyrus; 5, superior, posterior temporal gyrus. (From Waddington [1984], with permission.)

in the number of Heschl's gyri within individual brains. The mean length of Heschl's gyrus, however, was found to be larger in the left hemisphere (Musiek & Reeves, 1990).

The planum temporale is located on the cortical surface from the most posterior aspect of Heschl's gyrus continuing posteriorly to the end point of the sylvian fissure. In the human brain the planum temporale was shown to be significantly larger on the left side (3.6 cm) than on the right (2.7 cm) by Geschwind and Levitsky (1968). These researchers thought that the planum temporale may be an anatomical correlate to language (receptive) in man because the planum temporale is located in Wernicke's region and in the left hemisphere, which is dominant for speech. Musiek and Reeves (1990) supported these earlier findings (Geschwind & Levitsky, 1968) on the differences in the length of the left and right planum temporale. Musiek and Reeves proposed, however, that asymmetries in higher auditory and language function

may be related to anatomic differences of not only the planum temporale but also Heschl's gyrus.

The primary auditory area and a portion of the language area in humans are contained within the sylvian fissure. Rubens (1986) reviewed earlier anatomical work on the sylvian fissure, showing the left sylvian fissure to be larger than the right. Others have corroborated this finding, including Musiek and Reeves (1990), who found that asymmetry of the sylvian fissure was correlated with the greater length of the planum temporale on the left side.

Curving around the end of the sylvian fissure is the supramarginal gyrus, an area responsive to acoustic stimulation (Celesia, 1976). It is located in the approximate Wernicke's area region, along with the angular gyrus, which is situated immediately posterior to the supramarginal gyrus (Geschwind & Levitsky, 1968). These constitute a portion of a complex association area that appears to integrate auditory, visual, and somesthetic information, making it vital to the visual and somesthetic aspects of language, such as reading and writing.

Also responsive to acoustical stimulation are the inferior portion of the parietal lobe and the inferior aspect of the frontal lobe (Celesia, 1976; Galaburda & Sanides, 1980) (Fig. 3–8). The insula (a portion of the cortex located deep within the sylvian fissure medial to the middle segment of the temporal gyrus) is yet another acoustically responsive area. It appears that the most posterior aspect of the insula is contiguous with Heschl's gyrus. The only way to observe the insular cortex is by removing the temporal lobe or displacing it inferiorly (Figs. 3–9 and 3–10).

The insula contains fibers that respond to somatic, visual, and gustatory stimulation. Acoustic stimulation, however, causes the greatest neural activity (Sudakov et al, 1971). The posterior aspect of the insula, the section nearest to Heschl's gyrus, seems to possess the most acoustically sensitive fibers (Sudakov et al, 1971). Located just medial to the insula is a narrow strip of gray matter called the claustrum. The function of the claustrum is not well understood but seems to be highly responsive to acoustic stimulation (Noback, 1985; Sudakov et al, 1971).

People with dyslexia have been reported to have anatomical brain irregularities (Galaburda et al, 1985; Kaufman & Galaburda, 1989).

The findings just mentioned are interesting for two reasons. First, the areas of symmetry versus asymmetry and microdysgenesias appear to involve areas that in humans are mostly considered auditory regions of the cerebrum. Second, the reason for the high incidence of cortical dysplasias in people with learning disorders is unknown. One might speculate that these morphological abnormalities have functional or perhaps dysfunctional correlates. More studies are needed to relate these findings to behavioral consequences.

Thalamocortical Connections

Auditory fiber tracts ascending from the MGB to the cortex and other areas of the brain follow multiple routes. One of these groups of fibers supplies input to the basal ganglia,

---

> ### PEARL
>
> The planum temporale, normally significantly longer in the left hemisphere, was found to be symmetrical bilaterally in the brains of dyslexic patients which also had an unusually large number of cell abnormalities called cerebrocortical microdysgenesias, which are nests of ectopic neurons and glia in the first layer of the cortex. These ectopic areas are often connected with dysplasia of cortical layers (including focal microgyria), sometimes with superficial growths known as brain warts. Up to 26% of normal brains may contain these focal anomalies, but they are usually found in small numbers, often in the right hemisphere. A greater number of anomalies occur in patients with developmental dyslexia, frequently in the left hemisphere in the area of the presylvian cortex (Kaufman & Galaburda, 1989).

which is the large subcortical gray matter structure consisting of the caudate nucleus, putamen, and global pallidus (Figs. 3–7 and 3–10). The lenticular process, or nucleus, lies between the internal and external capsules, the white matter neural pathways, and contains the putamen and globus pallidus. In animal studies the MGB has been shown to transmit fibers that connect with the putamen, the caudate nucleus, and the amygdaloid body, a small almond-shaped expansion located at the tail of the caudate nucleus (LeDoux et al, 1983).

Two main pathways link the MGB and the cortex besides the aforementioned connections to the basal ganglia. The first pathway follows a sublenticular route through the internal capsule to the Heschl's gyrus and contains all auditory fibers emanating from the ventral MGB. The second pathway courses from the MGB through the inferior aspect of the internal capsule, ultimately under the putamen to the external

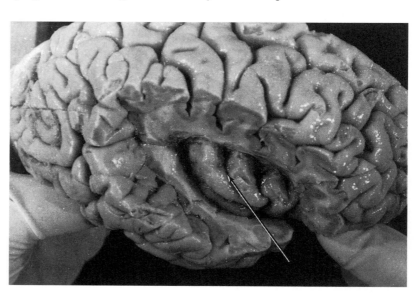

Figure 3–9 Right lateral view of the insula observed after removal of part of the parietal, frontal and temporal lobes. (Courtesy of W. Mosenthal, & F. Musiek, Anatomy Laboratory, Dartmouth Medical School, Hanover, NH.)

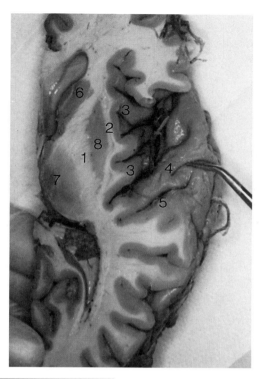

Figure 3–10 Transverse section of the right hemisphere cut along the sylvian fissure. 1, Internal capsule; 2, external capsule with claustrum coursing through it; 3, insula; 4, Heschl's gyrus; 5, anterior part of the planum temporale (posterior part is cut away); 6, caudate; 7, thalamus; 8, lenticular process (putamen, globis pallidus).

capsule, and consists of auditory, somatic, and possibly visual fibers. Beyond the external capsule, fibers connect to the insula (Musiek & Gollegly, 1985; Streitfeld, 1980). Further connections proceed from the MGB to the auditory cortex and most likely overlap the two pathways discussed here. These pathways represent the varied and complex connections of the thalamocortical auditory anatomy.

Intrahemispheric Connections

Intrahemispheric and interhemispheric connections are both present within the primary auditory cortex. Primary auditory area lesions in primates have produced degeneration of the caudal (posterior) aspect of the superior temporal gyrus and the upper bank of the adjacent superior temporal sulcus (Seltzer & Pandya, 1978). This pattern of degeneration suggests the existence of multisynaptic pathways in the middle and posterior areas of the superior temporal gyrus (Jones & Powell, 1970). Fibers from the superior temporal gyrus also connect to the insula and frontal operculum.

Few connections exist between the auditory area and the temporal pole (i.e., the anteriormost aspect of the temporal lobe) (Noback, 1985). Some audiological studies have investigated the validity of several central auditory tests by evaluating patients whose temporal poles had been removed. One would not anticipate these patients having central auditory deficits considering the anatomy of this region.

The arcuate fasciculus, one of the "long" association pathways, adjoins the auditory cortical areas and other sections of the temporal lobe with areas in the frontal lobe. This large fiber tract passes from the temporal lobe, up and around the top of the sylvian fissure, and extends anteriorly to the frontal lobe (Streitfeld, 1980). The arcuate fasciculus is coupled with the longitudinal fasciculus, a larger tract that travels in the same direction by means of comparable anatomical regions. Wernicke's area in the temporal lobe and Broca's area in the frontal lobe are two important regions connected by way of the arcuate fasciculus (Carpenter & Sutin, 1983).

In animals, reciprocal connections exist between the posterior auditory cortex and the claustrum, which is located in the external capsule. Although the claustrum's function is uncertain, it is clear that it is acoustically responsive (Rouiller, 1997). Given its location and its neural connections, the claustrum may have functions related to insular and Heschl's gyrus interactions.

Connections also exist from auditory regions to occipital and hippocampal areas of the brain, although the pathways are not anatomically defined. These connections provide memory and visual associations necessary for such functions as reading.

Interhemispheric Connections

The corpus callosum (CC), which is located at the base of the longitudinal fissure, is the primary connection between the left and right hemispheres (Figs. 3–1, 3–7, and 3–11).

The CC is covered by the cingulate gyri and forms most of the roof of the lateral ventricles (Selnes, 1974). It consists of long, heavily myelinated axons and is the largest fiber tract in the primate brain. In an adult the CC is approximately 6.5 cm long from the anterior genu to the posterior splenium and is approximately 0.5 to 1 cm thick (Musiek, 1986b). The CC seems to be larger in left-handed than in right-handed people, but it has significant morphological variability (Witelson, 1986).

The CC is not exclusively a midline structure (Musiek, 1986b) because it essentially connects the two cortices and thereby must span much of the intercortical space above the basal ganglia and lateral ventricles. Because it encompasses such a large portion of the cerebrum, it is probable that in many "cortical" lesions some region of the CC is involved.

Homolateral fibers (those that connect to the same locus in each hemisphere) are the primary fibers in the CC. The CC also contains heterolateral fibers, which are those connecting to different loci on each hemisphere (Mountcastle, 1962). Heterolateral fibers frequently have a longer and less direct route to the opposite side, which may necessitate a longer transfer time than required by their homolateral counterparts. The latency of an evoked potential recorded from one point on the cortex after stimulation of the homolateral point on the other hemisphere is referred to as the transcallosal transfer time (TCTT). The TCTT in humans decreases with age, and minimum values are achieved during teenage years (Gazzaniga & Sperry, 1962). These findings are consistent with increased myelination of the CC axons (Yakovlev & LeCours, 1967). The TCTT varies significantly, from a minimum of 3 to 6 msec to a maximum of 100 msec, in primates and humans (Bremer et al, 1956; Chang, 1953; Salamy, 1978). The concept

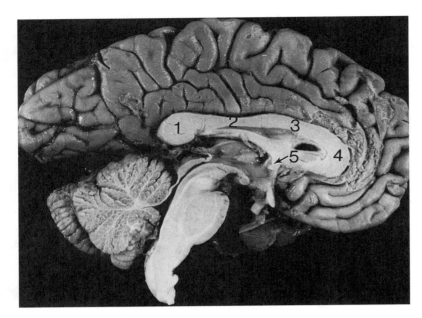

Figure 3–11   Sagittal cut separating the two hemispheres of the brain and sectioning the corpus callosum at its midline. Focus is the corpus callosum. 1, Splenium (visual); 2, sulcus (auditory); 3, trunk or body (somatic and motor); 4, genu (olfactory ? frontal lobe fibers), rostrum (olfactory ?); 5, anterior commissure. (Courtesy of W. Mosenthal, & F. Musiek, Anatomy Laboratory, Dartmouth Medical School, Hanover, NH.)

of inhibitory and excitatory neurons in the CC may be substantiated by this variability.

The anatomy of the CC subserves, and the neural connections correspond to, various regions of the cortex. The neural connections of the CC correspond to, and the anatomy subserves, various regions of the cortex. The genu, or anterior region of the CC, contains fibers leading from the anterior insula and the olfactory fibers (Pandya & Seltzer, 1986). The trunk comprises the middle section of the CC, where the frontal and temporal lobes are also represented. The posterior half of the trunk, called the sulcus, is thinner and contains most of the auditory fibers from the temporal lobe and insula. The splenium is the most posterior portion of the CC and contains mostly visual fibers that connect with the occipital cortex (Pandya & Seltzer, 1986).

Just anterior to the splenium in the posterior half of the CC is the auditory area of the CC at the midline. Although this information was obtained through primate research (Pandya & Seltzer, 1986), data on humans helped localize the auditory areas of the CC. Baran et al (1986) found little or no change in tasks requiring interhemispheric transfer (i.e., dichotic listening or pattern perception) after the sectioning of the anterior half of the CC. However, markedly poorer performance on these auditory tasks was shown in patients with a complete section of the CC (Musiek et al, 1984).

Lesions along the transcallosal auditory pathway may bring about interhemispheric transfer degradation. Although we have much information about the anatomy of the CC at midline, we know little about the course of the transcallosal auditory pathway. It is thought to begin at the auditory cortex and course posteriorly and superiorly around the lateral ventricles. It then crosses a periventricular area known as the trigone and courses medially and inferiorly into the CC proper. This information about the transcallosal auditory pathway comes from anatomical and clinical studies (Damasio & Damasio, 1979).

A recent study demonstrated size differences in the CC for children with attention deficits compared with control subjects. The auditory and the genu areas of the CC in the experimental group were smaller than those of the control group (Hynd et al, 1991).

The vascular anatomy of the CC is simple. The splenium, or posterior fifth, is supplied by branches of the posterior cerebral artery (Carpenter & Sutin, 1983). The remainder of the CC is supplied by the pericallosal artery, a branch of the anterior cerebral artery (Carpenter & Sutin, 1983).

Tonotopic Organization

As in the brain stem, distinct tonotopic organization exists in the auditory cortex. Tonotopic organization exists in the primary auditory cortex of the primate, with low frequencies represented rostrolaterally and high frequencies represented caudomedially (Merzenich & Brugge, 1973). Using PET to measure changes in cerebral blood flow, Lauter et al (1985) demonstrated a similar pattern in the human brain. Tones of 500 Hz evoked increased activity in the lateral part of Heschl's gyrus, whereas tones of 4000 Hz resulted in activity in the medial position. Most tonotopic information on the insular cortex has been obtained from studies of cats (Woolsey, 1960). In the cat insula the high-frequency neurons appear to be located in the inferior segment (Woolsey, 1960).

In the primary auditory area where cells are sharply tuned, highly definable tonotopic organization and isofrequency strips (contours) can be found (Pickles, 1985). "Columns" within the cortex appear to have similar characteristic frequencies (Phillips & Irvine, 1981). A spatial component to frequency representation also seems to be present in the auditory cortex; approximately 2 mm is required to encompass the frequency range of one octave. For extremely high frequencies less space is needed to represent an octave range (Mountcastle, 1968).

<table>
<tr><td>

SPECIAL CONSIDERATION

The tonotopicity of the auditory cortex has the plasticity to change if a lack of input is present at a given frequency range. Schwaber et al (1994) demonstrated in primates that if one frequency band of the auditory cortex was deprived of input, after about 3 months that frequency band shifted to the neighboring lower frequency for which there was input and stimulation, thus the cortical tissue remains active and viable even though its tonotopic arrangement was different. This type of finding has important clinical implications.

</td></tr>
</table>

Intensity Coding

The discharge or firing rate of cortical neurons in primates varies as a function of intensity and takes two forms: monotonic and nonmonotonic (Pfingst & O'Conner, 1981). Most neurons in the primary auditory cortex display rate-intensity functions similar to the auditory nerve (i.e., the firing rate is monotonic for increments of approximately 10- to 40-dB). Intensities greater than 40 dB do not increase firing rates. Many neurons in the auditory cortex are sharply nonmonotonic. In some cases the firing rate may be reduced to a spontaneous level, with a 10 dB increase above the threshold intensity (Pickles, 1988).

Phillips (1990) reported similar results with cats, identifying both monotonic and nonmonotonic profiles. For some nonmonotonic neurons, firing rates decreased precipitously, often to zero, at stimulus levels slightly above threshold. Phillips (1990) also found that the introduction of wide-band noise raised the threshold level of the cortical neurons. However, once threshold sensitivity was achieved in noise, the firing rate increased in a manner similar to the nonmasked condition, with the intensity profile remaining basically unchanged. With successive increments in the level of the masking noise, the tonal intensity profile is displaced toward progressively higher sound pressure levels. This phenomenon could be a way in which some cortical neurons can afford the auditory system an improvement in signal-to-noise ratio, perhaps permitting better hearing in noise. One may also hypothesize that if these cortical neurons are damaged, the signal-to-noise ratio is compromised and that hearing in noise may be more difficult.

Animal studies show some cortical neurons to be intensity selective. Certain cells respond only within a given intensity range, but collectively the neurons cover a wide range of intensities. For example, cortical cells may respond maximally, minimally, or not at all at a given intensity. When the intensity is changed, different cells may respond at a maximum level, and the previous neurons may respond minimally or not at all (Merzenich & Brugge, 1973).

Temporal Factors

Like the brain stem, the auditory cortex responds in various ways to the onset, presence, and offset of acoustic stimuli.

Abeles and Goldstein (1972) found four types of responses of cortical neurons to a 100-msec tone. One type of neuron sustained a response for the duration of the stimulus, although the firing rate was considerably less at the offset of the tone. "On" neurons responded only to the onset, and "off" neurons responded only after the tone was terminated. The fourth type responded to both the onset and the offset of the tone but did not sustain a response during the tone.

Additional information on timing or temporal processing in the auditory cortex can be found in the work of Goldstein et al (1971). These investigators studied cells in the primary auditory area (A1) of rats and found four categories of response to clicks presented at different rates. Approximately 40% of the A1 cells responded to each click at rates of 10 to 1000 per second, whereas 25% of the A1 cells did not respond at all. The third classification of A1 cells showed varying response patterns as the click rate changed. The fourth group of cells responded only to low click rates. Eggermont (1991) reported that several studies found click rates of auditory cortex neurons to be approximately 50 to100 per second or less. He also reported that recording methods may influence the quantification of the response rates of these neurons. However, it seems that cortical neurons have difficulty following high-rate periodic events.

The coding of transient events by the cortex is related to temporal resolution and is different from coding periodic events. Examples of transient events would be tasks such as click fusion or temporal ordering. For these kinds of tasks the cortex is temporally sensitive (Phillips, 1995). Only 2-msec to 3-msec differences were needed between two clicks to determine in humans that two stimuli were present and not one (Lackner & Teuber, 1973).

Timing within the auditory cortex plays a critical role in localization abilities. Many neurons in the primary auditory cortex are sensitive to interaural phase and intensity differences (Benson & Teas, 1976). In a sound field more cortical units fire to sound stimuli from a contralateral source than from an ipsilateral source (Eisenmann, 1974; Evans, 1968). This finding provided the basis for the initial clinical work on sound localization.

In 1958 Sanchez-Longo and Forster reported that patients with temporal lobe damage had difficulty locating sound sources in the sound field contralateral to the damaged hemisphere. Recently, Moore et al (1990) studied the abilities of both normal and brain-damaged subjects to track a fused auditory image as it moved through auditory space. The perceived location of the auditory image, which varies according to the temporal relationship of paired clicks presented one each from matched speakers, is referred to as the precedence effect. Although the normal subjects were able to track the fused auditory image accurately, two subjects with unilateral temporal lobe lesions (one in the right hemisphere, one in the left) exhibited auditory field deficits opposite the damaged hemispheres. Results of these investigations are consistent with other localization and lateralization studies that show contralateral ear effects (Liden & Rosenthal, 1981; Pinheiro & Tobin, 1969).

Electrical Stimulation of the Auditory Cortex

Various auditory stimulation experiments with humans during neurological procedures were performed by Penfield and associates (Penfield & Rasmussen, 1950; Penfield & Roberts, 1959). These investigators electrically stimulated areas along the margin of the sylvian fissure while the patient, under local anesthesia, reported what he or she heard. Numerous patients reported experiencing no auditory sensation during the electrical stimulation. Some patients, however, reported hearing buzzing, ringing, chirping, knocking, humming, and rushing sounds when the superior gyrus of the temporal lobe was stimulated. These sounds were directed primarily to the contralateral ear, but sometimes to both ears.

Penfield's patients frequently reported the impression of hearing loss during the electrical stimulation, although they heard and understood spoken words. Furthermore, patients claimed that the pitch and volume of the surgeon's voice varied during the electrical stimulation. In a later study, Penfield and Perot (1963) reported cases in which patients heard music and singing during electrical stimulation of the right auditory cortex. When the left posterosuperior temporal gyrus was stimulated, many patients who responded heard voices shouting and other acoustic phenomena.

Lateralization of Function in the Auditory Cortex

One important issue in central auditory assessment using behavioral tests relates to lateralization of the deficit. It is well known that behavioral testing often indicates deficiencies in the ear contralateral to the damaged hemisphere. The fact that each ear provides more contralateral than ipsilateral input to the cortex may explain this contralateral ear deficit. Solid physiological evidence upholds this theory. Mountcastle (1968) reported that contralateral stimulation of cortical neurons ordinarily had a 5- to 20-dB lower threshold for activation than did ipsilateral stimulation. Celesia (1976) also showed that near field potentials recorded from human auditory cortices during neurosurgery had larger amplitudes with contralateral ear stimulation than with ipsilateral stimulation. Studies of cats have also demonstrated comparable findings that indicate a stronger contralateral representation (Donchin et al, 1976).

Late auditory evoked potentials recorded with temporal/parietal region electrode placement in humans also revealed variances between contralateral and ipsilateral stimulation. The auditory evoked potentials recorded from contralateral stimulation were generally earlier and of greater amplitude than ipsilateral recordings (Butler et al, 1969). However, this may not always be the case, and these findings for far field evoked potentials are controversial (Donchin et al, 1976).

Behavioral Ablation Studies

Ablation experiments have served as the basis for the development of several auditory tests. By monitoring auditory behavior in animals the effects of partial or total ablation of the auditory cortex have been measured and have been valuable in the localization of function.

Differences among animal species are shown in studies with opossums (Ravizza & Masterton, 1972) and ferrets (Kavanagh & Kelly, 1988) in which auditory threshold recovery is almost complete after bilateral lesions of the auditory cortex. The effects of auditory cortex ablation on frequency

---

CONTROVERSIAL POINT

Kryter and Ades (1943) found little or no effect on absolute thresholds or differential thresholds for intensity in the CAT. These findings are consistent with data obtained from humans with brain damage or surgically removed auditory cortices (Berlin et al, 1972; Hodgson, 1967). However, some investigators (Heffner & Heffner, 1986; Heffner et al, 1985; Phillips, 1990) report that bilateral ablations of the primate auditory cortex result in severe hearing loss for pure tones. Bilaterally ablated animals demonstrated gradual recovery, but many retained some permanent pure tone sensitivity loss, especially in the middle frequencies (Heffner & Heffner, 1986). Unilateral cortical ablations resulted in hearing loss in the ear contralateral to the lesion and normal-hearing in the ipsilateral ear (Heffner et al, 1985). Permanent residual hearing loss also has been reported in humans with bilateral cortical lesions (Auerbach et al, 1982; Jerger et al, 1969; Yaqub et al, 1988).

---

discrimination in animals remains unclear, even after many years of research. Early studies (Allen, 1945; Meyer & Woolsey, 1952) reported that frequency discrimination was lost after ablation of the auditory cortex, whereas later studies (Cranford et al, 1976) contradicted these early findings. These discrepancies may be related to the difficulty of the discrimination tasks because each study used a different test paradigm to measure pitch perception. The complexity of the tasks, rather than the differences in frequency discrimination, is likely responsible for the discrepant findings (Pickles, 1988).

Lesion effects on frequency discrimination in humans may differ from those in animals. Thompson and Abel (1992) showed that patients with temporal lobe lesions have significantly poorer frequency discrimination for tones than do normal control subjects. Patients with lesions of the left temporal lobe yielded a greater deficit than did patients with right temporal lobe lesions (Fig. 3–12). Similar results of poor frequency discrimination in patients with central auditory lesions have been noted on a more informal test basis by the authors of this chapter.

Because ablation of the auditory cortex has debatable effects on absolute or differential thresholds for intensity or frequency, more complex tasks were sought to examine the results of cortical ablation. Diamond and Neff (1957) used patterned acoustical stimuli to examine the ability of cats to detect differences in frequency patterns after various bilateral cortical ablations. After ablation of primary and association auditory cortices, the cats could no longer discriminate different acoustical patterns, and despite extensive retraining they could not relearn the pattern task. On the basis of subsequent studies, Neff (1961) reported

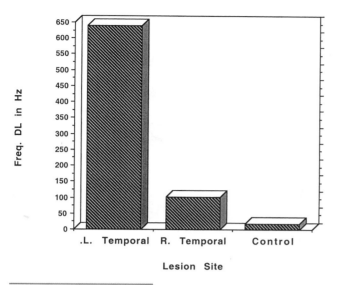

Figure 3–12 Column graph shows the mean difference limen (DL) in Hz obtained from subjects with left and right temporal lobe lesions compared with a control group. (Based on Thompson & Abel [1992].)

that the auditory cortex ablations affected primarily temporal sequencing and not pattern detection or frequency discrimination of the tones composing patterns. Colavita (1972, 1974) demonstrated in cats that ablation of only the insular-temporal region resulted in the inability to discriminate temporal patterns. The early research of Diamond and Neff influenced Pinheiro in her development of the frequency (pitch) pattern test, a valuable clinical central auditory test in humans (Musiek, 1985; Musiek & Pinheiro, 1987; Pinheiro & Musiek, 1985). Another pattern perception test, duration patterns, (see Chapter 17) has emerged as a potentially valuable clinical tool (Musiek et al, 1990). Temporal ordering appears to be a critical part of pattern perception, which in turn is affected by lesions of the auditory cortex.

Other studies show that the temporal dimension of hearing is linked to the integrity of the auditory cortex. Gershuni et al (1967) demonstrated that a unilateral lesion of the dog's auditory cortex resulted in decreased pure tone sensitivity for short but not long tones in the ear contralateral to the lesion.

In contrast, Cranford (1979) showed that cortical lesions had no effect on brief tone thresholds in cats. Cranford (1979) also demonstrated that auditory cortex lesions in cats markedly affected the frequency difference limen for short but not long duration tones presented to the contralateral ear. After the animal study, Cranford et al (1982) examined brief tone frequency difference limens in seven human subjects with unilateral temporal lobe lesions. Findings with human subjects were essentially the same as those with animals. Brief tone thresholds for subjects with temporal lobe lesions were the same as those of a normal control group, but the brief tone frequency difference limen was markedly poorer for subjects with lesions. The frequency difference limen was poorer for the contralateral ear for stimulus durations less than 200 msec.

Auditory Stimulation Influences on the Auditory Cortex

The auditory cortex appears to respond to acoustic stimulation and/or auditory training. This statement is associated with a number of important recent studies. One such study was conducted by Recanzone et al (1993) on owl monkeys. These animals were trained on a frequency discrimination task. After extensive training, each animal's auditory cortex was tonotopically mapped. The neural substrate matching the frequency of the training was two to eight times larger than the same region in a control group of animals that did not receive training. In addition, these animals' behavioral frequency discrimination improved markedly after training. Other studies, although differently oriented, have also shown changes (reorganization) in the auditory cortex as a result of stimulation and/or training (Hassmannova et al, 1981; Knudsen, 1988). This has changed our view on auditory training, especially its use with auditory processing disorders (for review see Chermak & Musiek, 1997; Musiek & Berge, 1998).

Imaging Techniques

Advanced imaging technology has made possible anatomical and physiological inspection of the human brain. This is important because at the subcortical and cortical levels animal brains are structurally and functionally different from the human brain, and it has been with concern that inferences have been made from animal models to humans on brain function related to audition. With imaging techniques it is possible to measure some functions of hearing in humans. Although it is too soon for these imaging techniques to replace the important animal studies, they have important potential.

Two types of imaging techniques will be discussed here: PET, and functional MRI (fMRI) (Elliott, 1994) (Fig. 3–13). The basis of PET is the decay of radioactive tracers that have been introduced into the body and emit positrons. These positrons undergo transformations that result in the release of photons that are detected by the scanning equipment. The radioactive tracer becomes perfused in the brain, and brain activity results in photon emissions that are measured. Two types of PET exist: one based on regional blood flow and one based on glucose metabolism. The blood-flow technique requires inhalation or injection of the radioactive tracer, which has a short half-life of about 2 minutes. Because the body clears the radioactive substance quickly, repeated tests are possible, but each test is obviously limited by time. The glucose metabolism technique uses fluoro-2-deoxy-D-glucose (FDG), which has a by-product linked to glucose, which in turn perfuses the brain differentially. The maximum perfusion is where the metabolism is greatest. The time window for measurement is 30 to 40 minutes after tracer injection, and multiple scans should not be performed because of risk to the patient.

The second imaging technique is fMRI. In fMRI, a strong magnetic field is used to align the body's protons, and a brief radio signal is then used to alter the tilt of the aligned protons. The energy released when the protons resume their original positions is measured. Because the blood acquires paramagnetic properties when the body is in a strong magnetic field, blood flow can be visualized by MRI. Blood flow is related to blood volume and oxygenation, which are

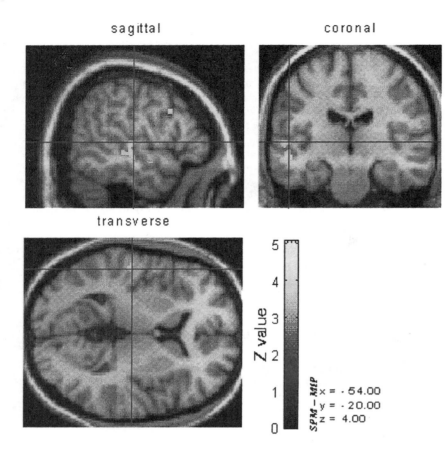

Figure 3–13 fMRI of the brain of a subject who was required to discriminate nonsense words as being alike or different. Note activity in the midportion of Heschl's gyrus and extending inferiorly into the supero-posterior midtemporal gyrus. Also note some frontal lobe activity on the sagittal view. All activity in these views seems to be limited to the left hemisphere. (Courtesy of Brain Imaging Laboratory, Dartmouth Medical School, Hanover, NH.) *(See Color Plate 1.)*

increased when certain areas of the brain are active. Hence, magnetic susceptibility of the blood changes with increased neural activity, and these changes are reflected in the MRI measurements (Elliott, 1994). With fMRI, no radioactivity is involved and its resolution is greater than that of PET. The noise present during fMRI testing is considerable, and this remains a factor in auditory studies.

Many contributions from imaging studies to auditory A&P exist, but we will highlight only a few studies. As mentioned, one early PET study investigated the tonotopic arrangement of Heschl's gyrus (Lauter et al, 1985). This showed low frequencies (500 Hz) to be anterior and lateral, whereas the high frequencies (4000 Hz) were posteromedial. Similar tonotopic results have been reported recently using fMRI (Talavage et al, 1996).

An fMRI study (Millen et al, 1995) using speech (context, reading passages) and tonal stimuli showed primarily activation at the superior temporal gyrus, with more activity on the left side than on the right. Activity appeared to occur in the insula as well. The regions that were active along the superior temporal gyrus varied. Interestingly, different intensities of the stimuli seemed to have no effect on activation patterns. In an fMRI study on word presentation rates, greater activation was seen on the left side than on the right, with activity increasing from 10 through 90 words/min and a drop in activity at 130 words/min. The superior temporal gyrus areas, including Heschl's gyrus, planum temporale, and a small area immediately anterior to Heschl's, were activated at high rates of word presentation. The posterior insula also became involved at high rates (Dhankhar et al, 1997). In

a PET study using words from a song for which pitch judgment of target words was required, the left cortex was more active than the right. Most activity was in the area of Heschl's gyrus but often extended both posteriorly and anteriorly beyond Heschl's gyrus. In this study the subjects were also asked to imagine performing the task. The auditory regions (though smaller and less intense) were activated for this type of task. This showed a way to activate the auditory cortex without external stimuli (Zattore et al, 1996).

Auditory Cortex Vascular Anatomy

The middle cerebral artery (MCA) branches directly from the internal capsule at the base of the brain and is the main artery supplying blood to the auditory cortex (Waddington, 1974). The length of the MCA varies. It can be only 2 cm long before its diffuse branching (Gershuni et al, 1967), or it can extend the full length of the sylvian fissure before becoming the angular artery and coursing posteriorly and laterally on the brain surface. Its route fluctuates greatly between species, but it courses primarily in an anterior-to-posterior direction within the sylvian fissure (Waddington, 1974).

Starting with an anterior view of the MCA, the fronto-opercular artery is the first major branch supplying an auditory region. This artery follows a superior route, supplying the anterior section of the insula. Just posterior to the fronto-opercular artery is the central sulcus artery that supplies the posterior insula and the anterior parietal lobe. Three arteries ascend from the MCA and course over the middle and posterior part of the temporal lobe (Waddington, 1974). These three are the anterior, middle, and posterior arteries and they supply the middle and superior temporal gyri. A combination of the MCA and angular artery presumably supply the primary auditory area along with the angular gyrus and a portion of the supramarginal gyrus. The posterior parietal artery supplies the remainder of the supramarginal gyrus.

Significant tissue damage to gray and white matter in the temporal-parietal regions of the brain may be caused by vascular insults involving the MCA. These lesions are devastating to both the structure and function of the auditory cortex and are among the most common anomalies affecting this region.

THE EFFERENT AUDITORY SYSTEM

The efferent auditory system likely functions as one unit, but the pathways are often viewed in two sections. The caudalmost part of the system, the olivocochlear bundle (OCB), has been studied, but little is known about the more rostral system. The rostral efferent pathway starts at the auditory cortex and descends to the medial geniculate and the midbrain regions, including the IC. A loop system appears to exist between the cortex and these structures, and fibers descend from the cortex to neurons in the brain stem. The IC also receives efferents from the medial geniculate (Pickles, 1988). The descending connections from the IC to nuclei in the SOC have not been well established. Sahley et al (1997) reviewed these connections and stated that connections exist from the IC to the ipsilateral trapezoid body nuclei and preolivary nuclei. Bilateral connections also appear to exist from the IC that are widespread to different areas of the SOC. Some areas of the descending pathway are not well studied, but a system is known to exist that allows neural communication from the cortex to the cochlea. In this regard it is known that electrical stimulation of the cortex results in the excitation or inhibition of single units in the lower auditory system (Ryugo & Weinberger, 1976). Physiological evidence exists for a descending train of impulses that eventually reaches the cochlea from the cortex (Desmedt, 1975).

The OCB is the best known circuitry of the efferent system. The OCB has two main tracts: the lateral and the medial (Sahley et al, 1997; Warr, 1980). The lateral tract originates from preolivary cells near the lateral superior olive and is composed mostly of uncrossed, unmyelinated fibers that terminate on the (ipsilateral) dendrites beneath the inner hair cells. These preolivary cells also send projections ipsilaterally to the cochlear nuclei by way of the ventral and dorsal acoustic stria. The medial tract of the OCB is composed of myelinated fibers that originate in preolivary nuclei in the area around the medial superior olive. Most fibers cross to the opposite cochlea, where they connect directly to the outer hair cells. Bilateral (mostly contralateral) connections to the CN also exist by way of both the dorsal and ventral acoustical stria. The lateral and medial OCB fibers after connecting to various divisions of the CN course along the vestibular nerves in the internal auditory meatus before terminating at the type I auditory nerve fibers below the inner hair cells and the base of the outer hair cells (see Sahley et al, 1997 for review; Pickles, 1988; Warr, 1980).

Early physiological studies show that stimulation of the crossed (medial) OCB fibers results in reduced neural response from the cochlea and auditory nerve (Galambos, 1956). Since then, the suppressive effect of the medial system has been shown in humans. In 1962 Fex showed that acoustic stimulation of the contralateral ear will trigger the medial OCB function. By stimulating the contralateral ear in humans, the action potential is reduced in amplitude as is the amplitude of the transient and distortion product otoacoustic emissions (Folsum & Owsley, 1987; Collet, 1993). It has also been shown that cutting the vestibular nerves in the internal auditory meatus (which is where the OCB fibers course) results in absent suppression of otoacoustical emissions (Williams et al, 1993). Hence, a procedure by which some facet of OCB function can be tested in humans exists by using otoacoustical emissions. This procedure is progressing toward clinical use.

Another important aspect related to function of the OCB is hearing in noise. Pickles and Comis (1973) showed that the application of atropine (a cholinergic blocker) in the region of the OCB resulted in poorer hearing in noise in animals. Other studies also show that the OCB has an important role for hearing in noise (Dewson, 1968; Kawase & Liberman, 1993; Nieder & Nieder, 1970). The mechanism underlying this facilitation for hearing in noise may be related to the ability of the medial OCB to trigger outer hair cell expansion/contraction, thereby enhancing or damping basilar membrane activity. This, in turn, may limit to low levels auditory nerve activity for unimportant (noise) stimuli, resulting in a larger dynamic range for the auditory nerve neuron to respond to other acoustic stimuli (see Sahley et al, 1997 for review). It is also important to consider that the OCB may sometimes enhance responses, even though data indicate many of its activities are related to suppression (see section on neurochemistry). Evidence shows that when an animal is surrounded by noise and the OCB is triggered (by electrical stimulation or by contralateral noise presented to the ear), a release of the auditory nerve from noise is accomplished, allowing better overall hearing in noise.

AUDITORY NEUROCHEMISTRY

Neurochemistry is reviewed as part of the discussion of auditory neuroanatomy and physiology because many known neurotransmitters are associated with the central auditory system. Neurotransmitters are neurochemical agents that convey information across the synapse between nerve cells. The type of synapse and particular neurotransmitters involved may influence many characteristics of auditory function and processing. Research on auditory neurotransmitters frequently has profound clinical implications.

The Anatomy of Neurotransmission

The synapse is the connecting link between nerve cells and the main structure in neurotransmission. It involves the synaptic button of the axon that communicates neurochemically with the dendrites, or in some cases the cell body, of another nerve cell. The neurotransmitters are released by vesicles and permeate the synaptic region to bind to proteins, called receptors, embedded in the adjacent cell membrane. Various events can take place as a result of this transmitter binding. One such event is a change in ions across the cell membrane, which may induce an alteration in a postsynaptic cell receptor potential. A number of neurotransmitter interactions occurring in a restricted time period will cause the postsynaptic cell to depolarize and fire its own impulse or action potential. An excitatory neurotransmitter is associated with this response (Musiek & Hoffman, 1990).

Hyperpolarization of the postsynaptic cell membrane is caused by inhibitory neurotransmitters making the cells less likely to fire an impulse or more difficult to excite (Musiek & Hoffman, 1990). The synapse can also be influenced by other biochemical actions of the cell that are beyond the scope of this review.

PEARL

Numerous therapeutic drugs are used to influence synaptic activity. Agonists can bind to and activate postsynaptic receptors, mimicking natural neurotransmitters. Antagonists can produce the opposite effect by binding to but not activating the receptor, thus blocking the natural neurotransmitter function.

Afferent Auditory Neurotransmission

If synaptic activity can be controlled by neurotransmitters, it may be feasible to control the functions that are based on these synaptic interactions. To accomplish this, neurotransmitters must first be localized and identified, keeping in mind that before a chemical can be considered as a neurotransmitter it must meet strict criteria (Musiek & Hoffman, 1990). New information on function and dysfunction of a system may be obtained through the use of agonists and antagonists once these neurotransmitters are identified.

It is not known which neurotransmitter operates between the cochlear hair cells and auditory nerve fibers, but one possibility is glutamate (Bledsoe et al, 1988). Glutamate or aspartate is believed to be involved in auditory nerve-to-CN transmission (Bledsoe et al, 1988; Guth & Melamed, 1982). Within the CN it is likely that several excitatory neurotransmitters exist, such as aspartate, glutamate, and acetylcholine (ACh) (Altschuler et al, 1984; Godfrey et al, 1985; Oliver et al, 1983). Inhibitory amino acids found at high levels within the CN are gamma amino butyric acid (GABA) and glycine (Godfrey et al, 1977). Gamma amino butyric acid and glycine are also both found in the SOC (Helfert et al, 1987; Wenthold et al, 1987). Also located in the SOC are excitatory amino acids including quisqualate, glutamate, and *N*-methyl-D-aspartate (NMDA) (Otterson & Storm-Mathison, 1984). Glycine and glutamate are likely neurotransmitters in the IC (Adams & Wenthold, 1987). Increased activity at the IC level has been shown from both NMDA and aspartate (Faingold et al, 1989).

Little information exists on auditory cortex transmitters. Evidence shows that ACh and opiate drugs affect auditory cortex activity or evoked potentials, but further research is needed before the neurochemistry of this brain region is understood fully (McKenna et al, 1988; Velasco et al, 1984).

Efferent Auditory Neurotransmission

More data are available about efferent neurotransmitters compared with afferent neurotransmitters. Neurotransmission within the OCB, for example, has been studied extensively. The OCB can be viewed as two systems. One system is lateral and originates from the outlying lateral superior olive region. The second system is medial and ascends from the medial olive region. Both systems are cholinergic, and the lateral system also contains the opioid peptides enkephalin and dynorphin (Altschuler & Fex, 1986; Hoffman, 1986). These efferent neurotransmitters can be found in the perilymph of the cochlea. The results of electrical stimulation on the OCB can be mimicked by applying ACh to this region (Bobbin & Konishi, 1971).

Auditory Function and Neurotransmitters

Several studies have examined neurotransmitter effects on auditory function that are measured electrophysiologically or behaviorally. Cousillas et al (1988) found that auditory nerve activity during sound stimulation was diminished when glutamatergic blockers were perfused through guinea pig cochleas. The application of aspartate, an excitatory amino acid, was also found to increase the spontaneous and acoustically stimulated firing rates of CN fibers. This effect was reversed when an antagonist drug was administered. Homogeneous neural modulating outcomes were shown in a similar study using antagonists and agonists such as glutamate, aspartate, and NMDA at the IC level (Faingold et al, 1989).

The late auditory evoked potential (P2) also showed an increased amplitude after administration of naloxone, an opioid antagonist, in humans. Fentanyl, an opioid agonist, was also found to reduce the P2 amplitude in the same study (Velasco et al, 1984).

Auditory function of the OCB and neurotransmission also have been studied. The OCB plays a role in enhancing hearing in noise (Pickles & Coomis, 1973; Winslow & Sachs, 1987). The chemical interaction of the OCB and the hair cells of the cochlea may mediate this role. The fact that outer hair cells can expand and contract might show a link to the OCB because neurotransmitters may control this hair-cell function. Regulation of this motor activity may in turn allow the OCB modulation of incoming impulses via the outer hair cells.

In recent studies on chinchillas the auditory nerve action potential was enhanced significantly by injecting the opioid agonist pentazocine (Sahley et al, 1991, 1997). Because opioids are found in the (lateral) OCB system, this effect, only noted at intensity levels near threshold, assuredly involves the OCB system.

The pharmacological means to enhance hearing may be furnished ultimately through the study of auditory function and neurotransmission. Neurochemistry's intrinsic role in auditory physiology is underscored by research in this important area.

MATURATION OF THE CENTRAL AUDITORY SYSTEM

Various segments of the brain and auditory system develop and mature at different rates. In a general sense the auditory system matures in a caudal-to-rostral manner. Maturation of the auditory system evolves around several mechanisms, including cell differentiation and migration, myelination, arborization, and synaptogenesis. We discuss the last three mechanisms.

Myelination

Myelin is white matter of the nervous system. It covers and insulates the axons of a nerve fiber. Generally, the amount of myelin on a nerve fiber indicates how fast the impulses are conducted. A heavily myelinated nerve fiber will conduct impulses quickly (some large fibers up to 100 m/s), whereas nerve conduction is slow in unmyelinated fibers (<2 m/s) (Mountcastle, 1968). Slow conduction limits the types of processing that take place. Examples come from the studies on the quaking mouse, a species that does not produce myelin because of a genetic disorder. Auditory brain stem response testing on these mice indicates that their interwave latencies are almost twice as long as in control mice (Shah & Salamy, 1980). In another study on myelination, the amount of myelin was measured in rats for 50 days postnatally. The study measured the amount of cerebroside (a lipid in the blood), which increases with the amount of myelin. As the rat pups grew older, the amount of myelin increased and the interwave latency of the ABRs decreased (Shah & Salamy, 1980).

Myelination of the brain occurs at different rates in different regions. It appears that the brain stem auditory tracts complete myelination before the subcortical regions of the brain. In humans most of the ABR indices reach adult values at around 2 years of age. However, the middle latency and late auditory evoked potentials do not reach adult characteristics until a child is 10 to 12 years of age (McGee & Kraus, 1996). The P1 component of the late potentials is thought by some investigators to be mature by 5 years of age (McPherson, 1996), but others believe full maturation of this potential occurs much later (Ponton et al, 1996). The P2 response of the late potentials appears to mature around 5 years of age (McPherson, 1996). The P300 auditory potential does not mature until the early teenage years (Musiek & Gollegly, 1988). Although present at birth, the mismatched negativity does not reach adultlike characteristics until the early school-age years (Kraus & McGee, 1994). What characterizes the evoked potentials at all levels of the auditory system during maturation is great individual variability. We have noted absent middle and late potentials in some early school-aged children with no apparent problems of any sort, whereas in other school-aged children these same potentials are well formed and easy to read. The development course of these evoked potentials is semiconsistent with the caudal-to-rostral myelination pattern in the brain.

Behavioral auditory tests also have an extended maturational course. Behavioral responses to sound involve more than the auditory system; therefore, maturation rates of the other systems involved may influence these measures. Auditory detection thresholds are 30- to 40-dB higher in 2- to 4-week-old infants than in adults. This difference decreases to 10- to 15-dB when the infant is 6 months old (Werner, 1996). These differences may be related to middle-ear and auditory pathway influences. More central type behavioral measures, such as masking level differences, are larger in preschoolers than in infants (Nozza et al, 1988). Jensen and Neff (1989) have shown that auditory frequency and duration discrimination is better in 6-year-old children than in 4-year-old children, but not as good as in adults. Dichotic listening and frequency pattern performance do not reach adult values until approximately 10 to 11 years of age. Although these behavioral measures do not depend only on the CANS, the central system does play a significant role in these functions.

What is the myelin (maturational) time course to which we refer and what is its foundation? Yakovlev and LeCours (1967) reported on years of study of human brains in regard to myelination at various ages and anatomical regions. Using a Loyez (silver) staining technique they quantified the amount of myelin in a given region of the brain. Their large collection of brains covered a wide range of ages. Yakovlev and LeCours (1967) showed that the optic tracts myelinated before the auditory tracts. The prethalamic auditory tracts are essentially myelin complete at 5 to 6 months after birth. However, postthalamic auditory tracts are not myelin mature until 5 to 6 years of age. The corpus callosum and certain auditory association areas may not have completed myelinogenesis until 10 to 12 years or older. The somatosensory-evoked potentials used to measure interhemispheric transfer time by comparing ipsilateral to contralateral stimulation latencies indicated that corpus callosum maturity ranges from about 10 to 20 years of age (Salamy et al, 1980). This was interpreted also as an index of myelination of the CC.

Another important factor of myelin maturation is the great variability in its rate (Moore, 1983; Yakovlev & LeCours, 1967). If the myelination rate varies, the processes it underlies may also vary. Therefore, if a certain amount of maturation is needed to complete a task but has not been achieved, the task cannot be completed. It is likely that the difference in children's performance on some auditory tests may be related to differences in the amount of myelination in critical regions of the brain.

Arborization and Synaptogenesis

The term *arborization* is used to mean axonal or dendritic branching. This is a maturational process of the nerve cell critical to the functioning of groups of neurons. Generally, as the cell matures arborization is greater; however, increased arborization may also be a result of certain types of continued stimulation after the nerve cell is mature.

A nerve cell is composed of three main parts: soma (cell body), axon, and dendrites. The cell body and axons change with maturity. Axonic and dendritic branching is one of the most dynamic maturational actions of the cell. In the very early maturational course, growing axons make their way to specific areas of the immature brain. After reaching its destination, the axon develops branching (i.e., arborization), and each branch has a bulbous terminal. These bulbs in turn make synapses with dendrites (Kalil, 1989). In the first year of life, one cortical neuron may connect with as many as 10,000 other neurons through axonal/dendritic branching (Crelin, 1973). Arborization continues to increase for several years (Crelin, 1973). It is difficult to determine when arborization reaches its maturational peak because it is influenced by environmental experience (Kalil, 1989). Arborization provides an anatomical basis for more complex interactions among neurons in the brain. Appropriate connections are needed for appropriate function; thus dendritic branching without connection to other cell bodies or axons is of little value. The course of dendritic maturation appears to show the greatest change in the first few years of life, but then extend well into adulthood and even into the elderly.

Recent information about synaptic development suggests an important role of action potentials. When young axons are prevented from generating action potentials, the synaptic structures (i.e., terminal bulbs) do not develop (Kalil, 1989). Therefore, these electrical impulses (most of which come from external stimulation) of the axon are crucial to synaptogenesis.

The synapse is the communication between neurons that involves the transfer of a neurotransmitter. Earlier we discussed this aspect of neurochemistry. Because dendrites are necessary for synapses, their maturity influences the overall amount of synaptic development. Studies on kittens show an increase in synapses at the IC until 14 days of age. Also, the number of synaptic terminals is considerably greater in an 8-day-old kitten than in a 3-day-old kitten (Reynolds, 1975).

Maturation is not the only influence on the synapse that can result in its change. Stimulation can alter the number of synapses and synaptic density after the system is mature. Conversely, a lack of stimulation (deprivation) may reduce the number of synaptic components.

CONCLUSIONS

Knowledge of the structure and function of the CANS is vital to the audiologist. Audiological procedures and related communication increasingly involve the CANS, and without an understanding of the way this system works, potential clinical insights will not be realized. The CANS is a complex system in which parallel and sequential processing takes place. In the brain stem ipsilateral, contralateral, and commissural connections exist to various auditory nuclei. Auditory nerve cells in the brain stem are composed of a variety of different cell types. These cell types respond in certain ways (often according to their structure) to alter or preserve the impulse pattern coming into the cell. This same type of processing takes place in the cells of the auditory cortex, but fewer cell types are present in the cortex than in the brain stem. This type of processing may provide a basis for increased information pertaining to complex acoustical stimuli. The brain stem and the cortex are both highly tonotopic and present with a variety of tuning curves. In regard to intensity coding, most cells in the brain stem and cortex have a range of 30- to 40-dB; however, some have severely reduced dynamic ranges. Of interest is that in a listening situation with background noise some cortical neurons will not respond until the target sound is above the noise floor, with apparently no restriction in their dynamic range. This relatively new information may provide an understanding of how we hear in noise that has not been considered previously.

In the cerebrum the auditory regions have intrahemispheric and interhemispheric connections to other auditory areas and to sensory, cognitive, and motor regions. At the cortical level seldom does a system function totally independently. This makes for an efficient processing of environmental input but also makes it difficult to design tests to isolate only auditory function. Much scientific study has been devoted to the afferent auditory system, and information on the efferent system is increasingly available. We have known for years that the efferent system—especially the OCB—can affect acoustical input . The OCB appears to play a role in allowing better hearing in noise. In a broader sense the OCB (and likely the entire efferent system) may have a modulatory effect on peripheral function. Some influences of the OCB can be measured in humans by using otoacoustical emissions or evoked potentials.

Contributions to the A&P of the CANS have been, and will continue to be, made by careful study of patients with lesions of the auditory system. This kind of study often involves the clinician and clinical tests. The study of patients with structural abnormalities of the auditory system can now be enhanced by the use of PET or fMRI studies. These imaging techniques can provide insight about the locus and degree of function in normal and abnormal states. The use of new functional imaging techniques will help solve two major problems in the study of the CANS. One is that now humans can be studied directly, the other is more complex and relevant stimuli such as speech can be used to study associated physiology.

A new area of study of the CANS is its neurochemistry or neuropharmacology. Surprisingly, the neurotransmitters of the OCB are better known than those of the afferent system. Neurotransmission takes place at the synapse of the nerve cell, and synaptic activity is governed largely by the type and amount of the neurotransmitter. Agonists are chemicals that can enhance the neural response and the synapse, whereas antagonists will shut down the response. Complex synaptic interactions among agonists and antagonists are the basis for complex auditory processing.

New information on the CANS is increasing on all fronts. More data on audition are available from audiologists, pharmacologists, physiologists, anatomists, and psychologists. The basic scientists have provided much knowledge that will enhance the diagnosis and treatment of central auditory disorders. However, this basic knowledge can be used to its greatest potential only if the clinician is well versed in the structure and function of the CANS.

REFERENCES

ABELES, M., & GOLDSTEIN, M. (1972). Responses of a single unit in the primary auditory cortex of the cat to tones and to tone pairs. *Brain Research, 42*;337–352.

ADAMS, J., & WENTHOLD, R. (1987). Immunostaining of GABA-ergic and glycinergic inputs to the anteroventral cochlear nucleus. *Neuroscience Abstracts, 13*;1259.

AITKIN, L.M., & WEBSTER, W.R. (1972). Medial geniculate body of the cat: Organization and response to tonal stimuli of neurons in the ventral division. *Journal of Neurophysiology, 35*;365–380.

AITKEN, L.M., WEBSTER, W.R., VEALE, J.L., & CROSBY, D.C. (1975). Inferior colliculus. I. Comparison of response properties of neurons in central, pericentral, and external nuclei of adult cat. *Journal of Neurophysiology, 38;*1196–1207.

ALLEN, W. (1945). Effect of destroying three localized cerebral cortical areas for sound on correct conditioned differential responses of the dog's foreleg. *American Journal of Physiology, 144;*415–428.

ALTSCHULER, R.A., & FEX, J. (1986). Efferent neurotransmitters. In: D.W. Hoffman, R.A. Altschuler, & R.P. Bobbin (Eds.). *Neurobiology of hearing: The cochlea,* (pp. 383–396). New York: Raven Press.

ALTSCHULER, R.A., WENTHOLD, R., SCHWARTZ, A., HASER, W., CURTHOYS, N., PARAKKAL, M., & FEX, J. (1984). Immunocytochemical localization of glutaminase-like immunoreactivity in the auditory nerve. *Brain Research, 29;*173–178.

AUERBACH, S., ALLARD, T., NAESER, M., ALEXANDER, M., & ALBERT, M. (1982). Pure word deafness. Analysis of a case with bilateral lesions and a defect at the prephonemic level. *Brain, 105;*271–300.

BARAN, J.A., MUSIEK, F.E., & REEVES, A.G. (1986). Central auditory function following anterior sectioning of the corpus callosum. *Ear and Hearing, 7(6);*359–362.

BARNES, W., MAGOON, H., & RANSON, S. (1943). The ascending auditory pathway in the brain stem of the monkey. *Journal of Comparative Neurology, 79;*129–152.

BENERENTO, L., & COLEMAN, P. (1970). Responses of single cells in cat inferior colliculus to binaural click stimuli: Combinations of intensity levels, time differences, and intensity differences. *Brain Research, 17;*387–405.

BENSON, D., & TEAS, D. (1976). Single unit study of binaural interaction in the auditory cortex of the chinchilla. *Brain Research, 103;*313–338.

BERLIN, C., LOWE-BELL, S., JANETTA, P., & KLINE, D. (1972). Central auditory deficits after temporal lobectomy. *Archives of Otolaryngology, 96;*4–10.

BLEDSOE, S., BOBBIN, R., & PUEL, J. (1988). Neurotransmission in the inner ear. In: A. Jahn, & J. Santo-Sacchi (Eds.). *Physiology of the ear* (pp. 385–406). New York: Raven Press.

BOBBIN, R.P., & KONISHI, T. (1971). Acetylcholine mimics crossed olivocochlear bundle stimulation. *Nature, 231;*222–224.

BORG, E. (1973). On the organization of the acoustic middle ear reflex. A physiologic and anatomic study. *Brain Research, 49;*101–123.

BOUDREAU, J.C., & TSUCHITANI, C. (1970). Cat superior olive S-segment cell discharge to tonal stimulation. In: W.D. Neff (Ed.). *Contributions to sensory physiology* (Vol. 4) (pp. 143–213). New York: Academic Press.

BREMER, F., BRIHAYE, J., & ANDRE-BALISAUX, G. (1956). Physiologie et pathologie du corps calleux. *Archives Suisses de Neurologic et de Psychiatrie, 78;*31–32.

BRUGGE, I.F., & GEISLER, C.E. (1978). Auditory mechanisms of the lower brain stem. *American Review of Neuroscience, 1;*363–394.

BUTLER, R., KEIDEL, W., & SPRENG, M. (1969). An investigation of the human cortical evoked potential under conditions of monaural and binaural stimulation. *Acta Otolaryngologica, 68;*317–326.

CAMPAIN, R., & MINCKLER, J. (1976). A note in gross configurations of the human auditory cortex. *Brain Language, 3;*318–323.

CARPENTER, M., & SUTIN, J. (1983). *Human neuroanatomy,* Baltimore: Williams & Wilkins.

CELESIA, G. (1976). Organization of auditory cortical areas in man. *Brain, 99;*403–414.

CHANG, H.T. (1953). Cortical response to activity of callosal neurons. *Journal of Neurophysiology, 16;*117–131.

CHERMAK, G.D., & MUSIEK, F.E. (1997). *Central auditory processing disorders.* San Diego: Singular Publishing Group, Inc.

CHIAPPA, K. (1983). *Evoked potentials in clinical medicine.* New York: Raven Press.

COLAVITA, F. (1972). Auditory cortical lesions and visual patterns discrimination in cats. *Brain Research, 39;*437–447.

COLAVITA, F. (1974). Insular-temporal lesions and vibrotactile temporal pattern discrimination in cats. *Psychological Behavior, 12;*215–218.

COLCLASURE, J., & GRAHAM, S. (1981). Intracranial aneurysm occurring as a sensorineural hearing loss. *Otolaryngology–and Head and Neck Surgery, 89;*283–287.

COLLET, L. (1993). Use of otoacoustic emissions to explore the medial olivocochlear system in humans. *British Journal of Audiology, 27;*155–159.

COUSILLAS, H., COLE, K.S., & JOHNSTONE, B.M. (1988). Effect of spider venom on cochlear nerve activity consistent with glutamatergic transmission at hair cell-afferent dendrite synapse. *Hearing Research, 36;*213–220.

CRANFORD, J. (1979). Detection vs. discrimination of brief tones by cats with auditory cortex lesions. *Journal of the Acoustical Society of America, 65;*1573–1575.

CRANFORD, J., IGARASHI, M., & STRAMLER, J. (1976). Effect of auditory neocortical ablation on pitch perception in the cat. *Journal of Neurophysiology, 39;*143–152.

CRANFORD, J., STREAM, R., RYE, C., & SLADE, T. (1982). Detection vs. discrimination of brief duration tones: Findings in patients with temporal lobe damage. *Archives of Otolaryngology, 108;*350–356.

CRELIN, E. (1973). *Functional anatomy in the newborn* (pp. 22–24). New Haven: Yale University Press.

CULLEN, J., & THOMPSON, C. (1974). Masking release for speech in subjects with temporal lobe resections. *Archives of Otolaryngology, 100;*113–116.

DAMASIO, H., & DAMASIO, A. (1979). Paradoxic ear extension in dichotic listening: Possible anatomic significance. *Neurology, 25(4);*644–653.

DESMEDT, J. (1975). Physiological studies of the efferent recurrent auditory system. In: W. Keidel, & W. Neff (Eds.). *Handbook of sensory physiology* (Vol. 2). (pp. 219–246). Berlin: Springer-Verlag.

DEWSON, J. (1968). Efferent olivocochlear bundle: Some relationships to stimulus discrimination in noise. *Journal of Neurophysiology, 31;*122–130.

DHANKHAR, A., WEXLER, B.E., FULBRIGHT, R.K., HALWES, T., BLAMIRE, A.M., & SHULMAN, R.G. (1997). Functional magnetic resonance imaging assessment of the human brain auditory cortex response to increasing word presentation rates. *Journal of Neurophysiology, 77(1);*476–483.

DIAMOND, I., & NEFF, W. (1957). Ablation of temporal cortex and discrimination of auditory patterns. *Journal of Neurophysiology, 20;*300–315.

DONCHIN, E., KUTAS, M., & MCCARTHY, G. (1976). Electrocortical indices of hemispheric utilization. In: S. Harnad, et al. (Eds.). *Lateralization in the nervous system.* New York: Academic Press.

DUBLIN, W. (1976). *Fundamentals of sensorineural auditory pathology.* Springfield: Charles C. Thomas.

DUBLIN, W. (1985). The cochlear nuclei-pathology. *Otolaryngology–Head and Neck Surgery, 93;*448–463.

DURRANT, J., MARTIN, W., HIRSCH, B., & SCHWEGLER, J. (1994). ABR analysis in a human subject with unilateral extirpation of the inferior colliculus. *Hearing Research, 72;*99–107.

EGGERMONT, J. (1991). Rate and synchronization measures of periodicity coding in cat primary cortex area. *Hearing Research, 56;*153–167.

EHRET, G., & MERZENICH, M.M. (1988). Complex sound analysis (frequency resolution, filtering and spectral integration) by single units of the inferior colliculus of the cat. *Brain Research Reviews, 13;*139–163.

EHRET, G., & ROMAND, R. (1997). *The central auditory system.* New York: Oxford University Press.

EISENMANN, L. (1974). Neurocoding of sound localization: An electrophysiological study in auditory cortex of the cat using free field stimuli. *Brain Research, 75;*203–214.

ELLIOTT, L.L. (1994). Functional brain imaging and hearing. *Journal of the Acoustical Society of America, 96*(3);1397–1408.

EVANS, E. (1968). Cortical representation. In: J. Knight, & A. de Reuck (Eds.). *Hearing mechanisms in vertebrates* (pp. 277–287). London: Churchill Livingstone.

FAINGOLD, C.L., HOFFMANN, W.E., & CASPARY, D.M. (1989). Effects of excitant amino acids on acoustic responses of inferior colliculus neurons. *Hearing Research, 40;*127–136.

FERRARO, J., & MINCKLER, J. (1977). The human lateral lemniscus and its nuclei. The human auditory pathways. A quantitative study. *Brain Language, 4;*277–294.

FEX, J. (1962). Auditory activity in centrifugal and centripetal cochlear fibers in cat. *Acta Physiologica Scandinavia 189*(55);5–68.

FOLSOM, R.L., OWSLEY, R.M. (1987). N_1 action potentials in humans. Influence of simultaneous contralateral stimulation. *Acta Otolaryngologica, 103;*262–265.

FRENCH, J. (1957). The reticular formation. *Scientific American, 66;*1–8.

GALABURDA, A., & SANIDES, F. (1980). Cytoarchitectonic organization of the human auditory cortex. *Journal of Comparative Neurology, 190;*597–610.

GALABURDA, A., SHERMAN, G., ROSEN, G., ABOITIZ, F., & GESCHWIND, N. (1985). Developmental dyslexia: Four consecutive patients with cortical anomalies. *Annals of Neurology, 18;*222–235.

GALAMBOS, R. (1956). Suppression of auditory nerve activity by stimulation of efferent fibers to cochlea. *Journal of Neurophysiology, 19;*424–437.

GAZZANIGA, M., & SPERRY, R. (1962). Some functional effects of sectioning the cerebral commissure in man. *Proceedings of the National Academy of Science, USA, 48;*1765–1769.

GERSHUNI, J. BARU, & KARASEVA, T. (1967). Role of auditory cortex and discrimination of acoustic stimuli. *Neurologic Science Transactions, 1;*370–372.

GESCHWIND, N., & LEVITSKY, W. (1968). Human brain: Left-right asymmetries in temporal speech region. *Science, 161;*186–187.

GODFREY, D., CARTER, J., BERGER, S., LOWRY, D., & MATSCHINSKY, F. (1977). Quantitative histochemical mapping of candidate transmitter amino acids in the cat cochlear nucleus. *Journal of Histochemistry and Cytochemistry, 25;*417–431.

GODFREY, D., PARK, J., DUNN, J., & ROSS, C. (1985). Cholinergic neurotransmission in the cochlear nucleus. In: D. Drecher (Ed.). *Auditory neurochemistry* (pp. 163–183). Springfield, IL: Charles C. Thomas.

GOLDBERG, J.M., & MOORE, R.Y. (1967). Ascending projections of the lateral lemniscus in the cat and the monkey. *Journal of Comparative Neurology, 129;*143–155.

GOLDSTEIN, M., DERIBAUPIERRE, R., & YENI-KOMSHIAN, G. (1971). Cortical coding of periodicity pitch. In: M. Sachs (Ed.). *Physiology of the auditory system.* Baltimore: National Education Consultants Inc.

GORDON, B. (1972). The inferior colliculus of the brain. *Scientific American, 227;*72–82.

GUTH, P., & MELAMED, B. (1982). Neurotransmission in the auditory system: A primer for pharmacologists. *Annual Review of Pharmacology and Toxicology, 22;*383–412.

HALL, J.W. III. (1985). The acoustic reflex in central auditory dysfunction. In: M.L. Pinheiro, & F.E. Musiek (Eds.). *Assessment of central auditory dysfunction: Foundations and clinical correlates* (pp. 103–130). Baltimore: Williams & Wilkins.

HASSMANNOVA, J., MYSLIVECEK, J., & NOVAKOVA, V. (1981). Effects of early auditory stimulation on cortical centers. In: J. Syka, & L. Aitkin (Eds.). *Neuronal mechanisms of hearing* (pp. 355–359). New York: Plenum Press.

HEFFNER, H., & HEFFNER, R. (1986). Hearing loss in Japanese Macaques following bilateral auditory cortex lesions. *Journal of Neurophysiology, 55;*256–71.

HEFFNER, H., HEFFNER, R., & PORTER, W. (1985). Effects of auditory cortex lesion on absolute thresholds in Macaques. *Proceedings of the Society for Neuroscience,* Annual Meeting, Dallas, TX.

HELFERT, R., ALTSCHULER, R., & WENTHOLD, R. (1987). GABA and glycine immunoreactivity in the guinea pig superior olivary complex. *Neuroscience Abstracts, 13;*544.

HODGSON, W. (1967). Audiological report of a patient with left hemispherectomy. *Journal of Speech and Hear Disorders, 32;*39–45.

HOFFMAN, D.W. (1986). Opioid mechanisms in the inner ear. In: R.A. Altschuler, D.W. Hoffman, & R.P. Bobbin (Eds.). *Neurobiology of hearing: The cochlea* (pp. 371–382). New York: Raven Press.

HYND, G.W., SEMRUD-CLIKEMAN, M., LORYS, A.R., NOVEY, E.S., ELIOPULOS, D., & LYYTINEN, H. (1991). Corpus callosum morphology in attention deficit-hyperactivity disorder: Morphometric analysis of MRI. *Journal of Learning Disabilities, 24;*141–146.

JEFFRESS, L., & McFADDEN, D. (1971). Differences of interaural phase and level of detection and lateralization. *Journal of the Acoustical Society of America, 49;*1169–1179.

JENSEN, J., & NEFF, D. (1989). *Discrimination of intensity, frequency and duration differences in preschool children: Age effects and longitudinal data.* Presented at the SRCH Biennial Meeting, Kansas City, MO.

JERGER, J., & JERGER, S. (1971). Diagnostic significance of PB word functions. *Archives of Otolaryngology, 93;*573–580.

JERGER, J., & JERGER, S. (1974). Auditory findings in brain stem disorders. *Archives of Otolaryngology, 99;*342–350.

JERGER, J., WEIKERS, N., SHARBROUGH, F., & JERGER, S. (1969). Bilateral lesions of the temporal lobe. A case study. *Acta Otolaryngologica, 258;*1–51.

JONES, E., & POWELL, T. (1970). An anatomical study of converging sensory pathways within the cerebral cortex of the monkey. *Brain, 93;*793–820.

JUNGERT, S. (1958). Auditory pathways in the brain stem. A neurophysiologic study. *Acta Otolaryngologica,* (Supplement), 138.

KALIL, R. (1989). Synapse formation in the developing brain. *Scientific American, 261;*76–87.

KAUFMAN, W., & GALABURDA, A. (1989). Cerebrocortical microdysgenesias in neurologically normal subjects: A histopathological study. *Neurology, 39;*238–243.

KAVANAGH, G., & KELLY, J. (1988). Hearing in the ferret (*Mustela putorius*): Effects of primary auditory cortical lesions on thresholds for pure tone detection. *Journal of Neurophysiology, 60;*879–888.

KAWASE, T., & LIBERMAN, M.C. (1993). Antimasking effects of the olivocochlear reflex. I. Enhancement of compound action potentials to masked tones. *Journal of Neurophysiology, 70(6);*2519–2532.

KEIDEL, W., KALLERT, S., KORTH, M., & HUMES, L. (1983). *The physiological basis of hearing.* New York: Thieme-Stratton.

KIANG, N.Y.S. (1975). Stimulus representation in the discharge patterns of auditory neurons. In: D.B. Tower (Ed.). *The nervous system* (Vol. 3). Human communication and its disorders (pp. 81–96). New York: Raven Press.

KNUDSEN, E. (1988). Experience shapes sound localization and auditory unit properties during development in the barn owl. In: G. Edelman, W. Gall, & W. Kowan (Eds.). *Auditory function: Neurobiological basis of hearing* (pp. 137–152). New York: John Wiley & Sons.

KNUDSON, E.I., & KONISHI, M. (1978). Space and frequency are represented separately in auditory midbrain of the owl. *Neurophysiology, 41;*870–884.

KRAUS, N., & MCGEE, T. (1994). Auditory event-related potentials. In: J. Katz (Ed.). *Handbook of clinical audiology* (4th ed.) (pp. 406–423). Baltimore: Williams & Wilkins.

KRYTER, K., & ADES, H. (1943). Studies on the function of the higher acoustic centers in the cat. *American Journal of Psychology, 56;*501–536.

KUDO, M. (1981). Projections of the nuclei of the lateral lemniscus in the cat. An autoradiographic study. *Brain Research, 221;*57–69.

LACKNER, J.R., & TEUBER, H.L. (1973). Alterations in auditory fusion thresholds after cerebral injury in man. *Neuropsychologia, 11;*409–415.

LAUTER, J., HERSCOVITCH, P., FORMBY, C., & RAICHLE, M. (1985). Tonotopic organization of human auditory cortex revealed by positron emission tomography. *Hearing Research, 20;*199–205.

LEDOUX, J., SAKAGUCHI, A., & REIS, D. (1983). Subcortical efferent projections of the medial geniculate nucleus mediate emotional responses conditioned to acoustic stimuli. *Journal of Neuroscience, 4;*683–698.

LEVINE, R.A., GARDNER, J.C., STUFFLEBEAM, S.M., FULLERTON, B.C., CARLISLE, E.W., FURST, M., ROSEN, B.R., & KIANG, N.Y.S. (1993). Binaural auditory processing in multiple sclerosis subjects. *Hearing Research, 68;*59–72.

LIDEN, G., & ROSENTHAL, V. (1981). New developments in diagnostic auditory neurological problems. In: M. Paparella, & W. Meyerhoff (Eds.). *Sensorineural hearing loss, vertigo and tinnitus.* Baltimore: Williams & Wilkins.

LYNN, G., GILROY, J., TAYLOR, P., & LEISER, R. (1981). Binaural masking level differences in neurological disorders. *Archives of Otolaryngology, 107;*357–362.

MASTERSON, B., THOMPSON, G.C., BECHTOLD, J.K., & ROBARDS, M.J. (1975). Neuroanatomical basis of binaural phase difference analysis for sound localization: A comparative study. *Journal of Comparative Physiology and Psychology, 89;*379–386.

MASTERTON, R.B., & GRANGER, E.M. (1988). Role of acoustic striae in hearing contribution of dorsal and intermediate striae to detection of noises and tones. *Journal of Neurophysiology, 60;*1841–1860.

MATKIN, N., & CARHART, R. (1966). Auditory profiles associated with Rh incompatibility. *Archives of Otolaryngology, 84;*502–513.

MATZKER, J. (1959). Two new methods for the assessment of central auditory functions in cases of brain disease. *American Journal of Otolaryngology, Rhinology & Laryngology, 68;*1188–1197.

MCGEE, T., & KRAUS, N. (1996). Auditory development reflected by the middle latency response. *Ear and Hearing, 17(5);*419–429.

MCKENNA, T., ASHE, J., HUI, G., & WEINBERGER, N. (1988). Muscarinic agonists modulate spontaneous and evoked unit discharge in auditory cortex of the cat. *Synapse, 2;*54–68.

MCPHERSON, D.L. (1996). *Late potentials of the auditory system.* San Diego: Singular Publishing Group, Inc.

MERCHAN, M., SALDANA, E. & PLAZA, I. (1994). Dorsal nucleus of the lateral lemniscus in the rat. Concentric organization and tonotopic projection to the inferior colliculus. *Journal of Comparative Neurology, 342;*259–278.

MERZENICH, M., & BRUGGE, J. (1973). Representation of the cochlear partition on the superior temporal plane of the Macaque monkey. *Brain Research, 50;*275–296.

MERZENICH, M.M., & REID, M.D. (1974). Representation of the cochlea within the inferior colliculus of the cat. *Brain Research, 77;*397–415.

MEYER, D., & WOOLSEY, C. (1952). Effects of localized cortical destruction on auditory discriminative conditioning in the cat. *Journal of Neurophysiology, 15;*149–162.

MILLEN, S.J., HAUGHTON, V.M., & YETKIN, Z. (1995). Functional magnetic resonance imaging of the central auditory pathway following speech and pure tone stimuli. *Laryngoscope, 105;*1305–1310.

MOLLER, A.R. (1983). *Auditory physiology.* New York: Academic Press.

MOLLER, A.R. (1985). Physiology of the ascending auditory pathway with special reference to the auditory brain stem response (ABR). In: M.L. Pinheiro, & F.E. Musiek (Eds.). *Assessment of central auditory dysfunction: Foundations and clinical correlates* (pp. 23–41). Baltimore: Williams & Wilkins.

MOLLER, M., & MOLLER, A.R. (1985). Auditory brain stem evoked responses (ABR) in diagnosis of eighth nerve and brain stem lesions. In: M.L. Pinheiro, & F.E. Musiek (Eds.). *Assessment of central auditory dysfunction: Foundations and clinical correlates* (pp. 43–65). Baltimore: Williams & Wilkins.

MOORE, C., CRANFORD, J., & RAHN, A. (1990). Tracking for a "moving" fused auditory image under conditions that elicit the precedence effect. *Journal of Speech and Hearing Research, 33;*141–148.

MOORE, D.R. (1983). Development of the interior colliculus and binaural audition. In: R. Romand (Ed.). *Development of auditory and vestibular system* (pp. 121–159). New York: Academic Press.

MOORE, D.R., & IRVINE, D.R.F. (1980). Development of binaural input, response patterns and discharge rate in single units of the cat inferior colliculus. *Experimental Brain Research, 38*;103–108.

MOORE, J.K. (1987). The human auditory brain stem: A comparative view. *Hearing Research, 29*;1–32.

MOREST, D.K. (1964). The neuronal architecture of medial geniculate body of the cat. *Journal of Anatomy, 98*;611–630.

MOUNTCASTLE V. (1962). *Interhemispheric relations and cerebral dominance.* Baltimore: Johns Hopkins Press.

MOUNTCASTLE, V. (1968). Central neural mechanisms in hearing. In: V. Mountcastle (Ed.). *Medical physiology* (Vol. 2). St. Louis: C.V. Mosby Co.

MUSIEK, F.E. (1985). Application of central auditory tests: An overview. In: J. Katz (Ed.). *Handbook of clinical audiology* (pp. 321–336). Baltimore: Williams & Wilkins.

MUSIEK, F.E. (1986a). Neuroanatomy, neurophysiology and central auditory assessment. Part II: The cerebrum. *Ear and Hearing, 7*;283–294.

MUSIEK, F.E. (1986b). Neuroanatomy, neurophysiology, and central auditory assessment: Part III: Corpus callosum and efferent pathways. *Ear and Hearing, 7*(6);349–358.

MUSIEK, F.E., & BARAN, J.A. (1986). Neuroanatomy, neurophysiology, and central auditory assessment. Part 1: Brain stem. *Ear and Hearing, 7*;207–219.

MUSIEK, F.E., BARAN, J.A., & PINHEIRO, M. (1990). Duration pattern recognition in normal subjects and patients with cerebral and cochlear lesions. *Audiology, 29*;304–313.

MUSIEK, F.E., BARAN, J.A., & PINHEIRO, M. (1994). *Neuroaudiology: Case studies.* San Diego: Singular Publishing Group, Inc.

MUSIEK, F.E., & BERGE, B. (1998). Neuroaudiological aspects of auditory training/stimulation and CAPD. In: J. Katz (Ed.). *Central auditory processing disorders: Mostly management.* Boston: Allyn and Bacon.

MUSIEK, F.E., & GEURKINK, N. (1982). Auditory brain stem response and central auditory test findings for patients with brain stem lesions. *Laryngoscope, 92*;891–900.

MUSIEK, F.E., & GOLLEGLY, K.M. (1985). ABR in eighth nerve and low brain stem lesions. In: J.T. Jacobson (Ed.). *The auditory brain stem response* (pp. 181–202). San Diego: College-Hill Press.

MUSIEK, F.E., & GOLLEGLY, K.M. (1988). Maturational considerations in the neuroauditory evaluation of children. In: F. Bess (Ed.). *Hearing impairment in children* (pp. 231–250). Parkton, MD: York Press.

MUSIEK, F.E., & HOFFMAN, D. (1990). An introduction to the functional neurochemistry of the auditory system. *Ear and Hearing 11*;395–402.

MUSIEK, F.E., KIBBE, K., & BARAN, J. (1984). Neuroaudiological results from split-brain patients. *Seminars in Hearing 5*(3);219–229.

MUSIEK, F.E., & KIBBE-MICHAEL, K. (1986). The ABR wave IV-V abnormalities from the ear opposite large CPA tumors. *American Journal of Otology, 7*;253–257.

MUSIEK, F.E., KIBBE-MICHAEL, K., GEURKINK, N., JOSEY, A., & GLASSCOCK, M. (1986). ABR results in patients with posterior fossa tumors and normal pure tone hearing. *Otolaryngology–Head and Neck Surgery, 94*;568–573.

MUSIEK, F.E., & PINHEIRO, M. (1987). Frequency patterns in cochlear, brain stem, and cerebral lesions. *Audiology, 26*;79–88.

MUSIEK, F.E., & REEVES, A.G. (1990). Asymmetries of the auditory areas of the cerebrum. *Journal of the American Academy of Audiology, 1*;240–245.

NEFF, W. (1961). Neuromechanisms of auditory discrimination. In: W. Rosenblith (Ed.). *Sensory Communication.* New York: John Wiley & Sons.

NIEDER, P., & NIEDER, I. (1970). Antimasking effect of crossed olivocochlear bundle stimulation with loud clicks in guinea pigs. *Experimental Neurology, 28*;179–188.

NOBACK, C.R. (1985). Neuroanatomical correlates of central auditory function. In: M.L. Pinheiro, & F.E. Musiek (Eds.). *Assessment of central auditory dysfunction: Foundations and clinical correlates* (pp. 7–21). Baltimore: Williams & Wilkins.

NODAR, R., & KINNEY, S. (1980). The contralateral effects of large tumors on brain stem auditory-evoked potentials. *Laryngoscope, 90*;1762–1768.

NOZZA, R., WAGNER, E., & CRANDALL, M. (1988). Binaural release for masking for speech sounds in infants, preschoolers and adults. *Journal of Speech and Hearing Research, 31*;212–218.

OH, S., KUBA, T., SOYER, A., CHOI, I., BONIKOWSKI, F., & VITER, J. (1981). Lateralization of brain stem lesions by brain stem auditory evoked potentials. *Neurology, 31*;14–18.

OLIVER, D.L., & MOREST, D.K. (1984). The central nucleus of the inferior colliculus in the cat. *Journal of Comparative Neurology, 222*;237–264.

OLIVER, D.L., POTASHNER, S., JONES, D., & MOREST, D. (1983). Selective labeling of spiroganglion and granule cells with D-aspartate in the auditory system of the cat and guinea pig. *Journal of Neuroscience, 3*;455–472.

OLIVER, D.L., & SHNEIDERMAN, A. (1991). The anatomy of the inferior colliculus: A cellular basis for integration of monaural and binaural information. In: R.A. Altschuler, R.P. Bobbin, B.M. Clopton, D.W. Hoffman (Eds.). *Neurobiology of hearing: The central auditory system* (pp. 195–222). New York: Raven Press.

OSEN, K.K. (1969). Cytoarchitecture of the cochlear nuclei in the cat. *Journal of Comparative Neurology, 136*;453–484.

OTTERSON, O., & STORM-MATHISON, J. (1984). Glutamate- and GABA-containing neurons in the mouse and rat brain, as demonstrated with a new immunocytochemical technique. *Journal of Comparative Neurology, 229*;374-392.

PANDYA, D., & SELTZER, B. (1986). The topography of commissural fibers. In: F. Lepore, M. Pitito, & H. Jasper (Eds.). *Two hemispheres—One brain: Functions of the corpus callosum.* New York: Alan R. Liss, Inc.

PENFIELD, W., & PEROT, P. (1963). The brain's record of auditory and visual experience: A final summary and discussion. *Brain, 86*;596–695.

PENFIELD, W., & RASMUSSEN, T. (1950). *The cerebral cortex of man.* New York: Macmillan and Company.

PENFIELD, W., & ROBERTS, L. (1959). *Speech and brain mechanisms.* Princeton, NJ: Princeton University Press.

PFEIFFER, R.R. (1966). Classification of response patterns of spike discharges for units in the cochlear nucleus. Tone burst stimulation. *Experimental Brain Research, 1*;220–235.

PFINGST, B., & O'CONNER, T. (1981). Characteristics of neurons in auditory cortex of monkeys performing a simple auditory task. *Journal of Neurophysiology, 45*;16–34.

PHILLIPS, D. (1990). Neural representation of sound amplitude in the auditory cortex: Effects of noise masking. *Behavioral brain Research, 37*;197–214.

PHILLIPS, D. (1995). Central auditory processing: A view from auditory neuroscience. *American Journal of Otology, 16*;338–350.

PHILLIPS, D., & IRVINE, D. (1981). Responses of single neurons in physiologically defined area AI of cat cerebral cortex: Sensitivity to interaural intensity differences. *Hearing Research, 4*(9);299–307.

PICKLES, J.O. (1982). *An introduction to the physiology of hearing.* New York: Academic Press.

PICKLES, J.O. (1985). Physiology of the cerebral auditory system. In: M. Pinheiro, & F. Musiek (Eds.). *Assessment of central auditory dysfunction: Foundations and clinical correlates.* Baltimore: Williams & Wilkins.

PICKLES, J.O. (1988). *An introduction to the physiology of hearing* (2nd ed.). New York: Academic Press.

PICKLES, J.O., & COMIS, S.D. (1973). Role of centrifugal pathways to cochlear nucleus in detection of signals in noise. *Journal of Neurophysiology, 29*;1131–1137.

PINHEIRO, M., & MUSIEK, F.E. (1985). Sequencing and temporal ordering in the auditory system. In: M. Pinheiro, & F. Musiek (Eds.). *Assessment of central auditory dysfunction: Foundations and clinical correlates* (pp. 219–238). Baltimore: Williams and Wilkins.

PINHEIRO, M., & TOBIN, H. (1969). Interaural intensity differences for intracranial lateralization. *Journal of the Acoustical Society of America, 401*;1482–1487.

PONTON, C.W., DON, M., EGGERMONT, J.J., WARING, M.D., & MASUDA, A. (1996). Maturation of human cortical auditory function: Differences between normal-hearing children and children with cochlear implants. *Ear and Hearing, 17*(5);430–437.

PORTMAN, M., STERKERS, J., CHARACHON, R., & CHOUARD, C. (1975). *The internal auditory meatus: Anatomy, pathology, and surgery.* New York: Churchill Livingstone.

RAVIZZA, R., & MASTERTON, R. (1972). Contribution of neocortex to sound localization in opossum (*Didelphis virginiana*). *Journal of Neurophysiology, 35*;344–356.

RECANZONE, G., SCHREINER, C., & MERZENICH, M. (1993). Plasticity in the frequency representation of primary auditory cortex following discrimination training in adult owl monkeys. *The Journal of Neuroscience, 13*;87–103

REYNOLDS, A. (1975). *Development of binaural responses of units in the intracolliculus of the neonate cat.* Unpublished undergraduate paper, Department of Physiology, Monash University, Clayton Victoria, Australia.

RHODE, W. (1985). The use of intracellular techniques in the study of the cochlear nucleus. *Journal of the Acoustical Society of Americans, 78*;320–327.

RHODE, W. (1991). Physiological-morphological properties of the cochlear nucleus. In: R. Altschuler, R. Bobbin, B. Clopton, & D. Hoffman (Eds.). *Neurobiology of hearing: The central auditory system* (pp. 47–78). New York: Raven Press.

ROSE, J.E., GALAMBOS, R., & HUGHES, J.R. (1959). Microelectrode studies of the cochlear nuclei of the cat. *Johns Hopkins Hospital Bulletin, 104*;211–251.

ROUILLER, E.M. (1997). Functional organization of the auditory pathways. In: G. Ehret, & R. Romand (Eds.). *The central auditory system* (pp. 3–96). New York: Oxford University Press.

RUBENS, A. (1986). Anatomical asymmetries of the human cerebral cortex. In: S. Harnad et al. (Eds.). *Lateralization in the nervous system.* New York: Academic Press.

RYUGO, D., & WEINBERGER, N. (1976). Corticofugal modulation of the medial geniculate body. *Experimental Neurology, 51*;377–391.

SAHLEY, T.L., KALISH, R., MUSIEK, F.E., & HOFFMAN, D. (1991). Effects of opiate drugs on auditory-evoked potentials in the chinchilla. *Hearing Research, 55*;133–142.

SAHLEY, T.L., NODAR, R.H., & MUSIEK, F.E. (1997). *Efferent auditory system: Structure and function.* San Diego: Singular Publishing Group, Inc.

SALAMY, A. (1978). Commissural transmission: Maturational changes in humans. *Science, 200*;1409–1410.

SALAMY, A., MENDELSON, T., TOOLEY, W., & CHAPLIN, E. (1980). Differential development of brain stem potentials in healthy and high risk infants. *Science, 210*;553–555.

SANCHEZ-LONGO, L., & FORSTER, F. (1958). Clinical significance of impairment of sound localization. *Neurology, 8*;118–125.

SANDO, I. (1965). The anatomical interrelationships of the cochlear nerve fibers. *Acta Otolaryngologica, 59*;417–436.

SCHUKNECHT, H.T. (1974). *Pathology of the ear.* Cambridge: Harvard University Press.

SCHWABER, M., GARRAGHTY, P., MOREL, A., & KAAS, J. (1994). Neuroplasticity of the adult primate auditory cortex following cochlear hearing loss. *American Journal of Otolaryngology, 14*(3);252–258.

SELNES, O.A. (1974). The corpus callosum: Some anatomical and functional considerations with special reference to language. *Brain & Language, 1*;111–139.

SELTZER, B., & PANDYA, D. (1978). Afferent cortical connections and architectonics of the superior temporal sulcus and surrounding cortex in Rhesus monkey. *Brain Research, 149*;1–24.

SHAH, S., & SALAMY, A. (1980). Brain stem auditory potential in myelin deficient mice. *Neuroscience, 5*;2321–2323.

SHEPERD, G. (1994). *Neurobiology.* (pp. 284-555). New York: Oxford Press.

STREITFELD, B. (1980). The fiber connections of the temporal lobe with emphasis on the Rhesus monkey. *International Journal of Neuroscience, 11*;51–71.

STROMINGER, N.L., & HURWITZ, J.L. (1976). Anatomical aspects of the superior olivary complex. *Journal of Comparative Neurology, 170*;485–97.

STROMINGER, N.L., & STROMINGER, A.L. (1971). Ascending brain stem projections of the anteroventral cochlear nucleus in the rhesus monkey. *Journal of Comparative Neurology, 143*;217–232.

SUDAKOV, K., MACLEAN, P., REEVES, A., & MARINO, R. (1971). Unit study of exteroceptive inputs to the claustrocortex in the awake sitting squirrel monkey. *Brain Research, 28*;19–34.

TALAVAGE, T.M., LEDDEN, P.J., SERENO, M.I., BENSON, R.R., & ROSEN, B.R. (1996). *Preliminary fMRI evidence for tonotopicity in human auditory cortex.* Paper presented at the 2nd International Conference on Functional Mapping of The Human Brain, Boston, MA.

TASAKI, I. (1954). Nerve impulses in individual auditory nerve fibers of the guinea pig. *Journal of Neurophysiology, 17*;97–122.

THOMPSON, M.E., & ABEL, S.M. (1992). Indices of hearing in patients with central auditory pathology. *Scandinavian Audiology, 21*(35);3–22.

TOBIN, H. (1985). Binaural interaction tasks. In: M. Pinheiro, & F. Musiek (Eds.). *Assessment of central auditory dysfunction: Foundations and clinical correlates* (pp. 151–171). Baltimore: Williams & Wilkins.

TSUCHITANI, C., & BOUDREAU, J.C. (1966). Single unit analysis of cat superior olive S-segment with tonal stimuli. *Journal of Neurophysiology, 29;*684–697.

TSUCHITANI, C., & JOHNSON, D.H. (1991). Binaural cues and signal processing in the superior olivary complex. In: R.A. Altschuler, R.P. Bobbin, B.M. Clopton, & D.W. Hoffman (Eds.). *Neurobiology of hearing: The central auditory system* (pp. 163–193). New York: Raven Press.

VAN NOORT, J. (1969). *The structure and connections of the inferior colliculus: An investigation of the lower auditory system.* Leiden: Van Corcum.

VELASCO, M., VELASCO, F., CASTANEDA, R., & SANCHEZ, R. (1984). Effect of fentanyl and naloxone on human somatic and auditory-evoked potential components. *Neuropharmacology, 23*(3);359–366.

WADA, S., & STARR, A. (1983). Generation of auditory brain stem responses III. Effects of lesions of the superior olive, lateral lemniscus and inferior colliculus on the ABR in guinea pig. *Electroencephalography and Clinical Neurophysiology, 56;*352–366.

WADDINGTON, M. (1974). *Atlas of cerebral angiography with anatomic correlation.* Boston: Little, Brown & Co.

WADDINGTON, M. (1984). *Atlas of human intracranial anatomy.* Rutland, Vt: Academy Books.

WARR, W.B. (1966). Fiber degeneration following lesions in the anterior ventral cochlear nucleus of the cat. *Experimental Neurology, 14;*453–474.

WARR, W.B. (1980). Efferent components of the auditory system. *Annals of Otology, Rhinology and Laryngology, 89*(Suppl. 74); 114–120.

WEBSTER, D.B. (1971). Projection of the cochlea to cochlear nuclei in Merriam's kangaroo rat. *Journal of Comparative Neurology, 143;*323–340.

WENTHOLD, R., HUIE, D., ALTSCHULER, R., & REEKS, K. (1987). Glycine immunoreactivity localized in the cochlear nucleus and superior olivary complex. *Neuroscience, 22;*897–912.

WERNER, L.A. (1996). The development of auditory behavior (or what the anatomists and physiologists have to explain). *Ear and Hearing, 17*(5);438–446.

WHITFIELD, I.C. (1967). *The auditory pathway.* Baltimore: Williams & Wilkins.

WILLIAMS, E.A., BROOKES, G.B., & PRASHER, D.K. (1993). Effects of contralateral acoustic stimulation on otoacoustic emissions following vestibular neurectomy. *Scandinavian Audiology, 22;*197–203.

WINER, J.A. (1984). The human medial geniculate body. *Hearing Research, 15;*225–247.

WINER, J.A. (1985). The medial geniculate body of the cat. *Advances in Anatomy, Embryology and Cell Biology, 86;*1–98.

WINSLOW, R., & SACHS, M. (1987). Effect of electrical stimulation of the crossed olivocochlear bundle on auditory nerve responses to tones in noise. *Journal of Neurophysiology, 57;*1002–1021.

WITELSON, S. (1986). Wires of the mind: Anatomical variation in the corpus callosum in relation to hemispheric specialization and integration. In: F. Lepore, M. Ptito, & H. Jasper (Eds.). *Two hemispheres—One brain: Functions of the corpus callosum.* New York: Alan R. Liss, Inc.

WOOLSEY, C. (1960). Organization of cortical auditory system: A review and synthesis. In: G. Rasmussen, & W. Windell (Eds.). *Neuromechanics of the auditory and visibility systems.* Springfield, IL: Charles C. Thomas.

YAKOVLEV, P., & LECOURS, A. (1967). Myelogenetic cycles of regional maturation of the brain. In: A. Minkowski (Ed.). *Regional development of the brain in early life.* Philadelphia: FA Davis.

YAQUB, B., GASCON, G., AL-NOSHA, M., & WHITAKER, H. (1988). Pure word deafness (acquired verbal auditory agnosia) in an Arabic-speaking patient. *Brain, 111;*457–466.

ZATORRE, R.J., HALPERN, A.R., PERRY, D.W., MEYER, E., & EVANS, A.C. (1996). Hearing in the mind's ear: A PET investigation of musical imagery and perception. *Journal of Cognitive Neuroscience, 8*(1);29–46.

## Chapter 4

Anatomy and Physiology of the Vestibular System

Charles G. Wright and Nathan D. Schwade

Outline

The vestibular sensory organs of the inner ear respond to physical stimuli related to movement and orientation of the head in three-dimensional space. In response to mechanical forces acting on the inner ear, neural messages regarding head motion and position are generated by the vestibular apparatus and relayed to the brain. That information, along with visual and proprioceptive input, is used by the central nervous system (CNS) to maintain clear vision during head movement, to control muscles responsible for upright posture, and to provide a sense of orientation of the body with respect to the surrounding environment.

Although the vestibular system is one of our major sensory modalities, it differs somewhat from other senses such as vision and hearing in that it operates largely in the service of motor reflexes, outside the field of conscious perception. Thus we are not ordinarily aware of vestibular sensory input unless the system is subjected to unusually high levels of stimulation or is compromised by disease, in which case the importance of vestibular function becomes acutely obvious. This chapter will present some fundamental aspects of vestibular anatomy and physiology, with emphasis on features of the system that provide the foundation for clinical testing of vestibular function.

STRUCTURAL AND FUNCTIONAL ORGANIZATION OF THE VESTIBULAR APPARATUS

As illustrated in Figure 4–1, the petrous portion of the temporal bone contains a series of interconnected cavities known as the osseous (or bony) labyrinth. The central cavity of the osseous labyrinth, the vestibule, is situated medial to the oval window. Anterior to the vestibule is the cochlea and posterior to it are the semicircular canals. The various sacs and ducts that make up the membranous labyrinth are enclosed within the osseous labyrinth, and they are surrounded by a clear fluid, called perilymph, which is quite similar in composition to cerebrospinal fluid. The membranous labyrinth itself is filled with endolymph, which contains high potassium and low sodium concentrations, much like intracellular fluid (Correia & Dickman, 1991). It is within the membranous labyrinth that the sensory receptors of the auditory and vestibular systems are found. Figure 4–2 depicts the membranous labyrinth isolated from the surrounding bone and provides some perspective regarding its actual size. As this illustration shows, the entire structure, including the cochlear duct and the vestibular apparatus, would easily fit within the circumference of a dime.

The position of the membranous labyrinth within the head is illustrated in Figure 4–3. The vestibular portion of the labyrinth includes five separate sensory organs (Figs. 4–1, 4–3, and 4–4). These are the saccule and utricle, located in the vestibule, and the three semicircular ducts, which occupy the canals of the osseous labyrinth (Schuknecht & Gulya, 1995). The sensory receptors within the vestibular organs are oriented at different angles with respect to the vertical and horizontal planes; they are therefore differentially affected by head movements in different spatial planes. These receptors are all stimulated by forces associated with acceleration (i.e., motion that involves a change in velocity). However, the sensory organs of the vestibule are functionally distinct from those of the semicircular canals. The neuroepithelia of the saccule and utricle are sensitive to linear acceleration and to gravitational force (which in physical terms is indistinguishable from linear acceleration). Because of this, they provide information relating to linear (i.e., straight line) motion and to head position within the earth's gravitational field. Because, on the earth's surface, these receptors are always acted on by gravity, they continuously monitor the position of the head in space even when the head is not in motion. On the other hand, the semicircular duct receptors are stimulated by angular acceleration (i.e., motion involving rotation); they are therefore influenced by rotational movement of the head. Under normal conditions, the semicircular duct receptors do not respond to static head position because they are not stimulated by gravitational force.

Audiology: Diagnosis. Edited by Roeser, Valente, and Hosford-Dunn. Thieme Medical Publishers, Inc., New York © 2000

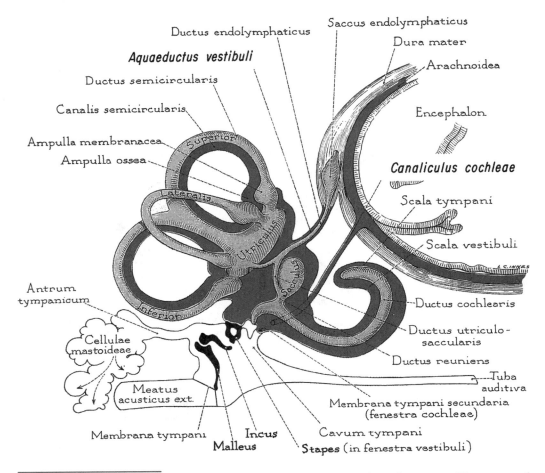

Figure 4–1   Schematic diagram of major components of the middle and inner ear. The organs of the membranous labyrinth *(in blue)* are shown enclosed within the various cavities of the bony labyrinth *(in red)*. (From Anson et al [1973], with permission.) *(See Color Plate 2.)*

The saccule is an ovoid membranous sac situated in a depression of the wall of the vestibule known as the spherical recess. It is located immediately adjacent to the basal portion of the cochlea and is connected with the cochlear duct by a narrow tube, the ductus reuniens (Fig. 4–4). The endolymphatic compartment of the cochlear duct is therefore in continuity with that of the saccule. The saccule does not have a direct fluid communication with the utricle; it does, however, give rise to the saccular duct that joins a smaller duct from the utricle to form the endolymphatic duct, which leads to the endolymphatic sac (Fig. 4–4).

The sensory neuroepithelium of the saccule, the macula sacculi (Fig. 4–4), is a specialized area of the membranous saccular wall that lies against the bony wall of the spherical recess and is oriented predominantly in the vertical plane. The macula is an oblong, platelike structure with a surface area of a little more than 2 mm[2]; the macular neuroepithelium contains approximately 16,000 sensory cells (Watanuki & Schuknecht, 1976). Its vertical orientation in the parasaggital plane makes it most sensitive to up-and-down translations of the head and to horizontal motion along the anteroposterior (front-to-back) axis.

The utricle is an irregularly shaped membranous tube that is considerably larger than the saccule (Igarashi et al, 1983). It has a superior-to-inferior orientation in the vestibule and lies behind (i.e., posterior to) the saccule. The macula of the utricle is a roughly circular thickening of the membranous utricular wall, which has a surface area of nearly 4 mm[2]. It contains about 31,000 receptor cells (Watanuki & Schuknecht, 1976). The macula is situated in the superior portion of the utricle (Fig. 4–4) and lies in approximately the horizontal plane. This orientation makes it most sensitive to linear movements in the horizontal plane.

The three semicircular ducts are thin, curved tubes that are attached to the utricle and open into it as shown in Figure 4–4. Each of the ducts forms about two thirds of a circle and each lies at right angles to the other two. As indicated in Figure 4–3, the three semicircular canals and the membranous ducts they enclose are named according to their relative positions in the upright head—superior (or anterior vertical), posterior (or inferior vertical), and lateral (or horizontal). The superior and posterior ducts are oriented vertically, whereas the lateral duct lies in an approximately horizontal plane. (The lateral duct is actually tilted upward by about 30 degrees located on a ridge of tissue called the crista ampullaris that extends transversely across the ampulla at right angles to the semicircular duct (Fig. 4–5). The neuroepithelium of each crista has a surface area of about 1 mm^2 and contains roughly 7,000 sensory cells (Watanuki & Schuknecht, 1976).

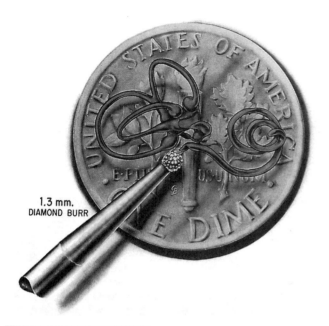

Figure 4–2 Drawing of the membranous labyrinth showing its size in relation to a dime and to a 1.3 mm dental burr. (From Anson et al [1973], with permission.)

from horizontal, a fact of importance for positioning the head during caloric testing [see Chapter 26].) Each of the semicircular ducts has a bulbous dilation at one end called the ampulla, which houses the sensory receptor organ. The non-ampullated ends of the superior and posterior ducts unite to form the crus commune, which joins the posterior aspect of the utricle (Fig 4–4). There are therefore five (rather than six) openings into the utricle associated with the semicircular ducts. The sensory neuroepithelium of each of the ducts is

---

PEARL
All five sensory organs of the vestibular apparatus are stimulated by acceleratory forces. *The maculae of the saccule and utricle respond to linear acceleration* (linear motion and gravity). *The cristae of the semicurcular ducts respond to angular acceleration* (rotational motion).

Microstructure of the Vestibular Neuroepithelia

Although the sensory receptors of the macular organs and the semicircular ducts are equipped with different types of accessory structures for stimulation of the vestibular sensory cells, the various neuroepithelia all have a very similar structural organization (Lindeman, 1969). As shown in Figure 4–6, which illustrates the saccular macula, the vestibular neuroepithelia are composed of sensory and supporting cells together with the neural structures that are associated with the sensory epithelium. The sensory cells are arranged in a single layer and are separated from one another by supporting cells. The receptor cells have clusters of hairlike cilia at their apical ends and, because of this feature, are often referred to as "hair cells." All vestibular hair cells have cilia of two types: stereocilia and kinocilia. The stereocilia are actually modified microvilli that are arranged in several rows

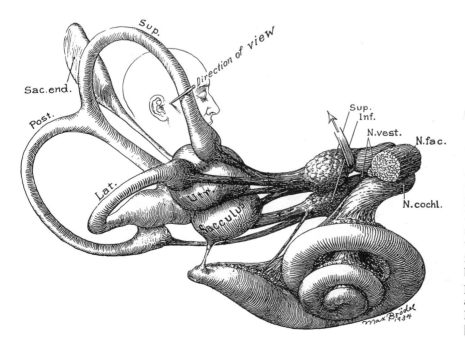

Figure 4–3 Orientation of the membranous labyrinth in the human head. The superior (*Sup.*) and posterior (*Post.*) semicircular ducts are vertically oriented and the lateral duct (*Lat.*) is tilted at about 30 degrees from the horizontal plane. Sac. end., endolymphatic sac; Utr., utricle; Sup./Inf., superior and inferior components of the vestibular nerve (*N. vest.*). The arrow indicates that the superior division has been slightly elevated to make the two parts of the nerve more distinctly visible as separate elements. N. fac., facial nerve; N. cochl., cochlear nerve. (From Brodel [1946], with permission.)

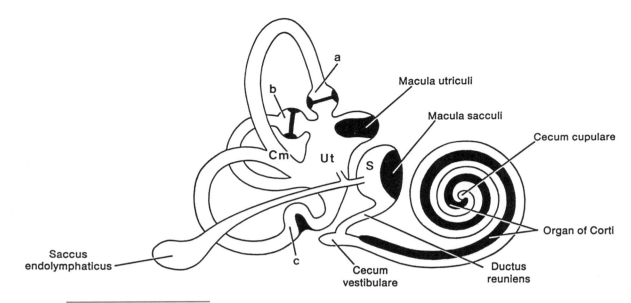

Figure 4–4 Diagram showing relationships between structures of the membranous labyrinth and location of the sensory epithelia within the vestibular apparatus. a, b, and c, Superior, lateral, and posterior ampullae with their sensory receptors (the cristae) shown in black. Cm, crus commune; Ut, utricle; S, saccule. (From Bloom & Fawcett [1962], with permission.)

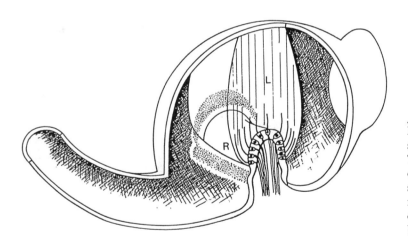

Figure 4–5 Schematic diagram of the sensory structures inside the ampulla of a semicircular duct. The crista (*R*), which extends across the ampulla, is covered by sensory epithelium. The cilia of the sensory cells project into the cupula (*L*), a gelatinous mass that fills the space between the surface of the crista and the opposite wall of the ampulla. (From Lindeman [1969], with permission.)

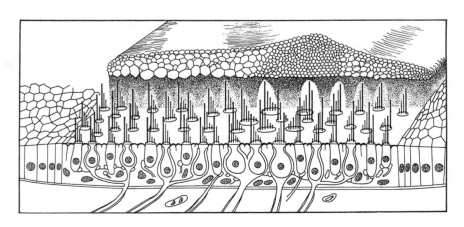

Figure 4–6 Drawing illustrating a cross section of the saccular macula. The stippled area above the macular surface represents the gelatinous layer of the otoconial membrane into which the stereocilia of the sensory cells project. Resting on the gelatinous layer are the otoconia. (From Lindeman [1969], with permission.)

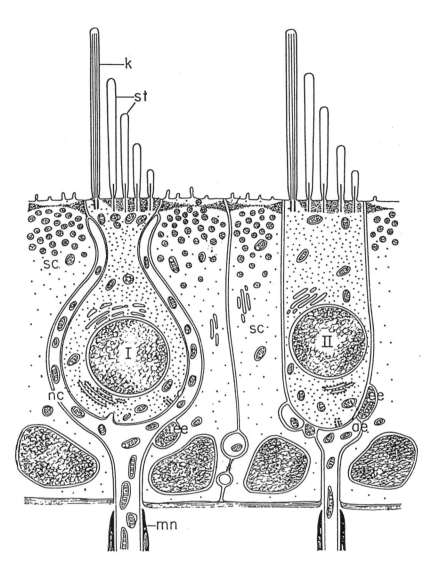

Figure 4–7   Diagrammatic cross section of vestibular neuroepithelium, illustrating type I and type II sensory cells surrounded by supporting cells (*sc*). The type I sensory cell is enclosed by an afferent nerve calyx (*nc*). Near its base, the type II cell receives small afferant (*ae*) and efferent (*ee*) nerve endings. Efferent endings are also found on the afferent nerve calyx. mn, Myelinated vestibular nerve fiber approaching the sensory epithelium. Kinocilia (*k*) and stereocilia (*st*) are prominent features on the apical surfaces of both type I and type II receptor cells. Note that the kinocilium is located immediately adjacent to the tallest of the stereocilia. (From Lindeman [1969], with permission.)

that increase in height across the top of the cell. They are thus configured in a stairstep pattern in which short stereocilia are postioned on one side of the hair cell and long ones on the other (Fig. 4–7). Situated near the tallest row of stereocilia is a single, longer process known as the kinocilium, which has a more complex internal structure like that of true, motile cilia found in other parts of the body. The orderly arrangement of stereocilia and kinocilia across the top of the vestibular sensory cell has important functional implications as discussed below.

The stereocilia and kinocilia of the macular hair cells project into a sheet of gelatinous material that blankets the surface of the neuroepithelium (Fig. 4–6). Resting on the gelatinous layer is a mass of tiny crystals called otoconia. The crystalline mass, together with the gelatinous layer, makes up the structure known as the otoconial membrane, which is responsible for stimulation of the macular hair cells in response to linear acceleration.

The otoconia are composed of calcium carbonate in the form of the mineral calcite, which has a density almost three times that of endolymph (Lim, 1984). As illustrated in Figure 4–8, individual otoconial crystals are cylindrical in shape and have pointed ends, somewhat resembling miniature grains of rice. The otoconia range from less than 1 μm to about 20 μm in length, with crystals of differing size arranged in a definite pattern across the otoconial membrane. Under the influence of gravitational force or linear head movement, the otoconial membrane undergoes minute shifts in position on the macular surface, thereby deflecting the cilia on the underlying sensory cells. This alters the electrical polarization of the hair cells, which controls the release of neurotransmitter onto the nerve endings making contact with the sensory cells. It is in this way that the discharge rate of vestibular nerve fibers is modulated by stimulation of the macular receptor cells (Goldberg & Fernandez, 1984).

In the ampullae of the semicircular ducts, the sensory cells are stimulated by the cupula, a gelatinous mass that rests on the crista and extends to the opposite wall of the ampulla, thus closing off the opening between the semicircular duct and the utricle (Fig. 4–5). The cupula envelops the cilia of the

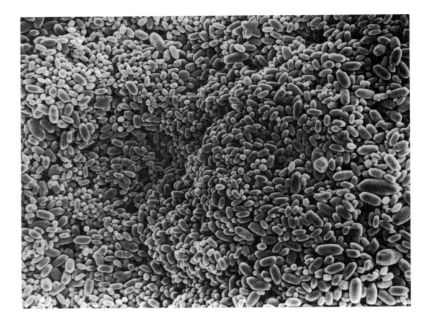

Figure 4–8   Scanning electron micrograph of utricular otoconia from a 10-month-old infant. At this magnification (approximately X 1,000) individual calcite crystals comprising the crystalline layer of the otoconial membrane are clearly seen.

hair cells and consists of material much like the gelatinous layer of the otoconial membrane, but it is without otoconia and so has the same density as endolymph. (It is therefore unresponsive to gravity.) Very small fluid displacements occurring in the semicircular ducts during angular acceleration deflect the cupula, resulting in deflection of the cilia on the receptor cells.

All the vestibular neuroepithelia contain sensory cells of two different morphological types (Lindeman 1969), which are illustrated diagrammatically in Figure 4–7. The type I receptor cell has a rather plump, gobletlike shape and is entirely surrounded by a single, large nerve ending, the so-called nerve calyx (or chalice). The calyceal endings are terminals of the large and medium-sized afferent fibers of the vestibular nerve (Correia & Dickman, 1991), that transmit information from the sensory cells to the CNS. The type II receptor cells are more slender and cylindrical in shape and they have clusters of small nerve endings at their basal ends. Both afferent and efferent nerve fibers terminate on the type II sensory cells.

The efferent terminals are the peripheral endings of nerve fibers with cell bodies located in the brain stem in the vicinity of the vestibular nuclei. Thus the efferent innervation projects from the CNS out to the periphery, where its fibers branch extensively and terminate in three locations: (1) on type II hair cells, (2) on afferent calyceal endings surrounding type I sensory cells, and (3) on afferent nerve fibers supplying both type I and type II hair cells (Correia & Dickman, 1991). Each labyrinth receives a total of 400 to 600 efferent fibers originating from neurons located on both the ipsilateral and contralateral sides of the brain stem (Gacek, 1980). The efferent innervation undoubtedly influences the flow of information transmitted from the vestibular neuroepithelia to the brain. However, the physiological significance of this innervation is not yet completely understood. Evidence exists that the efferent system may have both excitatory and inhibitory effects on afferent impulse transmission (Goldberg & Fernandez, 1984; Highstein, 1991).

Physiology of the Vestibular Neuroepithelia

The afferent nerve fibers that supply the vestibular neuroepithelia are activated by release of neurotransmitter from the sensory cells. Because some release of neurotransmitter apparently occurs even when the sensory cells are at rest, many of the afferent fibers transmit a steady stream of nerve impulses to the brain during periods when the neuroepithelia are not under active stimulation. As shown in Figure 4–9,

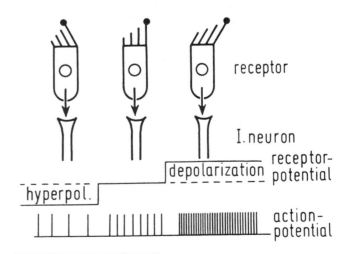

Figure 4–9   Effect of receptor cell stimulation on the activity of vestibular nerve fibers. In the absence of stimulation (*center*), vestibular neurons (*I. neuron*) show a continuous discharge of action potentials. Hair cell stimulation produces either depolarization (*right*) or hyperpolarization (*left*) depending on whether the stereocilia are deflected toward or away from the kinocilium (indicated here by the longest cilium with a beaded end). Hyperpolarization decreases the rate of action potential discharge, whereas depolarization increases the discharge rate. (From Leigh & Zee [1991], with permission.)

this "spontaneous" discharge rate may be increased or decreased by changes in transmitter release that occur when a stimulus is applied to the receptor cells (Goldberg and Fernandez, 1984; Leigh & Zee, 1991).

If the cupula or otoconial membrane moves so that the stereocilia on an underlying hair cell are deflected toward the kinocilium, the cell is depolarized. (Its membrane potential becomes less negative.) Depolarization increases the amount of neurotransmitter released onto the afferent nerve terminals, and the rate of neural discharge increases. If, on the other hand, the stereocilia are deflected away from the kinocilium, the cell's membrane potential increases (becomes more negative or hyperpolarized), resulting in reduced transmitter release and a decrease in afferent discharge rate. Because the spontaneous discharge rate can either be increased or decreased, the system shows directional sensitivity; movement of the cupula or otoconial membrane in one direction increases afferent discharge, and movement in the opposite direction decreases the discharge (Correia & Dickman, 1991).

In each of the vestibular neuroepithelia groups of sensory cells are oriented in such a way that all cells within a group are either depolarized or hyperpolarized by a given movement of the cupula or otoconial membrane (Lindeman, 1969). On the cristae of the semicircular ducts, all the receptor cells are oriented (or "polarized") in the same manner. In the case of the lateral crista each hair cell is situated so that its kinocilium is on the side of the cell nearest the utricle. (The cells are said to be oriented in such a way that their kinocilia "face" the utricle.) Thus, if the head moves so as to displace the lateral cupula toward the utricle (i.e., utriculopetal deflection), the stereocilia will be deflected toward the kinocilia, depolarizing the sensory cells and producing increased neural discharge (excitation). On the other hand, cupular deflection away from the utricle (utriculofugal displacement) will hyperpolarize the hair cells, resulting in reduction (inhibition) of neural discharge. The receptor cells of the superior and posterior cristae are polarized in a manner exactly opposite to those of the lateral crista. That is, they are oriented so that their kinocilia face away from the utricle. Therefore cupular deflection toward the utricle produces inhibition of neural output, whereas deflection away from the utricle results in excitation.

The arrangement of sensory cells on the two maculae is somewhat more complex. That is, each macula is divided into two areas of roughly equal size in which the hair cells are oppositely oriented. Therefore displacement of the otoconial membrane tends to excite cells on one half of the macula and inhibit those on the other half. The polarization patterns of sensory cells on the cristae and maculae are illustrated diagrammatically in Figure 4–10.

THE VESTIBULO-OCULAR REFLEX AND ITS ROLE IN EVALUATION OF VESTIBULAR FUNCTION

The reflex pathways connecting the vestibular system with the extraocular muscles of the eyes are important for maintaining clear vision during movement of the head and also

for clinical testing of vestibular function. Imagine an individual undergoing angular acceleration toward the right in the horizontal plane as diagrammed in Figure 4–11. As the head is rotated to the right, both lateral cupulae will be deflected toward the left. The lateral cupula on the right will therefore move toward the utricle and the left cupula will move away from the utricle. Because the hair cells of the lateral crista are oriented with their kinocilia facing the utricle, this stimulus will increase the rate of neural discharge from the right ear and reduce the discharge rate on the left. The change in neural activity will be relayed through the vestibular nerves to the vestibular nuclei of the brain stem. From there, neural pathways lead to the nuclei that control the extraocular muscles (in this case, the medial and lateral rectus muscles that move the eyes in the horizontal plane). As Figure 4–11 shows, the increased discharge from the right ear will be transmitted to the abducens and oculomotor nerves that control the lateral rectus muscle of the left eye and medial rectus muscle of the right eye. These muscles will then draw the eyes toward the left. Thus each labyrinth influences muscles that pull the eyes in a direction opposite to the direction of head rotation. When the head is rotated to the right, neural discharge from the right ear is increased and the eyes move to the left with velocity and amplitude equal to the velocity and amplitude of the head movement (Barber, 1984). This response is known as the vestibulo-ocular reflex (VOR). The VOR functions to stabilize the visual field on the retina as the head moves, thereby reducing visual blurring during head motion, which helps to maintain clear vision as the body moves.

PEARL

During head rotation, the extraocular muscles are stimulated so as to draw the eyes in a direction opposite to the direction of rotation. This reflex response (the *VOR*) is a result of vestibular stimulation, and it functions to stabilize the visual field on the retina as the head moves.

As the head moves to the right, the eyes move toward the left, but they can only move so far before they reach their limit of motion within the orbits. When that occurs, the eyes rapidly snap back to the midline position before moving left again. This repeated pattern of eye movement, in which the eyes move relatively slowly in one direction then quickly return to the midline, is called nystagmus. The initial, slower phase of the nystagmic beat is controlled by the vestibular system. The quick return to midline, on the other hand, is under control of the brain stem reticular formation. Because the quick return is the more obvious part of the nystagmic beat, it is the direction of eye movement during that phase that is said to be the direction of the nystagmus. Thus angular acceleration of the head to the right induces a right-beating nystagmus. The assessment of nystagmus is a very important tool for clinical evaluation of vestibular function. As described in Chapter 26, nystagmus may occur spontaneously in various disorders or it may occur when the head is placed in certain positions; it may also be induced in the clinic by rotational or caloric stimulation.

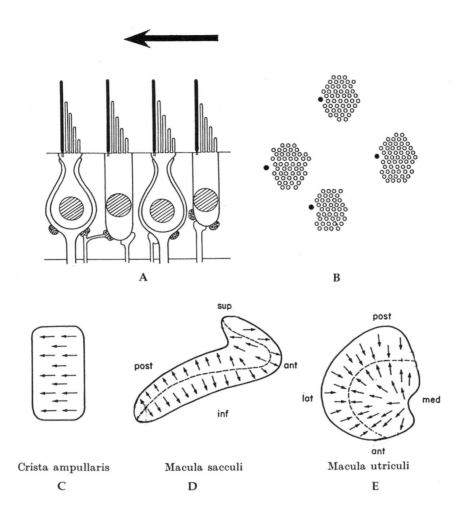

Figure 4–10 Diagram illustrating morphological polarization of the sensory cells and the polarization pattern of the vestibular sensory epithelia. The morphological polarization *(arrow)* of a sensory cell is determined by the postion of the kinocilium in relation to the stereocilia. **(A)** Cross section of the neuroepithelium. Note the increasing length of stereocilia toward the kinocilium *(shown in solid black).* **(B)** Section through the stereociliary bundles parallel to the epithelial surface. The solid black dots indicate the kinocilia. **(C)** The sensory cells of the crista ampullaris are all polarized in the same direction. The saccular **(D)** and utricular **(E)** maculae are each divided into two areas in which the sensory cells are oppositely polarized. Post (posterior), sup (superior), ant (anterior), and inf (inferior) indicate the orientation of the maculae. (From Lindeman [1969], with permission.)

PEARL

It is the *fast* component of the nystagmic beat that is used to designate the direction of nystagmus.

In some respects caloric stimulation is more informative than rotational testing because with caloric tests the two ears can be stimulated separately and their responses compared, thereby providing more diagnostically useful information. Caloric nystagmus is produced by irrigating the external ear canal with either warm or cool water or air, which changes the temperature of the middle ear cavity (Furman & Cass, 1996). The temperature change rather specifically affects the lateral semicircular duct because it lies close to the middle ear cavity. If the lateral duct is vertically oriented by appropriate tilting of the head, a warm stimulus to the right ear will increase the temperature of a portion of the endolymph in the lateral duct, causing it to rise and deflect the cupula toward the utricle. The resulting increase in neural discharge from the right side will then produce a right-beating nystagmus as described earlier. A cool stimulus, on the other hand, produces a response in the opposite direction. In that case endolymph in the lateral semicircular duct is cooled, becomes more dense, and sinks, so that the cupula will be deflected away from the utricle. This will reduce the discharge rate from the right ear, making the left ear dominant so as to provoke a left-beating nystagmus. The mnemonic COWS (Cold-Opposite; Warm-Same) is a helpful aid for remembering the side of the head toward which the nystagmic beat is directed during caloric stimulation.

THE VESTIBULAR NERVE AND CENTRAL VESTIBULAR SYSTEM

The sensory organs of the vestibular labyrinth are innervated by the vestibular component of cranial nerve VIII, which carries both afferent and efferent fibers to the vestibular apparatus. Afferent fibers of the vestibular nerve have their cell bodies located in Scarpa's ganglion, which occupies the internal auditory canal of the temporal bone. The vestibular nerve (including Scarpa's ganglion) is divided into superior and inferior divisions and together the two divisions contain between 18,000 and 20,000 nerve fibers (Schuknecht, 1993). As indicated in Figure 4–12, the peripheral portion of the superior division of the nerve innervates the utricular macula, the superior and lateral cristae, and the anterosuperior region of the saccular macula. Peripheral fibers of the inferior division supply the major portion of the saccular macula and the posterior crista. Central to Scarpa's ganglion, the vestibular nerve projects to the brain stem where most of its fibers enter the vestibular nuclei (Figs. 4–13 and 4–14). A small contingent of fibers, however, bypasses the vestibular nuclear complex and projects directly to the cerebellum (Brugge, 1991; Goldberg & Fernandez, 1984).

The vestibular nuclei are located in the dorsolateral portion of the brain stem near the junction of the medulla and pons (Fig. 4–13). They consist of four major nuclei (superior, lateral, medial, and inferior or descending) together with several closely associated minor nuclear groups (Gacek, 1980). As the vestibular nerve fibers enter the brain stem, they bifurcate into ascending and descending branches that distribute to the various nuclei in a highly organized fashion, with fibers from the cristae and maculae terminating in specific and, to some extent, independent areas of the vestibular nuclear complex.

In addition to the vestibular nerve fibers the vestibular nuclei receive input from various other sources, including the visual system, the cerebellum, the brain stem reticular formation, and the spinal cord. They therefore serve as much more than simple relay stations for peripheral input; these nuclei play a significant role in the complex interaction between the vestibular system and other major centers of the CNS (Brugge, 1991; Furman & Cass, 1996).

Certainly one of the most important central connections of the vestibular nuclei is with brain stem centers that control ocular motion (Barber, 1984; Goldberg & Fernandez, 1984; Leigh & Zee, 1991). As we described previously, the vestibular apparatus detects both static head position and head motion and through its central connections elicits compensatory eye movements that stabilize the visual image on the retina when the head moves or tilts (the vestibulo-ocular reflex). The vestibulo-ocular pathways involved in horizontal eye movements have been outlined earlier. In addition to input from the lateral crista, signals from the superior and posterior cristae and the maculae are also involved in reflex control of eye movement by means of connections through

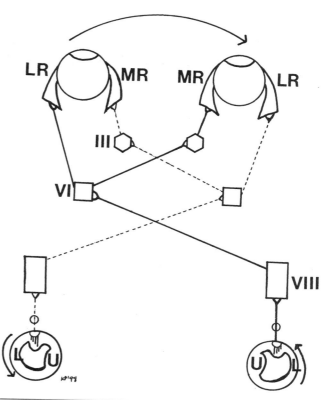

Figure 4–11 Simplified schematic drawing illustrating the basic neurocircuits that mediate the horizontal vestibular ocular reflex. The circular figures at the bottom of the diagram represent the right and left vestibular labyrinths, with "L" indicating the lateral semicircular duct and "U" indicating the utricle. From the cristae of the lateral ducts neural impulses are relayed through the vestibular nerve to the vestibular nuclei (*VIII*) and then to the nuclei of the abducens (*VI*) and oculomotor (*III*) nerves controlling the medial (*MR*) and lateral (*LR*) rectus muscles that move the eyes in the horizontal plane. These pathways involve relatively few neurons so that the stimulus-to-response time (latency) of the VOR is short. When the head undergoes angular acceleration to the right (*large arrow at top*), fluid displacement in the lateral duct deflects the stereocilia of the right crista toward the utricle and those of the left crista away from the utricle as indicated by the small arrows. This results in increased neural discharge in the pathway drawn in solid lines and decreased activity in the pathway shown in dotted lines, producing a leftward shift of the eyes because of contraction of the medial and lateral rectus muscles on the left side of each eye. Thus rotation of the head in one direction results in movement of the eyes in the opposite direction.

the vestibular nuclei to the oculomotor, trochlear, and abducens nuclei that are the primary cranial nerve nuclei responsible for control of eye motion in all spatial planes.

As a major CNS center for motor coordination, the cerebellum plays a significant role in regulation of vestibulo-ocular and vestibulospinal reflexes (Brugge, 1991; Goldberg & Fernandez, 1984). The vestibular system has quite substantial reciprocal connections with the cerebellum. Vestibular

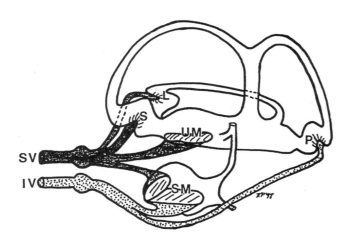

Figure 4–12 Diagrammatic sketch showing the peripheral distribution of the superior and inferior divisions of the vestibular nerve to the sensory organs of the inner ear. The superior division of the nerve (*SV, shown shaded*) supplies the cristae of the lateral (*L*) and superior (*S*) ampullae and the macula of the utricle (*UM*) and a portion of the saccular macula (*SM*). The inferior division of the nerve (*IV, stippled*) innervates the main portion of the saccular macula and the crista of the posterior ampulla (*P*).

input to the cerebellum includes a sizable projection from neurons in the vestibular nuclei and a direct input from the peripheral vestibular apparatus (Fig. 4–14). (The direct vestibular fibers are the only afferents that reach the cerebellar cortex directly from a peripheral sensory organ without an intervening relay.) Vestibular signals reaching the cerebellum are integrated with information from visual, oculomotor,

and proprioceptive pathways. The cerebellum, in turn, projects back to the vestibular nuclei and, after the vestibular nerve, supplies the second largest contingent of fibers to the vestibular nuclear complex. Although the cerebellum exerts excitatory and inhibitory effects on the vestibular nuclei, its major influence on vestibular nuclear activity is inhibitory. Interaction between the vestibular nuclei and cerebellum is of essential importance in coordination of eye and head movements and in control of balance and postural tone.

Vestibular influences on the spinal cord are mediated by two direct pathways from the vestibular nuclei and by indirect connections by way of the reticular formation of the brain stem (Brugge, 1991; Kevetter & Correia, 1997; Pompeiano, 1975). The first of the direct spinal pathways, which is of major importance with regard to postural control, is the lateral vestibulospinal tract that originates in the lateral vestibular nucleus, which receives sizable afferent input from the tilt-sensitive neurons innervating the utricular macula. The lateral vestibulospinal tract projects to all levels of the spinal cord and terminates in relation to motor neurons responsible for control of the antigravity muscles of the neck, trunk, and limbs. The second of the direct vestibulospinal pathways, the medial vestibulospinal tract, receives contributions from the medial, lateral, and inferior vestibular nuclei and descends to cervical (and probably upper thoracic) levels of the spinal cord. Reflexes mediated by the medial vestibulospinal tract operate to stabilize the head so as to provide a stable platform for the eyes during locomotion and also to maintain appropriate head position with respect to gravity.

In addition to the CNS regions just discussed, the vestibular nuclear complex makes functionally significant connections with other areas. These include the contralateral vestibular nuclei, brain stem centers controlling visceral reflexes, and the cerebral cortex.

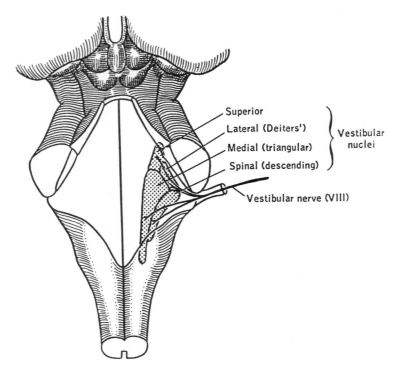

Superior
Lateral (Deiters') } Vestibular
Medial (triangular)   nuclei
Spinal (descending)

Vestibular nerve (VIII)

Figure 4–13 Drawing of the brain stem showing the location of the four major vestibular nuclei. For a detailed summary of the neuroanatomy of the vestibular nuclei and their connections with other brain stem centers, see Brugge (1991). (From House & Pansky [1967], with permission.)

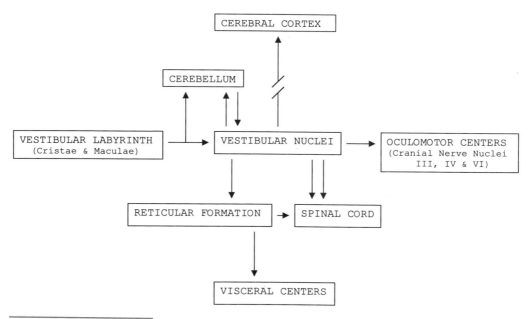

Figure 4–14 Highly simplified schematic drawing showing major CNS connections of the vestibular system. The interrupted arrow from the vestibular nuclei to the cerebral cortex is to indicate that this is a multisynaptic pathway whose exact connections are still under investigation. The two arrows from the vestibular nuclei to the spinal cord represent the medial and lateral vestibulospinal tracts. See text for discussion of central vestibular connections.

The distressing symptoms produced by unphysiological vestibular stimulation or inner ear disease can be a major consideration in clinical management of patients with vestibular disorders. In addition to vertigo and dysequilibrium, these patients may experience significant difficulty with autonomic/visceral upset because of high levels of vestibular system activity or markedly asymmetric vestibular input from the two ears. The neuroanatomical connections responsible for such symptoms are made by way of the reticular formation, which links the vestibular nuclei with various visceral reflex centers (Fig. 4–14), including the nuclei of origin of the vagus nerve, the phrenic nucleus, the salivatory nuclei, and the sympathetic chain ganglia (Crosby et al, 1962). These connections are responsible for the nausea, vomiting, sweating, and pallor that may result from intense vestibular stimulation or from disease processes affecting the vestibular system.

Although physiological evidence for vestibular input to the cerebral cortex exists, the anatomical connections underlying vestibular representation at the cortical level are not yet well understood. To a large extent, vestibular sensation comes to conscious awareness only when vestibular activity reaches unphysiological levels, as sometimes occurs in labyrinthine disease when patients may experience illusions of motion or body tilt. In addition, however, it is believed that vestibular input to the cerebral cortex is important for normal perceptual judgments regarding body orientation and motion (Furman & Cass, 1996; Leigh, 1994). Even though vestibular sensation is rather poorly defined at the cortical level, most investigators agree that one or more areas of the human cortex do receive vestibular impulses. However, their exact locations, as well as connections through the thalamus necessary for vestibular cortical representation, are not well agreed on (Brugge, 1991; Leigh, 1994). More research is therefore needed to better understand this important aspect of vestibular function.

ACKNOWLEDGMENT

We thank Karen S. Pawlowski for the artwork used in Figures 4–11 and 4–12.

REFERENCES

ANSON, B.J., & DONALDSON, J.A. (1973). *Surgical anatomy of the temporal and ear* (2nd ed.). Philadelphia: W.B. Saunders.

BARBER, H.O. (1984). Vestibular neurophysiology. *Otolaryngology–Head and Neck Surgery, 92*;55–58.

BLOOM, W., & FAWCETT, D.W. (1962). *A textbook of histology* (8th ed.). Philadelphia: W.B. Saunders.

BRODEL, M. (1946). *Three unpublished drawings of the anatomy of the human ear.* Philadelphia: W.B. Saunders.

BRUGGE, J.F. (1991). Neurophysiology of the central auditory and vestibular systems. In: M.M. Paparella, D.A. Shumrick, J.L. Gluckman, & W.L. Meyerhoff (Eds.), *Otolaryngology* (Vol. 1): *Basic sciences and related principles* (3rd ed.) (pp. 281–314). Philadelphia: W.B. Saunders.

CORREIA, M.J., DICKMAN, J.D. (1991). Peripheral vestibular system. In: M.M. Paparella, D.A. Shumrick, J.L. Gluckman, & W.L. Meyerhoff (Eds.), *Otolaryngology* (Vol. 1): *Basic sciences and related principles* (3rd ed.) (pp. 269–279). Philadelphia: W.B. Saunders.

CROSBY, E.C., HUMPHREY, T., & LAUER, W.L. (1962). *Correlative anatomy of the nervous system.* New York: Macmillan.

FURMAN, J.M., & CASS, S.P. (1996). *Balance disorders: A case-study approach.* Philadelphia: FA Davis.

GACEK, R.R. (1980). Neuroanatomical correlates of vestibular function. *Annals of Otolaryngology, Rhinology and Laryngology, 89;*2–5.

GOLDBERG, J.M., & FERNANDEZ, C. (1984). The vestibular system. In: J.M. Brookhart, V.B. Mountcastle, I. Darian-Smith, & S.R. Geiger (Eds.), *Handbook of physiology,* Section 1: *The nervous system* (Vol. III), *Sensory processes,* Part 2. (pp. 977–1021). Bethesda, MD: American Physiological Society.

HIGHSTEIN, S.M. (1991). The central nervous system efferent control of the organs of balance and equilibrium. *Neuroscience Research, 12;*13–30.

HOUSE, E.L., & PANSKY, B.P. (1967). *A functional approach to neuroanatomy* (2nd ed.). New York: McGraw-Hill.

IGARASHI, M., O-UCHI, T., & ISAGO, H., WRIGHT, W.K. (1983). Utricular and saccular volumetry in human temporal bones. *Acta Otolaryngologica (Stockholm), 95;*75–80.

KEVETTER, G.A., & CORREIA, M.J. (1997). Vestibular system. In: P.S. Roland , B.F. Marple, & W.L. Meyerhoff (Eds.), *Hearing loss* (pp. 54–70). New York: Thieme Medical Publishers.

LEIGH, R.J. (1994). Human vestibular cortex. *Annals of Neurology, 35;*383–384.

LEIGH, R.J., & ZEE, D.S. (1991). *The neurology of eye movements* (2nd ed.). Philadelphia: FA Davis.

LIM, D.J. (1984). The development and structure of the otoconia. In: I. Friedman, & J. Ballantyne (Eds.), *Ultrastructural atlas of the inner ear* (pp. 245–269). London: Butterworths.

LINDEMAN, H.K. (1969). Studies on the morphology of the sensory regions of the vestibular apparatus. *Advances in Anatomy, Embryology, and Cellular Biology, 42(1);*1–113.

POMPEIANO, O. (1975). Vestibulo-spinal relationships. In: R.F. Naunton (Ed.), *The vestibular system* (pp. 147–180). New York: Academic Press.

SCHUKNECHT, H.F. (1993). *Pathology of the ear* (2nd ed.). Philadelphia: Lea and Febiger.

SCHUKNECHT, H.F., & GULYA, A.J. (1995). *Anatomy of the temporal bone with surgical implications* (2nd ed.). New York: Parthenon Publishing Group.

WATANUKI, K. & SCHUKNECHT, H.F. (1976). A morphological study of human vestibular sensory epithelia. *Archives of Otolaryngology, 102;*583–588.

## Chapter 5

Disorders of the Auditory System

Jennifer A. Jordan and Peter S. Roland

Outline

The purpose of this chapter is to provide a brief overview of most of the common disorders seen by the otologist and audiologist, including diagnostic information and treatment options. A generalized knowledge of otologic pathological conditions is essential for the audiologist to render the appropriate testing necessary to help the physician properly diagnose and treat the patient with otologic complaints. The chapter will first review issues in the otologic examination. Disorders of the earcanal; tympanic membrane, middle ear, and mastoid bone; and inner ear and internal auditory canal are then covered. Because this chapter reviews a wide range of disorders in the auditory system, material is covered that is presented throughout the text. The chapter is meant to be an overview and will complement other chapters.

OTOLOGIC EXAMINATION

History

Children and adults are seen by the otologic physician with a limited number of complaints. Adequate evaluation of each patient requires complete explanation of their difficulties. The following information should be gathered for each presenting symptom:

1. When the symptom was first noted.
2. Whether the symptom is constantly present or intermittent.
3. If the symptom is intermittent, how often does the symptom occur and how long does it last with each occurrence? Do the symptoms come in clusters?
4. How severe is the symptom?
5. Whether, in general, the symptom is improving or worsening.
6. Is the symptom bilateral or unilateral? If bilateral and intermittent, does it occur in each ear simultaneously or independently? If bilateral, did it begin simultaneously in both ears?
7. If more than one symptom is troubling the patient, one must establish whether the symptoms occur independently or are clustered together to form a symptom complex (syndrome).

Patients seen by the otolaryngologist usually complain of one of several common symptoms. These include tinnitus,

Audiology: Diagnosis. Edited by Roeser, Valente, and Hosford-Dunn. Thieme Medical Publishers, Inc., New York © 2000

hearing loss, otalgia, otorrhea, and vertigo. Each of these common symptoms is discussed at length in the following sections.

Tinnitus

Tinnitis refers to a sound that appears to be coming from one or both ears, but is not related to an external stimulus; it is internally generated. Most tinnitus appears to be a consequence of hearing loss. The pitch of tinnitus is often related to the frequency of the hearing loss. High-frequency hearing loss is often associated with high-pitched tinnitus, and low-pitched tinnitus (often described as "roaring") is often related to low-frequency loss.

Millions of persons experience varying degrees of tinnitus; indeed, at some time or another almost everyone experiences brief episodes of tinnitus, usually in quiet environments. Most individuals are not bothered by such brief episodes, but when tinnitus remains sustained, they may experience considerable discomfort. Some persons find the symptom annoying. Others are kept awake at night and may have difficulty concentrating. A few individuals find the tinnitus disabling and are prevented from pursuing their usual daily activities. An occasional individual may find the experience so tortuous that suicide is contemplated to escape it.

In assessing the nature of the tinnitis it is necessary to establish whether the tinnitis is unilateral or bilateral, pulsatile or nonpulsatile, and constant or intermittent. Pulsatile tinnitis is often noted with vascular anomalies, such as vascular middle ear tumors (glomus tumors) or with carotid or temporal artery disease.

The same general considerations that apply to adults apply to children. One must take into account, however, that children may have much greater difficulty in expressing and describing their subjective sensations. On the whole, tinnitus seems to be a less bothersome symptom in the pediatric age group than it is among adults. Nonetheless, some children have their hearing loss first identified as part of an evaluation for tinnitus.

There is phenomenological evidence that tinnitus may be generated from more than one portion of the auditory or central nervous system. The tinnitus associated with salicylate intoxication appears to be generated in the cochlea and is associated with salicylate-induced hearing loss. Salicylate-induced hearing loss is thought to be related to reversible enzyme inhibition within cochlear tissues. On the other hand, experience with the cranial nerve VIII section for control of tinnitus has demonstrated that dividing the cochlear nerve may have little or no effect on tinnitus and may even worsen it. Such observations suggest a central origin. Both imaging and neurophysiological evidence exist to support a fairly widespread activation of the central nervous system in many cases of distressing or incapacitating tinnitus. Portions of the limbic and autonomic system appear to be involved. Individuals with tinnitus report with some uniformity that the tinnitus is exacerbated in quiet environments and in stressful situations. Stress may be psychological (anxiety, depression, anger) or physical (illness, physical exhaustion, arousal).

Pharmacological therapy includes the use of antidepressant medications for clinically depressed individuals. Antidepressants may be used for their neuroleptic effect and their antidepressant effect. Such neuroleptic effects appear to involve alteration of nerve transmission, and medications like amitryptyline are therefore useful for tinnitus and other chronic pain states. Hypnotic medications and anxiolytics generally provide some relief for most tinnitus sufferers. However, tolerance to these medications develops, and they have a significant potential for both psychological and physical addiction. Consequently, most physicians are reluctant to prescribe these medications for a condition that would require long-term therapy.

Because amplification partially remedies the hearing loss, it often has a beneficial effect on the underlying tinnitus. Tinnitus relief from amplification may persist for hours after the hearing aid has been removed.

Tinnitus masking techniques involve the use of narrow band noise generators, matched to the frequency of the patient's tinnitus. Noise is delivered at a sufficiently high intensity to "mask" the internally generated tinnitus signal.

Habituation therapy, on the other hand, uses broad-band, low-intensity noise generators to minimally elevate the level of ambient background noise. Habituation therapy does not seek to overwhelm or "mask" the tinnitus signal. It requires a relatively long time (12 to 18 months) and generally includes significant amounts of supportive therapy.

Biofeedback has also been shown to be effective for a significant number or patients. A variety of other "naturopathic" or "home" remedies have also been recommended with considerable enthusiasm, although documentation of their effectiveness is lacking.

Hearing Loss

Although formal audiometric testing is the most critical component in assessing hearing loss, it is often useful to gain some understanding of how much difficulty the individual experiences as a result of hypoacusis. One should establish in what circumstances he or she experiences difficulty and how troublesome these difficulties are. Such information can be helpful in determining the potential usefulness of amplification.

The time course of the hearing change is the most useful piece of historical information. Losses that have occurred many years before the current evaluation and are stable are not likely to require medical intervention. In making such determinations the availability of previous audiograms is extremely helpful, and every effort should be made to obtain them. Inquiries should be made into the circumstances of long-standing losses, and any association with febrile illness, antibiotic therapy, noise exposure, trauma, or surgery must be noted. Each patient should be specifically evaluated to see whether his or her hearing fluctuates and if so under what circumstances, how frequently, and with what severity. Any association of the hearing loss with vertigo or tinnitus, otalgia, otorrhea, upper respiratory infection, nasal stuffiness, headache, dysarthria, dysphagia, visual changes, numbness or tingling in the extremities, or focal motor weakness should all be established.

If other family members have hearing loss, the nature of such losses should be explored and audiograms obtained, especially if this loss occurred early in life. The time at which the patient first noted the loss, how he or she noted it, and its rate of progression should always be determined when possible. This can be somewhat difficult, especially in young children. In evaluating children consultation with family and teachers is critical. Parents are usually acute observers of their own child's hearing sensitivity and may be aware of fairly subtle changes. Although parents can be (and often are) manipulated by children, the parent's assessment should always be taken at face value even though subsequent information may sometimes demonstrate that the parent's assessment was inaccurate.

Otalgia

Otalgia (ear pain) precipitates many physician visits and has a myriad of causes. In a high percentage of adults, otalgia is not otogenic. It is estimated that in the primary care setting, only 50% of cases of ear pain in adults are caused by ear disease. Pain of otologic origin is usually dull, aching, and relatively constant. Pain that comes and goes frequently during the day is rarely otogenic.

Although nonotogenic otalgia is less common in children, the child or adult may experience ear pain as occurring within the structures of the ear when it is, in fact, referred from other embryologically related structures. Otalgia is commonly due to disorders affecting the larynx, pharynx, and tonsils. Tonsillitis and pharyngitis are two common causes of referred otalgia in children. Disorders of the muscles of mastication and the temporomandibular joint are also often perceived as ear pain.

Temporomandibular joint disease (TMJ) and myofascial pain dysfunction syndrome involving the muscles of mastication are important and common nonotogenic causes of ear pain. Most common is myofascial dysfunction syndrome involving the muscles of mastication. This disorder is characterized by inflammation, spasm, and tenderness of the muscles of mastication with pressure/pain transmitted to the TMJ. The joint itself, however, is relatively normal. In understanding this condition, it must be remembered that the glenoid fossa of the TMJ forms the anterior wall of the external auditory canal and portions of the anterior and lateral wall of the middle ear. Thus pain perceived in these areas will be localized to the ear and external canal.

Myofascial pain dysfunction syndromes are often related to teeth grinding, clenching, or gritting (bruxism). It is more common in individuals with an overbite. It may follow changes in occlusion associated with orthodontic treatments or the fitting of prostheses (dentures). Because teeth grinding, clenching, and gritting are frequently related to stress, this disorder is frequently a manifestation of stress. As such, it is often associated with or accompanied by tension headaches and inflammatory conditions of the posterior and lateral cervical muscles. Diagnosis depends on identifying tenderness over the joint or within the muscles of mastication. The temporalis muscles are frequently tender and bifrontal headache is a frequent accompaniment because of temporalis muscle inflammation and tenderness.

Occasionally, the disorder is characterized by degenerative or inflammatory processes arising from the TMJ itself. When the disease process is intrinsic to the joint, the condition is properly referred to as TMJ dysfunction. Popping, clicking, grinding, or crunching noises with mouth opening and mouth closure suggest intrinsic joint abnormalities. Definitive diagnosis generally depends on magnetic resonance imaging (MRI) scanning and/or endoscopic evaluation of the TMJ.

The pain of both disorders is generally characterized by sharp or aching pain described as either "deep in the ear" or epicentered around the tragus or TMJ. When asked to "point to where it hurts," patients often point directly into the external auditory canal, to the tragus, or to the joint. Pain commonly radiates inferiorly toward the hyoid bone along the ramus of the mandible. It generally lasts for several hours at a time. Individuals who grind and clench at night note that the pain is usually worse in the morning, although pain occasionally awakens them at night. In such circumstances the pain may be ameliorated or disappear completely during the day. Although uncommon, the pain can escalate to be so severe as to be completely incapacitating.

A high percentage of both individuals with myofascial pain dysfuction syndrome and true TMJ disease respond to nonsteroidal anti-inflammatory drugs (NSAIDs). Such agents should be prescribed regularly for a period of 10 to 14 days. In individuals who grit, grind, or clench their teeth at night, the use of a nocturnal bite splint is frequently helpful.

Many important otologic conditions such as cholesteatoma and other forms of chronic otitis media, Meniere's disease, and acoustic tumor are not associated with pain at all. Otogenic ear pain may be due to cerumen impaction, infection, and, quite rarely, neoplasms. The most common cause of otogenic ear pain is infection. Both external otitis and acute otitis media may cause excruciating pain that precipitates a physician visit, usually on an emergency basis. Because most cases are treated in the primary care setting, the incidence of ear pain caused by otologic disease is actually lower in a referral otologic practice than it is in a general practice.

PEARL

Palpation of the TMJ and muscles of mastication should be done when evaluating all patients with otalgia. Patients with joint or muscle tenderness should be referred to an oral surgeon for evaluation.

Otorrhea

With the rare exception of cases in which spinal fluid drains through the ear, otorrhea (drainage from the ear) is related to infection. The patient's history is especially important. Painless drainage is usually the result of chronic otitis media. This may be cholesteatoma, chronic mastoiditis caused by irreversible mucosal disease and tympanic membrane perforation, or chronic reflux through the eustachian tube. Otorrhea may occur sporadically as the result of an otherwise asymptomatic tympanic membrane perforation, especially if water has inadvertently entered the middle ear space. Patients with a history of painless drainage going back for months or years are highly suspect of harboring a temporal bone cholesteatoma. This is especially true if the drainage fails to resolve after vigorous treatment with systemic and topical antibiotics. Drainage associated with pain is more likely to be caused by an acute infectious process.

A perforation resulting from acute otitis media may be preceded by severe ear pain. Acute external otitis is frequently manifested by the simultaneous occurrence of aural drainage and acute ear pain. The prolonged use of antibiotic drops should alert the examiner to the possibility of fungal otitis, which occurs principally as a complication of broad-spectrum topical antibiotic treatment. Patients who routinely occlude the external auditory canal with hearing instruments or protective earplugs are much more difficult to treat because occlusion of the external auditory canal interferes with the normal cleansing mechanism of the ear.

Vertigo

Vertigo (dizziness) has a myriad of causes, many of which are entirely unrelated to the temporal bone and ear. A detailed history is the single most important piece of information in establishing a diagnosis. The following points should be clearly ascertained in every patient history:

- What exactly does the patient mean by "dizziness?"
- What does he or she experience?
- When did the symptom first occur, how often does it occur, and how long does it last when it does occur?
- What is the shortest and longest time the dizziness has lasted?
- Is the dizziness associated with nausea, vomiting, or sweating?
- Is the patient aware of any change in hearing before, during, or after the dizzy spell?
- Do any activities reliably bring on the dizzy spell?
- Is the dizzy spell associated with any difficulty in swallowing or speaking or any change in vision?
- Is consciousness ever completely lost during a dizzy spell?
- Is there associated tinnitus or a feeling of aural fullness?
- Can the patient tell when a dizzy episode is about to occur?

The answers to these questions vary dramatically. Vertigo arising from the vestibular system generally has as its principal component "the illusion of motion." This may be a sense of rotation or the sense of falling to one side or the other. When the patient uses such terms as "light-headed," "giddy," "confused," or "faint," the sensation is not likely to be labyrinthine in origin.

A special inquiry should be made into whether the patient has headaches before, during, or after each episode of vertigo or disequilibrium. It should be established whether a familial history of migraine exists. Migraine is a much more common cause of episodic vertigo in childhood than in adulthood and accounts for a substantial number of children with intermittent dizzy spells. It is important to inquire about the patient's other medical problems, especially visual difficulties, history of diabetes, stroke, or hypertension. Obtain a list of the patient's medications.

Elderly patients have a high incidence of balance complaints, many of which are exacerbated by medications. Antihypertensive medications can contribute to autonomic dysfunction, which may be attributed, in error, to the vestibular system. Careful evaluation of the history in light of basic audiometry will usually establish whether the vertigo is likely to be otogenic in origin and will probably suggest a diagnosis. Further diagnostic tests can then be ordered to confirm or deny these initial conclusions.

Physical Examination of the Ear

Examination of the ear begins with examination of the auricle. The size and shape of the auricle and its position should be carefully noted. Some children will have no auricle as a result of congenital aural atresia; some will have one that is abnormally small or poorly formed; other children may have an auricle placed either unusually low with respect to the remainder of the facial skeleton or unusually high (Fig. 5–1). The size and adequacy of the earcanal should be assessed. Some patients have collapsing earcanals with a slitlike opening, especially very young children. This should be noted before audiometry so that insert earphones can be used when hearing is tested.

To assess the earcanal, the auricle should be drawn backward and upward. This opens the lateral portion of the cartilaginous canal and permits assessment of the bony canal. An otoscope may then be used to examine the external auditory canal and tympanic membrane.

Preliminary examination of the size of the canal will allow the appropriate size speculum to be selected. The largest speculum that can be comfortably inserted into the patient's earcanal should be chosen. Specula for use in the earcanal are designed in such a way that they rarely protrude further into the ear than the cartilaginous portion of the canal. This portion can be stretched and manipulated with minimal or no discomfort. Should the speculum reach the inner third of the earcanal, even the slightest pressure will be extraordinarily painful. The patient's head needs to be tilted toward the opposite shoulder to account for the normal upward direction of the earcanal.

It will often be necessary to remove cerumen from the external auditory canal to examine the tympanic membrane (see Chapter 11 in *Treatment*). Cerumen that is deep in the canal or is impacted may be extraordinarily difficult to remove. Such patients should be referred to an otolaryngologist who can remove the cerumen by use of the operating microscope if irrigation techniques have failed. Occasionally, a general anesthetic will be required for cerumen removal in small children.

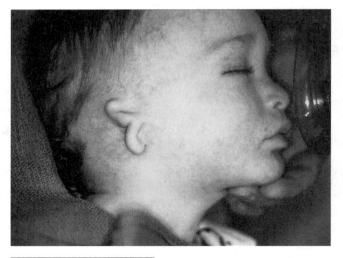

Figure 5–1   Young boy with unilateral microtia, or abnormal formation of the external ear.

Every attempt should be made to visualize the entire tympanic membrane. Otoscopic or microscopic examination of the ear cannot be considered complete until the entire tympanic membrane, including the pars flaccida, has been visualized. The anulus tympanicum should be followed anteriorly and posteriorly until it meets the anterior and posterior malleolar folds. The pars flaccida lies between these two folds (Fig. 5–2). Perforation or deep retraction of the pars flaccida is virtually diagnostic of a cholesteatoma. Both the long and short process of the malleus can be seen in the normal drum and their presence should be noted. The long process of the incus and chorda tympani can frequently, although not invariably, be seen through a normal tympanic membrane (Fig. 5–3). However, if the head of the malleus or body of the incus is seen, erosion of the superior external auditory canal and lateral wall of the middle ear space has occurred. This is seen almost exclusively in cholesteatoma.

Occasionally, a retracted drum lies directly on the incudostapedial joint, forming a "myringostapediopexy." In such circumstances, long-term retraction probably caused by eustachian tube insufficiency can be assumed. Surprisingly, hearing can often be near normal in such situations. The pneumatic otoscope is used to create positive or negative pressure on the tympanic membrane. Such pressure changes normally cause visible movement of the tympanic membrane. Using the pneumatic otoscope, the examiner can assess the degree of mobility of the tympanic membrane. Chronic middle ear effusion, for example, usually results in a sluggish or immobile tympanic membrane. In addition, brisk tympanic movements virtually exclude the possibility of tympanic membrane perforation.

Often a tympanic membrane perforation may heal without the middle fibrous layer of the eardrum, resulting in an extremely thin "secondary" membrane that is always translucent and often transparent. Such secondary membranes may be indistinguishable from perforations without

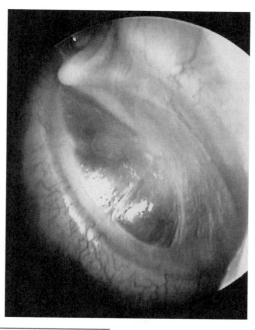

Figure 5–3 Normal tympanic membrane. Note that the short process of the incus and the malleus are well visualized. *(See Color Plate 3.)*

the use of the operating microscope. Pneumatic otoscopy using the handheld otoscopoe can sometimes induce movement in healed secondary membranes, which makes it apparent that the drum is indeed intact although quite thin. Immitance testing can also confirm the presence of an intact membrane with a type A tympanogram.

Masses behind the tympanic membrane may be caused by a variety of pathological processes. Color is important and may

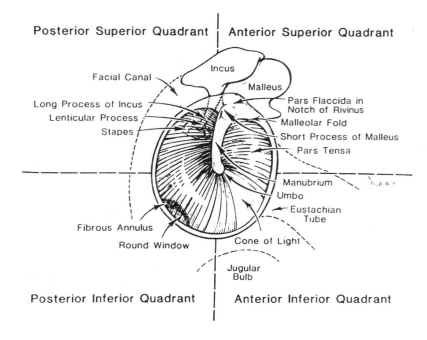

Figure 5–2 The landmarks of the tympanic membrane. (From Meyerhoff [1984], with permission.)

be a clue to the cause. White masses suggest cholesteatoma, tympanosclerosis, or, very rarely, middle ear osteoma (Fig. 5–4). Dark blue masses suggest venous vascular structures, such as a high jugular bulb. Dark red masses suggest highly vascular tumors such as glomus tympanicum tumors or granulation tissue. The presence of pulsations within a mass strongly suggests that it is arterialized and vascular in origin. This can sometimes be confirmed by applying positive pressure to the tympanic membrane with the pneumatic otoscope. Positive pressure reduces blood flow within the mass and causes blanching of the drum overlying the middle ear mass. Such blanching is referred to as a positive Brown's sign and strongly suggests a vascular neoplasm. Occasionally, a red blotch will be seen in the area of the oval window. This may not be a mass but may represent the hypervascular bone characteristic of an active focus of otosclerosis.

No otologic examination is complete without evaluation of facial nerve function. The patient should be asked to frown, smile, wrinkle his nose, whistle, show his teeth, and shut his eyes. Any asymmetry between sides or the inability to perform any of these motions should be clearly noted. The earliest and most subtle sign of facial weakness is lagophthalmos. The eyelid closes a bit more slowly on the affected side than on the normal, contralateral side. This is clearly evident when

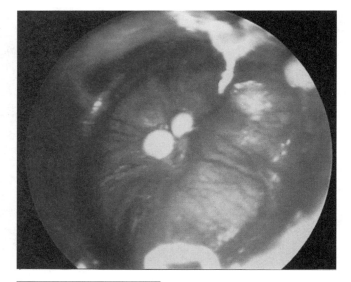

Figure 5–4 Two small white masses are visualized in the center of the tympanic membrane. These are cholesteatomas that have been implanted on the eardrum. *(See Color Plate 4.)*

the patient blinks spontaneously. The blink on the affected side appears to lag behind its normal contralateral partner.

DISEASES OF THE EARCANAL

Dermatitis

Two types of dermatitis affect the external auditory ear with some frequency. Seborrheic dermatitis is the most common type and is usually manifested by chronic itching of the external auditory canals and frequently, but not necessarily, associated with dry, flaky skin over the conchal bowl and medial portions of the external auditory canal. Careful physical examination often reveals the complete or near absence of cerumen. The condition is important not only because the itching is subjectively distressing but also because the chronic irritation of the skin of the external auditory canal reduces its effectiveness as a barrier to infection. Thus patients with chronic seborrheic dermatitis are much more susceptible to chronic bacterial external otitis (swimmer's ear) than are the unaffected, normal population. Indeed, after careful questioning, many patients who have recurrent episodes of external otitis will be discovered to have chronic, dry, flaking, and pruritic external auditory canals. In some patients the same condition waxes and wanes on an irregular and unpredictable basis. Many patients will have little or no difficulty for years, with sporadic "flare-ups" lasting weeks or months. Seborrheic dermatitis of the external auditory canal responds favorably to the use of very low dose steroid preparations at infrequent intervals. The use of 2% hydrocortisone cream applied to the conchal bowl and medial external auditory canal two or three times a week is frequently sufficient. In more difficult cases, a more potent steroid may be required. Some cases respond to the simple application of mineral oil or other emollient without the use of any medication whatsoever.

The other dermatitis that is seen with some frequency is allergic or atopic dermatitis. Most of these cases occur in response to exogenous materials placed in or around the external earcanal. Many allergic reactions are seen in response to topical antibiotic drops. Neomycin is especially likely to produce topical sensitization and result in allergic reaction. Allergic reactions to neomycin (and other topical antibiotics) occur in two somewhat distinct forms. A fulminant form is occasionally encountered that results in massive swelling of the earcanal and a dramatic drug eruption involving the conchal bowl, lobule, and frequently the skin of the neck. The eruption is associated with cutaneous weeping of serosanguinous fluid and is accompanied by intense pain and tenderness. Such reactions, of course, require the immediate discontinuation of the offending agent and often the use of both topical and systemic steroid medications. A more indolent form of hypersensitivity is manifested simply by the failure of a typical external otitis to resolve in response to what appears to be appropriate antibiotic therapy. Long-term drainage, edema of the external auditory canal, pain, and tenderness persist in the presence of both topical drops and mechanical cleansing. Such reactions can be adequately treated by discontinuing the offending agent and treating the external otitis with a nonantibiotic drop containing an antiseptic with or without a topical steroid. Atopic reactions occur to the materials from which both ear molds and earplugs are made. Again, the reaction may be fulminant with clear-cut swelling, pain, and tenderness or may be more indolent with only minimal swelling and moderate tenderness. The mainstay of treatment is replacement of the offending agent with a more hypoallergenic material.

External Bacterial Otitis

Acute external bacterial otitis is an infection of tissues of the earcanal and portions of the pinna. It is characterized by inflammation of the soft tissues of the canal with subepithelial edema and intense pain and tenderness. Erythema is variable; it may be intense or relatively absent. Severe cases of external otitis may have sufficient subepithelial edema as to cause blanching of the superficial tissues. Discharge varies from thick and mucopurulent to scanty and serous (Fig. 5–5).

The normal flora of the external auditory canal include diptheroids, gram-positive micrococci, and nonpathogenic staphyloccocal species, especially *Staphylococcus albus*. A large variety of fungi can be cultured from a normal earcanal. Indeed, fungi are more commonly cultured from normal earcanals than from infected canals. Only *Candida* species and species of *Aspergillus* have been associated with clinical infection.

Most external otitis is caused by bacterial organisms, generally gram-negative rods. Far and away the most common organism is *Pseudomonas aeruginosa*, which is the etiologic agent in more than 60% of cases. *Staphylococcus aureus* is the next most common pathogenic organism, followed by *Streptococcus* species. A minority of infections are caused by a fairly large variety of other gram-negative rods, among which *Proteus* species are featured prominently.

Pseudomonas is relatively ubiquitous in the environment and in the appropriate circumstances may be pathogenic. It is, however, extremely sensitive to the local acidity (pH) of

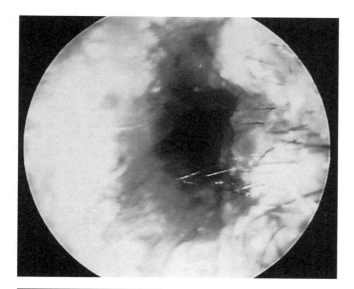

Figure 5–5 External bacterial otitis has led to a swollen earcanal with purulent debris. *(See Color Plate 5.)*

its environment. *Pseudomonas* is incapable of growing or reproducing in acidic environments. One of the functions of cerumen appears to be maintenance of a slightly acidic environment, which prevents the growth of *Pseudomonas*. Introduction of water into the earcanal by swimming (or other means) washes out the normal acidity of the canal and may substitute a slightly alkali environment. In such circumstances *Pseudomonas* may produce a purulent bacterial infection. The incidence of acute bacterial external otitis is significantly higher in June, July, and August because most swimming occurs during these months. As already mentioned, the presence of an impaired skin barrier, as can occur with seborrheic dermatitis, may significantly increase the chances of bacterial external otitis developing. The disorder is of relatively sudden onset and is characterized by severe pain localized to the affected external auditory canal. An important diagnostic feature is extreme sensitivity to any movement of the auricle or tissues surrounding the external auditory canal. Such tenderness is helpful in distinguishing external otitis from acute otitis media. The pain of acute otitis media is unaffected by even vigorous auricular movement.

Examination will show mucopurulent exudate (often thin or scant) accumulating in the external auditory canal, marked swelling of the tissues of the earcanal, and "weeping." Erythema is variable. It is often present and occasionally intense, but a severely swollen canal may be pale because of limited blood supply to the infected tissues. In many cases it is not possible to examine the tympanic membrane fully because of the exquisite tenderness of the canal and a marked amount of canal swelling. The disorder is rarely, if ever, associated with fever, malaise, or other signs of systemic infection. Treatment follows logically from the known cause of the infection. Reacidification of the earcanal is almost always sufficient to cure the disorder, unless the canal is so swollen as to prevent the acidifying fluids from entering or accumulated mucopurulent debris is so great that the drops do not come in contact with the infected tissues. An external canal that is swollen closed can be dealt with effectively by placing a small wick into the canal. The wick is made of an expandable material and draws the acidifying solution into the canal. When a large amount of mucopurulent debris has accumulated in the canal, mechanical removal of the debris using the operating microscope and suction is essential and often crucial to successful management. In severe cases such cleansing may need to be done two or three times on an every other day basis.

Antibiotic drops directed against *Pseudomonas* are effective in eliminating infection, but are often unnecessary. Antibiotic drops should be continued at least a week beyond remission of pain. The use of antibiotic drops carries with it the risk of producing a topical allergic reaction and the promotion of fungal external otitis.

Malignant Otitis Externa (Necrotizing External Otitis)

Malignant otitis externa (osteomyelitis of the temporal bone and skull base) is a rare, aggressive, and sometimes fatal infection that begins in the earcanal and proceeds to invade the bone of the skull base. The disease is almost always seen in elderly diabetic patients and is caused by *Pseudomonas aeruginosa.* Rarely, it develops in immunocompromised patients and, when it does, other organisms (gram-negative rods, fungi) may be the infecting organisms.

Traditionally, the treatment of malignant otitis externa consists of at least 6 weeks of intravenous therapy with a combination of an antipseudomonal penicillin and an aminoglycoside. Recently, evidence has been presented that the early stages of malignant otitis externa can often be successfully managed with oral quinolones. Careful follow-up is necessary so that treatment failures can be detected early and intravenous antibiotic therapy initiated. Gallium 67 scans can be followed to determine the effectiveness of therapy because they will normalize with resolution of the infection.

PEARL

Avoid deliberately placing water in the ear of a diabetic patient, even for cerumen removal. It could lead to necrotizing external otitis.

Fungal External Otitis

A wide variety of fungi colonize the normal earcanal. Fungal organisms are relatively more common in normal canals than abnormal canals. Most fungal growth that occurs within the earcanal is saprophytic (i.e., growing on dead material in the earcanal). The fungi grow on desquamated epithelium, cerumen, or the inspissated mucopurulent debris from a previous bacterial infection. True fungal external otitis with tissue invasion of fungal elements is uncommon and almost completely limited to individuals who are significantly immunocompromised. Individuals taking high-dose steroids, using immunosuppressive agents, or with immunodeficiency disorders are candidates for such infections. An exception to this general rule may be healthy individuals who have had long-term treatment with systemic antimicrobials or topical antibiotics. In such individuals fungi are sometimes cultured from a chronic draining external auditory canal, and they may be etiologically important.

Almost all clinically significant fungal otitis is caused by either *Candida* or *Aspergillus* species, the only fungi recovered more frequently from diseased than normal ears. Such fungal external otitis is best treated by withdrawal of the antibiotic therapy and the use of topical antiseptics like merbromin (Mercurochrome) or gentian violet. Antiseptics have the advantage of being fairly universal in their toxicity. Thus they are much less likely to select out resistant organisms, which can then grow unrestrained by their usual bacterial competitors. Acidifying agents are also useful in the treatment of fungal external otitis because many of the fungi are sensitive to ambient pH. Occasionally, especially in immunocompromised individuals, the use of topical or even systemic antifungal agents may become necessary.

Congenital Aural Atresias

Congenital aural atresias can involve the pinna, earcanal, middle ear space, or ossicles. Such malformations may occur alone or in association with other regional or distant malformations. A variety of different syndromes have been identified associated with malformations of the ear (Table 5–1).

TABLE 5–1 Syndromes associated with congenital aural atresia

Alport's syndrome	Crouzon's disease
Marfan syndrome	Osteogenesis imperfecta
Treacher Collins syndrome	Pierre Robin syndrome
Goldenhar's syndrome	Francheshetti syndrome
Nager's acrofacial dysostosis	Wildervanck's syndome
Sprengel's deformity	Pyle's disease
Paget's disease	Möbius' syndrome
Levy-Hollister's (LADD) syndrome	CHARGE syndrome
Alagille syndrome	Andersen's disease
Fraser's syndrome	Lenz's syndrome
Noonan's syndrome	

When gross malformation of the auricle is associated, the atresia is usually identified promptly, often on the day of birth. However, when the pinna is normal, identification of the stenotic or atretic earcanal may be delayed for a number of years. Identification may await the child's failure to meet developmental guidelines or failure of screening audiometric tests in school.

Malformations of the external and middle ears occur approximately once in every 10,000 to 20,000 births. It appears that a significant percentage of cases of atresia are not due to genetic causes. Fortunately, the malformation occurs unilaterally four times more frequently than it does bilaterally. The cause in unilateral cases often remains obscure, but many cases may be acquired as the result of vascular injury to the branchial arches, which can occur in utero. Because embryological development of the ear is finished by week 28 of gestation, injuries that occur in late pregnancy will not affect otologic development. Portions of the external auditory canal and middle ear develop from the same underlying embryological structures, so middle ear malformations are frequently associated with malformations of the earcanal. Fortunately, however, the cochlea, semicircular canals, and cranial nerve VIII are rarely affected. Most individuals with congenital aural atresia have a normally functioning neurosensory auditory system.

The anatomical course of the facial nerve is frequently altered in malformations of the ear and temporal bone, which makes surgical correction somewhat more hazardous, but facial nerve function is rarely affected by the malformation. The tympanic membrane is frequently replaced by a bony plate, and a large variety of identified malformations and deformities of the ossicles are present. Management of the child with congenital aural atresia should begin with a complete evaluation so as to detect any associated abnormalities. If an earcanal is present, an attempt should be made to see whether the canal is complete or whether it becomes stenotic or atretic medially. This is often difficult to do in the small child and may occasionally require radiographic imaging.

More important than radiographic assessment is accurate determination of hearing thresholds. Differentiation of conduction from sensorineural components is important but often difficult in the young child. The use of both air and bone conduction auditory brain stem response (ABR) for threshold assessment may be pivotal. Because hearing rehabilitation must occur long before these children are surgical candidates, amplification should be provided even in those children who may later benefit from reconstructive operations. The need for hearing restoration is immediate and should not be delayed even a few weeks beyond birth. Educational and social development can be retarded by hearing loss, and the restoration of hearing after the critical developmental period may not compensate for the handicapping effects of early hearing loss. The available options include the use of conventional amplification, externally applied bone conducting hearing aids, and implantable bone-conducting hearing aids. As a general rule, when conventional amplification can be used, it is the treatment of choice. We prefer the use of the implantable bone-conducting aid, when appropriate, in patients with bilateral maximal conductive hearing losses and normal bone levels if they cannot be successfully fitted with conventional hearing aids. In patients with only conductive hearing losses, even if maximal, the continued use of amplification may provide perfectly adequate hearing restoration. Surgical repair of the external auditory canal, tympanic membrane, and middle ear space can be accomplished by a variety of different surgical techniques. Favorable outcomes are more likely in individuals with the least severe abnormalities. Frequently, the air-bone gap can be closed to 30 dB or less, but failure to close the air-bone gap is the most common problem associated with reconstructive surgery. Restenosis of the external auditory canal is relatively common. Finally, although the rate remains low, facial nerve injury occurs significantly more commonly after repair of congenital lesions than after repair of acquired lesions.

SPECIAL CONSIDERATION

Whether surgical repair of unilateral atresia should be undertaken depends entirely on the patient and the parents. It is often useful to wait until the child is old enough to participate in the decision for surgical repair of the congenital atresia. Surgical intervention is not without risks and complications.

Osteomas and Exostoses

Osteomas and exostoses are two distinct lesions that may develop and cause obstruction in the earcanal. They are very frequently confused.

Exostoses are periosteal outgrowths that develop in the bony earcanal, usually in individuals who have done a great deal of swimming in cold water. They are often multiple and bilateral. Removal is only necessary if the lesion is causing a large conductive hearing loss or recurrent otitis externa.

Osteomas, on the other hand, usually are unilateral and occur at the bony-cartilaginous junction of the earcanal. The cause of this lesion is unknown. As with exostoses, treatment is indicated only for conductive hearing loss or recurrent infection.

Keratosis Obturans

Keratosis obturans is due either to an abnormality in epithelial migration or to increased production of keratin debris or a combination of both. Keratosis obturans presents as an accumulation of keratin debris (often mixed with cerumen) in the earcanal. It is accompanied by hearing loss, otorrhea, and a foul odor. Removal of the debris usually reveals a canal that is circumferentially expanded, especially medially. Keratosis obturans is often bilateral and occurs most commonly in patients in their 20s and 30s. It is associated with chronic sinusitis and bronchiectasis. The audiologist will occasionally see these patients in the evaluation of the patient's hearing loss.

Treatment involves aggressive and regular aural cleaning. Irrigation with acidic solutions can help reduce the quantity of debris.

PITFALL

Keratosis obturans is often confused with cholesteatoma of the external auditory canal. Cholesteatoma of the external canal is generally focal and usually occurs lateral in the canal and in older individuals. It can be deeply invasive. Shallow canal cholesteatoma can be treated by marsupialization of the cholesteatoma sac. Larger, deeper cholesteatomas require surgical excision.

DISORDERS OF THE TYMPANIC MEMBRANE, MIDDLE EAR, AND MASTOID PROCESS

Tympanic Membrane Perforations

Tympanic membrane perforations can arise either as a consequence of infection or trauma. Acute otitis media frequently results in perforation of the tympanic membrane. Generally speaking, such perforations heal spontaneously, but occasionally the perforation fails to heal and becomes a permanent feature of the tympanic membrane. Severe, acute, necrotizing otitis media (almost always streptococcal) has a much higher incidence of tympanic membrane perforation than the usual middle ear infections. Chronic infection with an unusual organism, such as tuberculosis, produces a much higher rate of permanent tympanic membrane perforation than occurs in the epidemic otitis media of school children.

A variety of different types of trauma can produce tympanic membrane perforation. "Blast" trauma is much more common than penetrating trauma. The results of a slap to the side of the head, which completely occludes the external auditory canal, forcing a column of air down onto the tympanic membrane and rupturing it, is one form of blast trauma. It is apparently this mechanism of injury that is most frequently responsible for the tympanic membrane perforations associated with water skiing. Injuries involving water or traumatic tympanic membrane perforations contaminated with water shortly after their occurrence are less likely to heal. When infection complicates an acute tympanic membrane perforation, the probability of spontaneous healing is significantly reduced. With those caveats in mind, most tympanic membrane perforations heal spontaneously and without significant or meaningful residue.

Perforations of the tympanic membrane diagnosed on physical examination should be first categorized as to their location. They may occur either in the pars tensa or the pars flaccida. Perforations of the pars flaccida may be assumed to be cholesteatomas and should be managed as such. Perforations in the pars tensa can be divided into those that are central and those that are marginal. A central perforation has at least a small rim of intact tympanic membrane around it (Fig. 5–6). Marginal perforations extend all the way to the bony anulus of the external auditory canal. It is often difficult and sometimes impossible to determine whether an anterior perforation is marginal because the anterior canal wall makes it difficult to see the most anterior portion of the tympanic membrane. The distinction between central and marginal perforations is important because marginal perforations have the potential to develop into cholesteatomas and, therefore, should be considered dangerous. Central perforations, on the other hand, are unlikely to develop into cholesteatomas and are sometimes referred to as "safe" perforations. Size can be recorded either in terms of an estimate of diameter in millimeters or estimate of the percentage of tympanic membrane involved in the perforation. The location should be identified in terms of which quadrant or quadrants of the tympanic membrane are involved. Both location and size are important factors in determining the amount of conductive hearing loss associated with a particular perforation.

Three sorts of difficulties arise from chronic perforations of the tympanic membrane: (1) formation of cholesteatoma, (2) significant conductive hearing loss, and (3) recurrent infection. Hearing loss caused by tympanic membrane perforations is highly variable. Small pinpoint perforations may have no associated hearing loss and larger perforations may produce

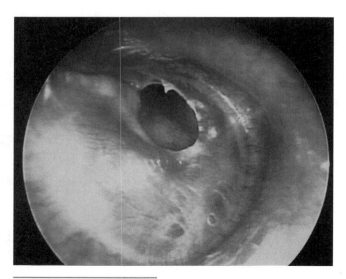

Figure 5–6   A small central perforation is seen involving the posterior superior portion of the tympanic membrane. (*See Color Plate 6.*)

losses up to 50 dB. Perforations directly over the round window niche may produce significant hearing loss because they eliminate phase cancellation. Conductive hearing losses greater than 40- to 50-dB suggest associated ossicular discontinuity or fixation. By permitting the ingress of bacteria from the external auditory canal into the middle ear space, perforations may lead to recurrent infections of the middle ear and mastoid process. If water is allowed to enter the earcanal, it is particularly likely to carry bacteria into the middle ear space (normally sterile) and further increase the likelihood of infection. Protection of the middle ear space from waterborne bacterial contamination is an essential part of management. Thus ear protection should be used for swimming or bathing.

Chronic obstruction of the external auditory canal also increases the likelihood of infections. Persons who use hearing aids or earplugs in an ear with a chronic perforation are much more likely to experience difficulty with recurrent mucopurulent infections and chronic otorrhea.

The treatment of tympanic membrane perforations is surgical repair. In individuals with marginal perforations, the propensity of these perforations to form cholesteatomas is sufficient to warrant surgical repair in most cases. Repair of central perforations, however, is entirely elective.

PEARL

All apparent perforations in the pars flaccida are cholesteatomas.

Tympanic Membrane Retractions

Tympanic membrane retractions occur almost exclusively as a result of eustachian tube dysfunction. The normally functioning eustachian tube remains closed at rest but should open episodically to equalize middle ear pressure with ambient barometric pressure. The eustachian tubes are opened by active muscular contraction of small palatal muscles during swallowing or yawning. If the tube remains chronically shut, negative pressure will develop in the middle ear. Negative middle ear pressure may result in the development of a retracted tympanic membrane, middle ear effusion, or both (Fig. 5–7).

Development of deep retractions in the pars flaccida or posterior superior quadrant of the tympanic membrane leads to cholesteatoma. Prolonged contact of the retracted tympanic membrane with the ossicles can cause ossicular erosion, ossicular discontinuity, and moderate-to-severe conductive hearing loss. Further atrophy will leave the tympanic membrane draped over the medial wall of the middle ear. This will produce functional elimination of the middle ear space. When the eardrum is left in this configuration for an extended time, fibrosis and scarring will occur, and the process will become irreversible (adhesive otitis media).

Treatment of retractions is difficult, especially in the pars flaccida region. A pressure-equalizing tube can be inserted in the region of the retraction if a middle ear space is still present. In cases of deep pars flaccida retractions that cannot be fully visualized, middle ear exploration to rule out the presence of cholesteatoma is warranted.

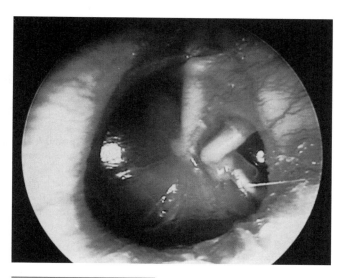

Figure 5–7   Marked retraction of the tympanic membrane is noted with a middle ear effusion. The incudostapedial joint is easily visualized. *(See Color Plate 7.)*

SPECIAL CONSIDERATION

Patients with poor eustachian tube function and tympanic membrane perforation may need to have a permanent tympanostomy tube placed at the time of tympanic membrane repair.

Otitis Media

Abnormal eustachian tube function appears to be a common pathological feature in the development of most forms of otitis media. If the eustachian tube is always open (patulous), bacterial-laden secretions from the nasopharynx may enter the middle ear and produce infection. By producing swelling of the mucous membranes of the eustachian tube and inhibiting normal ciliary function, middle ear effusions (either infected or uninfected) may themselves produce dysfunction of the eustachian tube and perpetuate their own condition. Infants and children are predisposed to otitis media because their eustachian tubes are more horizontal, shorter, and wider than those of adults. Palatal muscle function, as with muscle function generally, is less efficient in infants and small children than adults; therefore the active tubal opening is less reliable and vigorous.

Inflammation of the nasal end of the eustachian tube can produce sufficient swelling to obstruct it mechanically. Such inflammation may result from viral (a cold) or bacterial infection, chemical irritation (tobacco smoke, chlorinated pool water), or inhalant allergy. The consequences of long-term eustachian tube dysfunction include not only persistent or recurrent middle ear effusions with or without infection but also pathological alterations of the tympanic membrane and complications associated with the inner ear, mastoid process, or central nervous system, such as ossicular discontinuity, adhesive otitis media, or both.

Acute otitis media is one of the most common diseases of early childhood and affects at least 70% of children before the age of 3. It is the most common reason for the administration of antibiotics to children. Before the use of antibiotic medications, acute otitis media was the cause of significant mortality in infancy and childhood. Fortunately, current antimicrobials have significantly reduced (but not completely eliminated) the incidence of life-threatening complications. The peak incidence occurs between 6 and 24 months of age. It occurs more frequently during the winter months. Exposure to second-hand cigarette smoke and placement in day-care centers seem to increase the incidence of acute otitis media significantly. The disease is caused by infection with a number of different relatively common bacteria and generally responds to the institution of prompt antibiotic therapy. A worrisome new development is increasing resistance of these organisms to currently available antibiotics. Concern has recently developed that antibiotic resistance may increase in prevalence to the point where serious life-threatening complications are again common.

Acute otitis media is a purulent infection that begins with edema, hyperemia, and hemorrhage in the subepithelial space of the middle ear mucosa. These early changes are followed by the local infiltration of white blood cells and the accumulation of pus within the middle ear space (Fig. 5–8). Typically, acute otitis media is of relatively sudden onset. Because it represents the accumulation of pus within a closed body cavity, it is associated with significant systemic signs of infection, such as elevated temperature, malaise, and elevated white blood cell count. The ear is exquisitely painful, although no tenderness is present in the area of the auricle or periauricular tissues, as is seen with external otitis.

In untreated cases the condition resolves with spontaneous rupture of the tympanic membrane. The opening in the tympanic membrane allows the pus to drain out of the external auditory canal. Rupture of the tympanic membrane is

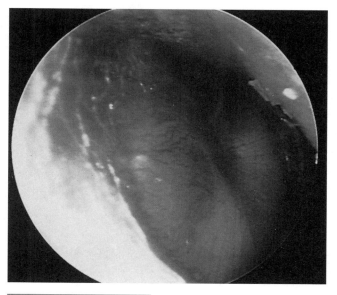

Figure 5–8   Purulent material is visualized behind a bulging tympanic membrane in acute otitis media. *(See Color Plate 8.)*

associated with very rapid relief of pain and prompt defervescence of fever. In more than 90% of cases, the tympanic membrane heals spontaneously and no residual perforation is present. Before the development of antibiotic therapy, most cases of acute otitis media resolved after spontaneous perforation. However, a significant minority did not resolve, and the affected child had chronic mastoiditis, sigmoid sinus thrombosis, facial nerve paralysis, labyrinthitis with complete neurosensory hearing loss, meningitis, or brain abscess develop. Many children died as a consequence of one or another of these complications.

A single episode of otitis media treated with appropriate antibiotics is generally followed by an effusion that clears within 1 month. In 90% of cases an effusion caused by an initial episode of acute otitis media clears within 3 months. When the middle ear space continues to harbor fluid for more than 3 months after an episode of acute otitis media, the condition is termed chronic middle ear effusion (Fig. 5–9). Although culture of such fluid shows that it does contain small numbers of viable bacteria, the condition is not an infection in the usual sense of the word. No associated pain, fever, or development of pus is present. Indeed, the condition is frequently asymptomatic and 50% of cases are "silent." Such cases can be diagnosed only on routine "well-baby" evaluations. The persistence of fluid behind the tympanic membrane presents difficulties if, and only if, it produces either significant conductive hearing loss or promotes frequently recurrent acute otitis media. The presence of this fluid in and of itself is of no great consequence. Therefore measurement of hearing threshold is crucial in the intelligent management of chronic middle ear effusion.

A child with normal-hearing thresholds who has relatively few middle ear infections need not be treated aggressively for the mere presence of middle ear fluid. When persistent middle ear fluid causes significant conductive hearing loss (greater than 15 dB in a child) or is associated with more than three episodes in 6 months or four episodes of acute otitis media per year, then treatment should be implemented. The use of prophylactic antibiotics has been advocated for many years. However, the rapid development of antimicrobial resistance in the organisms commonly responsible for acute otitis media now makes such protracted antibiotic treatment controversial.

Although otitis media is often a direct result of chronic eustachian tube dysfunction, several good clinical studies have shown that antihistamines and decongestants are of essentially no use whatsoever in the treatment of persistent middle ear fluid in children. The use of steroids remains controversial but can be effective. If effusions persist for more than 12 weeks and are associated with significant hearing loss, consideration should be given to the insertion of tympanostomy tubes (Fig. 5–10). In children with bilateral effusion who have conductive hearing losses greater than 15 or 20 decibels, justification for tympanostomy tube insertion is considerably reinforced. One must remember that the conductive hearing loss associated with middle ear effusions is variable, and audiometric evaluation may occur when a child is hearing relatively well. The observations of parents or teachers should be given great credence. When a documented or even suspected problem with the acquisition of speech and language skills or difficulty in school exists, insertion of tympanostomy tubes should be considered to eliminate the possibility of mild conductive hearing loss as an etiologic or confounding variable.

PEARL

The audiologist can often serve to reinforce the recommendations of tympanostomy tubes when parents appear hesitant by reviewing the effects of mild hearing loss on speech and language development.

Some children have special predisposing factors for otitis media with effusion. Children with cleft palate or Downs syndrome and patients with craniofacial syndromes such as

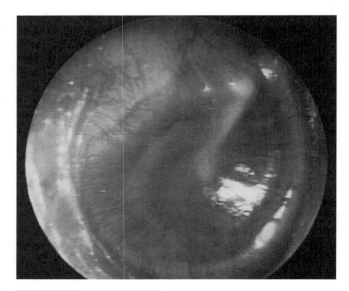

Figure 5–9   Tan-colored fluid is seen behind the tympanic membrane in chronic otitis media.

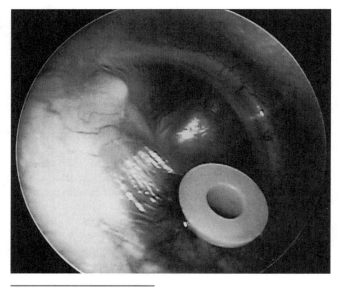

Figure 5–10   Otitis media with effusion has resolved with the placement of a tympanostomy tube. *(See Color Plate 9.)*

Treacher Collins or Crouzon's syndrome are especially predisposed to otitis. These patients should be evaluated individually, bearing in mind their congenital anomalies. Almost all will benefit from tympanostomy tubes. In children with concurrent sensorineural hearing loss, the use of tympanostomy tubes may be more urgent. If the sensorineural component is severe or profound, elimination of the conductive component may be the difference between aidable and unaidable hearing. Children with other medical problems that produce febrile conditions or with drug allergies may benefit from the early insertion of tympanostomy tubes. Children readily subject to febrile seizures may have little tolerance for the acute episodes of otitis media that most children deal with easily. In patients older than 4, a number of studies have now shown that hypertrophied adenoid tissue plays a significant etiologic role in the persistence of middle ear effusion.

In children older than 4 with persistent fluid, consideration should be given to simultaneous adenoidectomy at the time of tympanostomy tube insertion. The insertion of tympanostomy tubes is a relatively simple procedure. In many children older than 7 or 8 it can be performed as an outpatient office procedure, as is generally done with adults. However, in younger children, a short general anesthetic is necessary. The tympanostomy tubes act as prosthetic eustachian tubes. At the time of tympanostomy tube insertion, the fluid is mechanically aspirated from the middle ear space. The tympanostomy tube then permits effective pressure regulation, equalizing the ambient pressure between the earcanal and the middle ear space and draining middle ear fluid through the tube into the earcanal. The tubes are spontaneously extruded from the tympanic membrane after about 1 year. Complications related to the insertion of tympanostomy tubes are relatively infrequent.

Although the tympanic membrane heals completely after extrusion of tympanostomy tubes in 97 to 98% of cases, in 2 to 3% the tympanic membrane fails to heal after extrusion of the tube. This is somewhat more common with larger tubes and is more likely to occur when the tube is extruded in the presence of active infection. Even though the rate of permanent perforation related to tympanostomy tube placement is low, tympanostomy tube insertion has become sufficiently frequent so that iatrogenic perforation now accounts for a significant number of permanent tympanic membrane perforations in young children. Surgery to repair iatrogenic tympanic membrane perforation is successful greater than 90% of the time.

Ten to 25% of patients with tympanostomy tubes will develop an episode of otorrhea at some time. In most such cases, the infection can be effectively eliminated with a 5- to 7-day course of topical antibiotic drops placed into the external auditory canal.

Some cases of tympanosclerosis of the tympanic membrane appear to be related to the placement of tympanostomy tubes, but it is generally of no consequence. Such complications need to be compared with the rather serious complications of persistent otitis media and the developmental and educational consequences of persistent conductive hearing loss.

Tympanosclerosis and Myringosclerosis

Recurrent infection can deposit hyaline (a calcium-like substance) in the middle ear. These hyaline deposits termed

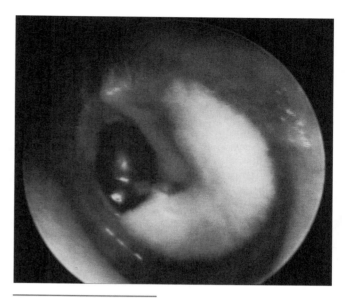

Figure 5–11 Tympanosclerosis is noted involving three fourths of the tympanic membrane. *(See Color Plate 10.)*

"tympanosclerosis," may be limited to the tympanic membrane or may involve the heads of the ossicles within the middle ear space. Tympanosclerotic plaques limited to the tympanic membrane are easily noticed but, although they may present a dramatic appearance, rarely produce hearing loss or other alteration of middle ear function (Fig. 5–11). On the other hand, tympanosclerotic deposition around the heads of the ossicles will produce fixation and maximum conductive hearing loss. Tympanometry will often show a type As tympanogram, indicating increased stiffness of the tympanic membrane. The development of tympanosclerosis of the tympanic membrane and middle ear space appears to be independent. Although good evidence exists that development of tympanosclerosis of the tympanic membrane is associated with injury to the drum (tympanic membrane perforation), the apparent cause of middle ear tympanosclerosis is entirely unknown. Fortunately, middle ear tympanosclerosis is uncommon.

PITFALL

Although it is tempting to attempt to remove tympanosclerosis from the ossicles, it is usually unsuccessful. Hearing aids are the best option for hearing rehabilitation in this group of patients.

Cholesteatoma

The lateral surface of the tympanic membrane consists of skin, and, like skin in other portions of the body, it sheds epithelial cells (desquamates). The normally functioning external auditory canal removes these shed components as they are produced. If a sufficient portion of the tympanic membrane is retracted far enough into the mastoid process, these shed epithelial cells can no longer escape out of the external auditory canal and they accumulate as a mass of dead skin within the temporal bone. Such collections of desquamated skin cells will erode bone slowly through a combination of pressure necrosis and enzymatic activity. Such a collection of dead skin trapped within the middle space or temporal bone and increasing slowly in size is termed a "cholesteatoma" (Fig. 5–12). The condition may also be referred to as a "keratoma" or "epidermoid inclusion cyst" or, in the older otologic literature, as a "pearly tumor." The dead skin components at the center of such skin-filled cysts are an excellent medium for bacterial growth and eventually infection will develop. Infection accelerates the process of bony destruction.

Infections in such cysts are difficult to eradicate because blood-borne antibiotics are not delivered to these nonvascular areas, and topical drops cannot penetrate to the core of the mass of dead skin. As cholesteatomas expand, they do so only

at the expense of surrounding normal structures (see Fig. 5–13). Thus cholesteatomas may result in any one of the following complications: (1) destruction of one or all of the ossicles producing conductive hearing loss; (2) erosion of the bone of the labyrinthine capsule with penetration of the membranous labyrinth, causing a severe or profound sensorineural hearing loss and overwhelming vertigo (labyrinthine fistula); (3) bacterial infection of the labyrinthine fluids producing bacterial labyrinthitis and total hearing loss. Because the fluids within the labyrinth are in direct communication with the cerebrospinal fluid, bacterial meningitis frequently develops as a consequence of bacterial labyrinthitis. Untreated bacterial meningitis may be fatal within a matter of only a few hours; (4) erosion into the cranial cavity producing either meningitis or brain abscess; (5) thrombosis or infection of the veins draining the brain, producing brain swelling, stroke, coma, and death; (6) thrombosis and infection of the major venous outflow tract (sigmoid sinus) may

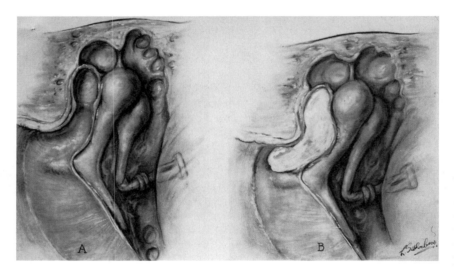

Figure 5–12 **(A)** Development of a retraction pocket in the pars flaccida region of the tympanic membrane. **(B)** Over time, the retraction pocket fills with squamous debris. (From Nager [1993], with permission.) *(See Color Plate 11.)*

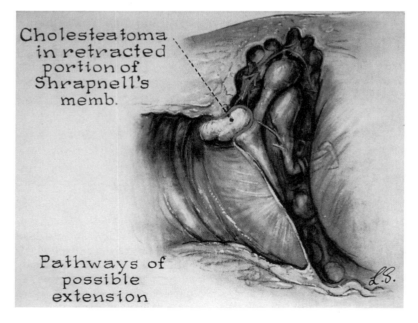

Figure 5–13 Cholesteatoma can take several paths of erosion into the middle ear. All routes usually result in ossicular erosion. (From Nager [1993], with permission.) *(See Color Plate 12.)*

produce metastatic infection, brain abscess, and death; and (7) erosion into and paralysis of the facial nerve.

Surgical removal is the only reliable treatment and requires mastoidectomy in virtually all cases. Because the complications of cholesteatoma may be fatal, surgical therapy has as its goal complete removal of cholesteatoma and creation of a "safe" ear not subject to recurrent disease. Mastoidectomy itself has no effect on hearing. However eradication of disease usually requires removal of one or more of the ossicles. Reconstruction of the disrupted middle ear transformer mechanism is of secondary importance. Even so, every effort is made to restore hearing when this is consistent with elimination of serious disease.

PEARL

A second-look procedure is recommended in most cases of cholesteatoma, 6 months after the initial surgery to check for residual disease that may have been missed at the initial operation. At this time, if no disease is found, ossicular reconstruction is usually performed.

Otosclerosis

Otosclerosis is more properly termed "otospongiosis." However, the term "otosclerosis" is so enshrined in the literature that its continued widespread use is irreversible. Otosclerosis is a disease process in which vascular spongy bone replaces the normally hard bone of the labyrinthine capsule. It occurs most frequently in the area of the oval window. In about 10% of affected individuals the otosclerotic process extends to involve the footplate and annular ligament. When this occurs, mobility of the footplate will be progressively reduced and a conductive hearing loss will develop slowly. Three quarters of all patients will develop disease in both ears. Evidence supports the notion that release of toxic enzymes into the perilymphatic spaces of the inner ear may cause progressive neurosensory hearing impairment and that this can be arrested by treatment of sodium fluoride. However, the diagnosis is difficult, especially in patients without concurrent stapes fixation, and the frequency with which "cochlear" otosclerosis occurs is not known.

Otosclerosis is hereditary in many (but certainly not all) cases. Although the exact mechanism of inheritance is unknown, a dominant pattern with variable penetrance is favored by most researchers. Definitive diagnosis depends on middle ear exploration with visualization of the otosclerotic focus and mechanical verification of stapes fixation. Presurgical diagnosis is based on the presence of slowly progressive conductive hearing loss in the absence of concurrent or preceding chronic ear disease. Presurgical diagnosis is accurate in about 90% of cases.

The cardinal audiometric finding in otosclerosis is a progressively increasing air-bone gap. Early in the course of the disease, when only the anterior portion of the stapes is fixed, a marked low-frequency air-bone gap is seen. As footplate fixation becomes complete, high frequencies become involved; and the loss becomes a flat, conductive hearing loss. Depression of bone conduction scores isolated to the 2000 Hz range

is characteristic of otosclerosis and referred to as "Carhart's notch." Tympanometry will often reveal a type A_S tympanogram despite a normal-appearing tympanic membrane.

When surgical correction is desired, the fixed stapes is completely or partially removed and replaced with a prosthesis. The operation takes about 45 minutes and may be performed with the patient under local anesthesia. It is a day surgical procedure and does not require hospitalization. A wide variety of different sorts of prosthesis and techniques have been used and most have produced excellent results. Indeed 95% of patients undergoing surgery for otosclerosis will experience a closure of the air-bone gap to within 10 dB. Three to 5% of patients will experience no improvement and will therefore continue to be good candidates for amplification. The biggest risk associated with stapedectomy is the 1 to 2% chance of complete and profound neurosensory hearing loss associated with the operative procedure. The reason for such catastrophic loss has never been completely clarified, but it does not seem to be necessarily related to technical intraoperative difficulties.

Ossicular Chain Discontinuity

Ossicular discontinuity may occur from a variety of causes. In children the most frequent cause is necrosis of the long process of the incus because of recurrent or persistent middle ear infection or effusion. In most such cases the ossicular discontinuity is not complete, but rather the necrotic distal segment of the long process of the incus is replaced by a thin band of fibrous tissue. The connection between the long process of the incus and the capitulum of the stapes thus becomes fibrous rather than bony. As such, it transmits sound inefficiently, and a significant conductive hearing loss is apparent. However, it is uncommon for the conductive hearing loss to be maximal. A significant percentage of these children have a rather interesting audiometric finding. The air-bone gap becomes larger in the higher frequencies than in the lower frequencies. This high-frequency accentuated air-bone gap is thought to be characteristic of fibrous union of the incudostapedial joint. A type A_d tympanogram is seen.

In adults trauma is one of the most common causes of ossicular dislocation. In general, trauma produces inferior dislocation of the incus. The long process loses contact with the capitulum of the stapes. The incudomalleolar joint can be disrupted at the same time. Less frequently, trauma produces subluxation of the stapes into the oval window. When this occurs, associated dizziness, neurosensory hearing loss, and conductive hearing loss may occur. If such a situation is suspected, then immediate surgical intervention should be recommended to limit the amount of neurosensory hearing loss and to close the opening between the inner and middle ear space (perilymph fistula).

Previous surgical procedures can leave discontinuities in the ossicular chain. Oftentimes, surgery for cholesteatoma requires removal of part or all of one or more of the ossicles. Most frequently, the incus needs to be removed because of irremediable involvement with cholesteatoma. The head of the malleus may also have to be removed and, frequently, the capitulum of the stapes. In many cases bony destruction of the ossicles by the cholesteatomatous process has occurred before surgical intervention.

Treatment of ossicular discontinuity or dislocation is called "ossiculoplasty." Repair of the ossicular chain is possible in most cases. Unfortunately, results are not as good with repair of defects involving the malleus and incus as stapes replacement is for repair of otosclerosis. Closure of the air-bone gap to 10 dB occurs in less than three quarters of all patients but depends somewhat on the nature of the hearing deficit. When the malleus and incus and stapes superstructure are gone and a total ossicular replacement prosthesis must be used, closure of the air-bone gap to within 25 dB is considered a good result. On the other hand, when the conductive hearing loss is caused by necrosis of the long process of the incus, complete closure can frequently be obtained.

Neoplasms

Glomus tumors are the most common benign neoplasms of the middle ear. They are vascular tumors derived from paraganglionic tissue in the middle ear and are more properly referred to as "paragangliomas" (Fig. 5–14). Glomus tumors can occur in all age groups but are most commonly found in middle-aged adults (Ogura et al, 1978). A subset of patients with glomus tumors have a genetic linkage, which is believed to be autosomal dominant with variable penetrance. In such families, individuals often have multiple glomus tumors of the skull base and neck.

The symptoms produced by glomus tumors are often related to its vascular nature and its tendency to erode surrounding structures. Most commonly patients present with conductive hearing loss, pulsatile unilateral tinnitus, and an observable middle ear mass. Tympanometry will reveal a type A tympanogram with tiny sawtooth variations, which occur as a result of changes in tympanic membrane compliance related to blood flow in the middle ear mass. Glomus tumors can grow to relatively large size before they are detected, and not infrequently cranial nerve palsies are noted.

Treatment is complete surgical excision. Radiation may be used for advanced lesions or those that extend intracranially, but glomus tumors are not very radiosensitive in general.

PEARL

Brown's sign refers to the blanching noted when applying positive pressure to the tympanic membrane of a patient with a glomus tumor.

DISORDERS OF THE INNER EAR AND INTERNAL AUDITORY CANAL

Sensorineural Hearing Loss

Sensorineural hearing loss has many causes, which can be roughly divided into congenital and acquired causes.

Congenital sensorineural hearing losses may be divided into genetic and nongenetic causes. A large variety of known genetic inner ear hearing loss syndromes exist. A variety of nongenetic sensorineural hearing losses that are congenital in nature have also been described. The most common is probably the maternal rubella syndrome in which deafness is associated with congenital cataracts and congenital heart disease. The availability of vaccines to prevent this disease has significantly reduced the incidence of hearing loss attributable to rubella. Toxoplasmosis, cytomegalovirus, and syphilis are other infections that can involve the developing embryo and produce postnatal hearing loss. Each of these processes can produce progressive sensorineural hearing losses of childhood. Ototoxic drugs given to the mother during pregnancy may produce congenital hearing loss. Hypoxia during intrauterine development may produce significant injury to the auditory system. Prenatal injury to the vascular system of the branchial arches can produce either unilateral or bilateral hypoplasia of the membranous labyrinth. Perinatal hypoxia caused by birth trauma may also result in sensorineural hearing loss, as may intracranial hemorrhage complicating delivery.

Acquired sensorineural hearing loss can also be divided into genetic and nongenetic forms (Fig. 5–15). The nongenetic causes are well known and probably consist most frequently of losses caused by infection, neoplasm, administration of ototoxic agents, noise, or trauma. A large variety of genetic causes for delayed neurosensory hearing loss exist. Cochlear

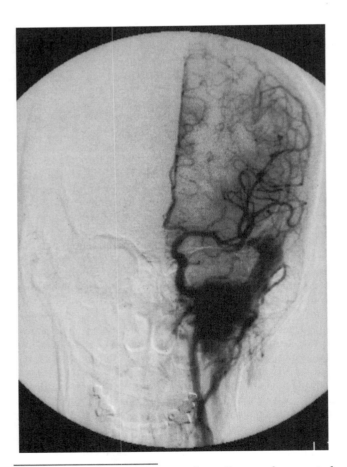

Figure 5–14   Glomus tumors can be quite vascular as noted in this angiogram showing a large glomus jugulare tumor with multiple feeding vessels.

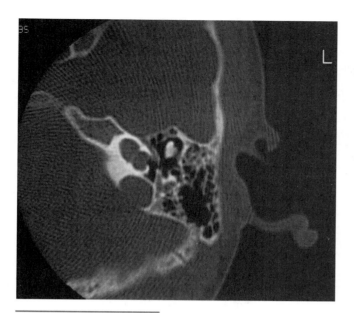

Figure 5–15 Genetic sensorineural hearing loss was noted in this patient with a common cavity deformity of the cochlea.

otosclerosis has already been mentioned as one such manifestation. Progressive sensorineural hearing loss can be attributed to a large variety of syndromes displaying musculoskeletal features. Among them are Paget's disease, van der Hoeve's syndrome, Alport's syndrome, and all of the mucopolysaccharidoses, such as Hunter's syndrome, Hurler's syndrome, Sanfilippo's syndrome, Morquio's syndrome, and Maroteaux-Lamy syndrome. Other well-documented syndromes are associated with visual problems, such as Alström's syndrome, Refsum's syndrome, and Cockayne's syndrome. However, the largest variety of delayed, genetically mediated sensorineural hearing losses occur sporadically as a consequence of a recessive inheritance pattern and are fortunately not associated with specific syndromes.

Hearing loss is often associated with meningitis, especially when caused by *Streptococcus pneumoniae*.

Progressive Sensorineural Hearing Loss

A large number of persons with hearing impairment have progressive losses. Many of these individuals have well-identified syndromes such as Alport's, renal tubular acidosis, branchio-otorenal syndrome, Archer's syndrome, Refsum's syndrome, Norrie's disease, Wallenberg's syndrome, osteogenesis imperfecta, osteopetrosis, or mucopolysaccharide storage diseases. Some will have familial tumors. The evaluation of individuals with progressive sensorineural hearing loss can identify a cause in as many as 50 to 60% of cases. This should include complete history and computed tomography scan to identify labyrinthine anomalies or neurofibromatosis. However, a significant number of persons with progressive sensorineural hearing loss have no obvious cause.

Inner ear fluid imbalance can result in progressive sensorineural hearing loss. It may involve perilymphatic fistula or Meniere's disease. Vertigo or disequilibrium may accompany the hearing loss about half the time. Epstein and Reilly

(1989) have documented that up to 6% of all children with sensorineural hearing loss had perilymph fistula. Perilymph fistula can be difficult to diagnose without surgical exploration. The likelihood of perilymph fistula is increased if a history of antecedent head trauma or barometric trauma or a history of Mondini's deformity exists. Abnormal electrocochleography (ECDG) certainly increases the possibility of perilymph fistula being the cause of the progressive sensorineural loss. If perilymph fistula is the cause, operative repair may prevent further deterioration and, although infrequently, in some patients may improve thresholds.

Noise-Induced Hearing Loss

Noise-induced hearing loss has become recognized as a significant problem, especially in industrialized societies. Occupational noise exposure has been well studied, but non-occupational noise exposure also accounts for a large amount of hearing loss in the general population.

Noise-induced hearing loss begins with selective loss at 4000 Hz, which is seen as a notch on the audiogram (Fig. 5–16). With continued exposure, the notch widens and will affect all the high frequencies. Eventually, hearing loss can be seen in the middle and lower frequencies.

Initial exposure to loud noise causes a threshold shift, which is reversible within the first 24 hours. The threshold shift may be associated with tinnitis. Continued exposure can lead to permanent shifts. Temporary threshold shifts may occur with the discharge of a firearm without hearing protection or even after attendance at a rock concert. Permanent threshold shifts are often seen in persons with occupations requiring continued exposure to loud noises, such as airline mechanics or artillary experts.

Brookhauser et al (1991) have reported on 114 children who showed progressive neurosensory hearing loss that appears to be noise induced. A striking male predominance exists. One quarter of these cases occurred before 10 years of age. Consequently, inquiry related to noise exposure must be made even in preadolescent children with high-frequency progressive types of losses. It is especially important to inquire whether any noise exposure occurred within the 24 hours before the onset of hearing loss, because it may be a temporary threshold shift only.

Evidence suggests that a great individual variability exists in susceptibility to noise-induced hearing loss. Occupational noise limits are designed to eliminate noise-induced hearing loss in the average person and therefore may not protect the most sensitive individuals.

Aging and Hearing Loss

Hearing loss resulting from the physiologic process of aging alone is known as "presbycusis." Most individuals will suffer increasing hearing loss with advancing age. Most authorities believe that at least a portion of this hearing loss occurs solely because of the aging process and is not related to cumulative noise or other environmental exposures. However, the Mabaan tribesman, who live in a remote area of the Sudan, have been found to have relatively normal-hearing even at advanced age. Identifying and studying presbycusis is difficult because of the effects of noise exposure, as well as diet, hypertension, diabetes, or smoking on hearing thresholds.

PURE TONE AUDIOGRAM

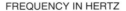

FREQUENCY IN HERTZ

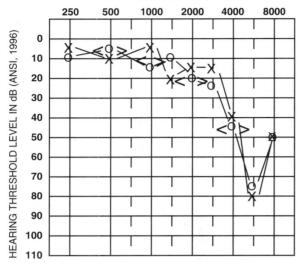

	RIGHT	LEFT
O	Air	X
△	Air Masked	D
<	Bone	>
[	Bone Masked	]
▶	No Response	◀

DNT: Did Not Test
CNT: Could Not Test

SPEECH

	RIGHT	LEFT
SRT	10 dB	10 dB
WRS	88 %	84 %

WRS Level 80 dB HL

| PTA | 13 dB | 10 dB |

Figure 5–16   Audiogram demonstrating noise-induced hearing loss. Note the notching present at 4000 Hz.

Schuknecht (1955), considered the father of modern temporal bone histopathology, has classified presbycusis into four distinct types: sensory presbycusis, neural presbycusis, metabolic presbycusis, and cochlear presbycusis.

- Sensory presbycusis is characterized by the loss of hair cells in the organ of Corti. The audiograms of individuals with sensory presbycusis typically reveal a high-frequency loss with a steep, sharp dropoff at 2000 Hz.
- Neural presbycusis occurs as a result of the loss of auditory neurons within the cochlea. This loss occurs evenly throughout the cochlear nerve and cochlea. Pure tone thresholds are not affected until approximately 90% of neurons are lost. Speech discrimination is often disproportionately worse than pure tone audiometry would suggest.
- Metabolic presbycusis is characterized by atrophy of the stria vascularis, which provides nutritional support to the labyrinth. The audiogram is characterized by a flat or slightly descending audiogram with good preservation of speech discrimination.
- Cochlear conductive presbycusis is still speculative but is believed to be caused by thickening of the basilar membrane, especially in the basal turn. This leads to high-frequency hearing loss.

PITFALL

Categorizing patients on the basis of audiograms is difficult because patients often have more than one pathological process occuring simultaneously.

Otoxicity

A great number of medications are known to cause damage to the ear with associated auditory and vestibular dysfunction. In general these drugs can be divided into distinct categories, including antiinflammatory drugs, aminoglycoside antibiotics, loop diuretics, antimalarials, chemotherapeutic agents, and ototopical medications.

Ototoxicity as a result of aspirin use was first recognized in 1877. Aspirin ototoxicity is manifest as a flat mild-to-moderate reversible sensorineural hearing loss accompanied by pronounced tinnitus. The serum level required to produce symptoms is between 35 and 40 mg. This correlates to approximately 6 to 8 g/day or 18 to 24 regular-strength aspirin tablets. The mechanism of action of salicylate ototoxicity has not been identified, but it is believed to be due to reversible enzyme inhibition. Other NSAIDs, specifically ibuprofen and naproxen, have been associated with a lesser incidence of associated hearing loss. However, the hearing loss associated with these medications is often permanent.

Aminoglycoside antibiotics are still the first-line treatment for a large variety of infectious processes despite their known side effects of nephrotoxicity and ototoxicity. The ototoxic effects of aminoglycosides correlate directly with the amount of drug delivered to the perilymph. The peak concentration of drug in the perilymph lags approximately 10 to 15 hours behind the serum peak levels. The ototoxic effects of the aminoglycosides are due to direct injury to the neural epithelial cells. This injury occurs primarily to the outer hair cells in the basal turn of the cochlea. This injury pattern is manifest as high-frequency sensorineural hearing loss on the audiogram. Inner hair cells may become damaged at high levels of toxicity. Within the vestibular system, type 1 hair cells are more sensitive to injury than type 2 hair cells.

Different types of aminoglycosides show different patterns of ototoxicity. Some are preferentially ototoxic, whereas others primarily affect the vestibular system. Streptomycin and gentamycin are primarily vestibulotoxic and have been used successfully to selectively destroy vestibular function as a part of the treatment of Meniere's disease. Streptomycin and gentamycin are sufficiently specific for the vestibular system so that hearing can often be preserved. Dihydrostreptomycin, neomycin, amikacin, and tobramycin are primarily cochleotoxic.

Prevention of the ototoxic effects of aminoglycosides is difficult. Monitoring of serum peak and especially trough levels is helpful, because toxicity is closely related to serum trough levels. Daily audiometric testing is usually not possible because of the gravity of illness typically present in patients receiving these drugs. When possible, high-frequency audiometry can be used to monitor the possibility of hearing loss during aminoglycoside treatment. Weekly or biweekly vestibular testing can detect vestibular injury before serious balance dysfunction becomes permanent.

Loop diuretics act by inhibiting reabsorption of electrolytes and water in the kidney. Toxicity is most likely in patients with preexisting renal dysfunction or patients receiving other potentially ototoxic medications such as aminoglycoside antibiotics. The toxic effects are manifest by direct injury to hair cells and damage to the stria vascularis. Hearing loss is usually temporary, resolving after cessation of the drugs. Toxic effects can be limited by avoiding rapid intravenous infusion.

Both quinine and chloroquine, commonly used to treat malaria, have been associated with hearing loss even at very small doses. Quinine, used for treatment of leg cramps, has also been associated with hearing loss. The hearing loss is usually temporary and primarily in the high frequencies because the basal turn of the cochlea is affected.

Many chemotherapeutic agents are known to have ototoxic effects. These include cisplatin, bleomycin, 5-flurouracil, and nitrogen mustard. The most studied drug is cisplatin, which is known to have its effects on the outer hair cells of the basal turn of the cochlea. The ototoxicity of cisplatin is dose dependent and permanent, as with aminoglycosides. There does appear to be individual genetic variability in susceptibility to toxicity.

Ototopical preparations have been shown to cause hair cell death and hearing loss repeatedly when instilled into the middle ear of experimental animals. Meyerhoff et al, (1983) have shown that a single application of commercial preparations containing neomycin, polymixin B, and propylene glycol (Cortisporin) can cause total hair cell destruction and significant vestibular injury in chinchillas. However, very few reports of ototoxicity from topically applied antibiotics have been reported in humans. Anatomical differences between experimental animal models and humans probably are responsible for the discrepancies. The round window niche of experimental animals is highly exposed, whereas in humans it lies deep within a bony niche. In addition, the round window membrane in humans is 6 to 10 times thicker than in experimental animals. Newer ototopical agents such as the fluroquinolones (ciprofloxacin, ofloxacin) have been shown to be effective in treating otitis externa without ototoxic effects.

Vestibular Neuronitis

Vestibular neuronitis is characterized by acute onset of unilateral peripheral vestibular dysfunction in the absence of auditory dysfunction. It becomes manifest as prolonged severe rotational vertigo with accompanying nausea. Early in the course of the disorder, spontaneous nystagmus can be detected beating toward the affected ear. The vertigo improves gradually over the first few days. However, the patient will often experience mild positional vertigo for weeks to months after the acute event. Symptoms commonly resolve completely within 6 months. Electronystagmography (ENG) will initially show hyporesponsiveness of the affected ear.

The cause is believed to be viral in nature, because up to 40% of affected patients had a preceding viral illness (Anttinen et al, 1983). Treatment is traditionally supportive, with antiemetics and vestibular suppressants. High-dose, short-term systemic steroids may also be helpful.

Benign Paroxysmal Positional Vertigo

Benign paroxysmal positional vertigo (BPPV) is a common disorder. Individuals with this disorder complain of brief rotational vertigo (15 to 30 sec) associated with head movement and rapid position change. Brief vertigo after rolling onto one side in bed at night is virtually pathognomonic, but symptoms also commonly occur with neck hyperextension (e.g. reaching for something on a high shelf) and bending over. Symptoms can be provoked when the patient's head is moved rapidly into a supine position with the head turned such that the affected ear is 30 to 45 degrees below the horizontal. This position is known as the Dix-Hallpike maneuver after the two individuals who fully defined the characteristics of BPPV. The vertigo has a brief latency (usually 1 to 5 seconds), limited duration, and is fatigable if the position is repeated. Characteristically, the nystagmus generated is predominantly rotatory with the fast component directed toward the affected ear.

Two theories exist regarding the cause of BPPV. The first, known as "cupulolithiasis" proposes that debris or fragments of degenerating otoconia from the utricle become adherent to the cupula of the posterior semicircular canal. This converts the canal from an organ sensitive to angular rotation to a gravity-sensitive organ. When the canal is in a plane parallel to the force of gravity, the cupula is inappropriately deflected producing vertigo.

The second theory is known as "canalithiasis." This hypothesis proports that the debris is free floating in the posterior semicircular canal. When the head is moved into the provoking position, the debris moves to the most dependent position of the canal, which causes the endolymph to move away from the ampulla, causing deflection of the cupulla and vertigo.

Treatment of BPPV focuses on several repositioning maneuvers designed to deposit the posterior semicircular canal debris into the vestibule. Epley's maneuver is based on the canalithiasis theory (Epley, 1992), whereas Semont's liberatory maneuver is based on the cupulolithiasis theory (Semont et al, 1988). A second treatment approach, designed by Norre and Beckers is based on vestibular habituation. Provoking positions are identified and repeated 5 to 10 times two to three times daily until the patient is symptom free for 2 days in a row (Norre & Beckers, 1988). The treatment approach is modified on the basis of patient factors, such as neck mobility, motivation and compliance of the patient, and anxiety level. All treatments appear equally effective at 6 weeks after treatment (Herdman, 1993).

BPPV is a specific pathological and clinical entity. A large number of other causes for positional vertigo exist. The brief disequilibrium and vertigo that follow labyrinthitis and post-traumatic vertigo are two good examples. Such conditions (there are others) are often referred to as benign positional vertigo and should not be confused with BPPV. Nomenclature is inconsistent and care should be exercised to ascertain which condition is being discussed.

Perilymph Fistula

Perilymph fistula (PLF) occurs when disruption of the barrier between the perilymphatic space of the inner ear and the middle ear occurs with loss of perilymph. This can occur in a variety of clinical situations, including head trauma, barotrauma, congenital malformations of the inner ear, post-stapedectomy or any situation that may increase cerebrospinal fluid pressure. PLF may also occur spontaneously (Paparella et al, 1991).

Common complaints include episodic vertigo, disequilibrium, and ataxia (Kohut et al, 1986). But presentation is highly variable and often includes some hearing loss. The clinical presentation is similar to Meniere's disease and may be indistinguishable from Meniere's disease (Table 5–2).

TABLE 5–2   Comparison of Meniere's disease and perilymph fistula

	Meniere's Disease	Perilymph Fistula
Age at presentation	Third to sixth decade	Any age
History of trauma	No	Often
Abnormal ECOG	Yes	Yes
Hearing loss	Usually low frequency fluctuating loss	Variable
Family history	Present in 20%	No
Vertigo	Episodic, rotational, lasts minutes to 1–2 h	Variable

No one test is diagnostic for PLF. Platform and ENG fistula tests, when positive, strongly suggest fistula if Meniere's disease and syphilis can be excluded. ECOG, which provides an electrophysiological measure of the cochlear microphonic, summating potential (SP), and action potential (AP) of the cochlear nerve has been shown to be sensitive in the diagnosis of PLF. Elevated SP/AP ratios are seen in up to 60% of patients with confirmed PLF (Roland & Marple, 1997). Even intraoperatively, diagnosis is difficult because irrigation, blood, or injected anesthetic are often present in the middle ear and cannot be distinguished from escaping perilymph. Perilymph fistulas may leak fluid only intermittently, adding to the diagnostic difficulty.

Diagnosis of PLF often depends on history. When hearing loss, disequilibrium, or vertigo closely follows head trauma, rapid external pressure change (aircraft descent, scuba diving), or interval increase in cerebrospinal fluid pressure (straining, sneezing, coughing), PLF should be considered.

When hearing levels are stable, initial treatment is usually medical and includes bedrest, head elevation, and avoidance of situations that may increase intracranial pressure such as

sneezing and straining. Surgical treatment is considered in patients with deteriorating hearing levels or with incapacitating or protracted vertigo. Surgical treatment consists of oval and round window grafting. Vestibular symptoms often resolve promptly after repair, but recovery of hearing is uncommon.

Meniere's Disease

Meniere's disease is characterized by four symptoms: (1) episodes of whirling vertigo lasting several minutes to several hours; (2) low-pitched roaring tinnitus occurring or worsening during a vertiginous attack; (3) fluctuating low-tone sensorineural hearing loss; and (4) a sense of fullness or pressure in the affected ear that can be very severe. The vertigo is frequently violent and associated with nausea and vomiting, diaphoresis, and pallor. The onset of symptoms is typically between the third and sixth decades, with a slight female preponderance. Only about 3 to 4% of patients with Meniere's disease are seen in the pediatric age group. Twenty to 40% of patients will eventually have bilateral involvement, and 20% have a positive family history.

The histological correlate of Meniere's disease is endolymphatic hydrops, which can only be confirmed by postmortem temporal bone examination. When endolymphatic hydrops or Meniere's disease is suspected, the use of ECOG and other vestibular testing may be helpful. ECOG will show an elevated SP/AP ratio. Consequently, although ECOG is helpful in establishing the inner ear cause of a patient's symptoms and can often pinpoint which ear is afflicted, it does not help distinguish between Meniere's disease and perilymph fistula. ENG and sinusoidal harmonic acceleration can be useful in documenting unilateral labyrinthine dysfunction and confirming the diagnosis of Meniere's disease. The disease is usually progressive. Early in the course of the disease, hearing often returns completely to normal between attacks, but over months or years a permanent hearing loss usually develops. This can often make early diagnosis difficult because by the time the patient is seen for evaluation, the symptoms have temporarily subsided. The hearing loss may follow any pattern, but low-frequency losses are more common in the early course of the disease. Patients with long-standing disease, on the other hand, are more likely to have flat losses (Figs. 5–17 to 5–19). It is not possible to predict the course of the disease in individual patients. Some individuals will experience a relatively indolent variety with attacks separated by years; others will lose all hearing and balance function over a period of several months. Most patients follow an intermediate course, with attacks coming in clusters lasting several weeks and separated by months or even years of symptom-free periods. The development of complete anacusis, loss of hearing, is uncommon: hearing loss usually stabilizes at a flat 50- to 70-dB level. Word recognition scores are variably affected but often well preserved. The definitive diagnosis is difficult and depends on the documentation of a fluctuating low-tone sensorineural hearing loss associated with abnormal vestibular function. The presence of abnormal ECOG strongly reinforces the diagnosis.

Most patients improve with medical management. Avoidance of caffeine and nicotine, which can exacerbate symptoms, is advised. The mainstay of treatment is the use of

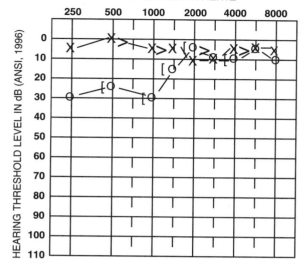

PURE TONE AUDIOGRAM
FREQUENCY IN HERTZ

	RIGHT		LEFT
	O	Air	X
	Δ	Air Masked	D
	<	Bone	>
	[	Bone Masked	]
	▲	No Response	▲

DNT: Did Not Test
CNT: Could Not Test

SPEECH

	RIGHT	LEFT
SRT	NA	NA
WRS	92 %	100 %

WRS Level 80 dB HL

PTA	20 dB	5 dB

Figure 5–17   Audiogram demonstrating the typical findings in a patient with early Meniere's disease. Note the mild low-frequency sensorineural hearing loss.

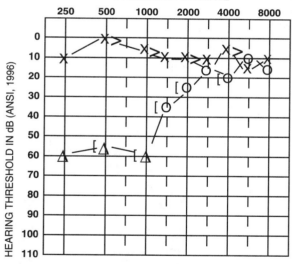
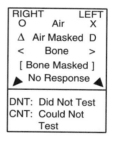

PURE TONE AUDIOGRAM
FREQUENCY IN HERTZ

	RIGHT		LEFT
	O	Air	X
	Δ	Air Masked	D
	<	Bone	>
	[	Bone Masked	]
	▲	No Response	▲

DNT: Did Not Test
CNT: Could Not Test

SPEECH

	RIGHT	LEFT
SRT	45 dB	10 dB
WRS	80 %	96 %

WRS Level 80 dB HL

PTA	47 dB	5 dB

Figure 5–18   Audiogram demonstrating the typical findings in a patient with middle-stage Meniere's disease. Note the increasing low-frequency sensorineural hearing loss.

diuretic therapy and a rigorous salt-restricted diet. If the patient does not respond to medical therapy, endolymphatic shunt procedures, labrinthectomy, or vestibular nerve sections should be considered. Selective vestibulotoxic aminoglycoside antibiotics can be infused into the middle ear to ablate the affected side in the most serious cases.

Autoimmune Inner Ear Disease

In 1979, McCabe first reported on a group of individuals with fluctuating sensorineural hearing loss responsive to immunosuppression, suggestive of an autoimmune cause. Harris demonstrated that a number of these patients possess antibodies to inner ear antigens (Harris, 1983). It is believed that an antigen of the inner ear exists, which is recognized as foreign, leading to antibody formation, immune complex deposition, and damage to the membranous labyrinth.

The diagnosis of autoimmune inner ear disease is difficult. Patients usually are seen with bilateral, asymmetric, fluctuating sensorineural hearing loss. About 50% of affected patients will complain of vestibular abnormalities. Age at presentation is usually in the 40s to 50s with a female preponderance. Approximately one third of patients will have evidence of a systemic autoimmune disorder such as lupus erythematosus, polyarteritis nodosa, rheumatoid arthritis, Behçet's disease, or Wegener's granulomatosus.

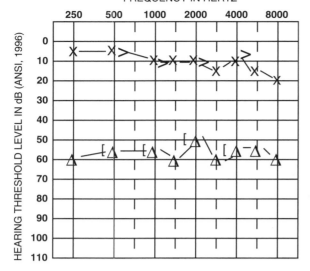

Figure 5–19 Audiogram demonstrating the typical findings in a patient with late Meniere's disease. Note the flat, moderate-to-severe sensorineural hearing loss.

In addition to standard audiometry and vestibular testing, all suspected patients should be screened with an antinuclear antibody test, erythrocyte sedimentation rate, rheumatoid factor, syphilis serological studies, thyroid function tests, and a test for the 68-kd protein, which is the best available test for inner ear antibodies.

Patients should be started on high-dose steroids, 1 to 2 mg/kg/d for 2 to 3 weeks. A dramatic response is often noted in the presence of an accurate diagnosis. Other immunosuppressive drugs such as cyclophosphamide are also successful in treating autoimmune inner ear disease. Rheumatology consultation is helpful in managing patients on long-term immunosuppression. The doses of immunosuppressive drugs may be tapered to keep symptoms at a minimum.

Tumors of the Internal Auditory Canal and Cerebellopontine Angle

Eighty percent of tumors arising in the cerebellopontine angle are acoustic neuromas (Fig. 5–20). The tumor arises from the Schwann cells, which surround the sheath of the eighth cranial nerve, not from the nerve itself.

Most patients present with a progressive, unilateral sensorineural hearing loss, which usually starts in the high frequencies and progresses to involve the lower frequencies. Twenty percent of patients, however, will present with sudden sensorineural hearing loss, and 20% will present with recurrent fluctuating hearing loss. Uncommonly, patients may have vertigo or other vestibular complaints. This is more common in patients with small tumors (<1 cm). As the tumor enlarges, neurological changes may be evidenced as decreased function of cranial nerves VII and V. Occasionally a patient may have hydrocephalus from brain stem compression.

Several findings on audiometry should alert the examiner to the possibility of an acoustic neuroma. The patient will often have a speech discrimination score that is reduced out of proportion to the level of hearing loss. Often "rollover"

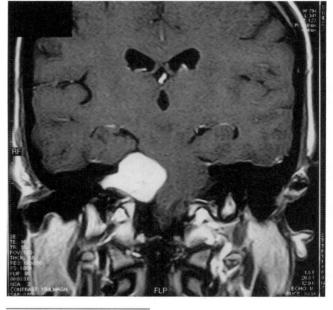

Figure 5–20 Coronal MRI scan with gadolinium showing a large acoustic neuroma.

(decreased ability to understand words as the volume increases) is present. Most (95%) patients will have absent stapedial reflexes. ABR will demonstrate an increased wave I to V interpeak latency, usually greater than 0.2 ms. ENG may be used as a screening tool, because up to 80% will have abnormal results. Because the ENG tests the function of the horizontal semicircular canal, which is innervated by the superior vestibular nerve, a normal test suggests that the tumor originates from the inferior vestibular nerve. Because of the location of the cochlear nerve, in this situation hearing preservation is less likely to be successful.

The best test for detecting acoustic neuromas is an MRI with gadolinium contrast. MRI scanning today allows the detection of tumors as small as 2 mm, increasing the likelihood of hearing preservation.

Individuals with neurofibromatosis type 2 will develop multiple schwannomas of the central nervous system and often present with bilateral acoustic neuromas at a young age. Unlike patients with spontaneous acoustic neuromas, tumors in patients with neurofibromatosis type 2 may grow to a very large size before becoming symptomatic. In addition, the tumors tend to be more infiltrative into the nerve, making hearing preservation more difficult.

The usual treatment for acoustic neuroma is surgery. The surgical approach depends on tumor size and location and the patient's audiometric results. In general hearing conservation surgery is considered when the patient has a small tumor (<1.5 cm) and a pure tone average of less than 50 dB with greater than 50% discrimination. Both the suboccipital and middle cranial fossa approaches allow for the possibility of hearing preservation. The most common approach to resection of acoustic neuromas is through the translabyrinth, which sacrifices hearing on the operated side. The risk of injury to the facial nerve increases with increasing tumor size and approaches 40% when tumor size increases beyond 3 cm.

Another treatment option is stereotactic radiation therapy (the "gamma knife"). Initially treatment using this modality was reported as having lower incidences of facial nerve injury, but longer follow-up studies have revealed a high incidence of late cranial nerve palsies. Radiation therapy is usually reserved for elderly patients, patients with medical problems that increase surgical risk, or individuals who refuse surgery. Radiation therapy does not eliminate the tumor but arrests growth in 80% for at least several years.

When tumors arise in elderly patients or patients who are poor candidates for surgery, a "wait and see" policy may be used. Serial MRI scans should be obtained every 6 months to detect changes in growth rate.

Most other tumors that can occur in the cerebellopontine angle are meningiomas. Rarely, lipomas, cholesterol granulomas, cholesteatomas or hemangiomas may present in the cerebellopontive angle.

Meningiomas may be confused with acoustic neuromas on MRI. Meningiomas should be suspected when an individual presents with a large tumor and relatively normal-hearing. In addition, meningiomas usually present eccentrically with respect to the internal auditory canal and fail to deform the bony auditory canal.

PEARL

Because acoustic neuromas may present with symptoms similar to Meniere's disease, all patients suspected of having Meniere's disease should have an MRI scan with gadolinium to look for the presence of an acoustic neuroma.

Vascular Compression Syndrome

Vascular compression of the eighth nerve in the internal auditory canal can cause vertigo and disequilibrium. Constant pulsations from a vessel lying on the nerve are believed to cause chronic irritation of the nerve and focal destruction of myelin. Usually the culprit vessel is a branch of the anterior inferior cerebellar artery.

The vestibular complaints of patients with vascular compression of the eighth nerve often include constant, chronic vertigo with marked exacerbation by motion and chronic nausea.

Audiometric and vestibular testing often reveal a low-frequency hearing loss or a 15 dB notch at one octave. The most common finding is an increased I to III interpeak latency on ABR.

Relief of symptoms can be provided by either section of the vestibular nerve or by vascular decompression. Symptoms seem to resolve more rapidly after nerve section.

CONTROVERSIAL POINT

Although vascular decompression is recommended for vertigo caused by vascular compression of the eighth nerve, it has not had the same results in relieving tinnitus. Only about one half of patients undergoing decompression for tinnitus improve, and no identifying preoperative factors predicting success have been found.

CONCLUSION

It is our hope that this chapter has provided fundamental background information on common otologic complaints and disease processes and that this information will enhance the reader's understanding of basic pathological diseases of the ear.

REFERENCES

ANNTTINEN, A., LANG, A.H., AANTAA, E., & MARTTILA, R. (1983). Vestibular neuronitis: A neurological and neurophysiological evaluation. *Acta Neurology Scandinavia, 67*;90–96.

BROOKHOUSER, P.E., WORTHINGTON, D.W., & KELLY, W.J. (1991). Noise-induced hearing loss in children. *Laryngoscope, 101*;1264–1272.

EPLEY, J.M. (1992). The canalith repositioning procedure: For treatment of benign paroxysmal postitional vertigo. *Otolarygology–Head and Neck Surgery, 107*;399–404.

EPSTEIN, S., & REILLY, J.S. (1989). Sensorineural hearing loss. *Pediatric Clinics North America, 36*(6);1501–1520.

HARRIS, J.P. (1983). Immunology of the inner ear: Response of the inner ear to antigenic challenge. *Otolaryngology–Head and Neck Surgery, 91*;17–23.

HERDMAN, S.J. (1993). Single treatment approaches to benign paroxysmal positional vertigo. *Archives of Otolaryngology–Head and Neck Surgery, 119*;450–454.

KOHUT, R.I., HINOJOSA, R., & BUDETTI, U.A. (1986). Perilymph fistula: A histopathologic study. *Annals of Otology, Rhinology, and Laryngology, 95*;466–71.

McCABE, B.F. (1979). Autoimmune sensorineural hearing loss. *Annals of Otology, Rhinology and Laryngology, 88*;585–589.

MEYERHOFF, W.F. (1984). *Diagnosis and management of hearing loss.* Philadelphia: W.B. Saunders.

MEYERHOFF, W.L., MORIZONO, T., WRIGHT, C.G., SHADOCK, L.C., & SHEA, D.A. (1983). Tympanostomy tubes and otic drops. *Laryngoscope, 93*;1022–1027.

NAGER, G.T. *Pathology of the ear and temporal bone.* Baltimore, MD: Williams and Wilkins.

NORRE, M.E., & BECKERS, A. (1988). Benign parosysmal positional vertigo in the elderly; treatment by habituation exercises. *Journal of the American Geriatric Society, 36*;425–429.

OGURA, J.H., CIRALSKY, G.J., & GADO, M. (1978). Glomus jugulare and vagale. *Annals of Otology, 87*;622.

PAPARELLA, M.M., DA COSTA, S.S., FOX, R., & YOON, T.H. (1991). Meniere's disease and other labyrinthine diseases. In: M.M. Paparella, D.A. Shumrick, & J.L. Gluckman, et al. (Eds.), *Otolaryngology* (3rd ed.) (pp. 1689–1710). Philadelphia: W.B. Saunders.

ROLAND, P.S., & MARPLE, B.F. (1997). Disorders of the inner ear, eighth nerve, and the CNS. In: P.S. Roland, B.F. Marple, & W.L. Meyerhoff (Eds.), *Hearing loss* (pp. 195–255). New York: Thieme Medical Publishers, Inc.

SCHUKNECHT, H.F. (1955). Presbycusis. *Laryngoscope, 65*;402.

SEMONT, A., FREYSS, G., & VITTE, E. (1988). Curing the BPPV with a liberatory manuever. *Advances in Otorhinolaryngology, 42*;290–293.

## Chapter 6

Radiographic Imaging in Otologic Disease

Debara L. Tucci and Linda Gray

Outline

Modern neuroimaging capabilities have revolutionized the practice of otology. The use of a combination of computerized tomography (CT) and magnetic resonance imaging (MRI) enable the otologist and neuroradiologist to define the nature and extent of most disease processes that affect the temporal bone and surrounding anatomical structures. With knowledge gained from interpretation of these images, the otologist can make an accurate diagnosis and plan an appropriate surgical procedure or other course of treatment. Proper use of neuroimaging can enhance patient care and reduce the risk of surgical or treatment-related complications.

This chapter will describe basic imaging techniques, discuss the use of these techniques in the diagnosis of otologic disease processes, and present a discussion of the specific uses of imaging in evaluation of patients in an otologic practice. This chapter is not meant to provide an exhaustive discussion of all otologic disease in which imaging could potentially be used. Rather, it is meant to give the reader a basic understanding of neuroimaging and of the most common uses of neuroimaging in the evaluation of the patient with otologic disease.

CONVENTIONAL RADIOLOGY

Conventional radiological techniques are rarely used for assessment of the temporal bone today. The ear is an extremely complex organ; many structures are located in a small space within the temporal bone. Conventional radiographic techniques do not permit the isolation of distinct anatomical structures, because each point on the film is a summation of all the points crossed by the x-ray beam travelling through the skull and temporal bone. These techniques have been abandoned, for the most part, in favor of CT, which offers a much higher resolution and a precise reconstruction of the entire area of interest in a series of images. Current use in an otologic practice is probably limited to the transorbital, or frontal, projection, which shows the otic capsule and may be used to confirm the position of cochlear implant electrodes.

COMPUTERIZED TOMOGRAPHY

CT (Grossman & Yousem, 1994) was first developed in the early 1970s and has continued to evolve over the years. This technique uses a highly collimated (or focused) x-ray beam that is differentially absorbed by various tissues within the body. The beam is rotated over many different steps so as to get differential absorption patterns through a single section of a patient's body. By mathematical analysis, one can obtain an absorption value for each point in a CT slice. The scale for CT absorption ranges from $+1000$ to -1000, with 0 allocated to water and -1000 to air. These units of absorption are termed *Hounsfield units* (HU) for the discoverer of CT. High-resolution CT techniques can provide slice thickness as narrow as .75 mm. Two or more projections are required for proper interpretation of a study. The most commonly used projections are the axial or horizontal and the coronal or frontal projections.

Special reconstruction algorithms can be used to highlight a particular tissue with CT. Bone algorithms are very useful for assessment of anatomy of the temporal bone. Iodinated contrast may be used to opacify blood vessels or vascular tumors, such as paragangliomas. However, small vascular tumors will not take up enough contrast to produce opacification. In general, contrast is not administered for routine temporal bone studies.

In most cases CT is the initial imaging study of choice for evaluation of patients with suspected otologic disease. The major exception to this statement is the evaluation of acoustic neuroma, for which MRI is most useful, as discussed below.

MAGNETIC RESONANCE IMAGING

MR is an imaging technique that does not expose the patient to ionizing radiation (Grossman & Yousem, 1994; Valvassori et al,

Audiology: Diagnosis. Edited by Roeser, Valente, and Hosford-Dunn. Thieme Medical Publishers, Inc., New York © 2000

PEARL

High-resolution temporal bone CT is typically used for preoperative assessment of a wide variety of otologic surgical problems, including cholesteatoma, tumors such as glomus tympanicum or glomus jugulare, cochlear implantation, and congenital atresia. CT may be helpful not only for diagnosis but also to delineate the surgical anatomy and aid in planning the operative procedure.

PEARL

MR cannot be used for patients with pacemakers or metallic implants, such as cochlear implants. Special nonferromagnetic cochlear implants are available for use for patients who might be expected to need MRI in the future (Heller et al, 1996). Otologic prostheses, such as for stapedectomy or stapedotomy, are generally MRI compatible.

1995). Although CT is a technique that relies on differential attenuation of an x-ray beam, MR relies on the unique response of various tissues to an applied magnetic field. For MR, images are generated by the interaction of hydrogen nuclei or protons, high magnetic fields, and radiofrequency pulses. The intensity of the MR signal to be captured on the image depends on the density of hydrogen nuclei in the tissue and on two magnetic relaxation times, called T1 and T2, which are tissue-specific. The appearance of both normal and pathological tissue will vary, depending on the relative contribution of the T1 and T2 relaxation times in the image generated. Variation of relaxation times is obtained by changing the time between radiofrequency pulses, TR or repetition time, and the time the emitted signal or echo is measured after the pulse, TE or echo time.

The signal intensity of various tissues is directly proportional to the amount of free protons present within the tissue. Soft tissue and body fluids contain large amounts of free proton and emit a strong MR signal. In contrast, air and bone contain few free protons and emit a weak MR signal. Pathological processes are recognizable when the proton density and relaxation times of the abnormal tissue are different from those of normal tissue. Some pathological processes are definable on the basis of the appearance on T1-weighted versus T2-weighted images. The recognition and differentiation of pathological processes is enhanced by the use of a ferromagnetic contrast agent, such as gadolinium, which may be taken up by abnormal tissue. MRI is most useful for detection of soft tissue tumors, such as acoustic neuroma and lesions of the petrous apex, and for detection of intracranial involvement by pathological processes such as cholesteatoma.

PEARL

MRI is most useful for imaging soft tissue in contrast to CT, which is most useful for imaging bony detail.

Magnetic resonance angiography (MRA) depends on creating intensity differences between flowing matter and stationary tissue. By suppressing background stationary tissue and focusing on the high-signal flowing blood, it is possible to depict vascular structures in three-dimensional space. Although this technique is useful for detecting vascular abnormalities such as intercranial aneurysms, its usefulness in temporal bone evaluation is limited.

NORMAL CT TEMPORAL BONE ANATOMY

A series of axial and coronal CT images showing normal temporal bone anatomy are shown in Figures 6–1 and 6–2. Some important structures and relationships to note include the following:

1. The internal auditory canal is located medial (or toward the middle of the head) to the external auditory canal (which is lateral, or toward the outside of the head). The internal auditory canals should be uniform in size, within 2 mm. An enlarged internal auditory canal raises the suspicion of an acoustic neuroma, although an MRI is a better method of assessment. The internal auditory canal transmits the facial nerve, superior vestibular nerve, inferior vestibular nerve, and cochlear nerve. An internal auditory canal that is less than 2 mm in diameter is suspected of transmitting only a facial nerve, without an normal auditory-vestibular nerve (Jackler et al, 1987a; Shelton et al, 1989).

2. The middle ear space is noted, with attention to the size and degree of aeration and the presence of a mass, soft tissue, or fluid. The ossicles are noted in the middle ear space, particularly the head of the malleus and the body of the incus in the epitympanum.

3. The ossicles are noted, including the head of the malleus and body of the incus superiorly. Their configuration should resemble that of an ice cream cone, with the head of the malleus representing the "ice cream" in the "cone" of the incus. The stapes is most inferior and best visualized in the coronal plane, lateral to the vestibule. The patency of the oval window can be assessed in this plane as well.

4. The otic capsule is noted, particularly the patency and morphology of the cochlea and the vestibule and semicircular canals. The cochlea is located most anterior and medial, and semicircular canals are more posterior and lateral. The cochlea is in proximity to the carotid artery, seen best in the coronal image.

5. The major vascular structures of the temporal bone include the carotid artery and jugular bulb. The jugular bulb is in continuity with the sigmoid sinus in the mastoid and is posterior and lateral to the carotid artery.

6. The facial nerve takes a complicated path through the temporal bone and may be visualized in a series of axial and coronal images. Segments include an internal auditory canal segment, a labyrinthine segment that is in proximity

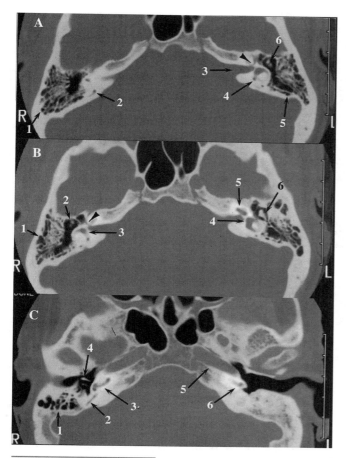

Figure 6–1 Series of axial CT images through the normal temporal bone. **(A)** Most superior; **(C)** Most inferior. **(A)** 1, Mastoid air cells; 2, posterior semicircular canal; 3, internal auditory canal; 4, posterior semicircular canal ampulla; 5, mastoid air cells; 6, ossicles. **(B)** 1, Mastoid air cells; 2, ossicles; 3, vestibule and horizontal semicircular canal; 4, vestibule; 5, cochlea (basal turn); 6, ossicles. **(C)** 1, Mastoid air cells; 2, common crus (posterior and superior semicircular canals); 3, basal turn of cochlea; 4, manubrium of malleus; 5, canal of the internal carotid artery; 6, basal turn of cochlea. *Arrowheads*, facial nerve, labyrinthine portion.

to the semicircular canals ending in the geniculate ganglion, a tympanic segment that travels horizontally through the middle ear just superior to the oval window, and a mastoid or vertical portion that extends from the level of the horizontal semicircular canal and oval window to the stylomastoid foramen near the mastoid tip. The nerve makes two sharp turns, one at the geniculate ganglion, which is the first genu, and another at the juncture of the tympanic and mastoid segments, which is called the second genu.

7. The vestibular aqueduct is seen posterior to the posterior semicircular canal, extending to the endolymphatic sac on the posterior aspect of the temporal bone. The cochlear aqueduct extends from the region of the round window to the subarachnoid space, inferior to the internal auditory

canal and medial to the jugular bulb at the level of the basal turn of the cochlea.

SPECIFIC USES OF IMAGING IN EVALUATION OF OTOLOGIC DISEASE

Neuroimaging is of critical importance in diagnosis of otologic disease in the modern otolaryngology practice. Patient populations for whom neuroimaging plays an especially important role in assessment of the disease process are described below.

Unilateral or Asymmetrical Sensorineural Hearing Loss

Because unilateral or asymmetrical sensorineural hearing loss (SNHL) and unilateral tinnitus are the most common presenting symptoms of acoustic neuroma, evaluation to rule out an eighth cranial nerve tumor is indicated in patients with these symptoms (Tucci, 1997). Gadolinium-enhanced MRI (MRIg) is considered the "gold standard" for detection of an acoustic neuroma (NIH Consensus Development Conference, 1991). Because the resolution of MRI is 500 µm, extremely small tumors, less than 1 mm, may be detected. Auditory brain stem evoked potential testing (ABR) has been used in the past to screen for abnormalities that require follow-up imaging. However, recent studies of detection rates with ABR and MRI have raised the concern that ABR is not adequately sensitive to diagnose small tumors (Telian et al, 1989). Although ABR sensitivity is reported by most authors as approximately 90% for all size tumors, the sensitivity for diagnosis of small, intracanalicular tumors is significantly lower (Wilson et al, 1997). In one prospective study (Ruckenstein et al, 1996) all patients with significant asymmetrical SNHL (defined in this study as asymmetry of ≥ 15 dB at two frequencies or asymmetry in speech discrimination scores of ≥ 15%) were evaluated with both ABR and MRIg. Preliminary data from this study, based on 47 patients, indicate that ABR sensitivity and specificity are both approximately 60%, which supports the contention by some authors (Chandrasekhar et al, 1995; Welling et al, 1990; Wilson et al, 1997) that MRIg be used as the preferred screening test for assessment of all patients with unilateral auditory-vestibular symptoms. It may be argued that an exception to this recommendation be made in the case of elderly patients for whom a small slow-growing tumor is not likely to create a health risk within their expected lifetime. In certain circumstances, such as in rural areas, access to MRI may be limited. In these situations ABR must be used for acoustic neuroma screening. In cases of asymmetrical hearing loss and a normal ABR, patient follow-up, every 6 to 12 months, is of critical importance. If hearing loss progresses or other symptoms such as tinnitus or vestibular dysfunction develop, repeated ABR is indicated (Tucci, 1997).

Appropriate MR imaging protocols will obtain adequately thin sections through the internal auditory canals (IACs) to rule out a small acoustic tumor. Gadolinium is used to increase the sensitivity of detection in the case of a small tumor. In the case of neuritis the nerve may enhance with gadolinium in the absence of a tumor mass. In this situation

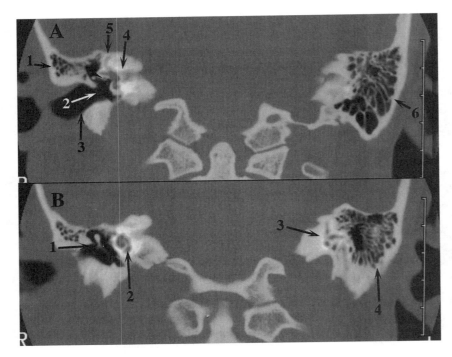

Figure 6–2   Series of coronal CT images through a normal temporal bone. **(A)** At the level of the semicircular canals, is posterior to **(B)** which is at the level of the cochlea. **(A)** 1, Mastoid air cells; 2, tympanic membrane; 3, external auditory canal; 4, internal auditory canal; 5, superior semicircular canal; 6, mastoid air cells. **(B)** 1, Scutum, or postero-superior external auditory canal, and Prussak's space, which is the space between pars flaccida of the tympanic membrane and the neck of the malleus in which cholesteatomas can form; 2, cochlea; 3, superior and horizontal semicircular canals; 4, mastoid air cells. *Arrowhead,* Facial nerve seen above the oval window, and inferior to the horizontal semicircular canal.

special MR techniques may facilitate the differential diagnosis (Syms et al, 1997). Some authors have advocated the use of abbreviated MRI techniques to screen for acoustic neuromas. These techniques have the advantage of reduced cost but the disadvantage of less comprehensive brain imaging, with the potential to miss other intracranial causes of auditory dysfunction such as multiple sclerosis or small vessel disease (Wilson et al, 1997).

The typical radiological appearance of an acoustic neuroma is that of a mass in the cerebellopontine angle (CPA) that extends into the IAC (Fig. 6–3). Tumor size may be described in terms of both an intracanalicular and an extracanalicular portion. The tumor tends to widen the most medial portion (or porous acousticus) of the IAC as it enlarges. However, small tumors may not erode the porous

acousticus. This is why small tumors are not easily or reliably detected by conventional CT. Most tumors in the CPA are acoustic neuromas. Meningiomas may also occur in this region and usually have a somewhat different appearance on MRI (Valvassori et al, 1995). In general, hearing is less affected by a meningioma in this region than by an acoustic neuroma. Surgical resection that preserves the potential for hearing conservation may be indicated in these cases, as well as for patients with small acoustic neuromas (McKenna et al, 1992; Rosenberg et al, 1987; Shelton et al, 1990; Tucci et al, 1994).

Other, less common causes of unilateral hearing loss of adult onset include other skull base tumors, particularly those located in the petrous apex. The petrous apex is the portion of the temporal bone that lies between the inner ear and the clivus, which is at the center of the skull base. The petrous apex

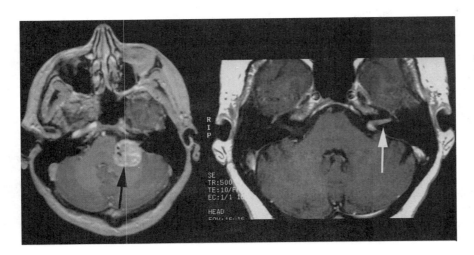

Figure 6–3   Axial MRI showing large *(left side)* and small *(right side)* acoustic ne uroma. On the left image, tumor fills the medial portion of the internal auditory canal (IAC), and expands the porus, or opening, of the canal. Tumor fills the cerebellopontine angle (CPA) and compresses the brain stem. The dark spaces within the tumor are indicative of small cysts within the tumor. The small tumor on the right is seen to fill the entire IAC and extend minimally into the CPA.

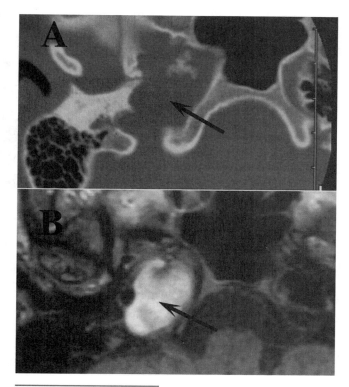

Figure 6–4 Lesion of the left petrous apex. **(A)** Axial CT demonstrating an expansile lesion of the petrous apex with associated calcification. **(B)** Axial T1-weighted MR scan demonstrating high signal intensity cholesterol cyst of petrous apex.

anteromedial petrous apex. MRI is very characteristic and shows a markedly hyperintense lesion on both T1-weighted and T2-weighted images, with no change after gadolinium administration. Cholesteatomas may arise in this location either from congenital squamous epithelial rests (a developmental anomaly) or, less typically, as a result of spread from cholesteatoma that occurred primarily in the mastoid. Cholesteatomas are much less common than cholesterol granulomas in this location and have a characteristic appearance on MRI, with low signal intensity on the T1-weighted images, high intensity on the T2-weighted images, and no enhancement with gadolinium. The T1-weighted images generally provide the information needed to make the diagnosis. Other, rarer tumors are also possible in this location (Jackler & Parker, 1992).

Sensorineural Hearing Loss in Children

In children, SNHL is less likely to be due to neoplasms or other pathological conditions as described for the adult and more likely to be the result of congenital anatomical or functional abnormalities. According to Jackler et al (1987b), about 20% of patients with congenital SNHL will have radiographic abnormalities that can be identified on temporal bone CT (Fig. 6–5). Jackler and colleagues developed a classification of cochlear malformation that is based on embryogensis. Abnormalities include: (a) complete aplasia of the inner ear—cochlea and labyrinth (Michel deformity); (b) cochlear aplasia; (c) cochlear hypoplasia, with a small cochlear bud; (d) incomplete partition, or a small cochlea with an incomplete interscalar septum (classic Mondini malformation); and (e) the common cavity malformation, in which the cochlea and vestibule form a common cavity without internal architecture. Malformations of the membranous portion of the cochlea are much more common than bony malformations; these are not detectable with currently available imaging techniques.

The radiographic finding of an enlarged vestibular aqueduct (Fig. 6–6) is known to be associated with SNHL, which can be progressive and profound (Jackler & De la Cruz, 1989). Enlargement of this structure may be due to developmental arrest of the endolymphatic anlage, much like arrest of cochlear development is thought to result in the malformations listed previously. This abnormality may also be associated with other malformations of the membranous cochlea.

is divided into two compartments by the IAC; the anterior compartment, which lies medial to the cochlea, is most frequently involved by disease processes. Patients may have unilateral hearing loss or other unilateral auditory-vestibular symptoms if lesions of the petrous apex involve either the inner ear or contents of the IAC. Although CT is very useful in delineating the extent of bony involvement of these lesions, MRI is most useful in defining the characteristics that help to make the differential diagnosis. One common lesion of the petrous apex is the cholesterol granuloma (Fig. 6–4), which is an expansile cystic mass that is typically located in the

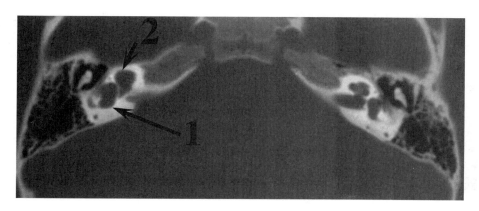

Figure 6–5 Cochlear malformation. Axial CT image at the level of the otic capsule. 1, Enlarged, malformed vestibule; 2, malformed cochlea. Normal anatomy is seen on the opposite side.

Children who have SNHL often undergo radiographic imaging, particularly if the hearing loss is profound or progressive. Children with profound hearing loss are often imaged in the course of evaluation for cochlear implant candidacy (see following). Children with malformations of the temporal bone may be at greater risk of progression of hearing loss resulting from head trauma (Jackler and De la Cruz, 1989). Recurrent meningitis has been documented in children with cochlear malformations, particularly in association with cerebrospinal fluid (CSF) leak and an oval window fistula (Ohms et al, 1990).

Cochlear Implant Evaluation

Radiographic imaging is an important part of the cochlear implant evaluation. A detailed temporal bone CT helps to define the surgical anatomy and alert the surgeon to potential abnormalities such as cochlear ossification and malformation (Figs. 6–7 and 6–8). Modifications of conventional surgical techniques permit implantation of patients with a variety of cochlear anomalies; surgical planning and patient counseling are enhanced by preoperative identification of these abnormalities. Bony malformations of the cochlea have been associated with absence of the oval and round windows and an aberrant course of the facial nerve. Free flow of CSF may occur into the cochlea from the IAC and may result in profuse flow of CSF on creation of the cochleostomy (Tucci et al, 1995). A narrow IAC may suggest absence of the auditory nerve, which is a contraindication to implantation in that ear (Jackler et al, 1987b; Shelton et al, 1989).

Pulsatile Tinnitus

The symptom of unilateral pulsatile tinnitus often warrants radiographic evaluation to rule out or diagnose abnormalities such as a vascular tumor of the temporal bone, vascular anomaly, or other rare disorders such as arteriovenous malformations or aneurysms. The two major blood vessels associated with the ear, the carotid artery and the jugular vein, both course along the floor of the middle ear, and either may demonstrate anomalous development. The carotid artery typically lies no further lateral in the temporal bone than the lateral wall of the cochlea. Because of a developmental abnormality, the carotid artery can course over the cochlear promontory and turn anteriorly under the oval window. Patients with an aberrant carotid artery may have pulsatile tinnitus

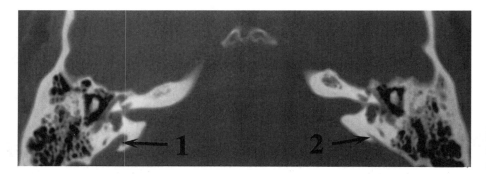

Figure 6–6 Axial CT image showing an enlarged vestibular aqueduct (*1*), and a normal vestibular aqueduct (*2*).

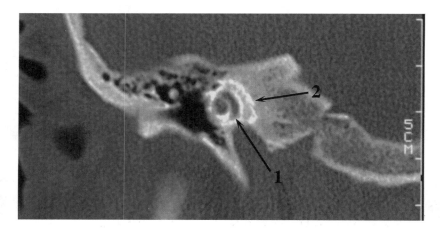

Figure 6–7 Coronal CT image showing the cochlea in a patient with otosclerosis. Sclerosis of the cochlea is evident, with narrowing of the cochlear lumen. 1, Cochlear lumen; 2, sclerotic bone

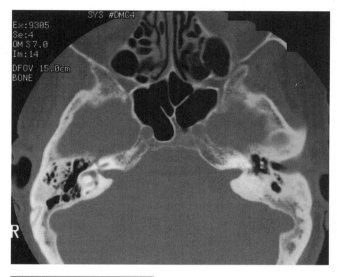

Figure 6–8 Axial CT showing complete labyrinthine ossification, left ear *(right side of figure)*. Right cochlea *(left side of figure)* is partially ossified, and the outline of a portion of the cochlea and semicircular canals is evident.

and conductive hearing loss (Fig. 6–9). Otoscopic examination may reveal a red retrotympanic mass that does not blanch on pneumotoscopy.

In about 6% of temporal bones the jugular bulb protrudes above the level of the floor of the external auditory canal. If the bony plate, which usually separates the jugular bulb and middle ear, is dehiscent, the bulb is exposed to the middle ear cavity. A "high-riding" jugular bulb may be visualized through the tympanic membrane as a bluish mass (Fig. 6–10); in severe cases it may cause a conductive hearing loss by interfering with the normal movement of the ossicular chain. Pulsatile tinnitus may be produced by a variety of mechanisms, including turbulent blood flow in the high-riding jugular bulb, transmission of intratemporal carotid artery pulsations, or retrograde transmission of atrial pulsations (Sismanis, 1997).

Other abnormalities that may be commonly associated with pulsatile tinnitus are not diagnosed by conventional imaging techniques. Sismanis (1997) argues that many young women with this disorder have benign intracranial hypertension. Atherosclerotic carotid artery disease is thought to be a common cause of pulsatile tinnitus in patients older than 50, particularly when they have risk factors for atherosclerosis (hypertension, angina, hyperlipidemia, diabetes mellitus, and smoking).

The most common vascular tumor affecting the temporal bone is the paraganglioma or glomus tumor (Fig. 6–11). Temporal bone paragangliomas originate most frequently from the jugular bulb (glomus jugulare) and less commonly over the promontory of the cochlea (glomus tympanicum). Either can grow to involve a large portion of the temporal bone, and tumors may extend intracranially. Glomus jugulare tumors are typically much more extensive than tympanicum tumors, which can be quite small on diagnosis. Tympanicum tumors can be easily seen through a translucent tympanic membrane and appear as a circumscribed, often pulsatile, cherry-red mass over the cochlear promontory. These patients may have conductive hearing loss as a result of ossicular involvement and pulsatile tinnitus.

Evaluation of Pediatric Conductive Hearing Loss

Conductive hearing loss in the pediatric patient may be due to an obvious cause, such as congenital aural atresia or cholesteatoma. However, if the otomicroscopic examination is normal, the diagnosis may be more subtle. Imaging is frequently used for evaluation of the pediatric patient. In the case of congenital anomaly or cholesteatoma, the scan will help define the anatomy and help with surgical planning and family counseling. In the case of conductive hearing loss of unknown cause, a detailed temporal bone study will help to determine whether an indication exists for early surgical intervention. A cholesteatoma that is not evident on physical examination may be evident on an imaging study and would require treatment, whereas the absence of such a problem should reassure the physician and family that surgical treatment may be scheduled electively.

In cases of congenital aural atresia, it is essential to perform a careful preoperative assessment to determine whether the

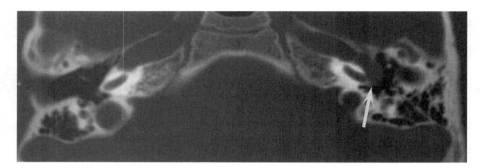

Figure 6–9 Axial CT showning an internal carotid artery malformation *(arrow)*. On the left side of the figure, the carotid artery is seen in its normal location medial to the cochlea. On the right side of the figure, the carotid artery courses lateral to the cochlea and extends over the cochlear promontory.

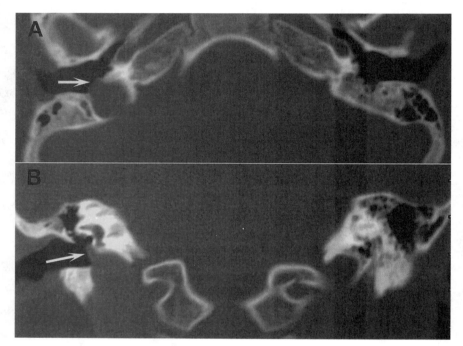

Figure 6–10 High-riding jugular bulb. **(A)** Axial image showing the jugular bulb at the level of the middle ear space, with dehiscence (lack of bone covering). **(B)** Coronal CT image showing dehiscence and extension into middle ear space. This could be visualized as a bluish mass behind the tympanic membrane on otoscopic examination. This patient also had a conductive hearing loss.

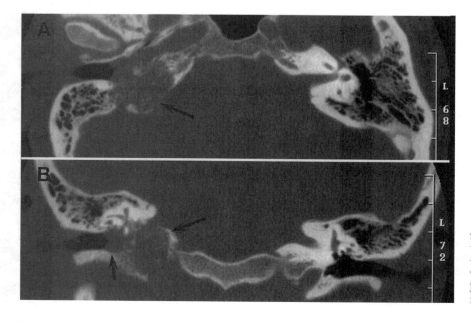

Figure 6–11 Glomus jugulare tumor. Axial **(A)** and coronal **(B)** CT scans demonstrating an erosive lesion of the jugular bulb, with extension of tumor into the middle ear (**B**, *vertical arrow*).

patient is a good candidate for reconstructive surgery. High-resolution CT of the temporal bone is used to assess the development of the temporal bone and anatomy of the middle ear space (Fig. 6–12). Jahrsdoerfer et al (1992) developed a guideline for assessment of the relevant anatomy and have made recommendations on the basis of surgical experience with a large number of patients with atresia. This grading system is based on the morphology of the ossicles, patency of the oval and round windows, size of the middle ear space, position of the facial nerve, degree of mastoid pneumatization, and appearance of the external ear. In general, surgery is not performed until a child reaches at least age 5, and canal reconstruction is preceded by auricular reconstruction if indicated (De La Cruz & Chandrasekhar, 1994; Jahrsdoerfer et al, 1992; Lambert, 1988). A CT scan may be performed long before the age at which surgery takes place to determine whether surgical intervention is appropriate and help with overall patient management decisions. In cases of bilateral atresia, surgical ear selection should be based both on middle ear and mastoid anatomy and, where possible, an assessment of cochlear integrity. This may be based on bony morphology of the cochlea as seen on CT and audiological assessment.

A number of other congenital abnormalities of the middle ear are described (Sando et al, 1990). These abnormalities may be diagnosed in children with known syndromic disorders, nonsyndromic dysmorphic features, or, most commonly, in otherwise normal children. In most cases diagnosis

of a specific ossicular problem cannot be made definitively on CT scan.

PEARL

CT may be useful in diagnosing conditions for which surgery is contraindicated. X-linked congenital mixed deafness is associated with a series of distinct morphologic features of the temporal bone that are evident on CT scan. Surgical treatment of the associated stapes fixation is likely to result in a CSF "gusher" during stapedectomy, with resultant profound SNHL (Talbot & Wilson, 1994). CT may also identify features such as an anomalous course of the facial nerve, which are important for surgical planning.

Evaluation of Chronic Ear Disease
(Glasscock et al, 1997; Hughes, 1997)

The term *chronic middle ear disease* reflects a wide range of pathological conditions, which can range in severity from chronic otitis media with effusion to extensive cholesteatoma with associated aural and intracranial complications. It is not always possible on physical examination to determine the exact nature or extent of the disease process. For this reason, imaging studies, particularly temporal bone CT, are an important component of patient evaluation.

The most common reason to obtain an imaging study in a patient with chronic ear disease is to determine the presence or absence and extent of cholesteatoma (Fig. 6–13). Aural cholesteatoma is defined as keratinizing squamous epithelium that is present in the middle ear, mastoid, or petrous apex. Cholesteatoma can be termed *primary acquired, secondary acquired,* or *congenital.* Primary cholesteatoma is caused by severe retraction of the tympanic membrane as a result of chronic eustachian tube dysfunction and resultant negative middle ear pressure. In this case the posterosuperior portion of the drum invaginates, forming an epithelial-lined cyst that accumulates keratin, enlarges, and destroys surrounding bone. This is commonly referred to as an "attic" cholesteatoma, because it occurs in the most superior portion of the middle ear. Areas of bone destruction can include the ossicles; scutum or posterosuperior earcanal wall; tegmen or bone separating the ear from the intracranial cavity; semicircular canals, particularly the horizontal canal, which is closest to the middle ear; and the fallopian canal, which houses the facial nerve and is particularly vulnerable as it travels through the middle ear just above the oval window. Cholesteatoma may extend into the mastoid cavity or even into the intracranial cavity. Secondary acquired cholesteatoma occurs when squamous epithelium from the surface of the tympanic membrane enters the middle ear through a perforation in the drum. This may occur as a result of trauma or infection.

Congenital cholesteatoma occurs as a result of a developmental abnormality. The typical patient is a young child with

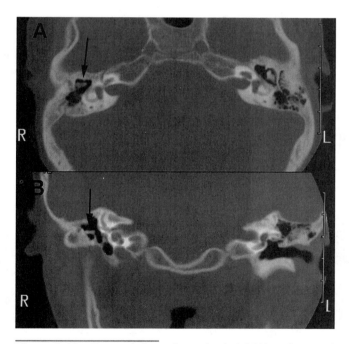

Figure 6–12 Congenital aural atresia. Axial **(A)** and coronal **(B)** CT images showing right ear *(left side of figure)* congenital atresia. Arrows indicate globular ossicular mass with adherence to atretic plate. Normal ossicles are seen for the left ear. The size of the middle ear space is similar on the right and left sides. An external auditory canal is seen on the coronal **(B)** image for the left ear.

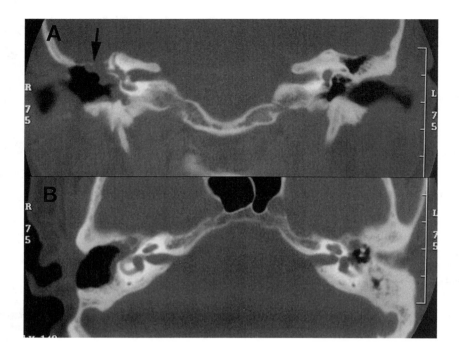

Figure 6–13 Cholesteatoma. **(A)** Coronal image demonstrates soft tissue in the middle ear space, a defect in the tegmen tympani *(arrow)*, and a horizontal semicircular canal fistula. **(B)** Axial image also demonstrates soft tissue in middle ear space and labyrinthine fistula. No ossicles are seen in the right middle ear space. (NOTE: Right ear is on left side of figure.)

a white mass visualized in the anterosuperior middle ear space, behind an intact, normal-appearing tympanic membrane. These patients have no history of tympanic membrane perforation, otorrhea, or otologic surgery to suggest a mechanism for acquired cholesteatoma. Disease can be extensive, regardless of the origin of the cholesteatoma.

Imaging is typically performed preoperatively for assessment of a known cholesteatoma only if clinically indicated (Blevins & Carter, 1998). Indications may include vertigo, or a suspected labyrinthine fistula, facial paresis or paralysis, SNHL, cholesteatoma in an only hearing ear, and planned revision surgery. Other extracranial complications can include labyrinthitis, mastoiditis, petrositis, and soft tissue abscesses.

MRI may be indicated in cases of suspected intracranial extension or other complications. Intracranial complications include extradural/perisinus abscess, lateral (sigmoid) sinus thrombosis, subdural abscess, cerebral abscess, otitic meningitis, otitic hydrocephalus, and brain herniation.

Temporal Bone Trauma

Temporal bone fractures (Swartz & Harnsberger, 1992) are described in terms of their predominant orientation with respect to the long axis of the petrous bone. Most fractures have either a longitudinal or transverse orientation. Complications associated with these fractures vary according to the orientation of the fracture and the temporal bone structures involved. Transverse fractures tend to be associated with more severe complications; fortunately, they are less common than longitudinal fractures.

About 70 to 90% of all temporal bone fractures are longitudinal (Fig. 6–14). These typically result from a blow to the

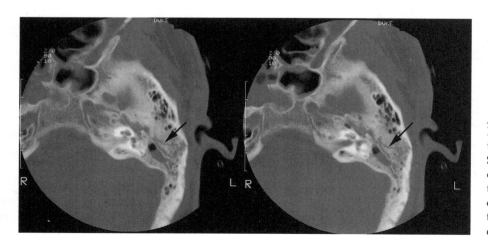

Figure 6–14 Longitudinal fracture through the temporal bone. Sequential axial CT images demonstrate the fracture line *(arrow)* that parallels the external auditory canal. The fracture line extends toward the middle ear space and ossicles. The cochlea is not involved.

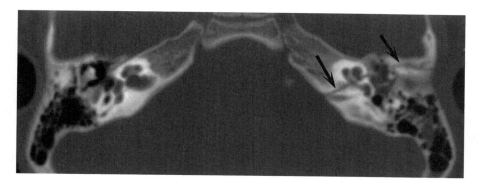

Figure 6–15 Transverse fracture of the temporal bone demonstrated on axial CT. Fracture line *(arrows)* extends through the cochlea.

temporal or parietal region. Fractures follow a path of least resistance, and because this fracture originates outside the dense bone of the otic capsule, it remains extralabyrinthine. The fracture line often involves the external auditory canal and middle ear. Involvement of the tympanic anulus usually results in a tympanic membrane tear. Hemotympanum is often identified on examination, and these patients typically have a conductive hearing loss. In the absence of a perforation the conductive hearing loss should resolve after several weeks. If it does not, ossicular dyscontinuity should be suspected. These fractures may result in facial paralysis or paresis. Cholesteatoma may form as a result of invaginating epithelium along the fracture line or through a perforation.

A transverse temporal bone fracture occurs less commonly (10 to 30% of the time) and usually results from a blow to the occiput. The fracture line typically begins in the vicinity of the jugular foramen or foramen magnum and extends to a foramen in the floor of the middle cranial fossa, often through the bony labyrinth (Fig. 6–15). When these fractures involve the otic capsule, deafness and severe vertigo usually result. Although the hearing loss is permanent, the vertigo is usually self-limited. Hearing loss and vertigo can result from

inner ear concussive injuries in the absence of fracture. In these cases head trauma produces mechanical disruption of the membranous components of the inner ear.

Facial nerve paralysis or paresis is a common sequela of temporal bone trauma. Facial nerve injury is associated with transverse fractures in as many as 50% of cases. Injury is less common with longitudinal fractures and occurs approximately 10 to 20% of the time. Patients with total paralysis and severely diminished responses on studies of facial nerve function (electroneuronography or electromyography) are candidates for facial nerve decompression surgery to reduce bony spicules or traction injuries and repair the nerve. CT imaging may be very useful in delineating areas of likely injury.

CONCLUSION

This chapter discussed the basic imaging techniques, normal CT temporal bone anatomy, the use of techniques in diagnosing otologic disease processes, and the specific uses of imaging in the evaluation of patients in otologic practice.

REFERENCES

ARRIAGA, M.A., & CARRIER, D. (1996). MRI and clinical decisions in cochlear implantation. *American Journal of Otology, 17;*547–553.

BLEVINS, N.H., & CARTER, B.L. (1998). Clinical forum: Routine preoperative imaging in chronic ear surgery. *American Journal of Otology, 19;*527–538.

CHANDRASEKHAR, S., BRACKMANN, D.E., & DEVGAN, K.K. (1995). Utility of auditory brain stem audiometry in diagnosis of acoustic neuromas. *American Journal of Otology, 16;*63–67.

DE LA CRUZ, A., & CHANDRASEKHAR, S.S. (1994). Congenital malformation of the temporal bone. In: D.E. Brackmann, C. Shelton, & M.A. Arriaga (Eds.), *Otologic surgery* (pp. 69–84). Philadelphia: W. B. Saunders.

GLASSCOCK, M.E. III, HAYNES, D.S., STORPER, I.S., & BOHRER, P.S. (1997). Surgery for chronic ear disease. In: G.B. Hughes, & M.L. Pensak (Eds.), *Clinical otology* (2nd ed.) (pp. 215–232). New York: Thieme Medical Publishers.

GROSSMAN, R.I., & YOUSEM, D.M. (1994). *Neuroradiology: The requisites* (pp. 1–22). St. Louis: Mosby.

HALL, J.W. III, GROSE, J.H., & PILLSBURY, H.C. (1995). Long-term effects of chronic otitis media on binaural hearing in children. *Archives of Otolaryngology–Head and Neck Surgery, 121;*847–852.

HELLER, J.W., BRACKMANN, D.E., TUCCI, D.L., NYENHUIS, J.A., & CHOU, C.K. (1996). *American Journal of Otology, 17;* 724–729.

HUGHES, G.B. (1997). Complications of otitis media. In: G.B. Hughes, M.L. Pensak (Eds.), *Clinical Otology* (2nd ed.) (pp. 233–240). New York: Thieme Medical Publishers.

JACKLER, R.K., & DE LA CRUZ, A. (1989). The large vestibular aqueduct syndrome. *Laryngoscope, 99;*1238–1243.

JACKLER, R.K., LUXFORD, W.M., & HOUSE, W.F. (1987a). Sound detection with the cochlear implant in five ears of four children with congenital malformation of the cochlea. *Laryngoscope, 97* (Suppl. 40); 15–17.

JACKLER, R.K., LUXFORD, W.M., & HOUSE, W.F. (1987b). Congenital malformations of the inner ear: A classification based on embryogenesis. *Laryngoscope, 97* (Suppl. 40); 15–17.

Jackler, R.K., Luxford, W.M., Schindler, R.A., & McKerrow, W.S. (1987c). Cochlear patency problems in cochlear implantation. *Laryngoscope, 97*;801–805.

Jackler, R.K., & Parker, D.A. (1992). Radiographic differential diagnosis of petrous apex lesions. *American Journal of Otology, 13*;561–574.

Jahrsdoerfer, R.A., Yeakley, J.W., Aguilar, E.A., Cole, R.R., & Gray, L.C. (1992). Grading system for the selection of patients with congenital aural atresia. *American Journal of Otology, 13*;6–12.

Lambert, P.R. (1988). Major congenital ear malformations: Surgical management and results. *Annals of Otology, Rhinology and Laryngology, 97*;641–649.

McKenna, M.J., Halpin, C., Ojemann, R.G., Nadol, J.B., Montgomery, W.W., Levine, R.A., Carlisle, E., & Martuza, R. (1992). Long-term hearing results in patients after surgical removal of acoustic tumors with hearing preservation. *American Journal of Otology, 13*;134–136.

NIH Consensus Development Conference (1991). Consensus Statement. *Acoustic Neuroma, 9*(4);1–24.

Ohms, L.A., Edwards, M.S., Mason, E.O., Igarashi, M., Alford, B.A., & Smith, R.J.H. (1990). Recurrent meningitis and Mondini dysplasia. *Archives of Otolaryngology–Head and Neck Surgery, 116*;608–612.

Pillsbury, H.C., Grose, J.H., & Hall, J.W. III. (1991). Otitis media with effusion in children. *Archives of Otolaryngology–Head and Neck Surgery, 117*;718–723.

Rosenberg, R.A., Cohen, N.L., & Ransohoff, J. (1987). Long-term hearing preservation after acoustic neuroma surgery. *Otolaryngology–Head and Neck Surgery, 97*;270–274.

Ruckenstein, M.J., Cueva, R.A., Morrison, D.H., & Press, G. (1996). A prospective study of ABR and MRI in the screening for acoustic neuromas. *American Journal of Otology, 17*;317–320.

Sando, I., Shibahara, Y., & Wood, R.P. II. (1990). Congenital anomalies of the external and middle ear. In: C.D. Bluestone, S.E. Stool, & M.D. Scheetz (Eds.), *Pediatric otolaryngology* (2nd ed.) (pp. 271–304). Philadelphia: W.B. Saunders Co.

Seidman, D.A., Chute, P.M., & Parisier, S. (1994). Temporal bone imaging for cochear implantation. *Laryngoscope, 104*;562–565.

Shelton, C., Hitselberger, W.E., House, W.F., & Brackmann, D.E. (1990). Hearing preservation after acoustic tumor removal: Long term results. *Laryngoscope, 100*;115–119.

Shelton, C., Luxford, W.M., Tonokawa, L.L., Lo, W.W.H., & House, W.F. (1989). The narrow internal auditory canal in children: A contraindication for cochlear implants. *Otolaryngology–Head and Neck Surgery, 100*;227–231.

Sismanis, A. (1997). Pulsatile tinnitus. In: G.B. Hughes, & M.L. Pensak (Eds.), *Clinical otology* (2nd ed.) (pp. 445–459). New York: Thieme Medical Publishers.

Swartz, J.D., & Harnsberger HR. (1992). *Imaging of the temporal bone* (2nd ed.) (pp. 247–267). New York: Thieme Medical Publishers.

Syms, C.A. III, De la Cruz, A., & Lo, W.W.M. (1997). Radiological findings in acoustic tumors. In: W.F. House, C.M. Luetje, & K.J. Doyle (Eds.), *Acoustic tumors: Diagnosis and management*. San Diego: Singular Publishing Group, Inc.

Talbot, J.M., & Wilson, D.F. (1994). Computed tomography diagnosis of X-linked congenital mixed deafness, fixation of the stapedial footplate, and perilymphatic gusher. *American Journal of Otology, 15*;177–182.

Telian, S.A., Kileny, P.R., Niparko, J.K., Kemink, J.L., & Graham, M.D. (1989). Normal auditory brain stem response in patients with acoustic neuroma. *Laryngoscope, 99*;10–14.

Tien, R.D., Felsberg, G.J., & Macfall, J. (1992). Fast spin-echo high-resolution MR imaging of the inner ear. *American Journal of Radiology, 159*;395–398.

Tucci, D.L. (1997). Audiological testing. In: W.F. House, C.M. Luetje, & K.J. Doyle (Eds.), *Acoustic tumors: Diagnosis and mangement*. San Diego: Singular Publishing Group, Inc.

Tucci, D.L., Telian, S.A., Kileny, P.R., Hoff, J.T., & Kemink, J.L. (1994). Stability of hearing preservation following acoustic neuroma surgery. *American Journal of Otology, 15*;183–188.

Tucci, D.L., Telian, S.A., Zimmerman-Phillips, S., Zwolan, T.A., & Kileny, P.R. (1995). Cochlear implantation in patients with cochlear malformations. *Archives of Otolaryngology–Head and Neck Surgery, 121*;833–838.

Valvassori, G.E. (1994). Update of computed tomography and magnetic resonance in otology. *American Journal of Otology, 15*;203–206.

Valvassori, G.E., Mafee, M.F., & Carter, B.L. (1995). *Imaging of the head and neck* (pp. 31–35, 113–115). New York: Thieme Medical Publishers.

Welling, D.B., Glasscock, M.E., Woods, C.I., & Jackson, C.G. (1990). Acoustic neuroma: A cost-effective approach. *Archives of Otolaryngology–Head and Neck Surgery, 103*; 364–370.

Wiet, R.J., Pyle, F.M., O'Connor, C.A., Russell, E., & Schramm, D.R. (1990) Computed tomography: How accurate a predictor for cochlear implantation. *Laryngoscope, 100*;687–692.

Wilmington, D., Gray, L., & Jahrsdoerfer, R. (1994). Binaural processing after corrected congenital unilateral conductive hearing loss. *Hearing Research, 74*;99–114.

Wilson, D.F., Talbot, J.M., & Mills, L. (1997). Clinical forum: A critical appraisal of the role of auditory brain stem response and magnetic resonance imaging in acoustic neuroma diagnosis. *American Journal of Otology, 18*; 673–681.

## Chapter 7

Functional Brain Imaging in Audiology

Lynn S. Alvord, Robert B. Burr, and Cynthia A. McCormick

For many years, scientists interested in the brain have longed to see it functioning "in vivo." New techniques, collectively termed *functional imaging*, allow this to be accomplished in a variety of modalities, including magnetic resonance imaging (MRI), positron emission tomography (PET), and magnetoencephalography (MEG). In functional imaging, areas of the brain that are active during mental processes, such as audition, may be "visualized" as computer-enhanced colored areas on the scan. This is made possible by advanced imaging techniques, whereby metabolic processes accompanying increased neuronal activation may be detected. Such changes are typically very small and must be determined by computer analysis post hoc.

Whereas previous attempts at "brain mapping" relied on injured, diseased, or indirect methods, functional imaging comes closer to direct determination of active cortical areas in normal and abnormal subjects. Terms such as "seeing the mind" depict the scope and future of this new technology that promises increased understanding of brain function.

Neuropsychologists, physicists, radiologists, and neurosurgeons are among those most often involved on the team. In the clinical setting a variety of stimulus types are used, including auditory and visual to determine location of critical language areas. This information helps the neurosurgeon predict the outcome of various surgical procedures. Because auditory stimuli are among the most often used, audiologists are becoming valuable members of the imaging team, bringing with them an in-depth knowledge of auditory neurophysiology and experience in stimulus design and delivery.

SPECIAL CONSIDERATION

Because scanner time is expensive and competitively sought after, researchers and clinicians are organized into "teams," thereby allowing more than one experiment to be performed on a given subject.

This chapter provides an overview of the principles, techniques, and recent findings using auditory stimuli for the various functional imaging modalities. Emphasis is given to functional magnetic resonance imaging (fMRI), including examples obtained at the University of Utah. The chapter assumes a working knowledge of cortical anatomy. The reader is referred to Fitzgerald (1992) for an excellent review. A review of auditory cerebral anatomy and physiology may be found in Musiek (1986).

FUNCTIONAL MAGNETIC RESONANCE IMAGING

Since its inception in the early 1990s, fMRI has rapidly become the most widely used modality in functional imaging (Binder et al, 1997; Lorberman et al, 1998). With greater temporal and spatial resolution than previous methods, fMRI is producing an ever-increasing number of studies in the auditory modality. The purpose of this section is to (1) provide a brief overview of the principles, technique, and instrumentation involved in the acquisition of fMRI images in the auditory mode; (2) describe general findings to date; and (3) discuss the role of audiologists in the future of fMRI.

General Principles
MRI Theory

Before discussing fMRI, a basic understanding of standard MRI is necessary. The reader is also referred to Sanders and Orrison (1995) for a more in-depth treatment of this subject. MRI differs from other imaging modalities such as x-ray imaging and computed tomography (CT) in that a magnetic field is used to produce images. MRI images are formed using radiofrequency (RF) magnetic measures of *water density* within tissue. Along with these density measures, various "weightings" (T1, T2, etc.) further affect the brightness of portions of the image and are chosen according to the desired goals of the scan.

Figure 7–1 shows a somewhat oversimplified explanation of how these weightings are achieved. A strong static magnetic field first aligns protons of hydrogen atoms (the most prevalent element in tissue) causing them to spin in synchrony. The spinning creates magnetic vectors, *L*, along the longitudinal axis of the body. A strong RF signal is next applied transversely to these protons (90 degrees), which realigns the magnetic vectors into the transverse position, *T*. This realignment causes the longitudinal magnetic vector, *L*, to lose strength while the transverse vector, *T*, gains strength. When the RF signal is switched off, these vectors assume their original positions and strengths over a very short period termed *relaxation time.*

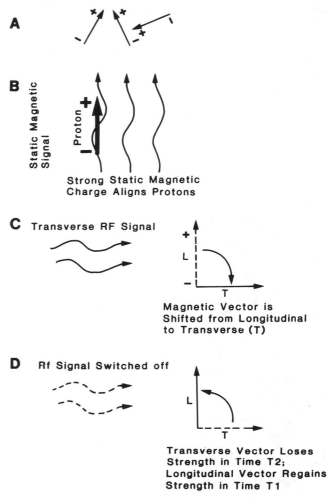

Figure 7–1 Derivation of *T1* and *T2* weightings of an MRI image. **(A)** Randomly aligned hydrogen protons. **(B)** Static magnetic signal aligns protons along the longitudinal axis of the body creating a net magnetic vector *(L)* in this axis. **(C)** Transverse radio frequency *(RF)* signal is applied, shifting the longitudinal vector *(L)*, creating a magnetic vector *(T)* in the transverse direction. **(D)** When RF signal is switched off, vectors return to their previous position. T2 is defined as the time in which vector T loses its strength. T1 is the time in which vector L regains its strength. Because T1 and T2 differ depending on tissue type, this information is used to produce T1- or T2-"weighted" images.

PEARL

In MRI, T1 is the time required for the longitudinal vector to *regain* strength, and T2 is the time required for the transverse vector to *lose* strength. Because time constants vary according to tissue type, the T1 and T2 information is used to *enhance* images into either T1- or T2-weighted images.

The time functions in which these vectors return to their original states are termed *T1*, the time in which the longitudinal vector *regains* strength, and *T2*, the time in which the transverse vector *loses* strength. Because these time constants vary according to tissue type, this information is used during image development to *enhance* the image into either a *T1*- or *T2*-"weighted image." Various weightings are best for particular tissue combinations needing to be imaged. For example, a T1-weighted image is particularly good for differentiating normal anatomic tissue boundaries. T2-weighted images are sensitive to most abnormal tissue, including tumors, abscesses, and infected areas. A variation of *T2*, termed *T2**, is optimally suited for *functional* imaging in normal, as well as abnormal individuals. Although a discussion of the difference between *T2* and *T2** is beyond the scope of this chapter, *T2** weighting is well suited for functional imaging because of its sensitivity to the status of deoxyhemoglobin concentration. This chemical affects MR signal intensity and forms the basis of the "BOLD fMRI" ("blood oxygenation level dependent") technique (Ogawa et al, 1990). "BOLD" fMRI is used in most current fMRI studies including those described in this chapter. For a more in-depth treatment of general MRI theory, the reader is also referred to Bronskill and Sprawls (1993). A simplified version of MRI theory is also published by Berlex Laboratories (1992).

BOLD Functional MRI

In BOLD fMRI, areas of the cortex that are active during mental tasks (such as listening) may be detected after computer analysis on the basis of the BOLD theory. According to this model (Fig. 7–2), increased neuronal activity in active cortical areas results in increased localized blood flow bringing greater concentrations of oxygenated hemoglobin relative to deoxygenated hemoglobin (deoxyhemoglobin). Because deoxyhemoglobin is paramagnetic, this chemical interferes with the magnetic processes producing the image; therefore lower concentrations of deoxyhemoglobin result in increases in the

BOLD Principle

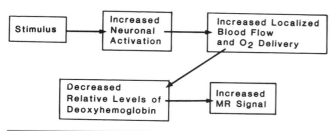

Figure 7–2 Sequence of events describing the "blood oxygenation level dependent" (BOLD) theory on which "BOLD fMRI" is based.

desired MR signal in the area. The above description is true particularly for *T2**-weighted images. A more detailed description of this theory may be found in Ogawa et al (1990). The increase in signal is not instantaneous but requires approximately 5 seconds to occur (Frahm et al, 1992). The small amount of increased brightness on the scan is not detectable to the naked eye but must be determined post hoc by computer analysis, which enhances active areas on the final version of the scan.

Stimulus Paradigm and Data Analysis

For analysis, the computer divides the cortical surface into tiny units ("pixels" if two dimensional, "voxels" if three dimensional). Analysis is made within each voxel to determine

whether the MR signal (1) exceeds a certain threshold, and (2) fluctuates in time with the on-off pattern of signal presentation (typically 30 seconds "on" alternated with 30 seconds "off").

An example fMRI scan performed in the University of Utah laboratory is shown in Figure 7–3. The normal, right-handed male subject was asked to listen and remember details of a story switched on and off every 30 seconds. The figure shows sagittal images with the right hemisphere on top. Note that primary auditory areas and more posterior language areas are activated. Additional information regarding this figure will be presented in the following sections. Figure 7–4 shows the on-off "boxcar" paradigm of signal delivery

---

PEARL

Besides correlation statistics, multiple *t* tests and other statistical procedures are used in some software to determine significance of the signal changes.

---

along with the change in MR signal for a particular voxel termed the *time-intensity profile*. For auditory stimuli, words, tones, or sentences are presented to the patient through non-metallic earphones consisting of a length of polyethylene tubing terminating in foam ear inserts (see Fig. 7–7).

Posthoc computer analysis is made within each voxel to determine whether fluctuations in signal strength exceed random variations. To be considered significant, these

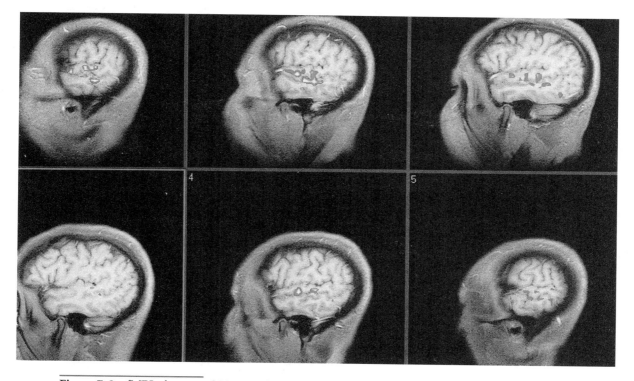

Figure 7–3 fMRI of a normal 34-year-old right-handed man. Stimulus was a narrative story delivered auditorily at the upper level of comfortable loudness. Top three sagittal slices are of the right hemisphere. Bottom three slices are of the left hemisphere. *(See Color Plate 13.)*

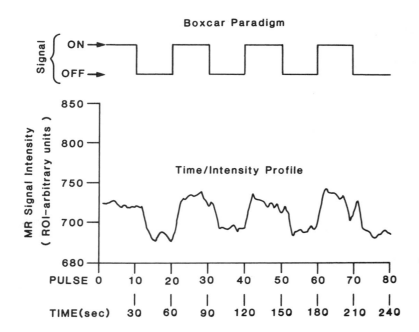

Figure 7–4 "Boxcar" stimulus delivery paradigm and "time/intensity profile" showing MR signal change in a single voxel, which fluctuates with the "on-off" pattern of the stimulus.

fluctuations must exceed a certain amount, as well as "wax" and "wane" correspondingly with the "on-off" cycles of the stimulus. To determine this second criterion, a correlation statistic is run comparing the curve of increasing and decreasing signal strength with an idealized "on-off" curve represented by a sine wave. A sine wave is assumed because the BOLD effect is not instantaneous in the tissues but gradually increases and decreases when the stimulus is turned on and off, respectively. If this correlation is found and if the signal changes also exceed a certain absolute value, the computer assigns a color depicting statistical significance (degree of activation) to the voxel being analyzed. Color schemes vary depending on the software.

Each voxel is analyzed independently in this manner to arrive at the final functional scan. Typically, correlation values of .35 or greater are necessary for significance. Although this value seems low, according to the mathematical models used in the analysis software, this value corresponds to p values much lower than .001. Changes in signal strength should typically increase by 2% to 6% (Rueckert et al, 1993). Signal changes greatly exceeding this amount (20 to 50% range) are likely caused by artifact such as when scanning directly over a blood vessel. Besides correlation statistics, multiple t tests and other statistical procedures are used in some software to determine significance of the signal changes.

Alternative Signal Paradigms

In a variation of the "boxcar" paradigm, instead of an "off" period, a second signal meant to activate a different area of the cortex (i.e., visual) is alternated with the auditory signal. By this "on-on method" (Fig. 7–5), two areas of the cortex may be analyzed in one session. The desired "off" period will still be achieved in the auditory cortex because visual stimuli, which do not activate auditory areas, will occur during the usual "off" cycle. For the visual area, the auditory stimulus serves as the "off" cycle. For example, the patient may receive auditory sentences for 30 seconds alternated with visually

presented words for 30 seconds, thereby stimulating both the auditory and visual areas of the cortex.

A third useful paradigm (Fig. 7–6) uses a type of subtraction technique to tease out a single feature within the same modality (for example, semantic area versus primary auditory area). The following example demonstrates this technique. If it were desired to determine the cortical location of receptive language among other cortical areas activated by sound, it would be necessary to subtract out the areas not involved in this specific process. To achieve this, meaningless sentences could be alternated with meaningful sentences. In areas sensitive to sound but not meaning, the message would be meaningless during both the "on" and the "off" cycles. Because no change is perceived, no activation would occur in this area. However, in the areas sensitive to meaning, "meaningful" words would be occurring every 30 seconds alternated with meaningless words. Thus an "on-off" activation pattern would be achieved only in the semantic areas affected by the meaningful words.

Image Acquisition and Equipment

Functional MRI may be performed either on research scanners designed specifically for this purpose or on high-quality scanners designed primarily for clinical use. Field strength of the magnet should be at least 1.5 tesla (Moonen, 1995). A "head coil" (Fig. 7–7), which better detects the magnetic signal focused on the head, is also highly beneficial. Custom-built "encapped" head coils are also available that further reduce noise. Studies at the University of Utah use a General Electric Medical Systems Signa Horizon Scanner (Milwaukee, WI) (Fig. 7–8). This model consists of a 1.5 tesla (magnetic field strength) "echo speed" scanner. Also shown in Figure 7–7 is the quadrature head coil (GE "three axis") ready to be positioned over the head. Pillows would then be packed inside the coil around the head to reduce the chance of head motion during the scan.

Final fMRI images are a composite of two sets of images, namely, functional images obtained during stimulus

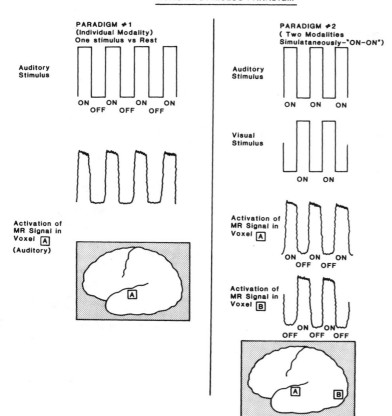

BOXCAR STIMULUS PARADIGM

PARADIGM #1
(Individual Modality)
One stimulus vs Rest

Auditory
Stimulus

ON   ON   ON   ON
   OFF   OFF   OFF

Activation of
MR Signal in
Voxel Ⓐ
(Auditory)

PARADIGM #2
(Two Modalities
Simultaneously-"ON-ON")

Auditory
Stimulus

ON   ON   ON

Visual
Stimulus

ON   ON

Activation of
MR Signal in
Voxel Ⓐ

ON   ON   ON
   OFF   OFF

Activation of
MR Signal in
Voxel Ⓑ

ON   ON
   OFF   OFF   OFF

Figure 7–5 Standard stimulus paradigm (No. 1) and alternative stimulus paradigm (No. 2) in which two areas of the cortex are stimulated during the same experiment.

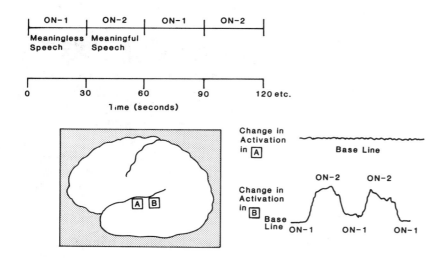

ON-1   ON-2   ON-1   ON-2

Meaningless Meaningful
Speech   Speech

0   30   60   90   120 etc.
        Time (seconds)

Change in
Activation
in Ⓐ

Base Line

Change in
Activation
in Ⓑ
Base
Line   ON-1   ON-1   ON-1

ON-2   ON-2

Figure 7–6 Subtraction paradigm used to tease out a subcategorical function (e.g., meaningful speech) within a broader category (e.g., "hearing" areas that include both meaningful and meaningless speech). Meaningful speech is alternated with meaningless speech. Because the software only determines areas in which *change* occurs, only the areas activated by meaningful speech will be shown in the final scan.

presentation, which are then overlaid on separately acquired anatomical images. The following procedure outlines the methods used at the University of Utah to obtain six sagittal fMRI images similar to those seen in Figure 7–3 (three images in the right and left hemisphere, respectively). A similar procedure may be used to obtain functional images in any other plane.

For the anatomical images, a "three-axis" T1 image is first acquired (axial then coronal and sagittal). Both the functional and anatomical images are acquired at slices set at the same

locations. Figure 7–9 shows how these locations are chosen. Slice locations are chosen using a different plane than the one in which the images are obtained. As seen in the Figure 7–9, locations are selected by first setting the sagittal slice locations in the *coronal plane* (19 vertical lines on Fig. 7–9B). Of these 19 slice locations, the outer three on each side were chosen (Fig. 7–9A) to obtain the final six sagittal images shown in Figure 7–3. Scanning for the functional imaging occurs sequentially in the six chosen slices with the scanner "seeing" each slice every 3 seconds.

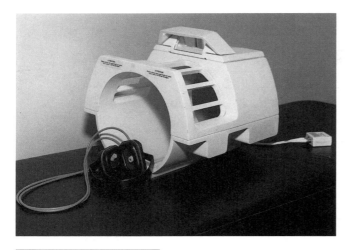

Figure 7–7   GE quadrature three-axis head coil used in fMRI scanning.

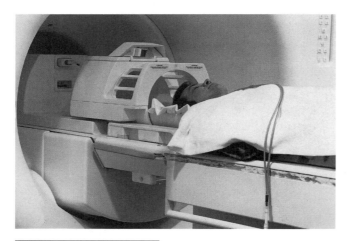

Figure 7–8   GE 1.5 tesla MRI high-speed "echo planar" scanner used in fMRI. Note the quadrature head coil ready to be positioned over the head.

From the computer analysis described previously, areas of functional activation (active voxels) are superimposed by the software onto the anatomical images to produce the final fMRI sagittal scans, an example of which is shown in Figure 7–3. The three top images of Figure 7–3 represent increasingly deeper sagittal slices (see Fig. 7–9B) for the *right hemisphere*, whereas the bottom three slices show increasingly *more lateral* slices of the *left hemisphere*. Right and left hemispheres must always be identified because right may not always be shown on top. Additional techniques allow transposition of the functional data onto one of the other planes (axial or coronal). However, this would require an additional step during the anatomical imaging termed a *whole head* acquisition.

Data Management

Images from both the anatomical and functional acquisitions represent a large amount of data requiring substantial computer disk space. Typically, these data cannot remain in the scanner's computer but are transferred to another computer

for analysis. Analysis requires commercially available software specifically written for this purpose. A typical analysis for a single patient requires approximately 1 to 2 hours, depending on user experience.

Variability Factors

Analysis Variables

Various analysis programs are available commercially, each resulting in slightly differing images, which is due to differences in underlying assumptions used in the software. For example, although an idealized "sine wave" is often used for correlation to the actual "on-off" signal changes, other idealized curves may be used. Software user variables also cause significant differences in the final image. During the analysis, various options may be used, including choice of statistical significance threshold values. Figure 7–10 shows the same scan shown in Figure 7–3 analyzed with the same software but using slightly higher statistical thresholds in the analysis. Note the result in a less "active"-looking scan. It would seem that a simple solution would be to use the same statistical values during analysis. However, clinical experience has shown that in cases of decreased patient motivation or alertness (discussed below), a slight lowering of the statistical threshold during analysis can result in a quite "normal"-looking scan, whereas using the typical thresholds may show no activation. Appropriate statistical values for use during analysis, as well as interaction with patient state, are topics in need of further study.

Subject State or Effort

Initial fMRI studies demonstrate that degree of activation is greatly affected by the conscious state of the subject. Similarly, motivation or degree of effort used by the subject can

---

PITFALL

Conscious state of the subject greatly affects the degree of activation. Sleeping or disinterested subjects may exhibit little or no activation.

---

affect scans. Sleeping subjects show little activation of cortical areas, which emphasizes the concept that areas of activity represent conscious thought processes. This is especially true when sensory stimuli are used or when the task involves memory or other cognitive abilities.

Head Movement and Muscle Artifact

Head movement at any time during the scanning process produces significant location errors and other artifact. Because the final fMRI scan is a composite of functional images superimposed on detailed anatomical images, head motion of as little as a few millimeters in either scan can greatly reduce the accuracy of the final image. Surrounding the head with towels tightly packed in the coil housing is a superior method to using a bite bar, which may also cause artifact because of active muscle clenching. Clenching of head or neck muscles may be particularly deceiving because this may occur in synchrony with "on" cycles. This timed head movement could conceivably cause areas on the cortex to appear active.

Choice of Slice Location

Functional images are acquired at predetermined slice locations in a particular plane (sagittal, coronal, or axial). Location of the slice can affect the degree of activation seen on the final scan; therefore it is best to observe activation at several different slice depths. In the sagittal plane three slice depths on each side such as shown in Figures 7–3 and 7–10 are utilized at the University of Utah. Having standard slice locations would aid in comparative studies, but unfortunately choice of slice location is somewhat arbitrary between laboratories or between subjects within the same laboratory. Arriving at standard slice locations is complicated by large variations in individual anatomy and head size. Until standardized methods can be achieved, small differences in slice location must be considered a possible source of error when comparing two data sets. However, the magnitude of this error may be quite small because studies of this issue report good correspondence between two such data sets having slight variations in slice location (DeYoe et al, 1994). Although

of less significance clinically, it is likely that small variations in slice location could lead to erroneous research conclusions. It is likely that a system based on an individual's own anatomical landmarks would have the greatest advantage for comparative studies.

Within and Between Subject Variability

Figure 7–11 shows test-retest results from a same-subject evaluated at the University of Utah. The subject, a right-handed, 24-year-old normal woman, was given two scans in succession on the same day. She received an auditorily presented taped story about the city of Chicago. The stimulus was binaurally balanced for loudness by the subject to her upper level of comfortable loudness prior to the test, and was alternated with 30-second periods of rest. Resulting sound levels as measured at the foam tip with a sound level meter were 92 dB(A) in the right ear and 91 dB(A) in the left. The subject was asked to pay close attention to the details of the story. Before the second scan, the patient was removed from the scanner, repositioned on the table, and asked to readjust the volume of the stimulus, resulting in levels of 93 dB(A) in the right

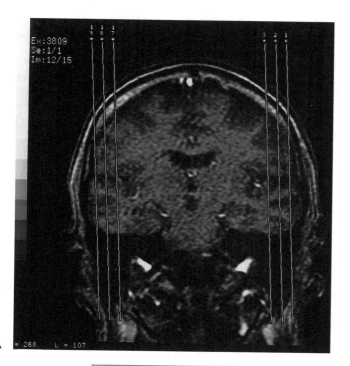

A

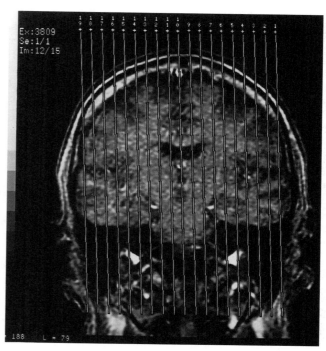

B

Figure 7–9 **(A)** Anatomical MRI locator scan (frontal radiologic view) with slice locator lines used to "set slices" for the sagittal plane for both the anatomical and fRMI acquisitions. **(B)** Six final slice locations chosen from the original 19 shown in **(A)**.

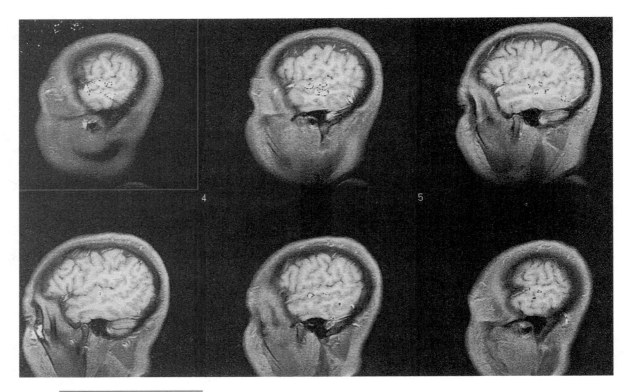

Figure 7–10 fMRI scan using same data from Figure 7–3 but a higher statistical cutoff during analysis. Note the apparent lesser degree of activation caused by the differing statistical choice made during analysis. *(See Color Plate 14.)*

ear and 90 dB(A) in the left (levels within 1 dB of those used in the first scan). Analysis of the two scans used the same software with the same statistical values (Z thresholds 3 to 7). Figure 7–11 shows results of the first and second scans, respectively. As seen, similar but not identical results were obtained with slightly more extensive activation occurring on the second scan. Although slices were chosen in the same manner for both scans (setting the outermost slice in the axial plane at the outer margin of the cortex), apparently some difference exists in slice depth between the two scans, which may account for much of the difference between scans. This is possibly caused by slight differences in head orientation in the scanner because the technologist noted the head being positioned slightly more forward (chin more downward) on the second scan (see earlier section on "Choice of Slice Location"). DeYoe et al (1994) also found minor differences in scans performed on the same individuals 1 week apart. Subject alertness or slight differences in slice locations were possible causes. Other possible variables are differences in head orientation, movement of the head, and lack of novelty when presenting the same stimulus twice.

PEARL

It is well established that individual differences exist in cortical organization for language.

When performing the same task on different subjects, considerable variability of results occurs. Using visual stimuli, Rombouts et al (1997) noted large variability in the size and location of the cortical area activated between subjects. However, a high degree of overlap of at least some portion of the areas being activated was noted. The greatest portion of this intersubject variability presumably comes from actual differences in individual cortical organization. It is well established that individual differences exist in cortical organization for language (Ojemann, 1983).

Validity

Validity of fMRI relates to several issues. fMRI provides an *indirect* measure of neural activity by use of measures in or around microvasculature, which is very close to neurons being activated. Therefore, it is possible that areas of blood pooling in larger veins could pose as sites of activation. This artifact may usually be determined because increase in MR signal strength in this case far exceeds the values typically achieved at true activation sites.

Another potential problem is encountered when scanning directly over a sulcus because signals at various levels may add together. Attempts are being made through software design to virtually "blow up" the cortical surface like a balloon during analysis, thus avoiding this problem. However, this approach may introduce other forms of artifact.

MR activation by the BOLD technique does not occur instantaneously. A time lag of approximately 5 seconds occurs

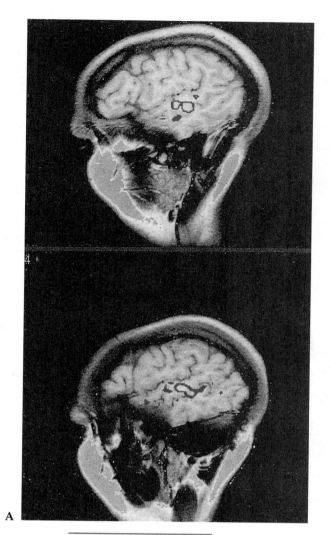

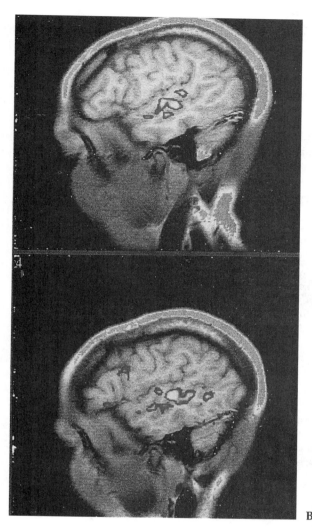

Figure 7–11 Two separate fMRI scans performed on the same subject 20 minutes apart using identical methodologies. **(A)** First scan performed. **(B)** Second scan performed 20 minutes later. Slice locations for the two scans were chosen to be nearly the same as possible (right hemisphere is shown on top for both acquisitions). *(See Color Plate 15.)*

between neural activation and the beginning of the BOLD effect (DeYoe et al, 1994). Use of a 30-second stimulus period allows amply for this factor.

Resolution

It should be recognized that the BOLD theory is only an indirect measure of neural activity at a location slightly remote from the neurons; that is, in or around the microvasculature. As mentioned in the previous section, the possibility exists that scanning near larger vessels where blood pooling may occur could result in an area of inactivity being identified as an active area. Notwithstanding this possibility, agreement with other more direct methods (magnetoencephalography or intraoperative electrode stimulation) is good and on the order of a few millimeters (Elliott, 1994). However, the degree of spread of the image beyond the actual point of neural activation is not known.

PEARL

The presence of activation on an fMRI scan provides evidence of some viable function in a particular area of the cortex.

Determining Degree of Activation

Another factor relating to validity is the unknown relationship between degree of activation on the fMRI scan and the degree of neural activity present. For example, whether greater neural activity is best represented by a wider area of activation (number of voxels activated) or greater percent increase in signal strength in response to the stimulus (percent change of signal strength of individual voxels) is unknown. Realizing that fMRI activation relates to conscious thought, exactly what a greater or lesser degree of response signifies is not known. For example, it is possible that a greater degree of response may occur in a brain that has some *loss* of function because the subject is trying to comprehend the stimulus harder. Therefore at present it is unclear whether greater amounts of activation represent greater cognitive ability, effort, tissue health, motivation, or a combination of the these and other factors. More studies are needed to clarify these issues. One thing that is clear is that the presence of activation on an fMRI scan provides evidence of some viable function in a particular area of the cortex.

Other fMRI Techniques

Alternative fMRI techniques fall under the heading "perfusion fMRI." These techniques that measure cerebral blood flow include "bolus tracking," which requires injection of a magnetic compound such as gadolinium (Belliveau et al, l991) and "spin-labeling" (Moseley et al, 1996). These techniques are somewhat limited in that they are either invasive ("bolus tracking"), which limits the number of times an individual may be scanned without risk of kidney damage, or are more time consuming ("spin-labeling"). However, spin-labeling can provide highly accurate results when only a specific area of the cortex is being examined.

Auditory Findings

Several centers have performed fMRI studies with auditory stimuli. The combination of functional images superimposed on high-resolution anatomical images provides an exciting view of auditory and language areas in normal and abnormal subjects. Studies have been conducted with a variety of stimulus types, including pure tones and passive speech (Millen et al, l995); nonspeech noise, single words, meaningless speech, or narrative text (Binder et al, l994); and native versus foreign language comprehension (Schlosser et al, 1998). This section summarizes general principles found both through earlier studies and those performed at the University of Utah. Schlosser et al (l998) provides a number of current references of fMRI studies by use of auditory stimuli. Although still under study, the following principles are apparent:

1. Sound stimuli that require little or no linguistic analysis such as noise, pure tones, or passive listening to uninteresting text, produce nearly symmetrical activity in or around the superior temporal gyrus of each hemisphere (Binder et al, l994).

2. When the task requires listening for comprehension, significant lateralization to the language-dominant hemisphere is present (Schlosser et al, l998). Meaningful, interesting speech produces activation in primary auditory areas and in more posterior language regions.

PEARL

When testing to determine language-dominant hemisphere, use tasks that are interesting or require linguistic analysis as opposed to passive listening tasks that tend to result in more symmetrical results.

3. When stimulating with meaningful speech, multiple additional areas of the cortex may be activated, the significance of which is not entirely understood. When the task is particularly difficult, such as listening in the presence of background noise, studies at the University of Utah have noted areas activated in the prefrontal cortex. This possibly represents decision-making processes for which the frontal lobe is particularly well suited. An alternative theory is that the frontal lobe, under difficult or noisy listening conditions, is playing its well-known role of selectively attending to the desired stimulus. Note the frontal lobe activation in the hearing-impaired subject in Figure 7–12 described later.

4. Stimuli of higher presentation rates or greater difficulty produce greater activation. When words are presented too slowly, allowing time for the subject to daydream between stimuli, activation is greatly reduced. Tasks that are uninteresting, although "language rich," may produce activation of primary auditory areas but little activation of language areas.

PEARL

Stimuli that are challenging or interesting produce greater activation.

fMRI In the Hearing-Impaired

Studies at the University of Utah have begun to evaluate activation of auditory areas in patients with hearing impairment. Such studies may be beneficial not only to basic research but also may prove helpful in predicting cochlear implant success. Figure 7–12 shows fMRI of a 73-year-old, severely hearing-impaired, right-handed male. The stimulus was the Davy Crockett story presented binaurally at the upper level of comfortable loudness (approximately 115 dB HL). The patient was "postlingually" deafened as a result of "hereditary factors" with the greater portion of the loss occurring around age 35. Hearing testing for the patient showed a nearly "corner audiogram" bilaterally. Pure tone hearing thresholds were right ear—55 dB at 250 Hz, 85 dB at 500 Hz, and no response at other frequencies; left ear—55 dB at 250 Hz, 50 dB at 500 Hz, 85 dB at 1000 Hz, and no response at other frequencies. Speech recognition thresholds were 95 dB with 0% word recognition bilaterally. Binaural amplification had been worn nearly constantly since the patient lost his hearing.

Figure 7–12 shows sagittal fMRI acquisitions superimposed on the anatomical images (right hemisphere on top). Note the strong, normal-appearing activation bilaterally in the temporal lobes. Also of interest is the lack of a strongly dominant hemisphere, a finding noted in most hearing-impaired subjects in our laboratory. The reason for this lack of dominance could be due to the stimulus sounding more like meaningless noise than a meaningful message. As noted earlier, meaningless sound often results in less lateral dominance in fMRI studies. Another explanation is that bilaterality is a "normal" characteristic of hearing-impaired subjects. Studies are ongoing to determine this possibility. Also of interest is the frontal lobe activation (middle bottom of Fig. 7–12). As

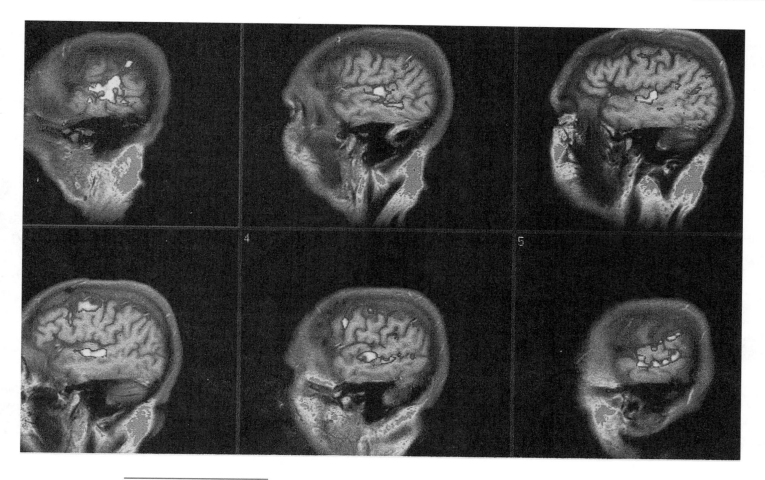

Figure 7–12 fMRI of severely hearing-impaired 73-year-old man (sagittal slices with right hemisphere on top). Note frontal lobe activation (*middle bottom*) in addition to normal areas of activation. (*See Color Plate 16.*)

noted in the previous section, this finding has sometimes been seen in normal individuals listening in difficult or noisy situations. The task for this subject would certainly be considered "difficult" because of the presence of the hearing loss.

The subject shown in Figure 7–12 received a cochlear implant following the imaging study and is reportedly doing well. It is hoped that such fMRI studies will prove useful in the prediction of cochlear implant success.

Role of Audiologists

The clinical applications for which fMRI is currently being applied include localization of the dominant language hemisphere in preneurosurgical patients (epilepsy, tumors, etc.), determining precise locations of hearing and language centers for determining effects of surgical removal of adjacent areas, and determining major anatomical landmarks such as the central sulcus before surgery.

Audiologists are well suited to the requirements of these clinical applications. The choice and delivery of auditory stimuli are important aspects of these case studies. For example, at the University of Utah, the "Davy Crockett" story from the SSI-ICM test has proven to be a very popular and robust stimulus for these clinical purposes. A special binaural version of the test was prepared by Auditek (St. Louis, MO) to avoid the intensity variations encountered in some portions of the standard SSI test. The educational background and clinical experience of audiologists in areas of neuroanatomy of the auditory system and neurological processing of sound make them welcomed participants on clinical and research teams. As stated earlier, teams are necessary and typical in this area because of the competition and large expense involved in the use of MRI scanners.

MAGNETOENCEPHALOGRAPHY

General Principles

Of all the functional imaging techniques, MEG provides the most direct assessment of neural events, detecting the tiny magnetic signals generated directly from traveling current along activated neurons. During functional MEG, cortical regions involved in sensory, motor, or cognitive functions experience increased neuronal activity. Because a traveling electrical charge always produces an accompanying magnetic field, these small magnetic signals are detected by a *magnetometer* or gradiometer positioned around the patient's head.

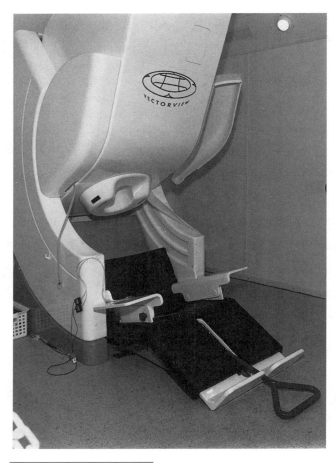

Figure 7–13 A 306-channel MEG scanner located at the Center for Advanced Medical Imaging, University of Utah.

The headpiece contains several discrete sensing transducers or "SQUIDs," (superconducting quantum interference devices), each sensing a small area of the cortex. The number of SQUIDs corresponds to the number of channels. Instruments are currently available having between 1 and 306 channels. Figure 7–13 shows a 306-channel device located at the Center for Advanced Medical Imaging at the University of Utah.

The various analysis programs that produce the final image operate under a variety of assumptions. According to the often used "single equivalent current dipole model (ECD)" or "single dipole" model, the mathematics used by the program assume that a discrete "group" of neurons is generating a "dipolelike" electrical field (Ganslandt et al, l997). Alternative models are also used in some software that result in slightly different looking images. A criticism of the single dipole model is that it tends to "see" areas of greatest neuronal activation while somewhat ignoring certain surrounding areas of lesser activation. Lewine and Orrison (l995) provide a more complete technical description of MEG technology and techniques.

Superimposing Anatomical Images

Once the areas of magnetic activation have been identified, they are superimposed on anatomical MRI images. These two

acquisitions need to have the same precise orientation. During MEG, this orientation is accomplished by placing four small coils on the scalp, one on the front, back, and each side of the head. Additional infrared sensors are aimed below the nose and into each ear just superior to the tragus. The computer "marks" these locations thereby determining head orientation. During the MRI anatomical scan, these locations are marked with small stickers placed on the head at the same locations so that the two final images may be aligned.

PEARL

"Evoked" MEG, in which a stimulus is delivered and analysis is time-locked to the stimulus, is of great usefulness in mapping cortical areas.

Types of MEG Scans

MEG may be obtained in either *spontaneous* or *evoked* format. In spontaneous mode the patient does nothing and receives no stimulus. Because effective spontaneous responses are only obtainable in the awake state, the patient is sometimes asked to read a passage from a book to maintain alertness, and a spontaneous sample is taken over a period of several minutes. Results of spontaneous MEG may be shown in a format similar to multielectrode electroencephalogram (EEG) tracings or may be "mapped" onto an anatomical grid such as seen in Figure 7–14. This figure shows results for a mildly autistic child having abnormal "epileptic" activity emanating from the location at the center of the left set of circles. Spontaneous MEG may be used to screen for abnormal cortical function such as may occur in schizophrenia or after head trauma in which case "slow" waves may be present. Other abnormal waveforms include altered "alpha" waves that are normally absent with the eyes open. Reading the raw data tracings of spontaneous multichannel MEG is a skill requiring

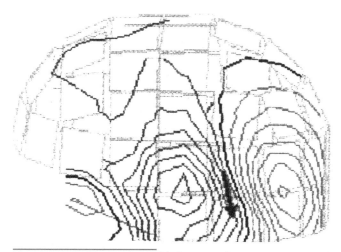

Figure 7–14 Posterolateral left view of spontaneous MEG scan of a mildly autistic child showing focus of epileptiform activity in left temporal lobe (*at center of left circles*). **(See Color Plate 17.)**

highly specialized training. At present, only a few individuals are qualified to perform these analyses.

Of greater usefulness in mapping cortical areas is "evoked" MEG, in which a stimulus is delivered and analysis is time-locked to the stimulus. For example, as a test of tonotopy, a pure tone may be delivered multiple times with a separation of 3 s between each tone. The magnetic signal is sampled during a short time period surrounding each tone (beginning 50 ms before the tone and extending 2 s after). The sampling period before the tone is used to establish baseline values. The individual magnetic responses are then averaged and displayed as an image.

PITFALL

A limitation of MEG is that any metal in the patient will greatly distort the signal as with MRI.

Strengths and Limitations

As with MRI, a limitation of MEG is that metal existing in the patient will greatly distort the signal. Compared with fMRI, perhaps the greatest limitation is the short time frame (a few seconds) in which the data must be gathered. Therefore, single words or sounds rather than sentences lend themselves best to MEG. Sentences may be used for stimuli if careful timing of the target words is maintained. These limitations may be overcome with careful stimulus planning. In addition, MEG has limited availability especially considering the paucity of centers possessing multichannel MEG devices. Finally, MEG only detects magnetic activity at or near the cortical surface as opposed to analyzing deeper structures.

A great strength of MEG compared with all other functional techniques is its unique ability to determine the temporal order of events as they occur in various locations of the cortex. This feature will undoubtedly offer exciting insights into the function of the brain. Functional MEG results, in the form of scans, also agree favorably with those of fMRI and intraoperative electrocortical stimulation mapping.

POSITRON EMISSION TOMOGRAPHY

PET, originally known as positron emission transverse tomography, or PETT, has been used as a radiological imaging technique in biomedical research since the 1970s. PET has been the pioneering technique of functional brain studies including those in the auditory mode. The reader is referred to Zatorre (1996) for a general review of PET and to Engelien et al (1995) who used PET to study sound categorization in normal individuals and a patient with auditory agnosia. These studies contain many pertinent references.

General Principles

PET uses positron-emitting radionuclides ("tracers") to detect biochemical or physiological processes involved in cerebral metabolism. These specially selected radiolabeled compounds are bound with biochemical substances and intravenously injected or inhaled into the body. The isotopes begin

to decay, producing positrons that interact with negative electrons. This process, termed positron-electron annihilation, produces two photons traveling colinearly (180 degrees) in opposite directions ("annihilation radiation"). In PET the positrons are then revealed in vivo by the detection of the annihilation radiation in a scanner encasing the head. The scanner reconstructs images on the basis of the distribution of the radioisotopes as they decay within tissue.

PEARL

Physiological activity that is affected by a disorder or pathological condition can be seen as a departure from normal biochemical processes and can be detected with PET.

PET relies on the assumption that all physiological activities including neural activation are associated with biochemical processes. These biochemical processes can be assessed with PET techniques, allowing function to be indirectly localized. Likewise, physiological activity that is affected by a disorder or pathological condition can be seen as a departure from normal biochemical processes and, therefore, can be detected with PET (Ter-Pogossian, 1995).

Functional PET, properly termed "stimulation PET" allows for localization of "functional" responses (detection of localized neuronal activity) on the basis of changes in metabolic activity associated with the delivery of the stimulus. These include changes in glucose metabolism or increased blood flow. PET was the first imaging modality by which successful functional studies were performed and a large volume of PET data forms the basis of modern functional imaging.

PET data are often overlaid onto anatomicalal images obtained with MRI or CT, which have better resolution than the PET scan itself.

Radionuclides

PET techniques developed from the understanding that a number of radiopharmaceuticals have chemical properties that give them the ability to enter into, and therefore trace, physiological processes. Radioactive isotopes (radionuclides) produced in a *cyclotron*, are used to (1) measure blood flow through the brain, (2) mark metabolic processes, or (3) bind to specific receptors (Ter-Pogossian, 1995). Table 7–1 lists some commonly used radionuclides indicating their half-lives (the amount of time required for half the atoms of the radioactive substance to undergo decay). The short half-life time (minutes) allows measurements to be repeated only at close intervals. This usually requires the cyclotron to be in the same building as the patient and scanner. A few radionuclides having longer half-lives have been used, eliminating the need for an on-site cyclotron (for example, N_4-methylthiosemicarbazone).

Instrumentation

For most PET applications, the detection of the annihilation radiation is accomplished with the use of a *scintillator*, an instrument that records flashes of light (scintillations) that

TABLE 7–1 Common radionuclides used in PET

Radionuclide	Symbol	Half-life (min)	Source
Oxygen-15	^{15}O	2.07	Cyclotron
Nitrogen-13	^{13}N	10	Cyclotron
Flourine-18	^{18}F	109.7	Cyclotron
Galium-68	^{68}Ga	68	^{68}Ge

occur when photons or high-energy particles bombard the transducer. Because the PET scanner must assess radiation at a particular region of the body, a *collimator* is also used. This device determines the location of the radioactive source in the body by detecting the presence and time of arrival of the photon emitted in the opposite direction (mentioned earlier). If no companion photon is found on the opposite side of the collimator, the signal is rejected as coming from a random source. Detection of the companion photon also allows for determination of the location of the generating source. This is done by comparing the time it takes the two photons to arrive at their respective transducers situated at opposing sides of the collimator (termed "time of flight" or "TOF") (Fig. 7–15). Distance from the source (hence location) can then be easily calculated by the computer from the TOF.

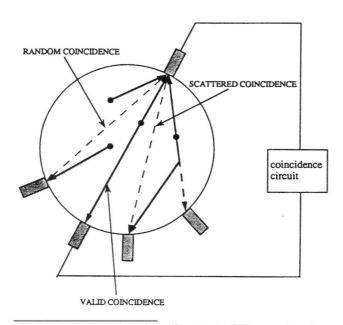

Figure 7–15 Function of a collimator in PET scanning. Random photons are detected by the *absence* of a "companion" photon arriving at the opposite end of the collimator. True photons emitted by radioactive nuclides in the body are detected by the presence of a companion photon at the opposite end of the collimator. Location of the emitting source is determined by comparing time of arrival of the two emitted photons.

Strengths and Weaknesses

A strength of PET is that scans may be obtained in patients having metal in their bodies including cochlear implants. Limitations are poorer resolution, both spatially and temporally, (when compared with fMRI or MEG), the need for injection or inhalation of a radionuclide and the paucity and high cost of available PET scanners. Figure 7–16 shows a posterolateral left view of a three-dimensional PET scan using auditory stimuli. The reader is also referred to Zatorre et al (1996) and Petersen and Fiez (1993) for examples of PET studies using auditory stimuli.

PEARL

The goal of SPECT is to determine the relative or absolute concentration of radionuclides as a function of time.

SINGLE PHOTON EMISSION COMPUTERIZED TOMOGRAPHY

General Principles

Single photon emission computerized tomography (SPECT), developed from emission CT (ECT), involves the detection of gamma rays emitted from radionuclides. SPECT is similar to PET in many ways. Both use radionuclides, which enter the body's metabolism and then emit radiation, which is detected to produce images (see comparison following). Janicek et al (1993) provide an example of how SPECT can be used for language analysis.

Radionuclides

As with PET procedures, radionuclides are necessary for producing SPECT images. SPECT uses radionuclides such as technetium-99m, xenon-133, and thallium-201. Several radionuclides used with SPECT are still in the experimental stage and are not approved by the U.S. Food and Drug Administration (FDA) (Hartshorne, 1995; Jaszczak & Tsui, 1995).

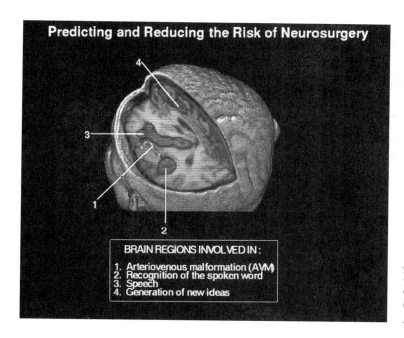

Figure 7–16   Posterolateral left view of a three-dimensional PET scan using auditory stimuli. (Courtesy of The Samaritan PET Center, Phoenix, Arizona.) *(See Color Plate 18.)*

Instrumentation

SPECT imaging requires the collimation (see PET section) of gamma rays emitted from the radionuclide distribution within the body. A scintillation (gamma) camera, containing a lead collimator, is placed in front of a crystal (usually of sodium iodide containing a small amount of thallium), which acts as a lens in an optical imaging system. The collimator consists of multiple channels that allow rays traveling within a desired angle to pass through the channels and interact with the crystal. An array of photomultiplier tubes at the back of the crystal view the scintillations produced by the interaction of the radiation with the crystal. Determination is then made as to the location of each gamma ray interacting with the crystal (Jaszczak & Tsui, 1995). Figure 7–17 shows a clinical SPECT scanner.

SPECT systems reconstruct images in two basic planes, parallel and perpendicular to the axis of the body. The detector arrays come in a variety of configurations, including discrete scintillation detectors, one or more scintillation cameras, and hybrid systems that combine the arrays.

PITFALL

Spatial resolution and noise are major factors that can affect the quality of SPECT images.

Strengths and Weaknesses

SPECT, like PET, has several weaknesses. Also, the attenuation and scatter of gamma ray photons in the patient's body can affect image quality. The size and location of the structure being imaged and the stillness of the patient during imaging affect quality and outcome. SPECT scans look similar to PET, with colored areas indicating degree of activation.

PEARL

Like PET and fMRI, SPECT has the ability to image deeper structures of the brain than MEG.

On the positive side, because SPECT systems are more widely available and less expensive to operate than PET, hospitals are more likely to have SPECT capabilities. Like PET and fMRI, SPECT has the ability to image deeper structures of the brain than MEG.

Comparison of PET and SPECT

Both PET and SPECT systems produce three-dimensional images of anatomical structures from digitally stored data,

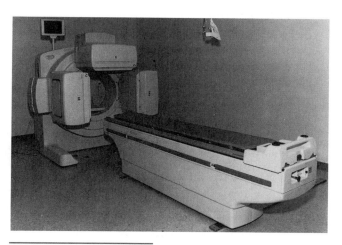

Figure 7–17   SPECT scanner at the Center for Advanced Medical Imaging, University of Utah.

which are then analyzed and displayed. Both procedures use radioactive isotopes injected into the body. PET uses two coincident annihilation photons from positron-emitting radionuclides, whereas SPECT uses gamma rays emitted from different types of radionuclides. Both procedures use the concepts of scintillation and collimation for imaging (Hartshorne, 1995).

PET is used in only about 100 centers around the world. Some of these systems are for clinical purposes, but most are used entirely for research. SPECT, on the other hand, is much more common, less expensive to use, and primarily for clinical purposes.

CONCLUSIONS

Functional imaging is an exciting new technology offering opportunities for audiologists to become involved in both clinical and research applications. Audiologists provide needed

expertise to the imaging teams, which is necessary in performing such studies. Although PET and MEG are not widely available, fMRI and SPECT can be performed on standard high-quality scanners. Especially in the case of fMRI, data analysis requires additional software and training and computer hardware capable of storing large amounts of data. Such instrumentation may already be available in many large hospitals or universities. Each of the imaging modalities described in this chapter has its own inherent strengths and weaknesses. MEG for example, has the distinct advantage of being able to determine the order of events as they occur in the cortex. However, fMRI, PET, and SPECT can probe into deeper areas of the brain.

The information gained in functional imaging is currently useful in surgical planning and postsurgical evaluation of language function. Future research in functional imaging will continue to provide new information on the basic mechanisms underlying central auditory and language function.

REFERENCES

Berlex Laboratories. (1992). MRI MADE EASY. Wayne, NJ: Berlex Laboratories.

Binder, J.R., Frost, J.A., Hammeke, T.A., et al. (1997). Human brain language areas identified by functional magnetic resonance imaging. *Journal of Neuroscience,* 17;353–362.

Binder, J.R., Rao, S.M., Hammeke, T.A., Yetkin, F.Z., Jesman-owicz, A., Bandettini, P.A., Wong, E.C., Estkowski, L.D., Goldstein, M.D., Haughton, V.M., & Hyde, J.S. (1994). Functional magnetic resonance imaging of human auditory cortex. *Annals of Neurology,* 35(6);662–672.

Bronskill, M.J., & Sprawls, P. (Eds.). (1993). *The physics of MRI.* Woodbury, NY: American Institute of Physics.

DeYoe, E.A., Bandettini, P., Neitz, J., et al. (1994). Functional magnetic resonance imaging (fMRI) of the human brain. *Journal of Neuroscience Methods,* 54;171–187.

Elliott, L.L. (1994). Functional brain imaging and hearing. *Journal of the Acoustical Society of America,* 96(3);1397–1409.

Engelien, A., Silbersweig, D., Stern, E., et al. (1995). The functional anatomy of recovery from auditory agnosia. *Brain,* 118;1395–1409.

Fitzgerald, M.J.T. (1992) Cerebral cortex. In M.J.T. Fitzgerald, *Neuroanatomy* (2nd ed.) (pp. 197–210). London: Bailliere Tindall.

Frahm, J., Bruhn, H., Merboldt, K.D., & Hanicke, W. (1992). Dynamic MR imaging of human brain oxygenation during rest and photic stimulation. *Journal of Magnetic Resonance Imaging,* 2;501–505.

Ganslandt, O., Steinmeier, R., Kober, H., et al. (1997). Magnetic source imaging combined with image-guided frameless stereotaxy: A new method in surgery around the motor strip. *Neurosurgery,* 41(3);621–628.

Hartshorne, M.F. (1995). Single photon emission computed tomography. In W.W. Orrison, J.D. Lewine, J.A. Sanders, & M.R. Hartshorne (Eds.). *Functional brain imaging* (pp. 213–238). St Louis: Mosby.

Janicek, M.J., Schwartz, R.B., Carvalho, P.A., et al. (1993). Tc-99m HMPAO brain perfusion SPECT in acute aphasia. *Clinical Nuclear Medicine,* 18(12);1032–1038.

Jaszczak, R.J., & Tsui, B.M.W. (1995). Single photon emission computed tomography (SPECT): General principles. In: H.N. Wagner, Z. Szaba, & J.W. Buchanan (Eds.), *Principles of nuclear medicine* (pp. 342–346). Philadelphia: W. B. Saunders.

Lewine, J.D., & Orrison, W.W. (1995). Magnetoencephalography and magnetic source imaging. In: W.W. Orrison, J.D. Lewine, J.A. Sanders, & M.R. Hartshorne (Eds.), *Functional brain imaging* (pp. 369–417). St Louis: Mosby.

Lorberbaum, J.P., Bohning, D.E., Shastri, A., et al. (1998). Functional magnetic resonance imaging (fMRI) for the psychiatrist. *Primary Psychiatry, March,* 60–70.

Millen, S.J., Haughton, V.M., & Yetkin, Z. (1995). Functional magnetic resonance imaging of the central auditory pathway following speech and pure-tone stimuli. *Laryngoscope,* 105;1305–1310.

Moonen, C.T.W. (1995). Imaging of human brain activation with functional MRI. *Biological Psychiatry,* 37;141–143.

Moseley, M.E., deCrespigny, A., & Spielman, D.M. (1996). Magnetic resonance imaging of human brain function. *Surgical Neurology,* 45:385–391.

Musiek, F.E. (1986). Neuroanatomy, neurophysiology, and central auditory assessment. Part II: The cerebrum. *Ear and Hearing,* 7(5);283–294.

Ogawa, S., Lee, T.M., Ray, A.R., & Tank, D.W. (1990). Brain magnetic resonance imaging with contrast dependent on blood oxygenation. *Proceedings of the National Academy of Science USA,* 87;9868–9872.

Ojemann, G.A. (1983). Brain organization for language from the perspective of electrical stimulation mapping. *Behavioral Brain Science,* 2;189–230.

Petersen, S.E., & Fiez, J.A. (1993). The processing of single words studied with positron emission tomography. *Annual Review of Neuroscience,* 16;509–530.

ROMBOUTS, S.A.R.B., BARKHOF, F., HOOGENRAAD, F.G.C., et al. (1997). Test-retest analysis with functional MR of the activated area in the human visual cortex. *American Journal of Neuroradiology, 18;*1317–1322.

RUECKERT, L., APPOLLONIO, I., GRAFMAN, J., et al. (1993). Functional activation of left frontal cortex during covert word production, Proceedings of 12th SMRM Annual Meeting, New York, p. 60.

SANDERS, J.A., & ORRISON, W.W. (1995). Functional magnetic resonance imaging. In: W.W. Orrison, J.D. Lewine, J.A. Sanders, & M.F. Hartshorne (Eds.), *Functional brain imaging* (pp. 239–326). St. Louis: Mosby.

SCHLOSSER, M.J., AOYAGI, N., FULBRIGHT, R.K., GORE, J.C., & McCARTHY, G. (1998). Functional MRI studies of auditory comprehension. *Human Brain Mapping, 6;*1–13.

TER-POGOSSIAN, M.M. (1995), Positron emission tomography (PET): General principles. In: H.N. Wagner, Z. Szabo, & J.W. Buchanan (Eds.), *Principles of nuclear medicine* (pp. 342–346). Philadelphia: W.B. Sanders.

ZATORRE, R.J., HALPERN, A.R., PERRY, D.W., et al. (1996). Hearing in the mind's ear: A PET investigation of musical imagery and perception. *Journal of Cognitive Neuroscience, 8*(1);29–46.

## Chapter 8

Pharmacology in Audiology Practice

Nathan D. Schwade

> ### PEARL
> The amount of drug given will often separate toxic from therapeutic effects.

At present, in the United States audiologists do not prescribe medications to patients. However, audiologists will examine and test patients taking a myriad of medications. Invariably, one of these medications will adversely effect an audiometric or vestibular test. Therefore it is important for audiologists to have an understanding of the untoward side effects associated with different classes of pharmacological agents. The audiologist may make changes in treatment and diagnostic regimens using this information regarding patients who, at the time of testing, are taking prescribed pharmacological agents.

Pharmacology can be defined as the study of chemical effects (toxic or therapeutic) on the human body. A *drug* is a chemical that is used for a therapeutic effect. The spectrum of undesirable effects of chemicals may be broad and ill defined. In therapeutics a drug typically produces numerous effects, but usually only one is sought as the primary goal of treatment. Most of the other nontherapeutic consequences are referred to as undesirable effects of that drug. *Side effects* of drugs are defined as *nondeleterious* and include effects such as dry mouth with tricyclic antidepressant therapy. A *toxic* response is a *deleterious* effect produced by the drug such as death or permanent liver damage. Paracelsus (1493-1541) noted that "All substances are poisons; there is none which is not a poison. The right dose differentiates a poison and a remedy." Mechanistic categorization of toxic effects is a necessary prelude to avoidance of them or, if they occur, to rational and successful management of them.

Within the past 25 years, an exponential growth has occurred in the number of drugs available to those who prescribe medication. Statistics have shown that 80% of all the drugs that were available in 1990 were obsolete 4 years later. This high turnover rate and the continuous development of new drugs presents a formidable challenge to students of pharmacology. One organizational approach to learning pharmacology is to group the drugs into functional classes. Drugs are usually categorized into groups and named by their therapeutic effects, anatomical effector organ, or by the chemical structure. The following are examples:

- The anxiolytics (psychological stress reduction) and the antihypertensives are named by therapeutic class.
- The loop diuretics are named for their anatomical effector organ, because these medications exert diuresis at the loop of Henle.
- The aminoglycoside antibiotics are named by the chemical structure they share.

It is much more important to understand *how* classes of drugs work and a prototypical example than to memorize long lists of drugs. To accomplish this goal one must understand the relationship of the different pharmacological classes to the following:

1. What is the normal anatomy and physiology of the organs affected?
2. What is the pathophysiology of the organ system?
3. How will the drug alter the physiology in the body?
4. What other body systems will be affected?

Each drug in a class is assigned a name. Most drugs have at least two names, a generic name and a trade name. For example, diazepam is the generic name for Valium, which is a trade name. Trade names are assigned by the pharmaceutical companies and are really marketing tools. It is not uncommon for a drug to have two or three trade names, but all drugs have only one generic name. Therefore, only generic names will be used for the drugs presented in this text. The *Physician Desk Reference* (PDR) is a good source of information on generic and trade names. Students should not use the PDR for information about side effects and complications

Audiology: Diagnosis. Edited by Roeser, Valente, and Hosford-Dunn. Thieme Medical Publishers, Inc., New York © 2000

because the PDR lists all possible effects associated with people and animals.

PHARMACOKINETICS

To arrive at a comprehensive understanding of the effect of a drug on the body, it is necessary to take into account the effects of the human body on the drug. *Pharmacokinetics* is the study of how drugs are absorbed, distributed, excreted, and metabolized in the body. A drug is administered to the body by a route of entry. These routes of entry include the following:

- The lungs (inhalation)
- The gut (pill or elixir)
- Mucous membranes other than the gut (suppository)
- Venous system (needle)
- Subcutaneous injection
- Intramuscular injection
- Intrathecal injection
- Sublingual
- Topical

The first pharmacokinetic stage of a drug before it has a physiological effect is for it to dissolve. Once the drug is in solution (air, blood, and water), the drug is absorbed into the bloodstream by one of several possible mechanisms. Because most medications are taken orally, they are usually absorbed from the intestine into the gastric venous system and then funneled to the portal vein, which carries blood directly to the liver. The liver is the primary organ of detoxification and may often modify the drug and thereby decrease the effectiveness of the medication. Loss of drug from the bloodstream as it

---

PEARL

Oral medications are primarily detoxified and often modified by the liver. This can decrease their effectiveness.

---

passes through the liver is called the *first-pass-effect*. *Parenteral* administration is defined as a route other then the gut. When drugs are administered through parenteral methods of delivery, the first-pass effect is avoided.

If a drug is injected into a vein over 5 to 30 seconds and blood samples are taken periodically and analyzed for unchanged drug, the results would be as follows. The concentration would be greatest a few minutes after injection, when the distribution of the drug throughout the circulatory system has equilibrated. This initial mixing up of the drug and the blood is essentially completed after several passes through the heart. The drug then disappears from the plasma by a variety of processes known as clearance. *Clearance* is the most important concept to be considered when a rational regimen for long-term drug administration is to be designed. The clinician usually wants to maintain steady-state concentrations of a drug within a known therapeutic range. Different types of clearance include the following:

- Slow distribution across membranes to tissue or other body fluids may occur across membranes.

- The drug may be eliminated unchanged by way of the renal or biliary routes.
- If the drug is volatile, it may be exhaled through the pulmonary pathway.
- The compound may undergo metabolism to other active or inactive species by hepatic enzymes.

SPECIAL CONSIDERATION

It is important to consider the concept of clearance when designing a rational regimen for long-term drug administration because the clinician usually wants to maintain a steady state concentration of the drug in a therapeutic range.

Many of these drugs will then be concentrated by the kidneys and excreted in the urine. In fact, during the early days of penicillin therapy, penicillin was extremely expensive, and it was learned that the drug was excreted in the urine virtually unchanged and could be extracted from the urine of patients. The patient's urine was collected, and the penicillin was extracted and then recycled into the patient during the entire course of treatment. Issues of clearance become extremely important with regard to susceptibility of patients to toxicity. *The serum levels of some drugs are also* strongly affected by a compromise in clearance, such as in the case of renal failure, which will lead to toxicity.

PITFALL

A compromise in clearance affects the serum levels of some drugs and can lead to toxicity.

Because of the clearance, an expected drop in plasma concentration occurs over time. The *half-life* is used to describe the reduction in plasma concentrations and is defined as the time required for the concentration to decrease to half the value at the start of the time interval. If a single dose is given, the plasma concentration will be approximately equal to zero after four to five half-lives. For example, if a 100 mg dose is given, after one half-life the concentration will drop to 50 mg, then to 25 mg after the second half-life, then to 12.5 mg, 6.25 mg, and 3.125 mg, respectively after consecutive half-lives.

Therefore multiple-dose therapy is required to maintain a steady-state concentration in the therapeutic range (see Fig. 8–1). Administering multiple doses of a medication allows plasma levels to rise to a desirable concentration range. Moreover, correctly spacing the time between repeat administration will prevent the plasma concentration from dropping below the therapeutic range. For some drugs, the effects are difficult to measure. Toxicity and lack of efficacy are both potential dangers when the therapeutic index is narrow. In these circumstances doses must be titrated carefully, and a target-level strategy is reasonable. A desired (target) steady-state concentration of the drug (usually in plasma) is chosen, and a dosage is computed that is expected to achieve this

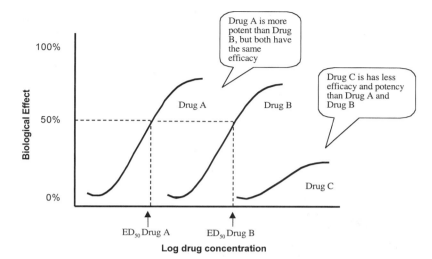

Figure 8–1 Dose-response curves representing the difference between potency and efficacy for three hypothetical drugs.

value. Drug concentrations are subsequently measured, and dosage is adjusted if necessary to approximate the target more closely.

PITFALL

Toxicity and lack of efficacy are potential dangers when the therapeutic index is narrow.

To apply the target-level strategy, the therapeutic objective must be defined in terms of a desirable range called the *therapeutic range*. For some drugs, the lower limit of the therapeutic range appears to be approximately equal to the drug concentration that produces about half of the greatest possible therapeutic effect. The upper limit of the therapeutic range (for drugs with such a limit) is fixed by toxicity, not by efficacy. For some drugs, this may mean that the upper limit of the range is no more than twice the lower limit. Of course, these figures can be highly variable, and some patients may benefit greatly from drug concentrations that exceed the therapeutic range, whereas others may suffer significant toxicity at much lower values. Barring more specific information, however, the target is usually chosen as the center of the therapeutic range.

SPECIAL CONSIDERATION

The upper limit of the therapeutic range is fixed by toxicity, not efficacy, and it should be such that no more than 5 to 10% of patients will experience a toxic effect.

Once the compound has entered the circulation, it will then have access to the cell receptors at the effector organ. Drugs that are not destroyed by the ligand receptor interaction will still be present in the bloodstream. In most clinical situations drugs are administered in a series of repetitive doses or as a continuous infusion to maintain a steady-state concentration of drug in plasma within a given therapeutic range. Thus calculation of the appropriate maintenance dosage is a primary goal. To maintain the chosen steady-state or target concentration, the rate of drug administration is adjusted such that the rate of input equals the rate of loss.

PHYSIOLOGICAL CONSIDERATIONS

Several anatomic barriers exist between the blood and certain organs of the body. The most common anatomical drug barrier is to the brain. Having a system to only allow certain molecules to enter into the brain is a protective measure developed by evolution. Because the brain is so important to our functioning, a selective evolutionary pressure has developed a system to exclude most molecules. These are very tight junctions between the endothelial cells that line the capillaries of the brain, which physically exclude molecules of larger sizes and accomplish this anatomical functionality. For a drug to have

---

PEARL

Tight endothelial junctions are responsible for the blood-organ barriers.

---

an effect on the neuron in the brain, it must first cross the blood-brain barrier. Therefore any drug that is psychoactive crosses the blood-brain barrier, which would include drugs such as alcohol, marijuana, amphetamines, and cocaine. Most often this selective effect is beneficial to the central nervous system. However, in some instances the blood-brain barrier can be a detriment as in the case of some antibiotic therapy. Many types of penicillin will not cross the blood-brain barrier, making treatment of brain abscesses extremely difficult with systemic therapy.

The blood-brain barrier is not the only anatomical barrier in the body. A similar obstacle to drug transport is known as the blood-placenta barrier, which protects the fetus. Most drugs that will cross the blood-brain barrier will also cross the blood-placenta barrier. Compounds capable of transversing the placental barrier are responsible for causing several types of birth defects, including fetal alcohol syndrome and the syndromes associated with cocaine use during pregnancy. Some antibiotics such as tetracyclines are known to produce damage to the enamel of the teeth in utero. These birth defects underscore the importance of drugs crossing anatomical barriers. Mothers who are lactating are also at risk for drugs that cross barriers. One of the barriers of paramount importance to this chapter is the blood-ear barrier. Before a drug may have a detrimental effect on the ear, it must cross the blood-ear barrier, which is another tight barrier. In addition to the vascular components of the ear, other anatomical issues are important to the pharmacology of this organ.

PITFALL

Drugs that cross the blood-placenta barrier may be highly concentrated in the womb, where they will become teratogens.

The ear has an extremely small fluid volume totaling less then 10 μl, which causes very small amounts of drug to be concentrated in the ear. Moreover, the clearance rate of the inner ear fluid is very slow, allowing drugs to be in contact with cells for a long time. Unlike other organs with high clearance rates, the ear is more susceptible to toxicity of certain drugs. The ear and kidney in tandem are often susceptible to toxic effects. In other words, drugs that are ototoxic are also often nephrotoxic and vice versa. Obviously, the kidneys have a high clearance rate, but they also concentrate drugs in the medulla of the kidney. This concentrating effect allows for a buildup of drug levels in the kidney setting the stage for nephrotoxicity.

SPECIAL CONSIDERATION

The clearance rate of the inner ear is very slow, allowing drugs to be in contact with cells for a long time; the ear is more susceptible to toxicity of certain drugs.

POTENCY AND EFFICACY

Potency and efficacy are important terms used in the discussion of pharmacology and deserve some attention in this chapter. A *dose* is the amount of drug given per amount of body weight (e.g., milligrams per kilograms); this is one of the reasons that the physician weighs the patient during an office visit. Using a dose allows standardization of the amount of medication given, taking into account the person's body weight. The average adult male weighs 70 kg (150 pounds), but ranges from 40 to 135 kg (90 to 300 pounds) are not uncommon. This dose system also allows for relative comparisons between individuals. If one administers 10 mg/kg and no effect is seen, the dose can be increased to 100 mg/kg in the same individual. To understand the definitions of potency and efficacy, one must first have an understanding of dose-response curves.

Dose-response curves are not difficult to comprehend if one thinks in terms of probability. Imagine an experiment of 100 subjects in which some physiological parameter is measured for each of the subjects. For simplicity, consider a binary (all or none) response: either the patients improve or they do not improve. For example, in an experiment in which the subjects are given a dose of 1 mg/kg of the drug; at this dose 10% of the population improves. Next, another 100 patients are given 10 mg/kg of the drug, and 35% of the patients improve. As the dose is increased, a point is reached where 100% of the patients are responding. When these data are graphed (log-linear), a graded *dose-response curve* is produced (see Fig. 8–2).

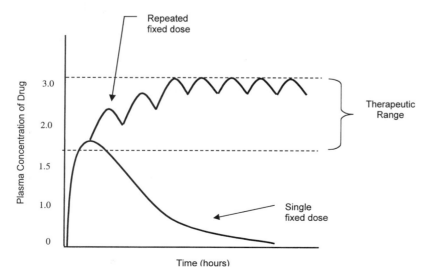

Figure 8–2   Graph of plasma concentration over time for an example drug. Note the difference between repeated fixed dose and a single fixed dose. The therapeutic range is also demonstrated in the graph.

Examining this graph, an investigator can interpolate the point at which the population is responding at 50% of the maximal response. This point is defined as the *ED50* or the effective dose for 50% maximal response. Dose-response experiments can be created for several different drugs and then compared.

Efficacy is the *maximal* response for a drug. In Figure 8–2, drug A has a higher efficacy than drug C. So when a drug is described as being more efficacious, this is always in reference to another drug. *Potency* is a measure of the concentration of a drug that is required to elicit a response. The ED_{50} is a good arbitrary point to compare two different drugs. As shown in Figure 8–1, drug A produces an ED_{50} at a lower concentration than drug B. Therefore drug A is more potent then drug B, but they both have the same efficacy. The important distinction is that increase in potency is defined as less of the drug required to produce the same response. An increase in efficacy is when the drug will actually be able to give a greater maximal response at the same concentration as another drug. The obvious question is why not give a dose that is several hundred times the ED50 to ensure a response from the entire population? The answer is that the most drugs produce unwanted dose-dependent side effects.

THERAPEUTIC INDEX

The *therapeutic index* is defined as the ratio of the dose that produces toxic effects to the dose that produces the desired clinical effect. One of the concepts of paramount importance to pharmacology is that drugs produce a dose-dependent effect. In other words, the *higher* the concentration in the body, the *greater* the effect. Conversely, after a reduction in plasma concentration a reversal of the effect is observed. A minimum concentration is required to produce the desired therapeutic effect. Below this concentration, the drug has no effect, and when levels rise above this point, toxic effects are produced. Therefore drugs that have a narrow therapeutic index have a low tolerance for dosing levels, and toxicity can be produced from plasma concentrations that are not much higher than the

dose required to produce the desired effect. For example, the dose of the aminoglycoside antibiotic streptomycin required to treat tuberculosis will produce hearing loss in most patients. Other drugs have a very high therapeutic index, and are much more forgiving with respect to plasma concentrations. For drugs with a high therapeutic index, toxic drug concentrations may be 10 times higher than the therapeutic concentration.

Recall that dose-response relationships describe dosages that are based on percentages of individuals responding. If a person is given an ED_{50} as a dose, a 50% chance exists that the drug will have the desired therapeutic effect. Most patients are not satisfied with 50% chance of improvement from taking a medication. Therefore drug regimens are adjusted to allow for the maximum benefits without crossing over into the toxic levels. All drugs have untoward side effects, so the potential risks must be weighed against the potential gains of the medication. The list of side effects associated with the various drug treatments can be daunting. However, identifying signs and symptoms of patients taking various medications will be a great asset to the healthcare team. Also many drugs will alter the physiology that is being tested in the diagnostic tests performed by audiologists. For example, the benzodiazepines have a profound effect on electronystagmograms and platform posturography (see Table 8–1 for a list). Therefore the remainder of this chapter will focus on the classes of drugs that will have direct effects on the diagnostic and therapeutic practices of audiology.

TABLE 8–1 **Partial list of pharmacological agents known to produce ototoxicity**

Action	Drug Class	Example
Supressant effect	Benzodiazepines Barbiturates Antihistamines (H_1 blockers) Anticholinergics	Diazepam Phenobarbital Diphenhydramine Ipratropium
Stimulatory effect	Alpha-adrenergic agonists	Pseudoephedrine

DRUGS THAT CAUSE OTOTOXICITY

Overview

Entire book chapters have been written on the subject of oto-toxicity, and this section is only designed to serve as a brief introduction. Should additional information be required the reader is referred to Stringer, Meyerhoff et al (1991). Ototoxicity has long been recognized as an undesirable side effect of medical treatment. *Ototoxicity* is defined as damage to the ear. The ear has two functional end organs: (1) the hearing system and (2) the vestibular system. Therefore ototoxic effects include both hearing and vestibular disturbances.

As early as the nineteenth century quinine* and salicylates[†], were noted to produce tinnitus, hearing impairment, and vestibular disturbances (North, 1880; Schwabach, 1884). Streptomycin was the first effective chemotherapeutic agent for tuberculosis, and with its use came the realization that the drug caused hearing impairment and vestibular disturbances (Hinshaw & Feldman, 1945). Other aminoglycoside antibiotics that subsequently came into clinical use were found to share streptomycin's potential for producing ototoxic side effects (Lerner et al, 1981). The susceptibility of the inner ear to injury by certain classes of drugs was further demonstrated after the introduction of the loop diuretics. Tinnitus, hearing loss, and vertigo are the cardinal symptoms of ototoxicity. Tinnitus usually accompanies acquired sensorineural hearing loss of any origin and frequently precedes and supersedes the hearing loss proper. The tinnitus associated with ototoxicity is typically described as intense and high pitched, ranging from to 4 kHz to 6 kHz.

In the presence of irreversible damage the tinnitus may become less severe but typically does not resolve. By way of example, loop diuretics may provoke intense tinnitus within minutes of intravenous injection. In less severe cases, however, they may produce an insidious, progressive sensorineural hearing loss. Transient hearing loss has also been reported with aminoglycoside antibiotics, but that loss is more commonly permanent. Hearing impairment caused by antibiotic administration usually occurs after 3 to 4 days but may become apparent after the first dose. Permanent drug-induced hearing loss may even be delayed days, weeks, or months after completion of therapy. Bilateral hearing loss predominates, but unilateral loss can occur.

Ototoxic hearing impairment is exclusively sensorineural, and patients typically present with audiometric evidence of a steeply sloping loss in the high frequencies (4 to 8 kHz), whereas some diuretic-induced ototoxicity results in a flat or slightly sloping audiometric pattern. Disequilibrium of ototoxic origin is most often associated with the administration of gentamicin and streptomycin. Its severity is directly proportional to the duration and quantity of the drug given and to the status of renal function. Disorders of gait and posture predominate, and patients often complain of an inability to stabilize ocular images (oscillopsia), particularly after positional changes. Aminoglycoside antibiotics and loop diuretics are two of the most commonly encountered and potentially dangerous classes of ototoxic drugs. In this chapter they are therefore discussed in depth, followed by other, less commonly encountered ototoxic agents.

Aminoglycoside Antibiotics

Both vestibular and auditory dysfunction can follow the administration of any of the aminoglycosides (see Table 8–2).

PEARL
If the drug name ends in *-micin* it could be ototoxic.

Studies of both animals and human beings have documented progressive accumulation of these drugs in the perilymph and endolymph of the inner ear (Huy & Meulemans et al, 1983). Accumulation occurs predominantly when concentrations in plasma are high. Diffusion back into the bloodstream is slow; the half-lives of the aminoglycosides are five to six times longer in the otic fluids than in plasma. Back-diffusion is concentration dependent and is facilitated when the concentration of drug in plasma reaches a trough. However, even a single dose of tobramycin has been reported to produce slight temporary cochlear dysfunction during periods when the concentration in plasma is at its peak (Wilson & Ramsden, 1977). The relationship of this observation to permanent loss of hearing is not known.

PITFALL
Ototoxicity is more evident in patients with persistently elevated concentrations of drug in plasma.

Ototoxicity is largely irreversible and results from progressive destruction of vestibular or cochlear sensory cells, which are highly sensitive to damage by aminoglycosides (Brummett & Fox, 1982). Studies in guinea pigs exposed to large doses of gentamicin reveal degeneration of the type I sensory hair cells in the central part of the crista ampullaris (vestibular organ) and fusion of individual sensory hairs into giant hairs (Wersall et al, 1973). Similar studies with gentamicin and tobramycin also demonstrate loss of hair cells in the cochlea of the organ of Corti (Theopold, 1977). Increasing the dosage of the drug and prolonged exposure cause damage that progresses from the base of the cochlea (where high-frequency sounds are processed) to the apex, which is necessary for the perception of low frequencies.

The association between aminoglycoside therapy and inner ear dysfunction became apparent during the earliest clinical trials, and this association has held true for every aminoglycoside antibiotic introduced. The usual hearing loss is bilateral and high in frequency, corresponding to hair-cell loss in the basal turn of the cochlea; however, either unilateral cochlear or vestibular disturbance is possible. The rapidity of onset and degree of hearing loss are usually dose-related and

---

*Quinine was used to treat malaria.
[†]Salicylates (aspirin) where used to treat pain and fever.

TABLE 8–2 Drugs that change electronystagmography and platform posturography

Drug Class	Generic Name	Comments
Aminoglycosides	Amikacin Neomycin Netilmicin Streptomycin Tobramycin Dihydrostreptomycin Gentamicin	Removed from market
Tetracyclines	Minocycline	
NSAID	Aspirin Naproxen	
Loop diuretics	Ethacrynic acid Furosamide	
Antineoplastic agents	Cisplatin	
Other	Erythromycin Buspirone Quinine Aztreonam Zalcitabine (2′,3′-dideoxycytidine) Polymyxin B	Used topically only

dependent on renal function, which are classic signs of untoward side effects caused by drugs. The onset of hearing impairment may be detected with high-frequency audiometry within 1 to 2 days of the initial dose, and the hearing loss is typically permanent. Although the various aminoglycoside antimicrobials are similar in many respects, each is distinct in its spectrum of antibiotic activity and in its ototoxic effect. Streptomycin was the first of the aminoglycosides to be clinically used, especially in the treatment of tuberculosis and it is primarily vestibulotoxic.

Although all aminoglycosides are capable of affecting both cochlear and vestibular function, some preferential toxicity is evident. Streptomycin and gentamicin produce predominantly vestibular effects, whereas amikacin, kanamycin, and neomycin primarily affect auditory function; tobramycin affects both equally. The incidence of ototoxicity is extremely difficult to determine. Data from audiometry suggest that the incidence may be as high as 25% (Moore et al, 1984). The relative incidence appears to be equal for tobramycin, gentamicin, and amikacin. Initial studies in laboratory animals and human beings suggested that netilmicin is less ototoxic than other aminoglycosides (Brummett & Fox, 1982; Lerner et al, 1983). However, the incidence of ototoxicity from netilmicin is not negligible and complications developed in 10% of patients in one clinical trial of netilmicin (Trestman et al, 1978). A definitive statement on relative ototoxicity awaits further clinical evaluation.

The incidence of vestibular toxicity is particularly high in patients receiving streptomycin; nearly 20% of individuals who received 500 mg twice daily for 4 weeks for enterococcal endocarditis had clinically detectable, irreversible vestibular damage (Wilson et al, 1984). In addition, up to 75% of patients who received 2 g of streptomycin for more than 60 days showed evidence of nystagmus or postural imbalance. It is recommended that patients receiving high doses or prolonged courses of aminoglycosides be monitored carefully for ototoxicity because the initial symptoms may be reversible; however, deafness may occur several weeks after therapy is discontinued.

Clinical Symptoms of Cochlear Toxicity

A high-pitched tinnitus often is the first symptom of impending difficulty. If the drug is not discontinued, auditory impairment may develop after a few days. The tinnitus may persist for several days to 2 weeks after therapy is stopped. Because perception of sound in the high-frequency range (outside the conversational range) is lost first, the affected individual is not aware of the difficulty and it will not be detected unless careful audiometric examination is carried out. If the loss of hearing progresses, the lower sound ranges are affected, and conversation becomes difficult.

PEARL

Classic signs and symptoms of ototoxicity include: tinnitus, hearing loss, vertigo, or balance disturbance.

Clinical Symptoms of Vestibular Toxicity

Moderately intense headache lasting 1 or 2 days may precede the onset of labyrinthine dysfunction. This is immediately followed by an acute stage, in which nausea, vomiting, and difficulty with equilibrium develop and persist for 1 to 2 weeks.

Vertigo in the upright position, inability to perceive termination of movement, and difficulty in sitting or standing without visual cues are prominent symptoms. Drifting of the eyes at the end of a movement so that focusing and reading are difficult, positive Romberg test, and rarely pendular trunk movement and spontaneous nystagmus are outstanding signs. The acute stage ends suddenly and is followed by the appearance of manifestations consistent with chronic labyrinthitis, in which, although symptomless while in bed, the patient has difficulty when attempting to walk or make sudden movements; ataxia is the most prominent feature. The chronic phase persists for approximately 2 months; it is gradually superseded by a compensatory stage, in which symptoms are latent and appear only when the eyes are closed. Adaptation to the impairment of labyrinthine function is accomplished by the use of visual cues and deep proprioceptive sensation for determining movement and position. Adaptation is better in the young than in the old but may not be sufficient to permit the high degree of coordination required in many special trades. Recovery from this phase may require 12 to 18 months, and most patients have some permanent residual damage. Although no specific treatment exists for the vestibular deficiency, early discontinuation of the drug may permit recovery before irreversible damage to the hair cells.

Pharmacological Labyrinthectomy

Mechanical destruction of the labyrinth has been efficacious in removing the symptoms of Meniere's disease. However, attendant with mechanical labyrinthectomy is hearing loss. Streptomycin has been applied for treatment of intractable Meniere's disease in an effort to chemically destroy the vestibular apparatus while preserving the cochlea (Schuknecht, 1950). Neomycin produces a high incidence of hearing loss with poor speech discrimination when administered parenterally and is therefore no longer recommended by that route. Additional predisposing factors to ototoxicity include any other coexistent form of deafness, acoustic trauma, and the simultaneous use of other ototoxic agents. As with all aminoglycoside antibiotics, hearing loss may occur early in therapy or have its onset several months after completion of drug treatment. Gentamicin has the potential to affect vestibular and cochlear sensory cells in a manner similar to streptomycin. The vestibular disturbances occur first and are more common clinically. Gentamicin is used widely as a potent antimicrobial against gram-negative bacterial infections. The potential ototoxicity of this drug was anticipated before clinical investigation and confirmed soon thereafter (Jackson & Arcieri, 1971). The incidence of ototoxicity is estimated to be 2%. Tobramycin may also cause vestibular and cochlear injury. Vestibular symptoms are less common, and high-frequency, steeply sloping hearing loss is more common than with gentamicin.

Clinical Studies

Hinshaw and Feldman reported deafness associated with streptomycin administration in 1945. Waisbren and Spink in 1950 were the first to coin the term *ototoxicity* with respect to aminoglycosides in a report of a neomycin trial. Hawkins (1951) subsequently used the term in the title of a paper on

hydroxystreptomycin. Vestibular disturbances in tuberculous patients treated with streptomycin were commonplace by 1948, and thorough clinical descriptions of the symptoms were published (Fowler & Seligman, 1947; Jongkees & Hulk, 1950; Northington, 1950). The first complaints by patients were usually blurred vision and motion-induced vertigo, with a sense of continued turning after the motion was terminated. Patients were noted to have a wide-based gait and to display difficulty walking on uneven surfaces or in the dark. Spontaneous and positional nystagmus were absent, and optokinetic nystagmus was normal. However, a fine nystagmus was commonly elicited on lateral gaze. Vestibular disturbance typically began after 3 to 4 weeks of intramuscular administration. The vestibular effects were also noted to begin earlier if the streptomycin was given intrathecally or in the presence of renal compromise. As compensation for vestibular loss occurred, particularly in young patients, symptoms were noted to slowly subside even with continued drug therapy. Subsequently, it was noted that the first signs of streptomycin ototoxicity might occur as late as 2 to 6 months after termination of therapy. Electronystagmographic and audiometric evaluation provided documentation of the retrospective clinical observation that the vestibular apparatus was usually affected before the cochlea. Rarely, the cochlear effects may be present before, and occasionally at the same time as, the vestibular disturbance (Serles, 1966). The vestibular and cochlear losses are typically permanent, although some hearing may be preserved if ototoxicity is detected early. Hearing loss has been reported after topical use of neomycin for burns and oral administration for bowel sterilization (Gibson, 1967). Ototoxic serum levels of neomycin have been demonstrated after peritoneal irrigation and topical irrigation of burn wounds and decubitus ulcers with 0.25% neomycin solutions (Masur et al, 1976; Myerson et al, 1970).

Tobramycin has been claimed to be less ototoxic than gentamicin in experimental animals, but evidence is not sufficient to substantiate this claim in humans. Prospective studies of aminoglycoside toxicity by Fee (1980) and Smith and colleagues (1980) revealed similar rates of cochlear injury (10 to 16%) for tobramycin and gentamicin, whereas the incidence of vestibular injury was found to be 5% for tobramycin and 15% for gentamicin. Lerner and associates (1984) described similar findings in a randomized, blind assessment of gentamicin, netilmicin, and tobramycin, with monitoring of serum levels and renal function. The risk of ototoxicity in newborns of mothers treated with aminoglycosides during pregnancy is uncertain. Streptomycin has been shown to cross the placental barrier and appear in fetal blood, although at a lower concentration than in maternal blood (Conway & Birt, 1965). Ototoxic deafness acquired in utero by children whose mothers have been treated with streptomycin and dihydrostreptomycin is said to be uncommon. However, case reports of congenital deafness associated with ototoxic drug administration during pregnancy do exist (Jones, 1973). Aminoglycosides should therefore be used with extreme caution in pregnant patients.

Pharmacology and Pharmacodynamics

Aminoglycosides consist of an amino sugar linked to another moiety by means of a glycoside bond. Neomycin is different from the remainder of the group in that it has three sugar rings rather than two. Structure activity variations in the chemical configuration (i.e., the number and placement of basic groups on the various sugars) affect the toxicity and the activity of these antibiotics (Yung, 1987). Aminoglycosides are usually applied topically or administered parenterally because only 3% of an oral dose is absorbed. Serum levels have been demonstrated to vary widely even among normal volunteers (Kaye et al, 1974). Tissue concentrations are typically one-third that of serum and are affected by many factors, including temperature, pH, electrolyte concentration, oxygen tension, and hematocrit. Penetration of the blood-brain barrier is negligible, except perhaps in neonates; therefore intrathecal administration is necessary to obtain sufficient cerebrospinal fluid levels.

The aminoglycoside antibiotics are not metabolized but rather are excreted almost completely by glomerular filtration, and urine concentrations may rise to 10 times that of the serum. Impaired renal function decreases the excretion of aminoglycosides, thereby increasing the level in the serum and perilymph and the risk of ototoxicity and nephrotoxicity (Naunton & Ward, 1959). The pharmacodynamics of aminoglycoside antibiotics vary somewhat among species, but the pattern is similar in animals and humans (Federspil et al, 1976).

SPECIAL CONSIDERATION

With decreased renal clearance, aminoglycosides are cleared more slowly from the perilymph than the serum, resulting in a prolonged perilymph half-life.

A single aminoglycoside injection results in a serum peak at 1 hour, which falls to negligible amounts at 6 hours. The perilymph level peak is reached slowly over 3 to 6 hours, and the aminoglycoside remains in the perilymph for a considerably longer period, reaching minimal levels in 24 to 36 hours. A definite correlation exists between the perilymph aminoglycoside level and the resultant ototoxic damage. The quantity of aminoglycoside in the perilymph is directly proportional to the serum level, allowing for a direct correlation of the extent of ototoxicity with the dose administered (assuming normal renal function). If the dosing interval does not allow for adequate renal excretion, then serum and perilymph levels continue to rise. Increases in kanamycin concentration in the perilymph have been demonstrated with repeated daily doses; however this has not been found to occur with gentamicin or tobramycin. Such accumulation and retention is not found in cerebrospinal fluid or aqueous humor. Aminoglycoside antimicrobials must reach the inner ear through capillary beds rather than through the cerebrospinal fluid because cerebrospinal fluid levels have been demonstrated to be low even with high serum plasma levels (Hawkins et al, 1950).

Mechanism of Action

Several proposals have been made regarding the mechanism of aminoglycoside ototoxicity. After streptomycin treatment, damage has been observed in the stria vascularis and in the neuroepithelia of the cochlea and vestibular apparatus. Hawkins (1973) proposed that aminoglycoside exposure results in injury to the secretory and reabsorptive tissues of the labyrinth, thereby disturbing microhomeostasis, with subsequent injury to the sensory cells. Some anatomical evidence also shows that degeneration in the lateral wall tissues may precede cochlear hair cell loss. In addition, the two-phase reduction in the human electrocochlear response after administration of tobramycin supports the hypothesis of an early strial effect (Wilson & Ramsden, 1977). The aminoglycoside antibiotics apparently exert an immediate physiological effect on the transduction of sensory input by reversibly blocking calcium-sensitive potassium channels on the apical aspect of the receptor cell (Lim, 1986). This short-term effect may explain the reversible suppression of cochlear microphonics produced by application of aminoglycosides. Eventual degeneration of the sensory cells is believed to be due to inhibition of the synthesis of structural proteins, or interference with cell membrane lipid metabolism, or both.

SPECIAL CONSIDERATION

Much available evidence points toward a direct influence of aminoglycosides in the hair cells of the cochlear and vesticular apparatus.

The antimicrobial effect of aminoglycoside antibiotics depends on their ability to inhibit protein synthesis by means of interaction with the 30S ribosomal subunit (Benveniste & Davies, 1973). Some evidence for an influence on protein synthesis in mammalian hair cells also exists on the basis of the ultrastructural findings indicating that ribosomal synthesis is disturbed by aminoglycosides (Lim, 1986). In addition, Schacht and colleagues have proposed interference with cell membrane lipids as a major factor underlying aminoglycoside injury of the inner ear. Specifically, these antibiotics have been shown to inhibit polyphosphoinositide metabolism, which is essential for control of cell membrane permeability and maintenance of membrane structure (Schacht, 1976, 1985; Stockhorst & Schacht, 1977).

Although these histological changes correlate with the ability of the cochlea to generate an action potential in response to sound, the biochemical mechanism for ototoxicity is poorly understood. Early changes induced by aminoglycosides have been shown in experimental ototoxicity to be reversible by Ca^{2+}. Once sensory cells are lost, however, regeneration does not occur; retrograde degeneration of the auditory nerve follows, resulting in irreversible hearing loss (Lietman, 1990). It has been suggested that aminoglycosides interfere with the active transport system essential for the maintenance of the ionic balance of the endolymph (Neu & Bendush, 1976). This would lead to an alteration in the normal concentrations of ions in the labyrinthine fluids, with impairment of electrical activity and nerve conduction. Eventually, the changes in electrolyte, or perhaps the drugs themselves, damage the hair cells irreversibly. Interest also has centered on the interaction of aminoglycosides with membrane phospholipids, particularly phosphatidylinositol and its phosphorylated derivatives, which are the precursors of the intracellular second messengers inositol 1,4,5-trisphosphate and diacylglycerol. Lim (1986) pointed out in a review on ototoxicity that it appears likely that aminoglycosides produce their effects on inner ear sensory cells by at least two different mechanisms. The first of these is reversible blockage of transduction channels on the apical portion of the hair cell; the second mechanism involves irreversible damage of the biochemical machinery necessary for cell maintenance and survival.

Recent studies have suggested that the ototoxic side effects of gentamicin may be caused by a metabolized or activated form of the drug. Song & Schacht (1996) have proposed that gentamicin may form an iron-gentamicin complex and that this complex may be responsible for generating free radicals. This theory is supported by experiments demonstrating that iron chelators protect against aminoglycoside-induced ototoxicity in experimental animals (Song & Schacht, 1996). The addition of specific iron chelators also does not decrease the serum levels of gentamicin and thereby does not affect the antimicrobial efficacy of the drug.

Nonsteroidal Anti-Inflammatory Agents

The anti-inflammatory, analgesic, and antipyretic drugs are a heterogeneous group of compounds, often chemically unrelated (although most of them are organic acids), which nevertheless share certain therapeutic actions and side effects. The prototype is aspirin; hence these compounds are often referred to as aspirin-like drugs; they also are frequently called *nonsteroidal anti-inflammatory drugs*, or *NSAIDs*, an abbreviation that will be used throughout the chapter to refer to these agents. The corticosteroids and their derivatives are the most potent and efficacious drugs to inhibit inflammation, and the NSAIDs are a distinctly separate group. These drugs are also often called salicylates because of their structural similarity to aspirin (acetylsalicylic acid).

Permanent aspirin ototoxicity is unusual because, unlike other ototoxic agents, its effects are largely reversible. In fact, its ototoxic manifestations were at one time used to titrate the dose of aspirin used in arthritis therapy. The endocochlear potential is not altered by aspirin, thus suggesting that it does not exert its effect by way of the stria vascularis. The severity of the symptoms seems to be dose dependent. Small occasional doses (e.g., one or two 300-mg tablets taken for headache) may induce noticeable tinnitus *without* appreciable hearing loss in many patients. At the other extreme, overdoses of aspirin have resulted in severe, albeit temporary, hearing losses. Intermediate losses may occur in situations that therapeutically use higher doses of aspirin, such as in the treatment of arthritis noted above.

Some patients also report that voices have a distorted sound quality, similar to a phonograph record played at excessive speed. Treatment consists primarily of withdrawal from the drug. Hearing thresholds gradually improve as the drug is metabolized and excreted. Acute and convalescent

audiometric thresholds should be measured to document resolution. It must be stressed that when hearing loss occurs as a result of an aspirin overdose, appropriate general medical treatment of the other aspects of the overdose is imperative, including psychiatric evaluation.

Loop Diuretics

Approximately 120 ml of ultrafiltrate is formed each minute, yet only 1 ml/min of urine is produced. Therefore greater than 99% of the glomerular ultrafiltrate is reabsorbed at a staggering energy cost. The kidneys consume 7% of total-body oxygen intake despite the fact that the kidneys make up only 0.5% of body weight. The kidney is designed to filter large quantities of plasma, reabsorb those substances that the body must conserve, leaving behind and/or secreting substances that must be eliminated. Approximately 25% of filtered solutes are reabsorbed in the loop of Henle, mostly in the thick ascending limb, which has a large reabsorptive capacity.

Inhibitors of Na^+-K^+-2 Cl^- symport are a group of diuretics that have in common an ability to block the Na^+-K^+-2 Cl^- symporter in the thick ascending limb of the loop of Henle; hence these diuretics also are referred to as *loop diuretics*. Although the proximal tubule reabsorbs approximately 65% of the ultrafiltrate, diuretics acting only in the proximal tubule have limited efficacy because the thick ascending limb has a great reabsorptive capacity and reabsorbs most of the rejectate from the proximal tubule. Diuretics acting predominantly at sites past the thick ascending limb also have limited efficacy because only a small percentage of the filtered load ever reaches these more distal sites. In contrast, inhibitors of Na^+-K^+-2 Cl^- symport are highly efficacious, and for this reason they often are called *high-ceiling* diuretics. The efficacy of inhibitors of Na^+-K^+-2 Cl^- symport in the thick ascending limb of the loop of Henle is due to a combination of two factors: (1) approximately 25% of the filtered solute load normally is reabsorbed by the thick ascending limb, and (2) nephron segments past the thick ascending limb do not possess the reabsorptive capacity to rescue the flood of rejectate exiting the thick ascending limb.

Because of blockade of the Na^+-K^+-2 Cl^- symporter, loop diuretics cause a profound increase in the urinary excretion of Na^+ and Cl^- (i.e., up to 25% of the filtered load of Na^+). Abolition of the transepithelial potential difference also results in marked increases in the excretion of Ca^{2+} and Mg^{2+}. Some (e.g., furosemide), but not all (e.g., bumetanide and piretanide), sulfonamide-based loop diuretics have weak carbonic anhydrase–inhibiting activity. Those drugs with carbonic anhydrase–inhibiting activity increase the urinary excretion of HCO_3^- and phosphate. The mechanism by which inhibition of carbonic anhydrase increases phosphate excretion is not known. All inhibitors of Na^+-K^+-2 Cl^- symport increase the urinary excretion of K+ and titratable acid. This effect is due in part to increased delivery of Na^+ to the distal tubule. The mechanism by which increased distal delivery of Na^+ enhances excretion of K^+ and H^+ is discussed in the section on inhibitors of Na^+ channels. Acutely, loop diuretics increase the excretion of uric acid, whereas chronic administration of these drugs results in reduced excretion of uric acid. The chronic effects of loop diuretics on uric acid excretion may be due to enhanced transport in the proximal tubule secondary to volume depletion, leading to increased uric acid reabsorption or to competition between the diuretic and uric acid for the organic acid secretory mechanism in the proximal tubule, leading to reduced uric acid secretion.

Hearing impairment and deafness are usually, but not always, reversible. Ototoxicity occurs most frequently with rapid intravenous administration and least frequently with oral administration. Ethacrynic acid appears to induce ototoxicity more often than do other loop diuretics. Loop diuretics also can cause hyperuricemia (rarely leading to gout) and hyperglycemia (rarely precipitating diabetes mellitus) and can increase plasma levels of low-density lipoprotein cholesterol and triglycerides while decreasing plasma levels of high-density lipoprotein cholesterol. Other adverse effects include skin rashes, photosensitivity, paresthesias, bone marrow depression, and gastrointestinal disturbances.

SPECIAL CONSIDERATION

Ototoxicity from loop diuretics is manifested as tinnitus, hearing impairment, deafness, vertigo, and a sense of fullness in the ear.

Antineoplastic Agents

Drugs that are used to treat cancer are called the antineoplastic agents. This is because cancers are known as neoplasms. Several of the medications used in the treatment of cancer have been identified as being capable of ototoxicity. They include bleomycin, 5-fluorouracil, and nitrogen mustard. The chemotherapeutic agent most commonly associated with ototoxicity is cisplatin, which can produce tinnitus, hearing loss, and otalgia. The platinum coordination complexes were first identified by Rosenberg and coworkers as cytotoxic agents in 1965. They observed that a current delivered between platinum electrodes produced inhibition of *Escherichia coli* proliferation. The inhibitory effects on bacterial replication were later ascribed to the formation of inorganic platinum-containing compounds in the presence of ammonium and chloride ions (Rosenberg et al, 1965, 1967). *cis*-Diamminedi-chloroplatinum (II) (cisplatin) was the most

active of these substances in experimental tumor systems and has proven to be of great clinical value (Rosenberg, 1973). More than 1000 platinum-containing compounds subsequently have been synthesized and tested. One of these, carboplatin, was approved for treatment of ovarian cancers in 1989; others are still being evaluated. Cisplatin has broad activity as an antineoplastic agent, and the drug is especially useful in the treatment of epithelial malignancies. It has become the foundation for curative regimens for advanced testicular cancer and has notable activity against ovarian cancer and cancers of the head and neck, bladder, esophagus, and lung.

SPECIAL CONSIDERATION

Ototoxicity from antineoplastic agents appears to be related to total cumulative dose.

Hearing loss is typically bilateral, beginning in the higher frequencies and then progressing to involve the lower octaves. As is true of the antibiotics, hearing loss may develop even after discontinuation of therapy. But the dose at which ototoxicity occurs has not been determined. Audiometric monitoring of patients receiving cisplatin over long periods may detect cisplatin ototoxicity early in its course. As with other ototoxic agents, the incidence of injury to the inner ear appears to be significantly enhanced when this drug is combined with other drugs known to have ototoxic effects. Research continues into combining medications with cisplatin that would stem some of the ototoxicity and nephrotoxicity.

CONCLUSIONS

This chapter is designed as an introduction into possible pharmacological explanations for changes in audiometric and vestibular tests. Several different drug classes that produce ototoxicity have been presented in this chapter. As with the undesirable side effects of most pharmacological agents, the effects have been determined by empirical observations. The mechanism of toxicity for each of these compounds is still elusive and remains an area of continued basic science research. The audiologist should be aware of the types of deleterious drug effects that may be encountered by their patients undergoing pharmacological treatment. Much of this information regarding a patient's current medication can be gleaned from a thorough patient history and review of the medical chart. In addition, diligent familiarity with the current literature will be required for delivering the best patient care regarding these issues.

REFERENCES

BENVENISTE, R., & DAVIES, J. (1973). Structure activity relationships among the aminoglycoside antibiotics: Role of hydroxyl and amino groups. *Antimicrobial Agents and Chemotherapy, 4;*402–409.

BRUMMETT, R., & FOX, K. (1982). Studies of aminoglycoside ototoxicity in animal models. *The aminoglycosides: Microbiology, clinical use, and toxicity, 14;* 419–451.

CONWAY, N., & BRIT, B.D. (1965). Strepotomycin in pregnancy: Effect foetal ear. *BMJ, 5456;*260–263.

FEDERSPIL, P., SCHATXLE, W., et al. (1976). Pharmacokinetics and ototoxicity of gentamicin, tobramycin and amikacin. *Journal of Infectious Diseases, 34;*5200–5205.

FEE, W., JR. (1980). Aminoglycoside ototoxicity in the human. *Laryngoscope, 90;*1–19.

FOWLER, E., & SELIGMAN, E. (1947). Otic complications of streptomycin therapy. *JAMA, 133;*87–91.

GIBSON, W. (1967). Deafness due to orally administered neomycin. *Archives of Otolaryngology, 86;*163–165.

HAWKINS, J. (1973). Ototoxic mechanisms: A working hypothesis. *Audiology, 12;*383–393.

HAWKINS, J.E., JR., BOXER, G.E., & JENINEK, V.C. (1950). Concentration of streptomycin in brain and other tissues of cats after acute and chronic intoxication. *Proc Soc Exp Biol, 75;* 759–761.

HAWKINS, J.E., JR. (1951). The ototoxicity of hydroxystreptomycin. In: *Transactions of the tenth conference on chemotherapy of tuberculosis* (pp. 224–226). Washington, DC: Veterans Administration.

HINSHAW, H., & FELDMAN W. (1945). Streptomycin in the treatment of clinical tuberculosis: A preliminary report. *Proceedings of the Mayo Clinic, 20;*313–318.

HUY, P., MEULEMANS, A. et al. (1983). Gentamicin persistence in rat endolymph and perilymph after a two-day constant infusion. *Antimicrobial Agents and Chemotherapy, 23;*344–346.

JACKSON, G.G., & ARCIERI, G. (1971). Ototoxicity of gentamicin in man: a survey and controlled analysis of clinical experience in the United States. *Journal of Infectious Diseases, 124;*Suppl. 124:130–135.

JONES, H.C. (1973). Intrauturine ototoxicity: A case report and review of lituature. *Journal of the National Medical Association, 65;*201–203.

JONGKEES, L., & HULK, J. (1950). The action of streptomycin on vestibular function. *Acta Otolaryngologica, 38;*225–232.

KAYE, D., LEVISON, M. et al. (1974). The unpredictability of serum concentrations of gentamicin: Pharmacokinetics of gentamicin in patients with normal and abnormal renal function. *Journal of Infectious Diseases, 130;*150–154.

LERNER, A., CONE, L. et al. (1983). Randomised controlled trial of the comparative efficacy, auditory toxicity, and nephrotoxicity of tobramycin and netilmicin. *Lancet, 1;*1123–1126.

LERNER, A., MATZ, G. et al. (1984). *Prospective, randomized blind assessment of nephrotoxicity and ototoxicity in patients treated with gentamicin, netilmicin, and tobramycin.* Twenty-Fourth Interscience Conference on Antimicrobial Agents in Chemotherapy. No. 488, Philadelphia, PA.

LERNER, S., MATZ, G. et al. (1981). *Aminoglycoside ototoxicity.* Boston: Little Brown & Co.

LIETMAN, P. (1990). Aminoglycosides and spectinomycin: Aminocyclitols. In *Principles and practice of infectious disease.* (3rd ed.) (pp. 269–284). Boston, MA: Little Brown & Co.

LIM, D. (1986). Effects of noise and ototoxic drugs at the cellular level in the cochlea: A review. *American Journal of Otolaryngology, 7;*73–99.

MASUR, H., WHELTON, P., et al. (1976). Neomycin toxicity revisited. *Archives of Surgery, 111;*822–825.

MEYERSON, M., KNIGHT, H. et al. (1970). Intrapleural neomycin causing ototoxicity. *Annals of Thoracic Surgery, 9;*483–486.

MOORE, R.D., SMITH, C.R., et al. (1984). Risk factors for the development of auditory toxicity in patients receiving aminoglycosides. *Journal of Infectious Diseases, 149;* 923–930.

NAUNTON, R., & WARD, P. (1959). The ototoxicity of kanamycin in the presence of compromised renal function. *Archives of Otolaryngology, 69;*398–399.

NEU, H., & BENDUSH, C. (1976). Ototoxicity of tobramycin: A clinical overview. *Journal of Infectious Diseases, 134;*S206–S218.

NORTH, A. (1880). Two cases of poisoning by the oil of chenopodium. *American Journal of Otology, 2;*197–200.

NORTHINGTON, P. (1950). Syndrome of bilateral vestibular paralysis and its occurrence from streptomycin therapy. *Archives of Otolaryngology. 52;*380–396.

ROSENBERG, B. (1973). Platinum coordination complexes in cancer chemotherapy. *Naturwissenschaften, 60;*399–406.

ROSENBERG, B., VAN CAMP, L., et al. (1967). The inhibition of growth or cell division in *Escherichia coli* by different ionic species of platinum (IV) complexes. *Journal of Biological Chemistry, 242;*1347–1352.

ROSENBERG, B., VAN CAMP, L., et al. (1965). Inhibition of cell division in *Escherichia coli* by electrolysis products from a platinum electrode. *Nature, 205;*698–699.

SCHACHT, J. (1976). Biochemistry of neomycin ototoxicity. *Journal of the Acoustical Society of America, 59;*940–944.

SCHACHT, J. (1985). Molecular mechanisms of aminoglycoside ototoxicity. *Abstracts of the Eighth Midwinter Meeting, Association for Research in Otolaryngology* (p. 68). St. Petersburg, FL: Association for Research in Otolaryngology.

SCHUKNECHT, H. (1950). Ablation therapy for the relief of Meniere's disease. *Laryngoscope, 66;*859–871.

SCHWABACH, D. (1884). Uber bleibende Storungen im Gehororgan nach Chinin und Salicylgebrauch. *Deutsche Medizinische Wuchenschrift, 10;*163–166.

SERLES, W. (1966). Streptomycinschaden im Elektronystagmogramm. *Wochenschrift Ohrenkeilk, 100;*251.

SMITH, C., LIPSKY, J. et al. (1980). Double-blind comparison of the nephrotoxicity and auditory toxicity of gentamicin and tobramycin. *New England Journal of Medicine, 302;*1106–1109.

SONG, B.B., ANDERSON, D.J., et al. (1997). Protection from gentamicin ototoxicity by iron chelators in guinea pig in vivo. *Journal of Pharmacology and Experimental Therapeutics, 282* (1);369–377.

SONG, B.B., & SCHACHT, J. (1996). Variable efficacy of radical scavengers and iron chelators to attentuate gentamicin ototoxicity in guinea pig in vivo. *Hearing Research, 94*(1-2);87–93.

SONG, B.B., SHA, S.H., et al. (1998). Iron chelators protect from aminoglycoside-induced cochleo- and vestibulo-toxicity [In Process Citation]. *Free Radical Biology and Medicine, 25*(2);189–95.

STOCKHORST, E., & SCHACHT, J. (1977). Radioactive labeling of phospholipids and proteins by cochlear perfusion in the guinea pig and the effect of neomycin. *Acta Otolaryngologica, 83*;401–409.

STRINGER, S.P., MEYERHOFF, W.L., et al. (1991). Ototoxicity. In: M.E. Paperella, D.A. Shumerick, J.L. Gluckman, & W.L. Meyerhoff. *Otolaryngology,* (Vol. 2) (pp. 1653–1670). Philadelphia, PA: W.B. Saunders.

THEOPOLD, H. (1977). Comparative surface studies of ototoxic effects of various aminoglycoside antibiotics on the organ of Corti in the guinea pig. A scanning electron microscopic study. *Acta Otolaryngologica, 84*;57–64.

TRESTMAN, I., PARSONS, J., et al. (1978). Pharmacology and efficacy of netilmicin. *Antimicrobial Agents and Chemotherapy, 13*;832–836.

WAISBREN, B., & SPINK, W. (1950). A clinical appraisal of neomycin. *Annals of Internal Medicine, 33*;1099–1119.

WERSALL, J., BJORKROTH, B. et al. (1973). Experiments on the ototoxic effects of antibiotics. *Advances in Otorhinolaryngology, 20*;14–41.

WILSON, P., & RAMSDEN, R.T. (1977). Immediate effects of tobramycin on human cochlea and correlation with serum tobramycin levels. *BMJ, 6056*;259–261.

WILSON, P., & RAMSDEN, R.T. (1977). Immediate effects of tobramycin on human cochlea and correlation with serum tobramycin levels. *BMJ, 1*;259–261.

WILSON, W., WILKOWSKE, C. et al. (1984). Treatment of streptomycin-susceptible and streptomycin-resistant enterococcal endocarditis. *Annals of Internal Medicine, 100*; 816–823.

YUNG, M. (1987). Comparative ototoxicity of kanamycin A and kanamycin B in the guinea pig. *Acta Otolaryngologica, 103*;73–80.

## Chapter 9

Acoustics and Psychoacoustics

Prudence Allen

PEARL

Psychoacoustics studies the physical parameters of sound and links them with the sensations and perceptions they evoke.

Psychoacoustics links the physical parameters of sounds with the sensations and perceptions that they evoke. Psychoacoustic findings have provided the foundation for behavioral testing in audiology and likewise hold the promise for future improvements and expansions in diagnostic audiology. The breadth of areas that have been studied using behavioral techniques is wide and more than can be considered, however briefly, in a single chapter. The focus of this chapter will therefore be on the psychoacoustic findings that provide the basis for current audiological practices, and those that hold promise for assessment and rehabilitation of hearing and hearing disorders in the future. Without clear and complete understanding of normal-hearing processes and how

those processes change throughout life, the evaluation of hearing disorders and their impact on communicative behavior will be limited.

The goal of this chapter is to provide an overview of auditory behavior and the limits of auditory ability. Whenever possible, current models of auditory processing will be discussed. It is through these models that researchers and clinicians may be better able to understand and predict the effect of a pathological process on overall auditory system functioning. The first part of the chapter provides an introduction to essential background information, including basic acoustics or how sound is quantified, and psychophysical methods or how behavioral responses to sound are measured. The second part of the chapter addresses how the auditory system processes level, spectral, and temporal information in relatively simple sounds. The goal is to provide a basic description of how acoustic features are encoded through discussion of the limits of detection and discrimination abilities and the perceptual correlates of physical acoustic features. The third part of the chapter deals with more integrative (and possibly higher level) functions, including the processing of binaural information for which information from both ears must be integrated into a single perceptual whole and the processing of complex sounds for which multiple features must be weighted and combined into a usable auditory image to which meaning can be assigned, often in the face of variability and uncertainty. The last part of the chapter summarizes the role of psychoacoustics in audiology, both historically and with a look to the future.

BASIC ACOUSTICS

The physical basis of sound is a large topic, complete discussion of which would exceed the bounds of this chapter. This section will therefore be limited to providing a definition of some basic terms and mathematical relationships. This should enable the reader to understand the essential elements of sound production and measurement. (For more detailed information, Hartmann [1998] is an excellent reference.)

Signal Magnitude

Instantaneous Magnitude

Sound is acoustic energy produced by a moving object. The movement of the object is transmitted through the medium in

Audiology: Diagnosis. Edited by Roeser, Valente, and Hosford-Dunn. Thieme Medical Publishers, Inc., New York © 2000

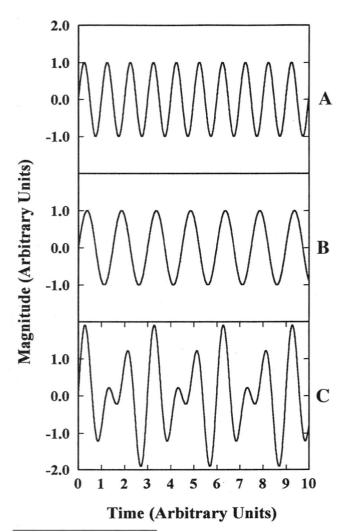

Figure 9–1 **(A–C)** Three signals displayed as a function of time in arbitrary units. All three are periodic within the time displayed. The signal in the lower panel is created by the addition of the signals in the upper and middle panels.

which the object lies, producing a pressure wave that varies over time and is propagated in all directions. When a sound is described in the time domain, x(t) denotes the *instantaneous pressure* of the signal at time t, and the sound is presumed to begin at t = 0.

Figure 9–1 shows a time domain representation of some simple signals. The *x* axis shows time, and the *y* axis shows instantaneous magnitude, both displayed in arbitrary units. When these signals are sounds traveling through air, three-dimensional condensations of air particles exist at the positive values and rarefactions at the negative values. Condensations and rarefactions are increases and decreases, respectively, in the density of air particles relative to that measured when the medium is in a state of rest. It is through this motion of particles in the air medium that sound is transmitted through space to arrive at and propagate through the external auditory meatus to a listener's tympanic membrane.

The magnitude of an acoustic waveform at any given moment will be determined not only by the instantaneous

pressure created by the moving force that is driving the disturbance but also by the characteristics of the medium in which the pressure wave is expected to travel. For example, a sound wave traveling through air will be very different from one traveling through water, even if they were created with the same force. The magnitude of the wave in a medium is the waveform *intensity*, I(t), and it is determined by the instantaneous pressure and the particle velocity, u(t), of the medium. Particle velocity is equal to the instantaneous pressure, x(t), divided by the *specific impedance*, ρc, of the medium in which the signal is transmitted: ρ refers to the density of the medium, measured in kilograms per square meter, and c is the speed of sound (343.2 m/s at 20 degrees C). The unit of measurement for intensity is watts per square meter. The relation between pressure and intensity is monotonic but nonlinear.

$$I(t) = x(t)*u(t) = x(t)*x(t)/\rho c = x^2(t)/\rho c$$

Note that sound intensity values will be positive for all time values, even though the pressure measurements from which they are derived may be both positive and negative.

Average Magnitude

It is often of interest to know not only the instantaneous magnitude of a signal (pressure or intensity) but also the average magnitude. This is calculated by averaging the instantaneous magnitudes over the duration of the signal (or some briefer time interval if the signal duration is very long).* The equation for computing average pressure is as follows:

$$\overline{P} = \frac{1}{T_D}\int_0^{T_D} dt\,P(t)$$

Where $P(t)$ is the instantaneous pressure at time, and t and T_D is the duration over which the average is taken. The typical measure of average pressure is the *root-mean-square* value, denoted as X_{RMS} and calculated as follows:

$$X_{RMS} = \sqrt{\frac{1}{T_D}\int_0^{T_D} dt\,x^2(t)}$$

The instantaneous pressures are squared, averaged over the time interval T_D, and the square root of the average is taken.

Peak Amplitudes and Crest Values

Sometimes, it is necessary to know how the instantaneous magnitudes and the average magnitude relate to one another (i.e., Is the instantaneous magnitude relatively uniform over time or does it vary throughout the signal's duration by a large amount?). A measure that relates *peak amplitude* to average magnitude is the *crest value* as follows:

$$Crest = \frac{max\,|x(t)|}{X_{RMS}}$$

---

*To obtain an adequate representation of signal magnitude the average must be taken over a time interval that is greater than the duration over which typical moment-to-moment variations occur. For very brief signals, the average should be made over the duration of the entire signal, but for longer signals a time period less than the total duration could be sampled as long as the interval is longer than the minor moment-to-moment fluctuations.

Large crest values suggest peaks in the signal will greatly exceed the RMS values, whereas small crest values suggest that magnitudes are more similar over time and thus similar to the average value.

Absolute and Relative Sound Levels

To this point, the discussion has been on the absolute values of sounds. But dealing with absolute values, particularly for acoustic signals, may easily become unruly. For example, the smallest pressure that can be detected by the human ear under ideal situations is $2*10^{-12}$ N/m^2. Intensity is related to pressure (squared) divided by the specific impedance of air that is commonly 415 Rayls, although it may vary with atmospheric pressure and temperature. Thus the smallest detectable intensity is $(2*10^{-5}$ N/m$^2)$ /415 = 0.964 $*$ 10^{-12} watt/m^2. For convenience, this is approximated by 10^{-12} watt/m^2. Listeners can also perceive, although perhaps painfully, intensities of 1 watt/m^2 or greater. This is a very large range, and discussion of magnitudes within that range requires the use of very large numbers. Signal magnitudes are therefore more commonly reported as relative levels computed with the log transformation. Signal level is equal to the log of a measured magnitude relative to a reference magnitude. The unit of measurement is the Bel or decibel (dB) (1 Bel is equal to 10 dB).

PEARL

Pressure is a force (measured in Newtons, N) applied over an area (square meters, m^2). Thus the standard unit of pressure in the MKS (meter-kilogram-second) system is the Newton/meter^2, N/m^2. Pressure may also be measured in Pascals (Pa): 1 Pa = 1 N/m^2.

$$Level \ (dB) \ = \ 10 \ log \left(\frac{Measured \ magnitude}{Reference \ magnitude} \right)$$

When level (in dB) is equal to 0, it does not suggest that no signal is present but that the magnitude of the measured signal is equal to the magnitude of the reference signal, 10 log(1) = 0.0. Although any reference value may be used in the measurement of sound levels, a standard reference is agreed on by the community of users (in audiology, hearing research, and engineering). The absolute reference for intensity is the minimum detectable, 10^{-12} Watt/m^2.

PEARL

Using this equation it can be seen that the range of human hearing (in dB) is large, 10 $*$ log(1 watt/m^2 /10^{-12} watt/m^2) = 120 dB.

The actual measurement of sound is most often made with pressure-sensitive microphones and sound level meters even though it is signal intensity that is the more relevant measure in practice as it reflects both waveform magnitude and the influence of the medium in which the waveform is transmitted. Because intensity is proportional to the square of the pressure, the computation for intensity levels computed from measured and reference pressure values is as follows:

$$L(dB) \ = \ 10 \ log \left(\frac{Measured \ pressure}{Reference \ pressure} \right)^2$$

By simple algebra [log(a/b)^x is equal to x log (a/b)]; the exponent can be moved to precede the log such that the computation of sound intensity from pressure values is as follows:

$$L(dB) \ = \ 20 \ log \left(\frac{Measured \ pressure}{Reference \ pressure} \right)$$

The absolute reference for sound pressures is the smallest pressure detectable ($2*10^{-5}$ Newtons/m^2, or 20 μPa). When this absolute reference value is used, the level is noted as dB sound pressure level (SPL).

Electrical Calibration

Sometimes sound measurement is performed electrically rather than acoustically. Knowing the sound pressure level that is produced when a given electrical magnitude is passed through a transducer enables the electrical calibration of acoustic signals. The unit of measurement is the volt. The standard, absolute reference is 1 volt. Likewise, because electric signals must also be transmitted through a medium, their magnitude can be noted as power that is similar to sound intensity. Power is equal to the instantaneous magnitude multiplied by the current flow, i(t). Current is equal to the instantaneous voltage, x(t) divided by the resistance of the medium, R. Thus power = x(t)*x(t)/R. When signal levels are computed in dB from voltage measurements, they are noted as dBV. It is common for transducer outputs in SPLs to be calibrated according to the output achieved with a 1 volt RMS signal passed across it.

Adding Signals

When signals are added in the time domain, their instantaneous pressures add linearly, thus, $x_{1+2}(t) = x_1(t) + x_2(t)$. The instantaneous pressure of the combined waveform is a sum of the instantaneous pressures of the components. Figure 9–1C shows the result of adding the signals shown in Figure 9–1A and B. Note that the magnitude of the waveform in C is produced by a linear addition of the magnitudes in A and B at each moment in time.

Unlike pressures, intensities do not add linearly. Intensity is related to pressure by squaring. Thus the intensity of a combined signal, I_{1+2} is as follows:

$$I_{1+2} \ = \ [x_1(t) \ + \ x_2(t)]^2$$

This expands algebraically to:

$$I_{1+2} \ = \ x_1^2(t) \ + \ x_2^2(t) \ + \ 2x_1(t)x_2(t)$$

Because $x_1{}^2$ is the intensity of signal 1 and $x_2{}^2$ is the intensity of signal 2, the equation for computing the average intensity of the combined signal will be as follows:

$$I_{1+2} \ = \ I_1 \ + \ I_2 \ + \ 2\frac{1}{T_D}\int_0^{T_D} dt x_1(t)x_2(t)$$

Therefore the combined intensity of two waveforms is equal to the sum of their individual intensities plus a sum that is related to the correlation between, or the cross-product of, the two waveforms. If x_1 and x_2 are uncorrelated, the integral is equal to 0 so that the intensity of the combined waveform reduces to the simple combination of the intensities in the two signals themselves. (This is the general assumption.) However, if the two waveforms are identical, their combined intensity is simply four times greater than that of one component because the integral would be equal to 1.0. Moreover, if the correlation between the two is equal to −1.0, that is they are exact opposites, 180 degrees out of phase with one another, their combined intensity would be 0 because the two signals would cancel one another out. If the correlation is other than 1, 0, or −1 as described in these examples, the computation is less simple.

Adding Sound Levels (Decibels)

The preceding examples show how to combine intensities when they are in absolute terms. However, it is more customary to add intensities that have been measured in decibels. The overall level of a combined signal in dB will be as follows:

$$L = 10 \, log\left(\frac{Intensity_1}{reference \; level}\right) + 10 \, log\left(\frac{Intensity_2}{reference \; level}\right)$$

Because the two signals have a common reference level, for example, 10^{-12} watts/m², the intensities of the individual waveforms can be computed from their dB values, $I(dB) = 10log(I/10^{-12})$. Solving for I, $= 10^{I(dB)/10}*10^{-12}$. The several values of I obtained for each signal to be added can then be combined. The overall level will be equal to:

$$10 \, log\left[\left(\sum_1^n I_n\right)/10^{-12}\right]$$

Periodic and Aperiodic Signals

When a signal repeats its pattern of vibration infinitely over time, it is said to be periodic. The time interval over which it repeats is the *period*. One of the simplest of periodic signals is the *sinusoid* or, in acoustics, the *pure tone*. (A gated pure tone, that is, one that is turned on and off and therefore not truly continuous in time, is the most common signal used in audiometric testing.) The pure tone or sinusoid is produced by a pattern of activity (voltage or pressure changes with time) that is defined according to the sine function such that:

$$x(t) = A \, sin(2\pi t/T + \phi),$$

where A is the maximum amplitude of the signal, T is the period (usually in seconds), and ϕ is the starting phase (in radians). The amplitude can take on any positive value. Because the sine function varies between 1 and −1, the signal magnitude will vary between A and $-A$. As can be seen in the definition of the sine wave, the magnitude will repeat with every cycle of the wave, that is, every 360 degrees or 2π radians. Assuming a starting phase of 0, (i.e. $\phi = 0$), x(t) will be equal to 0 whenever $2\pi t/T$ is equal to 0 or π because the sine of both are equal to 0.0. X(t) will reach a maximum, or peak amplitude, A, when the argument to the sine function is $\pi/2$ radians, or 90 degrees, and a minimum, $-A$, when the argument is $3\pi/2$

radians (or 270 degrees). As time, t, progresses, the pattern repeats. The frequency of the signal is $1/T$, noted in cycles per second, or *Hertz (Hz)*. The equation for the sinusoid can also be written as $x(t) = Asin(2\pi ft + \phi)$, where f is the frequency. If the starting phase is not zero, the function is identical in shape to one starting at zero phase but shifted in time by an amount corresponding to the phase shift. The signals shown in the upper and middle panel of Figure 9–1 are sine waves with starting phase of 0 degrees and are periodic over the time interval shown. If the time units were milliseconds, the period of the waveform in the upper panel would be 1 ms, and zero crossings would occur at t = 0.0, 0.5, and 1 ms, corresponding to phases of 0, π, and 2 π. The positive and negative maxima occur at 0.25 and 0.75, corresponding to $\pi/2$ and 3 $\pi/2$ radians. This pattern repeats for all successive replications of the period. (Note that the absolute magnitude shown in Figures 9–1A and B varies between + and −1.0. If this were a real signal, the magnitudes shown here would be multiplied by the peak amplitude, A.)

When sinusoids are added together, perceptible fluctuations may result in the amplitude, or envelope, particularly if the components are different frequencies. The envelope of the combined signal will be modulated at a frequency that coincides with the difference in the frequencies of the two constituent tones. This modulation frequency is often called the beat frequency. When one listens to the combined tones, the amplitude modulates at a rate corresponding to the beat frequency, which corresponds to the slow variations in the envelope of the combined signal that resulted from the orderly addition of instantaneous pressures. The effect on the envelope of signals produced by the addition of individual signals with other relations may be more complex. Note that the signal in Figure 9–1B is slightly different from that in Figure 9–1A. The addition of these two signals produces the waveform shown in Figure 9–1C. Note the slower variations in the overall amplitude of the envelope, which contrast with the constant envelope of the signals in Figures 9–1A and B.

PEARL

A beat frequency is the product of two simultaneous sinusoidal stimuli with different frequencies. The envelope of the combined signal modulates at the frequency that coincides with the differences in the frequencies of the two constituent tones.

Noise

Sounds that do not repeat in time are said to be *aperiodic*. A class of aperiodic sounds that are common in audiometry and hearing research are *noises*. A noise signal consists of frequency components that are not discrete, but continuous. That is, they contain energy at every frequency over a specific range, and therefore energy is represented as a continuous function of frequency. The noise is defined by the manner in which the amplitudes of the individual components are represented and by the bandwidth of frequencies represented. *Gaussian noise*, the most common type of noise used in hearing applications, is noise for which the amplitudes of the individual components are distributed normally. In contrast, *uniform noise* is that for which the amplitudes of the individual components are all the same.

The frequency composition of a noise is most often defined by its bandwidth. *Band-limited* noise refers to a noise consisting of components only over a range of frequencies. The bandwidth of the noise is defined as the difference between the upper (f_u) and lower (f_l) cut-off frequencies ($BW = f_u - f_l$). White noise is gaussian, with energy present as a continuous function of frequency. The bandwidth is limited only by the output characteristics of the transducer. Pink noise contains energy as a continuous function of frequency but the relative amplitude of components decreases at a rate of 3 dB/octave as frequency increases, thus biasing toward the lower frequencies. Other common noise types used in audiometric and hearing research are third-octave noise bands. These noises are defined by their center frequency and contain energy at frequencies only in the 1/3 octave wide region surrounding this center frequency. Other types of noise are also common in hearing research. For example, *band stop* noise refers to noise for which components are presented at all frequencies except those defined by the band stop region. This is also called *notched noise*.

Power Spectra of Signals

The overall power in a signal can be expressed as a function of the spectrum level of the individual components:

$$\overline{P} = \int_{f_l}^{f_u} df\, N_0(f).$$

The energy in each 1 Hz wide band of noise, N_0, is summed for each frequency component, f, over the entire bandwidth, noted by the integral with f_u and f_l representing the upper and lower cut-off frequencies, respectively. This measure is most often referred to as the *power spectrum*. When the power spectrum is noted in absolute units, dB relative to 10^{-12} watts/Hz, the *spectrum level*, or level of individual components, can be calculated from the overall level, L_0: $L_0 = 10\, log(N_0/10^{-12})$. When the power spectrum is constant with frequency, the spectrum level in dB, N_0, can be calculated from the total level, L: $N_0 = L - 10\, log(BW)$, where BW is the bandwidth of the noise.

Fourier Analysis

Most natural sounds are complex and consist of energy at multiple frequencies, although the energy distribution may not be as easily defined as in the preceding examples of pure tones and noises. A frequency domain representation, or spectral representation, is most useful for displaying the relative amplitudes of individual components. To obtain spectral information, signals are analyzed mathematically with the *Fourier transform*. The Fourier transform and the inverse Fourier transform enable movement back and forth between time and frequency domain representations of signals. Two types of Fourier transformations exist. The Fourier series,

which is applicable only to periodic signals, and the Fourier integral, which can be applied to all signals. (Although full treatment of this transform is not possible here, a brief introduction of the basic concepts will be provided. An excellent reference is Ramirez [1985].)

Fourier Series

The Fourier series is used to evaluate signals that are infinite, a requirement to be truly periodic. As periodic signals, all of the components must have a period that will fit exactly into the period of the waveform, T. The lowest frequency for which this is true is the fundamental frequency, f_0, which is equal to 1/T. Other components will be integer multiples of the fundamental and thus *harmonics* of it. The general form of the Fourier series states that a waveform, x(t), can be written as a sum of sine and cosine functions, each of which is weighted by a magnitude:

$$x(t) = A_0 + \sum_{n=1}^{\infty} A_n \cos(\omega_n t) + B_n \sin(\omega_n t)$$

where A_0 is a constant representing the average magnitude, such as the DC offset in an electrical signal, A_n and B_n are Fourier coefficients that weight each sine and cosine component; and ω_n is the frequency of each component. Note that ω is equal to $2\pi n/T$.

To solve for the Fourier coefficients, which are the magnitudes associated with each frequency component, two equations are needed, one to solve for the cosine components and one for the sine components:

$$A_n = \frac{2}{T} \int_{-T/2}^{T/2} dt\, x(t)\, \cos(\omega_n t)$$

and

$$B_n = \frac{2}{T} \int_{-T/2}^{T/2} dt\, x(t)\, \sin(\omega_n t) \text{, for n > 0}$$

To solve for the constant:

$$A_0 = \frac{1}{T} \int_{-T/2}^{T/2} dt\, x(t)^*$$

When signals are analyzed using the Fourier transform, a spectral representation of a signal can be visualized by plotting the Fourier coefficients (or frequency component magnitudes) and the starting phases as a function of frequency. Figure 9–2 shows the amplitude and phase spectra of the

---

*The equation for the series can also be represented in polar form such that:

$$x(t) = A_0 + \sum_{n=1}^{n} C_n \cos(\omega_n t - \phi_n),$$

where C_n represents the amplitude and ϕ_n is the phase of each component. By expansion using trigonometric identities:

$$x(t) = A_0 + \sum_{n=1}^{N} [C_n \cos(\omega_n t)\cos(\phi_n) + C_n \sin(\omega_n t)\sin(\phi_n)].$$

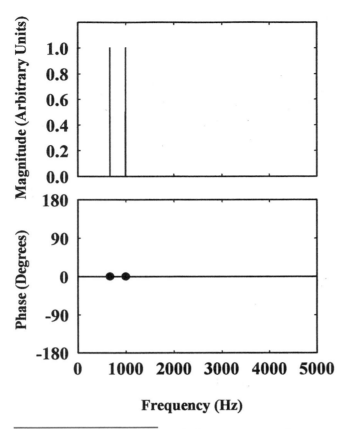

Figure 9–2   The amplitude and phase spectra, in the upper and lower panels, respectively, of the signal shown in the lower panel of Figure 9–1, assuming that the time units in Figure 9–1 are in milliseconds.

signal shown in Figure 9–1C, assuming of course that the signals in Figure 9–1 continue past the minimum and maximum time intervals shown.

Fourier Integral

The Fourier integral is more general than the Fourier series and can be used with signals that are not periodic. It states that from the frequency domain representation of a waveform, $X(\omega)$, a time domain representation, $x(t)$, can be written:

$$X(\omega) = \int_{-\infty}^{\infty} dt e^{-i\omega t} x(t)$$

The inverse integral to move from the frequency domain to the time domain is:

$$x(t) = \frac{1}{2\pi} \int_{-\infty}^{\infty} d\omega e^{i\omega t} X(\omega)$$

Discrete versus Continuous Fourier Transforms

Many signals used in hearing research laboratories and audiology clinics are not continuous analog signals but are produced digitally. As such, their instantaneous magnitudes do not occur as a continuous function of time but at discrete time intervals, the spacing of which is defined by the sampling rate (e.g., for a signal produced with a sampling rate of 10,000 points/s, an instantaneous magnitude will be available every 100 μs). To perform a spectral analysis on a discrete signal, the discrete fourier transform (DFT) is often used, as is the fast fourier transform (FFT). Because brief duration signals can never be truly periodic and not be continuous in time, it is often assumed that the period is equal to the duration of the signal itself. Another difference between the DFT and the Fourier series is that in the Fourier series the number of frequencies and coefficients extends infinitely, whereas in the DFT the components are limited by the Nyquist frequency, which is equal to 1/2 of the sampling frequency. (For a frequency to be represented, at least two samples must be present for the period.) Thus for a sampling rate of 10 kHz just suggested, only frequencies up to 5 kHz will be represented accurately.

Wave Propagation in Space

Acoustic signals are transmitted over space and time. A periodic signal will therefore repeat itself not only over the period but also over a distance in space. This distance is the wavelength, λ, and it is related to the period, $\lambda = cT$, and to the frequency $\lambda = c/f$, where c is the speed of sound. In general, sounds will move around objects if their size is smaller than the wavelength. Thus lower frequency sounds, with larger wavelengths, are less affected by objects in space because they are more likely to move around them. In contrast, higher frequencies with smaller wavelengths are more likely to bounce off objects in their path, thus producing differences in magnitudes on the two sides of the object, higher on the side facing the sound and lower on the opposite side.

PEARL

Lower frequency sounds, with larger wavelengths, are less affected by objects in space and more likely to move around them. In contrast, higher frequencies with smaller wavelengths are more likely to bounce off objects in their path.

Although sounds are propagated through a space, they lose intensity as the distance they travel increases, particularly if room reverberation is low. Signal intensity varies inversely with the square of the distance traveled. Because sound intensity is a function of force per unit area, as area increases with the space in which the sound is dispersed, the intensity decreases. The exact magnitude of the decrease will be proportional to the characteristics of the room itself. In a highly reverberant room the intensity may not be reduced at all because reflected sounds will add with direct sounds. But in a dead room, with little or no reverberation, sound intensity may be reduced quite rapidly with distance traveled. In general, sound waves propagate in all directions. However, some transducers and rooms cause sound to radiate in specific directions. This is called a directional sound, and the levels recorded will vary with the location of the recording microphone relative to the direction in which the source transmits.

PSYCHOMETRIC METHODS

Measurement of sound perception requires not only a working knowledge of the physical basis of sounds but also reliable methods for measuring listener's responses to those sounds.

Thresholds and Psychometric Functions

Audiologists focus much of their activity on *thresholds*. The measurement of absolute thresholds (or thresholds of audibility) is the most basic and agreed on audiometric measure. In more general terms threshold indicates the physical value of a stimulus at which a predetermined level of performance is obtained. It may apply to detection of, or discrimination between, events. It could be assumed that performance changes instantaneously from very poor to very good at the stimulus value corresponding to threshold. But in reality, a single value at which this change occurs does not exist. No level exists below which a sound is never audible or two sounds are never discriminable from one another and above which the sound is always audible and/or discriminable from others. Instead, perceptions change relatively gradually over a range of stimulus values.

> ## PEARL
>
> The function used to describe this gradual change in perception is the *psychometric function*. It relates performance, such as percent correct detection or discrimination, to measurable parameters of the stimuli.

In a task for which a listener is asked to detect a signal presented in quiet, the psychometric function would relate performance, possibly in terms of percent correct detections, to signal intensity. If threshold were a single value below which detection was not possible and above which the signal would be detected with 100% accuracy, the psychometric function would be a step function moving abruptly from 0 to 100% correct at a single value of the stimulus. But detection is probabilistic, changing gradually from 0 to 100% over a range of approximately 10- to 15-dB with adult listeners. (With young children the range may be somewhat larger and the functions may reach an asymptote at a performance level less than 100% correct [e.g., Allen & Wightman, 1994].) The shape of the function is nonlinear, often approximated by a logistic function. Because the rate of change in detection (or the slope of the psychometric function) is fairly constant for listeners under similar circumstances, performance is seldom measured in the clinic over a wide range of levels as would be needed to fit a psychometric function. Instead, performance is estimated at predetermined levels, generally corresponding to that at the inflection point on the psychometric function. That performance level is taken as threshold. When the psychometric function ranges from 0 to 100% correct, as in standard

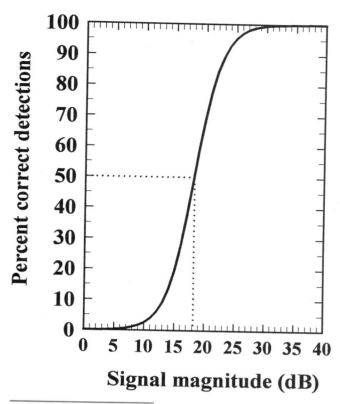

Figure 9–3 A theoretical psychometric function showing percent correct detections as a function of signal magnitude. The dotted line indicates the threshold magnitude corresponding to the 50% correct level.

clinical testing procedures, threshold corresponds to the 50% correct level. Figure 9–3 shows a sample psychometric function. The solid line shows a function that would best fit observed performance data.

> ## PEARL
>
> Often, when measuring an audiometric threshold, uncertainty may exist about whether a threshold value has actually been obtained. In those instances a signal at a level 5 dB above the suspected threshold may be presented. If the response to the signal is clear, it can be assumed that the level measured probably did correspond to the 50% correct threshold, and if the response at this 5 dB higher level is unclear, the threshold estimate is questioned and threshold-seeking procedures should continue because an individual's psychometric function ranges from 50 to 100% accuracy in approximately 5 dB as the whole function ranges over only 10 dB, thus performance 5 dB above a threshold value, if it represents the intercept in the function, should produce near perfect detection.

Note that predicted performance (detection accuracy) increases gradually as signal level increases from 10- to 25-dB. In this example threshold, taken as the 50% correct level, corresponds to a signal intensity of slightly greater than 18 dB.

Signal Detection Theory

In general, individuals try to make informed decisions when asked to do so. This concept extends to the detection and discrimination of auditory signals. When an individual is asked to listen to two sounds and decide which is louder, which is a tone plus noise versus a noise alone, or which of a set of sounds is higher in pitch, and so on, the listener will try to make the decision on the basis of the available sensory information and do so in a way that will maximize the probability of making a correct decision, weighted of course, by the costs and values associated with incorrect and correct decisions. *Statistical decision theory* and from that, *signal detection theory*, assists in explaining how these decisions are likely made (see Green & Swets, 1966).

In a simple detection task listeners have some sensory activity that they must judge as representing either the presence of a signal or simply random background activity. The evidence variable with which they must make their judgment, x, is in this case the amount of sensory activity in the system at the time of the observation. As signal intensity increases, so does the associated sensory activity. But, because some spontaneous activity in the system (noise) always exists, the listener must decide at what point the sensory activity is sufficiently high to warrant changing their description of it from that of "no signal" (or "noise") to "signal" (or "signal plus noise"). Where the criterion is set will vary with costs associated with the mistakes the listener is willing to make and the values of correct responses.

Assume that the random amount of activity that the listener experiences in the absence of a signal is normally distributed. Figure 9–4 shows a hypothetical distribution of this "evidence variable." The distribution representing the values of sensory activity present when noise alone or no signal is present, and the probability of each of those values occurring is labeled N. When a signal is added to this background activity, the mean of the distribution will increase but the variance will remain the same. The signal simply adds a constant value to the probable values of sensory activity present in general. This new distribution is labeled, *SN*, indicating that it is a signal-plus-noise distribution. On a given trial, listeners are asked whether it is believed that a signal was present. A decision is made to respond or not by examining the amount of sensory activity, x, that is present at the time of the trial. A decision must be made whether the value of x sampled at that time is more consistent with the existence of no signal, N, (i.e., that it is just random activity) or signal plus noise, *SN*. The only information the listener has to go on is the amount of activity sampled at that moment.

For a particular value of x two probabilities will exist: one that it came from the N distribution and another that it came from the *SN* distribution. Whenever N and *SN* overlap, as they will unless the signal level is very high, some error in the decision is bound to occur. All that the listener can do, according to statistical decision theory, is calculate the relative probabilities that the sensory experience was drawn from each of these two sensory states and compare them. This comparison is carried out by means of the *likelihood ratio (L)*. It compares the probability that the activity came from a signal state divided by the probability that the activity came from a noise alone state: $L = P(x/SN)/P(x/N)$. If the value of x is such that it is equally likely to have been drawn from either of the two distributions, that is, if it is equally probable to obtain this value of x in either state, the value of L is 1.0. In Figure 9–4, this would occur for values of x for which the N and SN distributions intersect. Higher values of L will occur for values of x that exceed this value and therefore indicate that it is more likely that the activity was produced by the presence of a signal and lower values of L indicate the opposite. The listener's task is to determine a critical value of the likelihood ratio above which they will say that a signal is present and below which they will say that none is present. This

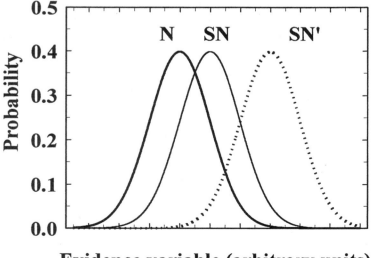

Figure 9–4   Three sample probability distributions of a hypothetical evidence variable used to make a decision in a signal detection or discrimination task. The heavy solid curve (*N*) shows the probability of each value of the evidence variable associated with a noise alone or no signal state. The lighter solid curve (*SN*) shows the distribution of values associated with the introduction of a low-level signal. The dotted line shows the distribution of values associated with the addition of a higher level signal.

value of the likelihood ratio at which their decision changes from no signal to signal is their *criterion*.

When the signal is very intense, it will drive the level of the activity way above that which is ever associated with simple, spontaneous activity and because the likelihood ratio will be large for nearly all the expressed values of x, the decision will be easily made. A change in activity resulting from the addition of such a signal to random background activity is suggested by the dotted line in Figure 9–4 labeled SN'. But when the signal is weak (e.g., SN in Fig. 9–4), it may only increase the background activity slightly, making the decision much harder and much more prone to error.

A correct response can be made in two ways: first the listener may judge that a signal is present when it in fact is (*hit*), and second the listener can judge that no signal is present when it is not (*correct rejection*). Similarly, two types of errors exist: one is that a signal will be judged to be present when it is not (*false alarm*), and the other that that no signal will be judged to be present when it is (*miss*). Obviously, for a block of trials the proportion of hits and misses can be calculated if only one of the two is known, because they sum to 1.0. (Measuring both therefore provides no more information than measuring only one of the two.) Similarly, if the rate of correct rejections is known, so also is the rate of false alarms, again these must sum to 1.0. To summarize, if the listeners say a signal is present, they are either right (hit) or wrong (false alarm), and if listeners say no signal is present, they are again either right (correct rejection) or wrong (miss). The key for understanding sensitivity is to know not only the rates at which correct and incorrect responses are made on signal trials, but also the rates of correct and incorrect responses on no-signal trials. It is only by measuring performance on both signal and no-signal trials that true sensitivity can be estimated.

For example, assume two listeners with equal threshold sensitivity. For a particular stimulus level the amount of sensory activity received is indicated by the *SN* distribution shown in Figure 9–4, and sensory activity with no signal is indicated by N. Suppose the first listener wants the examiner to think he or she has excellent hearing. A decision is made that no matter what is perceived a response will be made that a signal is present. Nearly every time when asked whether a sound is heard, the listener will respond that it was. This would give a hit rate near 1.0 and a miss rate near 0.0. To achieve this level of performance would require that the listener sets the criterion at a very low value of x. This listener would be described as having an extremely liberal response criterion. Suppose, in contrast, the other listener is much more conservative because concern exists about hearing/hearing loss. This listener would decide to respond only when absolutely sure that a sound is heard; that is, when it is fairly loud. This listener would set the response criterion at a very high value of x. The hit rate would be much lower than that of the first listener. Without knowing anything else one would be led to assume that this listener has poorer hearing than the more liberal listener. But the only difference between them is the bias in response patterns, not actual sensitivity. Only by also measuring the responses for no-signal trials would the difference become apparent. If the rate at which mistakes are made is examined, it will be seen that the liberal listener, because of the low criterion value, will often respond that a signal is present when it is not, that is when the listener

merely experiences a sample drawn from the N distribution. The false-alarm rate would be quite high and the correct-rejection rate would be very low. This would suggest that the listener's sensitivity may be much poorer than the very high hit rate had suggested. Conversely, the more conservative listener would have far fewer false alarms and many correct rejections, suggesting that perhaps sensitivity was better than the relatively low hit rate had indicated initially. Thus only by examining responses on signal and no-signal trials can an individual's true sensitivity be determined in a manner that is free of bias in the criterion.

Clearly, these extremes are rare in most settings. A listener is free to vary response criterion throughout the range of possible values of the likelihood ratio. Where listeners set their criterion will vary with the costs and values associated with both forms of incorrect and correct responses. If the value in a hit is high and the cost of a false alarm is low, the listener may set a more liberal criterion, but if the value of hits decreases and the cost of false alarms increases, listeners may choose to become more conservative. Evaluating true sensitivity requires an estimate of performance that includes responses on both signal and no-signal trials so that both hit and false alarm rates can be estimated.

SPECIAL CONSIDERATION

In the clinic, false alarm rates are seldom measured. When unsolicited responses occur, patients are reinstructed, encouraging them to be more conservative, "Press the button only if you are sure that there is a sound." The goal is to keep the false alarm rate as low as possible so that it will not bias the estimates of performance that are based solely on hit rates.

---

d-prime and Forced Choice Procedures

Many experimental measures of performance are reported as d-prime (d') values, not percent correct. d' is a bias free estimate of performance that incorporates both hit and false-alarm information. What is of interest in the measurement of performance is the relative detectability or discriminability of a particular stimulus. That is, how far does the distribution of *SN* values lie above the noise alone distribution. Does it lie only slightly above the *SN* distribution suggesting that sensitivity for this sound was quite low (SN), or does it lie substantially above it, suggesting that sensitivity must be quite high (SN')? To determine how far from the N distribution the *SN* distribution lies at each stimulus value, the mean of the *SN* distribution must be calculated relative to a normalized N distribution with a mean and $\sigma = 1.0$. In simple terms the mean of the *SN* distribution is calculated in standard deviation units relative to the mean and standard deviation of the N distribution: $d' = \text{Mean} ((SN) - \text{Mean} (N))/\sigma(N)$. Because the mean and standard deviation of the noise-alone distribution are 1.0, d' is actually the mean of the signal-plus-noise distribution in units normalized to the distribution of noise-alone values. So, for a $d' = 0$, the signal should not be discriminable at better than chance levels because the *N* and *SN* distributions must overlap completely. When $d' = 1.0$, it is assumed that the signal produced a mean value of x that lies 1 σ above the mean of the *N* distribution. Once d' values reach approximately 3.0, discriminability is near perfect because the *N* and *SN* distributions have little or no overlap.

In an experimental setting it is customary to measure performance in *forced-choice procedures*. Trials, usually consisting of multiple listening intervals, are well defined. Signals are presented in only one of the intervals of each trial. In this way performance is measured for both signal and no-signal options, simultaneously evaluating a combination of hit and false-alarm rates. The listener's task is to choose which of the intervals presented on each trial has the greatest likelihood of containing a signal (or being different from the rest, etc.). The listener must respond on every trial, even if unsure. In such a task performance can range from chance to a maximum that may or may not be associated with 100% correct levels.

PITFALL

Best performance will often, but not always, be associated with 100% correct, depending on the task, and the ability of the listener. Performance associated with chance performance will vary with the number of listening intervals. If two intervals are presented, chance performance will be 50% correct. If three intervals are presented, chance will be 33% correct. Yet in both cases, chance indicates a $d' = 0.0$. This makes it difficult to compare performance across several conditions using percent correct measures if the task was not identical. For quick reference, refer to tables presented in Swets (1964), Appendix I, Table II, that show d' values corresponding to a full range of percent correct values obtained in multiple-alternative forced-choice tasks.

Psychophysical Methods

Many psychophysical methods can be used to collect detection and/or discrimination data. Each has its own advantages and disadvantages and selection of an appropriate procedure must be made based on consideration of speed and efficiency in data collection, the nature of the experimental/clinical question being asked, and the capabilities of the listener. A few examples will be discussed.

Method of Limits

In the method of limits the listener is presented with a series of trials for which the physical value being tested is varied in an orderly and predetermined manner. For example, when the task is to determine an individual's threshold for the audibility of a signal, the signal level is presented in both ascending and descending series. In the ascending series the stimuli are initially presented at a very low intensity and as trials proceed, the stimulus level is increased. In descending series, the level begins high and is gradually reduced. The listener simply

responds if signals heard or not heard or, in a forced-choice task, which of n intervals is most likely to contain the signal. The lower and upper stimulus values tested are determined before the initiation of a trial block, usually requiring prior knowledge of the listener's overall response capabilities so that the desired levels of performance (i.e., chance to best performance) can be observed at the extreme values. Thresholds are determined by averaging the stimulus values associated with changes in listeners' responses obtained in both ascending and descending series. An advantage of this procedure is that a full range of performance levels can be estimated. However, a disadvantage, if only threshold estimates are of interest, is that many trials will be presented at stimulus values quite remote from threshold levels. This makes the procedure somewhat inefficient for threshold determinations.

Variations on the methods of limits are *adaptive procedures* that use algorithms to select stimulus values for each trial on the basis of the listener's responses on the preceding trial(s). These are also called staircase procedures. Rules are applied to the way stimulus values are chosen with the goal of concentrating trials at or near the desired percent correct (threshold) signal values. For example, in a 1-up 1-down procedure, the stimulus value is decreased every time a correct response is made and increased every time an incorrect response is made. The resulting threshold value tracked is that corresponding to 50% correct performance. This performance level is extrapolated from the midpoint between stimulus values for which a change in stimulus direction is noted (a reversal). If two correct responses are required before the stimulus value is decreased but the 1-up rule is kept (i.e., 2-down, 1-up rule), the threshold level that is estimated will correspond to a higher level of performance than that estimated from a 1 down, 1 up rule, approximately 70.7% correct (Levitt, 1971).

PEARL

On average, more trials will be presented at higher stimulus values with a rule requiring a greater number of correct responses before the stimulus value is decreased. Thus performance averaged across stimuli will be higher than when fewer sequential correct responses are required for a decrease in stimulus value. The performance level tracked in an n-down, 1 up procedure will be equal to $\sqrt[n]{0.5}$. In the audiology clinic a 1-down 1-up rule is generally applied to a task for which chance is 0% correct, thus tracking 50% correct performance levels.

Adaptive procedures have the advantage of placing nearly all trials in and around the region of the threshold, avoiding stimulus values that lie distant from the threshold value in either direction. The starting values in an adaptive procedure are usually set relatively high to ensure that the listener knows what to listen for. The stimulus values are then reduced, usually with a slightly larger step size than will be used for the remainder of the trial block. Once a reversal has occurred, the step size may be reduced. Generally, the first or second reversal values are not included in the calculation of the threshold estimate. (Stimulus levels at reversal points can be averaged or the stimulus levels midway between successive reversals can be calculated and averaged for the final threshold estimate.) The rule for stopping an adaptive track is that either a fixed number of trials has been completed or a predetermined number of reversals have occurred.

Method of Adjustment

In the method of adjustment the stimulus values are under the control of the listener, not the experimenter. For example, in the measurement of detection thresholds the level of the signal may gradually increase and decrease automatically with the direction of change under the control of the listener. Listeners are instructed to keep the signal level at a value that is just barely detectable by responding when the signal is heard and not heard. Signal intensity may gradually increase until the listener presses a response button to indicate that the signal is audible. At that point the intensity begins to decrease gradually. When the sound is no longer audible, the listener releases the response button signaling the system to now increase signal intensity. Threshold levels are determined from the average level, falling between successive responses indicating audible and inaudible signal values.

Method of Constant Stimuli

The experimenter may also select a variety of stimulus values that are both above and below the individual's threshold rather than estimate only a single threshold value. Several trials are presented at each of many stimulus values (often chosen randomly across a block of trials) and performance is calculated for each stimulus value. A psychometric function may then be fitted to those performance data. Threshold values can be extrapolated from these fitted functions if desired. This procedure is similar to the method of limits in that a wide range of signal values is tested but differs in the order in which those values are presented and perhaps in the interval between values.

Scaling

Often it is of interest how the magnitude of a psychological percept changes with changes in a physical parameter of a sound, rather than simply in an individual's ability to detect and/or discriminate between sounds. This information may be obtained by presenting listeners with a stimulus and asking them to rate the perceived magnitude of the stimulus (magnitude estimation) or by asking listeners to adjust a stimulus to match a magnitude that is presented (magnitude production). Listeners may also be presented with a signal and asked to adjust the magnitude of another signal to be a fraction or integer multiple of that first signal. Each of these procedures may be used alone or in combination with others to develop sensory scales.

Developing a scale relating a perception to a sensory magnitude must be carried out with care because many potential sources of *bias* exist in these tasks (e.g., Gravetter & Lockhead, 1973; Pradhan & Hoffman, 1963). For example, listeners often tend to limit or shorten the range of a parameter that is under their control when conducting matching tasks. This is called the *regression effect*. Thus when listeners are asked to estimate the loudness of a sound, the use of very small or very large numbers will be avoided. Conversely, when listeners are asked to adjust a stimulus magnitude to correspond to numbers that are given, extremely high and low signal values will be avoided. One way to limit the expression of this bias is to begin the task by presenting the listener with the full range of stimuli (or magnitude values) that will be presented during the task, thereby allowing the listener to adjust or calibrate the internal scale before the start of the task.

Another bias that is common in scaling procedures is the *sequential effect* in which listeners try to respond on each trial in a manner that is consistent with their previous responses. The effect of this bias can be observed over five to seven previous trials and occurs even if listeners are told to judge each stimulus independently of all others. Last, as with detection and discrimination procedures, listeners may be biased by costs and values associated with their responses or by their concerns about the subsequent use that will be made of the judgments they provide. One way to limit the biases commonly associated with scaling tasks is to use matching tasks for which a very strong correlation exists between the items to be matched. For example, in a task for which loudness is rated numerically, the biases will be strong because a perfect match does not exist between loudness levels and numbers. But, if loudness scales are created by matching similar stimuli, such as pure tones of slightly different frequencies as were used in the measurement of equal loudness contours, the biases will be much smaller.

PITFALL

Some rating procedures present stimuli to listeners in ascending or descending series rather than randomly. This can exacerbate the sequential effect. The listeners responses may appear to be more consistent (internal reliability will appear to increase), but the judgments may be less valid because each judgment is not independent but linked to previous judgments.

LEVEL, SPECTRAL, AND TEMPORAL ENCODING

Armed with a basic knowledge of the physical parameters of a sound and of the procedures used to measure a listener's responses to those sounds, the limits and abilities of humans to encode and use auditory information can be explored. As a first step toward understanding the perception of natural sounds, which are inherently complex, this section begins with an attempt to describe the perception of relatively simple sounds.

Intensity Encoding

Initial discussion of how the auditory system encodes intensity information will include a review of absolute detection thresholds, loudness growth functions and dynamic range, and intensity discrimination. Subsequent sections will address intensity encoding from the perspective of cross-frequency intensity processing or profile analysis.

Absolute Detection of Sounds in Quiet

Data describing detectability as a function of stimulus frequency provides the foundation of audiometric threshold testing. Absolute threshold data shown by the lower curve in Figure 9–5 show the average SPL required by young, healthy adult listeners to detect a signal of known frequency presented in quiet. Audiometric measures of hearing level (dB HL) are referenced to these threshold values noted in dB SPL (ANSI, 1989). Note that the human ear is most sensitive to frequencies in the 1- to 5-kHz range and that higher signal levels are required for the detection of signal frequencies above and below this range.

Calibration of Sound Levels: Effect on Threshold Estimates

In calibrating sound levels the method by which the calibration is obtained is important (see Chapter 10). For example, the values reflected in audibility curves (see Fig. 9–5) may vary slightly with the procedures used to calibrate the signals. When a listener is tested in a free field environment (i.e., with the sound presented through speakers in a room with no reflections), calibration of sound levels reaching the listener can be accomplished by removing the listener from the room and putting a measuring microphone in their place. The microphone is placed as close to the position of the listener's ear as possible, and measurements are made of the sound levels reaching the measuring microphone. These are *minimal audible field (MAF)* measurements. But the sound levels reaching the outer ear of the listener may not truly reflect the SPLs created in the earcanal. Because of the resonance characteristics of the outer ear, the sound reaching the tympanic membrane is often greater than that arriving at the entrance to the earcanal, which the MAF measurements most closely approx-

imate. One way to account for earcanal resonance measurements is to measure detection thresholds under headphones that are calibrated using a coupler that is approximately equal to the volume of the space created between the transducer and the tympanic membrane (approximately 6-cc for supraaural earphones and approximately 2-cc for insert phones). Measurements calibrated with earphones placed in a coupler are termed *minimal audible pressure (MAP)*. Threshold estimates referenced to these values will be slightly higher than those referenced to MAF measurements made in the sound field. (Thresholds calibrated with MAF techniques underestimate the intensity of the signal arriving at the tympanic membrane. For greater detail, see Robinson & Dadson [1956] and Sivian & White [1933].)

Although MAP measures provide a better approximation to the SPLs actually reaching the eardrum than do the MAF measures, they do not include the subtleties of individual differences in earcanal resonance, which are very different from that of a standard 2-cc coupler (see Shaw, 1997). The resonance characteristics of the outer ear are slightly different for every individual despite some general similarities (see Wightman & Kistler, 1997). Thus the best measure of sound pressure reaching the eardrum for an individual are made with *probe tube measurements*. A small probe microphone is placed deep within the earcanal of the listener and SPLs emitted by the transducer (which could be headphones or free field speakers) are measured directly as they arrive at the tympanic membrane. Care must be taken to place the probe microphone as close to the eardrum as possible. Probe placement must be identical with subsequent measurements to minimize error in repeated measures because even slight differences in probe placement could produce differences in sound levels measured at some frequencies.

Loudness

The psychological correlate of intensity is loudness. Near threshold level sounds are perceived as very soft, and loudness increases with increases in stimulus intensity. Through a combination of loudness estimation procedures it has been suggested that loudness grows exponentially with increases in signal intensity, $L = k\ I^{0.3}$, where L is loudness, k is a constant, and I is the signal intensity (Stevens, 1955, 1957, 1972). Thus loudness increases more slowly with increasing intensity at lower intensities and more rapidly at higher intensities. Loudness also grows most slowly in mid-frequencies and more rapidly at higher and lower frequencies. This is most clearly shown in the *equal loudness contours*, which were constructed by asking listeners to balance the loudness of sounds at several frequencies to that of a reference tone of predetermined frequency and level (Fletcher & Munson, 1933; Robinson & Dadson, 1956). Generally, the reference signal is a 1000 Hz tone whose level is systematically varied so that matches to different frequencies can be made at many intensities. Data from Fletcher and Munson (1933) are shown in Figure 9–5. Note that loudness growth is slowest for frequencies in the region of greatest sensitivity (i.e., smaller increments in intensity are required at very high or very low frequencies to match the loudness growth of much larger increments in the mid-frequencies). Note also that at threshold levels, sounds of different frequencies must be set at very different overall SPLs to achieve equal loudness, but at high signal levels, sounds of

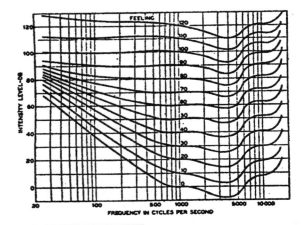

Figure 9–5 Equal loudness contours taken from Fletcher and Munson (1933). The lower curve, (*0*), reflects thresholds of audibility.

different frequencies are perceived as equally loud at very similar SPLs. The equal loudness curves become flatter with changes in frequency at very high levels, suggesting that dynamic range is narrower at frequency extremes than at mid-frequencies and that sound frequency is less of a determiner of loudness at high levels than at low levels. Small increments in intensity at extreme frequencies may be perceived as equivalent to larger increments at mid frequencies.

Dynamic Range

The human ear is capable of detecting and discriminating sounds across a very wide range of intensities. A listener's dynamic range is defined at the lower limit by detection thresholds and at the upper limit by thresholds of discomfort, feeling, and/or pain. For a normal-hearing listener, dynamic range may easily exceed 100 dB, but for a listener with a sensorineural hearing impairment, elevated thresholds and/or reduced thresholds of discomfort can combine to produce a reduced dynamic range.

PEARL

Listeners with cochlear hearing impairments typically perceive high-intensity sound levels in much the same way as do normal-hearing listeners. This, combined with their elevated detection thresholds, produces reduced dynamic ranges and faster than normal loudness growth functions (recruitment). Conversely, neural hearing losses are sometimes not associated with the normal perception of loudness at high intensities, regardless of whether thresholds are elevated or not. Conductive hearing impairments, while associated with elevated thresholds, are typically not associated with reduced thresholds of discomfort and so these listeners retain a relatively wide dynamic range.

Loudness and detection thresholds are not only affected by signal frequency and intensity but also by signal complexity and duration. Detection of a signal (d') varies approximately with the square root of the number of components (e.g., Green & Swets, 1966). When the bandwidth of the signal is less than a critical band, the loudness of the complex will be similar to that of a pure tone of equal intensity, at the center frequency. However, when the bandwidth exceeds a critical band, the loudness of the complex will increase (e.g., Zwicker et al, 1957). As with bandwidth, both detection and perceived loudness also vary with signal duration because signal energy is integrated over approximately 200 ms (temporal integration). Beyond 200 ms, energy is not fully integrated and loudness growth and detection thresholds remain stable.

In many modalities the magnitude of a percept may decrease over time. A decrease in the perceived loudness of a continuous sound is referred to as *loudness adaptation*. Simple adaptation is that which is attributable solely to the duration of the stimulation. Few studies have successfully demonstrated the presence of simple adaptation to signals that are

presented at moderate to high intensities (i.e., ≥ 30 dB SL). At these higher sensation levels loudness adaptation is likely to occur only if the measurement procedures involve matching the loudness of a continuous tone with that of an intermittent tone. Adaptation is measured for the loudness of the continuous tone, and the intermittent tone is used only to indicate the perceived loudness of that tone. The reference (intermittent) tone can be presented either to the ipsilateral or contralateral ear. Often, in these procedures the loudness of the continuous tone will appear to decrease. But this form of adaptation is most commonly referred to as induced and appears to be linked to the interaction between the two tones. The effect is largest at higher sound levels and at higher frequencies. It is greater for tones than for noise bands and for sounds that are steady state rather than modulated. When an intermittent tone is not used, little loudness adaptation has been observed at higher levels. However, at relatively low intensities a form loudness adaptation may be measurable. At lower levels the loudness of a signal may decrease such that the signal is no longer audible. This phenomenon is termed *threshold fatigue*. In a normal-hearing listener threshold fatigue is usually quite low (often < 10- to 15-dB SL). A fairly thorough evaluation of loudness adaptation and threshold fatigue was given by Scharf (1983).

PEARL

For individuals with retrocochlear hearing loss, threshold fatigue may be much higher than in normal-hearing listeners or listeners with a cochlear hearing loss. It is this observation that gave rise to the many tests of tone decay that became common in audiological practice beginning in the 1950s.

Intensity Discrimination

An important aspect of how the auditory system processes acoustic information is related to the ability to discriminate changes and/or differences in intensity. This ability can be evaluated by measuring the smallest intensity difference required for a listener to judge which of two sounds is more intense or the minimum intensity increment that can be detected when added to a continuous sound.

The ability of a listener to detect small changes in intensity is most often reported as a normalized value in the *Weber fraction*. This measure relates the minimum discriminable change in a stimulus parameter to the base value of that parameter. For intensity, the minimum detectable difference, or difference limen, ΔL, is equal to $10\log_{10}((I+\Delta I)/I)$, where I is the intensity of the sound and ΔI is the minimum detectable intensity increment. As with detection thresholds and loudness, the discrimination of intensity also varies with frequency. Sensitivity to intensity differences is greatest for the mid-frequencies (1 to 4 kHz) where the ear is most sensitive and poorest for frequencies both above and below the region. Discrimination accuracy also improves with increases in signal level and reaches values of less than 1 dB as base level reaches 40 dB HL. The ability to detect an intensity difference in a signal will also vary with signal duration. Progressively

SPECIAL CONSIDERATION

Weber's law holds that the just discriminable difference of a stimulus value will be a constant proportion of the base magnitude. For intensity processing, Weber's law holds true only if the signals are broad band. For narrower sounds, such as pure tones, discrimination of intensity increments/changes is better at higher levels than the law predicts, thus constituting the "near miss" to Weber's law.

larger increments are required for intensity discrimination if the signal duration decreases to less than 250 ms (Florentine et al, 1987; Jesteadt et al, 1977; Viemeister & Bacon, 1988).

PEARL

The short increment sensitivity index (SISI) was developed because it was observed that listeners with sensorineural impairments may be able to detect smaller intensity increments than listeners with normal-hearing (see Chapter 1). However, this observation is confounded by the sensation level at which individuals are tested. The SISI is typically administered at 20 dB SL. For a normal-hearing listener, this equates to hearing levels < 30 dB, regions where intensity discrimination may be reduced. Yet for an individual with significant sensorineural hearing loss, 20 dB SL could easily be well above the 40 dB level at which performance reaches asymptotic levels. For this reason high-level SISIs were developed. Only individuals with retrocochlear hearing losses will fail to discriminate intensity increments of at least 1 dB when presented at fairly high levels, in dB HL (or SPL).

Mechanisms of Intensity Encoding

Description of how processing of information changes with changes in stimulus level is important for better understanding of the differences in the processing abilities of normal-hearing listeners for whom a broad range of signal levels are audible and listeners with cochlear hearing impairments who must operate largely at mid-stimulus to high-stimulus levels. One way that intensity is encoded is by changes in the average firing rate of neurons. As level increases, so does average firing rate. But the dynamic range of the auditory system can be well over 100 dB in the normal-hearing listener and the average intensity range over which an individual auditory nerve fiber can increase its firing rate is typically ≤30 dB. Two other mechanisms that may contribute to intensity coding have been proposed: spread of excitation (e.g., Siebert, 1968; Lachs

et al, 1984) and the existence of high-threshold nerve fibers (Liberman, 1978).

At low intensities the movement of the basilar membrane is restricted to the regions representing the frequency composition of the signal, and displacement increases with signal level. But basilar membrane motion is nonlinear with respect to stimulus level. At high levels, intensity increments do not produce proportional increases in basilar membrane displacement as are observed at lower levels. Similarly, displacement may saturate. Associated with this saturation is a spread of excitation to adjacent areas. This spread of activity and the concomitant recruitment of more auditory nerve fibers that results may contribute to auditory processing at higher levels. Thus basilar membrane displacement and the firing rate of individual fibers may saturate at relatively low intensities, but a wider population of fibers is stimulated as intensity increases and the spread of excitation becomes less focal. These two findings alone cannot fully account for processing at high levels (e.g., Hellman, 1974; Viemeister, 1983). Other mechanisms must be involved. These may include differences in the spontaneous discharge rates of different nerve fiber populations and differences in their dynamic ranges. It has been suggested that many fibers in the eighth nerve have higher thresholds of excitation. The recruitment of these fibers may play a role in the encoding of intensity, especially at higher levels. The role of the olivocochlear system, the role of temporal processing in the form of coincidence detectors at higher levels of the auditory system, and the impact of external noise may also contribute (see Delgutte, 1996).

PEARL

Individuals with damage to the cochlea often perform poorest at low intensities, but as intensity is increased, performance is generally better. This may be because at low signal levels the place mechanisms are damaged but that at higher levels more temporal information is available. In contrast, individuals with damage to the auditory nerve often show reduced function predominantly at higher levels. For example, speech discrimination scores may be poor at high levels (rollover), listeners may be unable to detect intensity increments at high levels (reduced high-level SISI scores), and tone decay may be worst at the highest levels (e.g., suprathreshold adaptation test). This may result because at very low levels patients can use place mechanisms, but at higher intensities neural damage prevents relying on temporal mechanisms.

Frequency Encoding

Frequency Discrimination and Pitch Perception

Discrimination

One of the simplest ways to think of how the auditory system processes frequency information is to examine how well a listener can discriminate between frequencies. As with intensity difference limens, several methods exist for measuring frequency discrimination. A listener may be presented with a sequence of two sounds and asked to judge which is higher or lower in frequency; a listener may be presented with a steady tone of a given frequency and asked to discriminate between it and a similar signal whose frequency is modulated; or a listener may be asked to detect a small and transient change in the frequency of a continuous tone. The smallest difference that is discriminable at a predetermined level of accuracy is taken as the differential threshold, again most often expressed as a proportion of the base frequency, $\Delta F/F$. In general, difference limens for frequency are best for the mid-frequencies where the listener is most sensitive and tend to improve with increases in signal level (e.g., Sek & Moore, 1995; Weir et al, 1977). For mid-frequency sounds (around 1000 Hz) presented at moderate sound levels (e.g., 60 dB), differences of as little as 2 to 3 Hz are discriminable. When sound duration is reduced below about 200 ms, performance worsens.

Pitch

The psychological correlate of frequency is *pitch*. As with loudness, scaling procedures were used to develop a scale that relates perceived pitch to absolute frequency. The function describing the relation between frequency and pitch is nonlinear. Frequencies less than 1000 Hz are perceived as higher in pitch than their absolute frequency would suggest, and frequencies greater than 1000 Hz are perceived as slightly lower than their absolute frequency, thus compressing the range (Stevens & Volkmann, 1940). Similarly, pitch may not change linearly with changes in signal level. Higher level sounds are often perceived to be exaggerated in pitch such that at high intensities sounds less than 2 kHz are perceived to be lower in pitch than they are at lower levels and sounds greater than 4 kHz appear to be higher in pitch (Verschuure & van Meeteren, 1975).

Periodicity Pitch and the Missing Fundamental

The pitch of a signal is not always related only to the frequency of its components but may be related to the relationship between the components or the repetition rate. For example, the pitch of a sound may be related to the interval between the harmonics or the fundamental frequency of the signal even if no energy is present at the fundamental (i.e., missing fundamental). The specific frequency components or harmonics that are present give the signal its characteristic timbre, but the pitch is a function of the fundamental frequency. Also, when a signal is repeated at a relatively slow repetition rate, the pitch of the signal may correspond to the rate of the repetition more than to the specific spectral components of the signal. This phenomenon is called periodicity pitch.

Frequency Resolution

The ability of the ear to resolve the individual frequency components of a complex sound has a significant impact on a listener's ability to perceive the subtleties of spectral shape so important in nearly all sound discriminations and identifications. When frequency resolution is very good, all or most frequency components can be detected and the internal spectral representation of a signal will be faithful to the spectral characteristics of the sound itself, sharp and full of detail. But when resolution is poor, as is often the case in sensorineural hearing impairment, the internal spectrum of the signal may lack clarity and detail, making discrimination of similar signals difficult.

The encoding of spectral information is commonly modeled as though the periphery was composed of a bank of overlapping bandpass filters. Each hypothetical filter corresponds to the highly frequency-specific movement of the basilar membrane. The narrower these filters, the finer will be the internal spectral representation of sounds. Frequency resolving abilities, or estimates of the width and shape of the theoretical auditory filters, are most often studied behaviorally in humans through masking experiments. One sound, usually a pure tone, is presented in the presence of another sound, usually a noise masker, and the degree of interference from the masker on detection of the signal is measured. In a series of masking studies published first many years ago (Fletcher, 1940), it was noted that detection of a tonal signal decreases as the bandwidth of a noise masker, centered at the signal frequency, increases. This decrease in detectability continues until a critical masker bandwidth is reached, at which point, although masker loudness continues to grow, the masker has no additional effect on the detection of the tone. The bandwidth at which masking effects reach an asymptote is termed the *critical band*. Estimates of the critical band show that it increases with increases in signal frequency and is approximately 160 Hz at 1000 Hz (Scharf, 1970).

SPECIAL CONSIDERATION

Masking occurs when one sound interferes with a sensation evoked by another sound rendering it less audible. This can be effected through a variety of mechanisms. One sound may not evoke a perception because another sound, with similar spectral and temporal characteristics, is already stimulating the system. This is the most common way in which we think of masking, but others exist. Masking can occur through suppressive mechanisms that operate when the signal and masker occupy different frequency regions, but the presence of one necessitates that higher levels are needed to excite other regions (i.e., the level of a signal must be increased to be detected,) than would be required were the masker not present. Masking can also occur through adaptation, which occurs when the masker is of relatively long duration and the signal is either transient or at least much shorter than the masker. This would occur with a continuous masker and a briefer duration signal.

Recent studies and knowledge of basilar membrane mechanics suggest that the auditory filter is neither rectangular nor symmetrical as critical band data may lead one to believe. The shape of the auditory filter at low signal levels is more likened to a rounded exponential with very steep slopes above the signal and more shallow slopes below it. At higher intensities it becomes much more symmetrical and more broadly tuned (e.g., Patterson, 1976; Patterson et al, 1982).

The frequency-resolving ability of the auditory system and the shape of the auditory filter can be measured behaviorally by several methods. Two procedures, the measurement of psychoacoustic tuning curves and notched-noise masking procedures, will be discussed here. Although not all inclusive, they provide an example of ways in which frequency resolution can be measured with relative ease.

PITFALL

Maskers used to obtain psychoacoustic tuning curves are usually no more than 50 Hz wide, much narrower than the 1/3 octave narrow band noises available on an audiometer. Therefore to evaluate psychoacoustic tuning curves clinically would require specialized equipment or an external filter that could provide these very narrow spectra. Pure tone maskers, although significantly narrow, are poor choices for maskers because their temporal structure, when combined with the tonal signal, will produce audible beats that could be a useful cue to the listener that both a signal and masker are present.

Psychoacoustic Tuning Curves

The *psychoacoustic tuning curve* (Zwicker, 1977) is measured by asking listeners to detect a low-level signal, usually a pure tone at 10- to 20-dB SL in the presence of maskers, usually very narrow bands of noise that vary in both frequency and intensity. Masker frequencies will be at, above, and below the signal frequency, with level varied to determine the minimum masker level needed to render the signal inaudible. Results consistently show that maskers falling at or near the signal are most effective at masking the signal and do so at very low levels (see Fig. 9–6). As the frequency of the masker moves away from the signal, increasingly higher levels of masker are needed to obscure the signal. The relative increase in masker level required for masker frequencies higher than the signal frequency is greater than that for frequencies below the signal. This results in very steep high-frequency slopes and shallower low-frequency functions. Data obtained with this procedure are evaluated in terms of the bandwidth of the masking function, usually at an intensity 10 dB from the tip of the function, and in terms of efficiency, which reflects the overall level of the masked thresholds independent of the shape of the masking function. Narrower bandwidths and lower overall thresholds imply better resolution and efficiency than do wider bandwidths and higher thresholds.

Notched-Noise Masking

Another procedure for measuring the width and shape of the auditory filter is the notched-noise masking technique (e.g.,

---

CONTROVERSIAL POINT

In reference to psychoacoustic tuning curves, the term *efficiency* is often used to describe higher than normal thresholds or reduced performance levels. No well accepted definition of efficiency or of the elements that may contribute to it exist. However, it is generally agreed that efficiency is a result of processing beyond the cochlea itself, perhaps in the auditory nerve or higher centers of the brain.

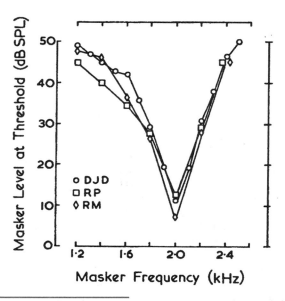

Figure 9–6 Psychoacoustic tuning curves obtained from three listeners. The signal was a 2000 Hz sinusoid. The masker was a 100 Hz wide band of noise. Data points show thresholds in dB spectrum level of the masker. Taken from Johnson-Davies & Patterson (1979).

Patterson, 1976). A listener is asked to detect a tonal signal in the presence of a noise masker with either a flat or notched amplitude spectrum. The masker level is fixed at a fairly moderate intensity, for example 30- to 40-dB spectrum level, and signal level is varied in a search for a detection threshold. Thresholds are obtained under several masker conditions, representing a variety of widths in the spectral notch. Sample data, shown in Figure 9–7, suggest that thresholds are highest when the masker spectrum is flat, with no spectral notch, and decrease as a notch in the masker is widened.

Thresholds should approach quiet detection levels when the notch is wide enough so that it no longer interferes with the detection of the tone (i.e., when the excitation pattern of the masker and the signal no longer interfere with one another). Results are analyzed in terms of the slope of the function relating threshold to notch width. If the function drops quickly as the notch is widened, it is assumed that the

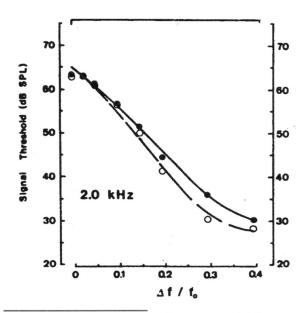

Figure 9–7 Threshold curves for a young adult listener plotted as a function of notch width in the masker. Open and filled symbols show right and left ears, respectively. The signal was a 2000 Hz sinusoid and the masker was a noise with a spectral notch at the signal frequency. Taken from Patterson et al (1982).

frequency-resolution of the listener is quite good. If instead the function is quite shallow with little change in threshold as notch width is increased, it is assumed that frequency resolving abilities are poor (or that the hypothetical filters are wide). Efficiency, as with the psychoacoustic tuning curve, is indicated by the overall threshold levels (intercept of the function) and is independent of the slope of the function.

When notched noise-masking procedures are used with the noise bands and spectral notches placed asymmetrically around the signal frequency, not only the width of the auditory filter but also its shape can be mapped. When this is done, it can be seen that the shape of the auditory filter is best approximated by a rounded exponential with steeper high-frequency sides and shallower low-frequency tails, consistent with data obtained using other masking procedures and with neural tuning curve data (Patterson, 1976).

Time Course of the Auditory Filter

Much speculation regarding the time course of the auditory filter exists. The question is whether frequency-resolving ability is instantaneously as sharp as possible or whether a time, however brief, exists over which frequency resolution reaches its maximum sharpness. Moore and colleagues (1987) examined this question by asking listeners to detect very brief (e.g., 20 ms) signals that were placed at the beginning, middle, and end of a slightly longer (400 ms) masker. Their results showed that thresholds did not vary with position of the signal relative to that of the masker and therefore concluded that auditory filters did not require time to develop to their maximum sharpness.

Frequency and Level Effects and Sensory Hearing Impairment

Frequency resolution is roughly proportional to center frequency. Thus as frequency increases, critical bands increase and the widths of measured auditory filters (in Hz) also increase. This likely reflects the frequency representation along the basilar membrane, which is roughly linear up to about 500 Hz, at which point representation becomes more logarithmic. Level also has a significant effect on frequency-resolving ability. Basilar membrane motion tends to saturate at very high intensities, and equal increases in signal intensity at high levels do not correspond to equal increases in basilar membrane amplitude as they do at lower levels. Also, as signal level is increased, the spectral representation on the basilar membrane is broader. Therefore when evaluated with signals or maskers at high sensation levels, even normal-hearing listeners show broader, more symmetrical filter shapes than at low sensation levels. Listeners with sensorineural hearing impairments, because of their sensitivity loss, can only be evaluated at relatively high-intensity levels. Thus it is not surprising that frequency-resolution estimates from these listeners generally show reduced ability (e.g., Florentine et al, 1980; Glasberg & Moore, 1986). However, damage to outer hair cells likely plays a significant role in exacerbating the problem (e.g., Evans, 1975; Evans & Harrison, 1976).

Mechanisms of Frequency Encoding

Analysis of the frequency composition of a sound is largely accomplished by basilar membrane mechanics and temporal firing patterns of auditory nerve fibers. The basilar membrane performs an initial spectral analysis of incoming sounds because of its unique structural properties. High-frequency sounds cause the membrane to vibrate at the base and lower frequency sounds cause vibration to localize at the more apical regions. The sharpness of the vibration pattern is facilitated through the active mechanisms of the outer hair cells. Because the auditory nerve is attached to the basilar membrane in an organized manner, the area of maximal vibration corresponds to a specific tonotopic map within the auditory nerve. Thus place of excitation contributes frequency information to higher level centers of the brain. In addition, as the basilar membrane vibrates, the pattern of auditory nerve responses also reflects temporal phase locking to signals that may be remote from the auditory nerve's characteristic frequency. As a result, auditory nerve fibers respond in a manner that reflects both the place of excitation on the basilar membrane and the temporal fine structure of the basilar membrane movement. This temporal information contributes useful frequency information to the central nervous system even though it often arises from regions adjacent to or remote from the place associated with the signal frequency. This means that frequency-specific information is encoded both by spatial place mechanisms and by temporal mechanisms. The existence of both mechanisms of encoding frequency information may facilitate frequency processing across a wide range of absolute levels and signal/noise ratios.

Temporal Coding

A primary source of information in every auditory signal lies in its temporal structure. Perhaps more than any other of the

---

SPECIAL CONSIDERATION

It could be hypothesized that listeners with cochlear damage are able to process frequency information at higher intensities through the use of temporal cues in the auditory nerve's firing patterns. However, individuals with neural lesions typically have difficulty with high intensity signals, potentially because of an inaccessibility of these temporal cues due to the auditory nerve damage.

---

human senses, temporal information is often critical to the discrimination and identification of signals. Aspects of temporal fine structure and the shape of the temporal envelope are encoded, and information about the order of acoustic elements or features is important.

Temporal Fine Structure: The Encoding of Periodicity

The auditory nerve will respond best to frequencies that vibrate maximally in the region of the basilar membrane to which the fiber is connected. However, remote frequency regions may be stimulated particularly at higher stimulus levels. The neural activity in these neurons may at first appear to be random. However, on closer inspection it can be seen that these neurons respond only at certain phases of the stimulus. The neurons may not respond to every cycle, but when they do respond the activity will be *phase locked* to the signal frequency, thereby providing information that encodes signal frequency, particularly when the activity of many fibers is summed. The phase-locked activity of neurons, both at and remote from the signal frequency, also provides listeners with information that enables them to discriminate periodic from aperiodic signals. Work that has attempted to uncover the psychological correlates of complex sounds has suggested that unfamiliar sounds are often differentiated on the basis of their temporal fine structure and their envelope (e.g., Allen & Bond, 1997; Howard, 1977; Howard & Silverman, 1976). Other studies have suggested that relative periodicity may be useful for detecting periodic signals presented in noise maskers, especially when other acoustic cues may be eliminated, although this information may typically be available only at high signal-to-noise ratios (Allen et al, 1998; Hartman & Pumplin, 1988).

Temporal Resolution: The Detection and Discrimination of Temporal Envelope

Gap Detection

Important temporal information is also provided by the shape of a signal's envelope, which reflects the slower fluctuations in a signal. The ability of a listener to encode temporal envelope is proportional to their temporal resolving ability. One very basic measure of temporal resolution is provided by *gap detection* thresholds. To measure these thresholds a listener is presented with a signal in which a temporal gap or silent period has been inserted. The listener's ability to detect

the presence of the gap is measured as a function of gap size. The minimum detectable gap is used to indicate temporal resolving ability. Generally, adult listeners can detect gaps of 2 to 3 ms if the signals containing the gaps are bands of noise (Fitzgibbons & Wightman, 1982; Penner, 1977; Plomp, 1964; Shailer & Moore, 1983). With sinusoidal signals, the estimates of gap detection thresholds are slightly higher, approximately 4 to 5 ms (e.g., Shailer & Moore, 1987).

PITFALL

Care must be taken when measuring gap detection thresholds in stimuli with very narrow spectral distributions, such as narrow bands of noise or pure tones. The introduction of a gap may produce spectral splatter in remote frequency regions, thus providing an additional cue to the listener that the gap is present. This cue can be masked by the use of a broad spectrum masker with a spectral gap at the signal frequency.

Temporal Modulation Transfer Functions

Another method for evaluating the temporal resolving capability of the auditory system is the *temporal modulation transfer function*. A listener is provided with a steady-state signal, usually a noise band, and asked to discriminate it from one for which the amplitude is sinusoidally modulated. Both the rate of modulation (modulation frequency) and the depth of modulation can be varied. Generally, the minimum detectable depth of modulation is measured as a function of modulation frequency. The function that relates threshold modulation depth to modulation frequency is the temporal modulation transfer function. With this technique it has been suggested that listeners are very good at perceiving modulation at relatively slow rates (e.g., < 50 Hz) but as the rate of modulation increases (i.e., the changes in amplitude occur more quickly over time), a greater depth of modulation is required for detection. Thresholds fall off slowly at first until approximately 100 Hz at which point threshold modulation depth increases (e.g., Bacon & Viemeister, 1985). Very slow rates of modulation, below 20 Hz, are perceptible largely as rhythm and often correspond to the rate at which words are spoken in continuous speech. Slightly faster rates of modulation (20 to 100 Hz) correspond to a sense of roughness or unpleasantness in a sound. These modulation rates often occur when two or more frequencies are combined in a complex signal if the two frequencies fall within a critical band (approximately 10 to 15% of the center frequency) so that they are not fully resolved (Pickles, 1988). The perception will be of roughness associated with the slower amplitude fluctuations produced by the combination of the components. Faster rates of modulation are more often associated with rates of vocal fold vibration and the perception of periodicity or voicing (Langner, 1992).

Duration Discrimination

Judgments about absolute duration, especially for speech sounds, are often used by listeners to infer something about speaker intent or emotion. Often, when speakers wish to emphasize a word or token, they may increase its overall duration, usually by increasing the duration of the steady-state portions of the sounds or the vowels. Yet, information derived from absolute duration is seldom useful for discrimination between tokens, at least in the English language. Small and Campbell (1962) showed that duration discrimination is good for very low-frequency signals but that performance may worsen for higher frequencies (e.g., 5000 Hz). In general listeners require proportionally larger changes to discriminate duration differences as the base duration of the signal increases (Abel, 1972). Thus for durations around 100 ms, a change of approximately 15 ms is required for discrimination, but for longer stimuli (1000 ms) approximately a 60 ms change is required. Discrimination of the duration of a silent interval is slightly better, approximately 15 ms for 320 ms base silences (Divenyi & Danner, 1977). These findings are roughly independent of the spectral content of the signals but may vary with overall intensity, being slightly poorer at lower levels than at higher levels.

Detection of Onset/Offset Asynchronies

For multiple-component signals, the onset/offset characteristics of the components may provide useful information to the listener. Listeners are quite good at detecting onset asynchronies, being able to discriminate onset disparities of 1 ms if the components are harmonically related (e.g., Zera & Green, 1993). If the components are not harmonically related, discrimination accuracy may be much poorer by factors as large as 50 times. The detection of offset asynchronies is somewhat poorer. Even with harmonically related components, 3 to 10 ms may be required. Sensitivity to onset/offset asynchronies may be important to listeners because it often indicates whether component frequencies arise from a single or multiple sources. Sounds arising from a single source often have simultaneous onsets and offsets.

Judgments of Temporal Order

Individuals are quite good at discriminating the temporal order of sounds, particularly if the sounds, when presented in a particular order, have meaning. For example, the order of sounds in some sequences of speech elements (morphemes or simple words) is important such that if the order of elements were to be changed, the item would no longer have the same meaning. In those instances listeners can discriminate order changes for sounds 7 ms or shorter (e.g., Divenyi & Hirsh, 1974). However, if the sounds are unrelated, the listener may require slightly longer durations, 10 to 20 ms for the same level of discrimination accuracy (Hirsh, 1959; Warren, 1974).

THE PERCEPTION OF COMPLEX SOUNDS

Much of what has been discussed so far has focused on the processing of discrete features of acoustically, relatively simple sounds. But this approach fails to capture the full range and intricacy of auditory processing. It is only when the issue

of how more complex sounds are processed is analyzed that the amazing capabilities of the human auditory system are evident. The topics selected for inclusion in this section are by no means inclusive, but it is hoped they will provide the reader with an introduction to the range of abilities and processes that contribute to the processing of complex auditory signals.

Profile Analysis

Many natural sounds have similar frequency content, but the relative distribution of energy within their bandwidth is different. Such differences in the shape of the amplitude spectra are useful in discrimination and identification tasks. Classic examples of listeners' use of spectral shape information can be found in the importance of formant ratios for the identification of vowels (Peterson & Barney, 1952) and the importance of frequency contours in the onset spectra of stop consonants (Stevens & Blumstein, 1978). To perceive spectral shape requires resolution of the primary frequency components and assessment of the relative amplitudes of those components, thus necessitating good frequency resolution and cross-channel level processing. The ability to perceive differences in spectral shape is termed *profile analysis*, and the theories surrounding this ability have led to a rethinking of how even simple tasks such as intensity discrimination are performed (Green, 1988).

For example, in a standard intensity discrimination task traditional models of intensity processing assume that the listener evaluates the relative energy levels arriving from the auditory filter centered at the signal frequency. Comparison is made between levels of sounds, and the listener decides which of the sounds is more or less intense than the other. This task is affected by the listener's ability to hold a representation of the sound intensity in memory. If the time between stimulus presentations is increased from 250 to 8000 ms, intensity discrimination thresholds can decrease by as much as 10 dB (Green et al, 1983), reflecting memory limitations. However, if the listener is provided with a background sound, such as a noise or other tones, performance may improve relative to that obtained with no background sound and will be unaffected by changes in the interstimulus interval (Green, 1988). Furthermore, a listener's ability to judge intensity changes remains high, even if the overall level of the background sound is varied randomly from presentation to presentation (thereby removing absolute level information) so long as the signal/background ratio is kept constant. This suggests that listeners make simultaneous within-signal comparisons of levels at different frequency regions rather than between signals at a fixed frequency in performing intensity discrimination tasks for which a background sound is present. Thus the overall shape of the signal spectrum is the important factor.

Models of Encoding Spectral Shape Information

At least two models of auditory processing have been suggested to explain listeners' discrimination of spectral shape. When the component frequencies lie within a critical band, it is likely that they compute an overall estimate of average frequency or pitch. For example, Feth and colleagues (Feth, 1974; Feth, O'Malley, & Ramsay, 1982) have shown that if two tonal complexes are presented to a listener, each of which is composed of two identical frequency components, but for which one component is more intense than the other, the listener can discriminate when the relative levels are reversed. For example, a listener is presented with two complexes, one consisting of frequencies f and f + Δf such that f is more intense than f + Δf and another such that f + Δf is more intense than f. If both f and f + Δf fall within one critical band, the two complexes will have the same overall RMS value and the same frequency components, yet be quite discriminable from one another. Feth proposed that the listener evaluates the complexes by computing a mean frequency that is weighted by the amplitude of each component. The overall average frequency and the corresponding pitch value will be higher when f + Δf is more intense than f and lower when their relative amplitudes are reversed. Thus this spectral shape discrimination is made on the basis of an extracted feature of the complex that corresponds to its overall pitch, which is computed from weighting the energy levels in the relative frequency components.

To explain spectral shape discrimination for components that are widely spaced in frequency may require some other model of auditory processing. Durlach et al (1986) proposed an excitation model in which peripheral processing occurs in multiple parallel filters. As a sound is heard, the listener performs a spectral decomposition of the sound, thus analyzing the relative energy levels in a range of frequencies. These theoretical filter outputs, each of which may contain some noise as a result of inaccuracies, for example in peripheral resolution, are combined at a more central level where a rough estimate of spectral shape is formed. This central representation may also have some error associated with it (often modeled as a form of central internal noise), but the error is in the way in which cross-frequency information is combined rather than in the quality of the analysis at each frequency. Internal correlation between the outputs of the independent frequencies is performed and the listener uses this information to compute the likelihood that it may or may not contain a signal.

Comodulation Masking Release

Another interesting phenomenon in auditory processing that reflects cross-channel processing is observed in comodulation masking release (Hall et al, 1984). The listener is asked to detect a masked signal. Usually the signal is a tone and the masker is a narrow band of noise centered at the signal frequency. Thresholds increase as the noise band is increased until the bandwidth of the masker exceeds the critical band as expected. Yet if the masker is amplitude modulated very slowly, thresholds will improve as the bandwidth of the masker is increased beyond the critical band contrary to critical band theory and inconsistent with our understanding of the mechanisms of masking. These results are obtained even though no energy in the masker surrounding the signal is removed and the overall level of the masker, because of its broader bandwidth, is much higher.

In similar experiments detection is evaluated for conditions in which the masker is a narrow band of noise placed at the signal frequency and a flanking noise masker is added at a remote frequency. When the flanking (off-frequency) masker is comodulated with the on-frequency masker, detection of the signal improves. However, if the flanking masker has an independent temporal structure from that at the signal frequency, detection thresholds show no change. These findings suggest that the auditory system is able to compare the temporal similarities in the masker at regions at, and remote from, the signal frequency in a manner similar to profile analysis. The amount of unmasking that occurs in the presence of temporally similar maskers at remote frequencies varies from 5- to 20-dB, depending on the specific stimulus and masker conditions. The theoretical explanations for comodulation masking release are many and outside the scope of this chapter, but the existence of comodulation masking release is a challenge to our understanding of how the auditory system processes complex sounds. A good review of comodulation masking release is provided by Green (1993).

PEARL

Detection of similarities in modulation patterns across frequencies may provide a useful cue to the perception of sound sources. A single vibrating source may produce many frequency components, but their temporal modulation patterns will be similar and will reflect the vibration of the source. Thus sounds that are not modulated with those produced by the source will not be perceived as part of it but as a separate source. As a result, modulation similarities and differences across frequencies may provide an essential cue for the separation of sound sources in space and may aid in the discrimination of signals in noise.

Classification of Complex Sounds

One of the primary goals of auditory processing is to assign meaning to sounds because without meaning sounds are of less value as sources of information. One of the ways in which meaning is assigned to sounds is through classification, which requires the perception of similarities in individual features or patterns of features. One method that has been used successfully to study the processing of complex sounds and reveal the acoustic features and feature patterns that listeners attend to when recognizing sounds is a multidimensional scaling (MDS) analysis of paired comparisons data. Listeners are asked to rate the relative similarity (or dissimilarity) of all possible pairs of a set of stimuli. The similarity ratings are used to place the stimuli in a multidimensional space (generally euclidean) of few dimensions. Stimuli that are rated as very similar are placed closer together in that space than are stimuli that are rated as dissimilar. The axes or dimensions in the space are assumed to represent the perceptual attributes of the sounds that were used in making the judgments. Each attribute may correspond to a single auditory feature or to a combination of features.

Howard and colleagues (Howard, 1977; Howard & Silverman, 1976) used an MDS analysis to evaluate listeners' processing of unfamiliar complex sounds. Their results suggested that encoding included both spectral and temporal characteristics of the sounds, but that the relative weighting given to features varied with the previous experiences and training of the listener. (Listeners with musical training were more likely to place greater weight on temporal cues than were listeners with no musical training who weighted spectral cues more heavily.) Recently, Christensen and Humes (1996) showed that individual differences in dimension weightings can be useful for predicting classification and categorization responses. In their study dimensions that were weighted most heavily by a listener in the paired comparisons task tended to be those used by that listener to form categories in a subsequent classification task. MDS analyses of similarity data are therefore useful tools for discovering the underlying structure of listeners' perceptions of complex sounds and can be used successfully with young children and adults (Allen & Bond, 1997).

Information Processing
Masking

The way that acoustic features are combined to form categories, particularly when variability in those features or in the context in which they are presented exists, has received much attention in psychoacoustics. Watson and colleagues were among the earliest investigators to study listeners' ability to detect subtle changes in acoustically well-controlled complex sounds. Their work showed that the perception of changes in the components of a complex sound is not easily predicted by a listener's ability to detect similar changes in an isolated sound. The presence of other sounds (context), even when they are irrelevant to the task, can reduce detection and discrimination accuracy, especially if they are similar to or more salient than the relevant features. For example, using word-length sequences consisting of approximately 10 brief duration tone pips (approximately 40 ms), Watson and colleagues found that listeners' ability to discriminate changes to the frequency, duration, or level of a target component in the sequence were approximately 10 to 20 Hz, 6 to 8 ms, and 2- to 3-dB, respectively (Watson & Kelley, 1981).

These measures are quite good and perhaps only slightly poorer than for sounds in isolation. Yet, if the acoustic features of the nontarget components, the context tones, are varied from trial to trial, performance becomes much worse. This variation in the context tones is termed *informational masking*. Because the auditory periphery is likely processing simple and complex sounds in a similar manner, changes in performance associated with context effects are most likely attributable to more central auditory processing abilities (Watson & Foyle, 1985). Similar effects of uncertainty associated with stimulus and context variance also extend to the processing of

components that are presented simultaneously (Green, 1988; Neff & Callaghan, 1988; Neff & Jesteadt, 1996).

Information Integration

Although variance can create uncertainty that is detrimental to the processing of complex sounds, it can also contribute to their encoding. Consider the task of learning a new word. If every time the word is heard it is exactly the same, as though it were a recorded signal, it would be difficult to recognize that same word if spoken by a different speaker, perhaps with a different accent or intonation pattern. It is only by hearing the word many times, in many contexts, and spoken by many speakers that the critical features of the item can be determined, enabling recognition in different contexts. Through the normal variability associated with a sound's repetition, the critical features are encoded. Thus variability or uncertainty can be equated to information. As another example, consider a task in which a set of items is to be organized. If the items are very similar this task will be very difficult because no features exist along which the items vary to provide dimensions along which the items can be grouped. Variability in the features of the items provides information that can be used to discriminate between them.

To resolve and make use of the uncertainty that naturally accompanies variability, listeners must attend to patterns in, and relationships between, features. This requires fine discriminations along each acoustic dimension, an ability that is related to peripheral resolving abilities, and integration of information from each feature into a meaningful whole, a process that is likely performed more centrally in the system. Both levels of processing can be tested auditorily with a sample discrimination paradigm (Berg & Robinson, 1987; Lutfi, 1989, 1990, 1992) in which a listener is asked to discriminate between two complex sounds. The components for each of the sounds are drawn from overlapping distributions of features such that some feature values may be equally likely to be drawn from either distribution, whereas other values have a higher probability of being drawn from one or the other. If only one sample of a feature is available, performance will be limited by the amount of overlap in the two distributions from which the features are selected. But as greater numbers of features or components are sampled, the listener's performance will improve. Results have shown that performance in a sample discrimination task will be limited by two factors: the listener's ability to discriminate between feature values (or components) sampled and the ability to combine, or integrate, information obtained from the total number of features sampled. If the components sampled are not discriminably different from one another, drawing more of them will provide no additional information. This limitation is related directly to peripheral resolving abilities.

In contrast, limits to the individual's ability to integrate multiple bits of information is likely a more central process. It is the limits to integration ability that prevent performance from increasing linearly as the number of sampled components increases. Performance will improve at a rate consistent with the individual's integration ability and will reach an asymptote that reflects their capacity for information processing. In general, d' in a sample discrimination task increases with the cubed root of the number of components sampled and will reach an asymptote at approximately 2 to 3 bits of information (see Lutfi, 1989). The sample discrimination technique holds promise for explaining the nature and magnitude of changes in complex sound processing that occur with maturation (e.g., Allen & Nelles, 1996) or hearing impairment (e.g., Doherty & Lutfi, 1996).

Weighting Functions and Attention

It is important to know when a listener makes a decision about a complex sound, what information was used in the decision. One way to perform such an analysis is through the use of COSS functions (e.g., Berg, 1989). With this technique, a listener's decision about a stimulus is analyzed according to the values of the individual components within the complex signal. Correlation functions are derived between the acoustic parameters of each component and the listener's response. In this way the relative weight the listener gives to each component in making the decision can be determined. With this technique it has been shown that listeners make comparisons of acoustic features across components within a stimulus, that they weight reliable information more heavily than unreliable information, and that when the intensity of a feature is increased, it may be weighted more heavily than lower intensity features, even if it is a less reliable parameter (Berg, 1990; Berg & Green, 1990). This form of analysis has the potential of being extremely useful in facilitating the understanding of what responses a listener makes when asked to perform a task involving complex signals and can provide useful information as to why those specific responses are made. It can tell far more about the features an individual listens to when performing a discrimination task than can be determined from a single estimate of performance such as percent correct or d'.

The weighting of various acoustic features of a complex sound, either derived from MDS analyses of dissimilarity data or from COSS analyses of discrimination data, is in many ways an indication of the salience of that feature or the attention given to it by the listener. An extension of research in feature salience is to evaluate the extent to which a listener can intentionally focus on a sound or on specific acoustic features of that sound, particularly in the presence of other sometimes irrelevant and often interfering and distracting features or sounds. One example of the role of auditory research in selective attention can be found in the study of auditory attention bands. This work asks questions about the extent to which listeners can focus attention on a single frequency region and how narrowly that auditory attention can be focused. The dominant technique used to study auditory attention is a probe-signal method (Greenburg & Larkin, 1969) in which a listener is led to expect a signal of a certain frequency. On an infrequent and randomly distributed percentage of the trials, the signal is of a slightly different frequency, but it is presented at a level that, if the listener were expecting it, would be detected with a high degree of accuracy. With this technique it has been shown that many listeners do not detect the off-frequency probes with the same degree of accuracy as the on-frequency expected signals. In fact, detection accuracy appears to decrease for the probes in a way that mirrors that derived in studies of frequency resolution, suggesting that listeners are able to focus attention on a very narrowly tuned region of the basilar membrane. Yet this performance is highly contingent on the stimulus (and masker) parameters. When the signals are presented in the presence of noise maskers, the attention bands appear to stay relatively focused, so long as the noise is not gated simultaneously with the signal. Usually, if the maskers are continuous, the measured attention bands are quite sharp (e.g., Scharf et al, 1987). However, if the signals and maskers are gated on and off together, much more individual variability exists and only some listeners show very sharply tuned functions (Dai & Buus, 1991). This suggests that with signals and gated maskers, listeners may not be able to focus frequency-specific attention as sharply as possible. Similarly, attention bands may vary with signal duration despite the gating characteristics of the masker. When the signals are of a very short duration (e.g., 5 ms), attention bands are wider than those measured in response to longer duration signals (e.g., 295 ms) even though auditory filter widths, as measured with notched-noise maskers, are equivalent at the two durations (Wright & Dai, 1994). Collectively, these results suggest that a listener is less likely to use a highly frequency-specific listening strategy for the detection and identification of very brief duration tones, but that as signal duration exceeds the temporal integration limits of the ear and as long as the signal and masker are temporally discrete from one another, listeners are capable of a very highly tuned, frequency-specific analysis.

In summary, many ways exist to study a listener's ability to process complex auditory signals that go beyond those used in traditional audiometry. Furthermore, strong evidence suggests that many of these information-processing abilities, including detection and discrimination in instances of uncertainty, information integration, and auditory attention, can be evaluated in children and do show strong age-related trends (Allen & Nelles, 1996; Allen & Wightman, 1995; Bargones & Werner, 1994). Therefore these tasks may be useful in evaluating the auditory processing abilities of children and adults and may ultimately shed light on the nature of auditory processing disorders.

Binaural Hearing and Sound Localization

How the auditory system combines information arriving at the two ears and the manner in which sounds are localized in space are areas of psychoacoustics for which tremendous advancements have been made very recently. In addition to the importance of understanding binaural hearing for completing our appreciation of the richness and complexity of auditory processing, binaural hearing research also has important technological applications relevant to the design and fitting of assistive listening devices and the creation of virtual spaces.

Much of what is known about binaural hearing comes from studies in which listeners are presented with stimuli under headphones. In this way the signals arriving at each ear can be well controlled acoustically and the effects of interaural disparities on sound perceptions can be studied. Yet binaural images produced by presenting dichotic sounds under headphones remain perceptually inside the listeners head and are not perceived as originating from sources external to the listener. It is only when sounds are perceived outside the head that localization, rather than lateralization, may be studied. This section will begin with an introduction to binaural hearing as observed in headphones studies and proceed to a discussion of listening in real (and virtual) three-dimensional auditory environments.

Discrimination of Interaural Time and Intensity Differences Presented Under Headphones

The human auditory system is very sensitive to even small interaural time and intensity disparities. When a signal is presented to the two ears at equal intensities, the image will be perceived in the center of the head. If the intensity at one ear is increased slightly, the image will shift toward the ear with the more intense signal (Blauert, 1983). As little as a 1 dB difference is sufficient to move the image off the center. When the interaural intensity differences are larger (on the order of 10 dB), the image will be fully lateralized to the ear receiving the more intense signal and the listener will be unaware that a signal is even being presented to the other ear. Similarly, the time of arrival of sounds at the two ears will also exert a strong influence on the perceived lateralization of the sound (Blauert, 1983). When the sounds are presented simultaneously, the perception will be of a sound located in the center of the head, but when one ear leads the other ear by as little as 10 μs, the image will be shifted toward the leading ear. With a 1 ms interaural time difference the image will be fully lateralized to the leading ear. Thus the binaural auditory system is highly sensitive to both interaural time and intensity differences.

PEARL

A useful technique for the biological calibration of earphones is to listen as a sound is presented binaurally at equal levels. If the sound appears lateralized away from the center of the head, it is possible that the output from the two earphones may not be perfectly matched and should be calibrated.

Interaural Disparities in the Free Field

When a sound is presented in the free field, the image arrives at both ears, but each receives a slightly different image in accordance with intensity and phase differences at the two ears. Intensity differences result as some sounds are diffracted when they reach the head such that the ear on the side opposite the sound source will receive a slightly less intense image. Sounds are most likely to be reflected off the head if their wavelength is small relative to the diameter of the head, producing a lower intensity representation at the far ear relative to that arriving at the near ear. This is termed the *head shadow* effect. Assuming that the diameter of the adult head is roughly 18 cm, sounds with frequencies greater than approximately 2000 Hz will be subjected to the head shadow and produce interaural intensity differences. (A wavelength, λ, of 18 cm corresponds to a frequency (f) of approximately 1907 Hz, given that the speed of sound (c) is 343.2 M/s ($f = c/\lambda$)). The magnitude of the head shadow will vary not only with the frequency of the sound but also with the position of the sound source. The greatest interaural intensity difference will be achieved when the sound source is located directly opposite to one ear and the signal is greater than 2000 Hz. It may

be as much as 20 dB for the higher frequencies. When the sound source is located directly in front of, above, or behind the listener, no interaural intensity differences will be observed. Interaural intensity differences are therefore useful for localizing a sound in space if the sound is high frequency and located sufficiently off the midline (see Wightman & Kistler, 1993).

Lower frequency sounds, with very long wavelengths that exceed the diameter of the human head, will arrive at each ear with little or no interaural intensity differences. At these frequencies the dominant cue for localization is provided by interaural time disparities. Sounds will arrive first at the leading ear and later at the lagging hear. This interaural time difference is, on average, slightly more than 650 μs in the adult when the sound is directly opposite one ear (see Wightman & Kistler, 1993). For lower frequency sounds this will be perceived as a phase lag. Higher frequencies will also be delayed in time of arrival to the lagging ear relative to the leading ear, but the differences are less likely to be discriminable to the listener, because phase coding is strongest at lower frequencies. At higher frequencies the interaural time delay is more likely to be perceived as a delay in the envelope of the sound rather than as a phase delay of the individual components.

In the free field, interaural time and intensity differences are available as cues to a sound's location. Recent studies examining the relative salience of these cues suggest that interaural time differences are generally the dominant cue used by listeners in determining the source of a sound (Wightman & Kistler, 1997) unless the cues are not plausible. For example, if an interaural difference is presented to a listener that is unreasonably large (i.e., greater than that possible in the space), and that cue is made to conflict with a plausible interaural intensity difference, the listener will ignore the time cue and bias their judgments toward the intensity cue even though intensity is generally a weaker cue (Hartmann, 1997).

Interaural time and intensity cues are often ambiguous. For example, when a sound is presented in the median sagittal plane, it will arrive simultaneously at the two ears with equal intensity. No interaural disparities will be present. The ambiguity produced is similar to that obtained for many other sound locations. Imagine an axis running through the two ears. As concentric circles are drawn around that axis, parallel to the direction in which the listener is facing, it can be seen that sound sources placed anywhere on one of those circles will provide equal interaural time cues, despite the fact that these points on the circle may be above, below, in front of, and behind the listener. This is commonly called the "cone of confusion," a region for which the binaural cues are ambiguous and could potentially lead to localization errors. However, listeners seldom make such confusions in the real world because most sounds are broadband. Thus ambiguities for individual components will not be as strong when considered within the context of the entire stimulus. Also, position-dependent, monaural spectral cues are available.

Monaural Cues to Sound Localization

The ability to correctly localize sounds is likely facilitated through the use of broadband, monaural cues provided by the filtering characteristics of the pinna. For example, when a sound is in front of a listener, the spectral representation arriving at the tympanic membrane will be different from that of a sound arriving from behind the listener, even if the interaural cues are the same (Shaw, 1974; Wightman & Kistler, 1989). The filtering characteristics of the pinna are position dependent, and this filtering likely provides strong information for localizing sounds in the free field. Many researchers (e.g., Middlebrooks, 1997; Wightman & Kistler, 1989; Wightman et al, 1991) have suggested that these spectral cues play an important role in the determination of elevation and in the resolution of front-back confusions arising from ambiguous interaural time and intensity differences.

It must also be noted that although interaural time and intensity disparities and spectral filtering by the pinna are the dominant cues used to position sounds in space, other nonauditory factors including vision, memory, and listener expectations also play a role. For example, the well-known ventriloquism effect is a strong example of how visual cues can override auditory cues in sound localization (Warren et al, 1981). Even though a listener may be well aware that a puppet or a figure on a movie or TV screen is not actually speaking, the sound is perceived as coming from those sources. A strong bias exists toward perceiving sounds as originating from a likely source. It is for this reason that many studies of sound localization are conducted in chambers where listeners' eyes are covered so that they will not see speaker locations and thus be biased to those locations in the localization of auditory signals with which they are presented.

The Precedence Effect

The free field condition is also complicated by the acoustics of the room, or space, in which the sound is presented. Most rooms are reverberant (i.e., sounds will be reflected off of hard surfaces in the room and back to the listener as secondary and delayed sources). The listener is thus faced with several waveforms from which to extract source localization information. The direct sound will come from the source, and the reflected waveforms that are highly correlated with the direct source come from locations that may be quite disparate from the source. If the reflected sounds arrive at the listener's ear with very little delay relative to the direct source, they may be integrated into the direct waveform and increase the sound level of the signal. However, if they arrive somewhat later and are significantly out of phase with the direct sound, they may produce an interference that degrades the quality of the signal. Furthermore, if the reflected sounds arrive quite late relative to the direct sound, they may be perceived as an echo. To localize a sound source, a listener must determine which of the many waveforms being received is the direct waveform, and therefore arises from the source, and which waveforms are reflected and arise from the surfaces of the room, thereby providing misleading localization information. It is the functioning of the binaural auditory system that tells the listener which waveform arises from the source, where that source is located, and that suppresses potentially interfering reflections (dereverberation).

The *precedence effect* states that a sound source location will be determined by the waveform that reaches the listener first, even if later arriving reflected waveforms may be more

---

PEARL

The *precedence effect* states that a sound source location will be determined by the waveform that reaches the listener first, even if later arriving reflected waveforms may be more intense.

---

intense. Consider a signal presented to a listener in a reverberant room. If the reflected waveform arrives after a very short delay (1 ms for a click) relative to the direct waveform, perception of the source location will be determined from an average of the acoustic cues provided by each waveform. However, the relative weight given to the lagging waveform will decrease as the magnitude of the delay increases. This is called *summing localization*.

When the reflected sound arrives slightly later (1 to 4 ms for a click stimulus) relative to the direct waveform, the perception of the source location will be affected only slightly by the reflected source, largely in terms of increasing error around the true location (localization blur) but not altering the location in the direction of the origin of the reflected source. The reflected sound will add to the direct source in a way that provides a sense of the room's acoustics or spaciousness. If the reflected sound arrives with a greater delay (5 to 10 ms for a click), it may be perceived as an additional sound, an echo. When signals are longer in duration than a click, such as would be the case for speech and music, much longer reverberation times produce integrated, single images than for clicks. The upper limit for reverberation before the reflected waves cause destructive rather than constructive interference is 10, 50, and 80 ms, for clicks, speech, and music, respectively (Blauert, 1983b).

A Note on Room Acoustics

Rooms with no reverberation, such as an anechoic chamber, are dead and sounds appear quite dull and flat in them. However, rooms with very long reverberation times may also sound poor, with reflected sounds adding to the direct sounds in an interfering and destructive manner. This is often the case in very large rooms with poor acoustics, such as school gymnasiums, for example. A room with good acoustics is one for which the reverberation time is sufficient to give a feeling of spaciousness, but not so long as to produce destructive interference. That only one image is perceived even though several waveforms are received at the listener's ear is attributable to the binaural hearing capabilities of the listener. These effects are not observed in the absence of binaural hearing. For example, when a recording is made in room through a single microphone, the quality of the sound will be quite poor. The reflected waves will interfere with the direct source making the sound appear distorted and possibly difficult to understand. It is only because of the "de-reverberation" provided by the precedence effect in the free field that clarity sound is maintained in highly reverberant rooms. Thus, binaural hearing plays an important role in sound source separation, location, and discrimination in noise.

Distance Perception

The perception of the distance of sound sources has received less attention than has the absolute location of sounds. Two cues are likely used by listeners. The first is related to the magnitude of a reverberated signal relative to the direct signal. When the direct signal is much more intense than the reflected signal, it is likely that the sound source is much closer than if the direct and reflected waveforms are more similar. Second, sounds that are farther away usually lose high-frequency energy before they reach the listener. Thus a bias toward lower frequency composition can suggest greater distance. This cue, of course, requires some prior knowledge of the sound's spectral characteristics (Mershon, 1997).

Audiological Implications of Complex Sound Processing

Assessment

Audiologists tend to focus on the listener's ability to detect (and sometimes discriminate between) relatively simple sounds. Yet most natural sounds are very complex and the ability to evaluate the processing of complex sounds has important implications for measuring the impact of a peripheral hearing loss and detecting and delineating the more elusive deficits found in central auditory processing disorders. One reason it is so difficult to detect and evaluate central auditory processing deficiencies is that as signals ascend the auditory system many factors impinge on its encoding and processing. Should a degraded image be present, occurring perhaps because of a pathological condition in the auditory periphery or somewhere along the auditory pathways, more central, cognitive processes such as learning, pattern recognition, restoration, and the like facilitate processing and render the sound understandable. This makes it difficult to determine the nature of a problem at higher levels within the system. It is often only when degraded signals are used in testing (either through the addition of background noise, the introduction of competing messages, filtering or time altering) that processing and encoding difficulties arising more centrally can be observed. With simpler sounds presented in a clear or undegraded way, it is often very difficult to detect anything but the most obvious and outstanding problems. Perhaps the tasks and abilities relevant to processing complex stimuli discussed in this chapter may hold promise for improved assessment and rehabilitation of central auditory processing disorders in addition to more peripheral disorders.

Auditory Training and Learning

The promise for rehabilitation/habilitation in auditory processing is clear. Psychoacoustic research has shown that many highly complex abilities, as well as more simple ones, can be trained. Improvements in performance are often observed, even in normal-hearing listeners over the course of repeated trials (Leek & Watson, 1984; 1988). Similarly, previous training and listening experience has been shown to have a significant impact on listeners' encoding of complex sounds (Howard, 1977; Howard & Silverman, 1976). Although auditory learning is expected and quite natural for children, it also occurs

with adult listeners. Sounds that are presented repeatedly become familiar and are therefore perceived with less effort than are unfamiliar sounds. Thus the usefulness of auditory training programs in habilitation and rehabilitation programs holds extensive promise.

CONCLUSIONS

Audiology has drawn significant knowledge from psychoacoustics and will likely continue to do so in the future. Much of the methodology in behavioral assessment was refined by psychophysicists enabling more precise hearing ability of individual listeners with efficiency and rigor. As well, the understanding of normal-hearing abilities and how those abilities may be impaired when there is damage or dysfunction in the auditory system comes largely from psychoacoustic study. Yet there have been limitations to extending psychoacoustic findings to the clinic.

One of those limitations was that most earlier research in psychoacoustics focused on understanding how normal listeners processed sounds. The aim was to define group, or average trends. For many tasks this was a reasonable goal because between-subjects variability is relatively low (e.g., quiet detection thresholds). However, for others, individual differences (and hence the between-subject variability) may be large. This is unfortunate because clinically a single individual rather than a group of individuals is faced and it must be decided whether the ability to perform an auditory task is within the acceptable range for normal-hearing listeners or whether it reflects an impairment of some sort. Thus individual variability and the extent to which data from an individual can be compared with that averaged across a group of listeners must be assessed. More recently, psychoacoustic studies have addressed issues of individual variance quite well, particularly as they relate to the processing of more complex sounds in which individual differences appear to be largest (Neff et al, 1993) and to the auditory processing ability of children (e.g., Allen & Wightman, 1994, 1995). Thus it is learned not only how people should perform on average but also what is the acceptable range of variability and how this variability changes with the task and with listener age.

Another limitation in the direct application of psychoacoustic research to clinical practice is that the psychoacoustic procedures are often lengthy and tedious, certainly not what is acceptable in a clinical practice. In many psychoacoustic studies the participants are trained listeners with hours and thousands of trials of practice and experience. Given that practice and training effects may sometimes be large, it is difficult to extrapolate from these highly practiced listeners what performance should be expected from a relatively naïve patient who is being seen for the first time. Similarly, it is unrealistic to expect that patients should perform thousands of trials before their hearing abilities can be assessed. Fortunately, some more recent studies have presented data from more naïve listeners and have attempted to develop procedures that enable quicker estimates of performance.

Also, many of our patients are either children or elderly individuals and much less is known about these populations than about the performance of young, healthy adult listeners. Until recently, relatively little was known about age-related changes in psychoacoustic abilities, often because few methods were available with which to test young children or very elderly listeners. Again, this pattern is changing, and recently interest and available data examining the psychoacoustic performance of a wide age range of listeners have increased.

Last, psychoacoustic studies have typically relied on advanced and often complicated equipment and computer software. The stimuli and techniques often required facilities, software, and equipment that were not available in the clinic. Audiologists have been, and sometimes continue to be, limited by what their clinical audiometer can do. However, the future is bright for bringing advanced psychoacoustic assessment to the clinic. The availability of small personal computers and highly sophisticated software that is now commercially available holds promise for the growth of behavioral testing and the further integration of psychoacoustics and audiology.

REFERENCES

ABEL, S. M. (1972). Duration discrimination of noise and tone bursts. *Journal of the Acoustical Society of America, 51,* 1219–1223.

ALLEN P., & BOND, C. (1997). Multidimensional scaling of complex sounds by school-aged children and adults. *Journal of the Acoustical Society of America, 102,* 2255–2263.

ALLEN, P., JONES, R., & SLANEY, P. (1998). The role of level, spectral, and temporal cues in children's detection of masked signals. *Journal of the Acoustical Society of America, 104,* 2997–3005.

ALLEN P., & NELLES, J. (1996). Development of auditory information integration abilities. *Journal of the Acoustical Society of America, 100,* 1043–1051.

ALLEN, P. & WIGHTMAN, F. (1994). Psychometric functions for children's detection of tones in noise. *Journal of Speech and Hearing Research, 37,* 205–215.

ALLEN P., & WIGHTMAN, F. (1995). Effects of signal and masker uncertainty on children's detection. *Journal of Speech and Hearing Research, 38,* 503–511.

AMERICAN NATIONAL STANDARDS INSTITUTE. (1989). *Specifications for audiometers. (ANSI S3.6).* New York: ANSI.

BACON S., & VIEMEISTER, N. (1985). Temporal modulation transfer functions in normal- and hearing-impaired ears. *Audiology, 24,* 117–134.

BARGONES, J., & WERNER, L. (1994). Adults listen selectively, infants do not. *Journal of the American Psychological Society, 5,* 170–174.

BERG, B. G. (1989). Analysis of weights in multiple observation tasks. *Journal of the Acoustical Society of America, 86,* 1743–1746.

BERG, B. G. (1990). Observer efficiency and weights in a multiple observation task. *Journal of the Acoustical Society of America, 88,* 149–158.

BERG, B. G., & GREEN, D. M. (1990). Spectral weights in profile listening. *Journal of the Acoustical Society of America, 88,* 758–766.

BERG, B., & ROBINSON, D. (1987). Multiple observations and internal noise. *Journal of the Acoustical Society of America, Suppl. 1, 81,* S33.

BLAUERT, J. (1983a). *Spatial hearing.* Cambridge, MA: The MIT Press

BLAUERT, J. (1983b). Review Paper: Psychoacoustic binaural phenomena. In: R. Klinke, & R. Hartmann (Eds.). *Hearing—Physiological bases and psychophysics.* Berlin: Springer-Verlag.

CHRISTENSEN, L. A., & HUMES, L. E. (1996). Identification of multidimensional complex sounds having parallel dimension structure. *Journal of the Acoustical Society of America, 99,* 2307–2315.

DAI, H., & BUUS, S. (1991). Effect of gating the masker on frequency-selective listening. *Journal of the Acoustical Society of America, 89,* 1816–1818.

DELGUTTE, B. (1996). Physiological models for basic auditory perceptions. In: H. L. Hawkins, T.N. McMullen, A.N. Popper, & R.R. Fay (Eds.). *Auditory computation.* New York: Springer-Verlag.

DIVENYI, P. L., & DANNER, W. F. (1977). Discrimination of time intervals marked by brief acoustic pulses of various intensities and spectra. *Perception and Psychophysics, 21,* 124–142.

DIVENYI, P. L., & HIRSH, I. J. (1974). Identification of temporal order in three tone sequences. *Journal of the Acoustical Society of America, 56,* 144–151.

DOHERTY, K. A., & LUTFI, R. A. (1996). Spectral weights for overall level discrimination in listeners with sensorimotor hearing loss. *Journal of the Acoustical Society of America, 99,* 1053–1058.

DURLACH, N. I., BRAIDA, L. D., & ITO, Y. (1986). Toward a model for discrimination of broadband signals. *Journal of the Acoustical Society of America, 80,* 63–72.

EVANS, E. F. (1975). The sharpening of frequency selectivity in the normal and abnormal cochlea. *Audiology, 14,* 419–442.

EVANS E. F., & HARRISON, R. V. (1976). Correlation between outer hair cell damage and deterioration of cochlear nerve tuning properties in the guinea pig. *Journal of Physiology, 252,* 43–44.

FETH, L. L. (1974). Frequency discrimination of complex periodic tones. *Perception and Psychophysics, 15,* 375–378.

FETH, L. L., O'MALLEY, H. & RAMSAY, J. (1982). Pitch of unresolved, two-component complex tones. *Journal of the Acoustical Society of America, 72,* 1408–1412.

FITZGIBBONS, P. J. & WIGHTMAN, F. L. (1982). Gap detection in normal and hearing loss listeners. *Journal of the Acoustical Society of America, 72,* 761–765.

FLETCHER, H. (1940). Auditory patterns. *Review of Modern Physics, 12,* 47–65.

FLETCHER H., & MUNSON, W. A. (1933). Loudness, its definition, measurement and calculation. *Journal of the Acoustical Society of America, 5,* 82–108.

FLORENTINE, M., BUUS, S., & MASON, C. R. (1980). Frequency selectivity in normally hearing and hearing impaired observers. *Journal of Speech and Hearing Research, 23,* 643–669.

FLORENTINE, M., BUUS, S., & MASON, C. R. (1987). Level discrimination as a function of level for tones from 0.25 to 16 kHz. *Journal of the Acoustical Society of America, 81,* 1528–1541.

GLASBERG, B. R., & MOORE, B. C. J. (1986). Auditory filter shapes in subjects with unilateral and bilateral cochlear impairments. *Journal of the Acoustical Society of America, 79*, 1020–1033.

GRAVETTER, F., & LOCKHEAD, G. R. (1973). Criterial range as a frame of reference for stimulus judgement. *Psychological Review, 80*, 203–216.

GREEN, D. M. (1988). *Profile analysis: Auditory intensity discrimination*. New York: Oxford University Press.

GREEN, D. M. (1993). Auditory intensity discrimination. In: W.N. Yost, A. N. Popper, & R. R. Fay (Eds.). *Human psychophysics*. New York: Springer-Verlag.

GREEN, D. M., KIDD, G. JR., & PICARDI, M. C. (1983). Successive versus simultaneous comparison in auditory intensity discrimination. *Journal of the Acoustical Society of America, 73*, 639–643.

GREEN, D. M., & SWETS, J. A. (1966). *Signal detection theory and psychophysics*. New York: John Wiley & Sons (reprinted Los Altos, CA: Peninsula Publishing, 1988).

GREENBERG, G. Z., & LARKIN, W. D. (1969). Frequency-response characteristics of auditory observers detection signals of a single frequency in noise: The probe signal method. *Journal of the Acoustical Society of America, 44*, 1513–1523.

HALL, J.W., HAGGARD, M.P., & FERNENDES, M.A. (1984). Detection in noise by spectro-temporal pattern analysis. *Journal of the Acoustical Society of America, 76*, 50–56.

HARTMANN, W. M. (1997). Listening in a room and the precedence effect. In: R. H. Gilkey, & T. R. Anderson (Eds.). *Binaural and spatial hearing in real and virtual environments*. Mahwah, NJ: Lawrence Erlbaum Associates.

HARTMANN, W. M. (1998). *Signals, sounds, and sensations*. New York: Springer-Verlag.

HARTMANN W. M., & PUMPLIN, J. (1988). Noise power fluctuations and the masking of sine signals. *Journal of the Acoustical Society of America, 83*, 2277–2289.

HELLMAN, R. P. (1974). Effect of spread of excitation on the loudness function at 250Hz. In: H.R. Moskowitz, B. Scharf, & S. S. Stevens (Eds.). *Sensation and measurement*. Dordredcht: Reidel.

HIRSH, I. J. (1959). Auditory perception of temporal order. *Journal of the Acoustical Society of America, 31*, 759–767.

HOWARD, J. H. (1977). Psychophysical structure of eight complex underwater sounds. *Journal of the Acoustical Society of America, 62*, 149–156.

HOWARD, J. H., & SILVERMAN, E. B. (1976). A multidimensional scaling analysis of 16 complex sounds. *Perception and Psychophysics, 19*, 193–200.

JESTEADT, W., WIER, C. C., & GREEN, D. M. (1977). Intensity discrimination as a function of frequency and sensation level. *Journal of the Acoustical Society of America, 61*, 169–177.

JOHNSON-DAVIES, D., & PATTERSON, R. D. (1979). Psychophysical tuning curve: Restricting the listening band to the signal region. *Journal of the Acoustical Society of America, 65*, 765–770.

LACHS, G., AL-SHAIKH, R., BI, Q., SAIA, R. A., TEICH, M. C. (1984). A neural counting model basin on the physiological characteristics of the peripheral auditory system. V. Application to loudness and intensity discrimination. *IEEE Trans, SMC-14*, 819–836.

LANGNER, G. (1992). Periodicity coding in the auditory system. *Hearing Research, 60*, 115–142.

LEEK, M. R., & WATSON, C. S. (1984). Learning to detect auditory pattern components. *Journal of the Acoustical Society of America, 76*, 1037–1044.

LEEK, M. R., & WATSON, C. S. (1988). Auditory perceptual learning of tonal patterns. *Perception and Psychophysics, 43*, 389–394.

LEVITT, H. (1971). Transformed up-down methods in psychoacoustics. *Journal of the Acoustical Society of America, 49*, 467–477.

LIBERMAN, M. C. (1978). Auditory nerve response from cats raised in a low-noise chamber. *Journal of the Acoustical Society of America, 63*, 442–455.

LUTFI, R. A. (1989). Informational processing of complex sounds. I: Intensity discrimination. *Journal of the Acoustical Society of America, 86*, 934–944.

LUTFI, R. A. (1990). Informational processing of complex sounds. II: Cross-dimensional analysis. *Journal of the Acoustical Society of America, 87*, 2141–2148.

LUTFI, R. A. (1992). Informational processing of complex sounds. III: Interference. *Journal of the Acoustical Society of America, 91*, 3391–3401.

MERSHON, D. H. (1997). Phenomenal geometry and the measurement of perceived auditory distance. In: R.H. Gilkey, & T.R. Anderson (Eds.). *Binaural and spatial hearing in real and virtual environments*. Mahwah, NJ: Lawrence Erlbaum Associates.

MIDDLEBROOKS, J. C. (1997). Spectral shape cues for sound localization. In: R.H. Gilkey, & T.R. Anderson (Eds.). *Binaural and spatial hearing in real and virtual environments*. Mahwah, NJ: Lawrence Erlbaum Associates.

MOORE, B. C. J., POON, P. W. F., BACON, S. P., GLASBERG, B. R. (1987). The temporal course of masking and the auditory filter shape. *Journal of the Acoustical Society of America, 81*, 1873–1880.

NEFF, D. L., & CALLAGHAN, B. P. (1988). Effective properties of multicomponent simultaneous maskers under conditions of uncertainty. *Journal of the Acoustical Society of America, 83*, 1833–1838.

NEFF, D. L., DETHLEFS, T. M., & JESTEADT, W. (1993). Informational masking for multicomponent maskers and spectral gaps. *Journal of the Acoustical Society of America, 94*, 3112–3126.

NEFF, D. L, & JESTEADT, W. (1996). Intensity discrimination in the presence of random-frequency, multicomponent maskers and broadband noise. *Journal of the Acoustical Society of America, 100*, 2289–2298.

PATTERSON, R. D. (1976). Auditory filter shapes derived with noise stimuli. *Journal of the Acoustical Society of America, 59*, 640–654.

PATTERSON, R. D., NIMMO-SMITH, I., WEBER, D. L., & MILROY, R. (1982). The deterioration of hearing with age: Frequency selectivity, the critical ratio, the audiogram, and speech thresholds. *Journal of the Acoustical Society of America, 72*, 1788–1803.

PENNER, M. J. (1977). Detection of temporal gaps in noise as a measure of the decay of auditory sensations. *Journal of the Acoustical Society of America, 61*, 552–557.

PETERSON, G. E., & BARNEY, H. L. (1952). Control methods used in a study of the vowels. *Journal of the Acoustical Society of America, 24*, 175–184.

PICKLES, J. O. (1988). *An introduction to the physiology of hearing*, New York: Academic Press.

PLOMP, R. (1964). The ear as a frequency analyzer. *Journal of the Acoustical Society of America, 36,* 1628–1636.

PRADHAN, P. L., & HOFFMAN, P. J. (1963). Effect of spacing and range of stimuli on magnitude estimation judgements. *Journal of Experimental Psychology, 66,* 533–541.

RAMIREZ, R. W. (1985). *The FFT: Fundamentals and Concepts,* Englewood Cliffs, N.J.: Prentice-Hall, Inc.

ROBINSON, D.W., & DADSON, R. S. (1956). A redetermination of the equal loudness relations for pure tones. *British Journal of Applied Physiology, 7,* 166–181.

SCHARF, B. (1970). Critical bands. In: J.V. Tobias (Ed.). *Foundations of modern auditory theory (Vol. 1).* New York: Academic Press.

SCHARF, B. (1983). Loudness adaptation. In: J.V. Tobias, & E.D. Schubert (Eds.). *Hearing research and theory (Vol. 2).* New York: Academic Press.

SCHARF, B., QUIGLEY, C., AOKI, N., PEACHEY, N., & REEVES, A. (1987). Focused auditory attention and frequency selectivity. *Perception and Psychophysics, 42,* 215–223.

SEK A., & MOORE, B. C. (1995). Frequency discrimination as a function of frequency, measured in several ways. *Journal of the Acoustical Society of America, 97,* 2479–2486.

SHAILER, M. J., & MOORE, B. C. (1983). Gap detection as a function of frequency, bandwidth, and level. *Journal of the Acoustical Society of America, 74,* 46–473.

SHAILER M. J., & MOORE, B. C. (1987). Gap detection and the auditory filter: Phase effects using sinusoidal stimuli. *Journal of the Acoustical Society of America, 81,* 1110–1117.

SHAW, E. A. G. (1997). Acoustical features of the human external ear. In: R.H. Gilkey, & T.R. Anderson (Eds.). *Binaural and spatial hearing in real and virtual environments.* Mahwah, NJ: Lawrence Erlbaum Associates.

SHAW, E. A. G. (1974). Transformations of sound pressure level from the free field to the eardrum in the horizontal plane. *Journal of the Acoustical Society of America, 56,* 1848–1861.

SIEBERT, W. M. (1968). Stimulus transformations in the peripheral auditory system. In: P.A. Kolers, & M. Edin (Eds). *Recognizing patterns.* Cambridge, Mass: MIT Press.

SIVIAN, L. J., & WHITE, S.D. (1933). On minimum audible sound fields. *Journal of the Acoustical Society of America, 4,* 288–321.

SMALL, A. M., & CAMPBELL, R. A. (1962). Temporal differential sensitivity for auditory stimuli. *American Journal of Psychology, 75,* 401–410.

STEVENS, S. S. (1955). The measurement of loudness. *Journal of the Acoustical Society of America, 27,* 815–829.

STEVENS, S. S. (1957). On the psychophysical law. *Psychological Review, 64,* 153–181.

STEVENS, S. S. (1972). Perceived level of noise by Mark VII and decibels (E). *Journal of the Acoustical Society of America, 51,* 575–601.

STEVENS, K. N., & BLUMSTEIN, S. E. (1978). Invariant cues for place of articulation in stop consonants. *Journal of the Acoustical Society of America, 68,* 836–842.

STEVENS, S. S., & VOLKMAN, J. (1940). The relation of pitch to frequency: A revised scale. *American Journal of Psychology, 53,* 329–353.

SWETS, J. A. (1964). *Signal detection and recognition by human observers.* New York: John Wiley & Sons (reprinted, Los Altos, CA: Peninsula Publishing, 1988).

VIEMEISTER, N. F. (1983). Auditory intensity discrimination at high frequencies in the presence of noise. *Science, 221,* 1206–1208.

VIEMEISTER, N. F., & BACON, S. P. (1988). Intensity discrimination, intensity detection and magnitude estimation for 1kHz tones. *Journal of the Acoustical Society of America, 84,* 172–178.

VERSCHUURE, J., & VAN MEETEREN, A. A. (1975). The effect of intensity on pitch. *Acustica, 32,* 33–44.

WARREN, D. H., WELD, R. B., & McCARTHY, T. J. (1981). The role of visual-auditory "compellingness" in the ventriloquism effect: Implications for transivity among the spatial senses. *Perception and Psychophysics, 30,* 557–564.

WARREN, R. M. (1974). Auditory temporal discrimination by trained listeners. *Cognitive Psychology, 6,* 717.

WATSON, C. S., & FOYLE, D. C. (1985). Central factors in the discrimination and identification of complex sounds. *Journal of the Acoustical Society of America, 78,* 375–380.

WATSON, C. S., & KELLEY, W. J. (1981). The role of stimulus uncertainty in the discrimination of auditory patterns. In: D.G. Getty, & J. H. Howard, Jr. (Eds.) *Auditory and visual pattern recognition.* Hillsdale, NJ: Erlbaum.

WEIR, C., JESTEADT, W., & GREEN, D. M. (1977). Frequency discrimination as a function of frequency and sensation level. *Journal of the Acoustical Society of America, 61,* 178–184.

WIGHTMAN, F. L., & KISTLER, D. (1989). Headphone simulation of free field listening II: Psychophysical validation. *Journal of the Acoustical Society of America, 85,* 868–878.

WIGHTMAN, F. L., & KISTLER, D. (1993). Sound localization. In: W.A. Yost, A.N. Popper, & R.R. Fay (Eds.). *Human psychophysics.* New York: Springer-Verlag.

WIGHTMAN, F. L., KISTLER, D., & ARRUDA, M. (1991). Monaural localization revisited. *Journal of the Acoustical Society of America, 89,* 1995.

WIGHTMAN, F. L., & KISTLER, D. (1997). Factors affecting the relative salience of sound localization cues. In: R.H. Gilkey, & T.R. Anderson (Eds.). *Binaural and spatial hearing in real and virtual environments.* Mahwah, NJ: Lawrence Erlbaum Associates.

WRIGHT B. A., & DAI, H. (1994). Detection of unexpected tones in gated and continuous maskers. *Journal of the Acoustical Society of America, 95,* 939–948.

ZERA, J., & GREEN, D. M. (1993). Detecting temporal onset and offset asynchrony in multicomponent complexes. *Journal of the Acoustical Society of America, 93,* 1038–1052.

ZWICKER, E. (1977). On a psychoacoustic equivalent of tuning curves. In: E. Zwicker, & E. Terhardt (Eds.). *Facts and models in hearing.* New York: Springer-Verlag.

ZWICKER, E., FLOTTORP, G., & STEVENS, S. S. (1957). Critical bandwidth in loudness summation. *Journal of the Acoustical Society of America, 29,* 548–557.

## Chapter 10

Basic Instrumentation and Calibration

Tom Frank

Outline

The practice of audiology requires that audiometers and acoustic immittance instruments produce accurate and controlled signals and that testing be conducted in an acoustically controlled environment. This is needed for making reliable and valid interpretations regarding a patient's peripheral hearing sensitivity, speech-processing ability, and middle ear status. Thus the extent to which audiometers and acoustic immittance instruments conform to standardized performance characteristics and that testing is done in an appropriate environment is a major concern to audiologists. Manufacturers are responsible for designing instruments that are accurate and reliable; however, audiologists are responsible for maintaining the accuracy of these instruments by conducting routine calibration measurements and daily inspection and listening checks.

The goal of this chapter is to provide an overview concerning the performance characteristics of audiometers and acoustic immittance instruments and the requirements for audiometric test rooms. To achieve this goal, the chapter has been divided into sections devoted to standards, audiometers, calibration instrumentation, performance characteristics of pure tone audiometers, automatic audiometers, speech audiometers, inspection and listening checks, acoustic immittance instruments, and audiometric test rooms. The sections concerning audiometers and acoustic immittance instruments contain information regarding the classification of instruments, transducers, calibration procedures, and standardized values. The audiometric test room section contains information regarding the measurement of ambient noise, standardized ambient noise levels, sources and ways to reduce ambient noise, and earphone attenuation values. Appendix A provides a list of standards used for the calibration of audiometers and acoustic immittance instruments and other standards having application to audiology. Appendix B contains several forms

Audiology: Diagnosis. Edited by Roeser, Valente, and Hosford-Dunn. Thieme Medical Publishers, Inc., New York © 2000

that can be used for recording calibration results for pure tone and speech audiometers, acoustic immittance instruments, and ambient noise levels in an audiometric test room.

STANDARDS

Purpose

A standard is a written document typically developed by a committee of national and international experts on the basis of scientific evidence and accepted practices. Standards related to audiology contain terms, definitions, and specifications concerning the measurement and the performance characteristics of various instruments used for testing hearing, transducers, and audiometric test rooms. Standards are developed as a public service for consumers, industry, and governmental agencies. The primary purpose of a standard is to provide uniformity among its users. For example, if all audiometers are calibrated to the same standard, intraclinic and interclinic hearing tests conducted for the same individual will result in equivalent results under comparable test conditions. Even though compliance with a standard is voluntary, audiologists should use audiometers, acoustic immittance instruments, and audiometric test rooms that meet specifications issued by the American National Standards Institute (ANSI). Only when standards are written into a law do they become mandatory. However, accreditation by the Professional Service Board of the American Speech-Language-Hearing Association (ASHA) and other accrediting agencies require that audiometric instrumentation and test rooms comply with ANSI standards.

Development of an ANSI Standard

In the United States, standards dealing with acoustics are the responsibility of four accredited standards committees of the Acoustical Society of America (ASA) known as S1-Acoustics, S2-Mechanical Vibration and Shock, S3-Bioacoustics, and S12-Noise. Standards dealing with audiometers, acoustic immittance instruments, audiometric test rooms, and calibration couplers fall under the jurisdiction of the S3-Bioacoustics committee. Each accredited committee is composed of several working groups (WGs) having an appointed chair and expert members. The purpose of each WG is to develop, maintain, and revise a standard(s). Once a WG has drafted a standard, it is reviewed and balloted by members of the accredited committee, individuals representing organizational members (e.g., ASHA, American Academy of Audiology, American Academy of Otolaryngology), and individual experts following procedures approved by ANSI. After the draft standard has been approved by the ASA accredited committee and ANSI, it is recognized as an American National Standard, called an ANSI standard, given a number, and published and distributed by the ASA.

PEARL

ANSI standards can be obtained from the ASA Standards Secretariat, 120 Wall Street, 32nd Floor, New York, New York 10005-3993.

ANSI requires that each standard be reviewed every 5 years. This is done so that any new scientific information, procedures, and equipment can be incorporated into the standard. When an ANSI standard is reviewed, the WG can recommend that the standard be revised, reaffirmed, or withdrawn. If a standard is revised, it typically retains its name and number, but the year changes to the year in which the revision was completed. For example, the ANSI standard S3.6-1989, *Specification for Audiometers*, was revised in 1996. The standard has kept its title but is now designated as ANSI S3.6-1996. If a standard is reaffirmed, the year in which the reaffirmation occurred preceded by an R appears in parentheses after the number and year that the standard was originally completed. For example, ANSI S3.39-1987 *Specifications for Instruments to Measure Aural Acoustic Impedance and Admittance (Aural Acoustic Immittance)* was reaffirmed in 1996 and is now designated as ANSI S3.39-1987 (R 1996).

International Standards

International standards have also been developed by the International Organization for Standardization (ISO) and the International Electrotechnical Commission (IEC). Since the early 1990s, ASA and ANSI have attempted to make all new standards and revisions of existing standards compatible and consistent with comparable ISO and IEC standards to promote international uniformity. For example, ANSI S3.6-1996 *Specification of Audiometers* is consistent with several ISO and IEC standards. This was done so that all audiometers would meet the same specifications, regardless of where in the world they were manufactured or used.

AUDIOMETERS

The standard governing audiometers is ANSI S3.6-1996, *Specification for Audiometers*, which was developed in 1969, revised in 1989, and revised again in 1996. As done in 1989, the 1996 standard includes terms and definitions, specifications for audiometers and transducers, signal sources, reference threshold levels, and calibration procedures. However, the 1996 revision is more complete than the 1989 version and was developed using some different principles (Frank, 1997).

Types of Audiometers

Historically, audiometers have been given names in reference to (1) the type of signal they produce (pure tone or speech); (2) the frequency range over which they operate (limited, normal, or high frequency); (3) the method in which hearing is measured (manual, automatic, or computer-controlled); (4) the purpose for which they are being used (clinical, diagnostic, industrial, or screening); (5) the number of independent audiometers contained in one unit (one-channel, two-channel, or channel-and-a-half); and (6) whether they are portable. ANSI S3.6-1996 classifies audiometers as pure tone, automatic, speech, extended high frequency, and free field equivalent on the basis of minimum required features, frequencies, and maximum hearing levels (HLs) they contain as shown in Tables 10–1 and 10–2.

TABLE 10–1 **Minimum required features for pure tone and speech audiometers (from ANSI S3.6-1996 with permission of the Acoustical Society of America, New York, NY)**

Minimum Required Features	Pure Tone 1	2	3	4	5	HF*	Speech A	B	C
Transducers									
Two earphones	Yes	Yes	Yes	Yes	No	Yes	Yes[†]	Yes[†]	Yes[†]
Insert earphones	Yes	No	No	No	No	No	No	No	No
Loudspeakers or electrical output‡	Yes	Yes	No	No	No	No	Yes	Yes	No
Bone vibrator	Yes	Yes	Yes	No	No	No	Yes	No	No
Hearing Levels, Test Frequencies									
(Table 10–2)	Yes	Yes	Yes	Yes	Yes	No	Yes	No	No
Test Signal Switching									
Presentation/interruption	Yes	Yes	Yes	Yes	Yes	Yes	Yes	Yes	Yes
Pulsed tone	Yes	Yes	No	Yes§	No	Yes	No	No	No
Frequency modulation (FM)	Yes	Yes	No	No	No	No	No	No	No
Reference Tone									
Alternate presentation	Yes	Yes[‖]	No	No	No	No	No	No	No
Simultaneous presentation	Yes	No	No	No	No	No	No	No	No
Speech Input									
Replay device or electrical	No	No	No	No	No	No	No	No	No
Input for recorded material[‖]	Yes	Yes	No	No	No	No	Yes	Yes	Yes
Microphone	No	No	No	No	No	No	Yes	Yes	No
Masking									
Narrow band noise	Yes	Yes	Yes	No	No	Yes	No	No	No
White noise	Yes	Yes	No	No	No	No	No	No	No
Speech spectrum noise	No	No	No	No	No	No	Yes	Yes	Yes
Routing of Masking									
Contralateral earphone	Yes	Yes	Yes	No	No	Yes	Yes	Yes	Yes
Ipsilateral earphone	Yes	No	No	No	No	No	Yes	No	No
Loudspeaker	Yes	Yes	No	No	No	No	Yes	Yes	No
Bone vibrator	Yes	No	No	No	No	No	No	No	No
Subject Response System	Yes	Yes	Yes	Yes§	No	Yes	Yes	No	No
Signal Indicator	Yes	Yes	No	No	No	Yes	Yes	Yes	Yes
Audible Monitoring	Yes	No	No	No	No	No	Yes	Yes	No
Operator to Subject Speech Communication	Yes	No	No	No	No	No	Yes	No	No
Talk Back System	No	No	No	No	No	No	Yes	Yes	No

*Type HF is for audiometers used for testing high-frequency pure tones from 8000 to 16000 Hz.
†Free field equivalent is recommended; where provided the audiometer shall be designated as type E.
‡If loudspeakers are not supplied with a speech audiometer, the manufacturer must specify how conformity will be achieved.
§Not required for manual audiometers.
¶Replay device is not always supplied by the manufacturer.
‖Not required for automatic recording audiometer.

TABLE 10–2 Minimum required frequencies and hearing levels for pure tone audiometers (from ANSI S3.6-1996 with permission of the Acoustical Society of America, New York, NY)

Frequency (Hz)	Hearing Levels (dB HL)*						
	Type 1‡		Type 2		Type 3		Type 4†
	Air	Bone	Air	Bone	Air	Bone	Air
125	70	—	60	—	—	—	—
250	90	45	80	45	70	35	—
500	120	60	110	60	100	50	70
750	120	60	—	—	—	—	—
1000	120	70	110	70	100	60	70
1500	120	70	110	70	—	—	—
2000	120	70	110	70	100	60	70
3000	120	70	110	70	100	60	70
4000	120	60	110	60	100	50	70
6000	110	50	100	—	90	—	70
8000	100	—	90	—	80	—	—

*Maximum HL shall be ≥ tabled value; minimum HL shall be ≤-10 dB for types 1 to 4; no minimum or maximum HL for type 5.
†Maximum HL shall be extended to 90 dB HL for type 4 if used for hearing conservation purposes.
‡Maximum HL may be 10 dB less than tabled values for type 1 using circumaural or insert earphones.

NOTE: Maximum HL for type HF shall be ≥90 dB HL from 8000 to 11,200 Hz and 50 dB HL from 12,000 to 16,000 Hz; minimum HL shall be −20 dB HL at all frequencies above 8000 Hz.

Pure Tone Audiometers

In its simplest form, a pure tone audiometer consists of a pure tone generator, interrupter switch, amplifier, attenuator, output selector switch, and earphones. The generator produces pure tones at discrete frequencies that are selected with a frequency control. The interrupter switch is used to turn the tone on and off before it is routed to the amplifier. Each pure tone is amplified to its maximum by the amplifier and directed to the attenuator. The tones are attenuated with the HL control, which is numbered in decibels relative to normal hearing. Turning the HL control from minimum to maximum decreases the amount of attenuation but increases the level of the tone delivered to the output selector switch. The output selector switch is used to direct the tone to either the right or left earphone.

ANSI S3.6-1996 classifies pure tone audiometers as type 1, 2, 3, 4, and 5, where the minimum required features, frequencies, and maximum HLs decrease as the type number increases as shown in Tables 10–1 and 10–2. For example, the minimum required features for a type 1 audiometer include four transducer types, frequencies from 125 to 8000 Hz for air conduction and 250 to 6000 Hz for bone conduction, and maximum HLs. On the other hand, a type 4 audiometer is only required to have supra-aural earphones and frequencies from 500 to 6000 Hz, with a maximum output of 70 dB HL at each frequency. For types 1 to 4, the minimum HL is ≤ −10 dB. If insert or circumaural earphones are used with a type 1 audiometer, the maximum HLs can be reduced by 10 dB. If a type 4 audiometer is used for hearing conservation purposes, the maximum HLs can be extended to 90 dB at each frequency. A type 5 audiometer has no required minimum or maximum features.

> ### PEARL
>
> Careful planning is needed before the purchase of an audiometer. Among other things, audiologist's must consider the audiometer's size, record of stability, computer interface capabilities, warranties, the use of a loaner, and most importantly user-friendliness. Typically, instrument suppliers will provide a complete demonstration and allow a trial period with an audiometer before its purchase.

Automatic Audiometers

Historically, automatic audiometers were used for diagnostic purposes (Brunt, 1985; Jerger, 1960); however, in current practice they are typically used to obtain air-conduction thresholds in industrial hearing testing programs. Automatic audiometers are also called Bekesy (Bekesy, 1947; Reger, 1952) or self-recording audiometers because they allow listeners to record their own hearing thresholds. This is done by allowing the listener to control the level of a pure tone by means of a hand switch. When the listener hears a tone, the hand switch is depressed and the audiometer automatically lowers the level of the tone. When the tone is no longer audible, the listener releases the hand switch and the audiometer automatically increases the level of the tone. Over a period of time, the listener has traced or bracketed his or her hearing threshold, which is recorded on an audiogram, on a form, or in a computer. ANSI S3.6-1996 types automatic audiometers using the same features, frequencies, and maximum HLs as done for pure tone audiometers.

Speech Audiometers

A speech audiometer has many of the same components as a pure tone audiometer, except the pure tone generator is replaced by a microphone and external inputs, and a monitoring meter is located between the amplifier and the attenuator (i.e., HL control). The microphone allows for live-voice speech testing and the external inputs allow for playback devices (e.g., cassette tape or compact disc [CD] player) to be connected into the audiometer for recorded speech testing. Historically, speech audiometers were stand-alone instruments; however, in current practice speech and pure tone audiometers are typically combined into one unit called a clinical or diagnostic audiometer.

ANSI S3.6-1996 classifies speech audiometers as type A, B, or C. Type A has the most required features, whereas a type C has the least (Table 10–1). All types are required to have an input for a playback device, but only types A and B are required to have a microphone input. Types A and B are required to have outputs for a supra-aural earphone and loudspeaker, whereas type C is only required to have an output for a supra-aural earphone.

Extended High-Frequency Audiometers

ANSI S3.6-1996 classifies extended high-frequency audiometers as type HF and defines these audiometers as instruments for measuring pure tone thresholds from 8000 to 16,000 Hz. An extended high-frequency audiometer contains the same components as a pure tone audiometer, except that the generator is capable of producing tones from 8000 to 16,000 Hz, and circumaural rather than supra-aural earphones are used. The standard specifies the minimum HL as −20 dB and the maximum HL as ≥90 dB from 8000 to 11,200 Hz and 50 dB from 12,000 to 16,000 Hz. Some commercially available stand-alone high-frequency audiometers exist; however, high-frequency testing capabilities are included in several audiometers typically used for testing from 125 to 8000 Hz.

Free Field Equivalent Audiometers

ANSI S3.6-1996 classifies a free field equivalent audiometer as type E and was included in the standard to be compatible with pending ISO and IEC audiometer standards. A free field equivalent audiometer is a pure tone and/or speech audiometer, whose transducer output levels are calibrated to be equivalent to sound field reference threshold levels. As such, hearing test results with an earphone or bone vibrator are equivalent to hearing tests done in a sound field at 0-degrees azimuth. Interested readers are referred to ANSI S3.6-1996 for detailed specifications.

CONTROVERSIAL POINT

The ANSI WG was reluctant to include the specifications for a free field equivalent audiometer in ANSI S3.6-1996. Many WG members questioned the need, and several manufacturers indicated that the circuitry for this type of audiometer would be very difficult to develop.

Types of Transducers

The function of a transducer is to convert one form of energy to another. A supra-aural, insert, or circumaural earphone and a loudspeaker convert the electrical output from the audiometer to acoustic energy, whereas a bone vibrator converts the electrical output to mechanical energy.

Supra-Aural Earphones

A supra-aural earphone consists of an earphone mounted in a circular cushion attached to a headband. The most common earphones are Telephonics TDH 39, 49, and 50. Figure 10–1 shows a Telephonics TDH type earphones, cushions, and a headband. These earphones have high sensitivity, low distortion, and the TDH 49 and 50 earphones have a relatively flat frequency response with limited output above 8000 Hz. Thus TDH-type earphones are only used for testing from 125 to 8000 Hz. ANSI S3.6-1996 specifies the characteristics of earphone cushions, which are met by a Telephonics Model 51 (shown in Figure 10–1) and MX-41/AR. Both cushions are made of molded rubber; however, the Model 51 is a one-piece cushion and the MX-41/AR is constructed from two pieces glued together. Headbands are produced by several manufacturers. Typically, the earphones are attached to the headband by a device consisting of a Y-shaped yoke. The Y-shaped ends of the yoke insert into the sides of the earphone to allow it to swivel vertically, and the other end of the yoke extends

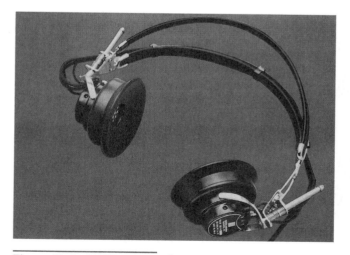

Figure 10–1 TDH-type earphones, model 51 cushions, and headband. (With permission of Telephonics Corporation, Huntington, NY.)

through a holding or spring-loaded clip on the headband to allow horizontal adjustments of the earphones.

When fitted, the cushion rests on and presses against the surface of the pinna. ANSI S3.6-1996 specifies that the static headband force should be 4.5 ± 0.5 N. The procedure for measuring static headband force requires that the supra-aural earphones be mounted on a test fixture, with the earphone diaphragms aligned and separated horizontally by 145 mm and positioned 129 mm from the top center of the headband. Once positioned on the test fixture, the static headband force can be measured with a calibrated strain gauge or with an electromechanical force transducer built into the test fixture.

PITFALL

Static headband force is rarely measured because very specialized instrumentation is required. Unfortunately, it is not unusual to find new headbands with a static force ranging from 2 to 12 N. Audiologists should purchase headbands only from suppliers that can guarantee that the static headband force is within 4.5 ± 0.5 N.

Insert Earphones

An insert earphone consists of a shoulder-mounted transducer coupled to the earcanal by means of a sound tube (240 mm long, 1.37 mm ID) attached to a connecting nipple (11 mm long, 1.37 mm ID) and then to an eartip tube (26 mm long, 1.93 mm ID), which runs through a foam eartip or a probe tip normally used for acoustic immittance measurements. The eartips are disposable and available in three sizes. Each size has the same length (12 mm) but different outside diameters to accommodate individuals with very large earcanals (17.8 mm), normal earcanals (13.7 mm), or small earcanals (9.7 mm). When fitted, the foam eartip is rolled and compressed and inserted into the earcanal so that its outer end is flush or just inside the bowl of the concha and held in place for at least 30 seconds to allow it to expand. Lilly and Prudy (1993) have reported the advantages and disadvantages of using an insert earphone.

Insert earphones manufactured by Etymotic Research (ER) are called ER-3A (Killion, 1984; Killion & Villchur, 1989) and by Aearo E-A-R Auditory Systems (formerly E-A-R Division of Cabot Corporation) are called E-A-RTONE 3A. The ER-3A and E-A-RTONE 3A are functionally equivalent because they are built to the same specifications. ER-3A insert earphones are shown in Figure 10–2. The frequency response of an ER-3A or E-A-RTONE 3A is relatively flat from 100 to 4000 Hz and then sharply decreases (Frank & Richards, 1991). Even though the ER-3A or E-A-RTONE 3A is used for testing from 125 to 8000 Hz, the available output at 6000 and especially at 8000 Hz is reduced compared with the output at 1000 Hz.

Circumaural Earphones

Circumaural earphones consist of an earphone, cushion, and headband. The earphone is typically attached or suspended to the inside of a plastic dome. The cushion on the plastic

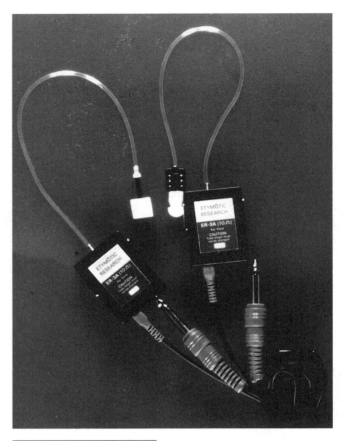

Figure 10–2   ER-3A insert earphones. (With permission of Etymotic Research, Elk Grove, IL.)

dome may be round or oval depending on the opening of the dome and may be detachable or glued to the dome. Examples of a circumaural earphone would include the Sennheiser HDA200 and Koss HV/1A. Sennheiser HDA 200 circumaural earphones are shown in Figure 10–3. When fitted, the cushion of a circumaural earphone fits over and around the pinna similar to an earmuff used for personal hearing protection. ANSI S3.6-1996 specifies that the static headband force should be 9 to 10 N with the same test fixture and procedures as done for supra-aural earphones. Circumaural earphones are most commonly used for testing hearing above 8000 Hz.

Loudspeakers

Loudspeakers used for audiometry should have a bandwidth between 100 and 10,000 Hz, a smooth frequency response, and be housed in an enclosure. To meet these requirements, typically two or more limited-range, frequency-response speakers are contained in the same enclosure. The output is controlled by an electrical crossover network(s) that minimizes overlap between the frequency response of each speaker to obtain an overall smooth frequency response. A loudspeaker should be capable of producing sounds from 0 to 120 dB sound pressure level (SPL) at a reference point in the sound field, be electrically isolated so that circuit or line noise is not amplified, and have very low distortion especially at very high output levels.

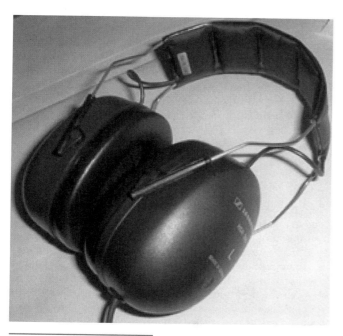

Figure 10–3 Sennheiser HDA 200 circumaural earphones. (With permission of Sennheiser Electronic Corporation, Old Lyme, CT.)

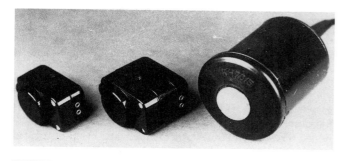

Figure 10–4 *Left to right*, Radioear B-71 and B-72 and Pracitronic KH 70 bone vibrators. (With permission of the American Speech-Language-Hearing Association, Rockville, MD.)

Bone Vibrators

A bone vibrator consists of an electromagnetic transducer having a plane circular tip area of 175 ± 25 mm^2 conforming to ISO (389(3)-1994) and ANSI (S3.6-1996) specifications. However, bone vibrators differ in size, shape, weight, input impedance, encapsulation, and frequency response. Figure 10–4 shows a Radioear B-71 and B-72 and a Pracitronic KH 70 bone vibrator. The B-71 weighs 20 g, whereas the B-72 weighs 48 g because it contains an added dynamic mass. Both the B-71 and B-72 have an input impedance of 10 ohms and are encapsulated in a plastic case. The KH 70 is manufactured in Germany, weighs 96 g, has an input impedance of 20 ohms, and is encapsulated in a cylindrical rubber housing.

The Radioear B-71 is the most commonly used bone vibrator in the United States. The electromagnetic transducer in the B-71 is connected to the inside back of its plastic case so that the entire case vibrates when the transducer is activated.

The frequency response of a Radioear B-71 is characterized by three resonant peaks at 450, 1500, and 3800 Hz that decrease in amplitude as frequency increases followed by a sharp drop in output above 4000 Hz (Richards & Frank, 1982). Thus bone-conduction testing with the B-71 is typically conducted from 250 to 4000 Hz. Like the B-71, the frequency response of a B-72 is characterized by three resonant peaks; however, the peaks occur at lower frequencies (250, 1350, and 3400 Hz) because of the added dynamic mass (Frank, et al, 1988). However, the B-72 presents several clinical problems because it tends to slip off the mastoid process as a result of its weight, especially with small children (Billings & Winter, 1977). The frequency response of the KH 70 is characterized by one major resonance at 200 Hz followed by a gradual decline in output. For the same input voltage, the overall output of the KH 70 is less than the B-71 and B-72 from 100 to 8000 Hz (Frank et al, 1988). However, the frequency response of a KH 70 is relatively flat from 8000 to 16,000 Hz and can be used for testing high-frequency (8000 to 16,000 Hz) bone-conduction thresholds (Richter & Frank, 1985).

When fitted, a bone vibrator can be placed on the mastoid or forehead using a headband. ANSI S3.6-1996 specifies the static headband force as 5.4 ± 0.5 N for either mastoid or forehead placement. The headband force can be measured with the same test fixture as done for supra-aural earphones, except the horizontal separation for forehead placement is 190 mm.

General Requirements

ANSI S3.6-1996 specifies that audiometers are required to have a stable output for temperatures ranging from 15° to 35°C (59° to 95°F) and for humidities from 30 to 90%. Furthermore, all audiometers must meet several safety requirements so that an electrical shock and external electrostatic or electromagnetic interference will not endanger the patient or audiologist or invalidate the test results. For battery-powered audiometers, manufacturers must provide an indicator showing if the battery is providing the appropriate voltage.

All audiometers are required to have several markings or labels. If an audiometer is calibrated to ANSI S3.6-1996 specifications, the marking *ANSI/ISO Hearing Level* must appear on the front panel or hearing level control. Furthermore, the standard requires that the audiometer type must be displayed on the front panel. It should be noted that one audiometer may meet several type designations. For example, the designation 1A would mean that the audiometer meets the minimum requirements for a type 1 pure tone and type A speech audiometer. If the audiometer also meets the minimum requirements for an extended high-frequency audiometer, the type designation would be 1HFA. If the audiometer also meets the minimum requirements for free field equivalent testing, the type designation would be 1HFAE. ANSI S3.6-1996 also requires that the maximum HL at each frequency should be marked on the frequency control if the audiometer does not automatically limit the HL output at each frequency. In addition, the name of the manufacturer, model number, serial number, transducers to be used with the audiometer, country of origin, and safety standards must be marked on the audiometer.

An instruction manual must be provided with each audiometer, and it is required that manufacturers include information as to how the audiometer and/or transducers meet several ANSI S3.6-1996 specifications. Interested readers should review ANSI S3.6-1996, Clause 10.2.

PEARL

Audiologists should read the instruction manual before using the audiometer. Then audiologists should reread the instruction manual as they are learning to use all the audiometer's features.

CALIBRATION INSTRUMENTATION

An electroacoustic calibration is conducted by measuring performance characteristics of an audiometer and each transducer with couplers and electronic instrumentation. If the measured values agree with the standardized values specified in ANSI S3.6-1996, the audiometer is said to be calibrated or operating within ANSI specifications. An electroacoustic calibration involves measuring output levels, attenuator linearity, frequency accuracy, distortion, tone switching, masking levels, frequency response, and other performance characteristics that could influence the test results.

All audiometers should (1) undergo an exhaustive calibration before they are used and thereafter at least once a year or sooner if there is reason to believe the output has changed, (2) be calibrated when the audiometer and transducers are in their customary locations, (3) be placed on a routine calibration schedule, (4) be calibrated quarterly for output level, and (5) be evaluated daily using inspection and listening checks. All of the calibration measurements, history of repair, and inspection and listening checks should be documented. This will assist in determining how well an audiometer remains in calibration and if a continual problem is occurring. Older audiometers, portable audiometers, and audiometers moved from one site to another (e.g., audiometers in a mobile testing unit) should be calibrated with more regularity because they are more susceptible to being damaged. Audiology clinics accredited by professional organizations or doing work regulated by law should check the time intervals for audiometer calibration required by these organizations or in the law.

The basic calibration instrumentation includes (1) couplers, (2) a sound level meter (SLM) having one-third octave band filters, (3) a voltmeter, (4) an electronic counter/timer, and (5) an oscilloscope. Other instrumentation such as an spectrum analyzer, distortion meter, and overshoot, rise/fall, and envelope detectors can also be used. Several manufacturers have developed audiometer calibration kits that include individual instruments or instruments packaged into an integrated unit. Unfortunately, the cost of calibration instruments may be prohibitive for most audiology clinics that would require purchasing a calibration service. However, an SLM having one-third octave band filters for measuring the output of a transducers and ambient noise levels and acoustic couplers used for measuring the output of supra-aural or insert earphones should be considered standard instrumentation for all audiology clinics. The following provides a discussion of couplers and calibration instruments. For a more in-depth discussion the reader is referred to Curtis and Schultz (1986) and Decker (1990).

Types of Couplers

Couplers are standardized devices used for measuring the output of transducers. They can be classified as acoustic or mechanical. Acoustic couplers are used for earphone measurements, have a standardized shape and volume, contain a calibrated microphone, and include the National Bureau of Standards (NBS) 9-A, IEC 318, Hearing Aid (HA) type 1 and 2, and an occluded ear simulator. A mechanical coupler has a standardized mechanical impedance and contains an electromechanical transducer for measuring the force level of a bone vibrator.

NBS 9-A Coupler

The NBS 9-A coupler (ANSI S3.7-1995) shown in Figure 10–5 is used to measure the output of a supra-aural earphone. Placing a supra-aural earphone on the top of the coupler creates an enclosed volume of air that *couples* the earphone to a calibrated microphone at the bottom of the coupler. The enclosed volume of air is 6 cc and was chosen to approximate the volume of air between the diaphragm of a supra-aural earphone and the tympanic membrane (Corliss & Burkhard, 1953). Thus the NBS 9-A coupler has been called a 6-cc coupler or an artificial ear. However, the NBS 9-A coupler does not simulate the acoustic impedance of a human ear over the entire frequency range (Corliss & Burkhard, 1953) and should not be considered as a true artificial ear. Several studies have demonstrated that the SPL developed in a NBS 9-A coupler is different than measured in real-ears (Hawkins, Cooper, & Thompson, 1990; Killion 1978; Zwislocki, 1970, 1971). Furthermore, because of its size, shape, and hard walls, the NBS 9-A coupler has a natural resonance around 6000 Hz and standing waves may occur within the coupler at frequencies higher than 6000 Hz (Rudmose, 1964). Despite its shortcomings, the NBA 9-A coupler is the accepted device for measuring the output of supra-aural earphones because it produces highly repeatable results. When measurements are obtained, a supra-aural earphone is positioned on the top of the coupler and a 500 g weight is placed on top of the earphone to simulate the static headband force.

PEARL

Placing a small circular level on top of a 500-g weight used to load a supra-aural earphone will help position the diaphragm of the earphone parallel to the diaphragm of the microphone in an NBS 9A coupler.

IEC 318 Coupler

To promote international uniformity, ANSI S3.6-1996 recognizes that the output of a supra-aural earphone can also be measured with an IEC 318 coupler (IEC 318-1970). The IEC 318 coupler contains three acoustically coupled cavities and a calibrated microphone. The acoustical properties of the IEC 318 coupler simulate the average human ear from 20 to 10000 Hz and can be used for measuring the output of physically dissimilar supra-aural earphones. When measurements are obtained, a supra-aural earphone is positioned on the top of the coupler and loaded with a 500-g weight.

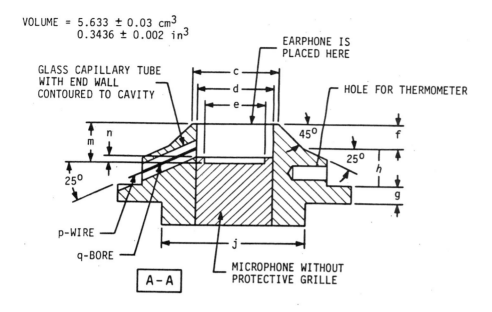

VOLUME = 5.633 ± 0.03 cm³
0.3436 ± 0.002 in³

		Dimensions			
	in	cm		in	cm
a	2.874	7.30	g	0.187	0.475
b	2.252	5.72	h	0.490	1.245
c	1.00	2.54	j	1.750	4.445
	+0	+0	m	0.528	1.3410
	−0.1	−0.025		±0.001	±0.0025
d	0.938	2.3825	n	0.077	0.195
	±0.0006	±0.0015			
e	0.728	1.85	p (dia)	0.016	0.041
f	0.295	0.75	q (dia)	0.024	0.061

Figure 10–5 National Bureau of Standards 9-A coupler used for the calibration of supra-aural earphones. (From ANSI S3.7-1995 with permission of the Acoustical Society of America, New York, NY.)

The IEC 318 coupler can be adapted to measure the output of a circumaural earphone by mounting either a type 1 or 2 flat plate adaptor on the top of the coupler as described in ANSI S3.6-1996, Annex C. When measurements are obtained, the circumaural earphone is positioned on the flat plate and loaded with a 900- to 1000-g weight. To differentiate between an NBS 9-A and IEC 318 coupler, ANSI S3.6-1996 refers to the NBS 9-A as an acoustic coupler and to the IEC 318 as an artificial ear.

Hearing Aid Couplers and Occluded Ear Simulator

A hearing aid type 1 coupler (HA-1) or a hearing aid type 2 coupler (HA-2) with rigid tube attachment (ANSI S3.7-1995) or an occluded ear simulator (ANSI S3.25-1989 [R 1995], IEC 711-1981) can used for measuring the output of an insert earphone. Both the HA-1 and HA-2 couplers contain an effective volume of air of 2 cc and a calibrated microphone; however, the HA-2 also contains an earmold substitute and tube adaptor. Thus these couplers are also called 2-cc couplers. An occluded ear simulator contains acoustically coupled cavities and a calibrated microphone. Figure 10–6 shows how an insert earphone is connected to these couplers. For the occluded ear simulator or the HA-2 with entrance through a rigid tube, the

insert earphone eartip is removed and the nipple is connected to the tube adaptor of the coupler through a 5-mm long piece of No. 13 tubing so that the nipple outlet will be held tightly and flush against the inlet of the tube adaptor. For the HA-1 coupler, the end of the eartip is sealed to the top of the HA-1 cavity so that the eartip opening is centered over the cavity inlet hole.

PEARL

The easiest and perhaps most efficient way to measure the performance characteristics of an insert earphone is to use an HA-2 coupler with rigid tube attachment.

Mechanical Coupler

A mechanical coupler is used for measuring the output of a bone vibrator. Because a bone vibrator is typically placed on the mastoid, a mechanical coupler is often called an artificial mastoid. However, a mechanical coupler is also called an artificial headbone because a bone vibrator can also be placed on

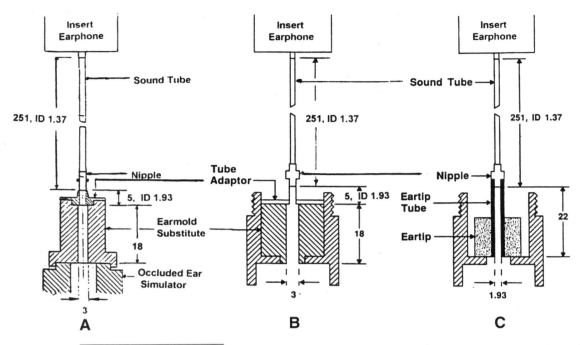

Figure 10–6 Couplers used for the calibration of insert earphones: **(A)** occluded ear simulator, **(B)** hearing aid type 2 coupler with rigid tube attachment, **(C)** hearing aid type 1 coupler. (From ANSI S3.6-1996 with permission of the Acoustical Society of America, New York, NY.)

the forehead. ANSI S3.13-1987 (R 1997) and IEC 373-1990 specify the design characteristics of a mechanical coupler that are met by a Bruel & Kjaer (B&K) 4930 artificial mastoid. Furthermore, the standards specify the mechanical impedance of the coupler that should be presented to a bone vibrator and a device for measuring the alternating force level produced by the bone vibrator. Figure 10–7 shows a schematic diagram of a B&K 4930 mechanical coupler. The original B&K 4930 had mechanical impedance values within the range specified in ANSI S3.13-1987 (R 1997) and IEC 373-1990, except around 3000 Hz. Unfortunately, the impedance of the coupler's rubber pad was found to be susceptible to aging and was replaced in 1975. The new pad had significantly higher mechanical impedance values than specified in ANSI S3.13-1987 (1997) and IEC 373-1990 (Dirks et al, 1979). Another problem with the B&K 4930 is that its output is temperature dependent, especially in the higher frequencies (Frank & Richter, 1985). Thus ANSI and IEC standards specify that the temperature of the mechanical coupler should be 23° ± 1°C (71.6° to 75.2°F) when it is used to calibrate the output of a bone vibrator. Even though the B&K 4930 does not conform to ANSI and IEC standards, it is still the most common device for measuring the output of a bone vibrator. When measurements are obtained, a circular-tipped bone vibrator is positioned on the top of the coupler and loaded with a 550-g weight.

Sound Level Meter

An SLM combines a microphone, amplifying circuits, and a meter into one unit and is used to measure the SPL developed in an acoustic coupler by earphones or in a sound field by a loudspeaker. ANSI S1.4-1983 (R 1994) specifies several types of

---

PITFALL

It cannot be assumed that the output of a mechanical coupler will remain stable from year to year. Like all measurement instrumentation, a mechanical coupler needs to be recalibrated to ensure that its output is stable.

SLM on the basis of features they contain. For audiometer calibration, a type 1 SLM having one-third octave band filters (re: ANSI S1.11-1986, R 1993) and a condenser microphone should be used. A type 1 SLM has two response integration times reflected by the ballistics of the meter called slow and fast. The slow response is useful for measuring signals that have level fluctuations typically greater than 4 dB as would be the case for masking signals or ambient noise. The fast response is used to measure signals having little or no level fluctuations such as pure tones. One-third octave band filtering is used because the filtering allows for measuring only the sounds contained within a very narrow frequency range and excludes the contribution of other sounds having frequencies outside the bandwith of the filter. A condenser microphone has low noise levels, a flat frequency response over a wide range of frequencies, and operates in a linear manner over a wide intensity range. A pressure condenser microphone should be used for all coupler measurements, whereas a sound field condenser microphone should be used for all loudspeaker measurements. Condenser microphones are sensitive to temperature and humidity, which must be taken into account

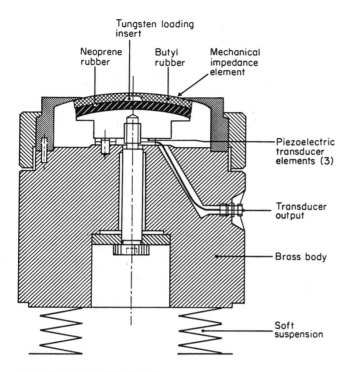

Figure 10–7   Bruel and Kjaer 4930 mechanical coupler used for the calibration of bone vibrators. (From ANSI S3.13-1987 [R 1997] with permission of the Acoustical Society of America, New York, NY.)

when an SLM is calibrated. An SLM is calibrated by placing a pistonphone, sound level calibrator, or acoustic calibrator over the microphone. These devices generate a known SPL output(s) at one or more frequencies (ANSI S1.40-1984 [R 1994]). The SLM reading should be adjusted to the output of the calibrator. Keeping track of the SLM calibration when done with a multiple-frequency calibrator is a very good idea. This provides a quick check of the frequency response of the microphone at two or more frequencies, which could change over time because of aging and variables associated with physically handling the microphone.

PEARL

When not in use, microphones should be stored in a low-humidity environment. This can be done by placing microphones in a sealed jar containing materials that act to reduce the humidity and eliminate condensation, which could influence the performance of the microphone.

Voltmeter

A voltmeter is used to measure the output of an electronic device. Because the acoustic output of a transducer follows the waveform and is directly proportional to the input voltage, except in nonlinear ranges, voltmeters can be used to determine whether a problem exists with a transducer, cord, or the audiometer. For audiometer calibration, a voltmeter should have a very high impedance (e.g., megaohm range) so that it will not influence the circuit load it is measuring, read the output in true root-mean-square, have a decibel scale, and have a sensitivity between 0.01 mV to 120 V. Some SLMs can also function as voltmeters.

When a voltmeter is used, the voltage is typically measured between the audiometer and transducer so that the audiometer continues to be loaded by the transducer. This can be done using a Y-patch cord where each end of the Y has a receptacle called a phone jack and the other end has a phone plug. In use, the patch cord phone plug is inserted into the appropriate audiometer output, the phone plug of the transducer is inserted into one of the patch cord phone jacks, and the voltmeter is inserted into the other phone jack. Whenever an electrical measurement is conducted, it is assumed that the transducer cord and transducer are functioning normally.

Electronic Counter/Timer

An electronic counter/timer is used to provide measurements of frequency and time. These devices typically measure frequency to within ±1 Hz and time intervals to within hundredths of a second.

Oscilloscope

An oscilloscope can be used for several purposes (e.g., as a voltmeter, timer, frequency monitor); however, its primary use is for measuring tone-switching performance characteristics, including rise/fall times, overshoot, and pulse durations. Because an oscilloscope is capable of measuring very low-level voltages, it can also be used for measuring whether a signal directed to one output crosses over to another output. However, this could also be done with a voltmeter using low-sensitivity settings. The most desirable oscilloscope would be one that has two channels capable of storing signals, a bandwidth from DC to 100 kHz, voltage sensitivity ranging from 0.5 mV to 10 V, time base from 1 ms to 1 s, and internal and external triggers. Unfortunately, an adequate oscilloscope is somewhat expensive. As an alternative, rise/fall time, overshoot, and/or envelope detectors are available from several manufacturers at a relatively low price. If these devices are used, they must be sensitive enough to measure the rise/fall times and overshoot specified in ANSI S3.6-1996.

SPECIAL CONSIDERATION

The instruments used for calibration must be calibrated to ensure that they have significantly less measurement error than the standardized tolerances for each performance characteristic.

PERFORMANCE CHARACTERISTICS OF PURE TONE AUDIOMETERS

Output Levels

The output levels of audiometer transducers must be calibrated to standardized reference threshold levels shown in Table 10–3. For air-conduction transducers, the reference

TABLE 10–3 Reference threshold levels for different transducer types (from ANSI S3.6-1996 with permission of the Acoustical Society of America, New York, NY)

Transducer Type, Coupler	\multicolumn{12}{c}{Frequency (Hz)}
	125	250	500	750	1000	1500	2000	3000	4000	6000	8000	Speech
TDH Type, IEC 318*	45.0	27.0	13.5	9.0	7.5	7.5	9.0	11.5	12.0	16.0	15.5	20.0
THD 39, NBS 9-A*	45.0	25.5	11.5	8.0	7.0	6.5	9.0	10.0	9.5	15.5	13.0	19.5
TDH 49/50, NBS 9-A*	47.5	26.6	13.5	8.5	7.5	7.5	11.0	9.5	10.5	13.5	13.0	20.0
Insert Earphone, OES*,†	28.0	17.5	9.5	6.0	5.5	9.5	11.5	13.0	15.0	16.0	15.5	18.0
Insert Earphone, HA-1*	26.5	14.5	6.0	2.0	0.0	0.0	2.5	2.5	0.0	−2.5	−3.5	12.5
Insert Earphone, HA-2*	26.0	14.0	5.5	2.0	0.0	2.0	3.0	3.5	5.5	2.0	0.0	12.5
Loudspeaker‡, Bin at 0 degrees	22.0	11.0	4.0	2.0	2.0	0.5	−1.5	−6.0	−6.5	2.5	11.5	14.5
Loudspeaker‡, Mon at 0 degrees	24.0	13.0	6.0	4.0	4.0	2.5	0.5	−4.0	−4.5	4.5	13.5	16.5
Loudspeaker‡, Mon at 45 degrees	23.5	12.0	3.0	0.5	0.0	−1.0	−2.5	−9.0	−8.5	−3.0	8.0	12.5
Loudspeaker‡, Mon 90 degrees	23.0	11.0	1.5	−1.0	−1.5	−2.5	−1.5	−6.5	−4.0	−5.0	5.5	11.0
Bone Vibrator§, Mastoid	—	67.0	58.0	48.5	42.5	36.5	31.0	30.0	35.5	40.0	40.0	55.0
Bone Vibrator§, Forehead	—	79.0	72.0	61.5	51.0	47.5	42.5	42.0	43.5	51.0	50.0	63.5

*In dB re: 20 μPa.
†Occluded ear simulator.
‡In dB re: 20 μPa at reference point at least 1 m from loudspeaker.
§In dB re: 1 μN using Bruel & Kjaer, 4930 mechanical coupler.

threshold levels are called reference equivalent threshold sound pressure levels (RETSPLs) and for bone-conduction transducers they are called reference equivalent threshold force levels (RETFLs). RETSPLs are the SPLs measured in an acoustic coupler, and RETFLs are the force levels measured on a mechanical coupler, that are equal to the mean hearing thresholds of otologically normal individuals of both genders from 18 to 30 years old. Stated another way, RETSPLs are the SPLs and RETFLs are the force levels that are equal to normal-hearing or 0 dB HL. However, RETSPLs and RETFLs are not measured at 0 dB HL. This occurs because air-conduction and bone-conduction transducers have very low output levels at 0 dB HL, which may exceed the lower limits of the measurement instrumentation, and ambient noise might influence the measurements for air-conduction transducers. Thus RETSPLs are typically measured at 70 dB HL so that the transducer output level will be within the range of the measurement instrumentation and well above the ambient noise level. RETFLs are typically measured at 20 dB HL at 250 Hz and 50 dB HL from 500 to 4000 Hz.

Because it is impossible and impractical for all transducers and measurement instruments to perform exactly the same, an acceptable variation, error, or tolerance is allowed for each performance characteristic. The tolerance for all reference threshold levels is ±3 dB from 125 to 5000 Hz and ±5 dB at 6000 Hz and higher. In theory, it would be possible to have an output level difference between earphones of 6 dB from 125 to 5000 Hz and 10 dB at 6000 Hz and above and still be within tolerance. However, this might be detrimental to interpreting differences between ears and for determining a change in

hearing sensitivity from one test to another. If this extreme situation occurs or if the transducer output is higher or lower than the tolerance, the output of the audiometer is too strong or too weak. However, the transducer phone plug, cord, or the transducer itself could be malfunctioning. All microprocessor-based audiometers have a calibration mode for changing transducer output levels. Older audiometers have adjustable potentiometers, or it may be necessary to replace some internal resistors to obtain the desired output level.

As a general rule, if the transducer output is greater than ±2.5 dB compared with the reference threshold level and cannot be changed during the calibration process, audiologists should develop a correction card as shown in Figure 10–8. This occurs even though the tolerance is ±3 from 125 to 5000 Hz and ±5 dB at 6000 Hz and higher. The correction card indicates adjustments, rounded to the nearest 5 dB at each frequency, that must be made to the HL setting when a patient is tested. If the transducer output is lower than the reference threshold level, the amount of deviation is subtracted from the HL setting. For example, the RETSPL at 1000 Hz for a TDH 49/50 earphone is 7.5 dB SPL (Table 10–3). If the HL control is set at 70 dB, the earphone output should be 77.5 dB SPL. If the measured output was 72.5 dB, the audiometer output is 5 dB too low. Testing a patient with a true threshold of 60 dB would have resulted in a threshold of 65 dB. To eliminate this inaccuracy, a correction of −5 dB is applied to the patient's threshold of 65 dB so that the patient's true threshold of 60 dB is recorded on the audiogram. If the transducer output level is higher than the reference threshold level, the amount of the deviation is added to the HL setting. Using the

Penn State University, Speech and Hearing Clinic, 110 Moore Building, University Park, PA 16802
Audiometer Output Level Correction Card

Audiometer: _____ Serial No: _____ Channel: _____ Date: _____

Frequency	Transducer Type					
	Right Earphone	Left Earphone	Right Insert Earphone	Left Insert Earphone	Bone Vib Mastoid	Bone Vib Forehead
125						
250						
500						
750						
1000						
1500						
2000						
3000						
4000						
6000						
8000						
Speech						

NEGATIVE table value means audiometer output is too weak; make threshold better/Hearing Level setting lowered by table value.

POSITIVE table value means audiometer output is too strong; make threshold worse/Hearing Level setting increased by table value.

Figure 10–8 Audiometer output level correction card.

previous example, if the measured output was 82.5 dB SPL instead of 77.5 dB SPL, the output is 5 dB too high. Testing the patient with a true threshold of 60 dB would have resulted in a threshold of 55 dB. Thus a correction of +5 dB is applied so that the patient's true threshold of 60 dB will be recorded on the audiogram. If a correction of more than 10 dB is needed, the audiometer should be repaired and recalibrated.

PITFALL

The danger of using a correction card is that it may get lost or the correction may not be applied to a patient's threshold. If a correction card is used, it should be tightly secured to the audiometer.

Supra-Aural Earphones

The output levels of a supra-aural earphone are measured by placing the earphone on either an NBS 9-A or IEC 318 coupler loaded with a 500-g weight. The coupler microphone is connected to a SLM. If the SLM has one-third octave band filters, the filter is adjusted to the frequency of the pure tone being measured. The position of the earphone is checked by directing a continuous 125 or 250 Hz tone at 70 dB HL to the earphone while it is adjusted to a position that produces the highest SPL. After this, the SPL is measured at each frequency for each earphone and recorded on a calibration form (Appendix B, Form 1). If the audiometer has two channels, the measurements are repeated using the other channel. After each individual measurement, the measured SPL is checked against the RETSPL plus 70 dB for the earphone type and coupler used during the measurements. This is done to determine whether the earphone output level is in calibration. For example, at 2000 Hz the RETSPL for a TDH 49/50 earphone measured in a NBS 9A coupler is 11.0 dB SPL. Because the HL was set at 70 dB, the measured SPL should be 81.0 dB SPL. If the measured SPL is not within ±2.5 dB of the RETSPL plus 70 dB (e.g., 81 dB SPL), the earphone output level should be adjusted using the audiometer's internal calibration mode. This is done so that the measured SPL is within ±2.5 dB of the

RETSPL plus 70 dB, even though the tolerance is ±3 dB from 125 to 5000 Hz and ±5 dB at 6000 Hz and higher. If this is not possible, a correction card (Fig. 10–8) should be developed.

Insert Earphones

The output levels of an insert earphone (Etymotic ER-3A or E-A-RTONE 3A) are measured by connecting the insert earphone to an occluded ear simulator, HA-1, or HA-2 coupler with rigid tube attachment as shown in Figure 10–6. The procedures used for measuring insert earphone output levels are the same as those for a supra-aural earphone and the coupler output SPLs should be recorded on a calibration form (Appendix B, Form 1). For example, at 1000 Hz the output level of an insert earphone measured in a HA-2 coupler with rigid tube attachment should be 70.0 dB SPL because the RETSPL is 0.0 dB SPL and the audiometer was set at 70 dB HL.

The insert earphone RETSPLs specified in ANSI S3.6-1996 (Table 10–3) were taken directly from the insert earphone RETSPLs specified in ISO 389(2)-1994. The ISO RETSPLs were based on the mean insert earphone threshold levels reported from three studies (Brinkman & Richter, 1990). The ANSI 1996 RETSPLs are not the same as the interim insert earphone RETSPLs specified in ANSI S3.6-1989 Appendix G. The interim ANSI RETSPLs were those suggested by the manufacturer and reported by Wilber et al, (1988). Table 10–4 shows the ANSI S3.6-1996 RETSPLs, the interim 1989 RETSPLs, and the threshold differences. The ANSI S3.6-1996 RETSPLs are lower than the interim 1989 RETSPLs, especially from 500 to 4000 Hz. Frank and Vavrek (1992) reported insert earphone thresholds and combined their results with eight other studies, including the three studies used to specify the ISO RETSPLs, to develop a nine-study database. They found that the mean threshold levels for the nine-study database were in closer agreement with the interim 1989 ANSI RETSPLs (e.g., manufacturer's levels) than the ISO RETSPLs used in ANSI S3.6-1996.

TABLE 10–4 **Insert earphone RETSPLs reported in ANSI S3.6-1996, interim RETSPLs reported in ANSI S3.6-1989 (Appendix G), and the threshold differences using a HA-2 coupler with rigid tube attachment**

Frequency (Hz)	ANSI S3.6-1996	ANSI S3.6-1989	Difference
125	26.0	27.0	−1.0
250	14.0	15.0	−1.0
500	5.5	8.0	−2.5
750	2.0	6.0	−4.0
1000	0.0	3.5	−3.5
1500	2.0	5.0	−3.0
2000	3.0	6.5	−3.5
3000	3.5	6.0	−2.5
4000	5.5	7.0	−1.5
6000	2.0	3.0	−1.0
8000	0.0	0.0	−1.0

> ### CONTROVERSIAL POINT
>
> Even though the ANSI S3.6-1996 insert earphone RETSPLs are lower than the interim ANSI 1989 RETSPLs and are not supported by a nine-study database (Frank & Vavrek, 1992), they were included in ANSI S3.6-1996 to promote international uniformity.

Type 1 pure tone audiometers are required to have insert earphones (Table 10–1). Thus the insert earphone output level can be adjusted to meet the ANSI S3.6-1996 RETSPLs using the audiometer's internal calibration mode. However, for other types of pure tone audiometers insert earphones are typically connected to the audiometer's output jacks normally used for supra-aural earphones. If this is done, the manufacturer has recommended *plug-in* correction values because the audiometer *thinks* that supra-aural earphones are still being used. Because the ANSI S3.6-1996 insert earphone RETSPLs are lower than suggested by the manufacturer, the use of the manufacturers *plug-in* correction values will no longer be valid for many frequencies. To be precise, audiologists should measure the coupler output of each insert earphone at each frequency and determine their own correction values, which should be listed on a correction card (Fig. 10-8) attached to the audiometer. Recall, if the measured level is lower than the reference level, the amount of deviation is rounded to the nearest 5 dB and subtracted. If the measured level is higher than the reference level, the amount of the deviation is added to the HL setting.

Circumaural Earphones

The output levels of a circumaural earphone are measured by placing the earphone on an IEC 318 coupler equipped with the appropriate flat plate coupler loaded with a 900 to 1000-g weight. The coupler microphone is connected to an SLM. At each frequency, the HL is set so that the measurements will not be influenced by environmental ambient noise. ANSI has not *officially* standardized hearing testing with circumaural earphones. However, ANSI S3.6-1996 Annex C provides interim RETSPLs for a Sennheiser HDA200 from 125 to 16000 Hz and for a Koss HV/1A at 1000 and 4000 Hz and from 8000 to 16,000 Hz. As done for supra-aural earphones, the measured SPL for each frequency and earphone is checked against the RETSPL plus the HL setting to determine whether the earphone output is in calibration. If the measured SPL is not within ±2.5 dB of the desired level (i.e., RETSPL plus HL setting), the earphone output level should be adjusted using the audiometer's internal calibration mode. If this is not possible, a correction card should be developed showing the HL adjustments for each frequency and earphone that will have to be made when a patient's threshold is recorded on an audiogram.

Bone Vibrators

The output levels of a bone vibrator are measured by placing the bone vibrator on a mechanical coupler loaded with a weight or spring-tension device that will produce a force of

5.4 N. The output of the mechanical coupler is connected to a voltmeter having a decibel scale calibrated in µN. Typically, bone vibrators are calibrated for mastoid placement and a correction (dB difference between forehead minus mastoid RETFLs, Table 10–3) is applied if testing is done using forehead placement. Furthermore, the audiometer HL is set to 20 dB HL at 250 Hz and 50 dB HL at higher frequencies. The force level is measured at each frequency and recorded on a calibration form (Appendix B, Form 1). After each individual measurement, the measured level is checked against the RETFL plus the HL setting. For example, at 1000 Hz with the audiometer set to 50 dB HL, the measured force level for mastoid placement should be 92.5 dB re: 1µN because the RETFL at 1000 Hz is 42.5 dB and the audiometer was set at 50 dB HL. If the measured force level is not within ±2.5 dB the desired output level (RETFL plus HL setting), the bone vibrator output should be adjusted using the audiometer's internal calibration mode or a correction card should be developed. The ANSI S3.6-1996 RETFLs are the same as those specified in ANSI S3.43-1992 and ISO 389(3)-1994. Because ANSI S3.6-1996 contains the same information as reported in ANSI S3.43-1992, ANSI S3.43-1992 has been withdrawn as a standard.

CONTROVERSIAL POINT

The ANSI S3.6-1996 RETFLs are for any bone vibrator having a plane circular tip with a nominal area of 175 ± 25 mm^2 applied with a static headband force of 5.4 ± 0.5 N. This occurred even though Frank et al (1988) reported that thresholds with a Radioear B-72 and Pracitronic KH 70 were about 10 dB higher at 250 Hz and about 5 dB lower at 500 Hz than a Radioear B-71 bone vibrator.

Loudspeakers

Before measuring the output levels of a loudspeaker, a decision has to be made as to whether to calibrate the loudspeaker output to RETSPLs for binaural or monaural listening. Historically, audiologists have used reference thresholds for monaural listening. In part, this is done so that sound field thresholds can be compared with monaural air-conduction thresholds. If the decision is made for monaural listening, then a decision is needed concerning the placement of a loudspeaker relative to the patient. Typically, if one loudspeaker is used, it should be located at 0 degrees azimuth. If two loudspeakers are used, the location for each loudspeaker should be 45 degrees azimuth on either side of the patient; however, some audiologists use a position of 90 degrees on either side of the patient.

ANSI S3.6-1996 specifies that the loudspeaker should be positioned to the head height of a seated patient and that output level measurements be done at a reference point at least 1 m from the loudspeaker. Typically, the reference point is permanently marked with a dot on the ceiling or floor or by hanging a plumb-bob from the ceiling. This is done because the reference point is where the middle of the patient's head would normally be located during testing. If two loudspeakers are used, they should have the same reference point.

Loudspeaker output levels are measured by substituting an SLM at the reference point so that sound from the loudspeaker will pass across the top of the SLM microphone. Furthermore, the audiometer is set to produce a test signal at 70 dB HL so that ambient noise will not influence the measurements. The SPL or one-third octave band SPL is measured at each frequency for each loudspeaker and each signal type to be used during testing and recorded on a calibration form (Appendix B, Form 2). After each individual measurement, the measured level is checked against the RETSPL plus 70 dB. For example, at 1000 Hz for monaural listening at 45 degrees the measured level should be 70 dB SPL because the RETSPL is 0.0 dB SPL and the hearing level was set at 70 dB. If the measured output level is not within ±2.5 dB of the RETSPL plus 70 dB, the loudspeaker output level should be adjusted using the audiometer's internal calibration mode or a correction card should be developed.

The ANSI S3.6-1996 RETSPLs for sound field testing (Table 10–3) were taken directly from ISO389(7)-1994. Because ANSI did not specify RETSPLs for sound field testing until 1996, audiologists have used reference threshold levels specified in the literature (Morgan et al, 1979; Walker et al, 1984) or the levels recommended in a 1991 ASHA tutorial. Table 10–5 lists the ANSI S3.6-1996 monaural sound field RETSPLs, the reference threshold levels recommended by ASHA in 1991, and the differences. The ANSI RETSPLs are lower than the ASHA 1991 reference threshold levels especially for 90 degrees azimuth.

CONTROVERSIAL POINT

Even though audiologists are using the sound field reference threshold levels recommended in a 1991 ASHA tutorial, the ANSI S3.6-1996 sound field reference thresholds are lower than the ASHA recommended levels. This occurs because the ANSI thresholds were taken from an ISO standard to promote international uniformity.

ANSI S3.6-1996 also specifies that measurements for each frequency, loudspeaker, and signal type must be done at several locations around the reference point. This is done to ensure that the SPL around the patient's head is stable. Specifically, measurements must be done at 0.15 m (6 inches) from the reference point on a left-right and up-down axis and must be within ±2 dB of the SPL at the reference point for any test signal. Furthermore, measurements must be done at 0.10 m (4 inches) in front and behind the reference point. The decibel difference between the front and behind measurements can deviate from the theoretical value given by the inverse square law by no more than ±1 dB for any test signal.

Attenuator Linearity

Measuring attenuator linearity is done to be sure that changes in the HL result in the same changes in the audiometer's output level. Attenuator linearity can be measured acoustically or electrically. For two-channel audiometers, the linearity of each attenuator must be measured. If attenuator linearity is

TABLE 10–5 Monaural sound field RETSPLs reported in ANSI S3.6-1996, ASHA-1991, and the threshold differences

Source	Frequency (Hz)											Speech
	125	250	500	750	1000	1500	2000	3000	4000	6000	8000	
Monaural at 0 degrees												
ANSI S3.6 (1996)	24.0	13.0	6.0	4.0	4.0	2.5	0.5	−4.0	−4.5	4.5	13.5	16.5
ASHA (1991)	32.0	16.0	9.5	7.5	5.5	4.5	2.5	.05	1.5	7.5	13.0	16.5
Differences	−8.0	−3.0	−3.5	−3.5	−1.5	−2.0	−2.0	4.5	6.0	−3.0	0.5	0.0
Monaural at 45 degrees												
ANSI S3.6 (1996)	23.5	12.0	3.0	.5	0.0	−1.0	−2.5	−9.0	−8.5	−3.0	8.0	12.5
ASHA (1991)	—	20.5	9.0	0.5	0.9	2.0	−0.5	−4.1	−3.1	3.8	—	12.5
Differences	—	−8.5	−6.0	0.0	−0.9	−3.0	−2.0	−4.9	−5.4	−6.8	—	0.0
Monaural at 90 degrees												
ANSI S3.6 (1996)	23.0	11.0	1.5	−1.0	−1.5	−2.5	−1.5	−6.5	−4.0	−5.0	5.5	11.0
ASHA (1991)	32.0	16.0	7.5	—	3.5	2.0	4.0	0.5	1.0	1.5	9.0	15.0
Differences	−9.0	−5.0	−6.0	—	−5.0	−4.5	−5.5	−7.0	−5.0	−6.5	−3.5	−4.0

SPECIAL CONSIDERATION

Once a sound field is calibrated, additional furniture, instrumentation, or other objects should not be moved or placed in the audiometric test room. If this is done, the sound field should be recalibrated.

measured acoustically, a supra-aural earphone is placed and loaded with a 500-g weight on a NBS-9A coupler connected to an SLM having a one-third octave band filter. The SPL is measured and recorded (Appendix B, Form 3) using a 1000-Hz tone and with the filter set to 1000 Hz, when the HL control is at maximum and for each 5 dB decrement or at 70 dB HL as a reference for each 5 dB step in both directions. At lower HLs, accurate measurements might not be obtained because the coupler SPLs might approach the noise floor of the SLM or the measurement may be influenced by the ambient noise in the room. However, switching to a 125 or 250 Hz test tone and filter setting typically allows for measurements to be completed over the entire HL range.

If attenuator linearity is measured electrically, it is necessary to connect a voltmeter between the output of the audiometer and earphone with a Y-patch cord so the audiometer is loaded with an earphone. Using a 1000 Hz tone, the voltage is measured over the entire HL range in 5 dB steps. This procedure assumes that measuring voltages will provide an accurate indication of the SPL output of an earphone. Thus a transducer having a nonlinear output will not be detected.

ANSI S3.6-1996 specifies that the output level difference between two successive HL settings no more than 5 dB apart cannot deviate by more than three tenths of the indicated difference or more than 1 dB, whichever is smaller. The cumulative error cannot exceed the output tolerance (i.e., ±3 dB from

125 to 5000 Hz and ±5 dB at 6000 Hz and higher). If the attenuator linearity does not meet the ANSI specifications, the cause of the problem should be determined and the audiometer should be repaired and recalibrated.

PEARL

Our experience has shown that some audiometers may exhibit an attenuator nonlinearity at lower HLs at 6000 Hz but demonstrate linearity at 1000 Hz. Thus we check attenuator linearity at both 1000 and 6000 Hz.

Frequency

Accuracy

Pure tone audiometers must accurately produce the frequencies indicated on the frequency control. If this does not occur, the patient would be responding to pure tones having different frequencies than those that the audiologist thought were being presented. Table 10–2 shows the required test frequencies for the different audiometer types; however, audiometers can also have additional frequencies located at one-third octave bands up to 8000 Hz and one-sixth octave bands up to 16,000 Hz. Frequency is measured by connecting an electronic counter/timer between the output of the audiometer and earphone using a Y-patch cord so that the audiometer is loaded with an earphone. The HL is set so that the audiometer's output is sufficient to activate the electronic counter/timer. Frequency is measured for each frequency control setting and is recorded on a calibration form (Appendix B, Form 3). ANSI S3.6-1996 specifies that the measured frequency compared with the frequency indicated on the audiometer must be within ±1% for type 1 and HF, ±2% for type 2, and ±3% for types 3, 4, and 5 audiometers. For example, the measured frequency at 1000 Hz for a type 1 audiometer should be between 990 and 1010 Hz.

Frequency-Modulated Signals

Type 1 and 2 audiometers are required to have frequency-modulated (FM) signals (Table 10–1). FM signals are most commonly used for sound field testing to avoid standing waves and other problems caused by use of pure tone signals. FM signals have three definable characteristics known as the carrier (i.e., center or nominal) frequency, modulation rate, and frequency deviation. ANSI S3.6-1996 specifies that the carrier may be modulated with either a sinusoidal or triangular waveform. The modulation or repetition rate is the number of times the FM signal changes per second and can range from 4 to 20 Hz with a tolerance of ±10% of the value stated by the manufacturer. Frequency deviation refers to the frequency range over which a change occurs for each modulation. ANSI S3.6-1996 specifies frequency deviation in percent around the carrier frequency, which can range from 5 to 25%, with a tolerance of ±10% of the value stated by the manufacturer. Most type 1 and 2 audiometers allow the audiologist to select the frequency deviation; which typically ranges from 1 to 5%. Measuring the characteristics of an FM signal is typically not done during a routine electroacoustic calibration. Interested readers are directed to Walker et al, (1984) and ASHA (1991) for more information.

Harmonic Distortion

Pure tone audiometers must present a *pure* signal that does not contain other frequencies so that the patient will only respond to hearing the frequency of the test tone and not its harmonics. For example, if a 500-Hz tone had excessive harmonics, the patient with an upward sloping audiogram might respond to the 1000 or 1500 Hz harmonic at a lower HL than responding to a 500 Hz tone that did not have excessive harmonics.

Harmonic distortion for each earphone type is measured by mounting the earphone on an appropriate coupler with the coupler microphone connected to an SLM having one-third octave band filters. ANSI S3.6-1996 specifies that harmonic distortion be measured at 75 dB HL at 125 Hz, 90 dB HL at 250 Hz and 6000 to 16,000 Hz, and 110 dB HL at 500 to 4000 Hz or the maximum hearing level, whichever is lower. With the audiometer adjusted to the appropriate HL and the SLM one-third octave band filter adjusted to the test frequency, the earphone SPL is measured and recorded. Then, without changing the audiometer settings, the SLM filter is changed to the second harmonic of the test frequency and the earphone SPL is measured and recorded. If the SLM filter center frequency does not correspond to the frequency of the harmonic, the next higher filter center frequency setting is used. This procedure is repeated until all of the higher frequency harmonics are measured. After this, measurements are obtained for the next frequency and all harmonics and the measurements continue until harmonic distortion has been measured at every audiometer test frequency for each earphone. For bone vibrators, harmonic distortion is measured

using similar procedures, except the bone vibrator is mounted on a mechanical coupler, the coupler output is directed to an analyzing instrument (which could be an SLM having one-third octave band filters) and the HL is set at 20 dB at 250 Hz, 50 dB at 500 and 750 Hz, and at 60 dB at 1000 to 5000 Hz. Harmonic distortion for loudspeakers will be discussed later in this chapter in the "Speech Audiometer" section. The standard recognizes that measurements of harmonics greater than 5000 Hz might be inaccurate because of limitations of acoustic and mechanical couplers and allows for electrical measurements greater than 5000 Hz. A form for recording the results of total harmonic distortion testing is shown in Appendix B as Form 4.

PITFALL

Octave-band filters are not suitable for measuring harmonic distortion because they do not have rejection rates sufficient to measure distortion products lower than 24- to 28-dB below the level of the test tone.

ANSI S3.6-1996 specifies the maximum total harmonic distortion for earphones as ≤2.5% from 125 to 16,000, ≤2% from 125 to 16,000 Hz for the second harmonic and from 125 to 4000 Hz for the third harmonic, ≤0.3% from 125 to 4000 Hz for the fourth and higher harmonics, and ≤0.3% from 250 to 16,000 Hz for all of the subharmonics. For bone vibrators from 250 to 5000 Hz, the maximum total distortion is ≤5.5%, ≤5% for the second harmonic, and ≤2% for third and higher level harmonics. Total harmonic distortion (THD) can be computed with the formula: $\%THD = 100 \sqrt{(p_2^2 + p_3^2 + p_4^2 + ... / p_1^2}$ where p_1 is the sound pressure of the test frequency and p_2, p_3, p_4,... are the sound pressures of the second, third, fourth, etc., harmonics. It is important to note that the "p's" in the formula are sound pressure, not SPLs. Sound pressure and SPL are related by the formula: $SPL = 20 \log_{10} (p/p_o)$, where p_o is the reference sound pressure of 20 μPa; conversely, $p = p_o$ antilog$_{10}$ (SPL/20). The following is an approximation of the percent of distortion corresponding to the decibel difference between the level of the test frequency minus the level of a harmonic: 5.5% = 25 dB, 5.0% = 26 dB, 2.5% = 32 dB, 2.0% = 34 dB, and 0.3% = 50 dB.

SPECIAL CONSIDERATION

Although ANSI S3.6-1996 requires measurements at fourth and higher harmonics and at all subharmonics, it is unlikely to have excessive distortion at these harmonics if the distortion for the second and third harmonics is acceptable. Measurements of distortion at all subharmonics is difficult and requires extremely sensitive measurement instrumentation.

Excessive harmonic distortion is typically due to a problem with the transducer and not the audiometer. Thus the first step to solve a problem with excessive harmonic distortion should be to replace the transducer with one of the same type and repeat the measurements. If the problem was due to the transducer, the audiometer should be completely recalibrated with the new transducer.

Signal Switching

For manual audiometers the pure tone is normally off and is turned on by pressing an interrupter or tone switch. Most audiometers also have another switch that turns the tone on continuously; pressing the interrupter switch turns the tone off. To ensure that the patient is responding only to a pure tone and not other sounds, ANSI S3.6-1996 specifies performance characteristics for on/off ratio, crosstalk, rise/fall times, and overshoot.

On/Off Ratio

Checking the on/off ratio is done to ensure that a tone will not be audible when it is turned off. ANSI S3.6-1996 requires that the earphone output must be 10 dB less than the RETSPL when the tone is off at HL settings ≤60 dB or at least 70 dB less than a HL setting ≤60 dB. The on/off ratio can checked acoustically or electrically. If done acoustically, the HL could be set to maximum and the coupler output should be measured with and without a tone directed to the earphone. If the measurements are done electrically, a Y-patch cord, voltmeter, and dummy resistive load would be required. The phone plug of the Y-patch cord would be inserted into the audiometer's earphone output jack, a voltmeter would be connected to into one jack of the patch cord, and the dummy load would be connected to the other patch cord jack. A dummy resistive load can be made by soldering a resistor equal to the impedance of the transducer at 1000 Hz across the terminals of a phone plug. The tone on minus the tone off one-third octave band SLM readings or voltmeter readings at each frequency should be ≥70 dB and recorded on a calibration form (Appendix B, Form 3).

Crosstalk

Crosstalk or crossover is another form of unwanted noise. Crosstalk occurs when a signal is directed to one earphone but is audible in the other earphone. Crosstalk can be measured acoustically or electrically as done to determine the on/off ratios. The measure is done by turning the tone on at an HL setting ≥70 dB and measuring the acoustical or electrical output in the other or nontest earphone. The measured signal must be at least 70 dB below the level of the signal directed to the test earphone.

Rise/Fall Times and Overshoot

Rise time is the time required for a tone to increase from a turned off to steady-state level. Fall time is the time required for a tone to decrease from a steady state to a turned off level. Overshoot occurs when a tone is turned on or off and temporarily exceeds its steady-state level. ANSI S3.6-1996 requires that the level of a tone that is off should be at least 60 dB less than the level when the tone is on. When the tone is turned on,

the rise time from −60- to −1-dB of the steady-state level cannot exceed 200 ms and from −20- to −1-dB cannot be less than 20 ms. When the tone is turned off, the fall time from 0- to −60-dB of the steady-state level cannot exceed 200 ms and from −1- to −20-dB cannot be less than 20 ms. Only 1 dB of overshoot above the steady state value is allowed when the tone is turned on or off. Verification of the rise/fall times and overshoot can be done electrically by connecting the audiometer output to an oscilloscope with a Y-patch cord so that the audiometer is loaded with an earphone. A calibrated rise/fall detector and/or an overshoot detector could be used in place of an oscilloscope. Typically, testing is done with a 1000 Hz tone; however, it is good practice to also do the measurements at 250 and 6000 Hz. Some older audiometers have switch mechanisms that might produce different rise/fall times as a function of frequency. The standard requires that overshoot should be measured acoustically. However, if overshoot is not observed during the electrical measurements, it is doubtful that it will occur acoustically. To be in compliance with the standard, an acoustic measurement of overshoot should be considered. If this is done, each transducer is placed on an appropriate coupler and the coupler output is connected to an SLM. The output of an SLM is connected to an oscilloscope to measure overshoot and possibly rise/fall times. The measurements for rise/fall time and overshoot should be recorded on a calibration form (Appendix B, Form 3).

> ### PITFALL
>
> **It cannot be assumed that signal switching characteristics will be the same at each frequency. This occurs because some audiometers use a nonoptical keying circuit to turn the tone on and off.**

Pulsed Tones

Type 1, 2, and HF audiometers are required to have a pulsed-tone feature that might be used to obtain threshold or for suprathreshold measures. Typically, a pulsed tone is activated by means of a switch that will automatically pulse a normally continuous tone. For pulsed tones, ANSI S3.6-1996 specifies that the rise time from −20- to −1-dB and the fall time from −1- to −20-dB of the steady-state level must be 20 to 50 ms. The plateau of the pulsed tone must be ≥150 ms and the time that a pulsed tone is on and off or the duty cycle must be 225 ±35 ms measured 5 dB below the steady-state level. Furthermore, the signal level during the off phase must be 20 dB lower than during the on phase. These measurements are typically done electrically with an oscilloscope and some can be done with an electronic counter/timer.

Masking

Narrow band and white noise signals are used to eliminate the possibility that a tone presented to one ear is heard in the other ear. The masking signals are adjusted by a masking level control marked in at least 5 dB steps. Regardless of the audiometer type, ANSI S3.6-1996 specifies that the masking output level must be sufficient to mask a tone of 60 dB HL at 250 Hz, 75 dB HL at 500 Hz, and 80 dB HL from 1000 to 8000 Hz.

Narrow Band Noise

Narrow band noise (NBN) is required for all audiometers equipped with a bone vibrator (types 1 to 3) and for HF audiometers (Table 10–1). This occurs because the RETFLs were standardized with 40 dB effective masking level (EML) presented to the nontest ear (Frank, 1982). ANSI S3.6-1996 specifies the bandwidth of each NBN from 125 to 16,000 Hz and requires that the output level be calibrated in EML. 0 dB EML is the SPL of a masking signal that masks a pure tone presented at 0 dB HL 50% of the time when the masking signal and pure tone are presented to the same ear. The standard specifies the SPL of each NBN equal to 0 dB EML using a correction factor added to the RETSPL of any earphone type from 125 to 8000 Hz. The correction factors for each NBN were taken from ISO 389(4)-1994 and were derived on the assumption that a NBN having a critical bandwidth (Scharf, 1970; Zwicker & Terhardt, 1980) will just mask a tone having the same frequency as the NBN at a signal-to-noise ratio of −4 dB.

The NBN output levels are measured the same way as pure tone output levels are measured with an SLM with one-third octave band filters. For each NBN, the measured SPL should be equal to the correction factor plus the earphone RETSPL plus the masking level setting. For example, at a masking control level setting of 70 dB EML, the SPL of a 1000-Hz NBN for a TDH 49 earphone measured in a NBS 9A coupler should be 83.5 dB SPL. This occurs because the 1000 Hz NBN correction factor is 6 dB, the TDH 49 RETSPL at 1000 Hz is 7.5 dB, and the masking control was set at 70 dB. Figure shows a calibration form for recording the measurements of masking signals and includes the NBN correction factors when the SPL of the NBN is measured with an SLM having one-third octave band filters. If the measured NBN SPLs are not within +5/−3 dB of the desired SPL (correction factor plus earphone RETSPL plus masking control level setting) at any frequency, the NBN output level should be adjusted with the audiometer's internal calibration mode to the desired SPLs. If this is not possible, a correction card should be developed showing the adjustments that will have to be applied to the masking level control when masked thresholds are obtained using NBN.

ANSI S3.6-1996 specifies that the NBN masking level control must range from 0 dB EML to the maximum air-conduction HL (Table 10–2) at each frequency but cannot exceed 115 dB SPL at any frequency. The linearity of the NBN masking level control is measured the same way as done for a pure tone.

White Noise

White noise (WN) is also called broadband noise and is required for type 1 and 2 audiometers. The sound pressure spectrum level for WN must be within ±5 dB of the level at 1000 Hz from 250 to 5000 Hz when measured in an acoustic coupler. The output of WN noise is typically calibrated in SPL; however, it can be calibrated in EML. If the WN is calibrated in SPL, the measured unfiltered SPL of the WN should be the same as the number on the masking level control

within +5/−3 dB and recorded on a calibration form (Appendix B, Form 5).

Reference Signals

Some audiometric tests require the use of a reference signal that is independently controlled by the use of a second channel on the audiometer. Type 1 and 2 audiometers are required to have a reference tone that can be alternately presented with the test tone, and type 1 audiometers are required to have a reference tone that can be simultaneously presented with the test tone (i.e., tone from the other channel) (Table 10–1).

ANSI S3.6-1996 specifies that the performance characteristics of signals generated from the second channel must meet the same requirements as those previously described for a single-channel audiometer, except for frequency range, HL range, increments, output level, and operation. The required frequencies of the reference signal must range from 250 to 6000 Hz rather than 125 to 8000 Hz, which are required test signal frequencies for a type 1 and 2 audiometer. The HL of the reference signal must range from 0 to no less than 80 dB HL at 250 Hz and to no less than 100 dB HL at 500 to 6000 Hz. The reference tone HL increments must be in 2.5 dB steps or less for a type 1 and 2 audiometer and in 5-dB steps if a reference tone is included on a type 3 audiometer. The output level of the reference tone must be calibrated to the same RETSPLs as normally done for the test tone. However, the output level of the reference tone must be within ±3 dB of the output level of the test tone from 500 to 4000 Hz and within ±5 at 250 and 6000 Hz. Finally, when the reference signal is on (second channel is operating), the output level of the test signal cannot change by more than ±1 dB.

PERFORMANCE CHARACTERISTICS OF AUTOMATIC AUDIOMETERS

Automatic audiometers are required to meet the same performance characteristics as pure tone audiometers. However, they are also required to meet additional performance characteristics related to the rate of signal level change, recording period, and frequency accuracy. The rate of signal level change is 2.5 dB/s for types 1 to 3 and 2.5 or 5 dB/s for types 4, 5, and HF with a ±20% tolerance. The rate of signal level change can be measured with a stopwatch simply by starting the audiometer and measuring the time it takes to change the signal level. The decibels per second rate can be determined by dividing the time into the decibel change. For example, a change in signal level of 40 dB should take 16 seconds for a 2.5 dB/s or 8 s for a 5 dB/s rate of signal level change. The rate of change should be measured for both increasing and decreasing signal levels.

If an automatic audiometer uses fixed frequencies, ANSI S3.6 requires a minimum recording period of 30 seconds at each frequency before the next fixed frequency begins. The frequency accuracy is the same as for a pure tone audiometer. If an audiometer uses a continuously variable or sweep frequency, the rate of frequency change is one octave per minute and the frequency accuracy must be within ±5% of the frequency indicated on the recording audiogram.

PERFORMANCE CHARACTERISTICS OF SPEECH AUDIOMETERS

Even though many of the performance characteristics for a speech audiometer are similar to the performance characteristics of a pure tone audiometer, additional measurements are needed. This occurs because speech signals cover a wider range of frequencies and have more amplitude and temporal fluctuations than a pure tone audiometer. Furthermore, a monitoring meter is used to adjust the input level of speech tests that can be presented live voice using a microphone (required for types A and B) or by presenting recorded material from a playback device (required for types A, B, and C). Thus additional measurements for speech audiometers include the performance characteristics of the monitoring meter, speech RETSPLs for each transducer, the frequency response of each transducer, playback device, and the microphone, harmonic distortion, and the masking signal.

Monitoring Meter

All speech audiometers have a meter to monitor the input level of the speech signal. Traditionally, the meter has been called a volume units or VU meter; however, ANSI S3.6-1996 refers to it as a monitoring meter. The scale of the monitoring meter is calibrated in decibels having a minimum value of −20 dB, maximum value of +3 dB, and a 0 dB reference position located between two-thirds and three-quarters of the full scale. Within the circuitry of a speech audiometer, the monitoring meter is located after the amplifier and before the attenuator (i.e., HL control). This is done so that a speech signal input can be monitored while the HL is increased or decreased when a patient is tested. The amplifier preceding the monitoring meter must have a gain control of at least 20 dB for adjusting the input speech level. It is important to note that the speech signal input level must be adjusted to 0 dB on the monitoring meter using the gain control so that the speech signal output level will be equal to the level indicated on the HL control. For example, if the 1000-Hz calibration tone preceding a recorded speech test is adjusted to 0 dB on the monitoring meter, the test will be presented to the patient at the level indicated on the HL control. On the other hand, if the level of the 1000-Hz calibration tone was adjusted to −10 dB on the monitoring meter, the test will be presented 10 dB lower than indicated on the HL control.

The monitoring meter must be accurate and stable so that undershoot and overshoot are at a minimum. The accuracy of a monitoring meter can be checked by directing a 1000-Hz tone from an external oscillator to a 1 dB step attenuator and then to the audiometer's microphone or playback input making sure that all impedances are matched. With the monitoring meter adjusted to +3 dB, increasing the attenuator output (more attenuation) in 1 dB steps should result in 1 dB decreases on the monitoring meter through its entire range. ANSI S3.6-1996 specifies the stability of a monitoring meter in reference to response time. Specifically, the time that it takes the monitoring meter to reach 99% of the 0 dB reference point

is specified as 350 ± 10% ms with an allowable overshoot of 1% but not more than 1.5%. Furthermore, the response time for frequencies from 250 to 8000 Hz can differ by no more than 0.5 dB compared with the response time for a 1000-Hz tone. One way to measure response time is to develop a calibration tape containing pure tones from 250 to 8000 Hz in octave intervals. At each frequency, a 10-second tone should be recorded for adjusting the monitoring meter to 0 dB followed by the same frequency tone having durations of 350 (standard time) and 315 and 385 ms (±10% of 350 ms). The test tape is directed into the audiometer through a playback device. After the adjustment of the monitoring meter to 0 dB for the 10-second tone, the level of the monitoring meter is visually observed for the 350 ms tone and for the tones of shorter and longer duration to ensure that the meter accurately deflects to 0 dB.

RETSPL for Speech

ANSI S3.6-1996 specifies the RETSPL for speech as 12.5 dB above the 1000-Hz RETSPL for any transducer when the monitoring meter and HL control are adjusted to 0 dB. Thus a 1000-Hz tone is the test signal used for measuring the RETSPL for speech. For measuring the RETSPL using the microphone, an external source can be used to generate a 1000-Hz test signal. For example, a calibrated pure tone audiometer could be set to produce a 1000-Hz tone through an earphone to deliver the test signal to the microphone. The level of the 1000-Hz tone should be at least 40 dB higher than the ambient room noise. For measuring the RETSPL using each playback device, a recording containing a 1000-Hz calibration tone at least 40 dB above the background noise of the recording can be used. With the monitoring meter adjusted to 0 dB for the 1000-Hz test signal and the HL at 70 dB, the coupler output level for each earphone should be 12.5 dB plus the RETSPL at 1000 Hz for the earphone being tested plus 70 dB. For a loudspeaker, the SPL at the reference test position should be 12.5 dB above the RETSPL at 1000 Hz for the listening condition (e.g., binaural or monaural at 0, 45, or 90 degrees azimuth) that will be used for sound field speech audiometry. Although not included in ANSI S3.6-1996, a 1000-Hz FM tone could be substituted for a 1000-Hz pure tone when measuring loudspeaker output levels.

The output levels for each transducer using the microphone and each playback device should be recorded on a calibration form (Appendix B, Forms 1 and 2). The measured SPL should equal 12.5 dB plus the transducer RETSPL at 1000 Hz plus the HL setting (e.g., 70 dB HL). The tolerance is ±3 dB. However, as with pure tone audiometer output calibration, the transducer output should be adjusted using the audiometer's internal calibration mode so that the measured SPL is within ±2.5 dB of the desired level. If this is not possible, a correction card should be developed.

Frequency Response

Because a speech signal covers a wide range of frequencies, ANSI S3.6-1996 has specified the frequency-response characteristics to ensure that each transducer, playback device, and the microphone has an acceptably flat response.

Output Transducers

For measuring the frequency response of each output transducer, ANSI S3.6-1996 specifies that the test signal should be WN directed to an input for an external signal (e.g., input normally used for a playback device). The source of the WN can be an external WN generator, where the output of the generator would be directed to an input for an external signal through a patch cord (making sure the impedances match). Another source would be the audiometer's internal WN generator. If the audiometer's WN generator is used as the source, the WN could be directed to a nontest earphone. The nontest earphone phone plug should be removed and replaced by one end of a patch cord, and the other end of the patch cord would be plugged into an input for external signals. Regardless of the source, once the WN has been directed into an input for external signals, the monitoring meter should be adjusted to 0 dB and the HL control set to 70 dB. The monitoring meter should not be readjusted during the measurements. For earphone measurements, each earphone is positioned on an appropriate coupler and for loudspeaker measurements, the SLM is positioned at the reference test position. One-third octave band coupler or sound field SPLs for each band from 125 to 8000 Hz are then recorded on a calibration form for each transducer and loudspeaker (Appendix B, Form 6). ANSI S3.6-1996 requires that the one-third octave band SPL for each band between 250 and 4000 Hz must be within ±3 dB of the average SPL for all the bands between 250 and 4000 Hz. Furthermore, the one-third octave band SPLs from 125 to 250 Hz must be within +0/−10 dB and from 4000 to 6000 Hz must be within ±5 dB of the average SPL for all the bands between 250 and 4000 Hz.

CONTROVERSIAL POINT

A one-third octave band analysis of the frequency response of a transducer may indicate a smooth frequency response. However, significant output level deviations may occur between the one-third octave bands. Thus, a one-third octave band analysis of the frequency response of a transducer, especially a loudspeaker, may not be sufficient to fully describe its frequency response.

Playback Devices

The frequency response of each playback device is also measured acoustically. This is done using the transducer normally used during the presentation of speech from a playback device. However, the recommended test signals are one-third octave bands of WN centered at one-third octave intervals from 125 to 8000 Hz (ANSI S3.6-1996, Annex B). This requires that a test signal tape or CD recording has to be developed or purchased. Each test signal should have a duration longer than 15 seconds, and any background noise in the recording should be at least 40 dB less than the level of the test signals. The same measurement procedures are done for each output transducer as previously reported, except the test signals are one-third octave bands of noise rather than WN. The frequency response requirements for playback devices are increased by ±1 dB from 250 to 4000 Hz and by ±2 dB for frequencies outside 250 to 4000 Hz but within 125 to 8000 Hz compared with those for the output transducers. Form 6 in Appendix B shows a calibration form for recording the frequency response of each transducer using playback devices.

Microphone

ANSI S3.6-1996 requires that the output voltage level of the microphone has to be within ±3 dB of the average level for all of the test signals from 125 to 8000 Hz when the signals are presented at 80 dB SPL under free field or equivalent conditions. The recommended test signals are the same as those used for measuring the frequency response of a playback device (i.e., one-third octave bands of WN centered at one-third octave intervals from 125 to 8000 Hz). These requirements create several problems in reference to delivering and acoustically measuring the test signals and the testing environment.

One method is to play the recorded test signals from a tape player to an external amplifier and then to an output transducer (e.g., loudspeaker or earphone). The audiometer microphone is positioned at the approximate distance and orientation from the output transducer as would normally occur during speech audiometry. The microphone of an SLM is placed into the *sound field* between the output transducer and as close as possible to the audiometer microphone without obstructing the sound pathway. The output of the microphone can be connected to a voltmeter using a Y-patch cord, where the microphone phone plug is inserted into one phone jack, the voltmeter into the other phone jack, and the patch cord phone plug is inserted into the audiometer microphone input. During the measurement, the output voltage level of the microphone is recorded in decibels after each test signal has been adjusted to 80 dB SPL as monitored with the SLM. If the audiometer has two channels, another method to deliver the test signals to the microphone is to route the tape player output to one channel and then to a supra-aural earphone. To obtain a constant 80 dB SPL at the audiometer microphone, the earphone output level could be adjusted using the HL control and/or adjusting the gain control of the monitoring meter to a level less than 0 dB.

The problem with each method is that the audiometer microphone may not be in a free field or may be picking up ambient noise during the measurements. One way to avoid these two problems is to place the test signal transducer and the microphone in a hearing aid test box using the reference microphone normally used during hearing aid measurements to monitor the SPL at the audiometer microphone. The ambient noise problem can also be addressed by measuring the ambient noise in the test environment before the measurements. This is done with the SLM placed in the position used for monitoring the test signals and with all of the instrumentation for delivering the test signals turned on. If the one-third octave band ambient noise SPL measurements from 125 to 8000 Hz are ≤40 dB SPL, it can be assumed that the ambient noise will not influence the microphone measurements because the input to the microphone is a constant 80 dB SPL. Form 6 in Appendix B shows a calibration form for recording the microphone frequency response.

Harmonic Distortion

Harmonic distortion for speech audiometers is tested with pure tones and measured acoustically for each transducer as done for pure tone audiometers. For this measurement, a 250-, 500-, and 1000-Hz pure tone from an external source is directed into the audiometer's microphone or playback device input and the monitoring meter is adjusted to 9 dB. It is important that the pure tone test signals do not have excess distortion (i.e., ≥ 1%) at each individual harmonic. If a calibrated portable pure tone audiometer is used as an external source, the monitoring meter can be adjusted to −1 dB. Then, increasing the portable audiometer's HL by 10 dB will drive the monitoring meter to 9 dB. For earphone measurements, the earphone is placed on an appropriate coupler and the HL control is adjusted to produce 110 dB SPL for each test frequency. After this, the coupler SPL is determined with one-third octave band filtering at each harmonic of the test tone frequency. ANSI S3.6-1996 requires that the THD should not exceed 2.5% for each test tone.

For loudspeaker measurements, the same test tones and procedures are used, except the SLM is positioned at the reference test position in the sound field and the output of each test tone is adjusted by the HL control to 80 dB SPL. The THD for each test tone frequency cannot exceed 3%. The procedure is then repeated with a loudspeaker output level of 100 dB SPL. At this level, the THD cannot exceed 10% for each test tone. Form 4 in Appendix B shows a calibration form for recording harmonic distortion of each loudspeaker.

Unwanted Noise

It is important to note that the internal background noise of transducers should be significantly lower than the speech signal. This can be measured acoustically for each transducer by turning the HL control to a relatively high level and turning the speech circuit on. Without an input into the speech circuit, the background noise level should be at least 45 dB less than the HL setting with the earphone mounted on the appropriate coupler and the SLM set to the A weighting frequency response. This measure should also be done with each loudspeaker because they are known to produce more amplifier hum, static, or internal noise than earphones. The background noise of a loudspeaker should be 45 dB less than the HL setting when measured at the reference test position using the A-weighting response of an SLM. However, a more precise measure of background noise from each earphone and loudspeaker would be to measure the one-third octave band SPLs from 125 to 8000 Hz in the appropriate coupler or at the reference test position when the HL control is set at 80 dB HL. With no signal directed to the earphones or loudspeakers, the SPL in each one-third octave band should be at least 45 dB below the HL control. If this does not occur, the source of the problem should be determined and corrected. For loudspeakers, a common cause of excessive background noise occurs because the amplifier is not properly grounded.

Masking

All speech audiometers are required to have masking (Table 10–1) called weighted random noise or speech noise because the sound pressure spectrum level is shaped to approximate the long-term pressure spectrum level of speech. ANSI S3.6-1996 specifies that the pressure spectrum level should be constant from 100 to 1000 Hz and decrease at a rate of 12 dB/octave from 1000 to 6000 Hz within ±5 dB. Furthermore, ANSI S3.6-1996 specifies that the speech noise output level must be calibrated in EML; however, the standard does not provide a correction factor as done for NBN. Instead, manufacturers are required to state the EML for speech noise in the instruction manual. Because the RETSPL for speech is measured with a 1000-Hz tone, several manufacturers use the EML correction factor for narrow band noise at 1000 Hz. If this is the case, 0 dB EML for speech noise is equal to the NBN correction factor at 1000 Hz plus the RETSPL for speech (12.5 dB above the RETSPL at 1000 Hz for any transducer). The EML for speech is measured for each transducer using the same procedures and tolerance (+5/−3 dB) as done for narrow band noise, except the SLM is adjusted to a linear frequency response. Form 5 in Appendix B shows a calibration form for recording the level of speech noise. As done for NBN, if the SPL of the speech noise is not within +5/−3 dB of manufacturer's reported value, the earphone output level should be adjusted using the audiometer's internal calibration mode. If this is not possible, a correction card should be developed showing the adjustments in masking level control that will have to be applied when speech noise masking is used.

INSPECTION AND LISTENING CHECKS

The operational status of an audiometer should be checked on a daily basis by completing several inspection and listening checks. These checks are not a substitute for the electroacoustic performance measurements; rather they are done to help ensure that the audiometer is functioning properly and to detect any problems that might require an immediate electroacoustic check. As is the case for electroacoustic measurements, inspection and listening checks are especially important for portable audiometers and audiometers transported to different testing sites (e.g., audiometers in a mobile van) because they are more susceptible to internal and transducer damage. The following are some daily inspection and listening checks. Figure 10–9 shows a form for recording inspection and listening checks.

PEARL

To save time, inspection and listening checks can be done at the same time by use of a procedure reported by Frank (1980) or Martin (1998).

Inspection Checks
Power Cord and Light

For audiometers that are consistently being plugged in and out of electrical outlets, the entire length of the power cord should be checked before it is plugged in, especially at each

Penn State University, Speech and Hearing Clinic, 110 Moore Building, University Park, PA 16802
Audiometer Inspection and Listening Checks

Audiometer Name/Model No: _____ Serial No.: _____ Location: _____

Inspection Checks		Date & Tester Initials (If Inspection and Listening Check are okay check box; if not report problem immediately)												
Power Cord															
Earphone Cords															
Insert Earphone Tubing															
Bone Vibrator Cord															
Headband and Cushions															
Controls and Switches															
Listening Checks															
Frequency	Right														
	Left														
Attenuator Linearity	Right														
	Left														
Tone Switch, Hum, Static	Right														
	Left														
Crosstalk	Right														
	Left														
Known Threshold	Right														
	Left														
Acoustic Radiation															

Figure 10–9 Audiometer inspection and listening checks.

end. If signs of wearing, cracking, or exposed wires are visible, the power cord should not be plugged in and should be replaced immediately.

Almost every audiometer has a light that comes on when the audiometer is turned on. There could be several reasons that the power light is not on once the power cord has been plugged in and the audiometer power switch has been turned on. One could be that the light is loose or burned out. If this is the case, the audiometer should still function normally, but the light should be checked and replaced. If the audiometer is powered by batteries, the battery indicator should be checked to see whether the batteries need to be replaced. Another reason could be that power to the electrical wall outlet has to be turned on (common in day care centers) by a wall switch or a circuit breaker. Yet another reason could be a burned-out fuse contained in some older audiometers as a protection from an excessive electrical input. Typically, the fuse is located next to the entrance of the power cord into the audiometer. To check a fuse, the audiometer must be unplugged and turned off. The fuse should be removed from its holder and inspected to see whether the filaments running through the fuse are intact. If the fuse is burned out, it must be replaced with one having the same size and ampere rating. The final, most likely reason is that the audiometer power switch has become defective and needs to be replaced.

Transducer Cords

Visual inspection should be made of each transducer cord along the entire length to look for signs of wearing and cracking, especially where the cord enters the transducer and the phone plug. A worn or cracked cord should be replaced with one of the same type and length. Although it is not a cord, the plastic tube of each insert earphone should be checked to be sure that it is tightly connected to the transducer and nipple and that there are no cracks along the entire length. Furthermore, the inside of the tube and nipple should be checked for moisture and debris.

Cushions and Headband

The earphone cushion should be tightly connected to the earphone or the plastic housing covering the earphone. This can be checked by holding the earphone or plastic housing and rotating the cushion. If the cushion can be easily rotated, it should be replaced. If a two-piece cushion (e.g., MX-41/AR) is being used, the connection between the two pieces should be inspected to be sure that the pieces are tightly glued together. A defective cushion should be replaced. Audiometer recalibration is not necessary. The earphone headband should have a certain tension to hold the earphones tightly against the pinna. This can be checked by positioning each post that connects the earphone to the headband to the mid-point position. When holding the top of the headband, the inside of the cushions should mate. If this does not occur, the headband should be bent (twisted) to restore its tension or be replaced.

Controls and Switches

All the dials, switches, and pushbuttons must be tightly connected, move through their entire function, and be in proper alignment. If a defect is found, the audiometer should be repaired and, depending on the problem, recalibrated, especially if an alignment problem was detected.

Listening Checks

Listening checks are done for many of the performance characteristics measured during an electroacoustic calibration. All listening checks should be done with a normally hearing listener and the audiometer and transducers in their customary locations. If an audiometer and transducers are located in separate rooms, two people are required to do listening checks, and a talk-over and talk-back system is typically required. However, in this situation many audiologists who work alone unplug the transducers from the audiometric test room jack box and plug the transducers directly into the audiometer after unplugging the patch cords that go from the audiometer to the control room jack box. The danger with this procedure is that the all the phone plugs that were removed have to be fully reinserted into the appropriate jacks, and it is assumed that the connections from the audiometer through the audiometric test room side of the jack box are functioning normally. If this procedure is used, the final check should be listening to a 1000 Hz tone at 60 dB HL through each transducer after it was reinserted into the audiometric test room jack box. An alternative procedure has been reported by Martin (1998) using a patch cord having a phone plug at each end. In this procedure the phone plug of the transducer to be checked is unplugged from the test room jack box and replaced by one end of the patch cord. The other end of the patch cord is inserted into an open jack on the jack box, which leads to an open jack on the control room jack box. The phone plug of the transducer to be checked is then inserted into the open jack on the control room jack box.

PEARL

Always be sure that a transducer phone plug is fully inserted into the output jack. If this does not occur, the transducer may have no or a reduced output, which could influence test results.

Audiometer Noise

If an audiometer is operated in the same room as the patient, the audiometer should not produce unwanted sounds that could invalidate the test results. That is, any sound that results from the operation of any control or sound radiated from the audiometer should not be audible. This does not apply to sound created by the movement of controls such as the frequency control or output selector when the patient is not actually being tested. This can be checked by disconnecting the earphones from the audiometer and terminating the earphone outputs with a dummy resistive load. A dummy resistive load can be made by soldering a resistor equal to the impedance of the transducer across the terminals of a phone plug. The listener wears the earphones, disconnected from the audiometer, while all of the controls on the audiometer that would normally be used during a test (e.g., interrupter switch, HL control) are manipulated. If the audiometer has a bone vibrator, the bone vibrator cord is disconnected and replaced by a dummy load. The listener wears the bone vibrator on one ear and an earphone occluding the other ear while the controls are manipulated. If unwanted sounds are detected, the audiometer needs to be checked to determine the source and repaired.

Frequency

Checking frequency is done by setting the frequency control to its lowest setting and directing a continuous 70 dB HL tone to one earphone. The frequency control is slowly moved through its entire range. This is repeated for the other earphone. A nonwavering tone should be heard at each frequency in each earphone. If this does not occur, the audiometer needs to be checked for frequency accuracy.

Attenuator Linearity

Checking linearity is done by setting the HL control to its lowest value and directing a continuous 1000 Hz tone to one earphone and moving the HL control through the entire range. This is repeated for the other earphone. The result should be hearing a tone that increases in loudness without any other noises at or between the HL steps. If this does not occur, the audiometer needs to be checked for linearity.

Transducer Cords

Transducer cords can be checked by directing a continuous 1000 Hz tone at 70 dB HL into each transducer. The cord should be twisted and flexed along its entire length, especially where it inserts into the transducer and the phone plug. The result should be hearing a steady-state 1000 Hz tone in each transducer. A defective cord will usually produce static or cause the tone to be intermittent. If a problem occurs at the transducer connection, tightening the screws that hold the cord into the earphone might solve the problem. If a problem occurs at the phone plug end, a wire(s) within the cord may be broken or the solder joint connecting a wire(s) to the phone plug may have broken loose and may need to be resoldered. However, many earphone cords have a plastic casing around the phone plug that cannot be removed. If a cord is defective, it should be replaced by one of the same type and length and a quick output level calibration should be considered.

Interrupter Switch and Static/Hum

This check can be done by directing a tone at 70 dB HL into one earphone at each frequency from 125 to 8000 Hz and pressing the interrupter switch. This is repeated for the other earphone. The result should be hearing a smooth tone on-set and off-set. When the tone is off, static, hum, or other noises should not be present. If turning the tone on and off does not produce a smooth tone on-set or off-set or when the tone is off if static, hum, or other noises are present, the audiometer should checked electroacoustically.

Crosstalk

As mentioned previously, crosstalk or crossover is a form of unwanted noise and occurs when a signal is directed to one earphone but is audible in the other earphone. Checking for crosstalk is done by wearing each earphone, but one earphone is disconnected from the audiometer and replaced with a dummy resistance load. With the audiometer set at 70 dB HL a tone is directed to the disconnected earphone while the frequency is changed over its entire range. The listener should not hear a tone in the earphone connected to the audiometer. The check is repeated in the same manner for the other earphone. If crosstalk occurs, the audiometer needs to be checked electroacoustically.

Acoustic Radiation

Unwanted sound from a bone vibrator can occur from sound leaking or radiating from the enclosure housing the electromagnetic transducer. This type of unwanted sound is called acoustic radiation and may cause an invalid high-frequency air-bone gap in patients who do not have a conductive pathological condition or collapsing earcanals. This occurs because the patients are responding by means of air conduction to the acoustic radiation at a lower HL than their true bone-conduction threshold (Bell et al, 1980; Shipton et al, 1980). Typically, acoustic radiation occurs in the higher frequencies, especially at 4000 Hz, and is greater for a Radioear B-72 than a B-71 bone vibrator (Frank & Crandall, 1986; Frank & Holmes, 1981). ANSI S3.6-1996 specifies an objective test for acoustic radiation that manufacturers must conduct to determine whether their bone vibrators produce acoustic radiation. The manufacturer must state the frequencies at which acoustic radiation may occur that would invalidate unoccluded bone-conduction thresholds. Acoustic radiation can be checked by obtaining bone-conduction thresholds at 2000 and 4000 Hz using mastoid placement. Then a foam earplug is placed between the surface of the bone vibrator and the mastoid. This is done to isolate the bone vibrator from the mastoid. The 2000 and 4000 Hz tones are then turned on individually at the HL that corresponded to the bone-conduction threshold. If acoustic radiation is present, the 2000 and/or 4000 Hz tone will be audible. If this occurs, the screws holding the bone vibrator together should be tightened and the test repeated. If acoustic radiation is still present, the bone vibrator should be replaced and bone-conduction calibrations must be completed.

Known Threshold

This check is done by obtaining air-conduction thresholds for each transducer on a listener (i.e., audiologist) and comparing them to previous thresholds. If the thresholds are not within ±5 dB of the previous thresholds, the output levels should be measured electroacoustically.

ACOUSTIC IMMITTANCE INSTRUMENTS

The term *acoustic immittance* refers to the reciprocal quantities of acoustic impedance or acoustic admittance, or to both quantities. Acoustic impedance refers to the opposition of the flow of energy, whereas acoustic admittance refers to the ease in which energy flows through a system. Historically, acoustic immittance instruments were used to measure acoustic impedance; however, all modern-day instruments measure the admittance of the ear. All acoustic immittance instruments require a method to deliver a sound, measure the resultant SPL, and control the air pressure in the earcanal. This is done by coupling the instrument to the earcanal using a probe having a reusable or disposable soft rubber tip so that an airtight seal is created when the probe tip is fitted in the earcanal. The probe contains several openings that are connected to different systems within the instrument. These systems typically include (1) a miniature loudspeaker(s) that produces a probe tone (e.g., 226 Hz) in the earcanal and activating signals for measuring the ipsilateral acoustic reflex, (2) a microphone that measures the earcanal SPL of the probe tone, and (3) an air pump for changing the air pressure in the earcanal. To learn more about the principles underlying acoustic immittance measurements, interested readers are directed to Lilly and Shanks (1981), Margolis (1981), Popelka (1984), Shanks (1984), and Wiley and Fowler (1997).

Acoustic immittance instruments are typically used to obtain a tympanogram and measure the acoustic reflex. A tympanogram is a measure of the acoustic immittance at the end of the probe tip (measurement plane) or at the eardrum (compensated) as a function of air pressure in the earcanal. The acoustic reflex is a measurement of stapedius muscle contraction to an activating stimulus (e.g., pure tones or noise) presented ipsilaterally through the probe or contralaterally using a supra-aural or insert earphone.

Terminology regarding acoustic immittance and the performance characteristics of acoustic immittance instruments using a 226 Hz probe tone have been specified in ANSI S3.39-1987 (R 1996) *Specifications for Instruments to Measure Aural Acoustic Impedance and Admittance (Aural Acoustic Immittance)* and IEC 1027-1991 *Instruments for the Measurement of Aural Acoustic Impedance/Admittance.* Form 7 in Appendix B shows a form that can be used for recording the results of an electroacoustic calibration of an acoustic immittance instrument.

Terminology, Plotting, and Symbols

Terminology used to describe acoustic immittance instruments and more importantly the test measurements has been inconsistent, confusing, and sometimes misleading (Popelka,

1984). In an effort to eliminate this problem and promote uniformity, ANSI S3.39-1987 (R 1996) provides standardized terms and their definitions and abbreviations for measured quantities. These terms have been accepted and are currently used throughout the literature.

ANSI S3.39-1987 (R 1996) has also standardized the tympanogram by defining labels and scale proportions known as an aspect ratio. This occurred because the morphological aspects of a tympanogram (height and width) are influenced by the aspect ratio. If the instrument measures acoustic admittance, the standard specifies that the vertical axis of a tympanogram must have a linear scale labeled "Acoustic Admittance (10^{-8} m^3/Pa $\times$ s [acoustic mmh])" or "Acoustic Admittance of Equivalent Volume of Air (cm^3)." If the instrument measures acoustic impedance, the label should be "Acoustic Impedance (10^8 Pa $\times$ s.m^3 [acoustic kohm])." The horizontal axis must be labeled "Air Pressure (daPa) [1 daPa = 1.02 mm H$_2$O]," where *0 daPa* represents the ambient air pressure at the test site. The aspect ratio for a 226 Hz tympanogram is defined as 300 dekapascals (daPa) on the horizontal scale equals the length to 1 acoustic mmho (1 cm^3) on the vertical axis. The standard also specifies symbols for plotting the threshold levels of ipsilateral and contralateral acoustic reflexes on an audiogram.

Types

As done for pure tone audiometers, ANSI S3.39-1987 (R 1996) classifies acoustic immittance instruments into types based on the features they contain and measurement capabilities (Table 10–6). In four types of instruments type 1 has the most features, functions, and capabilities, whereas type 4 has no

TABLE 10–6   Characteristic, function, or capability of acoustic immittance instruments (from ANSI S3.39-1987 (R 1996) with permission of the Acoustical Society of America, New York, NY)

Characteristic, Function, or Capability	Instrument Type 1	2	3
Probe Signal			
Sinusoidal, 226 Hz	Yes	Yes	Yes
Pneumatic System			
Manual control of air pressure	Yes	No	No
Automatic control of air pressure	Yes	No	No
Manual or automatic control of air pressure	No	Yes	Yes
Analog or digital output proportional to air pressure	Yes	No	No
Graphic display or indicator	Yes	Yes	Yes
Static Acoustic Immittance			
Measurement plane	Yes	No	No
Compensated	Yes	Yes	No
Proportional analog or digital output	Yes	No	No
Graphic display or indicator	Yes	Yes	Yes
Tympanometry			
Measurement plane	Yes	No	No
Compensated	Yes	Yes	No
Proportional analog or digital output	Yes	No	No
Graphic display or indicator	Yes	Yes	Yes
Acoustic-reflex Activating System			
Noise activating signal (stimulus)	Yes	No	No
Pure tone activating signals (stimuli)	Yes	Yes	No
Pure tone or noise activating signal	No	No	Yes
Contralateral presentation of stimulus	Yes	No	No
Ipsilateral presentation of stimulus	Yes	No	No
Contralateral and ipsilateral stimulus	No	Yes	Yes
Manual control of stimulus level	Yes	No	No

minimum requirements. Typically, type 1 or 2 is used for diagnostic testing, whereas type 3 is used for screening purposes. Type 4 instruments are usually those that have the capability for just one test such as tympanometry or acoustic reflex. Shanks (1987) has provided a detailed listing of the characteristics and specifications for each type of acoustic immittance instrument.

Range and Accuracy

All types of acoustic immittance instruments have a range of measurement capabilities. For those instruments designed to measure acoustic admittance the range is referenced to $m^3/Pa \times s$ or in acoustic mmho, and for those instruments that measure acoustic impedance the range is referenced to $Pa \times s/m^3$ or in acoustic ohms. The references can also be expressed in terms of an equivalent volume of air with units in cubic centimeters or cubic millimeters. If the instrument provides an assessment of the immittance at the frontal surface of the probe (i.e., measurement plane), the minimum range for all types is 0.2 to 5.0 acoustic mmhos or 200 to 5000 acoustic ohms. If the instrument corrects for the acoustic immittance in the earcanal (i.e., compensated measurement), the minimum range for types 1 and 2 is 0.0 to 2.0 acoustic mmhos or 500 to 10000 acoustic ohms and for type 3 is 0.0 to 1.2 acoustic mmhos and 833 to 10,000 acoustic ohms. The accuracy is specified as ±5% of the indicated value.

Calibration Cavities

An enclosed volume of air can be used to calibrate acoustic immittance instruments. This occurs because the acoustic immittance of a cavity is proportional to its volume for a 226-Hz probe tone if certain constraints regarding the dimensions of the cavity are met (Lilly & Shanks, 1981). ANSI S3.39-1987 (R 1996) requires that type 1 to 3 instruments have three calibration cavities having volumes of 0.5, 2.0, and 5.0 cm³ with a tolerance of ±2% or 0.05 cm³, whichever is greater. Additional cavities having volumes of 1.0, 1.5, 2.5, 3.0, 3.5, 4.0, and 4.5 cm³ are optional. For a 226-Hz probe tone, the admittance magnitude reading on the instrument in mmhos should be the same as the volume of each cavity. The impedance magnitude in acoustic ohms should be 2000, 500, and 200 for the 0.5, 2.0, and 5.0 cm³ cavity, respectively. Many instruments perform an automatic calibration once the probe is sealed in a cavity while others require an internal or external adjustment to obtain the desired value.

SPECIAL CONSIDERATION

It is important to note that acoustic immittance measures are influenced by atmospheric pressure and might require an adjustment. Lilly and Shanks (1981) and Shanks (1987) have provided correction factors for atmospheric pressure at different altitudes above sea level.

Probe Tone

All acoustic immittance instruments use a probe tone. The probe tone is calibrated for frequency, level, and distortion.

ANSI S3.39-1987 (R 1996) requires that types 1 to 3 instruments have a 226 Hz probe tone. If the instrument has additional probe tones, the manufacturer has to describe their acoustic characteristics. The SPL of a probe tone is below the threshold of the acoustic reflex but high enough to obtain a favorable signal-to-noise ratio. The manufacturer has to specify the SPL of the probe tone, which cannot exceed 90 dB SPL. The SPL of the probe tone is measured using an HA-1 coupler. This is done by sealing the end of the probe to a coupler, being careful to avoid any leaks between the end of the probe and the opening of the coupler cavity. Furthermore, the end of the probe must be flush with the cavity opening. The coupler SPL is measured with an SLM. If the SLM has a one-third octave band filter, the filter is set at 250 Hz. The measured SPL should be equal to the SPL stated by the manufacturer within ±3 dB. Typically, an internal calibration mode or external control changes the level of the probe tone level if the measured SPL is not within tolerance.

The frequency accuracy of any probe tone has to be within ±3% of the indicated value and can be measured with an electronic counter/timer. Harmonic distortion measurements of any probe-tone frequency are conducted with the probe coupled to an HA-1 coupler in the same manner as done for measuring the output level. To do this measurement, the coupler SPL is measured in one-third octave bands with a filter setting corresponding to the frequency of the probe tone and at filter settings corresponding to the harmonics of the probe tone. The total harmonic distortion cannot exceed 5% of the fundamental.

Air Pressure

Type 1 to 3 instruments must have the capability of changing air pressure in the earcanal and in the calibration cavities. The maximum limits are −800/+600 daPa measured in a 0.5 cm³ cavity; however, each type has a minimum air pressure range. For type 1 and 2 instruments the minimum range is −600/+200 daPa, for type 3 it is −300/+100 daPa, and for type 4 the range has to be stated by the manufacturer if provided. The tolerance in cavities from 0.5 to 2.0 cm³ for type 1 and 2 instruments cannot differ from the indicated reading on the instrument by ±10 daPa or ±10%, whichever is greater, and for type 3 and 4 instruments by ±10 daPa or ±15%, whichever is greater. The air pressure and the linearity of the air pressure scale can be measured by sealing the probe to a calibrated manometer or "U" tube water displacement device. Many instruments have the means to change the air pressure by an internal calibration mode or external control.

For some instruments, air pressure can be changed manually or automatically; however, most instruments automatically change air pressure once a seal is obtained. For these instruments, the manufacturer has to state the rate (daPa/s) and direction (positive to negative, negative to positive, or both) of the change.

Activating Signals for the Acoustic Reflex

Pure tone and noise signals can be used to activate the acoustic reflex. In addition, these signals can be presented contralaterally through a supra-aural or insert earphone and ipsilaterally through the probe.

Pure Tone Activating Signals

ANSI S3.39-1987 (R 1996) specifies that type 1 instruments must have 500, 1000, 2000, and 4000 Hz pure tones for both contralateral and ipsilateral stimulation and type 2 instruments must have at least 500, 1000, and 2000 Hz pure tones for contralateral or ipsilateral stimulation. The output levels for tones presented through a supra-aural earphone are referenced to HL using the RETSPLs listed in ANSI S3.6-1996 and must range from 50- to 90-dB at 250 Hz, 50- to 120-dB from 500 to 4000 Hz, and from 50- to 100-dB at 6000 Hz. For an insert earphone, the output can be calibrated in SPL or HL using the RETSPLs specified in ANSI S3.6-1996. The output level of the probe can also be calibrated in SPL or HL; however, the manufacturer has to provide the RETSPLs if the output level is calibrated in HL using the procedure outlined in Annex D of ANSI S3.6-1996 (formerly Appendix C in ANSI S3.6-1989). The insert earphone and probe output levels must range from 60- to 110-dB SPL from 500 to 2000 Hz and from 60- to 90-dB SPL at 4000 Hz.

PITFALL

Some manufacturers report that the output level of different frequency ipsilateral reflex activating signals are calibrated in HL when in fact all the frequencies have the same SPLs at 0 dB HL.

Noise-Activating Signals

A broadband noise-activating signal is required for type 1 immittance instruments and may be used instead of pure tone signals for type 3 instruments. When broadband noise is presented through a supra-aural earphone, the acoustic pressure spectrum level must be within ±5 dB relative to the level at 1000 Hz from 250 to 6000 Hz and must range from 50- to 115-dB SPL. For an insert earphone or the probe, the acoustic pressure spectrum level must be within ±5 dB relative to the level at 1000 Hz from 400 to 4000 Hz and must range from 50- to 100-dB SPL. Some acoustic immittance instruments also have low-pass, high-pass, band-pass noise signals. If this is the case, the manufacturer has to specify the acoustic pressure spectrum level of the noise, all other characteristics, and tolerances.

Measurement of Activating Signals

The performance characteristics of activating signals presented through a supra-aural or insert earphone are measured in the same manner and using the same couplers as done for a pure tone audiometer. For activating signals presented through the probe, the probe is sealed to an HA-1 coupler as previously described for measuring the characteristics of the probe tone. The required measures of activating signals include output levels, attenuator linearity, frequency accuracy, total harmonic distortion, and rise/fall times. The coupler output levels for pure tone signals from 250 to 4000 Hz have a tolerance of ±3 dB and a tolerance of ±5 dB for 6000 Hz and higher, as well as for any noise signal.

The attenuator linearity cannot differ from the indicated difference between intervals of 5 dB on the instrument or less by more than three-tenths or 1 dB, whichever is smaller. The cumulative error cannot be more than the output level tolerance. Frequency accuracy is ±3% of the indicated value. THD cannot exceed 3% for tones presented through a supra-aural earphone when the output is set at 90 dB HL at 250 and 8000 Hz and at 110 dB HL from 500 to 6000 Hz. For insert earphones and the probe, the total harmonic distortion cannot exceed 5% when the output is 85 dB HL or 95 dB SPL at 500 Hz, 100 dB HL or SPL from 1000 to 3000 Hz, and at 75 dB HL or SPL at 4000 Hz. The rise/fall time of an activating signal cannot exceed 50 msec or be less than 5 msec with 1 dB of overshoot.

Temporal Characteristics

The temporal characteristics of acoustic immittance instruments must be known if the instrument is going to be used for latency measurements of the acoustic reflex. For accurate measurements, the response time must be faster than the response of the acoustic reflex. ANSI S3.39-1987 (R 1996) requires that manufacturers specify the response time, which cannot exceed 50 ms. Interested readers are referred to a procedure for measuring the temporal characteristics of an acoustic immittance device provided in Appendix B of ANSI S3.39-1987 (R 1996). This procedure was reported by Popelka and Dubno (1978). Since then, Popelka (1979) reported a problem with the procedure, and Shanks et al (1985) have suggested an alternative procedure. Briefly, all the procedures involve a technique to simulate an instantaneous change in the acoustic immittance at the probe tip while measuring the temporal characteristics of the instrument to define initial latency, rise time, terminal latency, and fall time (Lilly, 1984). Initial latency is the time from the beginning of the instantaneous change in immittance to 10% of the measured change in the steady-state immittance. Rise time is the time from 10 to 90% of the change in the measured steady-state immittance. Terminal latency is the time from the end of the instantaneous change to 90% of the measured steady-state immittance change. Fall time is the time from 90 to 10% of the measured steady-state immittance change from the end of the instantaneous change.

Artifacts

ANSI S3.39-1987 (R 1996) does not address the need to be concerned about artifacts caused by an interaction of the activating signal and the probe tone during the measurement of the ipsilateral acoustic reflex. The presence of an artifact can be easily determined by placing the probe in the 0.5-cm^3 cavity and presenting each activating stimulus at increasingly higher levels. If no artifact is present, the needle or method of displaying the acoustic reflex on an acoustic immittance instrument should remain stationary for each activator signal at each output level. If an artifact is present, the needle will move when the activator signal is presented. The level at which each activator signal creates an artifact should be recorded, placed on the acoustic immittance device, and ipsilateral acoustic reflex measurements should not be measured at or above that level.

Inspection and Listening Checks

Daily inspection and listening checks of an acoustic immittance instrument are done in the same manner as for a pure tone audiometer. In addition, the probe should be checked to be sure that each opening is free of wax and debris. Furthermore, the instrument should be calibrated before its daily use by placing the probe in each calibration cavity. In addition, before daily use, the audiologist should obtain a tympanogram and ipsilateral and contralateral acoustic reflexes. These measures can then be compared with previous measures to be sure that the instrument is operating correctly.

AUDIOMETRIC TEST ROOM

An audiometric test room is also called an audiometric test booth or sound treated room. The purpose of an audiometric test room is to provide an acceptably quiet listening environment so that ambient noise will not elevate hearing thresholds caused by masking. Typically, audiometric test rooms are prefabricated with single-walled or double-walled construction. A double-walled room provides about 20- to 30-dB more attenuation of external ambient noise than a single-walled room, especially in the higher frequencies. Audiometric test rooms can range in size to accommodate a single person for earphone testing or be large enough to allow for sound field testing. The American Society for Testing and Materials has developed a standard (ASTM E596-1996) for measuring the amount of noise reduction of prefabricated audiometric test rooms. Before purchasing an audiometric test room, several

variables have to be considered. Information concerning these variables can be found in ANSI S3.1-1991, Appendix F.

ANSI Ambient Noise Levels

Because it is impossible to eliminate all ambient noise, ANSI has developed a standard (ANSI S3.1-1991) specifying maximum permissible ambient noise levels (MPANLs) allowed in an audiometric test room for testing hearing down to 0 dB HL. ANSI S3.1-1991 is a revision of an earlier standard (ANSI S3.1-1977 [R 1986]). Frank et al (1993) have provided an overview of ANSI S3.1-1991 that includes a discussion of the differences between the 1991 and the 1977 versions. The ANSI 1991 MPANLs are specified in octave and one-third octave band intervals for two test conditions and three test frequency ranges. The one-third octave band MPANLs are shown in Table 10–7. The octave band MPANLs are 5 dB higher for each MPANL shown in Table 10–7. One test condition is called *ears not covered* and applies when either one or both ears are not covered by a supra-aural earphone as would typically occur during bone-conduction or sound field audiometry. The other test condition is called *ears covered* and applies when both ears are covered simultaneously by a supra-aural earphone as would typically occur during air-conduction audiometry. The ears covered MPANLs exceed the ears not covered MPANLs by the attenuation provided by a supra-aural earphone. The supra-aural earphone attenuation values used in ANSI S3.1-1991 (see Table 10–9) were derived using the mean attenuation values averaged across three studies (Arlinger, 1986; Berger & Killion, 1989; Frank & Wright, 1990). The three frequency ranges are 125 to 8000 Hz, 250 to 8000 Hz, and 500 to 8000 Hz. The frequency ranges 125 to 8000 Hz and 250 to 8000 Hz are typically used for clinical testing

TABLE 10–7 One-third octave band maximum permissible ambient noise levels (from ANSI S3.1-1991 with permission of the Acoustical Society of America, New York, NY)

One-third Octave Band Intervals	Ears Covered			Ears Not Covered		
	125–8000 Hz	250–8000 Hz	500–8000 Hz	125–8000 Hz	250–8000 Hz	500–8000 Hz
125	29.0	31.5	42.5	23.0	27.5	37.5
250	17.5	17.5	28.5	13.5	13.5	23.5
500	14.5	14.5	14.5	9.5	9.5	9.5
800	16.5	16.5	16.5	7.5	7.5	7.5
1000	21.5	21.5	21.5	9.0	9.0	9.0
1600	21.5	21.5	21.5	5.5	5.5	5.5
2000	23.0	23.0	23.0	3.5	3.5	3.5
3150	28.5	28.5	28.5	3.5	3.5	3.5
4000	29.5	29.5	29.5	4.0	4.0	4.0
6300	33.0	33.0	33.0	9.0	9.0	9.0
8000	38.5	38.5	38.5	15.5	15.5	15.5

NOTE: Octave band maximum permissible ambient noise levels are 5 dB higher than each MPANL.

TABLE 10–8   Maximum permissible ambient noise levels specified by OSHA (1983) and ANSI S3.1-1991 for ears covered 500 to 8000 Hz and the differences

Octave-Band Interval	OSHA (1983)	ANSI (1991)	Differences
125	—	47.5	—
250	—	33.5	—
500	40.0	19.5	20.5
1000	40.0	26.5	13.5
2000	47.0	28.0	19.0
4000	57.0	34.5	22.5
8000	62.0	43.5	18.5

whereas the frequency range 500 to 8000 Hz is typically used for industrial testing and hearing screening.

The MPANLs are for monaural listening. When binaural listening occurs, 3 dB should be subtracted from the MPANLs to account for binaural summation. Binaural listening occurs when both ears are not covered for sound field testing or when both ears are covered by a supra-aural earphone and binaural thresholds or other binaural tests are conducted.

The MPANLs take into account the upward spread of masking because it is well known that excessive low-frequency noise can mask higher frequency thresholds. For the purpose of specifying MPANLs, the upward spread of masking was defined to have a slope of 14 dB/octave below the lowest test frequency (ANSI S3.1-1991). Thus the MPANL one octave below the lowest test frequency (125 Hz for the 250 to 8000 Hz range and 250 Hz for the 500 to 8000 Hz range) is equal to the lowest test frequency MPANL plus 14 dB and the MPANL two octaves below the lowest test frequency (125 Hz for the 500 to 8000 Hz range) is equal to the lowest test frequency MPANL plus 28 dB.

ANSI S3.1-1991 assumes that if the ambient noise levels in a test room are equal to or less than the MPANLs, hearing thresholds measured at 0 dB HL will not be elevated. However, when the level of a noise is near the level of a patient's unmasked threshold, the patient's masked thresholds might be elevated by as much as 2 dB. Thus the MPANLs have an uncertainty or negligible masking of 2 dB. That is, a maximum threshold shift of 2 dB may occur when thresholds are obtained at 0 dB HL in an audiometric test room having ambient noise levels equal to the MPANLs. Research by Berger and Killion (1989) and Frank and Williams (1993) has verified this assumption.

Measurement and Verification

Ambient noise levels are measured using an SLM having an octave or one-third octave band filter. Because some of the ears not covered MPANLs are very low, it is important that the noise floor of the SLM-filter combination does not interfere with the measurements. ANSI S3.1-1991 specifies that the SLM-filter combination must have an internal noise at least 3 dB below the MPANLs and describes ways that this can be measured. If this condition is not met, an SLM having lower internal noise must be used. During the measurements, the SLM microphone should be placed at the location(s) of the patient's head and all possible sources of noise should be operating. This would include the ventilation system, lights, and all instrumentation inside and outside the test room. Octave or one-third octave band SPL measurements are obtained within the inclusive range of 125 to 8000 Hz and should be recorded (Appendix B, Form 8). The measured SPLs are then compared with the MPANLs for the test condition and frequency range to be used in the test room. The test room is acceptable if the measured SPLs do not exceed the MPANLs at each octave or one-third octave band from 125 to 8000 Hz for the test condition and frequency range to be used in the test room. If the measured SPLs are equal to or less than the ears not covered MPANLs for the 125 to 8000 Hz range, the test room is acceptable for all test conditions and frequency ranges. Ambient noise should be measured annually and whenever a new noise source is operating inside or outside the test room.

If testing is going to be done at hearing levels other than 0 dB, the MPANLs can be adjusted using an equal trade-off between the hearing level to be used and the MPANLs. For example, if an air-conduction screening using supra-aural earphones is going to be conducted at 25 dB HL from 500 to 6000 Hz, then 25 dB can be added to each of the MPANLs for the ears covered and 500 to 8000 Hz range. To verify compliance, the ambient noise in the test room is measured from 125 to 8000 Hz in octave or one-third octave band intervals. The measured SPLs are compared with each MPANLs plus 25 dB for the ears covered test condition and 500 to 8000 Hz range. If measured SPLs are equal to or less than the MPANLs plus 25 dB, the test room is acceptable for screening at 25 dB HL from 500 to 6000 Hz.

Frank and Williams (1994a) reported the ambient noise levels for 136 audiometric test rooms used for clinical audiometry. Unfortunately, only about 50% had acceptable ears covered MPANLs for the 125 to 8000 Hz and 250 to 8000 Hz range and 82% for the 250 to 8000 Hz range. More unfortunately, only about 14% had acceptable ears not covered MPANLs for the 125 to 8000 Hz and 250 to 8000 Hz range and 37% for the 500 to 8000 Hz range. These results indicate that clinical audiometry is being conducted in test rooms having excessive levels of ambient noise.

OSHA Ambient Noise Levels

MPANLs have also been specified by the Occupational Safety and Health Administration (OSHA, 1983) for the purposes of industrial hearing testing. The OSHA MPANLs assume that ambient noise will be measured with an SLM in octave bands from 500 to 6000 Hz and testing will be done with supra-aural earphones. Table 10–8 shows the OSHA MPANLs and the ANSI 1991 octave band ears covered 500 to 8000 Hz range MPANLs for comparison. The OSHA MPANLs are much higher than the ANSI ears covered 500 to 8000 Hz MPANLs and do not take into account the upward spread of masking. For industrial testing, ANSI S3.1-1991 recommends using the ears-covered MPANLs for the 500 to 8000 Hz range.

Frank and Williams (1994b) reported ambient noise levels for 490 single-walled prefabricated audiometric test rooms used for industrial testing. All the rooms met the OSHA MPANLs, and 162 or 33% also met the ANSI MPANLs for ears covered testing from 500 to 8000 Hz. They recommended that the OSHA MPANLs be revised to the more stringent ANSI MPANLs so that hearing thresholds for baseline and annual audiograms could be measured down to 0 dB HL.

Sources and Reduction of Ambient Noise

Many sources of ambient noise exist. However, the primary source within a test room can be attributed to low-frequency (125 to 500 Hz) noise created by the ventilation system (Frank & Williams, 1994a,b). To determine whether the ventilation system is producing excessive noise, the ambient noise within the test room can be measured with the ventilation system on and off. If the test room meets the MPANLs with the ventilation system off but not on, steps should be taken to reduce the noise. This might include replacing worn-out fan parts, replacing the fan mounting gaskets, balancing or replacing the fan blade(s), or cleaning the air ducts. If the test room does not meet the MPANLs with the ventilation system off,

measures should be taken to increase the noise reduction of the test room. This would include replacing faulty door seals, truing the door, tightening the door latch, and installing acoustic insulation in and around the jack panel.

Passive Noise-Reducing Earphone Enclosures

The use of a passive noise-reducing earphone enclosure has been suggested as an alternative to a supra-aural earphone when hearing tests are conducted in excessive ambient noise (Benson, 1971; Stark & Borton, 1975; Wood & Fagundas, 1972). A passive noise-reducing earphone enclosure contains a supra-aural earphone mounted in a plastic dome that fits over and around the pinna like an earmuff used for hearing protection. Examples of these devices include an Audiocup, Auraldome II, AudioMate, and Madsen ME-70. The theory is that the enclosure will attenuate more excessive ambient noise than just a supra-aural earphone at the patient's ear, so that hearing thresholds will not be elevated as a result of ambient noise masking. However, the use of passive noise-reducing earphone enclosures has been strongly criticized for three reasons. The first reason concerns the calibration of the earphone output because ANSI S3.6-1996 does not have a provision or procedure specifying the output of a supra-aural earphone mounted in a passive noise-reducing enclosure. The second reason concerns hearing thresholds and threshold repeatability. Several studies (Billings, 1978; Cozad & Goetzinger, 1970) have demonstrated significant threshold differences between a supra-aural earphone and when the same earphone was mounted in an enclosure. Frank et al (1997) reported that when a supra-aural earphone cushion is recessed within the enclosure (e.g., AudioMate and Madsen ME-70), hearing thresholds are elevated and are less repeatable compared with a supra-aural earphone or when the cushion of a supra-aural earphone is flush with the enclosure's circumaural cushion (e.g., Audiocup and Auraldome II). The third reason concerns the amount of attenuation produced by a passive noise-reducing enclosure. Table 10–9 shows the amount of attenuation supplied by several

TABLE 10–9 Real-ear attenuation for a supra-aural and insert earphone and for passive noise-reducing earphone enclosure

One-Third Octave Band	Supra-aural Earphone	Insert Earphone	Earphone Types Passive Noise-Reducing Earphone Enclosures			
			Audiocup	Auraldome II	AudioMate	Madsen ME-70
125	6.0	29.9	4.1	4.4	14.6	9.1
250	4.0	31.4	1.6	10.1	13.4	15.6
500	5.0	33.7	15.6	13.0	21.6	18.3
1000	12.5	34.0	27.8	22.1	23.7	23.1
2000	19.5	34.1	32.0	32.2	28.8	30.4
3150	25.0	37.9	36.8	37.9	34.0	36.6
4000	25.5	38.6	38.5	34.3	37.7	38.5
6300	24.0	40.7	34.7	34.6	38.4	32.7
8000	23.0	42.7	34.0	35.7	37.4	31.0

enclosures reported by Frank et al (1997). Typically, enclosures having an oval cushion with a small opening (e.g., AudioMate and Madsen ME-70) supply more attenuation than those having a round cushion with a large opening (e.g., Audiocup and Auraldome II) because they have a more consistent and efficient enclosure-to-ear coupling. Because ambient noise is primarily contained in the low frequencies, the important aspect concerns the amount of low rather than high frequency attenuation supplied by the enclosure. Inspection of Table 10-9 reveals that some enclosures supply less low-frequency attenuation than a supra-aural earphone (e.g., Audiocup at 125 and 250 Hz; Auraldome II at 125 Hz).

PITFALL

Even though the theory of using passive noise-reducing earphone enclosures sounds very good, ample research indicates that passive noise-reducing earphone enclosures should not be used for testing hearing in excessive levels of ambient noise or, for that matter, even in quiet.

Insert Earphones

If hearing testing must be done in noise levels exceeding the ANSI MPANLs, perhaps the best alternative is to use insert earphones. This occurs because ANSI S3.6-1996 has provisions and procedures for specifying insert earphone RET-SPLs. More importantly, because an insert earphone is terminated by a foam eartip, similar to a foam earplug used for hearing protection, the attenuation provided by an insert earphone is significantly higher in the lower frequencies compared with a supra-aural earphone or enclosures. Table 10–9 shows the mean attenuation of an insert earphone averaged across three studies (Berger & Killion, 1989; Frank & Wright, 1990; Wright & Frank, 1992). From 125 to 500 Hz an insert earphone supplies about 27 dB more attenuation than a supra-aural earphone. Although not stated in ANSI S3.1-1991, the ears covered MPANLs for insert earphones would be equal to the ears not covered MPANLs for each frequency range (Table 10–7) plus the amount of attenuation (Table 10–9).

CONCLUSIONS

Audiometers and acoustic immittance instruments must produce accurate and controlled signals so that audiologists can make reliable and valid interpretations regarding a patients peripheral hearing sensitivity, speech processing ability, and middle ear status. Consequently, audiometers, acoustic immittance instruments, and the audiometric test room must conform to standardized performance characteristics. Furthermore, audiologists are responsible for maintaining the accuracy of the instruments they use by doing routine calibration measurements and daily inspection and listening checks. Hopefully, the information provided in this chapter will provide audiologists with a better insight into the development and usefulness of standards, calibration instrumentation, measurement of audiometer, acoustic immittance, and audiometric test room performance characteristics, and a greater appreciation of basic instrumentation and calibration.

Appendix A
ANSI Standards Used for the Calibration of Audiometers and Acoustic Immittance Instruments and other Standards Having Application to Audiology

S1.1-1994 Acoustical Terminology

S1.4-1983 (R 1997) Specification for Sound Level Meters

S1.4A-1985 Amendment to S1.4-1983

S1.9-1996 Instruments for the Measurement of Sound Intensity

S1.10-1966 (R 1997) Method for the Calibration of Microphones

S1.11-1986 (R 1993) Specification for Octave-Band and Fractional-Octave-Band Analog and Digital Filters

S1.13-1995 Measurement of Sound Pressure Levels in Air

S1.40-1984 (R 1997) Specification for Acoustic Calibrators

S1.42-1986 (R 1992) Design Response of Weighting Networks for Acoustical Measurements

S1.43-1997 Specifications for Integrating-Averaging Sound Level Meters

S3.1-1991 Maximum Permissible Ambient Noise Levels for Audiometric Test Rooms

S3.2-1989 (R 1995) Method for Measuring the Intelligibility of Speech over Communication Systems

S3.4-1980 (R 1997) Procedure for the Computation of Loudness of Noise

S3.5-1997 Methods For Calculation of Speech Intelligibility Index

S3.6-1996 Specification For Audiometers

S3.7-1995 Method For Coupler Calibration of Earphones

S3.13-1987 (R 1997) Mechanical Coupler for Measurement of Bone Vibrators

S3.20-1973 (R 1995) Bioacoustical Terminology

S3.21-1978 (R 1997) Method of Manual Pure Tone Audiometry

S3.25-1989 (R 1995) Occluded Ear Simulator

S3.39-1987 (R 1996) Specifications for Instruments to Measure Aural Acoustic Impedance and Admittance (Aural Acoustic Immittance)

Appendix B
Calibration Forms

Form 1: Calibration form for earphone and bone vibrator output levels.

Form 2: Calibration form for loudspeaker output levels.

Form 3: Calibration form for attenuator linearity, frequency accuracy, tone switching, and on/off ratio.

Form 4: Calibration form for total harmonic distortion.

Form 5: Calibration form for masking output levels.

Form 6: Calibration form for frequency response.

Form 7: Calibration form for acoustic immittance instrument.

Form 8: Calibration form for maximum permissible ambient noise levels.

Audiometer: _____ Serial No.: _____ Channel: _____ Date: _____ Calibrated by: _____

Transducer Type	Frequency in Hertz (Hz)											
	125	250	500	750	1000	1500	2000	3000	4000	6000	8000	Speech
1. Right TDH 49/50, SPL*												
2. Left TDH 49/50, SPL*												
3. RETSPL + 70 dB HL	117.5	96.5	83.5	78.5	77.5	77.5	81.0	79.5	80.5	83.5	83.5	89.5
Rt TDH 49/50, Error (1-3)†												
Lt TDH 49/50, Error (2-3)†												
4. Right ER-3A, SPL‡												
5. Left ER-3A, SPL‡												
6. RETSPL + 70 dB HL	96.0	84.0	75.5	72.0	70.0	72.0	73.0	73.5	75.5	72.0	70.0	82.5
Right ER-3A, Error (4-6)†												
Left ER-3A, Error (5-6)†												
7. Bone Vib, Mastoid, FL§												
8. RETFL		67.0	58.0	48.5	42.5	36.5	31.0	30.0	35.5			
9. Hearing Level Setting		20	50	50	50	50	50	50	50			
Bone Vib, Error (7-(8+9))†												

*One-third octave band SPL in NBS 9A coupler with an HL setting of 70 dB.

†Error equals measured output level minus RETSPL/RETFL plus HL setting; tolerance is ±3 dB from 125-5000 Hz and ±5 dB at 6000 Hz and above.

‡One-third octave band SPL in HA-2 coupler with rigid tube attachment with a HL setting of 70 dB.

§Force level using B&K 4930 mechanical coupler.

Form 1:   Calibration form for earphone and bone vibrator output levels.

Penn State University, Speech and Hearing Clinic, 110 Moore Building, University Park, PA 16802
Calibration Form for Loudspeaker Output Levels (re: ANSI S3.6-1996)

Audiometer: _____ Serial No.: _____ Channel: _____ Date: _____ Calibrated by: _____

Transducer Type	125	250	500	750	1000	1500	2000	3000	4000	6000	8000	Speech
1. Right Speaker, SPL*												
2. Left Speaker, SPL*												
3. RETSPL† + 70 dB HL	93.5	82.0	73.0	70.5	70.0	69.0	67.5	61.0	61.5	67.0	78.0	82.5
Right Speaker, Error (1-3)‡												
Left Speaker, Error (2-3)‡												
Rt Sp: Rt/Lt Error (±2 dB)	/	/	/	/	/	/	/	/	/	/	/	
Rt Sp: Up/Down Error (±2 dB)	/	/	/	/	/	/	/	/	/	/	/	
Rt Sp: Ft/Back Error (±1 dB)	/	/	/	/	/	/	/	/	/	/	/	
Lt Sp: Rt/Lt Error (±2 dB)	/	/	/	/	/	/	/	/	/	/	/	
Lt Sp: Up/Down Error (±2 dB)	/	/	/	/	/	/	/	/	/	/	/	
Lt Sp: Ft/Back Error (±1 dB)	/	/	/	/	/	/	/	/	/	/	/	

Frequency in Hertz (Hz)

*One-third octave band SPL at reference point with an HL setting of 70 dB.
†Monaural listening at 45 degrees azimuth.
‡Error equals measured output level minus RETSPL plus HL setting; tolerance is ±3 dB from 125-5000 Hz and ±5 dB at 6000 Hz and above.

Form 2: Calibration form for loudspeaker output levels.

Penn State University, Speech and Hearing Clinic, 110 Moore Building, University Park, PA 16802
Calibration Form for Attenuator Linearity, Frequency Accuracy, Tone Switching, and On/Off Ratio

Audiometer: _____ Serial No.: _____ Channel: ____ Date: _____ Cal by: _____

Attenuator Linearity			Frequency Accuracy			Tone Switching	
HL	Output	Error*	Freq.	Measured	Error†	Rise/fall‡	Overshoot§
120			125			/	
115			250			/	
110			500			/	
105			750			/	
100			1000			/	
95			1500			/	
90			2000			/	
85			3000			/	
80			4000			/	
75			6000			/	
70			8000			/	
65							
60							

On/Off Ratio‖				
	SA Phones TDH _____		Insert Phones _____	
Freq.	Right	Left	Right	Left

Attenuator Linearity (cont.)		
55		
50		
45		
40		
35		
30		
25		
20		
15		
10		
5		
0		
Total		

On/Off Ratio Freq.	Right	Left	Right	Left
125				
250				
500				
750				
1000				
1500				
2000				
3000				
4000				
6000				
8000				

*Error between 5 dB intervals is ≤ 1 dB, total error is ± 3 dB from 125 to 5000 Hz and ± 5 dB at 6000 Hz and above.
†Error is $\pm 1\%$ for type 1, $\pm 2\%$ for type 2, $\pm 3\%$ for types 3 to 5 of indicated frequency.
‡Error is <20 or >200 ms.
§Error is $>+1$ dB.
‖SPL output with tone switch off must be ≥ 70 dB less than with tone switch on.

Form 3: Calibration form for attenuator linearity, frequency accuracy, tone switching, and on/off ratio.

Penn State University, Speech and Hearing Clinic, 110 Moore Building, University Park, PA 16802
Calibration Form for Total Harmonic Distortion (re: ANSI S3.6-1996)

Audiometer: _____ Serial No.: _____ Channel: _____ Date: _____ Calibrated by: _____

Freq.	Supra-aural Earphone, TDH 49/50				Insert Earphone, ER-3A				Bone Vibrator, B-71		
	dB HL*	Allowed†	Right	Left	dB HL*	Allowed†	Right	Left	dB HL*	Allowed‡	Measured
125	75	≤2.5%			75	≤2.5%					
250	90	≤2.5%			90	≤2.5%			20	≤5.5%	
500	110	≤2.5%			110	≤2.5%			50	≤5.5%	
750	110	≤2.5%			110	≤2.5%			50	≤5.5%	
1000	110	≤2.5%			110	≤2.5%			60	≤5.5%	
1500	110	≤2.5%			110	≤2.5%			60	≤5.5%	
2000	110	≤2.5%			110	≤2.5%			60	≤5.5%	
3000	110	≤2.5%			110	≤2.5%			60	≤5.5%	
4000	110	≤2.5%			110	≤2.5%			60	≤5.5%	
6000	90	≤2.5%			90	≤2.5%					
8000	90	≤2.5%			90	≤2.5%					

Loudspeakers	Allowed§	250 Hz	500 Hz	1000 Hz	Loudspeakers	Allowed§	250 Hz	500 Hz	1000 Hz
Right, at 80 dB SPL	≤3%				Right, at 100 dB SPL	≤10%			
Left, at 80 dB SPL	≤3%				Left, at 100 dB SPL	≤10%			

*Or maximum HL, whichever is lower.

†Allowed percent for total harmonic distortion; ≤2% for second and third harmonic; ≤0.3% for fourth and higher harmonics; ≤0.03% for all subharmonics.

‡Allowed percent for total harmonic distortion; ≤5% for second harmonic; ≤2% for third and higher harmonics.

§Allowed percent for total harmonic distortion.

Form 4: Calibration form for total harmonic distortion.

Penn State University, Speech and Hearing Clinic, 110 Moore Building, University Park, PA 16802
Calibration Form for Masking Output Levels (re: ANSI S3.6-1996)

Audiometer: _____ Serial No.: _____ Channel: _____ Date: _____ Calibrated by: _____

Narrow Band Noise	125	250	500	750	1000	1500	2000	3000	4000	6000	8000
1. Right TDH 49/50, SPL*											
2. Left TDH 49/50, SPL*											
3. CF†+RETSPL+70 dBEML	121.5	100.5	87.5	83.5	83.5	83.5	87.0	85.5	85.5	88.5	88.0
Rt TDH 49/50, Error (1-3)‡											
Lt TDH 49/50, Error (2-3)‡											
4. Right ER-3A, SPL§											
5. Left ER-3A, SPL§											
6. CF†+RETSPL+70 dBEML	100.0	88.0	79.5	77.0	76.0	78.0	79.0	79.5	80.5	77.0	77.5
Right ER 3A, Error (4-6)‡											
Left ER-3A, Error (5-6)‡											

Frequency in Hertz (Hz)

	White Noise Setting	Error‡	Speech Noise Setting	CF‖	Error‡
Right TDH 49/50, SPL*	70		70		
Left TDH 49/50, SPL*	70		70		
Right ER-3A, SPL†	70		70		
Left ER-3A, SPL†	70		70		

*One-third octave band SPL in NBS 9A coupler with a setting of 70 dB EML.
†Correction factor for narrow band noise measured with one-third octave band filter.
‡Error equals measured output level minus CR plus RETSPL plus EML setting; tolerance is +5/-3 dB of indicated value.
§One-third octave band SPL in HA-2 coupler with rigid tube attachment with a setting of 70 dB EML.
‖Correction factor supplied by the manufacturer.

Form 5: Calibration form for masking output levels.

Penn State University, Speech and Hearing Clinic, 110 Moore Building, University Park, PA 16802
Calibration Form for Frequency Response (re: ANSI S3.6-1996)

Audiometer: _____ Serial No.: _____ Channel: _____ Date: _____ Calibrated by: _____

| Freq. | Supra-aural phones; TDH | | | | | | Insert phones; _____ | | | | | | Loudspeakers | | | | | | Mic‡ |
| | Earphones* | | Tape† | | CD† | | Earphones* | | Tape† | | CD† | | Speakers* | | Tape† | | CD† | | |
	Rt	Lt	Rt	Lt	Rt	Lt	Rt	Lt	Rt	Lt	Rt	Lt	Rt	Lt	Rt	Lt	Rt	Lt	
125																			
160																			
200																			
250																			
315																			
400																			
500																			
630																			
800																			
1000																			
1025																			
1600																			
2000																			
2500																			
3150																			
4000																			
5000																			
6300																			
8000																			

*One-third octave band SPL of WN; compared with average from 250 to 4000 Hz, tolerance is ±3 dB from 250 to 4000 Hz, 0/-10 from 125 to 250 Hz, ±5 dB from 4000-6300 Hz.

†One-third octave band SPL of one-third octave band test signals; compared with average from 250 to 4000 Hz, tolerance is ±4 dB from 250 to 4000 Hz, +2/-12 from 125 to 250 Hz, +7 dB from 4000 to 8000 Hz.

‡Output voltage level for constant 80 dB SPL of one-third octave band test signals; tolerance is ±3 dB from 125 to 8000 Hz.

Form 6: Calibration form for frequency response.

Penn State University, Speech and Hearing Clinic, 110 Moore Building, University Park, PA 16802
Calibration Form for Acoustic Immittance Instrument (re: ANSI S3.39-1987 (R 1996))

Instrument: _____   Serial No.: _____   Date: _____   Calibrated by: _____

| Source | Frequency Accuracy | | | SPL Output* | | | Harmonic Distortion* | | Attenuator Linearity | | |
	Freq.	Measured	Error[†]	Measured	Expected[‡]	Error[§]	SPL[‖]	Percent[¶]	Setting	Output	Error[#]
Probe Tone	226								120		
Ipsilateral Reflex Activating Signal	500				83.5		95		110		
	1000				77.5		100		105		
	2000				81.0		100		100		
	4000				80.5		75		95		
	Noise								90		
Contralateral Reflex Activating Signal	500				83.5		90		85		
	1000				77.5		110		80		
	2000				81.0		110		75		
	4000				80.5		110		70		
	Noise								65		
									60		
									55		
									50		

Linearity of Air Pressure System: _____   **Rise/Fall Time:** _____

On/Off Ratio	500	1000	2000	4000	Noise
Ipsilateral					
Contralateral					

*Measured in HA-1 or NBS 9A coupler.
[†]Error is ±3%.
[‡]SPL of probe tone, ipsi activating signal, and noise from manufacturer; SPL of contra activating signal equals RETSPL + 70 dB HL for TDH 49/50.
[§]Error is ±3 dB for tones, ±5 dB for noise.
[‖]SPL in HA-1 or NBS 9A coupler.
[¶]Percent of total harmonic distortion must be is ≤5% for probe tone and ipsi signals, ≤3% for contra signals from TDH 49/50.
[#]Error between 5 dB intervals is ≤1 dB.

Form 7: Calibration form for acoustic immittance instrument.

221

**Penn State University, Speech and Hearing Clinic, 110 Moore Building, University Park, PA 16802
Calibration Form for Maximum Permissible Ambient Noise Levels (re: ANSI S3.1-1991)**

Audiometric Test Room Number: _____   Date: _____   Calibrated by: _____

Source	One-third Octave Band Center Frequency in Hertz (Hz)										
	125	250	500	800	1000	1600	2000	3150	4000	6300	8000
1. One-third octave band SPLs											
2. Ears Covered; 250–8000 Hz	31.5	17.5	14.5	16.5	21.5	21.5	23.0	28.5	29.5	33.0	38.5
Difference (1 minus 2)*											
3. Ears Covered; 500-8000 Hz	42.5	28.5	14.5	16.5	21.5	21.5	23.0	28.5	29.5	33.0	38.5
Difference (1 minus 3)*											
4. Ears Not Covered; 250-8000 Hz	27.5	13.5	9.5	7.5	9.0	5.5	3.5	3.5	4.0	9.0	15.5
Difference (1 minus 4)*											
5. Ears Not Covered; 500-8000 Hz	37.5	23.5	9.5	7.5	9.0	5.5	3.5	3.5	4.0	9.0	15.5
Difference (1 minus 5)*											

[1]If the difference is a positive value (i.e., measured SPL higher than MPANL), the room should not be used for testing hearing down to 0 dB HL for that test condition and frequency range.

Form 8:   Calibration form for maximum permissible ambient noise levels.

REFERENCES

AMERICAN NATIONAL STANDARDS INSTITUTE. (1977). Criteria for background noise in audiometric test rooms (ANSI S3.1-1977 [R 1986]). New York: ANSI.

AMERICAN NATIONAL STANDARDS INSTITUTE. (1983). Specification for sound level meters (ANSI S1.4-1983 [R 1994]). New York: ANSI.

AMERICAN NATIONAL STANDARDS INSTITUTE. (1984). Specification for acoustic couplers (ANSI S1.40-1984 [R 1994]). New York:ANSI.

AMERICAN NATIONAL STANDARDS INSTITUTE. (1986). Specification for octave-band and fractional-octave-band analog and digital filters (ANSI S1.11-1986 [R 1993]). New York: ANSI.

AMERICAN NATIONAL STANDARDS INSTITUTE. (1987a). Mechanical coupler for measurement of bone vibrators (ANSI S3.13-1987 [R 1997]). New York: ANSI.

AMERICAN NATIONAL STANDARDS INSTITUTE. (1987b). Instruments to measure aural acoustic impedance and admittance (Aural acoustic immittance) (ANSI S3.39-1987 [R-1996]). New York: ANSI.

AMERICAN NATIONAL STANDARDS INSTITUTE. (1989). Occluded ear simulator (ANSI S3.25-1989 [R 1995]). New York: ANSI.

AMERICAN NATIONAL STANDARDS INSTITUTE. (1991). Maximum permissible ambient noise levels for audiometric test rooms (ANSI S3.1-1991). New York: ANSI.

AMERICAN NATIONAL STANDARDS INSTITUTE. (1995). Method for coupler calibration of earphones (ANSI S3.7-1995). New York: ANSI.

AMERICAN NATIONAL STANDARDS INSTITUTE. (1996). Specification of audiometers (ANSI S3.6-1996). New York: ANSI.

AMERICAN SOCIETY FOR TESTING AND MATERIALS. (1996). Standard method for laboratory measurement of the noise reduction for sound isolating enclosures (ASTM E596-1996). Philadelphia: ASTM.

AMERICAN SPEECH-LANGUAGE-HEARING ASSOCIATION. (1991). Sound field measurement tutorial. *ASHA, 33*(Suppl. 3); 25–37.

ARLINGER, S.D. (1986). Sound attenuation of TDH 39 earphones in a diffuse field of narrow band noise. *Journal of the Acoustical Society of America, 79*;189–191.

BEKESY, G.V. (1947). A new audiometer. *Acta Otolaryngologica (Stockholm), 35*;411–422.

BELL, J., GOODSELL, S., & THORNTON, A.R.D. (1980). A brief communication on bone conduction artifacts. *British Journal of Audiology, 14*;73–75.

BENSON, R.W. (1971). Auraldomes for audiometric testing. *National Hearing Aid Journal, 25*;14, 42.

BERGER, E.H, & KILLION, M.C. (1989). Comparison of the noise attenuation of three audiometric earphones, with additional data on masking near threshold. *Journal of the Acoustical Society of America, 86*;1392–1403.

BILLINGS, B.L. (1978). Performance characteristics of two noise-excluding audiometric headsets. *Sound Vibrations, 13*;20–22.

BILLINGS, B.L., & WINTER, M. (1977). Calibration force levels for bone conduction vibrators. *Journal of Speech and Hearing Research, 20*;653–660.

BRINKMAN, K., & RICHTER, U. (1990). Reference zero for the calibration of pure tone audiometers equipped with insert earphones. *Acoustica, 70*;202–207.

BRUNT, M.A. (1985). Bekesy audiometry and loudness balancing testing. In: J. Katz (Ed.), *Handbook of clinical audiology* (3rd ed.) (pp. 273–291). New York: Williams & Wilkins.

CORLISS, E.L.R., & BURKHARD, M.D. (1953). A probe tube method for the transfer of threshold standard between audiometer earphones. *Journal of the Acoustical Society of America, 25*;990–993.

COZAD, R.L., & GOETZINGER, C.P. (1970). Audiometric and acoustic coupler comparisons between two circumarual earphone and earphone-cushion combinations vs a standard unit. *Journal of Audiology Research, 10*;62–64.

CURTIS, J.F., & SCHULTZ, M.C. (1986). *Basic laboratory instrumentation for speech and hearing.* Boston: Little, Brown & Co.

DECKER, T.N. (1990). *Instrumentation: An introduction for students in speech and hearing sciences.* New York: Longman, Addison-Wesley Publishing Company.

DIRKS, D.D., LYBARGER, S.F., OLSEN, W.O., & BILLINGS, B.L. (1979). Bone conduction calibration status. *Journal of Speech and Hearing Disorders, 44*;143–155.

FRANK, T. (1980). Pure-tone audiometer inspection and listening checks. *Journal of National Studies of the Speech-Language Hearing Association, 10*;33–41.

FRANK, T. (1982). Influence of contralateral masking on bone-conduction thresholds. *Ear and Hearing, 3*;314–319.

FRANK, T. (1997). ANSI update: Specification of audiometers. *American Journal of Audiology, 6*;29–32.

FRANK, T., BYRNE, D.C., & RICHARDS, L.A. (1988). Bone conduction threshold levels for different bone vibrator types. *Journal of Speech and Hearing Research, 53*;295–301.

FRANK, T., & CRANDELL, C.C. (1986). Acoustic radiation produced by B-71, B-72, and KH 70 bone vibrators. *Ear and Hearing, 7*;344–347.

FRANK, T., DURRANT, J.D., & LOVRINIC, J.H. (1993). Maximum permissible ambient noise levels for audiometric test rooms. *American Journal of Audiology, 2*;33–37.

FRANK, T., GREER, A.C., & MAGISTRO, D.M. (1997). Hearing thresholds, threshold repeatability, and attenuation values for passive noise-reducing earphone enclosures. *American Industrial Hygiene Association Journal, 58*;772–778.

FRANK, T., & HOLMES, A. (1981). Acoustic radiation from bone vibrators. *Ear and Hearing, 2*;59–63.

FRANK, T., & RICHARDS, W.D. (1991). Hearing aid coupler output level variability and coupler correction levels for insert earphones. *Ear and Hearing, 12*;221–227.

FRANK, T., & RICHTER, U. (1985). Influence of temperature on the output of a mechanical coupler. *Ear Hearing, 6*;206–210.

FRANK, T., & VAVREK, M.J. (1992). Reference threshold levels for an ER-3A insert earphone. *Journal of the American Academy of Audiology, 3*;51–59.

FRANK, T., & WILLIAMS, D.L. (1993). Effects of background noise on earphone thresholds. *Journal of the American Academy of Audiology, 4*;201–221.

FRANK, T., & WILLIAMS, D.L. (1994a). Ambient noise levels in audiometric test rooms used for clinical audiometry. *Ear and Hearing, 14*;414–422.

FRANK, T., & WILLIAMS, D.L. (1994b). Ambient noise levels in industrial audiometric test rooms. *American Industrial Hygiene Association Journal, 55;*433–437.

FRANK, T., & WRIGHT, D.C. (1990). Attenuation provided by four different audiometric earphone systems. *Ear and Hearing, 11;*70–78.

FRANKS, J.R., ENGLE, D.P., & THEMANN, C.L. (1992). Real-ear attenuation at threshold for three audiometric headphone devices: implications for maximum permissible ambient noise level standards. *Ear and Hearing, 13;*2–10.

HAWKINS, D.B., COOPER, W.A., & THOMPSON, D.J. (1990). Comparisons among SPLs in real-ears, 2 cm^3 and 6 cm^3 couplers. *Journal of the American Academy of Audiology, 1;*154–161.

INTERNATIONAL ELECTROTECHNICAL COMMISSION. (1970). An IEC artificial ear of the wideband type for the calibration of earphones used in audiometry (IEC 318). Geneva: IEC.

INTERNATIONAL ELECTROTECHNICAL COMMISSION. (1990). Mechanical coupler for measurements on bone vibrators (IEC 373). Geneva: IEC.

INTERNATIONAL ELECTROTECHNICAL COMMISSION. (1991). Instruments for the measurement of aural acoustic impedance/admittance (IEC 1027). Geneva: IEC.

INTERNATIONAL ORGANIZATION FOR STANDARDIZATION. (1994). Acoustics-reference zero for the calibration of audiometric equipment—Part 1: Reference equivalent threshold sound pressure levels for pure tones and supra-aural earphones (ISO 389-1). Geneva: ISO.

INTERNATIONAL ORGANIZATION FOR STANDARDIZATION. (1994). Acoustics-reference zero for the calibration of audiometric equipment—Part 2: Reference equivalent threshold sound pressure levels for pure tones and insert earphones (ISO 389-2). Geneva: ISO.

INTERNATIONAL ORGANIZATION FOR STANDARDIZATION. (1994). Acoustics-reference zero for the calibration of audiometric equipment—Part 3: Reference equivalent threshold force levels for pure tones and bone vibrators (ISO 389-3). Genvea: ISO.

INTERNATIONAL ORGANIZATION FOR STANDARDIZATION. (1994). Acoustics-reference zero for the calibration of audiometric equipment—Part 4: Reference levels for narrow band masking noises (ISO 389-4). Geneva: ISO.

INTERNATIONAL ORGANIZATION FOR STANDARDIZATION. (1994). Acoustics-reference zero for the calibration of audiometric equipment—Part 5: Reference equivalent threshold sound pressure levels for pure tones in the frequency range 8 kHz to 16 kHz (ISO 389-5). Geneva: ISO.

INTERNATIONAL ORGANIZATION FOR STANDARDIZATION. (1994). Acoustics-reference zero for the calibration of audiometric equipment—Part 7: Reference threshold of hearing under free field and diffuse-field listening conditions (ISO 389-7). Geneva: ISO.

JERGER, J. (1960). Bekesy audiometry in analysis of auditory disorders. *Journal of Speech and Hearing Research, 3;*275–287.

KILLION, M.C. (1978). Revised estimate of minimal audible pressure: Where is the "missing" 6 dB. *Journal of the Acoustical Society of America, 63;*1501–1508.

KILLION, M.C. (1984). New insert earphones for audiometry. *Hearing Instruments, 35;*38,46.

KILLION, M.C., & VILLCHUR, E. (1989). Comments on "Earphones in audiometry" [Zwislocki et al., *J Acoust Soc Am* 83:1688-1689]. *Journal of the Acoustical Society of America, 85;*1775–1778.

LILLY, D.J. (1984). Evaluation of the response time of acoustic-immittance instruments. In: S. Silman (Ed.), *The acoustic reflex* (pp. 101–135). New York: Academic Press.

LILLY, D.J., & PRUDY, J.K. (1993). On the routine use of Tube-phone™ insert earphones. *American Journal of Audiology, 2;*17–20.

LILLY, D.J., & SHANKS, J.E. (1981). Acoustic immittance of an enclosed volume of air. In: G. Popelka (Ed.), *Hearing assessment with the acoustic reflex* (pp. 145–160). New York: Grune & Stratton.

MARGOLIS, R. (1981). Fundamental of acoustic immittance. In: G. Popelka (Ed.), *Hearing assessment with the acoustic reflex* (pp. 117–143). New York: Grune & Stratton.

MARTIN, F.N. (1998). *Exercises in audiometry: A laboratory manual* (pp. 1–5). Boston: Allyn and Bacon.

MORGAN, D., DIRKS, D.D., & BOWER, D. (1979). Suggested threshold sound pressure levels of modulated (warble) tones in the sound field. *Journal of Speech and Hearing Disorders, 44;*37–54.

OCCUPATIONAL SAFETY AND HEALTH ADMINISTRATION. (1983). Occupational noise exposure: Hearing conservation amendment. *Federal Register, 48;*9738–9785.

POPELKA, G.R. (1979). Effects of procedural variables on temporal measurements of acoustic immittance devices. Paper presented at the annual convention of the American Speech-Language-Hearing Association, Atlanta, GA.

POPELKA, G.R. (1984). Acoustic immittance measures: Terminology and instrumentation. *Ear and Hearing, 5;*262–267.

POPELKA, G.R., & DUBNO, J.R. (1978). Comments on the acoustic-reflex response for bone-conducted signals. *Acta Otolaryngologica, 86;*64–70.

REGER, S.N. (1952). A clinical and research version of the Bekesy audiometer. *Laryngoscope, 62;*1333–1351.

RICHARDS, W.D., & FRANK, T. (1982). Frequency response and output variations of Radioear B-71 and B-72 bone vibrators. *Ear and Hearing, 3;*37–38.

RICHTER, U., & FRANK, T. (1985). Calibration of bone vibrators at high frequencies. *Audiology Acoustics, 24;*2–12.

RUDMOSE, W. (1964). Concerning the problem of calibrating TDH-39 earphones at 6 kHz with a 9A coupler. *Journal of the Acoustical Society of America, 36;*1049.

SCHARF, B. (1970). Critical bands. In: J.V. Tobias (Ed.), *Foundations of modern auditory theory* (Vol. I) (pp. 159–202). New York: Academic Press.

SHANKS, JE. (1984). Tympanometry. *Ear and Hearing, 5;*268–280.

SHANKS, J.E. (1987). Aural acoustic-immittance standards. In: J.W. Hall (Ed.), *Seminars in hearing: Immittance audiometry, 8;*307–318.

SHANKS, J.E., WILSON, R.H., & JONES, H.C. (1985). Earphone-coupling technique for measuring the temporal characteristics of aural acoustic-immittance devices. *Journal of Speech and Hearing Research, 28;*305–308.

SHIPTON, M.S., JOHN, A.J., & ROBINSON, D.W. (1980). Air radiated sounds from bone vibrator transducers and its implications for bone conduction audiometry. *British Journal of Audiology, 14;*86–99.

STARK, E.W., & BORTON, T.E. (1975). Noise-excluding enclosure for audiometry. *Audiology, 14;*232–237.

WALKER, G., DILLION, H., & BYRNE, D. (1984). Sound field audiometry: Recommended stimuli and procedures. *Ear and Hearing 5;*13–21.

Wilber, L.A., Kruger, B., & Killion, M.C. (1988). Reference thresholds for an ER-3A insert earphone. *Journal of the Acoustical Society of America, 83*;669–676.

Wiley, T.L., & Fowler, C.G. (1997). *Acoustic immittance measures in clinical audiology.* San Diego, CA: Singular Publishing Group, Inc.

Wood, T.J., & Fagundas, K.W. (1972). Use of Amplivox "Audicup" in audiometry. *Journal of Audiology Research, 12*;313–317.

Wright, D.C., & Frank, T. (1992). Attenuation values for a supra-aural earphone for children and insert earphone for children and adults. *Ear and Hearing, 13*;454–459.

Zwicker, E., & Terhardt, E. (1980). Analytical expressions for critical-band rate and critical band-width as a function of frequency. *Journal of the Acoustical Society of America, 68*;1523–1525.

Zwislocki, J.J. (1970). *An acoustic coupler for earphone calibration.* Report LSC-S-7, Laboratory of Sensory Communication. Syracuse, NY: Syracuse University.

Zwislocki, J.J. (1971). *An ear-like coupler for earphone calibration.* Report LSC-S-9, Laboratory of Sensory Communication. Syracuse, NY: Syracuse University.

PREFERRED PRACTICE GUIDELINES

Expected Outcomes

- Audiometers calibrated to the performance characteristics specified in ANSI S3.6-1996 will produce accurate and controlled signals.
- Acoustic immittance instruments calibrated to the performance characteristics specified in ANSI S3.39-1987 (R 1996) will produce accurate and controlled signals.
- Audiometric test rooms having ambient noise levels less than or equal to maximum permissible ambient noise levels specified in ANSI S3.1-1991 are acceptable for testing hearing down to 0 dB HL.

Clinical Indications

- A complete electroacoustic calibration should be conducted on all new audiometers and acoustic immittance devices before they are used and thereafter on a yearly basis or sooner.
- An electroacoustic calibration should be conducted four times per year to check the output levels of each transducer.
- Audiometers transported to different testing sites should have a complete calibration at least two times per year.
- An electroacoustic check of an audiometer or acoustic immittance device should be conducted if a problem is detected during the daily inspection and listening checks.
- Ambient noise levels in an audiometric test room should be measured on a yearly basis and whenever any new noise source is operating inside or outside the test room.

Clinical Process

- Audiologists should read and understand all of the manual describing the operation of an audiometer or acoustic immittance instrument.
- Audiologists should conduct inspection and listening checks before the use of an audiometer and acoustic immittance device.
- Audiologists should conduct or be present when an audiometer or acoustic immittance device is calibrated.
- Audiologists should conduct or be present when ambient noise is measured in an audiometric test room.

Documentation

- Documentation includes all calibration records for each audiometer, acoustic immittance instrument, or audiometric test room in an audiology clinic.
- Documentation includes all information related to history of repair for each audiometer or acoustic immittance instrument.
- Documentation includes all records of daily inspection and listening checks.
- Documentation includes all purchase information and names and telephone numbers of instrument suppliers.

## Chapter 11

Pure Tone Tests

Ross J. Roeser, Kristi A. Buckley, and Ginger S. Stickney

Outline

The foundation of every audiological evaluation is the pure tone test. Results from pure tone audiometry are used to make the initial diagnosis of normal or abnormal-hearing sensitivity and help determine the intensity levels at which additional audiological procedures will be performed. When results are not within normal limits, pure tone tests are used to make the diagnosis of the type and degree of hearing loss. Pure tone test results also have value in determining (re)habilitation procedures for each patient. Because of the importance of pure tone data for the examination of each patient, performing pure tone testing is an important part of audiological diagnosis.

During pure tone testing, *thresholds* are obtained for test stimuli, consisting of single frequencies or pure tones. The term threshold is defined as the lowest intensity at which the patient is able to respond to the stimulus. Because it is impossible to measure the perception of hearing directly, the threshold is mathematically defined as the lowest intensity at which the patient responds to the stimulus in a given fraction of trials. The clinical criterion for threshold is typically based on 50%, which means the patient must respond to two out of four or three out of six trials. Pure tones are used because they are simple to generate and they provide valuable diagnostic information on the differential effects of lesions in the peripheral auditory system.

This chapter covers the topic of pure tone tests. Included are a physical description of pure tones, a description of the equipment used for pure tone testing, classification of test results (type and degree of loss), procedures followed, and interpretation and description of results. In addition, the use of pure tones for hearing screening is reviewed.

Audiology: Diagnosis. Edited by Roeser, Valente, and Hosford-Dunn. Thieme Medical Publishers, Inc., New York © 2000

PHYSICAL DESCRIPTION OF PURE TONES

The two basic physical measures associated with pure tones that should be understood by those performing pure tone audiometry are frequency and intensity.

Frequency

When sound is normally produced, molecules of air are forced to move back and forth by a vibratory source at different frequencies. This back-and-forth movement causes waves of compression and rarefaction to form. Frequency specifies the number of back-and-forth oscillations or cycles produced by a vibrator in a given time as molecular movement occurs and the sound is created. The term used to describe frequency is *hertz* (named after Heinrich Hertz), abbreviated Hz. This term specifies the number of cycles that occur in 1 second. For example, if a vibrator (tuning fork) was set into motion and completed 1000 back-and-forth cycles in 1 second, it would have a frequency of 1000 Hz. Frequency and pitch are related in that as the frequency of a sound increases, the listener perceives a tone of a higher and higher pitch. Pitch is the perceptual equivalent of frequency.

Because most sounds contain multiple frequencies, the oscillations that occur are complex. However, when pure tones are generated, only one frequency is present, so the oscillations produced are simple back-and-forth movements. Figure 11–1 shows the spectrum (intensity × frequency) for a pure tone at 1000 Hz. The only frequency represented in this figure is 1000 Hz, which is clearly shown as a narrow peak at the 1000 Hz nominal value. Pure tones lower in frequency than 1000 Hz would be shown as a similar narrow peak to the left of the 1000 Hz data and pure tones higher in frequency than 1000 Hz to the right.

The human ear responds to frequencies between 20 and 20,000 Hz. Frequencies that are less than this range are *infrasonic* and those greater than this range are *ultrasonic*. For example, a sound with a frequency of 10 Hz is infrasonic and

would not be perceived by the normal ear; a sound with a frequency of 30,000 Hz is ultrasonic and would also not be perceived. Although the ear responds to frequencies ranging from 20 to 20,000 Hz, only those frequencies between 300 to 3000 Hz are actually critical for the perception of speech. This means that it would be possible for an individual to have essentially no hearing greater than 3000 Hz and have only marginal difficulty hearing speech in a quiet environment. This observation explains why pure tones are important in a thorough assessment of the auditory system.

Pure tone thresholds are regularly assessed at *octave* and sometimes at *half-octave intervals* between the range of 250 and 8000 Hz. The 250 to 8000 Hz frequency range is generally the most audible to the human ear and provides guidelines on how well the individual is able to perceive speech because the speech frequencies of 300 to 3000 Hz fall within this range. In the typical pure tone test, thresholds are obtained for the frequencies 250, 500, 1000, 2000, 4000, and 8000 Hz. In addition, 750, 1500, 3000, and 6000 Hz are sometimes tested. More and more it is becoming customary to include 3000 and 6000 Hz in the standard audiometric evaluation, especially when hearing loss is present. Three thousand hertz is tested because of its importance in speech perception and because results from 3000 Hz are used to calculate the percent of hearing impairment as developed by The American Medical Association and the American Academy of Otolaryngology–Head and Neck Surgery. Six thousand hertz is tested because of its importance in diagnosing noise-induced hearing loss.

Intensity

The physical measurement of what is psychologically perceived as loudness is *intensity*. The intensity of a sound is determined by the amount of movement or displacement of air particles that occurs as a sound is created. The greater the amount of displacement, the more intense, or louder, the sound. Intensity is measured in units called *decibels*, abbreviated *dB*, a term that literally means one tenth of a bell (named after Alexander Graham Bell). The decibel is technically defined as the logarithmic ratio between two magnitudes of pressure or power.

As indicated by the technical definition, intensity is far more complicated than frequency. To understand the decibel fully requires knowledge of advanced mathematical functions. The decibel is based on a logarithmic function because the ear responds to a very large range of pressure changes. The use of logarithms allows these changes to be expressed by smaller numbers than would be required for a linear function. The interested reader may consult excellent references for additional information on how to compute decibels using logarithms such as Berlin (1967).

Although the concepts underlying the decibel are somewhat complicated and will not be covered in this chapter, a

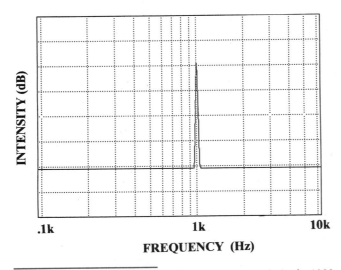

Figure 11–1   Spectrum (intensity × frequency plot) of a 1000 Hz pure tone.

less difficult concept is that the decibel is a relative unit of measurement. Simply stated, for example, 10 dB or 20 dB has no specific meaning without specifying the reference for the measure. Three reference levels exist for the decibel commonly used in audiometric testing: *sound pressure level (SPL), hearing level (HL), and sensation level (SL)* as follows.

dB SPL

Sound pressure level refers to the absolute pressure reference level for the decibel. The pressure reference used to determine dB SPL is .000204 dynes/cm². Therefore 0 dB SPL is equal to a pressure force of .000204 dynes/cm² and 10 dB or 20 dB SPL equals 10- or 20-dB above the .000204 dynes/cm² force. Because dB SPL is a physical measure, it is not affected by the frequencies present in sound.

dB HL

The reference for the decibel used to express deviation from normal-hearing sensitivity is dB HL. As will be pointed out in the following, the ear is not sensitive to all frequencies at the same intensity level. That is, hearing sensitivity changes as a function of the frequency of the sound. Therefore 0 dB HL represents an intensity equal to the threshold sensitivity of the normal ear at each frequency. Audiometers are calibrated in dB HL, so that any decibel value above 0 dB HL represents a deviation from normal-hearing levels. For example, 25 dB HL is 25 decibels above the normal-hearing threshold for that frequency.

Over the past 30 years, four standards have been used to define the absolute SPL levels at which the normal ear responds as a function of frequency (see Chapter 10). At present, all audiometers should conform to The American National Standards Institute (ANSI) 1996 standard.

In some instances dB hearing threshold level (HTL) will also be used. When dB HTL is used, it implies that the decibel value given was a measured threshold from a patient; that is,

the value was an actual level obtained during threshold assessment.

dB SL

Decibel sensation level is used to specify the intensity of stimuli presented to a given patient relative to the patient's threshold. That is, if a patient has a threshold of 45 dB HL, a signal presented at 20 dB SL would be 20 dB above 45 dB HL, or at 65 dB HL.

FREQUENCY AND INTENSITY FUNCTION OF THE HUMAN EAR

The ear responds to different absolute intensities, or different SPLs, as a function of frequency. Stated in another way, it takes a different SPL to reach the level at which the normal ear will perceive the sound (threshold level) at different frequencies. Figure 11–2 illustrates the threshold sensitivity function of the normal ear and gives the ANSI 1996 levels required to reach threshold at each frequency for normal ears (0 dB HL). As shown in this figure, the ear is most sensitive in the mid-frequencies, around 1000 to 1500 Hz. Because audiometers are calibrated in dB HL, it is not necessary to know the absolute dB SPL/HL difference at each frequency. The audiometer automatically corrects for the dB SPL/HL difference as the frequency is changed.

PURE TONE TEST EQUIPMENT— THE AUDIOMETER

Pure tone tests are performed with audiometers. Audiometers are electronic instruments used to quantify hearing sensitivity. Pure tone audiometers originated from tuning forks,

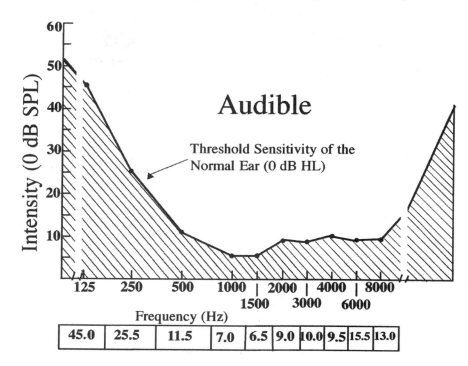

Figure 11–2 Threshold sensitivity of the normal ear as a function of frequency. The ANSI (1996) reference equivalent threshold sound pressure levels shown at the bottom of the figure are required to reach 0 dB HL for a TDH 39 supra-aural earphone.

and the frequencies produced by the first audiometers were similar to those produced by tuning forks. As an example, the frequencies 256, 512, and 1026 Hz were included on the first audiometers. However, today's standard pure tone audiometers have frequencies with a scale based on the octave and half-octave frequencies of 125, 250, 500, 750, 1000, 1500, 2000, 3000, 4000, 6000, and 8000 Hz.

Like any tool, audiometers vary in degree of sophistication, features offered, and configuration. The American National Standards Institute (1996) has developed a comprehensive classification system for audiometers that is reviewed in detail in Chapter 10. On the basis of their facilities, audiometers are classified into standard pure tone, speech, high-frequency or free-field equivalent. Figure 11–3 provides an example of a standard pure tone audiometer with the major components identified.

Audiometer Types

Standard Pure Tone and Automatic/Microprocessor Audiometers

Pure tone and automatic audiometers generate pure tone stimuli and are used for screening or basic threshold testing. Manual audiometers require the examiner to operate the controls, whereas automatic audiometers are controlled by a microprocessor that responds when the patient signals the system with a handheld switch. Automatic audiometers are commonly used for mass screenings, such as industrial hearing conservation programs. Although these instruments will save time in mass screening programs with cooperative adults, they have limited value in testing children and in diagnostic testing.

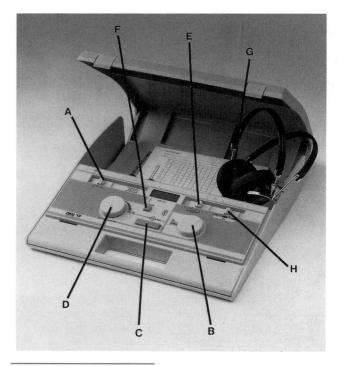

Figure 11–3   A standard pure tone audiometer with the external components labeled. (Courtesy of WelchAllen.)

Diagnostic Audiometers

Diagnostic audiometers include a wide variety of features such as controls for bone conduction testing, speech testing through monitored live voice or recorded presentation, and stimuli for masking and diagnostic (site-of-lesion) testing.

Extended High-Frequency Audiometers

Extended high-frequency audiometers are used for measuring pure tone hearing thresholds from 8000 to 16000 Hz. One of the main uses of this type of audiometer is to monitor the onset of possible high-frequency hearing loss from ototoxic medications. The individual susceptibility to ototoxic medication varies greatly (Park, 1996), making the prediction of damage from given dosages of any ototoxic medication virtually impossible; damage also may occur unilaterally (Fausti et al, 1994). Because the damage from most ototoxic medications begins in the very high frequencies and progresses to lower frequencies, monitoring of these very high frequencies can alert the treating physician to impending damage to the speech frequencies. More information regarding ototoxicity and monitoring protocols can be found in Park (1996) and Fausti et al (1994).

In rare cases patients may have hearing loss in the low to mid frequencies but show better hearing around 8000 Hz. In these cases it is important to test the ultra high frequencies, because the patient may have hearing in these frequencies. If this is the case, the patient may benefit from advanced technology, such as frequency transposition hearing aids.

Because of the acoustic variability encountered with high frequencies, the ANSI (1996) standard describes two circumaural earphone types to be used with high-frequency audiometers. Chapter 10 covers the calibration procedures and instrumentation for high-frequency audiometry.

SPECIAL CONSIDERATION

When a severe-to-profound hearing loss is present and thresholds at 8000 Hz show improvement greater than 15- to 20-dB, extended high-frequency audiometry (testing above 8000 Hz) should be considered.

Free Field Equivalent Audiometers

Free field equivalent audiometers are calibrated so that the output of the earphones or bone conduction oscillator can be expressed in terms of equivalent hearing as if the sound was presented at 0 degrees azimuth in the sound field. The output from free field equivalent audiometers is expressed in SPL, making it more adaptable to comparison of performance for hearing aids.

AUDIOMETER COMPONENTS

Regardless of the make or model, pure tone audiometers have certain basic controls and switches in common. These components may vary in appearance and location, but they perform the same basic functions. Table 11–1 lists and describes these components. They are shown in Figure 11–3.

TABLE 11–1 Summary of components and functions of pure tone audiometers

Label	Component	Function
A	Power (on-off) switch	Provides power to the audiometer circuit
B	Frequency selector dial (oscillator)	Selects the frequency of the stimulus
C	Tone interrupter (tone reverse) switch	Activates or inactivates the stimulus
Not shown	Amplifier	Increases the intensity of the signal
D	Attenuator (hearing level dial)	Adjusts the intensity of the stimuli
E	Signal router switch	Selects the device used to present the stimuli
F	Masking level controller	Adjusts the intensity of masking noise
G	Earphone(s)	Presents the stimuli by means of air conduction
Not shown	Bone oscillator	Presents the stimuli by means of bone conduction
H	Signal selector switch	Selects the type of stimuli to be delivered
Not shown	Loudspeaker	Presents the stimuli in the sound field

Power (On-Off) Switch (Labeled A in Figure 11–3)

Audiometers are equipped with standard three-pronged plugs for 120-volt power. After the audiometer has been plugged in, it should be turned on and allowed to "warm up" for approximately 10 minutes before testing. This procedure ensures that the proper current has reached all parts of the instrument for optimum functioning. The audiometer should remain in the "on" position for the remainder of the day when additional testing is to be performed, because there is less wear on the electrical components to leave it on all day than to turn it on and off several times during the day.

PEARL

Turning audiometers "on" and "off" throughout the day causes greater wear on the electronic components than turning them "on" each day and having them remain "on" during the entire day they are to be used.

Some portable pure tone screening audiometers are battery powered. Battery-powered audiometers are useful in situations in which conventional power is not available. However, the output from battery-powered audiometers is unstable, and they should be used only when necessary.

Frequency Selector Dial (Oscillator) (Labeled B in Figure 11–3)

The frequency selector dial changes the frequency of the stimuli in discrete octave and half-octave steps from 125 to 8000

Hz. On many audiometers, the frequency selector dial also shows, by use of smaller numerals on the dial, the maximum output (dB HL or dB HTL) that the audiometer is capable of producing at each test frequency.

Tone Interrupter (Tone Reverse) Switch (Labeled C in Figure 11–3)

The tone interrupter is a button, bar, or lever used either to present or interrupt the test stimuli, depending on the position of the tone reverse switch. The tone reverse switch allows the tone to be "normally on" or "normally off." In the "normally on" position the tone is turned off by depressing the tone interrupter. In the "normally off" position the tone is presented by depressing the tone interrupter. In standard pure tone testing, the tone reverse switch should always be in the "normally off" position. Serious errors can result if the tone reverse switch is in the "normally on" position. The "normally on" position is used only during calibration and for some diagnostic procedures.

Amplifier (Not Shown in Figure 11–3)

The amplifier, an internal component, increases the intensity of the electronic signal. Note that the amplifier delivers maximum intensity to the attenuator; the attenuator controls the output from the transducer (earphone, bone oscillator, or loud speaker) by reducing the signal from the amplifier.

Attenuator (Hearing Level Dial) (Labeled D in Figure 11–3)

The attenuator or HL dial controls the intensity of test stimuli. The amplifier delivers a constant level signal to the attenuator. The attenuator controls the intensity level of the output signal. Attenuators are resistive devices that control intensity in small steps; most attenuators are designed to operate in 5 dB steps, but some operate in steps of 1- or 2-dB. Because attenuators are resistive devices, the greater the attenuation, the less output is present at the earphone. Table 11–2 compares the relationship between the HL setting on the attenuator dial, the amount of attenuation, and the output at the audiometer earphone. As shown in this example, at maximum output (110 dB HL) the attenuator dial is at minimum attenuation (0 dB) and the output at the earphone is 116.5 dB SPL. The 6.5 dB difference between the audiometer dial and the output represents the dB HL/dB SPL correction specified by the ANSI 1996 standard (see Fig. 11–5) for the 1000 Hz tone used in this example. Also shown in Table 11–2 is that as the output decreases from 110 dB HL to 0 dB HL, the amount of attenuation increases until maximum attenuation is reached at 0 dB HL.

Attenuator (HL) dials have a range from 0- to 110-dB HL or 120 dB HL for air conduction testing. It should be noted that not all of the test stimuli are capable of being presented at intensities of 110 dB HL. Specifically, 250 and 8000 Hz have limited outputs. Bone conduction testing is limited to 0- to 40 or 0- to 60 to 70-dB HL, depending on the frequency. For bone conduction stimuli, the audiometer must deliver more energy to drive the bone conduction oscillator than to present the stimuli through earphones.

Signal Router Switch (Labeled E in Figure 11–3)

Test signals may be delivered to the right or left earphone, bone conduction oscillator, or (in the case of diagnostic audiometers) through loudspeakers. The signal router switch determines which of these devices is activated.

Masking Level Controller (Labeled F in Figure 11–3)

In some instances a masking sound must be applied to the nontest ear to ensure that crossover of the test signal to the nontest cochlea does not occur (see Chapter 10). The masking dial controls the level of the masking signal that is delivered to the nontest ear.

Earphone(s) (Labeled G in Figure 11–3)

Earphones are designed to transmit test stimuli to each ear individually. They are color-coded: red for the right ear and blue for the left ear.

Important points regarding earphones are (1) earphones are calibrated to one specific audiometer and should never be interchanged between audiometers unless the equipment is recalibrated, (2) the tension of the headband and resiliency of the earphone cushions are important factors for reliable test results, and (3) placement of the earphones on the patient is one of the most important procedures in audiometric testing.

Figure 11–4 shows schematics and photos of three types of earphones used in pure tone testing. As shown, in addition to the standard supra aural cushion, two other types of earphone systems are available: noise excluding (a combination-type system of a supra-aural cushion and a circumaural muff) and insert earphones. The use of noise-excluding earphones provides superior attenuation of ambient background

TABLE 11–2 Comparison attenuator setting, dB SPL and output (see note below)

Attenuator Setting (dB HL)	Amount of Attenuation	Output from Audiometer Earphone (dB SPL)
110	0	116.5
105	5	111.5
100	10	106.5
95	15	101.5
90	20	96.5
85	25	91.5
80	30	86.5
75	35	81.5
70	40	76.5
65	45	71.5
60	50	66.5
55	55	61.5
50	60	56.5
45	65	51.5
40	70	46.5
35	75	41.5
30	80	36.5
25	85	31.5
20	90	26.5
15	95	21.5
10	100	16.5
5	105	11.5
0	110	6.5

In this example a 1000 Hz pure tone is used and the HL/SLP correction is 6.5 dB (see Figure 11–5).

noise, which allows for accurate testing in environments having excessive noise. However, the size and complexity of noise-excluding earphones make them more difficult to use, thus they have not been endorsed for widespread use.

Insert-type earphones also have the advantage of increased attenuation of background noise. In addition, insert earphones provide increased interaural (between ear) attenuation, the elimination of earcanal collapse, increased comfort for long test sessions, and better approximate insertion measures when audiometric testing is conducted for hearing aid use. Clinicians should be aware that there is a small correction factor needed for calibrating insert earphones when used with an audiometer calibrated for standard supra-aural earphones. These values must be added to or subtracted from the threshold obtained at each frequency.

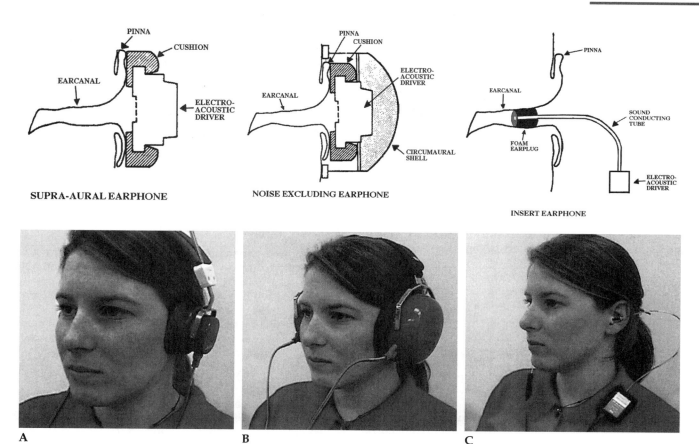

Figure 11–4   Schematic showing three types of earphones. **(A)** Standard supra-aural, **(B)** noise excluding (combination-type), and **(C)** Insert.

SPECIAL CONSIDERATION

Insert earphones eliminate the problem of collapsed earcanals experienced with supra-aural earphones.

Despite the advantages of insert earphones in audiometric testing, recent evidence indicates that only 24% of audiologists report their use in some clinical capacity (Martin et al, 1998). Nevertheless, their benefits certainly make insert earphones desirable for routine testing and some situations require their use, such as when the masking dilemma is encountered (see Chapter 12). If not used routinely, insert earphones are needed for at least part of standard audiometric testing.

SPECIAL CONSIDERATION

Removal of excessive/impacted cerumen may be necessary when insert earphones are used.

Bone Conduction Oscillator (Not Shown)

The bone conduction oscillator is used to obtain threshold measures of bone conduction sensitivity. Three types of bone conduction oscillators are used on audiometers: the Prac-itronic KH70 and the Radio Ear B72 and B71 (see Figure 10–4 in Chapter 10). The most common is the Radio Ear B71.

Signal Selector Switch (Labeled H in Figure 11–3)

In addition to generating pure tones, diagnostic audiometers are capable of presenting a variety of acoustic signals, including speech, masking noises, and frequency-modulated (warbled) tones. The signal selector switch provides a choice of signals to deliver to the patient.

Loudspeaker(s) (Not Shown)

Loudspeakers are used to present test stimuli in the sound field. One or more loudspeakers are mounted in a sound-treated room and test stimuli are presented to the patient at 0, 45, or 90 degrees off center to the right or left. As discussed in Chapter 14, pure tone stimuli should not be used with sound field tests; special considerations must be taken.

CALIBRATION OF AUDIOMETERS

The topic of audiometer calibration is covered extensively in Chapter 10. However, because of the importance of calibration in obtaining valid pure tone tests, the topic is reviewed in this chapter.

Over the past 45 years, five calibration standards have been adopted for audiometers: the American Standards Association (ASA) (1951), the International Standards Organization (ISO) (1961), and three different standards by the American National Standards Institute (ANSI, 1969, 1989, 1996). At present, all audiometers should conform to the ANSI (1996) standard (see Chapter 10). The Standard can be obtained for a fee by writing to the American National Standards Institute at 1430 Broadway, New York, NY 10018, or the Acoustical Society of America at 335 East 45th St., New York, NY 10005-3993.

The user of the audiometer is responsible for checking the equipment and providing for regular calibrations. Calibration is necessary to ensure that the audiometer is producing a pure tone at the specified frequency and intensity; that the stimulus is present only in the earphone to which it is directed; and that the stimulus is free from unwanted noise, interference, and distortion.

Four types of audiometer check/calibration schedules exist. These include a daily listening check, a monthly biological check, a periodic (annual) calibration, and an exhaustive calibration (every 5 years).

Daily Listening Check

After an appropriate warmup time (10 minutes), typically in the morning before the audiometer is put to use, the signal emitted from the audiometer is checked at various intensities and at all frequencies for transient clicks or distortion and to ensure that the signal is delivered to the correct earphone. In addition, the earphone opposite the activated earphone is checked to make sure no signal (*cross talk*) is present. It is far better to discover a malfunction in the equipment at the beginning of testing rather than to face inappropriate referrals.

Psychoacoustic (Biological) Check

At least once per month the output from the audiometer should be checked. This process can be performed with a psychoacoustic (biological) check or electroacoustical calibration check with a sound level meter. The psychoacoustic (biological) check involves obtaining baseline threshold measurements on three to five normal-hearing individuals who will be available for comparison testing throughout the year. If, on the monthly check, a threshold difference greater than 5 dB HL is found for one of the individuals for any test frequency between 500 and 6000 Hz, the other subjects should be checked. If a shift greater than 5 dB in the same direction is confirmed by the additional psychoacoustic checks, an electronic calibration of the audiometer is required. The results from each monthly psychoacoustic check should be recorded on a form that is kept in a calibration file maintained for each audiometer.

The electroacoustic calibration check is performed with a sound level meter and real-ear coupler. Measurements are obtained directly from the audiometer earphone at a fixed attenuator setting and compared with the expected ANSI 1996 reference equivalent threshold SPL value. If the difference is more than 3 dB, the audiometer would require electronic calibration. A recent survey by Martin et al (1998) found that 75% of respondents reported they used electroacoustical calibration checks as opposed to psychoacoustic (biological) measures to monitor their audiometric equipment.

PEARL

If access to a sound level meter and coupler is available, the monthly biological check can be replaced with an electroacoustic measurement of the audiometer output levels. The advantage of physical measurement is that if the outputs are found to be incorrect by more than 3 dB, it may be possible to correct them by changing the audiometer potentiometers.

Periodic Electronic Calibration

At least once each year, every audiometer should have an electronic calibration to ensure that it meets the minimum standards defined by ANSI S3.6-1996. For smaller programs that cannot afford the necessary equipment, calibration is provided by electronic or acoustic firms using specialized equipment. As soon as the audiometer is returned from calibration or repair, the user should perform a psychoacoustic check to re-establish new baseline thresholds as previously described.

Exhaustive Electronic Calibration

Every 5 years, each audiometer must have an exhaustive electronic calibration. This calibration is more comprehensive than the periodic electronic calibration and includes the testing of all settings on the frequency and intensity (HL/HTL) dials, as well as replacing switches, cords, earphone drivers, and cushions.

THE AUDIOGRAM AND AUDIOMETRIC SYMBOLS

The audiogram displays data from the audiological evaluation. As shown in Figures 11–5A and 11–5B, frequency is displayed on the abscissa (horizontal axis) and intensity, in dB HL , is displayed on the ordinate (vertical axis). Whenever an audiogram is constructed, one octave on the frequency scale should be equivalent in span to 20 dB on the HL scale. In addition, grid lines of equal darkness and thickness should appear at octave intervals on the frequency scale and at 10 dB intervals on the intensity scale. The ASHA audiogram form records both right and left ear information on one graph, as shown in Figure 11–5A. Forms with a graph for each ear, as shown in Figure 11–5B, are common in audiology practice.

Several audiometric symbol systems have been used by different clinics to record air and bone conduction thresholds. This diversity has resulted in confusion and possible misinterpretation when records are exchanged between clinics. For this reason, the American Speech-Language-Hearing Association (ASHA) has developed a standard symbol system for audiograms.

As shown, the symbols "O" and "X" are used for unmasked air conduction thresholds, and open arrows (carets) pointing with the open end facing to the right and to the left of the frequency indication line are used for unmasked bone conduction thresholds for the right and left ears, respectively. Triangles

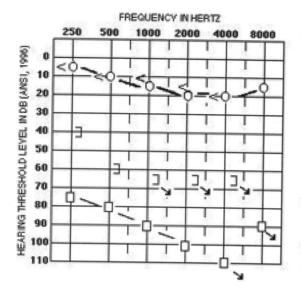

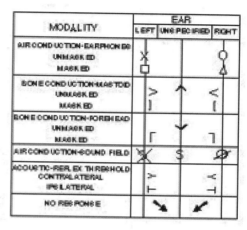

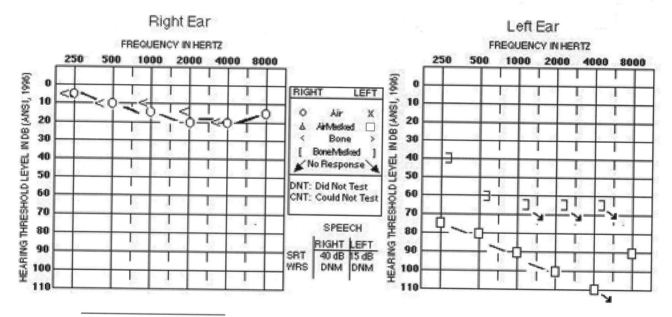

Figure 11–5 Example of on an ASHA audiogram form with symbol legend *(top)* and an audiogram form showing data for each ear separately with symbol legend *(bottom)* with the same audiometric data plotted on both.

and squares are used for right and left masked air conduction thresholds, respectively. Brackets with the open end facing to the right and to the left are used for masked bone conduction thresholds for the right and left ears, respectively. Positioning the symbols for bone conduction tests on the audiogram is easy to remember if the clinician imagines the patient's head on the audiogram facing forward; the open end of the bone conduction symbols fit over the ears like earphones. The symbol "S" is used to represent sound field testing.

When no response is obtained at the maximum output of the audiometer, the ASHA guidelines recommend the use of an arrow attached to the lower outside corner of the appropriate

symbol, about 45 degrees outward from the frequency axis (pointing down and to the right for left ear symbols and down and to the left for right ear symbols). The symbol system should appear on the audiogram form (see Fig. 11–5).

TYPES OF HEARING LOSS

Normal Findings

When no hearing loss is present, pure tone air and bone conduction thresholds will be at 0 dB HL at all frequencies. This

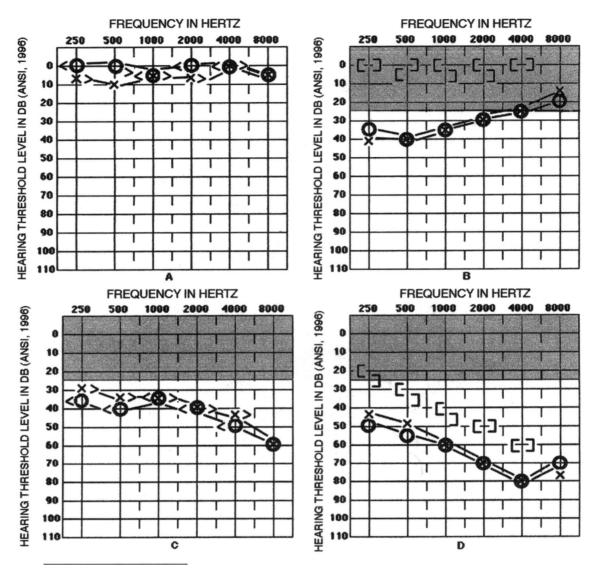

Figure 11–6   Audiometric results showing normal-hearing (**A**), conductive hearing loss (**B**), sensorineural hearing loss (**C**), and mixed hearing loss (**D**).

finding is shown in Figure 11–6A. It is possible to have all thresholds at 0 dB HL, but this finding is very rare. Typically, thresholds for patients with no communication difficulty fall between 0- and 15 or 0- and 25-dB HL. In a very few cases, it is possible to find thresholds less than 0 dB HL (-5 dB), which would suggest threshold sensitivity that is significantly better than the normal ear. However, since the acceptance of the ANSI standard, this is an extremely rare finding, and if it occurs frequently, calibration of the audiometer should be checked.

Although 0 dB HL is the value representing "perfect," normal-hearing sensitivity, a range of intensities is considered to be within normal limits (0- to 15-dB HL for children and 0- to 25-dB HL for adults). Those with thresholds in this range should have minimal or little difficulty hearing normal conversational speech, unless other audiological manifestations are present. However, it should be remembered that any deviation from 0 dB represents a decrease of hearing from the norm; a 10 dB threshold is a loss of 10 dB compared with the normal reference level.

As pointed out in Chapter 13, pure tone test findings should be in agreement with results from speech audiometry. The *pure tone average* (PTA), or the average threshold of 500, 1000, and 2000 Hz, should be within 5- to 10-dB of the speech reception threshold. If this is not the case, the clinician should first make sure the procedures used to perform the test were appropriate, check the equipment used to perform the tests and then reinstruct the patient. If the PTA and speech threshold results still do not agree it is possible that the patient is not cooperating (pseudohypoacusis; see the following).

By comparing air conduction thresholds to bone conduction thresholds, the three types of organic hearing loss can be defined: conductive, sensorineural, and mixed. Figure 11–7 shows the difference between these types of hearing loss on the basis of the anatomical site involved. In addition to these

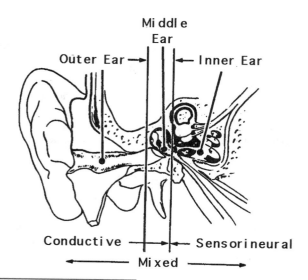

Figure 11–7 The three types of hearing loss classified according to anatomic site of involvement.

three organic types of hearing loss, two other classifications are pseudohypoacucis (nonorganic or functional hearing loss) and central auditory dysfunction.

Conductive Hearing Loss

The audiometric findings for conductive hearing loss are displayed in Figure 11–6B. As shown, both pure tone bone conduction thresholds are normal, and pure tone air conduction thresholds are abnormal with conductive loss. In addition, measures of middle ear functions (see Chapter 17) will be abnormal with conductive loss. Because the air conduction signals will actually set the skull into motion at levels of 60- to 70-dB HL, the maximum amount of hearing loss possible because of a pathological conductive condition is 60- to 70-dB. That is, losses greater than 60- to 70-dB cannot be exclusively conductive in nature.

Two behavioral symptoms may separate patients with conductive hearing loss from those with mixed or sensorineural hearing loss. Those with conductive hearing loss will demonstrate no difficulty discriminating speech for a sufficiently loud signal. Moreover, the individual's own speech may be spoken softly because the individual may hear his or her own voice louder than normal because of an "occlusion effect" resulting from the conductive hearing loss. This effect can be demonstrated easily to normal-hearing persons by having them close off their ears by placing their index fingers in their earcanals and speaking.

Sensorineural Hearing Loss

A pure tone audiometric pattern for sensorineural loss is shown in Figure 11–6C. With sensorineural hearing loss, air and bone conduction thresholds are both elevated and within 10 dB of each other.

Several symptoms characteristic of sensorineural hearing loss are shouting or talking in a loud voice, difficulty discriminating between speech sounds, and recruitment. Shouting or speaking in a loud voice may occur with sensorineural

loss because the impaired patient does not have normal-hearing by bone conduction. Hence, the patient's own voice or other voices may not be heard, causing these individuals to have difficulty regulating the intensity level of their voice. Not all patients with sensorineural hearing loss speak loudly, and not all patients with a conductive loss speak softly; many learn to regulate their voice levels appropriately. The frequent decrease in word discrimination ability associated with sensorineural hearing loss is due to distortion of the speech signal caused by auditory nerve fiber loss.

The typical sensorineural hearing loss is characterized by better hearing in the low frequencies than in the high frequencies. Consonants contain high-frequency information, whereas vowels are predominantly low in frequency. Therefore consonant sounds may not be heard or are easily confused. The clinician should keep in mind that, although the speech may be audible, it may not be intelligible.

Another symptom of sensorineural hearing loss, *recruitment,* refers to a rapid growth in loudness once threshold has been crossed. After the signal is intense enough to be perceived, any further increase in intensity may cause a disproportionate increase in the sensation of loudness. Thus the individual's *dynamic range* is limited. Dynamic range is the range of intensities between an individual's threshold and his or her uncomfortable listening level. Shouting at an individual with sensorineural hearing loss may result only in agitation rather than improved comprehension. Because of the combined effects of recruitment and word discrimination difficulty, individuals with sensorineural hearing loss experience greater difficulty in noisy surroundings than those with normal-hearing or a conductive hearing loss.

Mixed Hearing Loss

A pure tone audiometric pattern for a mixed hearing loss is displayed in Figure 11–6D. With a mixed loss, both air and bone conduction thresholds are elevated, but bone conduction thresholds are better (occur at a lower intensity) than air conduction thresholds by 10 dB or more. The difference between the two thresholds is referred to as the air-bone gap and represents the amount of conductive loss present.

Pseudohypoacusis

The diagnosis of pseudohypoacusis is made when an individual claims to have a hearing loss, but discrepancies in audiometric test findings and/or behavior suggest that the loss either does not exist at all or does not exist to the degree that is indicated by voluntary test results. Specific information on this classification of impairment and the diagnostic tests available are presented in Chapter 14 of this text.

Central Auditory Disorder

Central auditory processing disorders involve deficits in processing auditory information not attributed to impairment in the peripheral hearing mechanism or intellect. The processing of auditory information involves perceptual, cognitive, and linguistic functions. These functions and the appropriate interactions between these functions result in effective receptive communication. The following are examples of central auditory processing abilities (ASHA, 1993):

- Attending, discriminating, and identifying acoustic signals
- Transforming and continuously transmitting information through both the peripheral and central nervous systems
- Filtering, sorting, and combining information at appropriate perceptual conceptual levels
- Storing and retrieving information efficiently; restoring, organizing, and using retrieved information
- Segmenting and decoding acoustic stimuli using phonological, semantic, syntactic, and pragmatic knowledge
- Attaching meaning to a stream of acoustic signals through use of linguistic and nonlinguistic contexts.

Pure tone audiometric tests are severely limited in identifying central auditory disorders. As a result, specialized tests of central auditory function and central auditory processing have been developed. These specialized tests are covered in Chapters 15 and 16.

Auditory Neuropathy

Auditory neuropathy is a pathological condition of the auditory system. It is not a type of hearing loss but a dysfunction in the system. Auditory neuropathy describes a condition in which thresholds are in the mild-to-moderate hearing loss range, normal cochlear function is present (as evidenced by otoacoustic emissions and/or cochlear microphonic), and the auditory brain stem response (ABR) is abnormal or elevated beyond wave I. Speech perception abilities may be worse than suggested by pure tone data. Auditory neuropathy is a result of a lack of synchronous activity in the auditory nerve. For further information regarding auditory neuropathy, see Starr et al (1996).

DEGREE OF HEARING LOSS

The amount of hearing loss shown on the pure tone audiogram is used to classify the amount of hearing impairment. *Hearing impairment* is determined by results from audiometric data and is a function of the amount of abnormal or reduced audiological function. Hearing impairment is typically determined by the degree of loss, and results from pure tone tests are used as the primary means for classifying hearing impairment. No universal schemes are available for classifying the degree of hearing loss from pure tone tests. For this reason, a diversity exists from clinic to clinic in specifying the degree of loss. However, most classification systems are similar.

Because the effects of hearing loss vary according to age, separate systems are used for children and adults. Northern and Downs (1991) provide a common classification system for use with children as follows:

0- to 15-dB HL—Within normal limits
15- to 25-dB HL—Slight
25- to 30-dB HL—Mild
30- to 50-dB HL—Moderate
50- to 70-dB HL—Severe
70+—Profound

A classification system that is more appropriate with adults is as follows:

0- to 25-dB HL—Within normal limits
26- to 40-dB HL—Mild loss
41- to 55-dB HL—Moderate loss

56- to 70-dB HL—Moderate to severe loss
71- to 90-dB HL—Severe loss
91+ dB HL—Profound loss

These general guidelines for classifying hearing impairment become meaningful with respect to the communication difficulty a patient may experience when they are applied to the PTA of 500, 1000, and 2000 Hz. For example, if thresholds are 45-, 50-, and 65-dB HL at 500, 1000, and 2000 Hz, respectively, the PTA would be 53 dB and the loss would fall into the moderate range.

Hearing Disability and Hearing Handicap

Stating that a loss is mild, moderate, or severe on the basis of pure tone data provides assistance in describing the degree to which an individual will experience difficulty in communicating, but these simple terms do not detail the communicative, social, and emotional effects the loss may cause. In fact, it is impossible to predict the effects hearing loss will have on communicative and social function for an individual patient from pure tone data. However, the information presented in Table 11–3 is a general guide for estimating the communication difficulty presented by hearing losses of varying degrees.

The effect of the hearing loss on communicative function will depend on the type of loss and whether the loss involves one ear, both ears equally, or one ear to a lesser degree. For example, the patient with significant hearing loss in one ear and normal-hearing in the other will appear to hear normally, especially in a quiet listening environment. However, when noise is present, patients with unilateral hearing loss will have significant difficulty with speech intelligibility.

The terms *hearing disability* and *hearing handicap* are important in understanding the effects a hearing loss may have on an individual. Hearing disability refers to the limitation on function imposed by the hearing loss. Hearing handicap, on the other hand, is a measure of the effect the hearing loss has on psychosocial function. Seasoned audiologists realize that it is quite possible for one individual to have a severe hearing impairment, with only limited hearing disability or hearing handicap. On the other hand, some patients with mild hearing impairment may have severe hearing disability and hearing handicap.

Because the levels of disability and handicap are so variable between individuals, it is critical that audiologists make an assessment of these variables for each patient. Assessing these variables has the goal of defining the nature and extent of the hearing loss on the individual and providing appropriate strategies for rehabilitation.

Disability and handicap are measured with self-assessment scales. Patients are asked to fill out questionnaires addressing how the hearing loss affects them in a variety of listening situations and how it affects their self-perception. These scales are designed to assess the extent of the hearing disability, the social and emotional consequences on the individual, and the extent to which the hearing loss influences quality of life. It is only through this type of analysis that hearing disability and handicap can be determined.

Deaf versus Hard-of-Hearing

Sometimes the term *deaf* is used to describe individuals having severe or profound hearing loss. However, the term *deaf* is

TABLE 11–3 Degree of communication difficulty as a function of hearing loss

Communication Difficulty	Level of Hearing Loss (Pure Tone Average 500-1000-2000 Hz)	Degree of Loss
Demonstrates difficulty understanding soft-spoken speech; good candidate for hearing aid(s); children will need preferential seating and resource help in school.	25–40	Mild
Demonstrates an understanding of speech at 3–5 ft; requires the use of hearing aid(s); children will need preferential seating, resource help, and speech therapy.	40–55	Moderate
Speech must be loud for auditory reception; difficulty in group settings; requires the use of hearing aid(s); children will require special classes for hearing-impaired, plus all of the above.	55–70	Moderate-to-severe
Loud speech may be understood at 1 ft from ear; may distinguish vowels but not consonants; requires the use of hearing aid(s); children will require classes for hearing-impaired, plus all of the above.	70–90	Severe
Does not rely on audition as primary modality for communication; may benefit from hearing aid(s); may benefit from cochlear implant; children will require all of the above plus total communication.	90+	Profound

After Goodman (1965), with permission.

technically reserved for individuals with hearing loss whose auditory sensitivity is so severely impaired that only a few or none of the prosodic and phonetic elements of speech can be recognized. For these individuals, the primary sensory input for communication may be other than the auditory channel. Few individuals with hearing loss are truly "deaf."

On the other hand, the term *hard-of-hearing* refers to individuals with hearing loss that can identify enough of the distinguishing features of speech through hearing alone to permit at least partial recognition of spoken language. Individuals classified as hard-of-hearing rely on the auditory channel as the primary sensory input for communication. With the addition of the visual system (speechreading), individuals who are deaf or hard-of-hearing may understand even more language, provided the vocabulary and syntax are within the linguistic code.

PURE TONE AIR AND BONE CONDUCTION PROCEDURES

Pure tone tests are used to obtain air conduction and bone conduction thresholds that will determine the type and degree of the loss.

Pure Tone Air Conduction

In pure tone air conduction audiometry, threshold sensitivity is assessed with supra-aural or insert earphones. Pure tone air conduction thresholds are used to specify the degree of hearing loss but are not sufficient to determine the type of hearing loss (e.g., conductive, sensorineural, or mixed). That is, pure tone stimuli presented by the air conduction route stimulate both the conduction (outer and middle ear) and

sensorineural mechanisms (cochlea and the eighth cranial nerve), thereby making it impossible to isolate the site of damage to one area.

When performing air and bone conduction threshold audiometry, a possibility exists that the test signal will "crossover" to the nontest ear. Whenever the possibility of "crossover" exists, masking noise must be presented to exclude the nontest ear from participating in the test. The topic of masking is covered in detail in Chapter 12.

Reliable and valid pure tone data are critical in diagnostic audiology. Factors that can affect test results and/or should be considered as part of every pure tone test include case history/patient information, test environment, listener position, instructions to the patient, ear examination, earphone/bone conduction oscillator placement, ear selection, frequency sequencing, response strategy, threshold procedure, false negative and false positive responses, and infection control procedures.

Case History/Patient Information

Before testing begins, a complete case history should be completed and the patient's general communication impairment should be assessed. The importance of visual cues to comprehension can be determined by talking to patients outside their visual field or with the examiner's mouth covered. Preliminary information on the degree of hearing loss can be obtained by varying vocal intensity while the examiner's mouth is obscured. Answers to questions that could be helpful during pure tone threshold testing include whether the patient has tinnitus (a ringing sensation), which is the better ear (can the patient hear from each ear when using the telephone), and what types of sounds are the most difficult to hear.

It is important to realize that communicative impairment is complex, idiosyncratic, and does not always correlate with pure tone findings. For example, some patients with severe or profound losses, because they have learned to compensate with speechreading, may not demonstrate their severe impairment.

Test Environment

Pure tone threshold audiometry must be performed in a test environment that is free from visual distractions and that meets specifications for background noise levels as defined in ANSI (1991). To meet the standard it is virtually imperative that a commercially built sound-treated enclosure is used, although some custom-made environments are acceptable. If testing is performed outside sound-proofed enclosures, sound level measurements are required to determine whether the environment meets specifications. An important point is that even if a sound-proofed enclosure is used, a possibility exists that the environment will not meet minimum background noise specifications. Routinely finding elevated thresholds in the low frequencies (250 to 500 Hz) is one indication that the test environment is not appropriate for threshold audiometry.

Listener Position

The patient should be seated in such a manner that movements made by the examiner are not observable by the patient, yet gestures made by the patient are observable to the examiner. Some clinicians prefer to have the patient seated so that he or she is facing 90 degrees away from the audiometer. In sound field testing it is imperative that the listener be positioned correctly in reference to the calibration of the speakers (see Chapter 10).

Instructions to the Patient

Test instructions must be in a language appropriate to the patient and should include the following points:

1. The type of response (i.e., what the patients should do when they hear the stimulus).
2. That the objective is to respond even to the faintest stimulus.
3. To respond as soon as the stimulus is perceived and to stop immediately when the stimulus is not perceived.
4. That each ear will be tested separately and that tones with different "pitches" will be presented.
5. Finally, patients should be asked if they have any questions.

PEARL

After giving instructions, it is always helpful to ask patients whether they have any questions. This will give them the opportunity to ask for repetition or clarification of information that was not heard clearly and/or not understood.

Asking patients whether they have questions at the end of instructions is an important clinical protocol for any procedure because it opens the door to the patient to request repetition or clarification of information they may not have understood.

Ear Examination

Before earphone placement, the pinna should be examined to inspect for any active pathological conditions. In addition, the earcanal must be inspected with an otoscope for pathological conditions and occlusion and for the possibility of occlusion resulting from earcanal collapse. When the earcanal is impacted because of excessive cerumen, it must be cleaned or pure tone findings will be affected. An abnormal otologic finding during inspection of the ear requires that a medical referral be made.

Earcanal collapse during threshold audiometry results from the use of supra-aural earphones. The cartilage of the pinna and earcanal "close off" the opening to the earcanal when the earphones are placed over the ears. Audiometric findings show the presence of conductive pathological conditions when, in fact, none are present. This condition is present in as many as 10% of young children and older adults. Each time earphones are placed on a patient the possibility of earcanal collapse must be considered.

Depressing the pinna toward the mastoid and observing whether the pinna displacement causes the entrance to the earcanal to narrow or close is one method to check for the possibility of earcanal collapse. Having a supra-aural (doughnut) cushion without the driver mounted in it is helpful to perform this procedure. A simple technique to detect and remedy earcanal collapse during testing with supra-aural earphones is to have the patient hold his or her jaw or mouth wide open during testing (Reiter & Silman, 1993). The pulling forward and downward of the cartilaginous portion of the external earcanal increases the lumen and will eliminate the closure due to pressure on the pinna. Of course, insert earphones can be used whenever earcanal collapse is suspected.

Earphone/Bone Oscillator Placement

Supra-aural earphones are placed so that the diaphragm of the earphone is directly over the opening to the earcanal. When earphones are placed on the patient, eyeglasses must be removed and hair should be pushed away from the ear; a lifted earphone can result in a low-frequency transmission loss. With bone conduction testing the presence of eyeglasses could increase the likelihood of vibrotactile responses if the oscillator comes in contact with the eyeglass stems.

Earphones are always placed on the patient by the examiner; if the patient readjusts them the examiner should recheck them before testing proceeds. A small displacement of the earphone away from the earcanal entrance can result in a threshold shift of 25- to 30-dB, or more.

When using insert earphones, it is best to place them as comfortably deep into the earcanal as possible. Increased depth increases the real-ear and interaural attenuation and will help control problems associated with background noise, crossover, and collapsing earcanals.

When placing the bone oscillator on the mastoid, the clinician should make sure that the vibrator does not touch the pinna itself (Fig. 11–8). Before placing the bone vibrator on the mastoid, as much hair as possible should be pulled away and the oscillator placed on the most available part of the mastoid without hair.

Ear Selection

Testing should begin with the better ear as reported by the patient or from previous tests if they are available. Testing the better ear first allows the patient to respond to stimuli with the least possible distortion and may save time if masking is needed.

Frequency Sequencing

The most common frequency used to begin threshold testing is 1000 Hz. A 1000 Hz signal is used because as one of the mid-range frequencies to which the human ear is more sensitive to than lower or higher frequencies, it has a pitch that is more familiar to most listeners, it is less effected by background and physiological noise than low frequencies, and the wavelength in relation to the length of the earcanal makes test-retest reliability better than higher frequencies. After establishing a threshold for the 1000 Hz tone, the next highest octave frequency (e.g., 2000 Hz) is tested, then 3000 Hz, 4000 Hz, 6000 Hz, and 8000 Hz. Testing at 3000 and 6000 Hz is

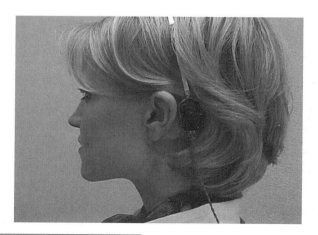

Figure 11–8 Bone conduction oscillator placed on the mastoid.

optional but is important when hearing loss is present at any adjacent frequency. After 8000 Hz is tested, 1000 Hz is tested for test-retest reliability and then threshold is established for the lower frequencies of 250 and 500 Hz.

Response Strategy

Two response strategies to signal the perception of the stimuli that are most commonly used with the cooperative adult patient are a handheld switch/button and hand/finger raising. Using a switch or button provides binary (yes/no) information. Hand or finger raising can provide the same level of information but can add quantitatively and qualitatively. Instructing the patients to raise their hands/fingers on the side corresponding to the ear in which they perceive the test signal helps to identify the location of the signal. In addition, the vigor and latency of the hand/finger response is often associated with the sensation level at which the patient is perceiving the signal. That is, at high sensation levels the response is more vigorous and has a shorter latency.

Threshold Procedure

The science of establishing the relationship between acoustic stimuli and the sensations that are produced by them is called psychoacoustics. Chapter 9 covers psychoacoustic principles in detail. When establishing threshold, the two choices are descending and ascending. With the descending technique, stimuli are first presented above the patient's threshold and the intensity is decreased until the patient no longer responds. The ascending technique, on the other hand, begins with stimuli that are below the patient's threshold and the intensity is increased until the patient responds.

The descending and ascending threshold techniques each have significant shortcomings. The descending technique is influenced by *perseveration* or continuing to respond when the stimuli are no longer perceived (false positive responses). The ascending technique is influenced by *inhibition* or failing to respond even when the stimuli are audible (false negative responses). Because of perseveration and inhibition, the use of an ascending or descending techniques alone for hearing threshold assessment can lead to high test-retest variability and inaccurate test results.

The modified Hughson-Westlake technique (Carhart & Jerger, 1959) was developed to reduce the influences of perseveration and inhibition. This procedure uses an ascending procedure to determine threshold. But each threshold search is preceded by a descending familiarization trial. A familiarization trial is used to reduce the effects of inhibition during the ascending threshold search. An ascending procedure was chosen for determination of threshold because it reduces the possibility that the patient may adapt to the signal or produce inappropriate responses on the basis of the rhythmical patterns of stimulus presentation.

Table 11–4 provides examples of the procedures followed with the modified Hughson-Westlake technique. Familiarization is accomplished by initially presenting a stimulus 1 to 2 seconds in length at a presumed suprathreshold level in the mid-range of hearing. This level, normally 40 dB HL, is determined by the audiologist during the pretesting interview with the patient. If a response is obtained, the intensity is decreased in 10- to 15-dB steps, and the stimuli are presented (1 to 2 seconds) until no response is obtained. If the patient

fails to respond at the initial setting of 40 dB HL, the intensity level is increased in 20 dB steps until a response is obtained (Table 11–4D). In Tables 11–4A to 11–4E familiarization is shown for each example from the initial presentation at 40 dB HL to the beginning of the threshold search. Broken lines denote the border between the two procedures.

Once familiarization has taken place, thresholds are established with an ascending technique in 5 dB steps. When the patient responds to a stimulus presentation, the signal is decreased by 10 dB and then increased in 5 dB steps until the patient responds once again. Threshold is defined as the lowest intensity level at which the patient responds to the stimuli for at least two out of three or three out of six trials.

ASHA's recommended procedure is similar to the modified Hughson-Westlake technique. Familiarization can be accomplished by one of two methods. The first method is to begin with the tone continuously on and increase the intensity until the patient responds. Alternately, the signal is presented at 30 dB HL. If a clear response occurs, threshold measurement should begin. If not, the level is increased to 50 dB HL, then in 10 dB increments until a clear response is elicited, after which the threshold search begins. This method of familiarization eliminates the need for the clinician to make assumptions regarding the patient's hearing ability before testing. Search for threshold begins 10 dB below the familiarization response.

TABLE 11–4   Examples of responses during pure tone threshold assessment (see text for further information)

A HL Dial dB HL	A Patient Response	B HL Dial dB HL	B Patient Response	C HL Dial dB HL	C Patient Response	D HL Dial dB HL	D Patient Response	E HL Dial dB HL	E Patient Response
40	+	40	+	40	+	40	−	40	+
35	+	30	+	25	+	60	−	25	+
20	+	15	+	15	+	80	+	10	−
10	−	5	+	5	−	70	−	15	−
15	−	0	+	10	−	75	+	20	+
20	+	0	+	15	−	65	−	10	−
10	−	0	+	20	−	70	−	15	+
15	−	Threshold = 0 db HL		25	+	75	+	5	−
20	+			15	−	65	−	10	+
10	−			20	+	70	−	0	−
15	−			10	−	75	+	5	−
20	+			15	−	Threshold = 75 dB HL		10	−
Threshold = 20 dB HL				20	+			15	−
				10	−			20	+
				15	−			10	−
				20	+			15	+
				Threshold = 20 dB HL				Threshold = ?????	

Each time the patient fails to respond, the level is increased by 5 dB. When a response is present, the level is decreased 10 dB. Threshold is defined as the lowest level at which responses were obtained in 50% of the trials, with a minimum of three responses.

The examples in Table 11–4 show the variety of responses that might be observed during threshold audiometry. Note that for example E the variability in the patient's responses made it impossible to establish a valid threshold. This patient would require reinstruction, retesting, and perhaps special testing.

Throughout testing, stimuli are presented with an on-time of 1 to 2 seconds and an off-time of at least 3 seconds. This technique takes advantage of the robust neural response to the onset of a stimulus and reduces the potential of auditory adaptation. Stimuli are not presented in regular temporal patterns during testing; the interval between tones is varied. Otherwise, the patient may simply respond in a rhythmic manner as opposed to attending to the stimuli.

False Negative and False Positive Responses

Two types of false responses can occur during threshold testing: the patient fails to respond when an audible stimulus is presented (a false negative) or the patient responds in the absence of the stimulus (a false positive). False negative and false positive responses are observed as part of the normal threshold procedure, especially when stimuli are presented at or near threshold. Stimuli near threshold are not easily perceived and when patients question the presence or absence of stimuli in the range near threshold, it is normal for them to respond incorrectly. For this reason, it is important that the patient be instructed to respond even when the stimuli are very faint and that it is acceptable to guess when unsure whether the tone was presented.

False negative responses are much less common than false positive responses during audiometric testing. Sometimes false negative responses reflect a lack of attention to the task. In this case the clinician may only need to reinstruct the patient. If simple reinstruction does not improve performance and the clinician has little faith in the responses obtained, this impression should be noted on the audiogram or examination report along with a note on the use of any nonstandard techniques.

False negative responses will occur when an individual is feigning a hearing loss (pseudohypoacusis). These individuals commonly exhibit unreliable responses because they have difficulty maintaining a consistent "threshold" level (they are unable to monitor their "loudness yardstick"). The special techniques outlined in Chapter 14 should be used for those patients demonstrating pseudohypoacusis.

False positive responses occur frequently when patients have tinnitus. That is, patients with tinnitus may mistake their tinnitus for pure tone stimuli and respond when no stimulus is present. These individuals typically have consistent responses but begin showing false positive responses for the frequencies at which tinnitus interference occurs, especially near threshold. Presenting a pulsed pure tone or warble tone signal for these patients helps them to differentiate the external signal from their constant internal tinnitus.

SPECIAL CONSIDERATION

Patients with tinnitus may exhibit a large number of false positive responses, especially when the test signal is near the tinnitus frequency. For these patients using a pulsed signal (200 ms on/off) or a warble tone will help them distinguish the test signal from the tinnitus.

Infection Control

Physical contact of any instrument used with the patient in the audiological evaluation can result in the spread of infection and/or disease. Supra-aural and, especially, insert earphones must be cleaned and disinfected between patients. Response switches/buttons should also be given the same attention. Because the clinician will come in physical contact with each patient during audiometric testing, handwashing should occur between patients.

PEARL

Handwashing is the most effective way to prevent the spread of infection and disease.

PURE TONE BONE CONDUCTION

Comparison of pure tone air conduction thresholds with pure tone bone conduction thresholds allows for the diagnosis of the type of hearing loss. With bone conduction testing, the conductive mechanism is bypassed, which provides for a measure of the integrity of the sensorineural mechanism in isolation. When air and bone conduction testing are used in combination, the difference between the air and bone conduction thresholds can be used to determine the magnitude of the conductive component. It is this difference that indicates whether the hearing loss is conductive, sensorineural, or mixed.

In bone conduction testing, thresholds are established in much the same manner as air conduction thresholds. However, instead of using earphones, a single bone conduction oscillator, secured in a standard headband, is placed on the skull. Before the development of audiometers with bone conduction capabilities, tuning forks were used to diagnose the type of hearing loss.

Tuning Fork Tests

Because they provide preliminary diagnostic information, require no special equipment, and are easy to administer, tuning forks continue to be used by many physicians in their everyday practice. As a result, audiologists must be aware of the tests that are used and their interpretations.

TABLE 11–5 Summary of commonly used tuning fork tests

Test	Purpose	Procedure	Results
Bing	Assesses the presence of conductive hearing loss	Tuning fork base is placed on the patient's mastoid, while the earcanal is alternately opened and closed by depressing tragus.	If louder when ear closed, the loss is sensorineural. If the same when the earcanal is open and closed, the loss is conductive.
Rinne	Compares air conduction to bone conduction sensitivity	Tuning fork is alternately held to the ear and then the base is placed on the mastoid process.	If louder when held to the ear, the loss is sensorineural (Rinne-positive result). If louder when base is placed on the mastoid process, the loss is conductive (Rinne-negative result).
Weber	Used for patients reporting unilateral hearing loss	Tuning fork base is placed midline on patient's forehead.	If lateralizes to the ear with loss, the loss is conductive. If lateralizes to the ear without loss, the loss is sensorineural or mixed.

The three tuning fork tests that continue to be used today are the Bing, Rinne, and Weber tests. Results from these tests are determined by the presence or absence of an occlusion effect (see Chapter 12). Because the occlusion effect depends on low frequencies, with each of these tests a low-frequency tuning fork (256 or 512 Hz) is used.

Table 11–5 provides a summary of three commonly used tuning fork tests.

As shown in Table 11–5, the *Bing test* is used for patients who have either a bilateral conductive or sensorineural hearing loss. In this test the tuning fork is set into vibration and the handle is placed on the mastoid process. With the tuning fork on the mastoid, the earcanal is alternately occluded and unoccluded by having the patient apply slight pressure on the tragus with his or her finger. The patient is asked whether the loudness increases when the earcanal is occluded (Bing positive) or whether no difference exists in the loudness of the tone for the occluded or unoccluded earcanal (Bing negative result). A Bing positive result means that the occlusion effect was evident and is responsible for enhancing the ear's sensitivity for bone conduction sounds. This result is seen in patients with normal-hearing or sensorineural hearing loss. If the occlusion effect is not evident (Bing negative result), the ear already has a conductive impairment.

PITFALL

Results from the Bing and Rinne tuning fork tests can be contaminated because of crossover of the bone-conducted test signal to the nontest ear.

With the *Rinne test*, the tuning fork is set into vibration and held close to the patient's ear. The patient is then asked to report when he or she can no longer hear the sound produced by the tuning fork. At this point, the handle of the tuning fork is quickly placed against the patient's mastoid process, and the patient is asked if he or she can again hear the tone. If the patient is able to hear the tone produced by the fork longer by bone conduction than by air conduction, the result is called Rinne negative. This finding is observed in patients with a conductive hearing loss. A positive Rinne test result occurs when the patient hears the tone longer by air than by bone conduction. This result is indicative of normal-hearing or a sensorineural hearing loss.

Care must be taken when interpreting results from the Rinne test because if the nontest ear has better bone conduction sensitivity than the test ear, the signal from the mastoid could crossover to the nontest ear and provide an inaccurate diagnosis of a conductive pathological condition.

The *Weber test* is a test of lateralization. It is used for patients who report unilateral hearing loss. The tuning fork is set into vibration, the handle is placed on the forehead, and the patient is asked to report where the signal is heard. Two possible responses are that the signal is heard in the ear with the hearing loss or is heard in the ear with the better hearing. If the signal lateralizes to the ear with the hearing loss, a conductive hearing loss is indicated because the improved bone conduction sensitivity is due to the occlusion effect. If the signal lateralizes to the ear with better hearing, a sensorineural hearing loss is indicated because the cochlea with the best hearing sensitivity will detect the signal. Patients with normal-hearing will report the sound in the midline position.

One more tuning fork test, the *Schwaback test*, was once popular but no longer is in general use. With this test, the tuning fork is used to quantify the magnitude of the hearing impairment. The tuning fork is set into vibration and is placed on the mastoid process. The patient is asked to report when he or she no longer hears the tone. At that point, the clinician quickly places the handle of the fork on his or her own mastoid and counts the number of seconds he or she continues to hear the tone. The main problem with this test is that it presumes that the clinician has normal-hearing. The results are expressed in terms of the time that the clinician heard the tone beyond that time that the patient's hearing diminished. For example, if the examiner can hear for 10 seconds longer than the patient, the test result is expressed as "diminished ten."

Audiometric tuning fork tests can replace standard tuning fork tests by placing a bone conduction oscillator set at 35- to 40-dB HL on the patient's forehead. The use of a bone conduction oscillator for these tests provides greater intensity control over the stimulus, increasing the reliability and validity of findings.

Pure tone bone conduction testing is significantly more sophisticated than tuning fork tests. However, tuning fork tests continue to be used regularly by many physicians to provide a preliminary diagnosis of the type of hearing loss. Although qualitative, tuning fork tests can provide a quick way to validate pure tone audiometric data. For example, the Weber test should lateralize to the impaired ear with a patient who has a unilateral conductive hearing loss. If it does not, the patient could have earcanal collapse during testing or masking might have not been used properly. Pure tone bone conduction tests provide both quantitative and qualitative information. As a result, tuning forks should never replace bone conduction audiometry.

Bone Conduction Tests

Signals from the bone conduction oscillator set the bones of the entire skull into motion, stimulating the cochlea in both mastoid bones. As a result, the cochleas of both ears are stimulated, and any responses obtained reflect the auditory sensitivity of the cochlea with the best hearing sensitivity. In bone conduction testing it is always important to be aware of the need to mask to prevent the nontest ear from participating in the test (see Chapter 12).

When the skull is set into motion by bone conduction stimulation, a complex mechanism occurs that involves osseotympanic, inertial, and distortional or compressional stimulation.

Osseotympanic Stimulation

The inertial properties of the bones composing the skull cause them to vibrate in response to the bone conduction oscillator. As the mandible moves, it distorts the cartilaginous portion of the external auditory meatus. As the cartilaginous portion is distorted, it alternately compresses the air in the meatus. In this manner skull vibrations radiate into the earcanal, and these vibrations are transmitted to the cochlea in the same manner as normal air conduction stimulation.

Inertial Stimulation

When the skull is set into motion with a bone conduction vibrator, the structures of the ossicular chain (including the malleus, incus, and stapes) are not rigidly attached, and a lag in their movement exists relative to skull movement. This lag causes the stapes to move in the oval window in a fashion similar to standard air conduction stimulation, thus transmitting the signal to the cochlea. This method of stimulation dominates in the low frequencies.

Distortional/Compressional Stimulation

When the skull is set into motion with a bone conduction vibrator, the compression of the bones of the skull gives rise to a distortion of the structures of hearing in the inner ear which, in turn, activate portions of the inner ear and electromechanical activity results in the sensation of hearing. The bony structures of the inner ear alternately compress the fluid-filled space of the inner ear. This compression forces the fluid contained within to move. Movement of the basilar membrane results from this compression and fluid movement, thereby stimulating the hair cells and resulting in the sensation of sound. This mode of stimulation is predominant in the high frequencies.

The procedure traditionally used for bone conduction testing is to place the bone oscillator behind the ear on the mastoid bone (see Fig. 11–8). However, some clinicians prefer forehead placement. Forehead placement increases test-retest reliability because frontal bone tissue is relatively homogenous compared with mastoid tissue. However, increased test-retest reliability is offset by the fact that 10- to 15-dB additional energy is required to stimulate the cochlea(s) with forehead placement, thereby reducing the dynamic range, or the amount of maximum output, achievable with bone conduction stimulation. Furthermore, ANSI standards for bone conduction are based on mastoid placement, and no forehead headband arrangements are commercially available that produce the necessary static force recommended by ANSI standards. These latter reasons explain why more than 90% of audiologists continue to use mastoid placement of the bone conduction vibrator (Martin et al, 1998).

CONTROVERSIAL POINT

Some advocate forehead bone conduction oscillator placement because test-retest reliability is increased. However, most audiologists continue to use mastoid placement because current ANSI standards are calibrated for mastoid placement, and forehead placement reduces the maximum output (dynamic range) for bone conduction tests.

PEARL

A routine procedure to improve intersubject and intrasubject reliability during bone conduction testing is to place the bone conduction vibrator on the mastoid at various locations while asking the patient to identify where the tone appears to be the loudest.

Although bone conduction testing is invaluable to the diagnostic test battery, inherent factors can affect bone conduction tests.

1. Variations in the size of the skull and thickness of the skin and bone of the skull are uncontrollable factors. As a

result, compared with air conduction testing, intersubject and intrasubject variability is high for bone conduction testing. With pure tone air conduction threshold audiometry, test-retest reliability for a cooperative adult is 5 dB. However, with pure tone bone conduction threshold audiometry, test-retest variability can often be 10 dB or even 15 dB.

2. Because it takes more energy to drive the bone conduction oscillator, maximum outputs from bone conduction signals are limited to 40 dB at 250 Hz, 50 dB at 500 Hz, and 60 to 70 dB at 1000 to 4000 Hz. The reduced output means that it is impossible use bone conduction results to determine the difference between a sensorineural and mixed loss when air conduction threshold sensitivity exceeds these values by more than 10- or 15-dB.

3. Tactile responses will be obtained for bone conduction stimulation at 250 and 500 Hz at intensities between 35- and 55-dB HL. Whenever low-frequency bone conduction thresholds are obtained in the 35- to 55-dB range, a high probability exists that the responses were a result of tactile, rather than auditory, stimulation.

4. The interaural (between ear) attenuation for bone conduction signals is 0- to 10-dB. As a result, crossover of a bone conduction signal from one ear to the other occurs even when a slight asymmetrical hearing loss is present, and masking must be used. Without the use of masking, it is quite possible to make serious errors in diagnosing the type and degree of hearing loss.

5. The effects of environmental noise are greater for bone conduction threshold testing because thresholds are obtained without occlusion of the external earcanals. With standard pure tone air conduction threshold audiometry, the earcanals are occluded with supra-aural earphones. The cushions of the earphones help attenuate the masking effects of ambient background noise in the environment. Bone conduction testing can be obtained with the earcanals occluded, which is referred to as *absolute bone conduction*. However, with standard bone conduction testing the earcanals are unoccluded, which is referred to as *relative bone conduction*. Because the ANSI calibration standard for bone conduction threshold testing is made on the basis of relative bone conduction thresholds (ANSI, 1996), it is not appropriate to occlude the test ear during threshold bone conduction testing.

PITFALL

Uncontrollable factors make the variability of bone conduction threshold testing considerably greater that air conduction testing. Clinicians must factor this into interpreting audiometric test results.

Although it is recognized that the preceding factors influence bone conduction testing, making test-retest reliability significantly greater than air conduction testing, bone conduction threshold audiometry is an integral part of the standard diagnostic audiological test battery. Clinicians must be aware that a greater variability exists in bone conduction measures and take this into consideration when interpreting diagnostic test results.

DESCRIBING PURE TONE FINDINGS

Table 11–6 lists terms that are commonly used to describe pure tone audiometric findings and graphically shows the general audiometric configurations they represent. Clinicians will have their own specific methods of describing audiometric findings, but the general protocol is to describe the degree of loss first, then state the ear(s) in which the loss is present, then use a descriptive term listed in Table 11–6 when applicable, and finally state the type of loss. Generally, the ear with the least amount of loss is described first.

Table 11–7 provides examples of pure tone audiometric findings from three different patients and verbal descriptions for each. Note in Example 1, when the term "high-frequency" is used, the implication is that the loss is above the upper limits for speech intelligibility (3000 Hz). In Example 2, two different types of losses are shown, and the symbols used indicate that masking was used to obtain right ear bone conduction thresholds and left ear air conduction thresholds. In Example 3, the term "presumed" sensorineural hearing loss was used for the left ear because the patient did not respond to bone conduction stimuli at the maximum limits of the audiometer, and it is possible that a conductive component is present.

HEARING SCREENING

The purpose of any screening program is to identify those individuals having a defined disorder as early as possible and refer for more comprehensive (diagnostic) testing. The objective is to accurately identify and refer those individuals with the condition (sensitivity) and dismiss individuals without the condition (specificity). This will avoid referring those individuals without the disease for further testing (false positive results) and missing those with the disease (false negative results). The goal of hearing screening is to identify those with hearing loss significant enough to interfere with communicative function and refer for medical and/or audiological follow-up, including rehabilitation.

Pure tone air conduction tests have been used for hearing screening of young children and adults for decades. Such tests have proven to be effective in identifying significant hearing loss for populations that are able to make voluntary responses to the pure tone signal. More recently, advanced audiological procedures have been developed that allow for testing noncooperative populations, such as neonates and infants. Table 11–8 provides guidelines for hearing screening from birth through 65+ years. Although the procedures for infants and young children do not use pure tone stimuli, they are included to show the capability that is now available for hearing screening throughout the life span. Chapters 21 and 19 cover the topics of otoacoustic emissions and ABR testing, respectively, and Chapter 22 is a detailed description of neonatal hearing screening.

TABLE 11–6   Common terms used to describe pure tone audiograms

Term	Description	Audiometric Configuration
Flat	Little or no change in thresholds (+ or −20 dB) across frequencies.	
Sloping	As frequency increases, the degree of hearing loss increases.	
Rising	As frequency increases, the degree of hearing loss decreases.	
Precipitous	Very sharp increase in the hearing loss between octaves.	
Scoop or trough shape	The greatest hearing loss is present in the mid-frequencies, and hearing sensitivity is better in the low and high frequencies.	
Inverted scoop or trough shape	The greatest hearing loss is in the low and high frequencies, and hearing sensitivity is better in the mid frequencies.	
High frequency	The hearing loss is limited to the frequencies above the speech range (2000–3000 Hz).	
Fragmentary	Thresholds are recorded only for low frequencies, and they are in the severe-to-profound range.	
4000–6000 Hz notch	Hearing is within normal limits through 3000 Hz and a sharp drop is seen in the 4000–6000 Hz range, with improved thresholds at 8000 Hz.	

Whether the hearing screening program is for infants or the elderly, common factors need consideration. These are background noise levels in the screening environment, pass-fail criteria, periodicity of testing, criteria for medical follow-up, criteria for audiological follow-up, and record keeping. These topics are covered in Roeser (1994) and ASHA (American Speech-Language-Hearing Association Panel on Audiologic Assessment, 1996).

CONCLUSIONS

Accuracy of pure tone tests is essential in audiometry because the pure tone test is the basis of diagnostic audiometry. The accuracy of testing depends on many factors the audiologist should understand. The stimulus is one such factor. The stimulus is composed of a wave of compression and rarefaction alternating at a given rate or frequency. This pure tone waveform has an intensity that is described in a logarithmic scale called decibels. The clinician must understand the equipment used to present the pure tone. The audiometer is a specialized piece of

TABLE 11–7   General format used to describe pure tone threshold findings

Degree	Ear	Description	Type
Mild	Right ear	Flat	Sensorineural
Moderate	Left ear	Sloping	Conductive
Moderately severe	Bilateral	Rising	Mixed
		Precipitous	
Severe		Scoop or trough shape	
Profound		Inverted scoop or trough shape	
		High-frequency	
		Fragmentary	
		4000–6000 Hz notch	

Example 1: Severe left ear precipitous high-frequency sensorineural hearing loss with normal right ear hearing.

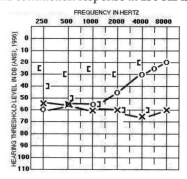

Example 2: Moderate-to-mild right ear rising mixed and a moderate left ear flat sensorineural hearing loss. (Note that the bone conduction response at 250 Hz is most likely tactile.)

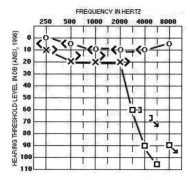

Example 3: Mild right ear rising conductive and profound (fragmentary) left ear (presumed) sensorineural hearing loss. (Note that the bone conduction responses at 250 and 500 Hz are most likely tactile.)

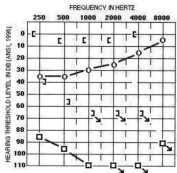

TABLE 11–8 Guidelines for hearing screening from birth through 65+ years

Age	Test Type	Opportunity To Screen	Referral Criteria
Birth to 4	Otoacoustic emissions (OAE) screen[1] Auditory brain stem response (ABR) screen	• All newborns not screened in hospital • Any child who presents with: ⇒ Parent concern ⇒ Speech delay ⇒ Language delay ⇒ Behavioral problems ⇒ Social problems ⇒ School performance problems	Those with high-risk criteria,[1] not already screened Those failing OAE or ABR screen Those with 3 continuous months of bilateral otitis media with effusion
4 to 18	Audiometric screen at 20 HL at 1000, 2000, and 4000 Hz[2]	• School hearing screening • Any child who presents with: ⇒ Parental concern ⇒ Speech delay ⇒ Language delay ⇒ Behavioral problems ⇒ Social problems ⇒ School performance problems ⇒ Excessive noise exposure	Rescreen those who fail at any frequency in either ear immediately Rescreen those who fail within 1 to 2 weeks Refer those who fail screen on second visit
18 to 65	Audiometric screen at 25 dB HL at 500, 1000, 2000, and 4000 Hz	• Periodic health assessment • Parent/family complaint • Poor or declining socialization or work habits • Excessive noise exposure	Rescreen those who fail at any frequency in either ear immediately Rescreen those who fail within 1 to 2 weeks Refer those who fail screen on second visit
65+	Audiometric screen at 25 dB or 40 dB HL at 500, 1000, 2000, and 4000 Hz (audioscope) Hearing Handicap Index	• Periodic health assessment • Patient/family complaint • Poor or declining socialization or work habits • Excessive noise exposure • Note that OSHA necessitates threshold testing (not screening)	Counsel those failing 25 dB screen that they have a problem Refer those failing 40 dB screen at any frequency except 4000 Hz Refer those failing Hearing Handicap Index

[1]Joint Committee on Infant Hearing (1991), with permission.
[2]ASHA (1996), with permission.

equipment that allows the clinician to control the intensity, frequency, and duration of the stimulus. The stimulus can be presented through earphones or speakers (air conduction) or through direct vibrational stimulus (bone conduction). By using both air and bone conduction signals, we are able to classify and describe the hearing of our patients. The clinician must have an understanding of the patient and of the response required. Another vital factor in testing accuracy is the procedure used to define the patient's thresholds. The presentation must follow standardized procedures to ensure the accuracy and reliability of the results. Results must be properly interpreted and classified. A careful record must be made to describe the hearing loss with standardized methods and recording techniques. Through knowledge of the nature of the test, the test equipment, the test procedures, and careful execution, an accurate assessment of the patient's hearing status can be made.

REFERENCES

ALLEN, G.W., & FERNADEZ, C. (1960). The mechanism of bone conduction. *Annals of Otology, 69;*5–29.

AMERICAN NATIONAL STANDARDS INSTITUTE. (1969). Specification for audiometers. *ANSI (S3.6-1969).*

American National Standards Institute. (1989). American national standard specification for audiometers. *ANSI (S3.6-1989).*

American National Standards Institute. (1991). American national standard maximum permissible ambient noise levels for audiometric test rooms. *ANSI (S3.1-1991).*

American National Standards Institute. (1996). American national standard specification for audiometers. *ANSI (S3.6-1996).*

American Speech and Hearing Association. (1974). Guidelines for audiometric symbols. *ASHA, 16;*260–264.

American Speech and Hearing Association. (1978). Guidelines for determining the threshold level for speech. *ASHA, 20;*297–301.

American Speech-Language-Hearing Association. (1990). Guidelines for audiometric symbols. *ASHA Supplement, 32,* 25–30.

American Speech-Language-Hearing Association Panel on Audiologic Assessment. (1996). *Guidelines for audiologic screening.* Rockville, MD: The Association.

American Standards Association. (1951). American standard specification for audiometers for general diagnostic purposes. *ASA Z24.5-151.*

Bell, J., Goodsell, S., & Thorton, A.R.D. (1980). A brief communication on bone conduction artifiacts. *British Journal of Audiology, 14;*73–75.

Berlin, C.I. (1967). Programmed instruction in the decibel. In: J.L. Northern (Ed.), *Hearing disorders.* Boston: Little, Brown & Co.

British Standard Institute. (1966). An artificial mastoid for the calibration of bone vibrators. In: British Standards House (Ed.), London.

Carhart, R. (1945). Classifying audiograms: An improved method for classifying audiograms. *Laryngoscope, 55;*640–662.

Carhart, R. (1950). Clinical application of bone conduction. *Archives of Otolaryngology, 51;*798–807.

Carhart, R. (1971). Observations on relations between thresholds for pure tones and for speech. *Journal of Speech and Hearing Disorders, 36;*476–483.

Carhart, R., & Jerger, J.F. (1959). Preferred method for clinical determination of pure-tone thesholds. *Journal of Speech and Hearing Disorders, 24;*330–345.

Chaiklin, J.B. (1967). Interaural attenuation and cross-hearing in air-conduction audiometry. *Journal of Audiological Research, 7;*413–424.

Corliss, E., & Koidan, D. (1955). Mechanical impedance of the forehead and mastoid. *Journal of the Acoustical Society of America, 27;*1164–1172.

Dirks, D. (1964). Factors related to bone conduction reliability. *Archives of Otolaryngology, 79;*551–558.

Dirks, D. (1985). Bone-conduction testing. In: J. Katz (Ed.), *Handbook of clinical audiology* (pp. 202–223). Baltimore: Williams & Wilkins.

Dirks, D., & Kamm, C. (1975). Bone vibrator measurements: Physical characteristics and behavioral thresholds. *Journal of Speech and Hearing Research, 18;*242–260.

Dirks, D., Lybarger, S.F., Olsen, W.O., & Billings, B.L. (1979). Bone conduction calibration. *Journal of Speech and Hearing Disorders, 44;*143–155.

Dirks, D., & Malmquist, C.M. (1964). Changes in bone-conduction thresholds produced by masking in the non-test ear. *Journal of Speech and Hearing Research, 7;*271–278.

Dirks, D., & Swindeman, J.G. (1967). The variability of occluded and unoccluded bone-conduction thresholds. *Journal of Speech and Hearing Research, 10;*232–249.

Fausti, S.A., Larson, V.D., Noffsinger, D., Wilson, R.H., Phillips, D.S., & Fowler, C.G. (1994). High-frequency audiometric monitoring strategies for early detection of ototoxicity. *Ear and Hearing, 15*(3);232–239.

Frank, T., Byrne, D.C., & Richards, L.A. (1988). Bone conduction threshold levels for different bone vibrator types. *Journal of Speech and Hearing Disorders, 53;*295–301.

Frank, T., & Holmes, A. (1981). Acoustic radiation from bone vibrators. *Ear and Hearing; 2,*59–63.

Goldstein, B.A., & Newman, C.W. (1985). Clinical masking: A decision-making process. In: J. Katz (Ed.), *Handbook of clinical audiology* (pp. 170–201). Baltimore: Williams & Wilkins.

Goldstein, D.P., & Hayes, C.S. (1965). The occlusion effect in bone-conduction hearing. *Journal of Speech and Hearing Research, 8;*137–148.

Goodman, A. (1965). Reference zero levels for pure tone audiometers. *ASHA, 7;*262–263.

Green, D.S. (1972). Pure tone air conduction thresholds. In: J. Katz (Ed.), *Handbook of clinical audiology.* Baltimore: Williams & Wilkins.

Hannley, M. (1986). *Basic principles of auditory assessment.* San Diego: College-Hill Press.

Harris, J.D. (1945). Group audiometry. *Journal of the Acoustical Society of America, 17;*73–76.

Hodgson, W.R. (1980). *Basic audiologic evaluation.* Baltimore: Williams & Wilkins.

Hood, L.J., Berlin, C.I., & Parkins, L. (1991). Measurement of sound. *Otolaryngology Clinics of North America, 24*(2);233–251.

Hudgins, C., Hawkins, J., Karlin, J., & Stevens, S. (1947). The development of recorded auditory tests for measuring hearing loss for speech. *Laryngoscope, 57;*57–89.

International Standards Organization. (1984). Acoustics: Pure tone audiometric test methods. *(ISO/DIS 8253),* Geneva: Switzerland.

Killion, M.C., Wilber, L.A., & Gudmundsen, G.I. (1985). Insert earphones for more interaural attenuation. *Hearing Instruments, 36;*34–36.

Kirikae, I. (1959). An experimental study on the fundamental mechanism of bone conduction. *Acta Otolaryngolagian Supplement, 145;*1–111.

Konig, E. (1957). Variations in bone conduction as related to the force of pressure exerted on the vibrator. Chicago: Beltone Translations.

Lybarger, S.F. (1966). Interim bone conduction thresholds for audiometry. *Journal of Speech and Hearing Research, 9;*483–487.

Martin, F.N. (1980). The masking plateau revisited. *Ear and Hearing, 1;*112–116.

Martin, F.N., Champlin, C.A., & Chambers, J.A. (1998). Seventh survey of audiometric practices in the United States. *Journal of the American Academy of Audiology, 9*(2);95–104.

Martin, F.N., & Wittich, W.W. (1966). A comparison of forehead and mastoid tactile bone conduction thresholds. *Ear Nose and Throat Month, 45;*72–74.

NAUTON, R.F. (1963). The measurement of hearing by bone conduction. In: J. F. Jerger (Ed.), *Modern developments in audiology* (pp. 1–29). New York: Academic Press.

NORTHERN, J.L., & DOWNS, M.P. (1991). Hearing and hearing loss in children. In: J. Butler (Ed.), *Hearing in children* (pp. 1–31). Baltimore: Williams & Wilkins.

PARK, K.R. (1996). The utility of acoustic reflex thresholds and other conventional audiological test for monitoring cisplatin ototoxicity in the pediatric population. *Ear and Hearing, 17*(2);107–115.

REGER, S.N. (1950). Standardization of pure-tone audiometer testing technique. *Laryngoscope, 60*;161–185.

REITER, & SILMAN. (1993). Detecting and remediating external meatal collapse during audiologic assessment. *Journal of the American Academy of Audiology, 4*(4);264–268.

ROBINSON, D.E., & WATSON, C.S. (1972). Psychophysical methods in modern psychoacoustics. In: J.V. Tobias (Ed.), *Foundations of modern auditory theory* (pp. 101–131). New York: Academic Press.

ROBINSON, D.O., & VAUGHAN, C.R. (1976). Relative efficiency of warble-tone and conventional pure-tone testing with children. *Journal of the Acoustical Society of America, 1*;252–257.

ROESER, R. (1994). Hearing loss and middle ear disorders in the schools. In: R. Roeser & M.P. Downs (Eds.), *Auditory disorders in school children.* New York: Thieme Medical Publishers, Inc.

SCHOW, R.L., & GOLDBAUM, D. (1980). Collapsed earcanals in the elderly nursing home population. *Journal of Speech and Hearing Disorders, 45*;259–267.

SHIPTON, M.S., JOHN, A.J., & ROBINSON, D.W. (1980). Air radiated sounds from bone vibrator transducers and its implications for bone conduction audiometry. *British Journal of Audiology, 14*;86–99.

STAAB, W.J. (1971). Comparison of pure tone and warble-tone thresholds. East Lansing: Michigan State University.

STARR, A., PICTON, T.W., SININGER, Y., HOOD, L.J., & BERLIN, C.I. (1996). Auditory neuropathy. *Brain, 119*;741–753.

STEPHENS, M.M., & RINTELMANN, W.F. (1978). Influence of audiometric configuration on pure-tone, warble tone and narrow band noise thresholds for adults with sensorineural hearing loss. *Journal of the Acoustical Society of America, 3*;221–226.

STREAM, R.W., & DIRKS, D. (1974). Effects of loudspeaker position on differences between earphone and free field thresholds (MAP and MAF). *Journal of Speech and Hearing Research, 17*;549–568.

STUDEBAKER, G.A. (1962a). On masking in bone-conduction testing. *Journal of Speech and Hearing Research, 32*;360–371.

STUDEBAKER, G.A. (1962b). Placement of vibrator in bone conduction testing. *Journal of Speech and Hearing, 5*;321–331.

STUDEBAKER, G.A. (1967). Clinical masking of the non-test ear. *Journal of Speech and Hearing Disorders, 32*;360–371.

STUDEBAKER, G.A. (1979). Clinical masking. In: W.F. Rintelmann (Ed.), *Hearing assessment* (pp. 51–100). Baltimore: University Park Press.

TONNDORF, J. (1972). Bone conduction. In: J.V. Tobias (Ed.), *Foundations of modern auditory theory* (pp. 84–99). New York: Academic Press.

VENTRY, I.M., CHAIKLIN, J.B., & BOYLE, W.F. (1961). Collapse of the earcanal during audiometry. *Archives of Otolaryngology, 73*;727–731.

VILLCHUR, E. (1970). Audiometer earphone mounting to improve intersubject and cushion-fit reliability. *Journal of the Acoustical Society of America, 48*;1387–1396.

WALKER, G., DILLON, H., & BYRNE, D. (1984). Sound field audiometry: Recommended stimuli and procedures. *Ear and Hearing, 5*;13–21.

WHITTLE, L.S. (1965). A determination of the normal threshold of hearing by bone conduction. *Journal of Sound Vibrations, 2*;227–248.

WILBER, L.A. (1979). Pure tone audiometry: Air and bone conduction. In: W. F. Rintelmann (Ed.), *Hearing assessment* (pp. 29–49). Baltimore: University Park Press.

WILBER, L.A., KRUGER, B., & KILLION, M.C. (1988). Reference threshold levels for the ER-3A insert earphone. *Journal of the Acoustical Society of America, 83*;669–676.

WILSON, W.R., & THOMPSON, G. (1984). Behavioral audiometry. In: J.F. Jerger (Ed.), *Pediatric audiology: Current trends.* (pp. 1–44). San Diego: College-Hill Press.

YANTIS, P.A. (1985). Pure tone air-conduction testing. In: J. Katz (Ed.), *Handbook of clinical audiology* (pp. 153–169). Baltimore: Williams & Wilkins.

ZWISLOCKI, J. (1953). Acoustic attenuation between ears. *Journal of the Acoustical Society of America, 25*;752–759.

ZWISLOCKI, J., KRUGER, B., MILLER, J.D., NEIMOELLER, A.F., SHAW, E.A., & STUDEBAKER, G.A. (1989). Earphones in audiometry. *Journal of the Acoustical Society of America, 83*;16.

ZWISLOCKI, J., MAIRE, R., FELDMAN, A., & RUBEN, A. (1958). On the effect of practice and motivation on the threshold of audibility. *Journal of the Acoustical Society of America, 30*;254–262.

## Chapter 12

Clinical Masking

Ross J. Roeser and Jackie L. Clark

Diagnostic audiology has the primary purpose of identifying etiological factors for hearing loss specific to each patient. To accomplish this goal, the auditory function of each ear must be assessed independent of the contralateral, or opposite, nontest ear (NTE).* That is, when an acoustic signal is presented to the test ear (TE), measures must be taken so that the contralateral, NTE, ear does not participate in the procedure. Stated differently, audiologists must be aware of prevailing circumstances that may allow the NTE to contribute to the evaluation of the TE because of *"crossover"* and be prepared to apply masking when necessary. Crossover occurs when an air-conducted or bone-conducted signal is presented to the TE at an intensity great enough to stimulate the NTE. Whenever the possibility of crossover exists, the application of appropriate clinical masking procedures is necessary.

Learning to apply masking principles regularly in clinical testing is one of the foremost challenges in audiology; students typically consider the topic of clinical masking a daunting undertaking. However, like all clinical skills the principles of clinical masking can be mastered easily if they are practiced regularly. To become part of routine clinical practice, masking principles must be studied thoroughly and then put into regular practice for several weeks or months.

This chapter provides readers with the principles of *clinical masking*. Specifically, clinical masking is defined and considerations for applying masking in clinical testing are covered. Applying masking in diagnostic audiology testing is based on two simple questions: When should masking be used? And, when needed, how much masking is necessary? Specific answers to these questions are provided, and examples demonstrate the principles of clinical masking.

WHAT IS MASKING?

Simply put, acoustic masking takes place when one sound (the masker) covers up, or makes inaudible, an acoustic signal (the primary auditory signal) a listener is attempting to hear. A more specific definition of masking is, "The process by which the threshold of hearing for one sound is raised by the

---

*The terms *nontest ear*, *contralateral ear*, and *opposite ear* will be used interchangeably throughout this chapter when referring to the ear opposite the test ear. During routine audiometric testing, when needed, masking is introduced into the nontest, contralateral ear.

Audiology: Diagnosis. Edited by Roeser, Valente, and Hosford-Dunn. Thieme Medical Publishers, Inc., New York © 2000

presence of another (masking) sound [and] the amount by which threshold of hearing for one sound is raised by the presence of another (masking) sound expressed in decibels" (ANSI, 1996, p. 5). In our everyday environment, as we listen to meaningful signals around us, we typically encounter masking in the form of unwanted, background noise. For example, during class lectures sounds from air-conditioning/heating systems, audiovisual equipment, conversations outside of the classroom, and so forth often interfere with (or mask) the instructor (the primary auditory signal). Masking in our everyday environment is considered interference; in this sense it is unwanted acoustic energy, an undesirable factor. However, when masking is applied properly during clinical audiometric testing, the masking signal is intentionally delivered to the NTE. Specifically, the appropriate use of masking prevents the inadvertent acoustic stimulation of the NTE resulting from a signal presented to the TE. This phenomenon is called crossover and will be discussed in detail later.

Masking versus Effective Masking

The definition of masking indicates that, like all other sounds, the intensity of a masking signal is measured in decibels (dB). For example, one could adjust the masking hearing level dial of an audiometer to 60 dB, and the specified level would then be 60 dB with regard to the audiometer dial for that particular audiometer.

Although the overall intensity of a masking signal can be specified in decibels, the decibel is a relative unit that becomes meaningful only if the reference is specified (see Chapter 10). For masking signals, the meaningful reference is *dB effective masking level (dB EM)*. The term dB EM specifies the ability of a masking noise to mask a signal of known frequency and intensity and is based on the spectrum (intensity and frequency) of the masking noise.

With the example from above, a masking signal delivered to an earphone with the masking dial of an audiometer set at 60 dB will provide 60 dB of masking noise to the specified transducer (earphone or loudspeaker). However, unless the audiometer has been properly calibrated, it is not clear how much acoustic energy can be masked by the masking signal at the 60 dB dial setting for each signal (pure tone or speech) the audiometer generates. That is, the 60 dB dial setting for the masking noise in the example might only mask a 1000 Hz pure tone at 45 dB HL, or a speech signal at 50 dB HL. If this were the case, at 1000 Hz the 60 dB setting on the masking dial would have an EM of 45 dB (i.e., 45 dB EM); for speech it would be 50 dB EM.

Clinicians should never assume that the masking dial settings on audiometers are calibrated in dB EM. Before masking is used with any audiometer, the effective masking levels of the masking signals must be measured. Measuring EM is also necessary when audiometers are modified as a result of calibration, especially when earphones or loudspeakers are replaced. The procedure for determining the effective masking level of masking signals will be discussed later in this chapter.

Clinical Masking

In routine audiometric testing, as shown in Figure 12–1A, acoustic signals delivered to one ear (the TE) can crossover

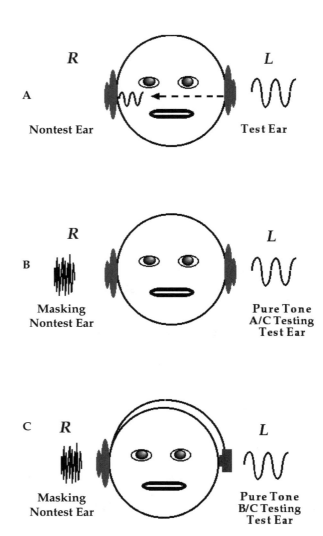

Figure 12–1 In routine audiometric masking **(A)** a signal delivered to the *(left)* TE will cross over to the NTE if presented at an intensity greater than the interaural attenuation level plus the B/C threshold of the NTE; when needed, the masking signal is delivered to the *(right)* NTE; **(B)** for A/C testing an earphone is placed over the *(left)* TE and masking is applied to the *(right)* NTE through an earphone; **(C)** for B/C testing with mastoid placement, the bone oscillator is placed on the mastoid of the *(left)* TE and masking is applied to the *(right)* NTE through an earphone.

to the NTE. When needed, the masking signal would be introduced into the contralateral, NTE. Figures 12–1B and 12–1C show how masking is applied during air conduction (A/C) and bone conduction (B/C) testing, respectively. Figure 12–1B shows an A/C signal being presented to the patient's left (TE) ear and a masking signal delivered to the patient's right (NTE) ear. In Figure 12–1C, a B/C signal is being presented with left mastoid placement of the B/C oscillator and masking is being delivered to the right ear with a standard supraaural earphone. When applying masking during B/C testing, the earphone on the nonmasked (TE) ear is placed anterior to the pinna. That is, during B/C testing the TE is *unoccluded*, and the masked ear (NTE) is occluded.

B/C thresholds obtained in the unoccluded condition are referred to as *relative B/C*, whereas B/C thresholds in the occluded condition are *absolute B/C*. Low-frequency differences between relative and absolute B/C thresholds result from reduction of background noise, changes in physiological noise, and a number of other factors. As a result, absolute B/C thresholds require less energy than relative B/C thresholds. B/C calibration procedures are based on relative (unoccluded) thresholds. Whenever the ear is occluded with an earphone during masking procedures for B/C testing, it is necessary to account for this difference by taking into account the *occlusion effect*. The occlusion effect is discussed in more detail later.

Central Masking

It has long been recognized that even with small-to-moderate amounts of masking noise in the NTE, thresholds of the TE shift by as much as 5- to 7-dB (Wegel & Lane, 1924). The term *central masking* is used to explain this phenomenon and is defined as a threshold shift in the TE resulting from the introduction of a masking signal into the NTE that is not due to crossover (Wegel & Lane, 1924).

Central masking results from an inhibitory response within the central nervous system, behaviorally measured as small threshold shifts in the presence of masking noises (Liden et al, 1959). As a result, the signal intensity level must be increased to compensate for the attenuation effect from the neural activity. Both pure tone and speech thresholds are affected similarly by the central masking phenomenon (Dirks & Malmquist, 1964; Martin & DiGiovanni, 1979; Studebaker, 1962).

Although the presence of central masking is unequivocal and averages about 5 dB, studies have shown variability in the magnitude of the central masking effect. Table 12–1 provides data showing the central masking effect for pure tone A/C and B/C stimuli for the frequencies 500 through 4000 Hz presented between 20- and 80-dB HL. As shown, the range is from 0.2- to 10.6-dB, with an overall average of 3.5 dB and 4.2 dB for A/C and B/C stimuli, respectively. On the basis of data from Dirks and Malmquist (1964) and data from other studies

(Martin, 1966; Studebaker, 1962), the average threshold shift from central masking has been estimated as 5 dB for pure tone A/C, B/C, and A/C speech testing.

However, some debate exists over a universal recommendation for a central masking correction applied during testing. It is argued by some that the general effect is about 5 dB, which would be considered well within test-retest tolerance for threshold measures. In addition, others find it difficult to recommend an exact correction simply because of the variability found by researchers. For these reasons, some clinicians do not correct for central masking during threshold testing. However, Martin (1966) suggests that compensation for central masking is wholly appropriate when testing suprathreshold speech recognition. As such, the presentation level would be set 5 dB greater than customary to account for the central masking effect. As with threshold measures, some clinicians believe that the 5 dB central masking effect is within test-retest tolerance and therefore do not include a correction factor for suprathreshold speech recognition testing.

THE NEED FOR MASKING

As stated previously, crossover occurs when the signal presented to one ear travels across the skull and stimulates the NTE. Crossover is encountered in routine testing with patients having unilateral or significant asymmetrical hearing loss, and the test signal must be presented at levels of 45- to 65-dB above the better ear. It is when patients with better hearing sensitivity in one ear are tested that masking is needed most. Crossover results when test signals "leak out" around the earphone cushions and travel around the head to the NTE or through the skull to the NTE (Chaiklin, 1967; Martin & Blosser, 1970).

A *shadow curve* may result when masking is not used and crossover occurs. Shadow curves are seen when thresholds from the ear with the greatest amount of hearing loss mimic thresholds from the normal or better hearing ear. Figure 12–2 provides an example of a shadow curve that would result

TABLE 12–1   Central masking effect for pure tone A/C and B/C stimuli between 500 and 4000 Hz presented at 20- to 80-dB HL*

| | Presentation Mode | | | | | | | |
	Pure Tone Air Conduction				Pure Tone (mastoid) Bone Conduction			
dB	500	1000	4000	Mean	500	1000	4000	Mean
20	0.2	1.2	0.6	0.7	0.5	0.9	0.6	0.7
40	1.8	3.0	2.2	2.3	2.9	4.5	1.6	3.0
60	3.6	4.5	3.1	3.7	5.0	5.9	2.1	4.3
80	7.2	8.8	6.2	<u>7.4</u>	7.8	10.6	7.3	<u>8.6</u>
Mean				3.5				4.2

*From Dirks & Malmquist, 1964.

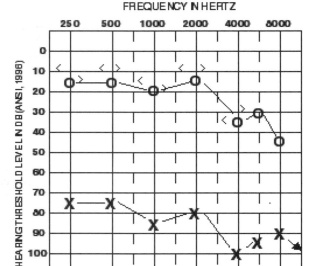

Figure 12–2 Example of a shadow curve. Note that the thresholds of the left ear are mimicking the B/C thresholds of the right ear at a level equal to 60- to 65-dB, which is the average interaural attenuation level.

from a patient with a mild-to-moderate right ear high-frequency sensorineural hearing loss and no hearing (a profound sensorineural hearing loss) in the left ear. As shown, right ear thresholds are consistent with a mild-to-moderate high-frequency sensorineural hearing loss, but thresholds from the left ear reveal a moderate-to-severe mixed hearing loss. For this audiogram, unmasked left ear A/C thresholds range between 50- and 65-dB poorer than those for the right ear. Because of crossover, A/C thresholds for the left ear are "shadowing" or mimicking the right ear by 50- to 65-dB. Note that the pattern of the left ear unmasked B/C thresholds are nearly identical to those for the right ear.

Figure 12–2 provides clear evidence for the need to mask in audiometric testing. Unmasked A/C and B/C thresholds from the left ear are highly inaccurate. The spurious finding of a conductive component in the left ear suggested medical treatment, when, in fact, a profound loss is present in the left ear. With the application of appropriate masking, the profound sensorineural loss in the left ear would be properly identified.

CONSIDERATIONS IN CLINICAL MASKING

Two basic considerations in clinical masking include interaural attenuation for A/C and B/C stimuli and the occlusion effect.

Interaural Attenuation

Attenuation of acoustic signals refers to the reduction or weakening of the force or value of energy (intensity) transmitted within some medium. As such, *interaural attenuation* is the amount of energy lost during the transmission of sound

by A/C or B/C across or through the skull to the contralateral ear. Interaural attenuation is measured as a level difference (in decibels) in the signal between ears. For example, if a pure tone signal is presented through a supra-aural earphone at an intensity of 95 dB HL to the right TE, and 45 dB HL reaches the cochlea of the left NTE, the interaural attenuation would be (95 dB − 45 dB) 50 dB. High interaural attenuation levels are desirable because the possibility for crossover is reduced. Interaural attenuation values are significantly different for A/C and B/C stimuli.

Air Conduction Interaural Attenuation

Interaural attenuation during A/C testing varies according to three factors: subject variability, frequency spectrum of the test signal, and earphone transducer type. Subject variability should not be surprising because it is known that interaural attenuation increases as the area of head exposed to the sound waves decreases (Zwislocki, 1953). The amount of sound vibration ultimately transmitted to the cochlea depends on individual skull properties, including thickness, density, and other such physical features. In addition to physical skull variations, there is also the ever present test/retest variability naturally occurring in individual subjects.

Table 12–2 lists means and ranges of interaural attenuation values for pure tone A/C stimuli between 250 and 8000 Hz using standard supra-aural earphones. As shown, the mean values for A/C interaural attenuation values are from 45- dB to 70-dB at octave frequencies from 250 to 8000 Hz, with a range of 40- to 80-dB. To prevent the possibility of crossover contaminating test results and in recognition of the large inter-subject variability, the recommended minimal interaural attenuation value for masking during A/C testing is 40 dB (ASHA, 1978; Martin 1994; Studebaker 1967). With the conservative interaural attenuation value, the possibility of not masking will be reduced or eliminated when it is called for. However, it should be realized that basing the need for masking during A/C testing on the minimal interaural attenuation value of 40 dB presents the likelihood of applying masking during clinical testing when, in fact, it may not be needed.

PEARL

The need for masking for A/C testing is based on the *minimum* interaural attenuation level of 40 dB for A/C. However, it should be realized that the *average* interaural attenuation level for A/C is 60- to 65-dB. This conservative approach will result in masking being used when it may not be needed. However, the application of this rule also implies that clinicians will never fail to use masking when it is needed.

Until recently, virtually all studies on interaural attenuation were performed with supra-aural earphones because supra-aural earphones have been the standard for audiometric testing. However, the use of insert earphones for routine audiological testing is becoming more commonplace (see

TABLE 12–2 Mean and ranges of interaural attenuation values for pure tone air conducted signals using standard supra-aural earphones (in dB)

Study	Transducer		Frequency (Hz) 250	500	1000	2000	3000	4000	6000	8000	Mean
Chaiklin, 1967	TDH-39	Mean	51	59	69	61	68	70	65	57	62.5
		Range	44–58	54–65	57–66	55–72	56–72	61–85	56–76	51–69	
Coles & Priede, 1970	NA	Mean	61	63	63	63		68			63.6
		Range	50–80	45–80	40–80	45–75		50–85			
Killion et al, 1985	TDH-39	Mean	50	60	60	60	60	65			59.1
		Range	45–65	52–65	52–65	50–68	50–68	52–74			
Liden et al, 1959	NA	Mean	58	60	57	60		61		63	59.2
		Range	45–75	50–70	45–70	45–75		45–75		45–80	
Sklare & Denenberg, 1987	TDH-49	Mean	54	59	62	58	57	65	65		60.0
		Range	—	45–60	45–75	60–65	45–70	45–70	60–75	50–80	
Zwislocki, 1953	NA	Mean	45	50	55	60		65			55.0
		Overall Mean	55	59	61	60	62	66	65	60	

TABLE 12–3 Mean interaural attenuation for insert earphones for pure tone stimuli between 250 and 6000 Hz (in dB)

Study	Frequency 250	500	1000	2000	3000	4000	6000	Mean
Killion et al, 1985	95	85	70	75	80			81
Konig, 1962	95	90	83	75	80	82	70	82
Sklare & Denenberg, 1987	100	94+	81	71	69	77	75+	81+

Chapter 10). One of the primary advantages of insert earphones related to clinical masking is that they provide increased interaural attenuation. Table 12–3 displays data showing mean interaural attenuation values for insert earphones for pure tones from 250 to 6000 Hz. As indicated, the range is from 70- to 100-dB, with mean values across frequency of 80- to 82-dB. The increased interaural attenuation for insert earphones will benefit clinicians during masking procedures. If insert earphones are not used in routine testing, they should be available to clinicians for difficult masking situations, such as the masking dilemma, described later.

Bone Conduction Interaural Attenuation

Interaural attenuation for B/C stimuli is dramatically less than A/C stimuli because both cochleas are encased within each temporal bone of the same skull. Once the skull is set into vibration, both cochleas are stimulated. The B/C oscillator may be placed directly on one mastoid process during unmasked B/C testing, but it should not be assumed that the response originates from the TE or even from one ear. As a result, clinicians cannot be certain which cochlea is being tested during unmasked B/C audiometry. In B/C testing the

minimum interaural attenuation is conservatively defined as 0 dB, and crossover should always be considered as likely during unmasked B/C testing.

The Occlusion Effect

Covering (occluding) the ear by any means can lead to a significant improvement in low-frequency B/C threshold sensitivity. This phenomenon is termed the *occlusion effect*. The occlusion effect is present at 1000 Hz or less and results from occluding the earcanal with an earphone, earplug, earmold, or any other object or substance. Although threshold sensitivity appears to improve during the occlusion effect, the hearing sensitivity of the cochlea does not change. Instead, the signal intensity received at the cochlea is increased. When the skull is set into vibration through osseotympanic bone-conducted sound transmission, sound waves are subsequently generated at the external earcanal and tympanic membrane. These sound waves reach the cochlea through the normal air-conducted route (Martin & Fagelson, 1995). Some radiated energy, especially low frequencies, will escape through the unoccluded external auditory meatus, but when the canal is

TABLE 12–4 Mean occlusion effect (dB) for normal-hearing subjects

Study	Mean Occlusion Effect Frequency (Hz)				
	250	500	1000	2000	4000
Elpern & Naunton, 1963	30.0	20.0	10.0		
Goldstein & Hayes, 1965	12.2	13.1	4.9	0.0	0.0
Hodgson & Tillman, 1966	22.0	19.0	7.0	0.0	0.0
Dirks & Swindeman, 1967	23.7	19.3	7.5	−0.6	0.0
Martin et al, 1974	20.0	15.0	5.0	0.0	0.0
Berger & Kerivan, 1983	20.3	21.6	7.5	−1.3	0.0
Mean	21.3	18.0	6.9	−0.3	0.0
Recommended occlusion effect values	**20.0**	**15.0**	**5.0**		

occluded (as with a supra-aural earphone) low-frequency bone-conducted sound transmission increases.

Individuals with sensorineural hearing loss or normal hearing are most likely to experience an occlusion effect, whereas those individuals with conductive hearing loss will not. This seeming lack of occlusion effect in patients having conductive hearing loss can be attributed to the occlusion effect resulting from middle ear pathology.

Table 12–4 shows the mean occlusion effect (dB) from several studies for normal-hearing subjects. Occlusion effect data shown in Table 12–4 were derived by subtracting B/C thresholds obtained from occluded and unoccluded conditions.

Because the occlusion effect is implicated as influencing thresholds during B/C testing, it is advisable to keep the TE unoccluded, thereby only covering the NTE with the earphone when preparing for masking. However, an occlusion effect can also be found with the earphone placed over the NTE during masked B/C testing. Overmasking, imprecise thresholds, or both could result if inadequate or no consideration is given to the occlusion effect.

TYPES OF MASKING NOISES

Effectiveness and efficiency of a masking signal depends almost entirely on the critical bandwidth. *Critical bandwidth* of a masking signal determines the masking efficiency or effectiveness of the signal. The goal is to mask test stimuli with a minimum amount of energy in the masking signal.

Fletcher (1940) was able to calculate a critical bandwidth to determine the necessary range of frequency components in the masker that would surround the test signal. His observations were that some outlying frequency components comprising the masker could be eliminated while still maintaining maximum masking efficiency. It was shortly thereafter that Hawkins and Stevens (1950) investigated dimensions of masking intensity level and the interaction with frequency band. They found that for a test signal to be at a just barely audible level, the overall energy of the masker's

critical band had to be equal to the test signal energy. Moreover, they found that those frequencies at and near the test signal had the greatest masking effect. As a result, they concluded that masking effectiveness is decreased when using a broad band masking signal because of the presence of unnecessary masking energy. As a result, masking noise effectiveness depends on the signal to be masked and the type of masking noise used.

The early diagnostic audiometers were equipped only with *complex masking noise*. Considered efficient for its time, the complex noise spectrum was made up of a fundamental signal at 120 Hz and all of the harmonics at multiples of the fundamental. Listeners could hear "beating" or pulsating sounds within the ear because of the discreet frequencies comprised within the signal. Complex noise provided inconsistent frequency and energy levels across frequency. Because of the restricted usefulness of complex noise, today's audiometers are not built with complex noise generators for use in masking.

Three types of masking noises are now available on most audiometers: broad band or white (thermal) noise; narrow band noise; and speech (spectrum) noise. Any of these noise signals can effectively mask a variety of test stimuli when presented at an appropriate intensity. However, to be most effective, a masking signal should be chosen with a spectrum as close as possible to the test signal. A basic masking principle is that the most efficient masker produces the greatest threshold shift with the least amount of energy.

Descriptions of each type of masking noise used in audiometric testing follow. Typical spectral plots for these masking noises are illustrated in Figures 12–3A to 12–3C.

Broad Band or White (Thermal) Noise

Broad band and white (thermal) noise are terms referring to masking signals having a wide band of frequencies within the range of 100 to 10,000 Hz at approximately equal intensities. However, as shown in Figure 12–3A, the typical acoustic spectrum of white noise maintains a relatively flat frequency response only from about 200 to 6000 Hz, at which point the

A

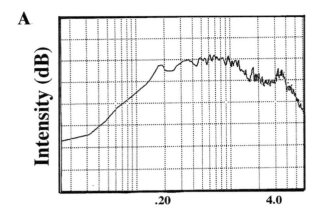

B

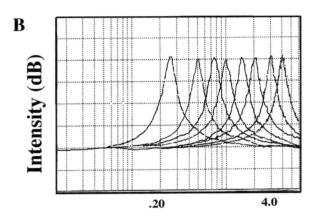

C

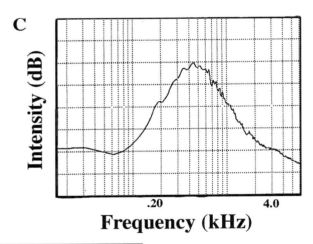

Frequency (kHz)

Figure 12–3 Types of masking noise used in audiometric testing. **(A)** broad band or white (thermal) noise; **(B)** narrow band noise; and **(C)** speech noise.

energy is dramatically diminished. For newer supra-aural transducers and insert earphones the response can extend to about 8000 Hz. The sudden drop in acoustic energy results from the limited frequency response of the transducer; frequency response characteristics vary from transducer to transducer. Despite limited high-frequency response, white noise is still considered a reasonably efficient masker for both pure tone and speech stimuli.

Narrow Band Noise

Narrow band noise is a type of filtered white noise. That is, narrow band noise is a band-pass–filtered white noise that allows for discrete shaping of the masking signal into defined bands. Specific noise bands are chosen during testing to contain only the frequencies surrounding the test signal to be masked. ANSI (1996) has provided the standard for the acceptable range of upper and lower cutoff frequencies for narrow band maskers for each test frequency. Filters are adjusted so that the noise band is centered on the same frequency as the pure tone test signal. As a result, narrow band noises are described by each center frequency; if the narrow band noise is centered at 1000 Hz, it would be defined as a 1000 Hz narrow band noise.

Figure 12–3B shows the acoustic spectrum for narrow band noise signals from 250 to 8000 Hz. This figure clearly illustrates how the center frequency of a narrow band masking signal is changed from low to high frequencies. During pure tone testing the center frequency of the masking signal is adjusted to correspond to the pure tone signal being tested. Use of narrow band noise during pure tone testing increases the efficiency of the masking signal, thereby requiring less energy to mask the test signal effectively. The increased effectiveness of narrow band noises reduces the intensity of the masked signal, which increases patient comfort during the masking procedure.

Speech Noise

Speech noise is a type of a narrow band masking signal that has center frequencies within the speech range. Because the primary acoustic energy responsible for speech intelligibility is in the 300 to 3000 Hz range, speech noise is shaped to correspond to this range (see Figure 12–3C).

CALIBRATING MASKING SIGNALS

One might incorrectly assume that the calibration reference of the relative average hearing level (i.e., dB HL), used with pure tone signals is equivalent for masking signals. However, it is not. A more meaningful reference for the effect a masking stimulus will have on a test signal is the EM. ANSI (1996) defines the EM level of a masking signal as the intensity of the masking required to shift the threshold of a test signal during simultaneous presentation with 50% probability of detection (p. 5). ANSI (1996) provides the necessary parameters for narrow band noise signals to establish EMs between 125 to 16,000 Hz. As shown in Table 12–5, specific critical bandwidths are designated with a lower and upper cutoff frequency for each center frequency specified. In addition, correction factors to add to the reference equivalent threshold sound pressure levels are included (see Chapters 9 and 10) to establish EMs for each narrow band noise masking signal. Of course, to establish physical measures of EMs would require sophisticated equipment, including a precision sound level meter, spectral analyzer, and an acoustic coupler, artificial ear, ear simulator, or mechanical coupler.

For most clinicians it is not feasible to purchase and maintain the necessary calibration equipment to establish EMs for

TABLE 12–5   Narrow band masking noise calibration standards (ANSI, 1996) with bandwidths, center frequencies, and corrections to determine reference test sound pressure level (dB)

Center Frequency (Hz)	Low Cutoff Frequency (Hz) Min	Low Cutoff Frequency (Hz) Max	Upper Cutoff Frequency (Hz) Min	Upper Cutoff Frequency (Hz) Max	Critical Bandwidth (Hz)	One-third Octave Correction to RETSPL (dB)*	One-half Octave Correction to RETSPL (dB)*
125	105	111	140	149	100	4	4
160	136	143	180	190	100	4	4
200	168	178	224	238	105	4	4
250	210	223	281	297	105	4	4
315	265	281	354	375	105	4	4
400	336	356	449	476	110	4	5
500	420	445	561	595	115	4	6
630	530	561	707	749	125	5	6
750	631	668	842	892	135	5	7
800	673	713	898	951	140	5	7
1000	841	891	1120	1190	160	6	7
1250	1050	1110	1400	1490	190	6	8
1500	1260	1340	1680	1780	225	6	8
1600	1350	1430	1800	1900	240	6	8
2000	1680	1780	2240	2380	300	6	8
2500	2100	2230	2810	2970	385	6	8
3000	2520	2670	3370	3570	480	6	7
3150	2650	2810	3540	3750	510	6	7
4000	3360	3560	4490	4760	685	5	7
5000	4200	4450	5610	5950	915	5	7
6000	5050	5350	6730	7140	1150	5	7
6300	5800	5610	7070	7400	1250	5	6
8000	6730	7130	8980	9510	1700	5	6
9000	7570	8020	10100	10700			
10000	8410	8910	11220	11890			
11200	9420	9980	12570	13320			
12500	10510	11140	14030	14870			
14000	11770	12470	15710	16650			
16000	13450	14250	17960	19030			

*Reference effective masking levels are calculated by adding the appropriate values to the reference equivalent threshold sound pressure levels (RETSPLs) at each frequency.
Reprinted with permission from the Acoustical Society of America.

masking signals. Fortunately most audiometers manufactured within the past few years have masking signals calibrated in EM. However, variability in audiometer masking signals makes it important to verify the EM of masking signals before they are used. The responsibility of verifying and monitoring masking stimuli used during testing lies with the clinician. An alternative to physical calibration of EM is the biological method.

Biological Method of Calibrating Effective Masking Levels

Calibrating EM with the biological method relies on responses from human ears. Because the biological method is relatively simple to perform, it is commonly used by most clinicians. With the biological method, EMs for normal hearing subjects are established by calculating the amount (in dB) that a masking signal is able to shift threshold for a test signal, either pure tones or speech, presented at a known hearing level. To determine the EM of a masking signal, the test signal is presented simultaneously with the masking signal through the same (ipsilateral) earphone. The EM of a masking signal is established at the intensity that the test signal is just barely masked by the masking noise. Threshold shifts are recorded for each test signal at a number of intensities (e.g., 10, 20, 30 dB) until the threshold shifts are linear. The difference between the masker dial setting and the test signal HL level are noted as a correction factor (CF), if needed, to establish the EM. This procedure is completed with three to five subjects. Results are averaged and made available for reference during testing, usually by posting them on the front of the audiometer.

Table 12–6 provides an example of results obtained with the biological method using three types of test stimuli: pure tones at 500 Hz, pure tones at 2000 Hz, and speech. Taking 500 Hz as an example, when the test signal was presented at 10 dB HL, a masking dial level of 15 dB was required to just barely mask the signal in the same earphone. At 20 dB HL, the masking dial level required to mask the 500 Hz signal was 30 dB. Above 20 dB HL a linear relationship was found between the increases in the amount of test signal and the amount of masking dial increase necessary to mask the test signal. That is, as the test signal was increased in 10 dB steps, the required masking increases were the same. In this case a correction factor of 10 dB was calculated at 500 Hz. Using this procedure at 2000 Hz and with speech, CFs of 15 dB and 10 dB were calculated for this audiometer, respectively. All additional test signals (250, 500, 750, 2000, 3000, 4000, 6000, and 8000 Hz, and speech) would be evaluated in a similar manner, and mean correction factors would be posted on the audiometer.

Speech noise is calibrated with reference to the speech recognition thresholds (SRTs). Therefore EM for speech noise can be calibrated with speech stimuli, as described previously, or are estimated by use of the average EM with speech noise at 500, 1000, and 2000 Hz. Calibration of spondee masking signals would assume average masked thresholds of three pure tones (500, 1000, and 2000 Hz) are equivalent to the SRT. Research has shown that when these three pure tones are combined, they best reflect major speech components (Sanders & Rintelmann, 1964). As a result, mean difference values for the average of 500, 1000, and 2000 Hz pure tones can be used for the calibration reference for spondees.

An alternative biological method, the *minimum EM level method (MEML)*, bases mean values from subjects with hearing impairment (Veniar, 1965). The MEML procedure assumes that ears with pathological conditions respond differently to masking than normal ears. Both test and masking signals are presented as in the biological method for pure tones. However, the noise that just barely masks the pure tone in these hearing-impaired subjects is defined as 0 dB MEML.

Certainly, the relative simplicity of obtaining EM with human subjects is an attractive alternative to other methods requiring specialized, and sometimes costly, equipment. However, as demonstrated in Table 12–6, the biological method can be time consuming because it requires evaluating a number of volunteers to implement the calibration procedure. Some degree of intersubject and intrasubject variability known to occur is tolerated while establishing threshold, but other threshold variations intrinsically occur as a function of the number of subjects tested. Intersubject threshold variability becomes more pronounced when the subject base is small or unskilled listeners are used. Skilled listeners are preferred because they have less variability in their responses.

THE APPLICATION OF CLINICAL MASKING

Consideration of several factors is required when the decision is made to use masking during the audiometric evaluation. To this point, underlying theories and principles to conduct audiometric masking have been covered. Because each mode of threshold testing (i.e., A/C, B/C, SRTs, and word recognition testing) has been dealt with individually, the application of masking procedures will be considered for each separate test procedure. During routine audiometric testing the first decision is to ask the question, "When is masking needed?" Once it is determined that masking is needed, it becomes necessary to calculate the amount of masking required.

WHEN IS MASKING NEEDED?

Through the years clinical practice has established basic rules that guide clinicians in making decisions regarding the application of clinical masking. The following describes masking rules for the essential test battery, including pure tone A/C, pure tone B/C, SRT, and word recognition testing.

PEARL

Masking principles are based on the *minimum interaural attenuation levels of 40 dB for A/C and 0 dB for B/C*. Consequently, when they are applied, masking will always be used whenever the *possibility* of crossover is present. Because of the conservative nature of masking rules, strict adherence to them will result in the use of masking when, in fact, it may not be necessary.

TABLE 12–6 Demonstration of the procedure for calibration of effective masking levels for pure tones at 500 and 2000 Hz and for speech stimuli (see text for description)

500 Hz

Hearing level dial	Masking dial
10	15
20	30
30	40
40	50
50	60
60	70

10 dB

2000 Hz

Hearing level dial	Masking dial
10	20
20	35
30	45
40	55
50	65
60	75

15 dB

Speech

Hearing level dial	Masking dial
10	25
20	30
30	40
40	50
50	60

10 dB

Correction Factors

Frequency	250	500	1000	2000	3000	4000	6000	Speech
CF		10		15				10

Pure Tone Air Conduction Testing

In pure tone A/C testing the determination of when to mask is made on the basis of the *minimum* interaural attenuation for A/C signals. Recall that for supra-aural earphones, the average interaural attenuation level for pure tones is 55 to 65 dB. However, the minimum interaural attenuation level for pure tone A/C signals with standard supra-aural earphones is 40 dB (see Table 12–2). Therefore to prevent the possibility of crossover during pure tone A/C testing, masking is needed when the pure tone A/C threshold of the TE exceeds the pure tone *B/C threshold* of the NTE by 40 dB or more. This is a conservative rule in most instances because crossover will not occur until the difference between the two ears is 55- to 65-dB. However, when using 40 dB as the criterion to determine the need for masking, it will ensure that masking will be used especially for those few patients with small interaural attenuation levels. However, with this conservative rule, it is possible that masking will be used when, in fact, it is not necessary. However, the use of masking should not affect test results, and it is better to err by masking unnecessarily than by not masking when it is necessary.

Comparing the unmasked pure tone A/C threshold of the TE to the unmasked pure tone *B/C threshold* of the NTE is *always* the fundamental procedure followed to determine the need for masking in pure tone A/C testing. The principle underlying the fundamental rule is simply that the pure tone A/C signal of the TE will crossover to the pure tone B/C sensitivity of the NTE.

PEARL

A corollary to the basic rule of when to use masking for pure tone A/C testing is as follows: Masking is needed when the pure tone A/C threshold of the TE exceeds the pure tone A/C threshold of the NTE by 40 dB or more.

Although the need for masking in pure tone A/C testing is based on a comparison of unmasked *A/C thresholds* of the TE to the *B/C sensitivity* of the NTE, a corollary to the rule allows for a shortcut in testing. That is, the need for masking can be determined by comparing the pure tone A/C thresholds for each ear. When a difference of 40 dB or more exists between the two pure tone A/C thresholds, masking is needed to obtain the threshold of the poorer ear. This corollary applies to A/C testing because B/C thresholds cannot be poorer than A/C thresholds. As a result, when the two A/C thresholds differ by 40 dB or more, the A/C threshold of the poorer ear and the B/C threshold of the better ear likewise will differ by 40 dB or more.

Clinicians must be acutely aware of the fact that it is not possible to assess the need for masking by comparing only the A/C thresholds of the two ears. It is only when thresholds differ by 40 dB or more that the need for masking is inadvertently made known. The ability to determine the need for masking when the two A/C thresholds differ by 40 dB or more is a clinical shortcut that may save time during routine testing. That is, it may be the case during the initial portion of

the audiological evaluation that only A/C thresholds are available. In such instances the need for masking can be established when the thresholds from the two ears differ by 40 dB or more.

Figure 12–4A provides an example of when to mask for pure tone A/C testing; for this example, the masking signal from the audiometer calibrated in Table 12–6 is used. As shown in Figure 12–4A, the patient's unmasked A/C and B/C thresholds at 1000 Hz are 10 dB HL for the right ear, respectively; for the left ear pure tone A/C and B/C thresholds are 60 dB HL and 10 dB HL, respectively. It is possible that left ear A/C threshold (as well as the left ear B/C threshold—see following) could be a result of crossover because a difference exists between the A/C threshold of the left ear and B/C threshold of the right ear (60 dB − 10 dB) of 50 dB. For this patient, masking would be needed when testing the left ear A/C threshold. That is, masking would be introduced into the right ear while obtaining the threshold at 1000 Hz for the left ear.

The masking corollary for A/C testing also applies to this example. Because the pure tone A/C threshold of the left ear (60 dB HL) differs from the pure tone A/C of the right ear (10 dB) by 40 dB or more (60 dB HL − 10 dB HL = 50 dB), masking would be needed when testing the left ear threshold. This corollary could be applied if only A/C thresholds were available during the test session.

Pure Tone Bone Conduction Testing

When deciding whether crossover has occurred during pure tone B/C testing, unmasked A/C thresholds of the TE are compared with unmasked B/C thresholds of the *same* ear; masking is needed if the difference is greater than 10 dB. That is, masking is needed whenever unmasked results indicate the presence of a conductive component greater than 10 dB.

PEARL

Masking is needed for pure tone B/C testing when the B/C threshold differs from the A/C threshold of the same ear by more than 10 dB.

Recall that the minimum interaural attenuation for B/C stimuli is 0 dB. Assuming that A/C and B/C threshold sensitivity is the same (± 5- to 10-dB) for each ear, B/C thresholds for each ear will be within 10 dB. However, as the degree of B/C threshold sensitivity of the TE differs from the threshold sensitivity of the NTE, crossover becomes more and more a possibility. When a difference in sensorineural sensitivity is present between the two ears of more than 10 dB, B/C stimuli presented to the poorer hearing ear will crossover to the better hearing ear before they are perceived by the ear with poorer hearing. In fact, when testing B/C and the threshold sensitivity of the NTE is better than the TE by 15 dB or more, crossover to the TE is likely.

Figure 12–4A provides an example of when masking is needed for pure tone B/C testing. As shown in this figure, when comparing the unmasked A/C threshold of the left ear (60 dB HL) with the unmasked B/C threshold of the left ear

A

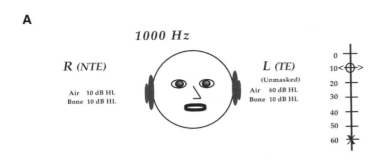

B

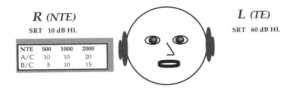

C

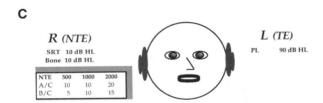

Figure 12–4 Audiometric data showing when to mask for **(A)** pure tone A/C and B/C testing; **(B)** SRT testing; and **(C)** word recognition testing.

(10 dB HL), the threshold difference (i.e., air-bone gap) is 50 dB. The criterion of an air-bone gap (ABG) of 10 dB or greater is not only met but is also exceeded by 40 dB, suggesting that crossover is likely. For this example, it is obvious that crossover affects the test results. With this patient, masking would be introduced into the right ear when testing the left ear B/C threshold at 1000 Hz.

Speech Recognition Threshold Testing

> ### PEARL
>
> **Masking is needed for SRT testing when the presentation level in the TE exceeds the best B/C threshold in any of the speech frequencies (500, 1000, or 2000 Hz) by 45 dB or more.**

Similar to pure tone A/C and B/C testing, crossover is possible when speech is used as the stimulus. The interaural attenuation level for spondees varies between 45- and 55-dB. On the basis of this, the minimum criterion on which to base the need for masking has been established as 45 dB (Konkle &

Berry, 1983). As a result, the decision to mask the NTE when obtaining the SRT in the TE is based on a 45 dB difference between the presentation level (PL) in the TE and the best B/C threshold in the speech range (500, 1000 and 2000 Hz) for the NTE. In practice, clinicians must consider the unmasked PL of the SRT in the TE and compare it with the B/C thresholds of the NTE at 500, 1000, and 2000 Hz. If any of the comparisons reveals a difference of 45 dB or greater, masking would be introduced into the NTE and a masked SRT would be obtained.

> ### PEARL
>
> **A corollary to the basic rule of when to mask for the SRT is that the need for masking exists when the SRT of the TE exceeds the SRT of the NTE by 45 dB or more.**

A masking corollary for SRT testing is that masking is needed whenever a 45 dB or more difference exists between the SRT of the TE and the NTE. This corollary is similar to the 40 dB rule used to determine the need for masking in pure tone A/C threshold testing. As with pure tone testing, this corollary applies to SRT testing because B/C thresholds cannot be poorer than A/C thresholds. Therefore when the two SRTs differ by 45 dB or more, the difference between the A/C threshold of the ear with the greater hearing loss (the TE) and the best B/C threshold in the speech frequencies (500, 1000, and 2000 Hz) in the NTE must be 45 dB or more. This corollary has a clear practical application. Some clinicians obtain SRTs for each ear before B/C threshold testing. As a result, if the two SRTs are found to differ by 45 dB or more, the need for masking would be evident without examining B/C threshold test results. An important point is that if the two SRTs do not differ by 45 dB or more, it is not possible to conclude that masking may or may not be needed; the corollary applies only if the SRTs, in fact, differ by 45 dB or more.

Figure 12–4B provides an example of test results requiring masking for SRT testing. In this case an unmasked SRT of 60 dB is obtained for the left TE, and pure tone B/C thresholds are 5 dB, 10 dB, and 15 dB for the right NTE at 500, 1000, and 2000 Hz, respectively. Because the 60 dB unmasked SRT in the left ear differs from the best B/C threshold of 5 dB at 500 Hz for the right ear by 55 dB, masking would be required to obtain the SRT in the left ear.

The SRT masking corollary also applies to the data in Figure 12–4B. Note that the unmasked SRT in the left ear differs from the SRT of the right ear by 50 dB. Although the B/C thresholds are also available in Figure 12–4B, it is apparent that masking would be necessary before B/C testing because the two SRTs differ by more than 45 dB.

Word Recognition Testing

Because word recognition testing is undertaken at suprathreshold presentation levels, an increased risk for crossover exists during word recognition testing. In fact, masking is used during word recognition testing more often than not.

PEARL

Masking is needed for word recognition testing when the presentation level in the TE exceeds the best B/C threshold in any of the speech frequencies (500, 1000, or 2000 Hz) by 35 dB or more.

Interaural attenuation levels for monosyllabic words have been reported between 35- and 50-dB. On the basis of these data, the criterion on which masking is based for word recognition testing is 35 dB (Konkle & Berry, 1983). To determine the need for masking during testing, clinicians would compare the presentation level in the TE to the best B/C thresholds in the speech range for the NTE (500, 1000, and 2000 Hz). Masking would be needed if the difference at any one frequency was 35 dB or greater.

As with other masking rules, a word recognition corollary exists: masking is needed when the presentation level in the TE exceeds the SRT in the NTE by 35 dB or more. Once again, this corollary applies because B/C thresholds cannot exceed

---

PEARL

A corollary to the basic rule of when to mask for word recognition testing is that the need for masking exists when the PL in the TE exceeds the SRT in the NTE by 35 dB or more.

A/C thresholds, which implies that a 35 dB difference exists between the PL in the TE and the best B/C threshold in the NTE at 500, 1000, and 2000 Hz.

Figure 12–4C provides an example of when masking would be needed for word recognition testing. As shown in this example, a 90 dB HL PL was chosen. A PL of 90 dB HL exceeds the best B/C threshold of the NTE by 85 dB, which is a clear indicator for masking. In addition, the PL exceeds the SRT of the NTE by 80 dB HL, also indicating the need for masking. For this patient, the right NTE would receive the masking signal when testing word recognition in the left TE.

HOW MUCH MASKING IS NEEDED: GENERAL PRINCIPLES

Over the years, psychoacoustic masking procedures have been developed to address the effects of threshold shifts in the TE resulting from various masking levels in the NTE. The plateau method, described by Hood (1960), provides clear definitions of three important masking levels (see Figure 12–5): the minimum amount of masking needed to prevent the possibility of crossover "minimum necessary masking;" the range of acceptable effective masking levels in the NTE "plateau;" and the point at which any additional masking is too much, "the maximum permissible masking." Any masking that is less than the minimum necessary masking is undermasking; masking greater than the maximum permissible masking is overmasking. Because of their importance in

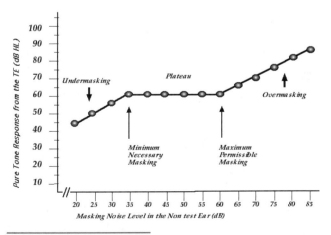

Figure 12–5 Example of the masking plateau showing undermasking, minimum necessary masking, the plateau, maximum permissible masking, and overmasking.

determining the amount of masking to be used, undermasking, the plateau, and overmasking are discussed in more detail in the following.

Undermasking

Considerable variation in terminology for the minimum or sufficient masking levels exists. Examples are "minimum effective masking level" (Liden et al, 1959), "minimum effective masking" (Lloyd & Kaplan, 1978), or "minimum masking level" (Studebaker, 1962). All terms refer to the minimum amount of masking in the NTE that would prevent the possibility of crossover occurring in the TE, or the *minimum necessary masking*. Any intensity less than the minimum necessary masking level is undermasking.

When undermasking occurs, a danger exists that the test signal will still be perceived in the NTE because of an insufficient amount of masking noise presented to the NTE. This situation may inadvertently occur because of equipment calibration errors resulting from an underestimation of the EM or clinician calculation error that underestimated the potential interaural attenuation. Obviously, either of these errors can render invalid audiological results.

An undermasking situation will continue to occur during testing as long as it is possible for test stimuli to be perceived in the NTE. For example, Figure 12–5 shows a case where masking noise presented below 35 dB in the NTE is at a level that undermasking occurs. For this masking situation a level of at least 35 dB is required to reach the plateau.

The Plateau

The masking plateau is the intensity range between the minimum necessary masking level and the maximum permissible masking level. The plateau begins at the intensity where the threshold in the TE remains stable when the masking noise in the NTE is increased. This is the point at which the minimum necessary masking level has been reached. Above this level, threshold in the TE begins to increase linearly while the intensity of the masking noise in the NTE is increased and the maximum permissible masking level has been reached. The masking plateau is the range of intensities at which effective masking of the NTE can be achieved while obtaining valid thresholds in the TE.

Figure 12–5 provides data from a hypothetical case where the width of the masking plateau is 25 dB (35 dB to 60 dB). As indicated in this figure, introducing less than 35 dB into the NTE would be undermasking, and introducing more than 60 dB would be overmasking. Intensities between 35 dB and 60 dB would effectively mask the NTE ear without affecting the TE threshold; this range of intensities is the patient's masking plateau. Establishing the plateau during masked threshold assessment provides solid evidence of the TE's true masked response for the test signal.

Masking plateau width will vary from patient to patient. The primary determining factor is the patient's interaural attenuation level. That is, the width of the plateau cannot exceed the magnitude of the interaural attenuation for each patient. From Table 12–2 it can be seen that the average interaural attenuation level for standard supra-aural earphones ranges between 55- and 65-dB, depending on the test frequency. These data imply that the average masking plateau will be within this range. However, during clinical testing the interaural attenuation value for a given patient is not known; an assumption is made that it may be as little as 40 dB, but will average between 55- and 65-dB.

Factors that can reduce the masking plateau for a given patient include reduced interaural attenuation values, reduced A/C thresholds in the NTE (a conductive component), or an increased occlusion effect (Gelfand, 1997). In fact, masking situations exist in which no masking plateau is present. That is, the minimum necessary masking and the maximum permissible masking are the same, and obtaining a masked threshold is not possible. This situation presents a masking dilemma because the level required to just mask the threshold of the masked ear will result in overmasking. The masking dilemma is discussed in more detail below.

As pointed out earlier in this chapter, the use of insert earphones has the advantage of increasing the interaural attenuation from 55- to 65-dB to 75- to 100-dB. By increasing the interaural attenuation, the maximum width of the masking plateau is also increased.

Overmasking

Overmasking occurs when the masking noise in the NTE is at an intensity great enough to influence thresholds in the TE. Figure 12–5 demonstrates the effects of overmasking. As shown, when the masking noise level in the NTE increases from 60- to 85-dB, the pure tone threshold in the TE increases linearly. Clearly, beginning at the 65 dB masking noise level, crossover from the masked NTE to the TE causes poorer thresholds in the TE. Any time the masking noise level in NTE is equal to or exceeds the interaural attenuation plus the B/C threshold of the TE, overmasking becomes a certainty (Martin, 1997).

HOW MUCH MASKING IS NEEDED: SPECIFIC PROCEDURES

At this point it should be clear that when the need for masking in the NTE exists, clinicians have a range of intensities at which the masking signal can be presented. The primary question, then, is at what intensity should masking begin, or for each masking situation what is the *starting level* for masking.

PEARL

To be certain that patients are clear about their expected task, it should be pointed out that they will hear a number of noises; regardless of their "loudness," the patient's task is to continue to respond only to the very soft pure tone (i.e., "note" or "beep") signals.

Establishing the Starting Level

The minimum intensity necessary to mask the NTE has to be at the level that will just affect the threshold of the NTE. This minimum intensity would be at an effective masking level equal to the threshold of the masked ear, or 0 dB effective level, and, as described above, is referred to as the minimum necessary masking. Starting level for masking is set at an intensity slightly above the minimum necessary masking. As a safety factor, 10- to 15-dB is added to the minimum necessary masking to account for the normal threshold sensitivity variability. By adding the 10- to 15-dB safety factor, one ensures that the masking signal is at an effective level just above the threshold of the masked ear. During testing, the factors needed to calculate the starting level for pure tone A/C testing are the threshold of the NTE (the masked ear) and the safety factor of 10- to 15-dB. In addition, unless the audiometer masking signals are calibrated in EM, a CF is included in the calculation. When masking is needed, the examiner begins by introducing the masked signal into the NTE at an effective level 10- or 15-dB above the threshold of the NTE. As described in the following, the patient's response to the masked signal presented at the starting level determines the procedures to be followed.

The same basic principle is followed for pure tone B/C testing. However, because B/C threshold calibration is based on unoccluded ears, and one ear is occluded with an earphone during B/C testing with masking, the occlusion effect is factored into the formula to determine starting level for B/C testing.

Two possible outcomes exist once the starting level of masking is introduced into the NTE. The two are illustrated in Figures 12–6A and 12–6B. First, it is possible that unmasked thresholds do not change significantly when the masking starting level is introduced into the NTE. This finding would indicate that the unmasked threshold was, in fact, not a result of crossover (a "crossover threshold") or that the unmasked threshold was valid. In Figure 12–6A the starting level of masking was determined to be 40- to 45-dB. The 40- to 45-dB level was found to be greater than the intensity required for the minimum necessary masking and within the masking plateau. In this case the threshold of the TE did not increase when the starting level of masking was introduced into the NTE.

Another possibility is that the starting level chosen is inadequate to prevent crossover. Stated differently, the possibility

A

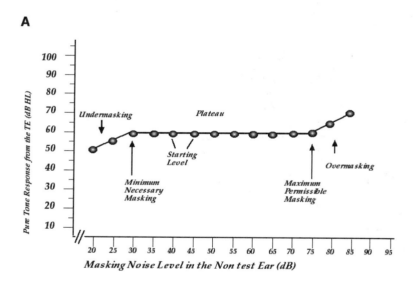

B

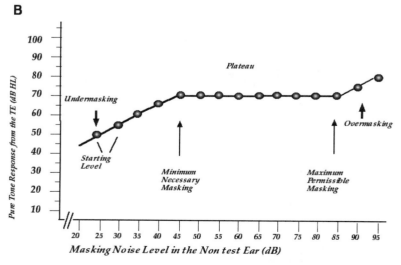

Figure 12–6 Examples of two possible outcomes when masking: **(A)** when the starting level exceeds the minimum necessary masking and is within the masking plateau; and **(B)** when the starting level is less than the minimum necessary masking.

exists that the starting level is not within the masking plateau. Figure 12–6B shows that when a starting level of 25 to 30 dB was introduced into the NTE, it was necessary to continue increasing the masking intensity above the starting level to find the masking plateau. In this case responses from the TE shifted to 45 dB HL before the minimum necessary masking was achieved and the masking plateau was found.

Specific procedures to establish the starting levels and necessary follow-up protocols for each of the basic audiological tests is discussed in more detail in the following.

Determining Masking Levels for Pure Tone A/C Testing

Figure 12–7(A to C) provides an example of when masking would be needed for pure tone A/C testing and the three possible outcomes for masked findings. As shown, for each of the three examples the unmasked right ear A/C threshold at 2000 Hz is 55 dB HL; left ear A/C and B/C thresholds are 10 dB HL and 5 dB HL, respectively. The 50 dB difference between the A/C threshold of the right ear and the B/C threshold of the left ear is greater than the 40 dB minimum criterion to establish the need for masking when the right ear A/C threshold is obtained. For this patient, when testing the right ear A/C threshold, the starting level for the left ear (NTE) would be at an effective level equal to 10- to 15-dB above the threshold of the left ear. Because the NTE A/C threshold is 10 dB HL for this patient, the starting level for masking would be at an effective level of 20- to 25-dB (10 dB HL threshold plus the 10- to 15-dB safety factor).

PEARL

To calculate the starting level for pure tone A/C threshold testing, add the threshold of the NTE, plus the CF (if needed), plus a safety factor of 10 to 15 dB.

Starting level (PT A/C) = threshold of the NTE + CF + Safety factor (10- to 15-dB)

Assuming the same audiometer used to calculate the correction factors in Table 12–6 was used to test this patient, the factors required to calculate the starting level are:

A/C NTE + Safety factor (SF) + CF = Starting level
 (10 dB) + (10–15 dB) + (15 dB) = 35–40 dB dial
                                             setting

The correction factor was calculated by use of the procedures described earlier in this chapter.

Once the starting level of masking is introduced into the NTE, the procedure then is to determine whether the unmasked threshold of the TE was affected by introducing masking noise into the NTE. That is, while masking is introduced into the NTE threshold sensitivity is assessed in the TE. Recall that central masking will affect thresholds in the TE by an average of 5 dB. The implication of this factor is that when masking is used in the NTE, it is likely that thresholds in the TE will change by 5 dB as a result of central masking.

PEARL

During masking patients may occasionally need reinstruction. Some indicators are frequent positive responses (both false and true); pure tone thresholds continue to increase and never reach plateau; or the patient ceases to respond to the audible pure tone stimulus because the masking noise is "annoyingly" loud.

Three outcomes are possible when masking is used: (1) masking does not affect thresholds in the TE by 5 dB or more; (2) masking does affect thresholds in the TE by 5 dB or more and a plateau is found; and (3) masking does affect thresholds in the TE by 5 dB or more and it is not possible to find a plateau.

Outcome 1: Masking does not affect the A/C threshold in the TE by 5 dB or more (Fig. 12–7A). If the unmasked pure tone A/C threshold does not vary from the masked threshold by more than 5 dB, the unmasked threshold is assumed to be valid and is recorded as a masked threshold. In this case, if the masked threshold is either 55 dB or 60 dB, this level would be accepted and recorded as a valid threshold and recorded as a masked threshold (as shown in Fig. 12–7A).

Outcome 2: Masking does affect the A/C threshold in the TE by 5 dB or more and a plateau is established (Fig. 12–7B). If the masked threshold shifts by 10 dB or more when the masking starting level is introduced into the NTE, it becomes necessary to find the masking plateau. When masking is used and the threshold in the TE shifts by 10 dB or more, the masking plateau is established as follows:

1. The threshold in the TE is reestablished by increasing the test signal in 5 dB increments.

2. Once a response to the pure tone signal is obtained, the masking noise in the NTE is increased in 5 dB steps and the threshold of the TE is reestablished.

3. This procedure is followed until the threshold in the TE does not change while the masking noise is increased in three consecutive 5 dB steps (the plateau is reached).

4. Once the plateau is reached, the masked threshold has been found. To account for the central masking effect, 5 dB is subtracted from the masked threshold and this value is recorded on the audiogram form as a masked threshold.

CONTROVERSIAL POINT

Some clinicians use 5 dB steps to reach the plateau, whereas others prefer 10 dB steps.

As seen in Figure 12–7B the initial unmasked threshold of 55 dB HL shifted to 70 dB HL by introducing a starting level of 35 dB masking (35 dB dial/20 dB EM). With successive increases of masking in the left ear (NTE), the right ear (TE) threshold increased to 75 dB HL and was unchanged when the masking signal in the NTE was increased from 40- to 55- dB. At this point, the plateau had been reached and the masked threshold is 75 dB HL. The correction of −5 dB for

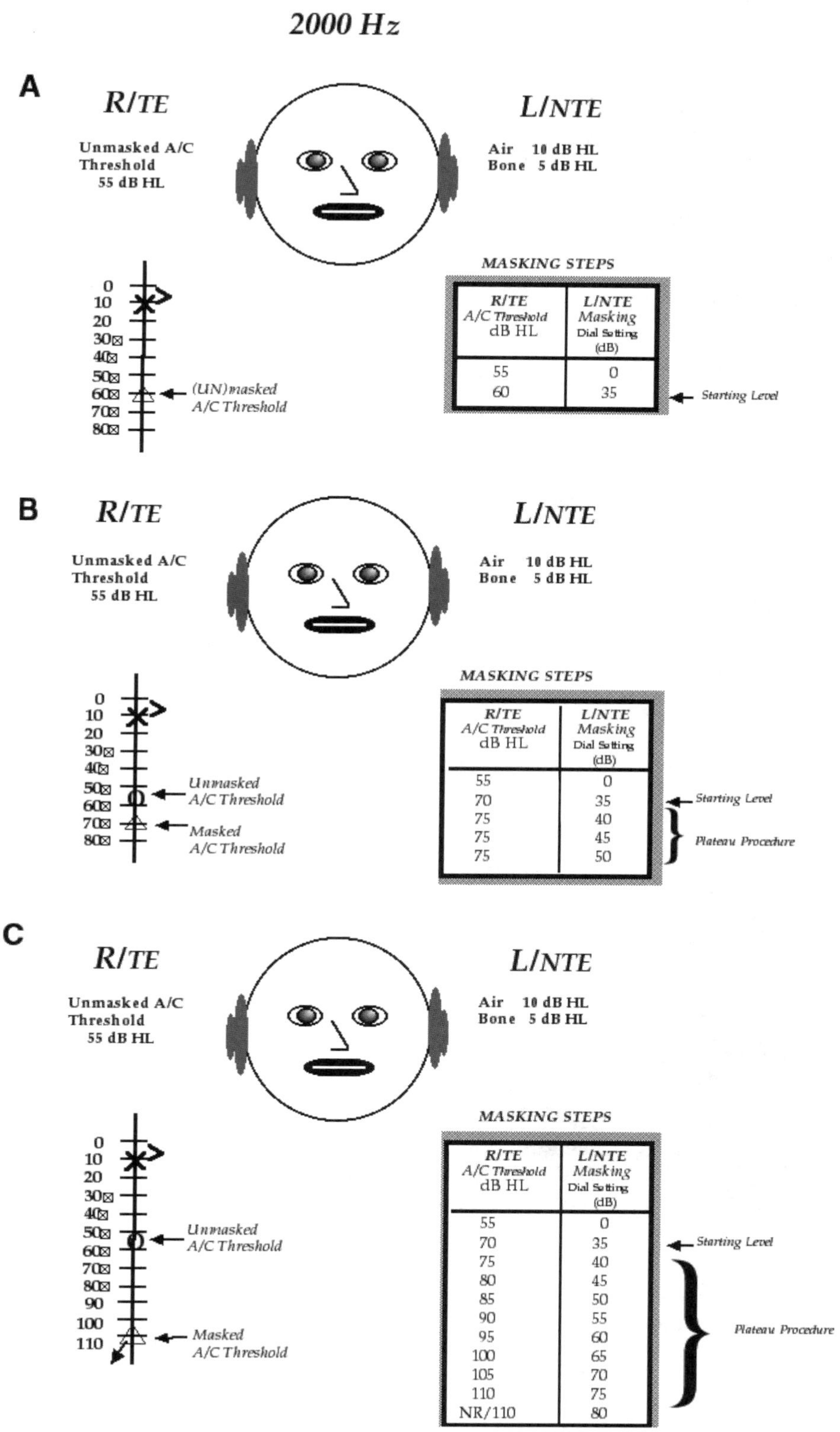

2000 Hz

A

R/TE

Unmasked A/C
Threshold
55 dB HL

L/NTE

Air   10 dB HL
Bone 5 dB HL

0
10
20
30⊠
40⊘
50⊠
60⊠ ← (UN)masked
70⊠   A/C Threshold
80⊠

MASKING STEPS

R/TE A/C Threshold dB HL	L/NTE Masking Dial Setting (dB)	
55	0	
60	35	← Starting Level

B

R/TE

Unmasked A/C
Threshold
55 dB HL

L/NTE

Air   10 dB HL
Bone 5 dB HL

0
10
20
30⊠
40⊘
50⊠ ← Unmasked
60⊠   A/C Threshold
70⊠ ← Masked
80⊠   A/C Threshold

MASKING STEPS

R/TE A/C Threshold dB HL	L/NTE Masking Dial Setting (dB)	
55	0	
70	35	← Starting Level
75	40	
75	45	} Plateau Procedure
75	50	

C

R/TE

Unmasked A/C
Threshold
55 dB HL

L/NTE

Air   10 dB HL
Bone 5 dB HL

0
10
20
30⊠
40⊘
50⊠ ← Unmasked
60⊠   A/C Threshold
70⊠
80⊠
90
100
110 ← Masked
       A/C Threshold

MASKING STEPS

R/TE A/C Threshold dB HL	L/NTE Masking Dial Setting (dB)	
55	0	
70	35	← Starting Level
75	40	
80	45	
85	50	
90	55	} Plateau Procedure
95	60	
100	65	
105	70	
110	75	
NR/110	80	

Figure 12–7 Example of when masking would be needed for pure tone A/C testing and the three possible outcomes: **(A)** masking *does not* affect thresholds in the TE by 5 dB or more; **(B)** masking *does* affect thresholds in the TE by 5 dB or more and a plateau is found; and **(C)** masking *does* affect threshold in the TE by 5 dB or more and plateau is not found.

central masking is accounted for and the masked threshold is recorded at 70 dB HL.

Outcome 3: Masking does affect A/C thresholds in the TE by 5 dB or more and a plateau is not established (Fig. 12–7C). A possible masking outcome is that successive increases in the masking signal increase the threshold in the TE to the limits of the audiometer without establishing a plateau. The implication is that stimuli in the TE were consistently crossing over to the NTE and the increases in masking made them imperceptible in the NTE. When this finding occurs, it is assumed that the TE threshold is beyond the limits of the audiometer and a "no response" symbol is recorded at the audiometer's limits (as shown in Figure 12–7C).

Determining Masking Levels for Pure Tone B/C Threshold Testing

Factors that are used to calculate the starting levels for pure tone B/C testing are the same as for pure tone A/C, with the exception that the occlusion effect must be added when applicable. Recall that the occlusion effect is the enhancement of B/C thresholds when the external earcanal is occluded. Because a masking earphone is placed over the NTE during the masking procedure and because the minimum interaural attenuation level for B/C is 0 dB, thresholds obtained with masking can be influenced by the occlusion effect. Table 12–4 shows the mean occlusion effect within the mid-intensity range of 60 dB to be 20 dB, 15 dB, and 5 dB at 250 Hz, 500 Hz, and 1000 Hz, respectively. These values are added to the masking levels whenever pure tone B/C testing is performed at these frequencies.

PEARL

To calculate the starting level for pure tone B/C threshold testing add the threshold of the NTE, plus the CF (if needed), plus a safety factor of 10 to 15 dB, plus the occlusion effect (when applicable).

Starting level (PT B/C) = threshold of the NTE + CF + Safety factor (10- to 15-dB) + Occlusion effect

---

Figure 12–8 (A to C) provides examples of when masking would be needed for pure tone B/C testing and the three possible outcomes for masked findings. For each of the three examples the right ear masked A/C threshold at 500 Hz is 70 dB HL with an unmasked B/C threshold of 5 dB HL; left ear A/C and B/C thresholds are 10 dB HL and 5 dB HL, respectively. The 65 dB difference between the A/C threshold of the right ear and the B/C threshold of the right ear is greater than the 10 dB minimum criterion required to establish the need for masking when the right ear B/C threshold is obtained. (An unmasked conductive component greater than 10 dB is present.)

Assuming the same audiometer used to calculate the correction factors in Table 12–6 was used to test this patient,

factors required to calculate the starting level when testing the right ear B/C thresholds at 500 Hz are:

A/C	Safety	Correction	Occlusion	
NTE	+ Factor (SF)	+ Factor (CF)	+ Effect (OE)	= Starting Level
(10 dB) +	(10–15dB) +	(10 dB) +	(15 dB)	= 45–50 dB dial setting

As shown in Table 12–6, 15 dB was added to the calculation for the occlusion effect because the test frequency is 500 Hz.

As with A/C testing, when the starting level is introduced into the NTE, the procedure is to determine whether the unmasked threshold in the TE is influenced by the introduction of masking in the NTE. Three possible outcomes may occur.

Outcome 1: Masking does not affect the B/C threshold in the TE by 5 dB or more (Fig. 12–8A). If the unmasked threshold does not shift by more than 5 dB, the unmasked threshold is assumed to be valid and is recorded as a masked threshold. In this case a masked B/C threshold of either 5- or 10-dB HL would be accepted as valid and recorded as a masked threshold. This result is shown in Figure 12–8A.

Outcome 2: Masking does affect the B/C threshold in the TE by 5 dB or more and a plateau is established (Fig. 12–8B). When masking is introduced at the starting level into the NTE and B/C thresholds shift by 10 dB, the plateau is found in the same manner described previously. In the example in Figure 12–8B, the 5 dB HL unmasked B/C threshold shifts to 20 dB HL when the starting level is used. Subsequent 5 dB increases in the masking level result in threshold shifts in the TE to a level of 45 dB HL. With two 5 dB incremental increases of the masking noise, the TE threshold remains constant at 45 dB HL, indicating that the plateau has been established. To account for central masking, the masked threshold is recorded as 40 dB HL.

Outcome 3: Masking does affect the B/C threshold in the TE by 5 dB or more and a plateau is not established (Fig. 12–8C). One additional outcome is that the B/C thresholds in the TE do not plateau at the maximum levels of the audiometer. Figure 12–8C provides an example of this finding. The unmasked B/C threshold of 5 dB shifts as the masking levels increase from the initial starting level of 40- or 45-dB to 90 dB. At the masking level of 90 dB the patient does not respond to the test signal at the maximum limits of the audiometer for B/C at 60 dB HL. In this case a "no response" B/C symbol is recorded at 60 dB HL.

Determining Masking Levels for Speech Recognition Threshold Testing

Principles for calculating masking levels for speech stimuli are the same as for pure tones, with a slight variation in the procedure. An acoustic method using a subtraction procedure is recommended for speech stimuli (Studebaker, 1979). To use the subtraction procedure, the minimum interaural attenuation levels for the speech stimuli must be taken into account. The subtraction procedure is based on the assumption that speech in the TE can be prevented from crossing to the NTE effectively if the level of noise in the NTE is above the minimum interaural

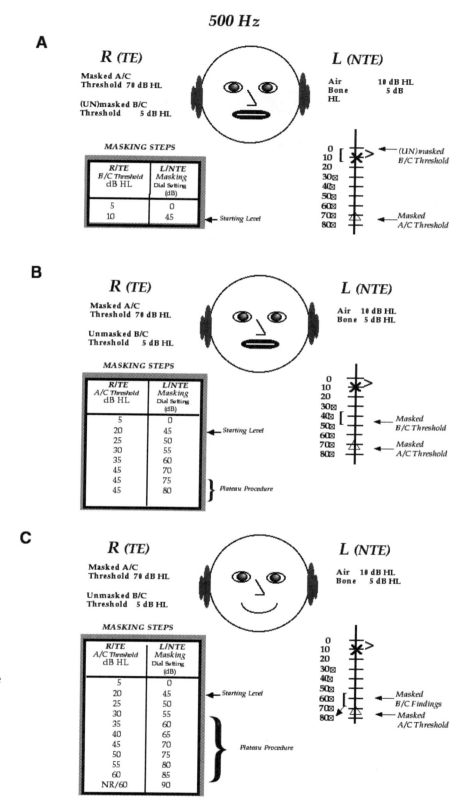

500 Hz

Figure 12–8 Example of when masking would be needed for pure tone B/C testing and the three possible outcomes: **(A)** masking *does not* affect B/C thresholds in the TE by 5 dB or more; **(B)** masking *does* affect B/C thresholds in the TE by 5 dB or more and a plateau is found; and **(C)** masking *does* affect B/C threshold in the TE by 5 dB or more and plateau is not found.

attenuation level. A safety factor of 10 dB is added to the noise to account for patient variability. For SRT testing the starting level is determined by subtracting 35 dB from the presentation level of the unmasked SRT (45 dB minimum interaural attenuation level − 10 dB safety factor).

PEARL

To calculate the starting level for SRT testing subtract 35 dB from the PL of the unmasked SRT in the TE and add the ABG in the speech frequencies of the NTE (if any).

Starting level (SRT) = PL (TE) − 35 dB*
                      + Average ABG (NTE)

*(45 dB minimum interaural attenuation level − 10 dB safety factor)

The acoustic method is quite adequate as long as no conductive component is present in the NTE. If a conductive component exists, the masking signal must be increased by the average level of the conductive component (the ABG). Otherwise the intensity of the masking signal will be inadequate and undermasking will result.

Figure 12–9A and B provides examples of masking for SRT testing without and with air-bone gaps present in the NTE, respectively. For each example the audiometer used to calculate the correction factors in Table 12–6 was used to test this patient. For Figure 12–9A no significant air-bone gaps are present in the NTE. The factors required to calculate the starting level are:

(PL (TE)   − IA SRT) + CF + NTE Avg. ABG = Starting level (SRT)

(75 dB HL − 35 = 40) + 10 +   0   = 50 dB dial setting

This starting level would be introduced into the NTE, and the masked threshold would be established in the same manner as for pure tone thresholds. That is, with masking, either the unmasked threshold would change by 5 dB or less, a plateau would be found, or the SRT would shift to the maximum limits of the audiometer. When the masked SRT is found, the result would be recorded on the audiogram form.

Speech Recognition Threshold Testing

A WITHOUT Air-Bone Gap

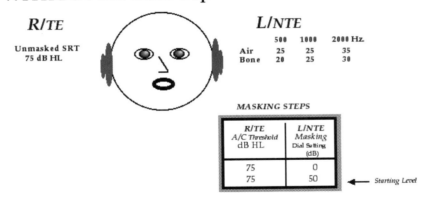

B WITH Air-Bone Gap

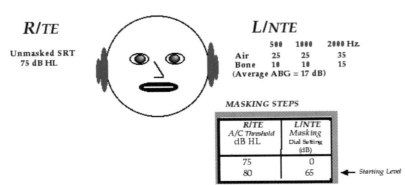

Figure 12–9 Example of when to mask for SRT testing when (**A**) an ABG in the speech frequencies is *absent* in the NTE; and (**B**) an ABG in the speech frequencies is *present* in the NTE.

When an ABG is present in speech frequencies of the NTE, calculating the starting level for SRT testing must factor in the conductive component. Figure 12–9B provides an example when an ABG is present. The factors required to calculate the starting levels for SRT testing when an ABG is present are:

$$(\text{PL (TE)} - \text{IA SRT}) + \text{CF} + \text{NTE Avg. ABG} = \text{Starting level (SRT)}$$

$$(75 - 35 = 40) \quad + 10 + \quad 15 \quad = 65 \text{ dB dial setting}$$

Once again, this starting level would be introduced into the NTE. With masking, either the unmasked threshold would change by 5 dB or less, a plateau would be found, or the SRT would shift to the maximum limits of the audiometer. Results would be entered on the audiogram form.

Determining Masking Levels for Word Recognition Testing

As with SRT testing, masking levels during word recognition testing use the acoustic method. However, unlike threshold procedures, the PL of test stimuli during word recognition testing remains constant. Consequently, the intensity of the masking stimulus is the same throughout the procedure. Another difference between masking for SRT and word recognition testing is that the recommended safety factor is increased to 20 dB (Studebaker, 1979). The intensity level of the masking in the NTE is based on subtracting 25 dB from

the PL of the monosyllabic words in the TE. The 25 dB level is derived from the minimum interaural attenuation level for speech (45 dB) minus the safety factor of 20 dB.

PEARL

To calculate the starting level for word recognition testing, subtract 25 dB from the PL in the TE and add the ABG in the speech frequencies of the NTE (if any).

Starting level
(word recognition tests) = PL (TE) − 25 dB*
+ Average ABG (NTE)

*(45 dB minimum interaural attenuation level − 20 dB safety factor)

Similar to SRT testing, when a conductive component is present in the speech range of the masked (NTE) ear, the average difference (ABG) between the A/C and B/C thresholds at 500, 1000 and 2000 Hz is added to the masking level.

Figures 12–10A and B illustrates examples of masking for word recognition testing with and without ABGs present in the NTE, respectively. For each example the audiometer used to calculate the correction factors in Table 12–6 was used to test this patient.

Word Recognition Testing

A WITHOUT Air-Bone Gap

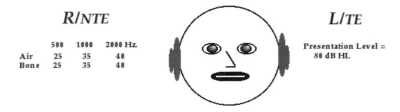

	500	1000	2000 Hz.
Air	25	35	40
Bone	25	35	40

R/NTE   L/TE

Presentation Level = 80 dB HL

Masking Level in NTE = 65 dB

B WITH Air-Bone Gap

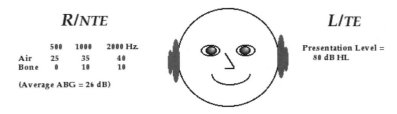

	500	1000	2000 Hz.
Air	25	35	40
Bone	0	10	10

(Average ABG = 26 dB)

R/NTE   L/TE

Presentation Level = 80 dB HL

Masking Level in NTE = 90 dB

Figure 12–10 Example of when to mask for word recognition testing when: **(A)** an ABG in the speech frequencies is *absent* in the NTE; and **(B)** an ABG in the speech frequencies is *present* in the NTE.

No ABGs are present in the speech frequencies for the NTE for the patient in Figure 12–10A. The factors required to calculate the starting level are:

(PL (TE) − IA SRT) + CF + NTE Avg. ABG = Masking level
(word intel)

(80 dB HL − 25 = 55) + 10 +   0   = 65 dB dial
setting

This 65 dB masking level would be presented to the right (NTE) ear throughout the test procedure. When the masked word recognition score is established, the result would be recorded on the audiogram form as a masked score.

Figure 12–10B provides an example of masking for word recognition testing when an ABG is present. Those factors required to calculate the starting level for word recognition testing when an ABG is present are:

(PL (TE) − IA SRT) + CF + NTE Avg. ABG = Masking level
(word intel)

(80 dB HL − 25 = 55) + 10 +   25   = 90 dB dial
setting

The 90 dB masking level would be introduced into the NTE. Once completed, the masked word recognition score is entered on the audiogram form.

The Masking Dilemma

A masking dilemma occurs when it is impossible to mask the NTE effectively without achieving the minimum necessary masking level. Whenever bilateral conductive hearing loss of 35 dB or more is present, a masking dilemma is possible. As the extent of conductive hearing loss increases in the NTE, the likelihood of the masking dilemma becomes greater until the point at which the patient's interaural attenuation level is reached. Because the average interaural attenuation ranges between 55- and 65-dB, the masking dilemma is a certainty for most patients when a conductive component is present in the masked (NTE) ear in the 55-65 dB range. Recall that some patients will have interaural attenuation levels lower than the average 55 to 65 dB range, possibly as low as 40 dB. This implies that the masking dilemma will be present for a few patients when the masked (NTE) ear has a conductive component as low as 40 dB.

Figure 12–11 displays audiometric results from a patient with a moderate to severe bilateral conductive hearing loss. Because the bilateral conductive components exceed 50 to 55 dB, a masking dilemma is posed in this case. As an example, the starting level when testing the right ear pure tone A/C threshold at 1000 Hz (masking the left [NTE] ear) would be:

A/C NTE + Safety factor (SF) +   CF   = Starting level
(55 dB)   +   (10–15 dB)   + (15 dB) = 80–85 dB dial
setting

Masking presented to the NTE at 80 to 85 dB dial setting is at an effective level of 65 to 70 dB (80 to 85 dB dial setting minus the 15 dB correction factor). If this patient had an average interaural attenuation level between 55 and 65 dB, a masking noise in the NTE would cross to the TE and overmasking would result. For this patient, the result of introducing masking into either ear will shift thresholds in the TE when attempting to find the plateau. In fact, thresholds will be

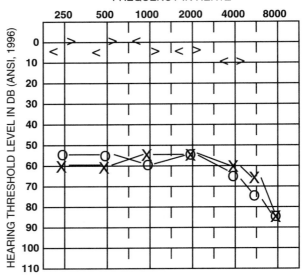

AUDIOGRAM

FREQUENCY IN HERTZ

Figure 12–11   Example of a masking dilemma with a patient having a moderate-to-severe bilateral conductive hearing loss.

shifted to the maximum limits of the audiometer, a finding that is impossible because the unmasked results on the audiogram must reflect the threshold sensitivity of at least one ear. Thresholds for both ears cannot shift when masking is used.

When confronted with a masking dilemma, clinicians should use insert earphones to obtain thresholds. Insert earphones increase the interaural attenuation levels from an average of 55- to 65-dB to an average of 80 dB (see Table 12–3). Increased interaural attenuation will allow for the use of greater masking levels in the NTE without crossover to the TE.

CASE STUDIES

Case Study No. 1

Results from three patients are presented in Figures 12–12 through 12–14 to illustrate the masking principles presented in this chapter. Unmasked results for the data in Figure 12–12 show a moderate-to-severe right ear mixed hearing loss and a moderate-to-severe left ear high-frequency sensorineural hearing loss. Although many of today's audiometers do not require correction factors, to become familiar with factoring them into the calculation the two examples will use the following correction factors (in dB):

250	500	1000	2000	3000	4000	6000	8000	Hz Speech
10	5	15	5	10	15	20	5	0

The starting levels for masking required for the data in Figure 12–12 are as follows:

- When obtaining right ear pure tone A/C thresholds, no masking is needed.
- When obtaining left ear pure tone A/C thresholds, no masking is needed.

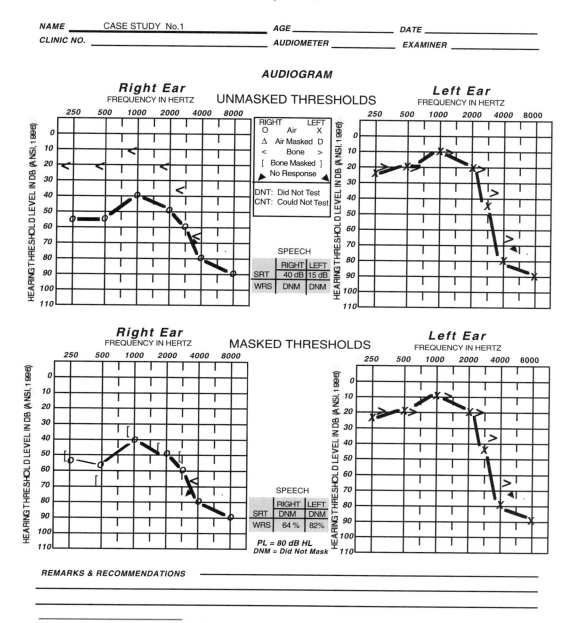

Figure 12–12 Case Study No. 1.

- When obtaining right ear pure tone B/C thresholds:

	A/C NTE	+	Safety factor (SF)	+	CF	+	Occlusion effect	=	Starting level
250 Hz =	25	+	10–15	+	10	+	20	=	65–70
500 Hz =	20	+	10–15	+	5	+	15	=	50–55
1000 Hz =	10	+	10–15	+	15	+	5	=	40–45
2000 Hz =	20	+	10–15	+	5	+	0	=	35–40
3000 Hz =	45	+	10–15	+	10	+	0	=	65–70
4000 Hz =	No masking is needed								

- When obtaining left ear pure tone B/C thresholds, no masking is needed.
- When obtaining the right ear SRT, no masking is needed.
- When obtaining the left ear SRT, no masking is needed.
- When obtaining the right ear word recognition score:

$$\text{PL (TE)} - 25 \text{ dB} + \underset{\text{(500, 1k, 2k)}}{\text{Avg ABG NTE}} + \text{CF} = \text{Masking level}$$
$$80 \text{ dB HL} - 25 \text{ dB} + 0 + 0 = 55 \text{ dB}$$

- When obtaining the left ear word recognition score:

Callier Center for Communication Disorders

University of Texas at Dallas
1966 Inwood Road; Dallas, Texas 75235
phone (214) 905-3000

NAME _____CASE STUDY #2_____   AGE _____   DATE _____

CLINIC NO. _____   AUDIOMETER _____   EXAMINER _____

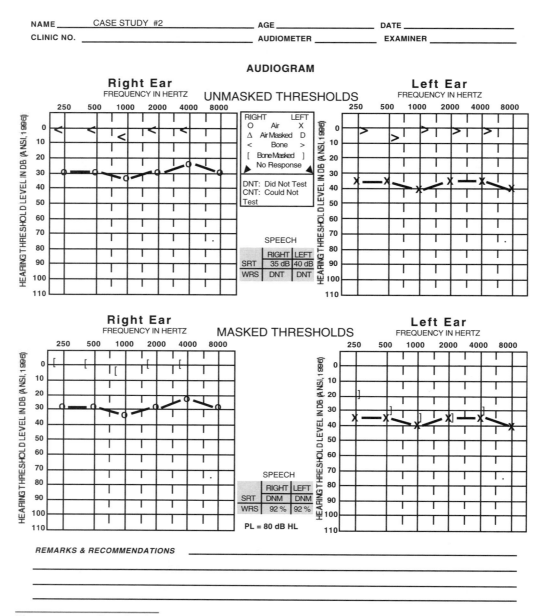

Figure 12–13   Case Study No. 2.

	Avg ABG NTE*	Masking
PL (TE) − 25 dB	+ (500, 1k, 2k) + CF =	level
80 dB HL − 25 dB	+ 30 + 0 =	85 dB

Once masking is introduced into the NTE for threshold measures and the patient's responses do not change by more than 5 dB, the threshold is accepted as valid and recorded on the audiogram form as masked results. For

*The average ABG at 500, 1000, and 2000 Hz is based on unmasked findings. If masked findings were available, there would be no ABG at 500, 1000, and 2000 Hz and the masking level would be 55 dB.

word recognition tests the level is held constant throughout the procedure.

Case Study No. 2

In Figure 12–13 unmasked findings suggest a mild bilateral conductive hearing loss. For this patient the starting levels would be as follows:

- When obtaining right ear pure tone A/C thresholds, no masking is needed.

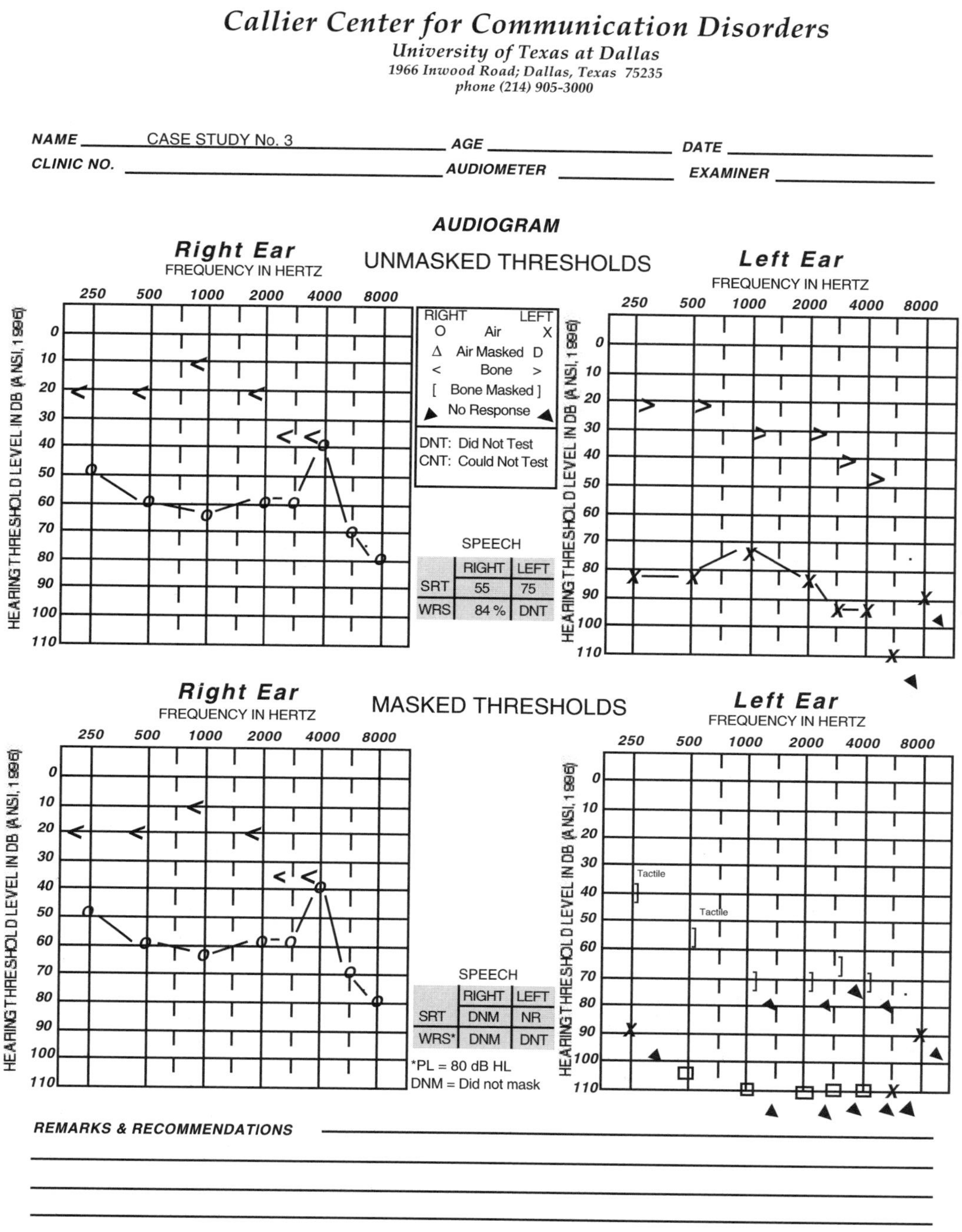

Callier Center for Communication Disorders
University of Texas at Dallas
1966 Inwood Road; Dallas, Texas 75235
phone (214) 905-3000

NAME _____ CASE STUDY No. 3 _____   AGE _____   DATE _____

CLINIC NO. _____   AUDIOMETER _____   EXAMINER _____

AUDIOGRAM

Figure 12–14   Case Study No. 3.

- When obtaining left ear pure tone A/C thresholds, no masking is needed.
- When obtaining right ear pure tone B/C thresholds:

	A/C NTE +	Safety factor (SF) +	CF +	Occlusion effect =	Starting level
250 Hz =	35 +	10–15	+ 10 +	20	= 75–80
500 Hz =	35 +	10–15	+ 5 +	15	= 65–70
1000 Hz =	40 +	10–15	+ 15 +	5	= 70–75
2000 Hz =	35 +	10–15	+ 5 +	0	= 50–55
4000 Hz =	35 +	10–15	+ 15 +	0	= 60–65

- When obtaining left ear pure tone B/C thresholds:

	A/C NTE +	Safety factor (SF) +	CF +	Occlusion effect =	Starting level
250 Hz =	30 +	10–15	+ 10 +	20	= 70–75
500 Hz =	30 +	10–15	+ 5 +	15	= 60–65
1000 Hz =	35 +	10–15	+ 15 +	5	= 65–70
2000 Hz =	30 +	10–15	+ 5 +	0	= 45–50
4000 Hz =	25 +	10–15	+ 15 +	0	= 50–55

- When obtaining the right ear SRT, no masking is needed.

- When obtaining the left ear SRT, no masking is needed.
- When obtaining the right ear word recognition score:

	Avg ABG NTE*		Masking
PL (TE) − 25 dB	+ (500, 1k, 2k) + CF =		level
80 dB HL − 25 dB	+ 35 + 0 =		90 dB

- When obtaining the left ear word recognition score:

	Avg ABG NTE		Masking
PL (TE) − 25 dB	+ (500, 1k, 2k) + CF =		level
80-dB HL − 25 dB	+ 30 + 0 =		85 dB

Case Study No. 3

Unmasked audiometric results in Figure 12–14 show a moderate-to-severe right ear and severe-to-profound left ear mixed hearing loss. This case is presented to illustrate that if masked results from one ear shift significantly, there is no need to mask findings from the other ear. For this patient masking would be used when testing left ear thresholds first, because the severity of the loss in the left ear makes the likelihood of crossover greater for the left ear than the right ear.

PEARL

When masked results from one ear shift significantly, there is no need to mask findings from the other ear.

The starting levels used when testing the left ear are as follows:

- When obtaining left ear pure tone A/C thresholds:

A/C NTE	Safety factor (SF)	CF	=	Starting level
250 Hz = 50	+ 10–15	+ 10	=	70–75
500 Hz = 60	+ 10–15	+ 5	=	75–80
1000 Hz = 65	+ 10–15	+ 15	=	90–95
2000 Hz = 60	+ 10–15	+ 5	=	75–80
3000 Hz = 60	+ 10–15	+ 10	=	80–85
4000 Hz = 40	+ 10–15	+ 15	=	65–70
6000 Hz = No masking needed				
8000 Hz = No masking is needed				

- When obtaining left ear pure tone B/C thresholds:

A/C NTE	Safety factor (SF)	CF	Occlusion effect	=	Starting level
250 Hz = 50	+ 10–15	+ 10	+ 20	=	90–95
500 Hz = 60	+ 10–15	+ 5	+ 15	=	90–95
1000 Hz = 65	+ 10–15	+ 15	+ 5	=	95–100
2000 Hz = 60	+ 10–15	+ 5	+ 0	=	75–80
3000 Hz = 60	+ 10–15	+ 10	+ 0	=	80–85
4000 Hz = 40	+ 10–15	+ 15	+ 0	=	65–70

- When obtaining the left ear SRT:

	Avg ABG NTE		Masking
PL (TE) − 35 dB	+ (500, 1k, 2k) + CF =		level
75 dB HL − 35 dB	+ 45 + 0 =		85 dB

- When obtaining the left ear word recognition score, this test cannot be performed because of the severity of the loss.

As illustrated in Figure 12–14, the use of masking when testing the left ear caused pure tone and speech thresholds to shift to the profound level. Consequently, even though the masking rules would suggest the need for masking when testing the right ear, data from the right ear are known to be valid. That is, unmasked findings always reflect the performance of the better ear. When one ear is eliminated through the use of masking, the resulting unmasked data must reflect findings from the remaining ear.

Data in Case Study No. 3 represent an advanced masking concept. This and others will become secondhand once the masking principles outlined in this chapter become familiar to the clinician.

CONCLUSIONS

The proper use of masking during clinical audiometry ensures the examiner that test results reflect the performance of the test ear only. This chapter describes the principles used in clinical masking. The questions of when to mask and how much masking to use are addressed. By following the masking principles in this chapter, one is assured that the diagnostic test results from the test ear are valid.

REFERENCES

AMERICAN NATIONAL STANDARDS INSTITUTE (ANSI 53.6, 1996). Specifications for Audiometers.

AMERICAN SPEECH-LANGUAGE-HEARING ASSOCIATION (ASHA) (1978). Guidelines for manual pure-tone audiometry. *ASHA, 20*;297–301.

BERGER, E.H., & KERIVAN, J.E. (1983). Influence of physiological noise and the occlusion effect on the measurement of real-ear attenuation at threshold. *Journal of the Acoustical Society of America, 86*;1392–1403.

CHAIKLIN, J.B. (1967). Interaural attenuation and cross-hearing in air conduction audiometry. *Journal of Auditory Research, 7*;413–424.

COLES, R.R.A., & PRIEDE, V.M. (1970). On the misdiagnosis resulting from incorrect use of masking. *Journal of Laryngology and Otology, 84*;41–63.

*The average ABG at 500, 1000, and 2000 Hz is based on unmasked findings. If masked findings were available, there would be no ABG at 500, 1000, and 2000 Hz and the masking level would be 55 dB.

DIRKS, D.D., & MALMQUIST, C. (1964). Changes in bone conducted thresholds produced by masking in the non-test ear. *Journal of Speech and Hearing Research, 7*;271–278.

DIRKS, D.D., & SWINDEMAN, J.G. (1967). The variability of occluded and unoccluded bone-conduction thresholds. *Journal of Speech and Hearing Research, 10*;232–249.

ELPERN, B., & NAUNTON, R.F. (1963). The stability of the occlusion effect. *Archives of Otolaryngology, 77*;376–384.

FLETCHER, H. (1940). Auditory patterns. *Review of Modern Physics, 12*;47–65.

GELFAND, S.A. (1997). Clinical masking. In: *Essentials of audiology*. New York: Thieme Medical Publishers, Inc.

GOLDSTEIN, D.P., & HAYES, C.S. (1965). The occlusion effect in bone-conduction hearing. *Journal of Speech and Hearing Research, 8*;137–148.

HAWKINS, J.E., & STEVENS, S.S. (1950). Masking of pure tones and of speech by white noise. *Journal of the Acoustical Society of America, 22*;6–13.

HODGSON, W.R., & TILLMAN, T. (1966). Reliability of bone conduction occlusion effects in normals. *Journal of Auditory Research, 6*;141–153.

HOOD, J.D. (1960). The principle and practice of bone-conduction audiometry: A review of the present position. *Laryngoscope, 70*;1211–1228.

KILLION, M.C., WILBER, L.A., & GUNDMUNDSON, G.I. (1985). Insert earphones for more interaural attenuation. *Hearing Instruments, 36(2)*;34.

KONIG, E. (1962). On the use of hearing aid type earphones in clinical audiometry. *Acta Otolaryngologica, 55*;331–341.

KONKLE, D.F., & BERRY, G.A. (1983). Masking in speech audiometry. In: D.F. Konkle, & W.F. Rintleman (Eds.), *Principles of speech audiometry* (pp. 285–319). Baltimore: University Press.

LIDEN, G., NILSSON, G., & ANDERSON, H. (1959). Masking in clinical audiometry. *Acta Otolaryngologica, 50*;125–136.

LITTLER, T.S., KNIGHT, J.J., & STRANGE, P.H. (1952). *Proceedings of the Royal Society of Medicine, 45*;783.

LLOYD, L.L., & KAPLAN, H. (1978). *Audiometric interpretation: A manual of basic audiometry*. Baltimore: University Park Press.

MARTIN, F.N. (1966). Speech audiometry and clinical masking. *Journal of Auditory Research, 6*;199–203.

MARTIN, F.N. (1997). Pure-tone audiometry. In: *Introduction to audiology* (6th ed.). Boston: Allyn & Bacon.

MARTIN, F.N. (1994). *Introduction to audiology* (5th ed.). Needham Heights, MA: Allyn & Bacon.

MARTIN, F.N., BAILY, H.A.T., & PAPPAS, J.J. (1965). The effect of central masking on threshold for speech. *Journal of Auditory Research, 5*;293–296.

MARTIN, F.N., & BLOSSER, D. (1970). Cross hearing air conduction or bone conduction. *Psychonomic Science, 20*;231.

MARTIN, F.N., BUTLER, E.C., & BURNS, P. (1974). Audiometric Bing test for determination of minimum masking levels for bone conduction tests. *Journal of Speech and Hearing Disorders, 39*;148–152.

MARTIN, F.N., & DI GIOVANNI, D. (1979). Central masking effects on spondee thresholds as a function of masker sensation level and masker sound pressure level. *Journal of the American Audiology Society, 4*;141–146.

MARTIN, F.N., & FAGELSON, M. (1995). Bone conduction reconsidered. *Tejas, 20*;26–27.

MARTIN, F.N., & WITTICH, W.W. (1966). A comparison of forehead and mastoid tactile bone conduction thresholds. *The Eye, Ear, Nose, & Throat Monthly, 45*;72–74.

SANDERS, J.W., & RINTELMANN, W.F. (1964). Masking in audiometry. *Archives of Otolaryngology, 80*;541–556.

SKLARE, D.A., & DENENBERG, L.J. (1987). Interaural attenuation for Tubephone insert earphones. *Ear and Hearing, 8*;298–300.

STUDEBAKER, G.A. (1962). On masking in bone conduction testing. *Journal of Speech and Hearing Research, 5*;215–227.

STUDEBAKER, G.A. (1967). Clinical masking of the nontest ear. *Journal of Speech and Hearing Disorders, 32*;360–371.

STUDEBAKER, G.A. (1979). Clinical masking. In: W.F. Rintelmann (Ed.), *Hearing assessment* (pp. 51–100). Baltimore: University Park Press.

VENIAR, F.A. (1965). Individual masking levels in pure-tone audiometry. *Archives of Otolaryngology, 82*;518–521.

WEGEL, R.L., & LANE, G.I. (1924). The auditory masking of one pure tone by another and its probably relation to the dynamics of the inner ear. *Physiological Review, 23*;266–285.

ZWISLOCKI, J. (1953). Acoustic attenuation between ears. *Journal of the Acoustical Society of America, 25*;752–759.

Speech Audiometry

Linda M. Thibodeau

Outline

recognition scores contribute to decisions regarding site of lesion and development of rehabilitation programs.

Over time, the terminology used for speech audiometry has changed as speech perception research with patients has expanded from a clinical to psychoacoustic framework. Consequently, a discussion of speech audiometry must begin with a clear taxonomy of terminology followed by a review of those critical aspects of speech in relation to diagnostic information that uses various evaluative techniques. Although this chapter will focus on the diagnostic application of speech audiometry, it must be realized that just as speech processing is an important step in the diagnostic process, it is equally important in the rehabilitative process. Therein lies the ultimate challenge for audiologists: To provide technology and behavioral strategies that will allow the patient with impaired hearing to maximize his or her communicative functioning.

To assess speech processing adequately, several decisions regarding the signal, presentation format, and response task must be made. These decisions have an impact on the analysis and interpretation of the results. Factors influencing such decisions include age of the patient, purpose of the evaluation, and available time for testing. Clinicians must evaluate the relative importance of these variables for each patient and determine the most efficient means of obtaining the desired information.

Information presented in this chapter will provide the framework for decisions regarding the signal, presentation format, and response task, with evidence supporting the most efficient and sensitive procedures that can be used both diagnostically and rehabilitatively. In addition, common problems in the evaluation of speech processing will be addressed with suggestions for avoiding those pitfalls. Typically, these problems arise from a mismatch between the selected materials, procedure, or response task and patient capabilities. Therefore it is imperative to begin with a clear rationale for why evaluation of speech processing is necessary followed by a review of how the various evaluation procedures can have an impact on results before a review of the possible tests and procedures available for different age groups.

TERMINOLOGY

Traditionally, evaluation of speech processing at threshold levels has resulted in obtaining a "speech awareness or detection threshold" or "speech reception threshold," and evaluation at suprathreshold levels has resulted in obtaining a "speech discrimination score" or "word discrimination score."

Evaluation of speech processing is an important component of the diagnostic audiological evaluation for variety of reasons. First, speech thresholds provide validating data for pure tone thresholds. In addition, at suprathreshold levels, speech

Audiology: Diagnosis. Edited by Roeser, Valente, and Hosford-Dunn. Thieme Medical Publishers, Inc., New York © 2000

However, as the many facets of speech processing are considered, it becomes apparent that more precise terminology is needed. Ideally, the same taxonomy would apply to both diagnostic and rehabilitative services. A clearly established hierarchy of four levels of auditory processing used by Erber (1982) in auditory training can be applied to the diagnostic battery. The four levels of processing are awareness, discrimination, identification/recognition, and comprehension. Currently available tests in speech audiometry fall into either awareness or identification/recognition. A brief review of how the clinical measures fall into this hierarchy is provided in the following, and greater discussion is provided in the section entitled "Level of Auditory Ability Assessed."

Awareness: Those tests that require the patient to simply indicate that a sound was detected such as the "SAT" or "SDT."

Discrimination: Those tests that require the patient to detect a change in the acoustic stimulus. At present, no true tests of discrimination are used in traditional speech audiometry.

Identification/recognition: Those tests that require the patient to attach a label to the stimulus either by pointing to a corresponding picture or object or repeating the stimulus orally or in writing. Routine clinical assessments in speech audiometry include measures of the threshold for speech [Speech Recognition Threshold (SRT)], and measures at suprathreshold levels using words [Word Recognition Score (WRS)] or sentences [Sentence Recognition Score (SRS)].

Comprehension: Those tests that require the patient to attach meaning to the stimulus by answering questions verbally, in writing, or pointing to a picture that conveys the associated meaning. Auditory comprehension is not assessed in traditional speech audiometry.

Appendix A lists common abbreviations used in speech audiometry.

RATIONALE FOR EVALUATING SPEECH PROCESSING

Typically, speech-processing evaluations are included in the routine audiological examination to determine the extent to which altered thresholds disrupt perception of complex signals. Evaluation of responses to pure tone information does not allow for complete understanding of a patient's deficit. Consequently, evaluation of speech processing should be included not only in the diagnostic battery but also in the hearing aid fitting process. Indeed, in some pathological conditions, abnormal speech processing may be the most significant diagnostic factor. Furthermore, it is often the case that two patients with the same degree of hearing loss demonstrate very different speech-processing ability. In other words, two patients may have the same reduction in absolute sensitivity (i.e., thresholds) but vary in their differential sensitivity or processing of suprathreshold information. This would not necessarily lead to different hearing aid fittings for these two patients because at present no hearing aids are available to compensate for suprathreshold processing deficits. However, rehabilitation for these two patients would differ in that the one with the greater speech-processing deficit would require more emphasis on repair strategies and possible environmental modifications. Thus the rationale for the evaluation of speech processing includes three areas: (a) relative effects of reduced absolute and differential sensitivity, (b) contributions of speech evaluations to differential diagnosis, and (c) application of speech evaluations to the hearing aid fittings.

Relative Effects of Reduced Absolute and Differential Sensitivity

When audibility of the signal is reduced, the effects on recognition of specific speech features are generally well predicted by the absolute thresholds for pure tones (Bilger & Wang, 1976; Dubno & Levitt, 1985; Miller & Nicely, 1955). The reduction in absolute sensitivity is routinely represented on the audiogram and may be interpreted relative to the long-term speech spectrum commonly referred to as the "speech banana." The relationship of thresholds to the "speech banana" shown in Figure 13–1 is often used in counseling the patient with hearing loss regarding the speech sounds that will be difficult to perceive. However, speech processing involves more than just audibility of the signal as illustrated in two case studies presented by Skinner et al (1982). They identified two patients with hearing loss and similar thresholds but very different SRSs and attributed the difference in scores to differences in suprathreshold processing.

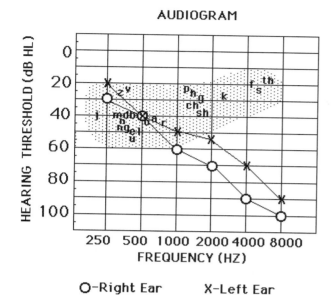

AUDIOGRAM

O-Right Ear   X-Left Ear

Figure 13–1 Relationship of a patient's threshold to the speech banana.

The relationship between differential sensitivity and threshold sensitivity varies widely. Evaluation of differential sensitivity is not routinely included in the clinical audiological battery. Psychoacoustic studies have shown moderate-to-strong correlations between speech recognition and frequency resolution (Stelmachowicz et al, 1985; Thibodeau & Van Tasell, 1987; Tyler et al, 1982) and temporal resolution (Dreschler & Plomp, 1985; Festen & Plomp, 1983; Tyler, Summerfield et al, 1982). Therefore, when speech-processing performance is lower than expected on the basis of threshold information, the reduced performance might be related to a reduction in differential sensitivity.

PEARL

Differential sensitivity refers to the ability to detect changes in intensity, frequency, and temporal aspects of the signal, all of which are potential cues for speech recognition.

In the typical clinical assessment of speech processing, the effects of reduced absolute and differential sensitivity cannot be separated. Unless measures are taken to ensure complete audibility of the signal, the combined effects of these deficits will be represented in a single score. The degree to which amplification can compensate for reduced speech recognition is based in part on improvements in speech recognition with increased audibility.

One way to account for changes in absolute sensitivity is through a procedure known as the Articulation Index (AI) (French & Steinberg, 1947; Pavlovic, 1984). By comparing one's performance to that predicted by the AI, one can gain an estimate of the speech-processing problems that may exist even after audibility is restored, and thereby provide more appropriate counseling.

Contributions of Speech Evaluations to Differential Diagnosis

In addition to determining the effects of reduced absolute and differential sensitivity, evaluation of speech processing is a critical part of the differential diagnostic battery. Although a wide range of speech processing abilities exist across auditory pathological conditions, the assessment is particularly useful in the diagnostic process when performed at more than one intensity level (Jerger & Jerger, 1971). When evaluating speech processing, the type and degree of the hearing loss, age of the patient, and linguistic sophistication are considered. Because of the variety of speech materials and assessment procedures, an absence of normative data exists across these variables of age, type, and degree of loss for interpretation of a single score. Some argue that speech audiometry is of limited diagnostic value because of the wide dispersion of performance scores (Bess, 1983). General trends are reported in the literature, which contribute to the differential diagnostic process of general site of lesion rather than specific cause. For example, it has been shown that patients with conductive losses have excellent recognition of single words (>90%) when presented at comfortable listening levels. However, patients with losses of the same degree but sensorineural in nature will generally have reduced speech recognition (Hood & Poole, 1971).

To evaluate the significance of reduced speech recognition scores, audiologists should compare speech recognition performance with that expected for patients with similar degrees of hearing loss. Dubno et al (1995) determined the 95% confidence limit for maximum recognition of specific speech materials for patients with sensorineural hearing loss of varying degrees as discussed later. When speech recognition is outside the 95% confidence limit for that degree of loss, it may be indicative of a retrocochlear pathological condition.

Perhaps the greatest diagnostic significance of speech audiometry is the reduction in speech recognition with increases in intensity or the "rollover effect" that occurs with retrocochlear pathological conditions (Dirks et al, 1977; Jerger & Jerger, 1971). A discrepancy in performance between scores from a patient's two ears or between word and sentence recognition is also suggestive of a retrocochlear pathological condition. To increase the diagnostic significance of speech audiometry, the test battery must be expanded to include testing across different intensity levels, types of materials, or competing backgrounds.

PEARL

Rollover occurs when the speech recognition score decreases more than 20% from the maximum performance at a lower intensity level and is consistent with a retrocochlear pathological condition (Jerger & Jerger, 1971).

Application of Speech Evaluations to the Hearing Aid Fittings

Speech audiometry plays a significant role in the recommendation for amplification. Pure tone thresholds may unquestionably indicate the need for amplification, and it can quickly be determined that average conversational speech is not completely audible by use of techniques such as the AI (Mueller & Killion, 1990) described later. However, the evaluation of speech processing as part of the hearing aid fitting also involves examining the relationship of average conversational speech to a patient's dynamic range as shown in Figure 13–2. For this patient exhibiting a flat hearing loss of 70 dB HL and uncomfortable listening levels of 90 dB HL, the gain required to amplify average conversational speech so that it is suprathreshold yet below his or her uncomfortable listening levels is only 25 dB at 2000 Hz. This results in the speech information at 2 KHz being about 9 dB SL and less than the 90 dB HL discomfort level. If, instead, a half-gain rule were applied at 2000 Hz, this patient

would receive 35 dB of gain that would result in the speech information being amplified to the discomfort level.

However, unless patients and their significant others indicate through informal discussion or formal handicap measures that the loss of hearing interferes with their daily communication, a hearing aid evaluation may not be warranted. When daily communication is affected, the results of speech audiometry help to determine potential hearing aid benefit. For example, if speech recognition improves when stimuli are presented at a more intense level than typical conversational speech, the patient is likely to benefit from amplification. Conversely, if the speech recognition deteriorates at increased intensity levels, perhaps resulting from a reduced dynamic range, the prognosis for successful use of amplification is more guarded.

Once it is determined that amplification will be of potential benefit, the perception of speech through the hearing aid(s) must be assessed. It is possible to provide amplification that restores audibility of the signal but results in reduced recognition (Van Tasell & Crain, 1992). To provide benefit, patients

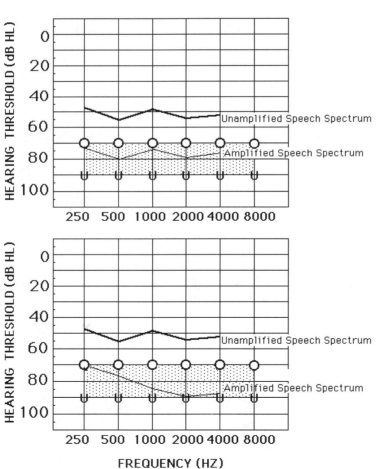

Figure 13–2 Relationship of unamplified *(heavy line)* and amplified *(thin line)* average speech spectrum to a patient's dynamic range *(shaded region)*. Speech spectrum is from Pascoe (1975). The upper audiogram illustrates 25 dB gain and the lower one represents application of a half-gain rule.

must be assured that speech is as intelligible as it was without amplification and that perceptible and significant gains in recognition in quiet or in noise are achieved. Such gains may not be realized at the initial fitting (Gatehouse, 1993) but should be assessed during a trial period.

Audiologists must document gains in speech recognition performance to patients to justify the fitting of amplification. Improved performance relative to no amplification can easily be documented except perhaps in cases of mild high-frequency hearing loss. Showing the benefits of new technology, compared with the patient's present hearing aid(s), may be more difficult. Recent research with new hearing aid circuits including digital signal processing has often failed to show clinically significant differences in speech recognition over traditional amplification, despite patients' subjective preference for the newer technology (Newman & Sandridge, 1998). As hearing aid technology has moved beyond the basic premise of restoring audibility in the past 10 years, the demands for more sensitive speech assessment procedures will increase. For example, the benefits of circuits designed to address poor frequency resolution may not be evident by measuring percent correct recognition of word lists but require a more sensitive measure such as discrimination of high-frequency second-formant transitions (Thibodeau & VanTasell, 1987). Perhaps the greatest challenge and impetus for change in speech audiometric practices will be the development of more sophisticated speech materials to allow assessment of hearing aid benefit.

VARIABLES IN SPEECH EVALUATION PARADIGMS

Speech Acoustics

To select appropriate speech materials and evaluate the results obtained, the importance of the acoustics of the signal being presented must be considered. A brief review of the long-term and short-term characteristics of the speech signal will be provided; an in-depth review of speech acoustics relative to hearing loss may be found in Van Tasell (1986). When assessing speech processing, one must know the typical level of conversational speech that a patient will encounter in everyday life. By averaging conversational speech levels over time, the long-term speech spectrum can be determined (Dunn & White, 1940; Olsen et al, 1987) as shown in Figure 13–2. It is important to note, for reasons given later, that the most intense portion of the spectrum is in the 500 Hz region. The average overall level of speech is approximately 74 dB SPL (Benson & Hirsh, 1953), which corresponds to 54 dB HL on the audiometer for TDH 39 earphones (ANSI, 1996). When a measure of speech processing at conversational levels is desired, 50 dB HL is the typical level used.

Regarding the short-term characteristics of speech, the intensity range from the weakest to the most intense phoneme is about 30 dB (Fletcher, 1970). Vowels are more intense and longer than consonants, consequently more intelligible. During the typical speech assessment, the weak consonants are often inaudible for persons with hearing loss of moderate or greater degree. Particularly, patients with high-frequency hearing loss may find low-intensity fricatives

and sibilants inaudible even at an overall presentation level of 80 dB HL as shown in Figure 13–3. For a patient with a severe sensorineural loss greater than 1000 Hz, the high-frequency consonants in the shaded region will not be audible when speech is delivered at 80 dB HL from the audiometer. Therefore true maximum speech recognition may not be observed in the typical clinical evaluation.

Knowing the types of speech cues most likely to be misperceived is useful when analyzing error types. Through analysis of consonant confusion matrices obtained from normal-hearing persons who listened to speech through a variety of filtering conditions, it was determined that voicing and manner cues are carried across the frequency spectrum. However, place of articulation is cued primarily in high-frequency information (Dubno & Levitt, 1985; Miller & Nicely, 1955). Therefore one would expect a patient with a high-frequency hearing loss to have the most difficulty with place information. These error patterns were confirmed by Olsen and Matkin (1979), who also reported that consonant errors were likely to be substitutions rather than omissions. When omissions did occur, they were most likely for final consonant sounds.

Recent advances in hearing aid technology have affected the temporal characteristics of the speech signal (e.g., adaptive compression), making it important to know the temporal characteristics of sounds, syllables, and pauses between words in sentences. To evaluate the effects of technology that alter the signal in the temporal domain, the duration of the stimuli must be considered in relationship to temporal processing. For example, to evaluate the effects of a compression system that is designed to vary the release time relative to the duration of the signal that set it into compression, speech stimuli must be used that would allow observation of this effect. It is unlikely that presenting lists of monosyllabic words of relatively equal duration would reveal the effects of such a circuit. However, presenting connected speech in the presence of background noise where the average duration between words is 200 ms would be more likely to reveal differences between an adaptive release time circuit and one with a fixed release time less than 150 ms.

Temporal characteristics of importance to these decisions include not only the durations of speech sounds but also duration of pauses between words and syllables. Pickett (1999) provides an overview of how the duration of individual sounds depends on position relative to pauses, syllables, stress, linguistic content, and acoustic features. For example, vowels can range from 52 to 212 ms, but average 130 ms when in a stressed syllable and 70 ms in an unstressed syllable (Klatt, 1976). In addition, vowels are about 20 ms shorter when followed by a voiceless stop consonant (Umeda, 1975). Consonants vary from 25 ms for a stop consonant such as /t/ preceding a stressed vowel to 86 ms for a nasal consonant such as /m/ in the initial stressed syllable of a word. As with vowels, consonant duration is about 20 to 40 ms longer in

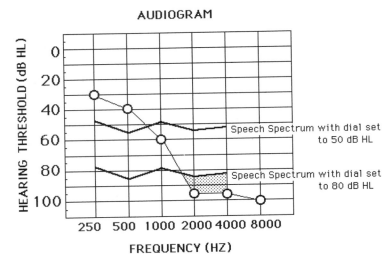

AUDIOGRAM

O-Right Ear   X-Left Ear

Figure 13–3 Audibility of speech for a patient with a severe high-frequency hearing loss. Speech spectrum is from Pascoe (1975). The shaded region represents the portion of the speech spectrum that is not audible even at a higher presentation level on the audiometer.

words having higher content meaning (Umeda, 1977). Consonants such as /s/ can range from a duration of more than 200 ms at the end of a phrase to 50 ms in a consonant cluster.

Syllable duration is also influenced by stress and proximity to pauses. Initial syllables range from 130 to 483 ms, whereas final syllables preceding a pause range from 243 ms to 516 ms (Crystal & House, 1990). Pauses that occur between syllables, words, and sentences are related to speaking rate. For conversational speech, the rate is typically 200 words per minute. When speakers are instructed to speak "clearly," the rate is typically 100 words per minute (Picheny et al, 1989). Pauses account for about 20% of the time during reading and up to 50% of the time in conversation (Klatt, 1976).

Given a speaking rate of 200 words per minute and a pause rate of 50%, the average word and pause duration would be 150 ms each. It is argued that compression circuits with release times of 40 to 50 ms would potentially allow background noise to be amplified during pauses (Teder, 1993). Therefore evaluation of such circuits or adaptive release time circuits must include speech stimuli of appropriate durations for the electroacoustic effect or lack thereof to be used.

Level of Auditory Ability Assessed

Unfortunately, speech processing is often assessed without regard for the level of auditory processing that is being required by the task. This is particularly important when testing children so that low scores are not interpreted as poor performance when a child is not capable of performing at that level of auditory processing. As mentioned earlier, evaluation of speech processing can be considered in terms of a hierarchy of auditory processing that is often used as a guide for establishing auditory training activities (Erber, 1982). It is necessary to relate traditional audiological tests to the hierarchy to illustrate the misconceptions associated with the typical speech test erroneously called *word discrimination*.

Audiological tests at the simplest level of processing, awareness, are known as speech awareness or detection threshold (SAT or SDT). In an infant this may be a change in

some observable behavior such as eye widening, sucking, or general body movement. For the toddler, the awareness response may be a turn to the sound source, which is then reinforced by a visual stimulus. Preschoolers may respond to speech through play audiometry, where a block is dropped in a bucket on hearing speech.

PEARL

Assessment of speech processing can be performed at various levels of processing, including awareness, discrimination, identification or recognition, and comprehension.

Although auditory discrimination, the next level of auditory processing proposed by Erber (1982), can be evaluated in many ways, no procedures are routinely used in the audiological battery. The evaluation of discrimination (i.e., one's ability to detect a change in the acoustic stimulus) is accomplished in young infants by using a dishabituation response recorded as a change in sucking or heart rate (Eimas et al, 1972). In toddlers, the dishabituation response may be a head turn. When paired with appropriate visual training, children's speech discrimination may be tested with the oddity paradigm as young as 4 years of age. By age 5 or 6, a same or different paradigm is often used to evaluate discrimination. For adults, discrimination of speech features has most often been measured using an ABX procedure in which the listener determines whether the first (A) or second (B) stimulus is the same as the last one (X). In all these procedures the patient is required to respond only when a change has been perceived in some acoustic dimension of the stimulus such as the intensity, frequency, or timing. Patients may respond by changing an ongoing response when an auditory change is noted, by indicating which item in a stimulus sequence is different, or by comparing two stimuli and indicating whether they were identical or not.

Therefore when assessing auditory discrimination, the patient is merely comparing stimuli. Use of the terminology *word discrimination* to refer to the evaluation of speech processing during the audiological examination is not accurate because the typical clinical procedure requires the patient to repeat what is heard, which is the next level of auditory processing, identification, or recognition.

The next level, auditory identification or recognition, may be done by selecting an object, pointing to a picture, or producing the stimulus in written or verbal form. Patients must recognize the sequence of sounds and then associate it with some previous experience. Recognition tasks differ from the next level of processing in that no semantic processing is required. That is, the patient may be able to imitate the word *laud* but not be able to define it or use it in a sentence. Typical audiological speech assessments at the recognition level of processing include the SRT, WRS, and SRS. It is important to note that audiologists typically perform recognition tests as a function of intensity level. A recognition test is usually administered at threshold level and at one or more suprathreshold levels. It is becoming increasingly common to include another recognition test at a suprathreshold level, which is speech recognition in the presence of background noise.

Auditory comprehension, the final level of auditory processing in Erber's (1982) hierarchy, is not routinely assessed during the clinical audiological battery. However, in some cases, assessment of auditory comprehension may be accomplished most efficiently in a sound-treated room with the precise presentation level known to be audible for the patient. Because evaluation of auditory comprehension is not within the scope of this chapter, the reader is referred to Johnson et al (1997), who discuss this level of auditory processing and associated materials in detail.

Response Format

Two general types of response formats exist: open or closed set. For closed-set tasks, the patient will have objects, pictures, or printed stimuli from which to choose. For open-set tasks, three response options exist: repeat the stimuli orally, write the stimuli on paper, or type the stimuli on a keyboard. Response formats largely depend on the age of the patient because younger children are more likely to respond in closed-set formats as a result of limited vocabulary and oral or graphic skills, whereas older patients with normal speech production are likely to repeat the stimuli, which is the most time-efficient format.

A closed-set task results in the greatest scoring accuracy because the response is clearly indicated. If time permits, obtaining a written response can be more accurate than receiving a verbal one. Interpretation of the verbal response may be influenced by the articulation of the patient and by the bandwidth and signal/noise ratio of the monitoring system. Furthermore, a tendency exists for the examiner to err in favor of accepting an incorrect verbal response (Merrell & Atkinson, 1965). When testing young children whose articulation skills are still developing, two examiners may be needed: one to deliver the stimuli and monitor responses through the talkback system and the other to manipulate response choices and monitor responses from within the test room (see Chapter 14).

Speech Stimuli

Possible types of speech stimuli range from nonsense syllables to connected speech. Table 13–1 contains a summary of the relative advantages and disadvantages of the types of speech materials as presented by Tyler (1994). Two major factors influencing selection of the material are patient age and the purpose of the evaluation.

PEARL

Foremost in selecting speech evaluation materials, the vocabulary level must be appropriate; otherwise the test will reflect the effects of language as well as hearing abilities.

Once the vocabulary level is determined, the purpose of the assessment will dictate the materials to be used. If the goal is to determine which acoustic features can be identified, a representative sample of speech sounds that is not influenced by phonemic or syntactic constraints is necessary. For example, a patient may hear "boke" and respond that the word is "broke" or "boat" because these phonemic combinations are possible in English as opposed to "bsoke" or "bopke." Because familiarity with the language and one's ability to guess have an impact on responses when whole words are used, a true assessment of "hearing" speech features must be done using nonsense syllables such as the Nonsense Syllable Test (Levitt & Resnick, 1978).

When evaluating a patient's ability to use context, speech stimuli that differ in semantic relationships will be needed. One such test is the Speech Perception in Noise (SPIN) (Bilger et al, 1984), which is composed of sentences with the final word either semantically related (high probability) or not related (low probability) to the remainder of the sentence. Differences in the scores on the high-probability and low-probability lists reflect the degree to which the patient benefits from semantic context.

Another purpose of a speech assessment may be to determine the minimum intensity level required for 50% speech recognition (i.e., the Speech Recognition Threshold or SRT). This preferred term is synonymous with the traditional terminology Speech Reception Threshold (ASHA, 1988). For this test, it is necessary for the stimuli to be as homogeneous as possible with respect to time and intensity so that intelligibility is equivalent across the words in the list. A recommended list of 15 spondaic words that were determined to be homogeneous in sound-pressure level (Young et al, 1982) is provided in Appendix B.

To predict real-world performance, ideally the stimuli must have great face validity but are a subset of what the patient will

---

PEARL

A common purpose for assessing speech recognition performance is to predict how much difficulty that person may have in the real world as a result of the hearing loss.

TABLE 13–1   Relative merits of different types of speech materials

Speech Stimulus	Advantages	Disadvantages
Nonsense syllables	Examine phonetic errors Use of closed set Linguistic knowledge not an influence	Perceived poor face validity No evaluation of context Limited coarticulation effects
Words	High face validity Relatively easy to adapt to closed-set requiring picture-pointing response Short administration time	Some words may be over-used and not truly open set Familiarity with language may be an influence
Sentences/phrases	High face validity Includes coarticulation effects Evaluation of temporal effects of pauses between words	Influenced by linguistic sophistication and memory More time to administer/score
Paragraph	Highest face validity Can be used for judgments of intelligibility and quality	More time to administer Possible confound if familiar with the topic

Adapted from Tyler (1994).

encounter in the real world. Much effort has been spent on developing word lists that are phonetically balanced representative lists of words encountered in English. For historical reviews of these studies, the reader is referred to Bess (1983) and Penrod (1994). Recently, the question of whether a sample of single words will be predictive of performance with sentences has been raised. Boothroyd and Nittrouer (1988) and Olsen et al (1997) have shown that the scores on tests of single word recognition are predictive of performance on sentence recognition. Their results support the notion that speech recognition is a generalized skill and that scores on all speech recognition tests are related. Therefore audiologists may choose from a variety of available speech stimuli to assess speech recognition, but such decisions will be influenced by a tradeoff between time and reliability.

A recent survey of 218 audiologists across the United States by Martin et al (1998) revealed that word lists, rather than sentence lists, were used by 92% of the respondents. Common speech recognition lists were the Central Institute for the Deaf W-22 (CID W-22) lists (48%) and the Northwestern University 6 (NU6) lists (44%), the origins of which are described in depth by Penrod (1994). Interestingly, comparison with similar surveys conducted since 1985 showed that the use of CID W-22 lists was declining, whereas the NU6 lists were increasing in popularity. Most audiologists (56%) administer half lists (25 words) to each ear. Bess (1983) reviews the controversy in the literature in the 60s and 70s regarding the issues surrounding using half lists, including disruption of the phonetic balance of the list and reduced reliability with fewer stimulus presentations. However, the size of the list to present must be determined according to the purpose of testing. If a half list is presented to determine a general estimate of speech recognition ability, one must interpret the score according to the critical difference range for a

25-word list as described later. When a pathological condition results in slight changes in speech recognition, percent correct measures at a fixed intensity level are probably not as sensitive as an adaptive procedure.

Thornton and Raffin (1978) have shown that the sensitivity of a speech measure is proportional to the number of trials administered. They developed a probabilistic model on the basis of speech recognition as a binomial distribution; that is, the variability in performance is highest in the middle range of scores and lowest at the extreme ranges of scores (0 and 100%). If a recognition test stimulus is scored as correct or incorrect and the total score reflects the percentage of the items perceived correctly, test scores may be compared with the critical differences determined by Thornton and Raffin for a given number of test items as shown in Table 13–2. For example, if an initial test score was 80% on a 50-item list, a subsequent score would have to fall outside the range of 64 to 92% to be considered significantly different at the 95% confidence level. In other words, a 95% probability exists that on repeated tests, a patient having a score of 80% will receive a score between 64 and 92%. However, if a 25-item list were presented, the subsequent score would have to be lower than 56% or higher than 96% to be significantly different. If a 10-item list were presented the critical difference range increases to 40 to 100%.

One solution to the tradeoff dilemma has been proposed by Olsen et al (1997), who suggest the use of isophonemic word lists made up of 10 consonant vowel consonant syllables that are scored by phonemes rather than whole word correct. Two lists of 10 words each can be presented monaurally in approximately 2 minutes, less time than required for 25 monosyllables. If the two scores are not significantly different according to the Thornton and Raffin (1978) critical differences, the two can be averaged to represent the speech

TABLE 13–2   Critical differences for speech recognition scores

Initial Speech Recognition Score (%)	100 Items	50 Test Items	25 Test Items	10 Test Items
90	81–96	76–98	72–100	50–100
80	68–89	64–92	56–96	40–100
70	57–81	52–86	48–92	30–90
60	47–73	42–78	36–84	20–90
50	37–63	32–68	28–76	10–90
40	27–53	22–58	16–64	10–80
30	19–43	14–48	12–56	10–70
20	11–32	8–36	4–44	0–60
10	4–19	2–24	4–32	0–50

Based on Thornton and Raffin (1978).
For a given number of test items, values within each range are not significantly different from the initial speech recognition score (p >.05).

recognition performance for that ear. If variability is high and the two scores are different, additional lists will be required.

Presentation Mode

Speech audiometry stimuli can be presented by monitored live voice or recorded voice. Use of live voice is convenient and allows for flexibility and reduced administration time. Live-voice presentation is typically used for determination of the SRT, despite the ASHA (1988) recommendation to use recorded materials. Fewer audiologists use live-voice presentation for suprathreshold speech recognition testing (82 vs. 94% of surveyed audiologists, Martin et al, 1998). Live voice may be more acceptable for threshold testing because the patient is responding primarily to the intense vowel sounds that are generally equated by monitoring the peaks on the volume unit (VU) meter. However, for suprathreshold recognition testing, performance depends more on receiving less intense consonant information that cannot be monitored by fast action of the VU meter. Furthermore, the SRT contributes less to the differential diagnosis and is primarily used to confirm the pure tone testing results. However, the speech recognition score contributes to the site-of-lesion determination such that greater precision is required.

PEARL
For determining the SRS, it is imperative that prerecorded stimuli are presented that have been equated for intensity so that scores reflect true performance of the patient and not variations in the speaker.

Increased reliability of performance with taped rather than live-voice presentation has been consistently demonstrated (Brandy, 1966; Hood & Poole, 1980) yet warrants reiteration according to the results of a recent current practice survey. Martin et al (1998) reported that 82% of audiologists responding to the survey are still using monitored live-voice presentation. Reasons for this most likely include the greater flexibility for the examiner and perhaps lack of equipment. It is hoped that the move toward recorded presentation will increase as manufacturers are more likely to include compact disc players with audiometers that facilitate access to particular lists.

A study that clearly illustrates the problems associated with live-voice testing for speech recognition was performed by Brandy in 1966. Speech recognition scores for 25-word lists were obtained from 24 patients with normal-hearing. Half of the patients listened to three different recordings from the same talker and the other half listened to three randomizations of one recording of the same talker. Variation in scores across the three different recordings by the same talker was significant (9.76%), whereas variation in scores for the same recording was nonsignificant (3.3%). Given the inherent variability in speech recognition testing even when recorded materials are used as illustrated by Thornton and Raffin (1978), monitored live-voice testing must be done only in last resort situations. Such situations would include (1) equipment limitations so great that even a cassette player or compact disc player cannot be added, or (2) testing patients that demand frequent interaction to maintain attention and complete the test.

Often live-voice testing is performed with the explanation being that it is more expedient. However, stretching this logic, the time argument could also be used to rationalize the use of tuning forks for pure tone audiometry. Audiologists would agree that this would not be a very sensitive or reliable measure of hearing. In addition, it would be difficult to determine the degree of hearing loss without reference to some calibrated standard for normal-hearing. The same criterion for precision is also required for reliable speech processing measures.

PEARL

It has been argued that if limited time precludes the use of taped speech materials, time should be preserved by not administering speech tests at all (Stach, 1998).

Presentation Level

Depending on the purpose of the speech recognition assessment, the stimuli may be presented at (a) the level of average conversation, (b) the most comfortable listening level for the patient, or (c) the level necessary to achieve maximum performance. To contribute to the differential diagnostic process, several presentation levels may be necessary to determine which one affords the patient the maximum opportunity for clear recognition and to determine whether performance declines with increased intensity (i.e., rollover).

PEARL

Evaluation of speech recognition at several intensity levels is referred to as a performance-intensity (PI) function.

The shape of the PI function is unique not only for a given patient but also for the type of material used. PI functions for words and sentences are shown in Figure 13–4. The function for sentences is the steepest where each dB of intensity results in approximately 10% increase in recognition. However, for words each dB results in about a 4% increase.

By obtaining a PI function, audiologists can determine the maximum performance for each patient, referred to as PB Max, when phonetically balanced monosyllabic word lists are used. To evaluate the significance of the PB Max score, it may be compared with data obtained from patients with similar degrees of sensorineural hearing (Dubno et al, 1995; Yellin et al, 1989) as described later in "Interpretation of Results." If

the PB Max is disproportionately low relative to others with similar hearing loss, it is suggestive of a retrocochlear pathological condition.

It is often not clinically feasible to evaluate speech processing at several intensity levels. Therefore in an attempt to achieve PB Max and determine whether rollover is present, testing may begin at a high level such as 80 dB HL, unless this level is less than the SRT + 30 dB (80 dB HL <SRT + 30). If the 80 dB HL level is adequate, and the measured score is 84% or higher when a half-list is used, further testing to determine PB Max is not necessary. The reason is that even if the maximum possible score of 100% was obtained at a lower intensity, the difference score of 16% is less than the 20% criterion difference to be considered rollover (Jerger & Jerger, 1971). However, if a score less than 84% is achieved, it could mean one of two things: (1) higher presentation level is needed to achieve PB Max because of reduced audibility of the signal, or (2) a lower presentation level is needed because the score reflects rollover.

The decision to present a second list at an intensity level above or below 80 dB HL will be determined by the pure tone average (PTA). If the PTA is above 40 dB HL, it is likely that a higher presentation level is necessary to achieve PB Max because the AI predicts that the entire spectrum may not have been audible at 80 dB HL presentation level. However, if the PTA is less than 40 dB HL, the AI predicts that the speech information should have been audible and a lower presentation level would determine if the low score was suggestive of rollover.

PITFALL

When using a high-intensity presentation level during speech audiometry, the probability for crossover is high and masking may be needed (see Chapter 12).

Evaluation of speech recognition for rehabilitation purposes should include presenting stimuli at an average conversational level (50 dB HL) to demonstrate to the patient the effects of reduced audibility and potential for improvement received from amplification. It may also be helpful to determine the recognition performance at the most comfortable

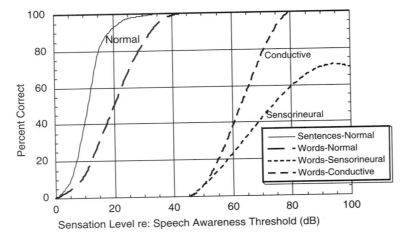

Figure 13–4 Performance intensity functions for sentences and words for patients with normal hearing and for words for patients with conductive and sensorineural hearing loss. (Adapted from Hood and Poole [1971].)

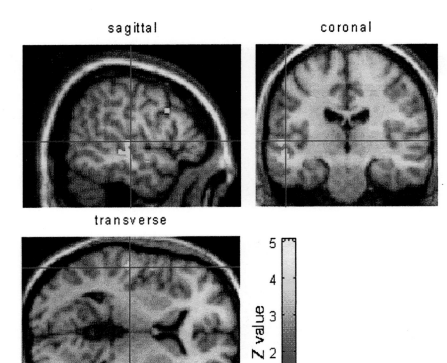

sagittal

coronal

transverse

$$x = -54.00$$
$$y = -20.00$$
$$z = 4.00$$

Z value

Color Plate 1. fMRI of the brain of a subject who was required to discriminate nonsense words as being alike or different. Note activity in the midportion of Heschl's gyrus and extending inferiorly into the superoposterior midtemporal gyrus. Also note some frontal lobe activity on the sagittal view. All activity in these views seems to be limited to the left hemisphere. (Courtesy of Brain Imaging Laboratory, Dartmouth Medical School, Hanover, NH.) *(See Chapter 3, Figure 3–13.)*

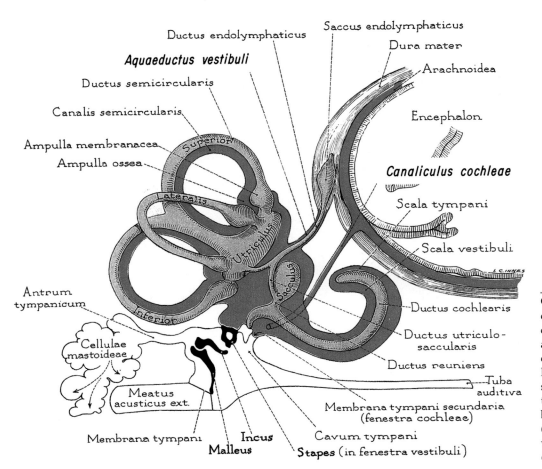

Ductus endolymphaticus

Saccus endolymphaticus

Aquaeductus vestibuli

Dura mater

Arachnoidea

Ductus semicircularis

Canalis semicircularis

Encephalon

Ampulla membranacea

Canaliculus cochleae

Ampulla ossea

Scala tympani

Superior

Lateralis

Scala vestibuli

Utriculus

Sacculus

Antrum tympanicum

Inferior

Ductus cochlearis

Cellulae mastoideae

Ductus utriculo-saccularis

Ductus reuniens

Meatus acusticus ext.

Tuba auditiva

Membrana tympani secundaria (fenestra cochleae)

Membrana tympani

Incus

Cavum tympani

Malleus

Stapes (in fenestra vestibuli)

Color Plate 2. Schematic diagram of major components of the middle and inner ear. The organs of the membranous labyrinth *(in blue)* are shown enclosed within the various cavities of the bony labyrinth *(in red).* (From Anson et al [1973], with permission.) *(See Chapter 4, Figure 4–1.)*

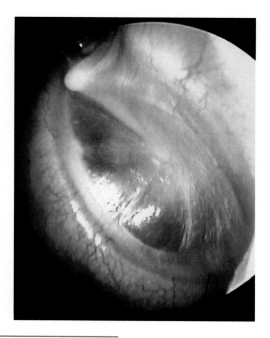

Color Plate 3. Normal tympanic membrane. Note that the short process of the incus and the malleus are well visualized. *(See Chapter 5, Figure 5–3.)*

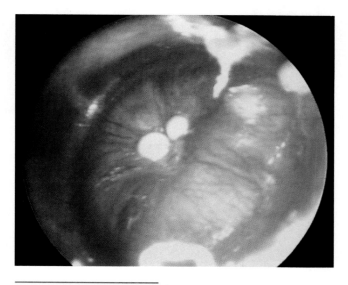

Color Plate 4. Two small white masses are visualized in the center of the tympanic membrane. These are cholesteatomas that have been implanted on the eardrum. *(See Chapter 5, Figure 5–4.)*

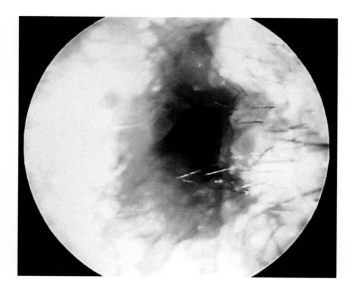

Color Plate 5. External bacterial otitis has led to a swollen earcanal with purulent debris. *(See Chapter 5, Figure 5–5.)*

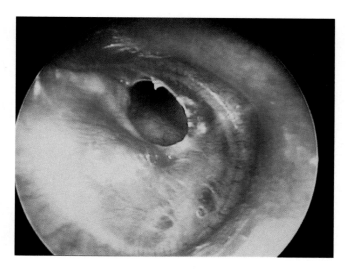

Color Plate 6. A small central perforation is seen involving the posterior superior portion of the tympanic membrane. *(See Chapter 5, Figure 5–6.)*

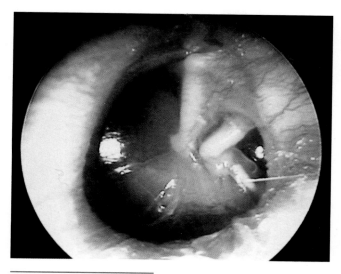

Color Plate 7. Marked retraction of the tympanic membrane is noted with a middle ear effusion. The incudostapedial joint is easily visualized. *(See Chapter 5, Figure 5–7.)*

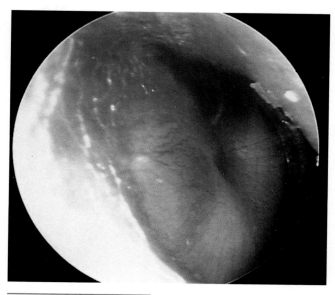

Color Plate 8. Purulent material is visualized behind a bulging tympanic membrane in acute otitis media. *(See Chapter 5, Figure 5–8.)*

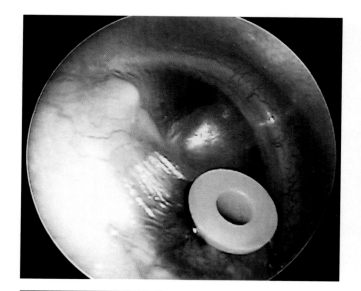

Color Plate 9. Otitis media with effusion has resolved with the placement of a tympanostomy tube. *(See Chapter 5, Figure 5–10.)*

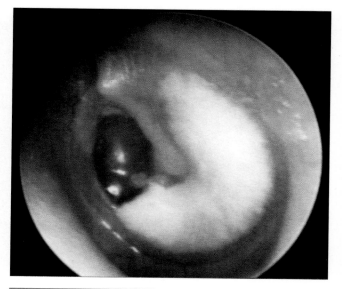

Color Plate 10. Tympanosclerosis is noted involving three fourths of the tympanic membrane. *(See Chapter 5, Figure 5–11.)*

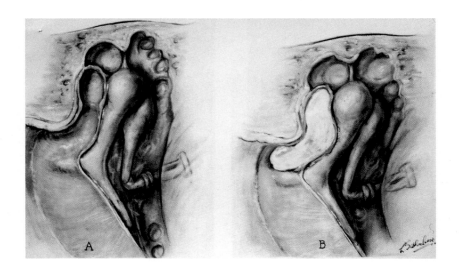

Color Plate 11. **(A)** Development of a retraction pocket in the pars flaccida region of the tympanic membrane. **(B)** Over time, the retraction pocket fills with squamous debris. (From Nager [1993], with permission.) *(See Chapter 5, Figure 5–12.)*

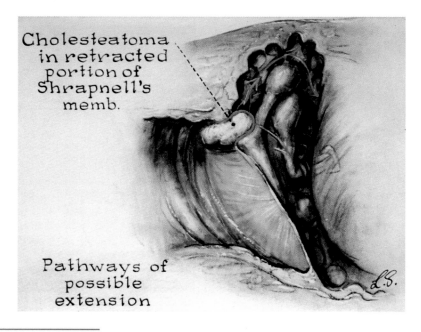

Cholesteatoma in retracted portion of Shrapnell's memb.

Pathways of possible extension

Color Plate 12. Cholesteatoma can take several paths of erosion into the middle ear. All routes usually result in ossicular erosion. (From Nager [1993], with permission.) *(See Chapter 5, Figure 5–13.)*

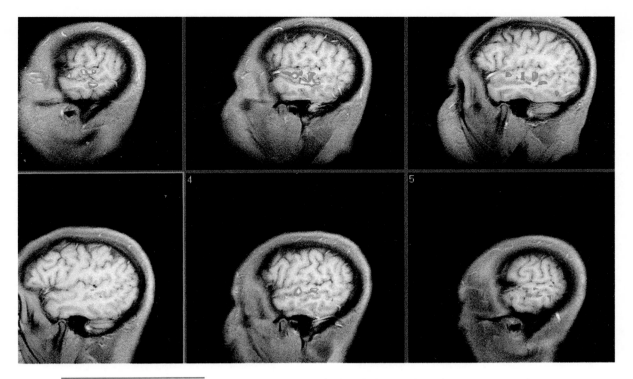

Color Plate 13. fMRI of a normal 34-year-old right-handed man. Stimulus was a narrative story delivered auditorily at the upper level of comfortable loudness. Top three sagittal slices are of the right hemisphere. Bottom three slices are of the left hemisphere. *(See Chapter 7, Figure 7–3.)*

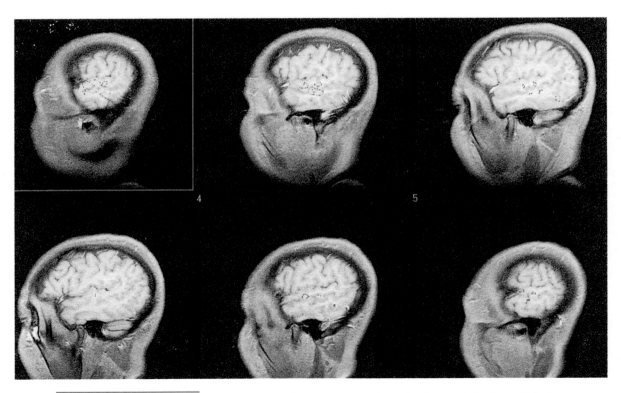

Color Plate 14. fMRI scan using same data from Figure 7–3 but a higher statistical cutoff during analysis. Note the apparent lesser degree of activation caused by the differing statistical choice made during analysis. *(See Chapter 7, Figure 7–10.)*

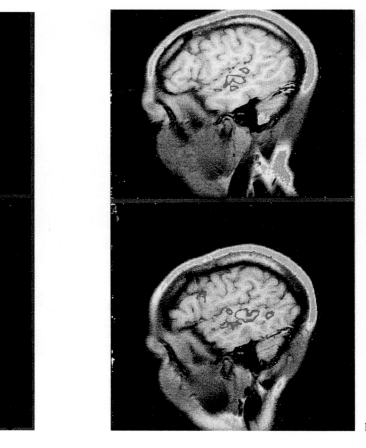

A   B

Color Plate 15.   Two separate fMRI scans performed on the same subject 20 minutes apart using identical methodologies. **(A)** First scan performed. **(B)** Second scan performed 20 minutes later. Slice locations for the two scans were chosen to be nearly the same as possible (right hemisphere is shown on top for both acquisitions). *(See Chapter 7, Figure 7–11.)*

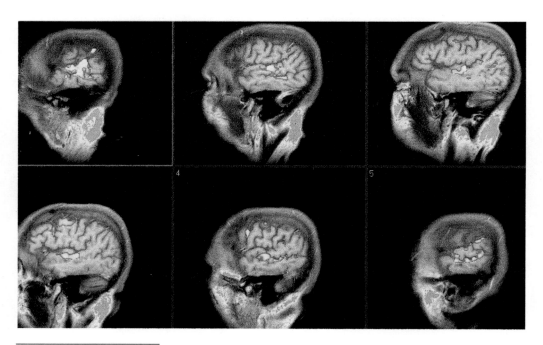

Color Plate 16.   fMRI of severely hearing-impaired 73-year-old man (sagittal slices with right hemisphere on top). Note frontal lobe activation (*middle bottom*) in addition to normal areas of activation. *(See Chapter 7, Figure 7–12.)*

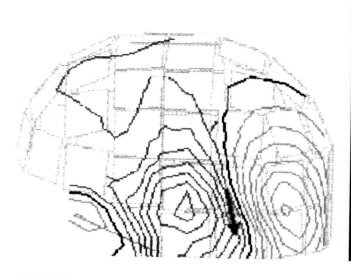

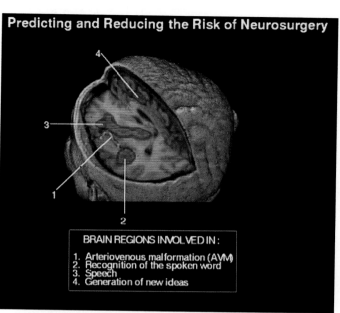

Color Plate 17. Posterolateral left view of spontaneous MEG scan of a mildly autistic child showing focus of epileptiform activity in left temporal lobe *(at center of left circles)*. *(See Chapter 7, Figure 7–14.)*

Color Plate 18. Posterolateral left view of a three-dimensional PET scan using auditory stimuli. (Courtesy of The Samaritan PET Center, Phoenix, Arizona.) *(See Chapter 7, Figure 7–16.)*

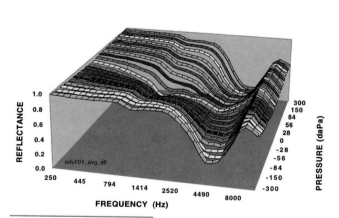

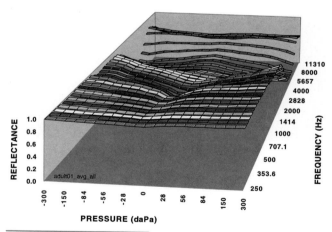

Color Plate 19. Energy reflectance for normal subjects at various earcanal air pressures. *(See Chapter 17, Figure 17–23.)*

Color Plate 20. Average reflectance tympanograms for 20 normal adult subjects. As the test frequency progresses from low to high, tympanometric patterns progress from V-shaped, to inverted V, to flat. *(See Chapter 17, Figure 17–24.)*

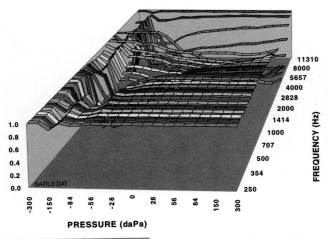

Color Plate 21. Reflectance tympanograms for the left ear of patient SR. *(See Chapter 17, Figure 17–31.)*

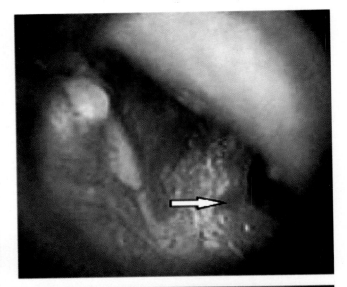

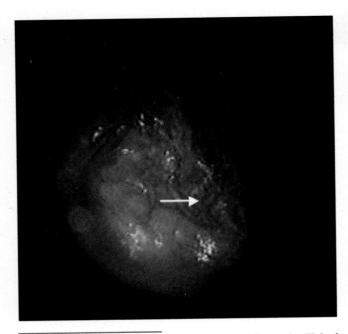

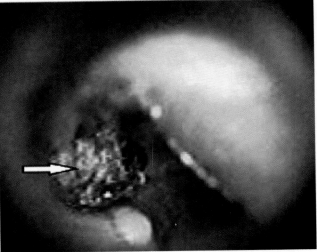

Color Plate 23. Otomicroscopic image of the right TM of patient JT. Identifiable landmarks were completely absent. A deep retraction pocket was present anteriorly and a tympanosclerotic region was present in the anterosuperior region. Most of the drum was retracted against the promontory of the middle ear and was immobile on pneumatic stimulation. Only a small portion of the drum was mobile. *(See Chapter 17, Figure 17–36.)*

Color Plate 22. Otomicroscopic image of the right TM of patient SP. The image shows two areas of squamous debris, one on pars tensa and one on pars flaccida. A cholesteatoma in the middle ear originated from the squamous debris on pars tensa. *(See Chapter 17, Figure 17–32.)*

level (MCL) preferred by the patient. These results may facilitate patient counseling regarding the gradual adjustment to amplification of the signal to levels above their MCL that may be required to receive maximum benefit.

Calibration for Speech Stimuli

Presentation of complex signals requires different calibration procedures than those used for pure tone testing. Because speech is a dynamic signal that results in difficulty determining a precise level, a 1000-Hz tone is used to set the audiometer level so that the output from the earphone is 20 dB above the HL dial value for a TDH50 earphone. That is, 0 dB HL or normal-hearing for speech is equivalent to 20 dB SPL (ANSI, 1996). SPLs for normal-hearing for speech are provided in Table 13–3. When recorded materials are produced, a calibration tone precedes the stimuli. This tone is generally recorded at a level that is equivalent to the frequent peaks of the speech signal unless otherwise specified. The calibration tone should be set to peak at 0 on the VU meter.

When calibrating for sound field testing, many factors must be accounted for that include: (1) distance from the speaker, (2) azimuth, (3) earcanal resonance, (4) head shadow, and (5) standing waves. Reference levels for speech recognition at 0 and 45 degrees azimuth are 16.5 dB SPL and 12.5 dB SPL, respectively (ASHA, 1991). Because pure tone signals can combine and cancel when presented in rooms with reflective surfaces resulting in standing waves, the calibration stimulus for speech in the sound field is speech-weighted noise. Even though the threshold for speech will be lower in the sound field than under phones because of the advantages of earcanal acoustics, the calibration values are such that the sound field and earphone testing are equated. In other words, when the audiometer is calibrated properly for sound field and earphone testing, the average SRTs obtained monaurally under phones and in the sound field should be essentially equal given normal test-retest variability.

TABLE 13–3 Sound pressure levels (SPLs) for normal hearing of speech for various transducers

Transducer*	dB SPL for Normal Hearing†	dB HL equivalent
Earphone-TDH 39	19.5	0
Earphone-TDH 49	20.0	0
Earphone-TDH 50	20.0	0
Insert phone	12.5	0
Sound field speaker— 0 degrees azimuth	16.5	0
Sound field speaker— 45 degrees azimuth	12.5	0

From (ANSI, 1996).
* All TDH earphones mounted in MX-41/AR cushions.
†All earphone values determined in an NBS 9A 6-cc coupler with the exception of the insert phone value which was measured in a dB-0138 2-cc coupler.

Procedures

A variety of measures are used in speech audiometry. If assessing awareness of speech, the procedure will be an adaptive one to determine the level at which speech is just barely audible. For assessment of speech recognition, at least three choices exist: (1) present speech stimuli at a fixed presentation level and measure the percent correctly identified, (2) present running speech at a fixed presentation level and measure intelligibility in percent, and (3) present words or sentences in an adaptive paradigm and determine the intensity level necessary to achieve 50% correct recognition. The first method to assess speech recognition has been used by most audiologists since at least 1972 (Martin et al, 1998). More recently, equivalent passages have been developed for patients to rate intelligibility, but these have been used primarily for hearing aid comparisons (Cox & McDaniel, 1989). Adaptive procedures have been shown to be sensitive measures of the effects of hearing loss configuration or selective amplification (Van Tasell & Yanz, 1987). One advantage of adaptive tests over a fixed presentation level is reducing ceiling and floor effects. Only one clinical test of speech recognition with normative data using an adaptive procedure is commercially available. The Hearing in Noise Test (HINT), in which the patient repeats sentences presented with a background noise, was originally designed for the assessment of binaural hearing in noise in the sound field. This test has not been used as a routine clinical assessment of monaural speech recognition (Nilsson et al, 1994).

Other procedures are required for the determination of the loudness of speech, which include most comfortable loudness (MCL) and uncomfortable loudness level (ULL or UCL). These levels are typically determined with an adaptive procedure where the patient is asked to judge the loudness of running speech as the level is adjusted. Hawkins (1984) recommends using an ascending method of limits to determine the UCL as that level between the patient's judgments of "loud, but OK" and "uncomfortably loud."

Analysis of Results

For suprathreshold measures of speech recognition, percent correct scores are generally reported. However, if a closed set is used, the probability of guessing must be considered. For example, chance performance on a test with a response set of four is 25%. Rather than whole-word scoring for open-set testing, Olsen et al (1997) suggest scoring by phonemes. Perhaps a more useful summary of performance would be to analyze error patterns by means of a confusion matrix. Error patterns associated with various configurations of hearing loss as reported in the literature (Bilger & Wang, 1976) could be used for comparison purposes to determine whether one's error patterns were typical for their loss. If not, additional counseling may be needed.

If an adaptive procedure is used, some average value will be determined on the basis of a given number of reversals. For example, the HINT (Nilsson et al, 1994) involves varying the level of the sentences and averaging the levels at which the response changed from correct to incorrect or vice versa. If a simple up-down procedure is used, the threshold represents the level at which 50% correct performance would be achieved.

Interpretation of Results

Regardless of presentation, stimuli, response format, and analysis, the results are most valuable if they can be compared with normative values for interpretation. To compare results, one must use procedures identical to those used with the standardization sample. It is evident from performance intensity functions (Fig. 13–4) that considerable variation in performance occurs across presentation level and speech stimuli. Therefore standardized procedures are needed against which to compare speech recognition scores. Despite the variety of clinical materials available for assessing speech recognition, few exist with normative data based on standardized procedures. It is often assumed that the norm for comparison is that achieved with normal-hearing. If testing were performed in quiet using common English vocabulary, the predicted norm would be 100%. This may be acceptable if test conditions allow the entire speech spectrum to be audible, but generally this is not the case. Therefore it is important to assess how missing high-frequency information would have an impact on a speech recognition test score. Two simplified clinical procedures are described later to facilitate interpretation of speech recognition by accounting for audibility: (1) a Count-the-Dot Audiogram, and (2) a Speech Recognition Interpretation (SPRINT) chart.

SPECIAL CONSIDERATION

Some speech recognition materials are available in Spanish and French (see Table 13–4); however, normative data to aid interpretation of results are limited. Further information regarding issues in cultural diversity is found in Chapter 14.

One way to compare speech performance on the basis of audibility of the signal is to use the Count-the-Dot Audiogram, which is based on the AI developed by French and Steinberg (1947) and modifications by several for clinical applications (Humes, 1991, Mueller & Killion, 1990; Pavlovic, 1989). This Index ranges from 0 to 1 and represents the proportion of the speech spectrum that is available to convey information to the patient. It is computed from acoustical measurements of the speech spectrum, the effective masking spectrum of any noises, and the auditory dynamic range of the patient. These measurements can be made in each of 15 one-third octave bands throughout the speech range.

Formally, the AI is defined as follows:

$$AI = P \sum_{i=1,15} BI(i) \, BE(i)$$

PEARL

The Articulation Index reflects the audibility of the speech spectrum by representing the proportion that is available to the patient from 0 to 1.

---

where P is a proficiency factor considered to represent practice effects of the patient and precision with which test materials are enunciated, BI (band importance) is a weight chosen to represent the relative contribution of a given frequency band (i) to speech transmission under ideal conditions, and BE (band efficiency) is a measure of the proportion of the speech signal in a given band (i) that is above the patient's masked threshold and below loudness discomfort level. Initial validation studies showed that the effects on speech recognition performance of varying frequency/gain characteristics by filtering or adding noise to the signal were well predicted by the AI for normal-hearing persons (French & Steinberg, 1947; Kryter, 1962). Standard normal curves (ANSI, 1998) relating speech recognition to the AI are shown in Figure 13–5.

Clinical adaptations of this procedure were developed so that the AI could be easily determined by plotting one's hearing thresholds on an audiogram that had the relative weights of the speech information across the frequency range represented by dots. An example of the Count-the-Dot Audiogram is shown in Figure 13–6. This may be used as a reference against which to compare one's performance and determine whether effects of the hearing loss on speech recognition are beyond those accounted for by loss of audibility. Because the AI accounts for reduced absolute sensitivity, one may predict a speech recognition score after calculating the AI and by using the function in Figure 13–5. The degree to which one's score deviates from that predicted by the AI reflects difficulties resulting from reduced differential sensitivity. For example, an AI of .2 predicts that the normal-hearing persons would achieve only about 50% correct speech recognition for single words. If the person with hearing impairment achieves less than this, it may be concluded that the person was not able to use suprathreshold speech information as efficiently as normal-hearing individuals. This might be the result of reduced differential sensitivity, such as poor frequency or temporal resolution (Pavlovic, 1984).

Another way to evaluate performance is to use the SPRINT charts shown in Figures 13–7 and 13–8. As mentioned earlier, performance can be compared within a patient through the use of the binomial distribution for speech developed by Thornton and Raffin (1978). They determined the degree to which a second speech recognition score must vary from an initial score to be significantly different at various confidence levels; the data in Figures 13–7 and 13–8 are based on a 95% confidence level. To ease interpretation in the audiological setting, the SPRINT charts may serve as a quick reference sheet. The two charts were developed to quickly interpret the significance of the difference between two scores for 25-word and 50-word lists. Vertical arrows represent the 95% confidence differences for percentage scores (Thornton & Raffin, 1978). If the intersection of the plot of the two scores, using the abscissa for the first score and the right ordinate for the second score, falls within the bounds of the arrow, the two scores are not significantly different. It can easily be seen in both figures that the critical difference ranges are largest in the midrange of scores (40 to 60%) and decline at the upper and lower ranges of performance. For example, in Figure 13–7, by looking at the arrow above the 40% score, it can be seen that a second score on a 25-word list would have to be less than 16% or greater than 64% to be significantly different (a range of 48%). However, for a score of 88%, the critical difference

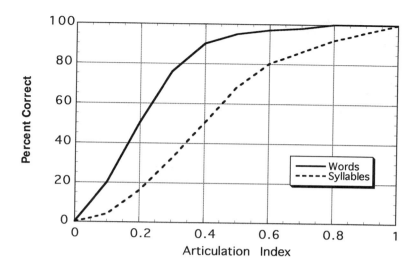

Figure 13–5 AI function for words and syllables. (Adapted from French and Steinberg [1947] and ANSI [1998].)

range is only 68 to 96% (a range of 28%). In addition, it is clear that the range of differences is greater for 25 words than 50 words. For example, if the score is 40% and 25 stimuli are used (Fig. 13–7), the range within the 95% level of confidence is 48% (16 to 64%), but if 50 stimuli are used (Fig. 13–8), the range is 36% (22 to 58%).

> **PEARL**
>
> Audiologists can interpret speech recognition scores through the use of tools such as the Count-the-Dot Audiogram or the SPRINT chart.

COUNT-THE-DOT AUDIOGRAM

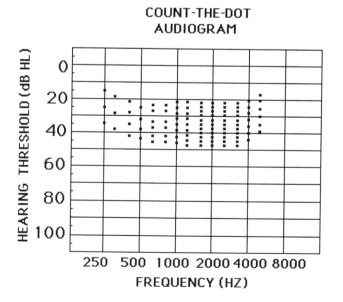

Figure 13–6 Count-the-Dot Audiogram. (Adapted from Mueller and Killion [1990].)

> **PEARL**
>
> Scores obtained using 50-word lists that differ by 20% or more will always be significantly different relative to 95% confidence limits established by Thornton and Raffin (1978). For 25-word list use 25%.

Figures 13–7 and 13–8 can also be used to estimate whether a single WRS agrees with expected values according to pure tone sensitivity for 25-word and 50-word lists, respectively. Data for these comparisons were based on the 95% confidence limits of the PB Max for NU6 word lists from a sample of 407 ears with a wide range of pure tone averages (PTAs) (500, 1000, and 2000 Hz) (Dubno et al, 1995). When a patient's PB Max is less than that predicted for their PTA, it may be concluded that word recognition is significantly impaired relative to most patients with equivalent hearing loss. To determine this on the SPRINT chart, the score represented on the abscissa is plotted as a function of the PTA represented on the left ordinate. If it falls within the shaded region, the percent correct score is considered disproportionately low for that degree of hearing loss. For example, if the patient's PTA is 52 dB HL and a 25-word list was used (Fig. 13–7), the 95% confidence limit is 48%. Any score less than 48% would fall in the shaded region and be considered abnormally low for that PTA. For PTA values not listed in the SPRINT chart (such as 62 dB HL), round up to the next higher PTA (64 dB HL) for a conservative interpretation. When speech recognition scores fall below expected values, further diagnostic testing is warranted and specific counseling during the rehabilitation process regarding coping strategies is needed.

One may also want to compare group speech recognition scores. If the dependent variable is a percent correct score, an arc-sine transform is necessary before any statistical analysis of the results (Studebaker, 1985). On the basis of the number of words in the list, the scores ranging from 0 to 100% may be transformed from 0 to 120%. This transform adjusts for the disparate variances that exist in perception scores in which less variability is observed at the extremes than in midrange of performance.

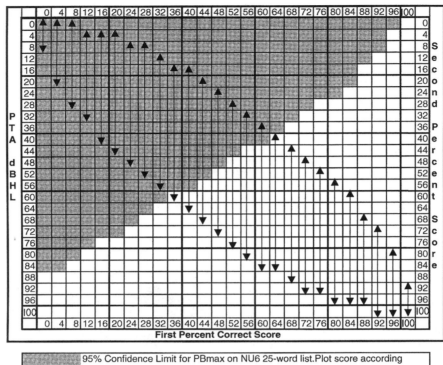

95% Confidence Limit for PBmax on NU6 25-word list. Plot score according to PTA on left ordinate and percent correct score on the abscissa. If it falls in the shaded area, it is considered disproportionately low. (Adapted from Dubno et al., 1995)

95% Critical differences for 25-word list. Plot first and second score according to the abscissa and right ordinate. If it falls within the arrow, the two scores are not significantly different (Adapted from Thornton & Raffin, 1978)

Copyright by Linda M. Thibodeau, 1999

Figure 13–7 Speech Recognition Interpretation (SPRINT) chart for 25-word NU6 lists. (Adapted from Thornton and Raffin [1978] and Dubno et al [1995].) See text.

Interpretation of results also involves comparison across measures for accuracy checks and predictive purposes. Examining the interrelationships among speech measures can be helpful in determining whether performance falls within expected ranges. For example, the SDT is generally 10- to 12-dB less than the SRT (Eagan, 1948).

PEARL

SDT is within ± 10 dB of the 500-Hz threshold unless the audiogram rises in the higher frequencies in which case the SDT will be ± 5 dB of the best threshold (Frisina, 1962).

Appropriate tests for each age level are presented in the following section with consideration of the factors mentioned previously. Only those tests for which normative data are available are included so that interpretation of performance is possible.

SPEECH AUDIOMETRY MEASURES

Audiological assessments involving speech will be discussed according to the hierarchy of auditory processing beginning with awareness followed by discrimination and identification. Following this general discussion, typical patterns of results by pathological condition and assessment options by age group will be presented. Table 13–4 contains the hierarchy of speech perception measures of interest. For the suprathreshold tests, only those that have recorded versions available and have published data to which results can be compared are discussed. For a comprehensive review of speech recognition tests, the reader is referred to Roeser (1996) and Mendel and Danhauer (1997). Measures used to assess auditory comprehension level are not included in this review because this assessment at this level of performance does not exclusively lead to a differential diagnosis of a certain auditory pathological condition. Although a central auditory processing problem may contribute to difficulties in auditory comprehension, such problems may be identified through more commonly used testing at the identification

Speech Recognition Interpretation Chart
(SPRINT)

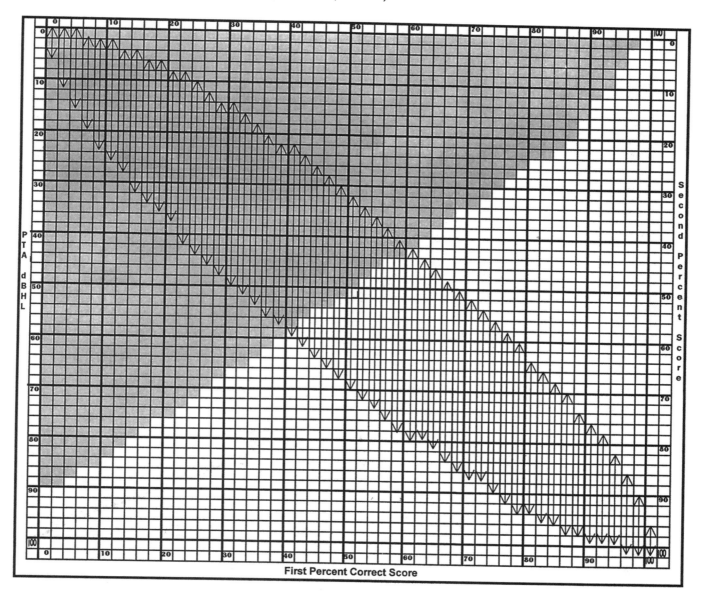

95% Confidence Limit for PBmax on NU6 50-word list. Plot score according
to PTA on left ordinate and percent correct score on the abscissa.
If it falls in the shaded area, it is considered disproportionately low.
(Adapted from Dubno et al.,1995)

95% Critical differences for 50-word list. Plot first and second score
according to the abscissa and right ordinate. If it falls within the arrow, the two
scores are not significantly different. (Adapted from Thornton & Raffin, 1978)

Copyright by Linda M. Thibodeau, 1999

Figure 13–8   Speech Recognition Interpretation (SPRINT) chart for 50-word NU6 lists. See text.

TABLE 13–4 Hierarchy of speech perception measures

Code	Test	Author	Recommended Age	Stimuli	Presentation Format	Response	Norms
Awareness							
SDT	Speech Detection Threshold	ASHA (1988)	Birth to 3 yr	Monosyllabic words	Live voice	Behavioral change	Northern & Downs (1991)
Discrimination							
ADT	Auditory Discrimination Test	Wepman (1973)	5–8 yr	Monosyllabic word pairs	Live voice	Respond verbally, same/different	Yes
Identification							
SRT	Speech Recognition Threshold	ASHA (1988)	3–adult	Spondees	Tape or CD[+†]	Repeat the word or point to pictures	ANSI (1998)
GFW	Goldman Fristoe Woodcock Diagnostic Auditory Discrimination Test	Goldman et al (1974)	3–adult	Monosyllabic words presented in quiet	Tape[‡]	Point to one of 2 pictures	Included in manual based on age
WIPI	Word Intelligibility by Picture Identification	Ross & Lerman (1970)	4–6 yr	Four equivalent lists of 25 monosyllabic words each	Tape or compact disc (CD)[*]	Point to one of 6 pictures	Papso & Blood (1989), Sanderson Leepa & Rintelmann (1976)
NU-CHIPS	Northwestern University Children's Perception of Speech	Elliott & Katz (1980)	3–5 yr	50 Monosyllabic words	Tape or CD[*]	Point to one of 4 pictures	Included in manual
PSI	Pediatric Speech Intelligibility Test	Jerger & Jerger (1982)	3–6 yr	20 Monosyllabic words and two sentence formats in two lists of 10 sentences each	Tape or CD[*]	Point to 1 of 5 pictures	Jerger & Jerger (1982)
TAC	Test of Auditory Comprehension	Trammell (1981)	4–17 yr	Environmental sounds, words, stereotypic messages arranged in 10 subtests	Tape[§]	Point to 1 of 3 pictures	Included in manual, based on PTA and Age
PBK	Phonetically Balanced Kindergarten Word Lists	Haskins (1949)	6–12 yr	50 Monosyllabic words	Tape or CD[*]	Repeat the words	Sanderson-Leepa & Rintelmann (1976)

TABLE 13–4 (continued) Hierarchy of speech perception measures

Code	Test	Author	Recommended Age	Stimuli	Presentation Format	Response	Norms
HINT-C	Hearing in Noise Test for Children	Nilsson et al (1996)	6–12 yr	Sentences	CD°	Repeat the sentence	Included in manual
HINT	Hearing in Noise Test	Nilsson et al (1994)	13 yr and up	Sentences	CD°	Repeat the sentence	Included in manual
PAL PB 50	Psychoacoustics Laboratory, Phonetically Balanced 50-word Lists	Eagan (1948)	12 yr and up	Monosyllabic words	Tape or CD*	Repeat the words	Yellin et al (1989)
CID W-22	Central Institute for the Deaf W-22	Hirsh et al (1952)	12 yr and up	Monosyllabic words	Tape or CD*	Repeat the words	See text re: using Yellin et al (1989)
NU6	Northwestern University	Tillman & Carhart (1966)	12 yr and up	Monosyllabic words	Tape or CD*	Repeat the words	Dubno et al (1995)
SPIN	Revised Speech Perception in Noise	Bilger et al (1984)	12 yr and up	High and low predictability sentences	Tape$^{\|}$	Repeat the final word of the sentence	Included in manual
SSI	Synthetic Sentence Identification	Speaks and Jerger (1965)	12 yr and up	Sentences that do not convey meaning	Tape or CD*,†	Identify the sentence from a list of 10	Jerger (1973)

* Available from Auditec of St. Louis, 2515 S. Big Bend Blvd., St. Louis, MO 63143; 314-781-8890, http://www/auditec.com.
† Comparable materials in Spanish and French are available from Auditec of St. Louis, 2515 S. Big Bend Blvd., St. Louis, MO 63143; 314-781-8890, http://www/auditec.com.
‡ Available from American Guidance Service, 4201 Woodland Rd., Circle Pines, MN 55014-1796; 800-328-2560.
§ Available from Forewords Publications, Box 82289, Portland, OR; 503-653-2614.
$\|$ Available from Robert C. Bilger, 901 South Sixth St., Champaign, IL 61820; 217-333-2230.
° Available from Starkey Laboratories, Inc., 6700 Washington Ave. S., Eden Prairie, MN 55344; 800-733-2596.

level of processing. Speech measures used to assess loudness perception of speech are also reviewed as they relate to hearing aid fitting.

Awareness

The intensity level at which one becomes aware of the presence of speech is determined in the much same way as for pure tone thresholds. An SDT is usually obtained for patients who are not able to repeat words, a skill that is necessary for the SRT. Although referring to the same threshold, the preferred term is SDT because it is a more accurate description of the task (ASHA, 1988). Assessment of SDT can be useful to confirm the validity of pure tone thresholds on the basis of the relationships that have been observed. SDTs reflect hearing abilities primarily in the 250-Hz to 500-Hz region because that is the most intense region in the speech signal to which a patient first responds. Frisina (1962) reported that the SDT was highly correlated with the threshold at 500 Hz in students with significant hearing loss ($r = .84$ to $.98$ across age groups). Average SDT was 2- to 6-dB better than the average threshold at 500 Hz. He advised that if the difference exceeded 10 dB, the validity of either measure should be questioned. However, if the audiogram rises in the higher frequencies, one would expect the SDT to be within ±10 dB of the best threshold.

SDT may be determined by presenting speech in an ascending or descending manner. A descending approach is preferable, but if response validity is questionable, an ascending approach may be used as an exploratory search for the first response to speech. Generally, the level is changed by 20 dB per presentation until a reversal is observed (i.e., no response if descending and a positive response if ascending). Familiar words, nonsense syllables, or connected speech may be presented at each level. When a reversal is noted, the intensity level is also changed in the reverse direction and a bracketing procedure is initiated using 10 dB down, 5 dB up (descending approach) and 10 dB up, 5 dB down (ascending approach). Bracketing around threshold continues until the lowest level is determined at which a response is obtained on half the trials presented.

Discrimination

Despite numerous procedures to evaluate discrimination in the research setting, only one test of true discrimination exists in which the patient is asked to detect a change in auditory information. First developed for children in 1958, then revised in 1973 by Wepman, the Auditory Discrimination Test (ADT) includes 40 pairs of monosyllabic words in two forms. The pairs are presented orally to children ages 5 to 8 years old who are instructed to respond verbally whether the pairs are the same or different. Ten of the 40 pairs are the same, and the remaining word pairs contain phonemes within the same phonetic category. For example, monosyllables with stop consonants were paired with monosyllables with stops to assess discrimination of primarily spectral cues rather than spectral and temporal cues. Performance may be compared with a chart where a "rating scale" value is determined ranging from +2, which indicates "very good development," to −2, which means below the "level of the threshold of adequacy."

Identification

Most of the speech tests routinely used in the audiological test battery assess performance at the identification level. Typically, the patient is asked to repeat nonsense syllables, words, or sentences or to point to pictures in response to standardized stimuli. Speech recognition performance at three intensity levels is of interest: at threshold, at 30- to 40-dB SL, and at 80- to 90-dB HL.

Speech Recognition at Threshold Level

ASHA (1988) recommended a procedure for assessment of SRT that includes presenting spondee words without a carrier phrase. Martin and Weller (1975) found no effect of using a carrier phrase on the SRT. Patients should be familiarized with the test list so that the effects of audibility of the signal are being measured and not familiarity of the vocabulary (Tillman & Jerger, 1959). Testing is begun at a level 30 to 40 dB above the estimated SRT. Words are presented at decrements of 10 dB or increments of 20 dB for correct and incorrect responses, respectively, until a level is reached at which two consecutive words are missed. Intensity level is then increased by 10 dB to begin the threshold determination. Two spondees are presented at each 2 dB decrement until five of six words are repeated incorrectly. Testing may also be done using 5 dB decrements until both words at a given intensity level are missed. Threshold is determined by subtracting the number of correct responses from the starting level and adding a correction factor of 1 dB (2 dB if 5 dB decrements were used) necessary when estimating threshold at the 50% point on the psychometric function with 2 dB steps. Martin et al (1998) reported that approximately 90% of audiologists are using 5 dB decrements and 60% do not use the ASHA-recommended criterion of missing five of six words. Instead they follow an abbreviated procedure shown by Martin and Dowdy (1986) to yield results similar to the ASHA procedure. They recommend presenting one spondee starting at 30 dB HL and at 10 dB decrements thereafter until an incorrect response is obtained. If the response is incorrect or absent at 30 dB HL, increase to 50 dB HL, and use 10 dB increments thereafter until a correct response is obtained. Bracketing techniques require presenting one word at each level by incrementing in 5 dB steps for incorrect responses and decrementing in 10 dB steps for correct responses until three correct responses have been obtained at a given level. Threshold is the lowest level at which a minimum of three correct responses were obtained. The SRT is generally 10- to 12-dB greater than the SDT (Eagan, 1948).

Speech Recognition at Suprathreshold Levels

Tests that have been developed and can be interpreted relative to normative data include the NU6 and PAL PB 50 monosyllabic word lists, the Goldman-Fristoe-Woodcock (GFW) Test of Auditory Discrimination, and the revised SPIN, HINT, and Synthetic Sentence Identification (SSI) sentence lists (see Table 13–4 for references). For comparison with normative data, recorded materials for specific presentation levels must be used as described for each test. When prescribed procedures cannot be used, the modification must be noted, and cautions regarding interpretation should be stated.

PAL PB 50 monosyllabic word lists were created by Eagan (1948) in an attempt to have all the phonetic elements represented in proportions as they exist in English. Although not commonly used clinically (Martin et al, 1978), the 20 lists of 50 words each were used by Yellin et al (1989) with 324 patients. By presenting lists at increasing intensity levels, the maximum percent correct score (PB Max) was determined. Interpretation of the PB Max scores for 25-word, PAL PB 50 lists according to high-frequency PTA (HF-PTA: 1, 2, and 4 kHz) can be made by using tables provided by Yellin et al (1989). For HF-PTAs between 20- and 80-dB HL, the following formula based on the Yellin et al data can be used to determine the lower limit of performance for PAL-50 word lists:

$$\text{Lower limit score} = 89.15 + (\text{HF-PTA})(-1.03)$$

If a word recognition score falls below this limit, it is considered disproportionately low for that degree of hearing loss, and further testing to rule out a retrocochlear pathological condition and an otologic referral are warranted.

PEARL

PB Max is the highest speech recognition score determined on a PI function.

Although normative data are not available for the most-often used speech recognition test, CID W22s (Martin et al, 1998), data provided by Yellin et al (1989) with PAL PB 50 lists may be used for interpretation of CID W-22 scores with limitations. Because the more difficult words were eliminated (resulting in four lists of 50 words each), the scores on the CID W22 lists will generally be higher than those obtained with PAL PB 50 lists (Hirsh et al, 1952). Therefore, if the speech recognition score obtained with W22 words falls below the 95% lower boundary determined for the PAL-50 word lists, it is surely disproportionately low for that degree of hearing loss based on HF-PTA. If the score falls at the 95% confidence limit or above, interpretation is compromised.

In an attempt to improve the phonetic balance of the lists, Tillman and Carhart (1966) developed the NU6 word lists, which also consist of 200 monosyllabic words divided into four phonemically balanced lists. These lists are the second most frequently used material for assessing speech recognition (Martin et al, 1998). Interpretation of PB Max scores obtained using 25-word, NU6 lists, as a function of three-frequency PTA (.5, 1, and 2 kHz) can be done by using Table 5 of Dubno et al (1995). For PTAs between 20- and 72-dB HL, the following formula based on the Dubno et al data can be used to determine the lower limit of performance for NU6 25-word lists:

$$\text{Lower limit score} = 110.05 + (\text{PTA})(-1.24).$$

If a word recognition score falls below this limit, it is considered disproportionately low for that degree of hearing loss.

As described earlier, the SPRINT charts in Figures 13–7 and 13–8 may be used to interpret NU6 scores obtained with 25 and 50 words, respectively. The PB Max scores that are less than the 95% confidence limit are represented by the shaded bar for each PTA value.

Although not traditionally used in the audiological evaluation, the GFW Diagnostic Auditory Discrimination is another test of auditory recognition that is designed for ages 3 to adult, which can be very useful because of the extensive normative data. This test consists of three parts that are administered by audiocassette tape and earphones (Goldman et al, 1974). Part 1 consists of a closed-response task of 100 monosyllabic stimuli, each pictured with a perceptually similar foil. If performance is poor on Part 1, the next two parts are given, which allows for more specific description of sound confusions. Although normative data for the Test of Auditory Discrimination was not obtained in a sound suite at a specified presentation level, the performance levels for normal-hearing patients would allow the clinician to assess the relative effects of reduced absolute and differential sensitivity. If the taped stimuli are presented at a comfortable level for the patient and the score is within two standard deviations of the mean value for that age group, it can be concluded that the patient does not have significant deficits in differential sensitivity. However, if the score is significantly less than that of the normative sample, it may be concluded that the performance was the result of the combined effects of reduced absolute and differential sensitivity. One way to attempt to parcel out these effects would be to conduct the test with amplification that has been adjusted to maximize the AI (Rankovic, 1995).

Three tests of speech recognition using sentence stimuli that have normative data include the SPIN, HINT, and SSI. Bilger et al (1984) developed the revised SPIN test to assess the patient's use of semantic context by comparing final-word recognition scores from high-predictability and low-predictability sentence lists presented with a 12-talker babble competing signal. Stimuli consist of eight lists of 50, five-word to eight-word sentences in which the final word is a monosyllabic noun. Sentences are presented at a fixed signal/babble ratio of +8 dB with the sentences 50- to 55-dB above a patient's threshold for the babble. Norms were developed on 128 persons, ages 19 to 69, with sensorineural hearing loss ranging from mild to severe. A table is provided in the manual with the range of acceptable number correct scores for the high-context sentences as a function of the low-context sentences. One's ability to use the context information was found to be independent of the degree of hearing loss. The 95% confidence limits for the low-predictability and high-predictability sentences are ±0.95 and ±0.68, respectively, which suggests that this test is very sensitive to changes in performance.

The HINT consists of 25 equivalent lists of 10 sentences comprised of four to six words each, that are presented in an adaptive procedure to determine reception thresholds for sentences (RTSs) (Nilsson et al, 1996). Norms were developed for sound field testing with speech always at 0 degrees azimuth and the speech-spectrum noise at 0, 90 or −90 degrees azimuth. Currently, no norms are available for testing under headphones. Speech noise is presented at 65 dB A, while the level of the sentences is decreased or increased if the sentence was repeated correctly or incorrectly, respectively. To use the HINT normative data, the results of the test administered with a particular soundroom, audiometer, and loudspeakers must be compared with the norms collected in a laboratory setting. Results may vary because of differences in room acoustics resulting from size and the reflective surfaces. For adult normal-hearing patients, the mean RTS in quiet is 16.62 dB A and the mean signal/noise ratios are −2.82, −9.07, and −10.42 for RTS in noise at 0, 90, and −90 degrees, respectively. To compare two scores, the 95% confidence limit values are ±1.48, ±1.2 and ±1.42 dB in quiet, noise at 0 degrees, and noise at each side, respectively.

The SSI test was developed to overcome some of the problems with single-word tests, such as the lack of a dynamic signal resembling connected speech, and with sentence tests, such as the influence of nonauditory factors like memory and context. Speaks and Jerger (1965) developed a set of 10, seven-word sentences in which every successive three words are related syntactically but not semantically to be presented in a closed-set format in the presence of a competing single talker. The competing message can be presented ipsilateral to the sentences (SSI-ICM) or contralateral to the sentences (SSI-CCM). Sentences are presented at 50 dB above the PTA or SRT. For SSI-ICM a series of message-to-competition ratios (MCR) beginning at +10 and decreasing until the percent correct identification drops to 20%. Jerger (1973) reported that adults with normal-hearing will achieve 100, 80, 55, and 20% identification on the SSI-ICM with MCRs of 0, −10, −20, and −30 dB, respectively. However, on the SSI-CCM, persons with normal-hearing perform very well with MCRs as high as 40 dB. SSI-CCM has been most useful in differential diagnosis of a retrocochlear pathological condition.

LOUDNESS PERCEPTION

Two common tests of loudness judgments contribute useful information to the differential diagnostic and rehabilitative process. Unusual sensitivity to loud sounds is consistent with recruitment observed with cochlear pathological conditions. Judgments of loudness are also important in hearing aid fitting strategies. For example, one strategy is to amplify speech to the patient's MCL level. A patient's UCL level or LDL must always be considered when fitting amplification so that the output limiting of the hearing aid can be set to a level that allows maximum receipt of the dynamic range of speech without sacrificing maximum comfort.

> ### PITFALL
> **Measuring UCL with running speech will reflect loudness perception primarily in the 500-Hz region, where the most intense energy in the speech signal is contained. Frequency-specific UCL measures, particularly in the region of the hearing loss, may provide more useful diagnostic information.**

MCL and UCL are typically determined with running speech so that the patient judges the loudness of the fluctuating intensities in the speech signal. Presentation usually begins approximately 20 dB above the SRT, and the patient is asked to judge the loudness of the stimuli. Hawkins (1984) suggested a 9-point rating scale to provide the patients help define the ranges of responses they may use. Choices range from "very soft" to "comfortable, but slightly loud" to "painfully loud." At each presentation level, one of the descriptions is selected that best describes the loudness. Hawkins recommends a bracketing procedure using 10 dB steps to increase intensity and 5 dB steps to decrease intensity until the desired loudness level (MCL or UCL) is determined in two of four trials. Cox (1981) has shown that UCLs are typically 3 dB lower on first trial compared with subsequent measures of UCL. Therefore, if a single estimate is obtained, one may consider it a conservative estimate of the patient's true UCL.

SPEECH AUDIOMETRY IN DIFFERENTIAL DIAGNOSIS

An overview of characteristic patterns of speech recognition for words and sentences and expectations for uncomfortable listening levels for patients with conductive, sensorineural, and retrocochlear pathological condition is presented. These patterns are summarized in Table 13–5 by pathological condition and typical speech test. The reader is referred to Figures 13–7 and 13–8 for more specific interpretations of word recognition scores and to Chapter 1 for more discussion of differential diagnosis of retrocochlear pathological conditions.

Normal-Hearing

For persons with normal-hearing, predictable relationships exist among various measures of speech processing as shown in Table 13–5. The SDT should agree with pure tone thresholds at 500 Hz, and SRT should agree with PTA within ±10 dB. For all suprathreshold speech recognition measures, persons with normal-hearing are expected to perform near 100% correct when age-appropriate materials are used. Speech recognition with words and sentences should be relatively equal. The UCL should be approximately 100 dB above the SRT.

Conductive Hearing Loss

Patients with conductive hearing losses perform similarly to normal-hearing persons once the intensity of the signal is increased to overcome the reduction in audibility. Recognition of words and sentences should be near 100%. The UCL will also be about 100 dB above the SRT.

Sensorineural Hearing Loss

Patients with sensorineural hearing loss generally have reduced speech recognition consistent with the degree of loss. Expected performance on NU6 lists is illustrated in Figures 13–7 and 13–8. No significant decline (>20%) exists in speech recognition as intensity level is increased. However, there are characteristic patterns of PB Max and SSI Max depending on the configuration of the hearing loss as outlined in Table 13–5.

TABLE 13–5 Diagnostic significance of speech audiometry*

Hearing Status	SRT	WRS (NU6 Lists)	SRS (SSI)	PB Max versus SSI Max	PI Function	UCL for Speech
Normal hearing	SRT ± 10 dB = PTA	88% or higher on 25-word list presented at 30 dB above SRT	100% at MCR of 0 dB	PB Max = SSI Max	No decline >20% in performance as intensity is increased	UCL – SRT = 80–100 dB
Conductive hearing loss	SRT ± 10 dB = PTA	88% or higher on 25-word list presented at 30 dB above SRT	100% at MCR of 0 dB	PB Max = SSI Max	No decline >20% in performance as intensity is increased	UCL – SRT = 80–100 dB
Cochlear hearing loss	SRT ± 10 dB = PTA	Reduced re: that expected for PTA (Figs. 13–7 and 13–8)	Flat: Reduced by same degree as WRS; Sloping: Reduced by same degree as WRS	Flat: PB Max = SSI Max; Rising: PB Max-SSI Max = 2%; Sloping 2 kHz: PB Max = SSI Max; Sloping 1 kHz: PB Max-SSI Max = –12%; Sloping .5 kHz: PB Max-SSI Max = –20%	No decline >20% in performance as intensity is increased	UCL – SRT = 30–50 dB
Retrocochlear hearing loss	SRT ± 10 dB = PTA	Disproportionately low re: that expected for PTA (Figs. 13–7 and 13–8)	Eighth nerve: Rollover—decline in PI function >20% on affected side; Central: Rollover can be present on side opposite lesion	Eighth nerve: PB Max = SSI Max; Central: PB Max-SSI max >2% in the side opposite the lesion	Eighth nerve: Rollover—decline in PI function >20% on affected side; Central: Rollover can be present on side opposite lesion	UCL – SRT = 80–100 dB
Presbycusis	SRT ± 10 dB = PTA	Disproportionately low re: that expected for PTA (Figs. 13–7 and 13–8)	Reduced usually more than PB Max	PB Max-SSI Max >10%	Rollover: decline in PI function >20%	UCL – SRT = 30–100 dB

*Classifications based on Thornton & Raffin (1978); Dubno et al (1995); Jerger & Jerger (1971); Jerger et al (1968).
NOTE: *SRT*, Speech Recognition Threshold; *PTA*, Pure tone average; *WRS*, Word Recognition Score; *SRS*, Sentence Recognition Score; *MCR*, Message-to-Competition Ratio; *PB Max*, Highest score on phonetically balanced word list; *SSI Max*, Highest score on Synthetic Sentence Identification in the ipsilateral competing condition at 0 dB message/competition ratio; *PI function*, Performance intensity function; *UCL*, Uncomfortable loudness level.

301

Retrocochlear Hearing Loss

Patients with retrocochlear hearing loss have three significant characteristics in their speech performance. Their speech recognition for single words is poorer than that expected on the basis of their PTA (see Figs. 13–7 and 13–8). Recognition performance declines with increased intensity, and a discrepancy exists between recognition of words and sentences. Typical patterns for eighth nerve and central lesions are provided in Table 13–5.

SPEECH AUDIOMETRY FOR SPECIAL AGE GROUPS

Toddlers (2 to 4 Years)

Speech Awareness

Speech audiometry is often administered first in the young pediatric assessment because the toddler is more likely to respond to speech than pure tones (Eagles & Wishik, 1961). Discussion will be divided into two sections, depending on whether the child has imitation skills. The test format will be more informal for the child who is not yet able to repeat words because the vocabulary will be more restricted and individually tailored. Because of the nature of this test, presentation must be live voice, and, if possible, ear-specific responses should be obtained. Insert earphones may be preferable for ear-specific information because of their small size. If earphones are not tolerated, the child should be seated at the calibrated location from the loudspeaker (ASHA, 1991) at zero degrees azimuth.

Often, the first measure for the toddler who cannot yet repeat words is the SDT. Some audiologists prefer to start below threshold calling the child's or caregiver's name with 10 dB increases in intensity until an observable response is obtained. A carrier phrase should be used such as "Where is . . ." or "Show me the . . ." Starting below threshold, presentations should continue until the minimum level is determined at which an observable response was obtained twice.

If conditioned orientation reflex (COR) audiometry procedures can be used (see Chapter 14), the clinician would start with names at a suprathreshold level. Although this would normally be 40 dB HL, if hearing loss is present or suspected, initial stimuli should be presented at 70 dB HL or higher until a response is obtained. When it is determined that the child is conditioned to the task, the level is lowered in 20 dB steps until no response exists, at which time it is raised in 5 dB steps until a response is obtained again. Bracketing then begins where the level is reduced in 10 dB steps and increased in 5 dB steps until the lowest level is determined at which a response is obtained twice. Minimum response levels for speech may be interpreted relative to that reported by Northern and Downs (1978) in Table 13–6.

Speech Recognition at Threshold Levels

A measure of speech recognition would be completed with vocabulary familiar to the child as reported by the caregiver. Most likely this will involve asking the child to point to body parts or get familiar objects or toys using live-voice presentation at a 30- to 40-dB SL. If possible, it is desirable to use spondees, two-syllable words presented with equal stress. Griffing et al (1967) developed the Verbal Auditory Screening for Preschool

TABLE 13–6 Minimum response levels for speech and warbled pure tones

Age (mo)	Speech (dB HL) (SD)	Warbled Pure Tones (dB HL) (SD)
0–1	40–60	78 (6)
1–4	47 (2)	70 (10)
4–7	21 (8)	51 (9)
7–9	15 (7)	45 (15)
9–13	8 (7)	38 (8)
13–16	5 (5)	32 (10)
16–21	5 (1)	25 (10)
21–24	3 (2)	26 (10)

Reported by Northern and Downs (1978).

Children (VASPC), a screening procedure involving determining the SRT on the basis of 12 spondaic words that are pictured on a board. Although the identification of 12 common words, easily recognizable in pictures, was a useful contribution to the pediatric test battery, the VASPC was not found to be a sensitive screening tool (Mencher & McCulloch, 1970; Ritchie & Merklein, 1972).

In some instances when a child cannot be tested with headphones, speech awareness or recognition may be evaluated through the use of the bone-conduction vibrator. Calibration of speech through the bone vibrator should be verified from audiometer manufacturer's documentation. When calibrated properly, high correlations exist between the bone-conducted pure tone average threshold (500, 1000, and 2000 Hz) and bone-conducted speech recognition threshold (Merrell et al, 1973). Comparison of speech processing through the bone vibrator and through the earphones may be necessary to approximate the air-bone gap when pure tone thresholds cannot be obtained.

Speech Recognition at Suprathreshold Levels

As with the SRT procedure, speech recognition at suprathreshold levels must be performed with words within the child's receptive vocabulary. Besides using a closed set of familiar words, such as body parts, toys, objects, or pictures, at least two formal measures are designed for children younger than 4.

Elliott & Katz (1980) designed the Northwestern University Children's Perception of Speech (Nu-Chips) test for preschoolers ages 3 to 5. Four randomizations of a 50-word list are used with two picture books of 50 monochrome plates of four pictures each. Book A is used for forms A and B and book B for C and D. Some of the foils on each page are phonemically similar to the test stimulus. Commercially available monosyllabic word lists are presented by tape at 30- to 40-dB SL with either a male or female talker.

Another test for young children is the Pediatric Speech Intelligibility (PSI) test by Jerger and colleagues (Jerger & Jerger, 1982; Jerger et al, 1980, 1981). This closed-response test for children ages 3 to 6 includes one list of 20 monosyllabic words and two lists of 10 sentences in two syntactic formats ("Show me the rabbit putting on his shoes" and "The rabbit is putting on his shoes"). The child is instructed to choose one of five pictures of animals that corresponds to the stimulus. Unlike the word test, performance on the sentence test varies with receptive language age with format 2 being reserved for children with higher language functioning. The test may be presented with competition using a +4 message/competition ratio (MCR) for the word test and 0-dB MCR for the sentence tests. Jerger and Jerger (1982) reported that the performance intensity functions for the words and sentences in quiet was 8- to 10-dB and for words and sentences in competition was 10- to 12-dB. At a presentation level of 50 dB SPL (30 dB HL), normal-hearing children achieve 100% performance on the words and the sentences in both quiet and in noise.

Children (4 to 12 Years)

Speech Recognition at Threshold Levels

By age 4, children should be able to imitate words and complete a traditional SRT procedure by pointing to familiar pictures. Testing may be performed by live voice to tailor the spondees to the child's vocabulary. Testing should follow the ASHA (1988) recommended procedures or Martin and Dowdy (1986) modification as described earlier.

PEARL

A procedure to use for the occasional child who presents a nonorganic hearing loss is to begin presenting spondees at the intensity level that elicits imitation from the child. For each spondee that is repeated correctly, the intensity is lowered 1 dB. Usually the child is unable to discern that the intensity level is changing and shortly, he or she is responding at a level expected for children with normal hearing. At that point, the child should be congratulated on having excellent hearing and encouraged to maintain the excellent attention to the task.

Speech Recognition at Suprathreshold Levels

As mentioned earlier, the Nu-Chips test is appropriate for children through age 5. A widely used test with children ages 4 to 6 is the Word Intelligibility by Picture Identification (WIPI) (Ross & Lerman, 1970); however, limited normative data are available to assist in interpretation of these scores. Sanderson-Leepa and Rintelmann (1976) presented the WIPI in the sound field to 12 normal-hearing children in each age group 3.5, 5.5, 7.5, and 9.5 years old. At a 32 dB sensation level re: SRT, the mean percent correct was 91.7, 97.3, 98.7, and 99.0, respectively. Standard deviations ranged from 6.26 for the youngest to 1.8 for the oldest. Papso and Blood (1989) also evaluated the WIPI in the sound field with 30 normal-hearing children

from 4 to 5 years old. In quiet, the average percent correct was 94.3 (SD = 4.5) compared with an adult control group who achieved 100%. However, in multitalker noise at a +6 signal/noise (S/N) ratio, the children scored 67.6% (SD = 12.0) and the adults scored 94.9% (SD = 3.5). These data document that children as young as 3.5 years old should be able to perform near 90% (±6%) correct on the WIPI. Furthermore, if the WIPI is administered in the presence of babble (+6 S/N) , one would expect approximately a 30% decline in performance.

For children older than 6, the Phonetically-Balanced Kindergarten (PBK) lists are most often used. Similar to the open-set format used with adults, these lists have vocabulary from the spoken vocabulary of kindergartners (Haskins, 1949). Sanderson-Leepa and Rintelmann (1976) found that normal-hearing preschoolers performed significantly lower than 5- to 6-year-olds verifying the appropriateness of the PBKs for use with kindergartners.

The only auditory processing test with normative data on children with hearing loss is the Test of Auditory Comprehension (TAC). Designed to complement an auditory training curriculum, the TAC includes 10 subjects ranging from awareness to comprehension in background noise. A profile of performance is provided in the areas of discrimination, memory sequencing, and figure-ground perception. Tape-recorded stimuli are presented at a comfortable listening level, and the child responds by selecting the corresponding monochrome picture from a set of three choices. Performance can be interpreted against normative data provided in the manual according to degree of hearing loss from moderate to severe-profound and age from 4 to 17 years.

Clinicians are often seeking a measure of speech recognition in noise for the school-aged child because referrals for suspected auditory processing problems are frequently made at this age. As mentioned earlier, normative data exist for the PSI and WIPI for children up to age 6 listening to speech in noise. Rupp (1980) provided data for recognition of PBK lists presented in white noise at a 0 dB S/N ratio at most comfortable listening levels for children in kindergarten through fifth grade. Performance in the sound field ranged from 34 to 49% correct for kindergartners and fifth graders, respectively.

More recently, the HINT was adapted for use with children ages 6 to 12 (Nilsson et al, 1996). Results from testing 84 children revealed that a more favorable S/N ratio was needed for children to achieve the same performance level as adults. Average differences between children's scores and adult scores are provided in the manual for testing in quiet and with noise at 0 and 90 degrees azimuth. For example, at 0 degrees azimuth, an average adult achieves a reception threshold for sentences (RTS) of −2.82 dB. The average difference for a 7-year-old child is 2.18 dB, so one would

---

PITFALL

Limited materials with normative data are available to assess speech recognition in children. Audiologists must carefully select the most sensitive materials with normative data that are appropriate for the child.

expect an RTS of 0.64 dB ($-2.82 + 2.18 = 0.64$). In other words, the average adult can repeat sentences correctly 50% of the time when the speech is 2.82 dB below the noise, but the average 7-year-old needs the speech to be just above the noise to perform at the same level.

Geriatric Patients (65+ Years)

Evaluation of speech recognition in the elderly involves the same procedures as for adults with two considerations: shorter stimuli may be necessary because of memory difficulties and comparison with normative values will be different to account for the normal reductions in audibility with aging. Clinical experience has shown that the elderly are more successful with monosyllabic stimuli than sentence materials. NU6 lists are appropriate to use with the elderly and can be interpreted according to the Dubno et al (1995) values for disproportionate speech recognition. Of their subject pool, 86% were older than 60 years of age, with the oldest being 82 years of age. If a closed-set response task is needed, the GFW Test of Auditory Discrimination includes normative data up to age 70 years and the GFW Auditory Discrimination Test includes normative data up to age 87 years. These two tests require the patient to choose one of two pictures that corresponds to the stimulus. One advantage of these latter two tests is the sound confusion analysis that may be particularly helpful to assess benefits of an auditory training program or monitor hearing aid adjustment.

CONCLUSIONS

At least three objectives of speech audiometry exist: (1) to determine the effects of hearing loss on absolute and differential sensitivity, (2) to contribute to the differential diagnostic process, and (3) to facilitate the hearing aid fitting process. To accomplish these objectives several decisions regarding the evaluation process must be made, including the level of processing to be assessed, response format, stimuli, presentation mode and level, calibration, procedures, and analysis and interpretation of results. Because these choices may dramatically influence the results, audiologists must have a clear understanding of the options and the resulting information that may be obtained.

When choosing the appropriate procedures for speech audiometry, it is imperative to consider sensitive and valid measures of performance. In addition, there is no benefit to the patient to evaluate speech recognition if performance is not evaluated relative to a normative database. It is no longer acceptable to report that "word recognition was poorer than expected on the basis of pure tone thresholds" without indicating how such a conclusion was reached. Tools such as the Count-the-Dot Audiogram and the SPRINT charts should be readily available for the audiologist's use in the interpretation of test scores. Certainly a need exists for further development of more sensitive assessment procedures with normative data across a wide range of hearing impairments.

Appendix A
Common Abbreviations Used in Speech Audiometry

ADT	Auditory Discrimination Test
AI	Articulation Index
XANSI	American National Standards Institute
ASHA	American Speech, Language, and Hearing Association
CCM	Contralateral Competing Message
CD	Compact Disc
CID	Central Institute for the Deaf
COR	Conditioned Orientation Reflex
dB	Decibel
GFW	Goldman Fristoe Woodcock
HF-PTA	High Frequency Pure Tone Average
HINT	Hearing in Noise Test
HINT-C	Hearing in Noise Test for Children
HL	Hearing Level
ICM	Ipsilateral Competing Message
LDL	Loudness Discomfort Level
MCL	Most Comfortable Level
MCR	Message to Competition Ratio
mo	Months
NU	Northwestern University
Nu-Chips	Northwestern University Children's Perception of Speech
p	Probability
PAL	Psychoacoustics Laboratory
PBmax	Maximum score obtained with a Phonetically Balanced word list

PBK	Phonetically Balanced Kindergarten
PI	Performance Intensity
PSI	Pediatric Speech Intelligibility
PTA	Pure Tone Average
RTS	Reception Threshold for Sentences
S/N	Signal to Noise Ratio
SAT	Speech Awareness Threshold
SD	Standard Deviation
SDS	Speech Discrimination Score
SDT	Speech Detection Threshold
SIR	Speech Intelligibility Rating
SL	Sensation Level
SPIN	Speech Perception in Noise
SPL	Sound Pressure Level
SPRINT	Speech Recognition Interpretation
SRS	Sentence Recognition Score
SRT	Speech Recognition Threshold
SSI	Synthetic Sentence Identification
TAC	Test of Auditory Comprehension
UCL	Uncomfortable Loudness Level
ULL	Uncomfortable Loudness Level
VASPC	Verbal Auditory Screening for Preschool Children
VU	Volume Unit
WDS	Word Discrimination Score
WIPI	Word Intelligibility by Picture Identification
WRS	Word Recognition Score

Appendix B
Homogeneous Spondee Words

Inkwell
Playground
Sidewalk
Railroad
Woodwork

Baseball
Workshop
Doormat
Grandson
Eardrum

Toothbrush
Northwest
Mousetrap
Drawbridge
Padlock

From Young et al (1982).

REFERENCES

AMERICAN NATIONAL STANDARDS INSTITUTE. (1996). American National Standards specifications for audiometers, *ANSI S3.6-1996*. New York: American National Standards Institute.

AMERICAN NATIONAL STANDARDS INSTITUTE. (1998). American National Standards methods for the calculation of the articulation index, *ANSI S3.5-1998*. New York: American National Standards Institute.

AMERICAN SPEECH-LANGUAGE-HEARING ASSOCIATION. (1988). Guidelines for determining threshold level for speech. *ASHA, 30,* 85–89.

AMERICAN SPEECH-LANGUAGE-HEARING ASSOCIATION. (1991). Sound field measurement tutorial. *ASHA, 33,* 25–37.

BENSON, R.C., & HIRSH, I.J. (1953). Some variables in audio spectrometry. *Journal of the Acoustical Society of America, 2,* 449–453.

BESS, F. (1983). Clinical assessment of speech recognition. In: D. Konkle, & W. Rintelmann (Eds.), *Principles of speech audiometry* (pp. 127–201). Baltimore, MD: Academic.

BILGER, S., NUETZEL, J.M., RABINOWITZ, W.M., & RZECZKOWSKI, C. (1984). Standardization of a test of speech perception in noise. *Journal of Speech and Hearing Research, 27,* 32–48.

BILGER, S., & WANG, M. (1976). Consonant confusions in patients with sensori-neural hearing loss. *Journal of Speech and Hearing Research, 19,* 718–740.

BOOTHROYD A., & NITTROUER, S. (1988). Mathematical treatment of context effects in phoneme and word recognition. *Journal of the Acoustical Society of America, 84,* 101–114.

BRANDY, W. T. (1966). Reliability of voice tests of speech discrimination. *Journal of Speech and Hearing Research, 9,* 461–465.

COX, R. (1981). Using LDL to establish hearing aid limited levels. *Hearing Instruments, 32,* 16–20.

COX, R.M., & MCDANIEL, D.M. (1989). Development of the speech intelligibility rating (SIR) test for hearing aid comparisons. *Journal of Speech and Hearing Research, 32,* 347–352.

CRYSTAL, T.H., & HOUSE, A.S. (1990). Articulation rate and the duration of syllables and stress groups in connected speech. *Journal of the Acoustical Society of America, 88,* 101–112.

DIRKS, D., KAMM, D., BOWER, D., & BETSWORTH, A. (1977). Use of performance intensity functions for diagnosis. *Journal of Speech and Hearing Disorders, 27,* 311–322.

DRESCHLER, W.A., & PLOMP, R. (1985). Relations between psychophysical data and speech perception for hearing-impaired subjects. II. *Journal of the Acoustical Society of America, 78,* 1261–1270.

DUBNO, J., & LEVITT, H. (1985). Predicting consonant confusions from acoustic analysis. *Journal of the Acoustical Society of America, 69,* 249–261.

DUBNO J.R., LEE F.S., KLEIN A.J., MATTHEWS L.J., & LAM C.F. (1995). Confidence limits for maximum word-recognition scores. *Journal of Speech and Hearing Research, 38,* 490–502.

DUNN, H.K., & WHITE, S.D. (1940). Statistical measurements on conversational speech. *Journal of the Acoustical Society of America, 11,* 278–288

EAGAN, J. (1948). Articulation testing methods. *Laryngoscope, 58,* 955–991.

EAGLES, E., & WISHIK, S. (1961). A study of hearing in children. *Transactions of the American Academy of Opthalmology and Otology, 65,* 261–282.

EIMAS, P., SIQUELAND, E., & JUSCYZK, P., et al. (1972). Speech perception in infants. *Science, 171,* 303.

ELLIOTT, L., & KATZ, D. (1980). *Development of a new children's test of speech discrimination.* St. Louis: Auditec.

ERBER, N. (1982). *Auditory training.* Washington, DC: The Alexander Graham Bell Association for the Deaf.

FESTEN, J., & PLOMP, R. (1983). Relations between the auditory functions in impaired hearing. *Journal of the Acoustical Society of America, 73,* 652–662.

FLETCHER, S.G. (1970). Acoustic phonetics. In: F.S. Borg, & S.G. Fletcher (Eds.), *The hard of hearing child* (pp. 57–84). New York: Grune & Stratton.

FRENCH, N.R., & STEINBERG, J.C. (1947). Factors governing the intelligibility of speech sounds. *Journal of the Acoustical Society of America, 19,* 90–119.

FRISINA, R. D. (1962). Audiometric evaluation and its relation to habilitation and rehabilitation of the deaf. *American Annals of the Deaf, 107,* 478–481.

GATEHOUSE, S. (1993). Role of perceptual acclimatization in the selection of frequency responses for hearing aids. *Journal of the American Academy of Audiology, 4,* 296–306.

GOLDMAN, R., FRISTOE, M., & WOODCOCK, R. (1974). *G-F-W Diagnostic Auditory Discrimination Test.* Circle Pines, MN: American Guidance Service, Inc.

GRIFFING T.S., SIMONTON K.M., & HEDGECOCK, L.D. (1967). Verbal auditory screening for preschool children. *Transactions of the American Academy of Ophthalmology and Otolaryngology. 71,* 105–11.

HASKINS, H. (1949). *A phonetically balanced test of speech discrimination for children.* Unpublished master's thesis, Evanston, IL: Northwestern University.

HAWKINS, D. (1984). Selection of a critical electroacoustic characteristic: SSPL90. *Hearing Instruments, 35,* 28–32.

HIRSCH, I., DAVIS, H., SILVERMAN, S., REYNOLDS, E. ELDERT, E., & BENSON, R. (1952). Development of materials for speech audiometry. *Journal of Speech and Hearing Disorders, 17,* 321–337.

HOOD, J.D., & POOLE, J.P. (1971). Speech audiometry in conductive and sensorineural hearing loss. *Sound, 5,* 30–38.

HOOD, J.D., & POOLE, J.P. (1980). Influence of the speaker and other factors affecting speech intelligibility. *Audiology, 19,* 434–455.

HUMES, L. (1991). Understanding the speech-understanding problems of the hearing impaired. *Journal of the American Academy of Audiology, 2,* 59–69.

JERGER, J. (1973). Audiological findings in aging. *Annals in Otorhinology and Laryngology, 20,* 115–124.

JERGER, J. & HAYES, D. (1977). Diagnostic speech audiometry. *Archives of Otolaryngology, 103,* 216–222.

JERGER, J., & JERGER, S. (1971). Diagnostic significance of PB word functions. *Archives of Otolaryngology, 93,* 573–580.

JERGER, J., SPEAKS, C., & TRAMMEL, J. (1968). A new approach to speech audiometry. *Journal of Speech and Hearing Disorders, 33,* 318–328.

JERGER, S., & JERGER, J. (1982). Pediatric Speech Intelligibility Test: Performance-intensity characteristics. *Ear and Hearing, 3,* 325–334.

JERGER, S., JERGER, J., & LEWIS, S. (1981). Pediatric Speech Intelligibility Test II. Effect of receptive language age and chronological age. *International Journal of Pediatric Otorhinolaryngology, 3,*101–118.

JERGER, S., LEWIS, S., HAWKINS, J., & JERGER, J. (1980). Pediatric speech intelligibility test. I. Generation of test materials. *International Journal of Pediatric Otorhinolaryngology, 2,* 217–230.

JOHNSON, C., BENSON, P., & SEATON, J. (1997). *Educational audiology handbook.* San Diego: Singular Publishing Group, Inc.

KLATT, D. (1976). Linguistic uses of segmental duration in English: Acoustic and perceptual evidence. *Journal of the Acoustical Society of America, 59,*1208–1221.

KLATT, D. (1980). Software for a cascade/parallel formant synthesizer. *Journal of the Acoustical Society of America, 67,*971–995.

KRYTER, K. (1962). Methods for the calculation and use of the articulation index. *Journal of the Acoustical Society of America, 43,*1689–1697.

LEVITT, H., & RESNICK, S.B. (1978). Speech reception by the hearing impaired: Methods of testing and the development of new tests. *Scandinavian Audiology, 6,*107–130.

MARTIN, F. N., CHAMPLIN, C.A., & CHAMBERS, J.A. (1998). Seventh survey of audiometric practices in the United States. *Journal of the American Academy of Audiology, 9,*95–104.

MARTIN, F.N., & DOWDY, L. K. (1986). A modified spondee threshold procedure. *Journal of Auditory Research, 26,*115–119.

MARTIN, F.N., & WELLER, S.M. (1975). The influence of the carrier phrase on the speech reception threshold. *Journal of Communication Pathology, 7,*39–44.

MENCHER, G.T., & MCCULLOCH, B.F. (1970). Auditory screening of kindergarten children using the VASC. *Journal of Speech and Hearing Disorders, 35,*241–247.

MENDEL, L., & DANHAUER, J. (1997). *Audiologic evaluation and management and speech perception assessment.* San Diego: Singular Publishing Group, Inc.

MERRELL, H.B., & ATKINSON, C.J. (1965). The effect of selected variables on discrimination scores. *Journal of Auditory Research, 5,*285–292.

MERRELL, H.B., WOLFE, D.L., & MCLEMORE, D.C. (1973). Air and bone conducted speech reception thresholds. *Laryngoscope, 83,*1929–1939.

MILLER, G., & NICELY, P. (1955). An analysis of perceptual confusions among some English consonants. *Journal of the Acoustical Society of America, 27,*338–352.

MUELLER, H.G., & KILLION, M.C. (1990). An easy method for calculating the articulation index. *Hearing Journal, 43,*14–17.

NEWMAN, C.W., & SANDRIDGE, S.A. (1998). Benefit from, satisfaction with, and cost-effectiveness of three different hearing aid technologies. *American Journal of Audiology, 7,*115–128.

NILSSON, M., SOLI, S., & GELNETT, D. (1996). *Development and Norming of a Hearing in Noise Test for Children.* House Ear Institute Internal Report.

NILSSON, M. , SOLI, S., & SULLIVAN, J. (1994). Development of the Hearing in Noise Test for the measurement of speech reception threshold in quiet and in noise. *Journal of the Acoustical Society of America, 95,*1085–1099.

NORTHERN, J., & DOWNS, M. (1978). *Hearing in children.* Baltimore: The Williams & Wilkins Company.

OLSEN, W.O., HAWKINS, D., & VAN TASELL, D.J. (1987). Representations of the long-term spectra of speech. *Ear and Hearing, 8,*100S–108S.

OLSEN, W.O., & MATKIN, N. (1979). Speech Audiometry. In: W. Rintelmann (Ed.), *Hearing assessment.* Baltimore, MD: University Park Press.

OLSEN, W.O., VAN TASELL, D.J., & SPEAKS, C.E. (1997). The Carhart Memorial Lecture, American Auditory Society, Salt Lake City, Utah 1996. Phoneme and word recognition for words in isolation and in sentences. *Ear and Hearing, 18,*175–88.

PAPSO, C., & BLOOD, I. (1989). Word recognition skills of children and adults in background noise. *Ear and Hearing, 10,*235–236.

PASCOE, D. (1975). Frequency response of hearing aids and their effects on the speech perception of hearing-impaired subjects. *Annals of Otorhinology and Laryngology, 84,*5–40.

PAVLOVIC, C.V. (1984). Use of the articulation index for assessing residual auditory function in listeners with sensorineural hearing impairment. *Journal of the Acoustical Society of America, 75,*1253–1258.

PAVLOVIC, C.V. (1989). Speech spectrum considerations and speech intelligibility predictions in hearing aid evaluations. *Journal of Speech and Hearing Disorders, 54,*3–8.

PENROD, J. (1994). Speech threshold and word recognition/discrimination testing. In: J. Katz (Ed.), *Handbook of clinical audiology.* Baltimore, MD: Williams & Wilkins.

PICHENY, M., DURLACH, N., & BRAIDA, L. (1989). Speaking clearly for the hard of hearing III: An attempt to determine the contribution of speaking rate to differences in intelligibility between clear and conversational speech. *Journal of Speech and Hearing Research, 32,*600–603.

PICKETT, J. M. (1999). *The acoustics of speech communication, fundamentals, speech perception theory, and technology* (pp. 86–89). Boston, MA: Allyn and Bacon.

RANKOVIC, C.M. (1995). Derivation of frequency-gain for maximizing speech reception. *Journal of Speech and Hearing Research, 38,*913–929.

RITCHIE, B.C., & MERKLEIN, R.A. (1972). An evaluation of the efficiency of the Verbal Auditory Screening Test for Children (VASC). *Journal of Speech and Hearing Research, 15,*280–286.

ROESER, R. (1996). *Audiology desk reference.* New York: Thieme Medical Publishers, Inc.

ROSS, M., & LERMAN, J. (1970). A picture identification test for hearing-impaired children. *Journal of Speech and Hearing Research, 13,*44–53.

RUPP, R. (1980). *Discrimination of PB-K's in Noise (PBKN).* St. Louis: Auditec.

SANDERSON-LEEPA, M.E., & RINTELMANN, W.F. (1976). Articulation functions and test-retest performance of normal hearing children on three speech discrimination tests: WIPI, PBK-50, and NU Auditory Test No. 6. *Journal of Speech and Hearing Disorders, 41,*503–519.

SKINNER, M., KARSTAEDT, M., & MILLER, J. (1982). Amplification bandwidth and speech intelligibility for two listeners with sensori-neural hearing loss. *Audiology, 21,*251–268.

SPEAKS, C., & JERGER, J. (1965). Method for measurement of speech identification. *Journal of Speech and Hearing Research, 8,*185–194.

STACH, B. (1998). Word-recognition testing: Why not do it well? *The Hearing Journal, 51,*10–16.

STELMACHOWICZ, P., JESTEADT, W., GORGA, M., & MOTT, J. *(1985).* Speech perception ability and psychophysical tuning curves in hearing impaired listeners. *Journal of the Acoustical Society of America, 77,*620–627.

Studebaker, G. (1985). A "Rationalized" arcsine transform. *Journal of Speech and Hearing Research, 28,*455–462.

Teder, H. (1993). Compression in the time domain. *American Journal of Audiology. 2,*41–46.

Thibodeau, L.M., & Van Tasell, D.J. (1987). Tone detection and synthetic speech discrimination in band-reject noise by hearing-impaired listeners. *Journal of the Acoustical Society of America. 82,*864–73.

Thornton, A.R., & Raffin, M.J.M. (1978). Speech discrimination scores modified as a binomial variable. *Journal of Speech and Hearing Research, 21,*507–518.

Tillman, T.W., & Carhart, R. (1966). An expanded test for speech discrimination utilizing CNC monosyllabic words. Northwestern University Auditory Test No. 6. *Technical Report No. SAM-TR-66-55.* USAF School of Aerospace Medicine, Brooks Air Force Base, Texas.

Tillman, T.W., & Jerger, J. (1959). Some factors affecting the spondee threshold in normal-hearing subjects. *Journal of Speech and Hearing Research, 2,*141–146.

Trammell, J. (1981). *Test of auditory comprehension.* Portland, OR: Foreworks Publications.

Tyler, R. (1994). The use of speech-perception tests in audiological rehabilitation: current and future research needs. In: J.P. Gagne, & N. Tye-Murray (Eds.), *Research in audiological rehabilitation: Current trends and future directions* (pp. 47–66). Monograph, *Journal of the Academy of Rehabilitative Audiology, 27.*

Tyler, R., Summerfield, A., Wood, E., & Fernandes, M. (1982). Psychoacoustic and phonetic temporal processing in normal and hearing-impaired listeners. In: G. van den Brink, & F. Bilsen (Eds.), *Psychophysical, physiological, and behavioural studies in hearing* (pp. 458–465). Holland: Delft University Press.

Tyler, R., Wood, E., & Fernandes, M. (1982). Frequency resolution and hearing loss. *British Journal of Audiology. 16,*45–63.

Umeda, N. (1975). Vowel duration in American English. *Journal of the Acoustical Society of America, 58,*434–445.

Umeda, N. (1977). Consonant duration in American English. *Journal of the Acoustical Society of America, 61,*846–858.

Van Tasell, D.J. (1986). Auditory perception of speech. In: J. Davis, & E. Hardick (Eds.), *Rehabilitative audiology for children and adults* (pp.13–58). New York: Macmillan Publishing Company.

Van Tasell, D.J., & Crain, T.R. (1992). Noise reduction hearing aids: Release from masking and release from distortion. *Ear and Hearing, 13,*114–121.

Van Tasell, D.J., & Yanz, J.L. (1987). Speech recognition threshold in noise: Effects of hearing loss, frequency response, and speech materials. *Journal of Speech and Hearing Research, 30,*377–386.

Wepman, J.M. (1973). *Auditory discrimination test: Manual of administration, scoring, and interpretation.* Chicago, IL: Language Research Associates.

Yellin, M.W., Jerger J., & Fifer R.C. (1989). Norms for disproportionate loss in speech intelligibility. *Ear and Hearing, 10,*231–234.

Young, L., Dudley, B., & Gunter, M. (1982). Thresholds and psychometric functions of the individual spondaic words. *Journal of Speech and Hearing Research, 25,*586–593.

## Chapter 14

Audiologic Evaluation of Special Populations

Angela G. Shoup and Ross J. Roeser

Outline

Audiologists provide diagnostic assessments for a wide variety of patient populations. For example, in a typical day or week, in addition to evaluating normally developing children and normal adults, an audiologist may provide diagnostic assessment for newborns only hours of age, infants who are days or weeks old, children or adults who are mentally challenged, elderly patients with dementia or even Alzheimer's disease, patients who have had strokes, and patients with pseudohypoacusis* or hyperacusis. This chapter covers the topic of diagnostic tests for patients with special needs, namely, those in special populations. For the purposes of this chapter, patients who require extra consideration or extraordinary means for diagnostic audiological assessment make up "special populations." The following special population areas are covered:

- Infants and young children (0–5 yr)
- The elderly
- The mentally/physically challenged
- Those with dementia
- Those with visual impairment
- Adults with cognitive deficits (aphasia and Alzheimer's disease)
- Those with pseudohypoacusis
- Those with hyperacusis

For each patient having special needs, specific knowledge of the most successful protocols to use and a unique set of clinical skills for successful application of diagnostic tests are required.

CONSIDERATIONS IN EVALUATING SPECIAL POPULATIONS

Each patient entering the audiology clinic should be thought to have special needs. For example, patients with normal-hearing sensitivity at all frequencies and normal word/speech intelligibility in quiet who still report difficulty in adverse listening situations are special. These patients seek help for listening problems in their personal or professional lives that they consider debilitating. Rather than ignoring the patient's complaints after establishing normal performance on standard audiological testing, assessment with central auditory processing tests should be considered (see Chapters 15 and 16). Although these patients do have special problems, many are capable of completing traditional audiological test procedures with little difficulty. However, for other patients the standard audiological test environment and procedures may be unachievable. Skilled clinicians will recognize when changes are needed and modify diagnostic test protocols appropriately within acceptable clinical guidelines.

It is incumbent on all clinicians to view each patient as an individual, making careful behavioral observations,

---

*The term *pseudohypoacusis* is sometimes spelled pseudohypacusis. The more accurate spelling is pseudohypoacusis.

Audiology: Diagnosis. Edited by Roeser, Valente, and Hosford-Dunn. Thieme Medical Publishers, Inc., New York © 2000

asking questions when necessary, and truly listening to responses. Clinician flexibility in the testing session may translate into redesigning the environment for optimum results, changing the order in which tests are completed, and obtaining nontraditional responses during the diagnostic procedures. This approach to the evaluation process is even more important when the patient has multisensory deficits or handicaps in addition to hearing loss. Consideration is given in this chapter to evaluating normally developing patients across the lifespan and patients who present challenges because of existing medical/cognitive/developmental/psychological conditions. It is often difficult for clinicians to develop proficiency in testing patients with special needs, because of the heterogeneity of patient populations and infrequency in encountering these patients in the traditional audiology clinic. For these reasons, it is important for clinicians to have a thorough understanding of the deviations in test protocols that are acceptable and how these acceptable deviations may impact test results and their interpretation.

Cognitive Status

Chronological age is an important factor when selecting appropriate testing techniques for patients with special needs, but mental age and neurological status are also key factors. When assessing infants, gestational age is calculated in order to determine the "corrected" age. This will allow accurate estimation of whether the infant is responding in a developmentally appropriate manner. Physiological responses, such as the auditory brain stem response (ABR), can also be more accurately interpreted when the corrected age is used. Clinicians who have a "feel" for the mental age of the patient can select test procedures and interpret responses more accurately. Finally, even if a patient can function at an age-appropriate mental age in some areas, other impairments may impede the mode of expected responses, indicating the need to modify testing. For example, a patient with cerebral palsy may be capable of understanding traditional adult test procedures, but physical limitations may make traditional response modes unsuitable.

Cross-Check Principle

A test battery approach is especially useful with special populations. When limited information is obtained from traditional tests, converging evidence acquired from a carefully selected test battery helps in developing a "picture" of the patient's auditory capabilities so that appropriate recommendations can be made. Obtaining valid information through this approach was first proposed by Jerger and Hayes (1976) and was labeled the "cross-check principle." This principle takes into consideration that many patients may be able to provide only limited behavioral audiometric information, and the validity may be questioned. When this occurs, clinicians may use another test procedure such as an objective measure (i.e., immittance, otoacoustic emissions, ABR) to verify the behavioral results or to provide additional information about auditory status.

PATIENTS FROM DIVERSE CULTURAL BACKGROUNDS—A GROWING NEED

Although most patients from diverse cultural backgrounds are not mentally or physically challenged, language barriers and differences in rules of interaction may influence testing protocols. When faced with evaluating or treating culturally diverse patients, most clinicians readily consider concerns about difficulty caused by language differences. Appropriate communication with patients from diverse cultural backgrounds requires understanding not only of spoken language but also accepted mannerisms and behaviors (cultural pragmatics). For example, many cultures consider direct eye contact to be rude. Other cultures, such as Hinduism and Islam, consider the head to have special religious significance, so the clinician should seek approval before touching the head in any way (Nellum-Davis, 1993). However, language and basic rules for interaction are not the only barriers to successful service delivery; more important barriers may include a lack of recognition and understanding of varying values and beliefs.

Ethnocentrism has been defined as "an attitude or outlook in which values derived from one's own cultural background are applied to other cultural contexts where different values are operative" (LeVine & Campbell, 1972, p. 1). In many cases, this is taken even a step further when an individual considers all cultural values or beliefs that are different to be wrong or unacceptable. Clinicians can become impatient and develop negative impressions about parents who hesitate to follow through with recommendations for amplification or specific intervention strategies. Before judging too harshly, clinicians should try to learn about and understand the patients' cultural beliefs about healthcare and disease. For example, some Asian-American patients may believe that the hearing loss or other disease or disorder is due to a curse or a gift from God (Cheng, 1993). Many cultures, including American Indians and Hispanics, may believe in folk remedies or religious ceremonies for treatment and be hesitant to pursue "Western medicine."

PITFALL

Although in many cases the patient will have a friend or family member with him who speaks English as well as the patient's language, the use of informal interpreters such as family or friends is generally discouraged for many reasons. First, when an acquaintance of the patient serves as interpreter, the patient's privacy may be violated. Furthermore, the clinician cannot verify the competence of an informal interpreter. Finally, when a child is used the resulting "role reversal" may "jeopardize traditional family values" by undermining "parental respect and authority" (Smart & Smart, 1995).

When a non–English speaking patient enters the clinic for diagnostic assessment, the issue of procuring the services of a language interpreter should be considered. The rules for communicating through a language interpreter are the same as for when a sign-language interpreter is needed for hearing-impaired patients. Clinicians should remember to speak to the patient—not the interpreter, pause after statements to allow the interpreter to present the information to the patient, and allow the patient time to ask questions.

INFANTS AND YOUNG CHILDREN (0-5 YR)

By far, the largest group of special needs patients seen by audiologists are neonates, infants, and young children. The topic of neonatal hearing screening, diagnostic assessment, and follow-up is covered in Chapter 22. This section covers diagnostic assessment of infants and young children.

Test environment and test stimuli are two important factors in assessing infants and young children. Moreover, test protocols are determined on the basis of the chronological/mental age of the child, with the procedures falling within the following categories: 0 to 6 months, 6 to 24 months, and 2 to 5 years. The following sections discuss diagnostic procedures with consideration to the above factors.

Test Environment

Audiological test environments for infants and young children must meet the same criteria as for adults. These include adequate lighting, ventilation, and ambient noise levels that meet ANSI standards (ANSI, 1991). In addition, when designing an audiological test environment for infants and young children, special attention must be paid to safety. Furniture details, such as rounded edges rather than sharp corners and chairs that are "child height" to avoid having the child sit in a caregiver's lap during testing, should be used. Speakers mounted securely will prevent accidental displacement by a playful child. A nonthreatening environment is the foremost concern when selecting furniture and decorations for testing young children.

SPECIAL CONSIDERATON

Brightly colored chairs and tables, and child-friendly wall hangings are more inviting to a child than a dark, formal test room. Readily recognizable popular children's characters can help make a child feel less afraid of the test situation.

Test rooms will need to be larger for testing children than those used for testing adults only. The sound room should be large enough to accommodate not only a chair for the caregiver to hold the child but also a pediatric table and chairs for conducting play audiometry. Flexibility is important; thus the ability to arrange the testing booth for procedures with the clinician in or out of the room is required.

Test Stimuli

Each test procedure has a choice of stimuli, which may include warbled pure tones; speech; filtered speech; white,

---

PEARL

For difficult-to-test patients it is helpful to have immittance and otoacoustic emission equipment available in the sound room so that the test order can be modified quickly. Once the child is comfortable in a specific test environment, time can be saved and the possibility of acquiring more complete information can be enhanced if the child is not moved to a different location.

---

narrow band or speech noise; or environmental sounds. Obviously, for frequency specificity, warbled pure tones are preferable. However, for some patients, obtaining valid responses to pure tones is not achievable, and the clinician must use other types of stimuli that will be successful in evoking a response from the infant.

The auditory behavior index (ABI) in Table 14–1 can be used as a simple guideline that summarizes development of auditory behavior from birth to 24 months. It should be noted that the minimal response levels improve with age. Between 0 and 6 weeks of age speech stimuli in the range of 40- to 60-dB are required to elicit gross behavioral responses, but at 21 to 24 months sound localization can be seen at intensities as low as 3- to 5-dB HL. Table 14–1 also shows that the type of stimuli needed to elicit a response will vary depending on the developmental level of the infant or toddler. More common types of stimuli used are noisemakers, warbled pure tones, and speech. It is not surprising that responses to speech stimuli are consistently at lower intensities than any other types of stimuli.

PEARL

The ABI may also be useful in identifying infants at risk for developmental delay (Northern & Downs, 1984). Because the ABI provides developmentally appropriate responses to sound, the type of response observed may be used as an indication of the child's physiological or cognitive status.

Although some general information can be inferred when using stimuli other than pure tones, caution must be used in interpretation. For example, when narrow band noise is used, the spectral characteristics must be known. Some audiometers produce narrow band noises that have very wide filter skirts, which may provide spurious data when precipitous hearing losses are found, usually in the high frequencies. In addition, the type of stimulus used should be clearly noted on the audiogram and the limitations on interpretation of stimuli that are not frequency specific should be stressed. Because other professionals may not be aware of the importance of frequency-specific information, it is the responsibility of the audiologist to ensure that clinical data are presented properly for interpretation. For example, some physicians may assume

TABLE 14–1 Auditory behavior index for infants: stimulus and level of response

Age	Noisemakers (approx. dB SPL)	Warbled Pure Tones (dB HL)	Speech (db HL)	Expected Response
0–6 wk	50–70	78	40–60	Eye widening, eye blink, stirring or arousal from sleep, startle
6 wk–4 mo	50–60	70	47	Eye widening, eye shift, eye blinking, quieting, beginning rudimentary head turn by 4 mo
4–7 mo	40–50	51	21	Head turn on lateral plane toward sound; listening attitude
7–9 mo	30–40	45	15	Direct localization of sounds to side, indirectly below ear level
9–13 mo	25–35	38	8	Direct localization of sounds on side, directly below ear level, indirectly above ear level
13–16 mo	25–30	32	5	Direct localization of sound on side, above and below
16–21 mo	25	25	5	Direct localization of sound on side, above and below
21–24 mo	25	26	3	Direct localization of sound on side, above and below

Adapted from Northern and Downs (1984).

no reason exists for concern about hearing impairment if a child responds to speech within normal limits. Whenever the only data available are a speech threshold (SRT or SAT), it should be made clear that information is not sufficient to rule out a significant hearing loss. Speech awareness thresholds (SATs) can be obtained at normal levels for a child with severe or even profound hearing loss above 500 Hz.

When reporting test results in pediatric patients, a distinction exists between threshold and minimal response level. Because of developmental improvement in responses to sound (see Table 14–1), the term *minimal response level* was recommended by Matkin (1977) for describing audiological test results in young children. At an early age, the softest level to which an infant responds may not, in fact, be the infant's threshold. Attention, motivation, and other factors influence when an infant chooses to respond and impact test results.

SPECIAL CONSIDERATION

When testing infants and young children, speech stimuli should be presented initially because the likelihood of a response is greater. When using pure tones, 500 and 2000 Hz are presented first so that if the child habituates, information is available about threshold sensitivity in the low-frequency and high-frequency speech range.

Order of stimulus presentation is determined by the child's responsiveness. Children usually respond more readily to speech stimuli. Consequently, when evaluating infants and young children, speech is used as the initial stimulus in testing to obtain a general idea of auditory sensitivity. It is usually used first when conditioning a child for a specific type of response.

Quite often a child may not participate for a complete audiometric examination. For this reason, once speech testing is finished, high-frequency (2000 Hz) and low-frequency (500 Hz) stimuli are presented so that responses in the speech range are confirmed. If the child is willing to continue with testing, other frequencies can then be evaluated. Similarly, if the child will wear earphones, then ear-specific responses can be obtained. With this hierarchical approach, if the child becomes uncooperative, sensitivity for speech and some ear-specific data is available, depending on the amount of data collected.

0 to 6 Months

Appropriate audiological evaluation of the very young infant has become increasingly important with the advent of universal newborn hearing screening programs. In the past, infants would be evaluated over a period of time, often delaying recommendations for habilitation of hearing loss until the infant could be fully assessed with traditional behavioral measures. This is no longer an acceptable practice. In 1993 the NIH consensus statement on early identification of hearing impairment in infants and young children recommended that all newborns be screened for hearing impairment to initiate early intervention as soon as possible. Early identification of hearing impairment and subsequent early intervention is of great importance in alleviating developmental delays accompanying such a handicapping condition. Studies have shown that the first 2 years of life are critical for language development and communication skills. Children who do not receive intervention within the first 2 years are less likely to overcome associated delays than those who have received intervention (Dennis, 1973; Greenstein et al, 1976; Lach et al, 1970; Ling, 1971).

Recent data reported by Robinshaw (1995) have shown that severely and profoundly hearing-impaired infants identified and subsequently amplified by 6 months of age acquire vocal communicative and linguistic skills at an age comparable to, or more typical of, their normal-hearing peers than infants identified later. Robinshaw concluded that reduced auditory stimulation for periods of only 3 to 6 months can delay the normal course of language acquisition.

Apuzzo and Yoshinaga-Itano (1995) reported that infants with hearing loss who were identified and provided with amplification/intervention before the age of 6 months performed at age level on language tasks at 40 months of age. However, infants who were identified and received remediation after 12 months of age were not. In a more recent study Yoshinaga-Itano et al (1998) evaluated factors including the degree of hearing loss, cognitive ability, and socioeconomic status as related to the contribution of time of identification and intervention in hearing-impaired children. They found that regardless of degree of hearing loss or socioeconomic status, infants who were identified as hearing-impaired before 6 months of age had better expressive and receptive language abilities than those identified later. This was true regardless of normal or delayed cognitive developmental status. The language abilities of early identified hearing-impaired children, regardless of degree of hearing loss, were more closely related to overall cognitive ability than for the later identified children. On the basis of such data, it has been recommended that amplification and early intervention be initiated before 6 months of age.

In evaluating pediatric patients, knowledge and understanding of auditory and other areas of development are important. Other areas of development to be evaluated include gross motor, fine motor, self-help, and social skills. Not only can this information facilitate interacting with the child and selecting appropriate tests, but the clinician can also be alerted to possible concerns that may require referral to another professional.

A clear understanding of appropriate age-specific behaviors can be obtained from subjective observation, and the parent or caregiver. Questions should be asked about auditory behavior and general development either through a case history or asking the parent to complete a simple questionnaire or checklist. Table 14–2 provides an example of a parent checklist that can be helpful in obtaining information about a child's auditory behaviors.

Diagnostic Testing

Selection of the appropriate test procedure depends on the developmental age. Table 14–3 summarizes test procedures for evaluating infants and children. Many of these procedures also assess auditory sensitivity in developmentally delayed older patients. Information about technique, appropriate developmental age, and advantages or disadvantages of each procedure is shown in Table 14–3.

TABLE 14–2 Parent checklist of auditory behavior

Age (mo)	Yes	No	Auditory Development
0–3			Does your baby quiet for a moment when you talk to him/her?
			Does your baby act startled or stop moving for a moment when there are sudden loud noises?
4–6			Does your baby turn his/her eyes or head to the sound of your voice if he/she can't see you?
			Does your baby smile or stop crying when you or someone else he/she knows speaks?
7–9			Does your baby stop and pay attention when you say "no" or call his/her name?
			Does your baby move his/her head around to try to find out where a new sound is coming from?
			Does your baby make strings of sounds ("ba ba ba, da da da")?
10–15			Does your baby give you toys or other objects (bottle) when you ask, without your having to use a gesture (holding out your hand or pointing)?
			Does your baby point to familiar objects if you ask ("dog," "light")?
16–24			Does your child use his/her voice most of the time to get what he/she wants or to communicate with you?
			Can your child go get familiar objects that are kept in a regular place if you ask him/her ("Get your shoes.")
25–36			Does your child answer different kinds of questions ("when . . . ," "who . . . ," "what . . . ")?
			Does your child notice different sounds (telephone ringing, shouting, doorbell)?

From the Program for Amplification of Children in Texas, Texas Department of Health, Austin, Texas (with permission).

TABLE 14–3 Summary of audiological evaluation procedures for infants and young children

Test	Technique	Developmental Age Range	Advantages	Disadvantages
Behavioral Observation Audiometry (BOA)	*Conditioning:* None *Reinforcement:* None	0–6 mo	No specialized equipment needed. Can be used with children who cannot be conditioned.	Rapid habituation. Only sensitive to patients with severe to profound hearing losses. Not sensitive to unilateral hearing loss. Large intersubject and intrasubject variability.
Conditioned Orienting Response (COR)/ Visual Reinforcement Audiometry (VRA)	*Conditioning:* Head turn *Reinforcement:* Lighted/animated toy and social	6–30 mo	Can present stimuli through speakers, earphones, or bone oscillator. Less intersubject and intrasubject variability. Can obtain minimal response to levels close threshold. Sensitive to even mild hearing losses.	Some infants cannot be conditioned until about 12 mo of age. Many infants will not tolerate earphones or will not turn their heads with earphones on. Specialized equipment is required.
Tangible Reinforcement Operant Conditioning Audiometry (TROCA)	*Conditioning:* Press button/lever *Reinforcement:* Candy, cereal, small toys, etc.	30 mo–4 yr	Accurate thresholds can reliably be obtained. Stimuli can be presented through speakers, earphones, or bone oscillators.	May require numerous sessions. Patient habituates when satiated by reinforcer. Reinforcers may not be appropriate/safe.
Conditioned Play Audiometry (CPA)	*Conditioning:* Play activity *Reinforcement:* Play activity and social May also use visual reinforcement	30 mo–4 yr	Accurate thresholds can be reliably obtained. Can be accomplished with traditional equipment. Stimuli can be presented through speakers, earphones, or the bone oscillator.	May have to change activities many times to keep child's interest. Child may need to be reconditioned when activities change.

Auditory sensitivity has traditionally been difficult to assess behaviorally in newborns. Research in older infants (6 to 18 months) suggests that behavioral thresholds, or minimal response levels, are 20- to 40-dB higher than adults. However, results obtained by Olsho and colleagues (1987, 1988) with the observer-based psychoacoustic procedure (a carefully controlled type of behavioral observation audiometry) with 3, 6-, and 12-month-old infants indicate that the auditory sensitivity of infants is not as decreased as previously reported. They also suggest that the extent of the reported decreased auditory sensitivity does not correspond to physiological assessment of the infant auditory system (Werner et al, 1993).

Behavioral Observation Audiometry

The sensitivity of behavioral observation audiometry (BOA) is low and will usually only identify infants with a severe-to-profound hearing loss (Downs, 1978). Infants do not perform reliably in a conditioned head-turn procedure until at least 5 months of age (Moore & Wilson, 1978). Once an infant reaches this stage, visual reinforcement audiometry (VRA) may be used. However, infants who are developmentally delayed or are premature may be unable to complete such an assessment until much later (Moore et al, 1992). Older children can be evaluated with conditioned play audiometry (CPA) (Table 14-3). The intersubject and intrasubject variability for VRA and CPA is much better than for BOA.

BOA uses various types of sounds to elicit generalized responses. Newborn hearing screening programs once used a form of BOA using loud stimuli (90 dB SPL) presented to sleeping babies (Downs, 1978). A requirement was that the baby be completely still at least 15 seconds before stimulus presentation. Any generalized body movement after sound presentation (movement of more than one limb or some eye movement) was counted as a response. Two independent observers had to agree on the presence of a response, and it had to be repeatable. Other behavioral observation techniques include the use of noisemakers of various frequencies and intensities. Although noisemakers are useful for obtaining a general idea of auditory responsiveness, they lack frequency specificity and control of intensity.

BOA can also be accomplished with an audiometer. For this type of evaluation, the infant is positioned in sound field between two speakers. The infant may be held in the caregiver's lap with a second audiologist positioned closely to observe changes in behavior. Test stimuli are presented through loudspeakers beginning at 0 dB and ascending until a response is observed. Behavior changes may include an increase or decrease in sucking on a pacifier, eye movement, and body movement. This response must be repeated, and the evaluation also includes elicitation of a startle reflex. No reinforcement is used and, unfortunately, the response rapidly habituates. Advantages of BOA include the lack of need for specialized equipment and the time required for the evaluation is minimal. A step-by-step procedure for BOA is as follows:

1. The child is seated between two speakers, preferably in a calibrated sound-treated room. If children will not separate from their parent(s), they may sit on either parent's lap. The parent(s) are instructed not to prompt the child by their own movement. It is preferable for the child to sit alone in a small chair or high chair to restrict excessive movement.

2. To keep the test room quiet, conversation and ambient noises should be at a minimum. The child is distracted by looking at pictures or playing with quiet toys. The audiologist with the child directs the child's activity.

3. Stimuli (speech, warbled tones, or narrow band noise) are presented first at 0 dB HL. If no response (behavioral change) is observed, the intensity is increased in 10 dB steps until a response is observed. This procedure is repeated

until two to three reliable responses are observed. When using tonal stimuli, 500 Hz and 2000 Hz are tested first. If the child does not fatigue, 1000 Hz and 4000 Hz are tested.

4. Behavioral changes include head turning or localization, initiating activity or cessation of activity, eye widening or blinking, increased or decreased sucking, increased respiration, verbalization, or searching. Time intervals between stimulus presentation should be varied to avoid patterning. It is important to observe the child between stimuli to determine how often the behavior occurs without stimulus presentation. If it is uncertain that the child is responding, the intensity should be increased and the behavior should be more pronounced if the child is responding.

5. To avoid fatigue, testing should proceed as rapidly as possible. If no responses are observed at low intensities, an intense stimulus should be presented to elicit a startle response.

Unfortunately, with BOA the audiometric information obtained is limited. Because the stimuli are presented through speakers, responses provide insight into the status of the better ear only. In addition, a wide range of behaviors are accepted as "responses" and likely are obtained using a wide range of intensities, even in normal-hearing infants. Consequently, intersubject and intrasubject variability of BOA is high (Thompson & Wilson, 1984). Such variation may be due to differences in rate of development among infants. Examiner bias can introduce error because of the subjective nature of judging the presence or absence of a response. As stated earlier, the major limitation of BOA is that the minimal response levels are usually suprathreshold, and it is infants with severe-to-profound hearing loss who are identified with BOA. The procedure is subjective and the test/retest variability is high.

6 to 24 Months

Visual Reinforcement Audiometry and Conditioned Orientation Reflex

Infants between 4 and 7 months will begin to turn their heads (localize) on a lateral plane in response to sound (see Table 14–1). When developed, this skill can become part of a protocol to obtain more reliable behavioral test procedures with infants. Two audiometric tests that rely on the localization response are (VRA) and conditioned orientation reflex (COR) audiometry. VRA requires the infant to respond with a head turn toward a sound source. These head turns are then reinforced by presenting an attractive three-dimensional animated toy so that the child can see it. Only one sound source is required for VRA, but two are needed for COR.

To respond successfully for COR, the infant must hear the stimulus, localize the source, and make a head turn in the correct direction. Learning to respond to the appropriate speaker may be especially difficult for infants with middle ear disease and unilateral hearing loss.

Some special equipment is needed for VRA and COR testing. For VRA, the sound room must have at least one speaker for sound field presentation of test stimuli. For COR, the sound room has to be designed with two speakers, usually placed at 90 and 270 degrees (Hayes & Northern, 1996). To provide visual reinforcement, animated toys are mounted on

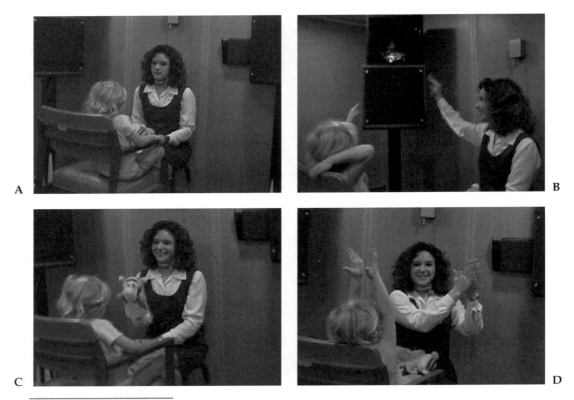

Figure 14–1   Example of COR/VRA being carried out in a sound field (see text for explanation).

top of the speakers (Fig. 14–1A). Ideally, boxes with dark Plexiglas covers are placed over the toys so that the toys are invisible until lighted. A control switch is available to light the box and provide reinforcement when the child localizes the sound to the speaker.

A step-by-step procedure for COR is as follows:

1. A sound field test room is set up with a darkened box placed on each speaker (Fig. 13-1A). In the boxes are animated toys that can be illuminated by the audiologist by activating a switch (Fig. 14–1B).

2. The child is seated alone in a chair, high chair or on a parent's lap between the two speakers. The child's attention is distracted by looking at pictures or playing with a quiet toy (Fig. 14–1C).

3. An auditory stimulus (speech, warbled pure tone, or narrow band noise) is presented at approximately 70 dB above the child's expected threshold and the box containing the toy is illuminated. If the child localizes the toy visually, he or she is reinforced by the audiologist in the sound room by praise (Fig. 14–1D). This conditioning continues and the auditory stimuli are alternated between speakers, with the auditory and visual stimuli presented simultaneously for a period of 3 to 4 seconds.

4. Once the child is conditioned, the auditory stimuli are presented without visual reinforcement. The illuminated toy in the box is activated only as a reward to the child when a response is observed. This procedure is continued,

decreasing the intensity of the auditory stimuli until the child does not respond and the minimal response level is obtained.

Appropriate positioning of the infant in the sound room is critical for VRA/COR to be conducted properly. Calibration of the sound presented from the speakers is affected by position in the room. The infant must be seated between the two speakers as close to the point of calibration as possible. Providing earplugs for the parent or caregiver helps eliminate unwanted participation in the test at low intensities and protects their ears at high intensities when eliciting startle responses. An option for cueing is to place earphones on the caregiver and present a low-level masking noise during the test session.

Two clinicians are preferred for standard VRA/COR testing: one audiologist remains in the sound room with the child and one in the control room at the audiometer. Communication between examiners during testing is imperative and can be accomplished through a microphone/earphone talk-forward system between the two rooms. The bone oscillator can also be placed on the clinician inside the test room, and communication between the two audiologists can take place by presenting speech through the bone oscillator.

The audiologist working with the child in the test room has the responsibility for conditioning the infant to respond to the signal; controlling the child's attention by providing distraction to keep the child looking at midline between trials; indicating when a response has occurred; and offering social reinforcement as needed. The audiologist in the booth can indicate when the infant has responded with a handheld signaling switch.

PEARL

When two audiologists are not available for testing young children with behavioral measures, the child's caregiver or a volunteer can be the observer in the sound room.

When two audiologists are not available, it is possible to carry out COR/VRA by using the child's caregiver or a volunteer in the sound room to control attention and observe the child. This modification requires a short training session before testing is carried out, reminding the observer to be careful not to inadvertently give the child any cues.

Results obtained with VRA and COR are more reliable than with BOA due to less intersubject and intrasubject variability. As a result, comparison of individual test results can be made to normative clinical data.

Some of the disadvantages of VRA and COR include the need for specialized equipment (i.e., speaker configuration and reinforcement/centering toys), two examiners (preferably audiologists) are required, and examiner bias is not eliminated. Parents usually hold the infants during VRA and COR and they may cue them to respond. Because VRA and COR are usually conducted in sound field, ear-specific information is not obtained with traditional methods; results will reflect hearing sensitivity of the better ear when differences exist. Some children have "neck freeze" develop when earphones are set in place. These children will not turn their heads to the sound until the earphones are removed. With many children, however, successful ear-specific testing with VRA/COR can be accomplished with the use of insert earphones. The use of insert earphones can also be advantageous in avoiding collapsed earcanals during testing. The benefit of having an audiologist in the sound room adds confidence to test results, although not all clinics can afford the cost of this luxury.

2 to 5 Years

Conditioned Play Audiometry

Conditioned play audiometry (CPA) is the method of choice for children from approximately 30 months to 5 years of age. From approximately 25 months to 30 months, infants are often more difficult to test. They habituate rapidly to VRA and typically are not yet ready to participate in CPA. Clinicians must be flexible and patient when attempting to obtain valid information about auditory sensitivity in this age group.

CPA involves conditioning children to engage in some activity whenever they perceive a sound. Often, the tasks are organized in a hierarchical fashion from simple to complex. This enables the child to be conditioned with a fairly simple task, and then increase task difficulty as the child becomes restless or bored. For example, the audiologist may first condition the child to place blocks in a bucket until interest is lost. Then, the task can be changed to a more difficult one, such as stacking rings on a stick. Perhaps after this, the task may

change to placing pegs in holes on a board or other increasingly more interesting/difficult games. When selecting these games, the composition of the game pieces are an important consideration. The pieces need to be the appropriate size for a child to manipulate easily and also not too visually interesting. Testing becomes more difficult and lengthy if the child spends excessive time inspecting attractive objects.

Part of the condition for CPA requires holding the child's hand to assist in conditioning (such as placing or throwing the block in the bucket) as soon as the sound is presented. Assistance stops once the child begins responding independently. A step-by-step procedure is as follows:

1. With the help of the audiologist, the child holds an object, such as a block close to, but not touching, his or her ear (Fig. 14–2A).
2. An auditory stimulus that is known to be above the child's threshold is presented, and the audiologist directs the child's hand to make a response, such as dropping an object (a block) in a container (a bucket; Fig. 14–2B). Initially, the stimulus can be a high-intensity pure tone delivered from the headset of a portable audiometer placed on a table near the child. Reinforcement through praise is given once the child performs the response.
3. The conditioning continues until the child performs the behavior (dropping the block in the bucket) on his or her own.
4. Earphones are then placed on the child and testing proceeds with 500 Hz and 2000 Hz first, then 1000 Hz and 4000 Hz for each ear (Fig. 14–2C).

It may be difficult to condition some children to sound. If this is the case, the child may first be conditioned to a stimulus in another sensory modality. Thorne (1967) suggested presenting a somatosensory stimulus, such as having the child hold the bone vibrator in one hand and a block in the other with the two objects touching. When a 500 Hz stimulus is presented through a bone oscillator at the limits of the equipment, the child will feel the vibration with his or her hand. The child is then taught to drop the block in the bucket each time this sensation occurs (Fig. 14–3A). After the child begins responding consistently, the bone vibrator is transferred to the mastoid and the child is conditioned to drop the block in response to the auditory stimulus (Fig. 14–3B). Finally, earphones are placed on the child and responses are obtained to pure tone air-conducted stimuli (Fig. 14–3C).

A similar procedure called play audiometry reinforcement using a flashlight (PARF) is easily accomplished in the traditional setting with a flashlight or otoscope (Roeser & Northern, 1981). For PARF, the child is given an object, such as plastic block, and a flashlight or otoscope is held next to it (Fig. 14–4A). Each time the light is turned on for a second or two the child is conditioned to drop the block in the bucket by holding his or her hand and directing it to the bucket (Fig. 14–4B). Once the child is able to carry out the task with the light, earphones are placed on a table and a 1000-Hz stimulus is presented at a high intensity (Fig. 14–4C). The child is then reconditioned to provide the appropriate response to the sound. Finally, earphones are placed on the child and testing with pure tones is carried out (Fig. 14–4D).

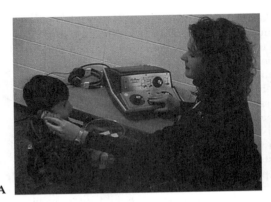

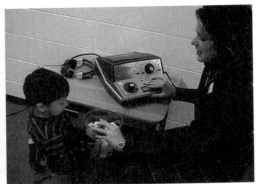

B

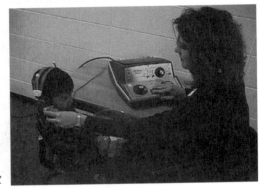

A

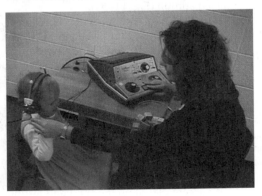

C

Figure 14–2 **(A–C)** CPA is carried out by conditioning the child to perform a motor task, such as dropping a block in a bucket, when the auditory stimuli are perceived. Note that the audiometer is located outside the child's peripheral vision (see text for explanation).

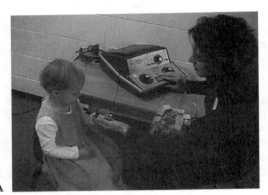

A

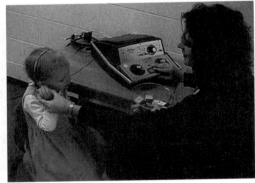

B

C

Figure 14–3 **(A–C)** Tactile stimulation using a low-frequency (250 or 500 Hz) bone-conducted stimulus at high intensities can assist in conditioning a child during CPA (see text for explanation).

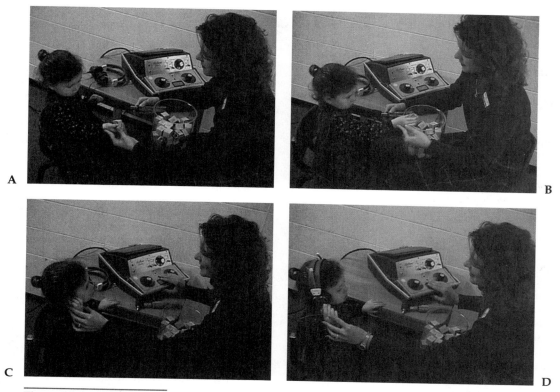

Figure 14–4   PARF is carried out by having the child initially respond to a visual stimulus (flashlight or otoscope light; **A,B**). After the child is conditioned to the visual stimulus, conditioning to an auditory stimulus is attempted **(C,D)**.

Use of visual and tactile stimuli for CPA is beneficial because they are more concrete than auditory stimuli and children will condition more readily when they are used. This allows the examiner to determine whether the child can be conditioned to the tasks involved in CPA. If a child can be conditioned to respond to light or tactile stimuli but cannot be conditioned to an auditory stimulus, hearing loss is probable.

Tangible Reinforcement Operant Conditioning Audiometry

Tangible reinforcement operant conditioning audiometry (TROCA) has also been recommended for use with children from 3 to 5 years of age and for use with developmentally disabled patients. TROCA has some similarities to CPA, but the primary reinforcement is automatically given when the child makes a correct response. The reinforcer is one desired by the child, often in the form of food, such as cereal or candy.

TROCA is rarely used in the traditional audiological clinic for a variety of reasons. A primary disadvantage is that numerous short test sessions are required, during which time the child is conditioned. Most clinical situations do not afford the luxury of this type of conditioning, and test results are delayed, often for weeks or even months, while the child is conditioned. Edible reinforcers can contain sugar that will increase hyperactive behavior. To avoid these difficulties,

some audiologists have used small toys or coins as reinforcers. However, small toys or coins may inadvertently be swallowed by the child.

CONTROVERSIAL POINT

TROCA is a viable behavioral procedure for obtaining reliable audiometric results with young children and other special populations. However, this procedure is rarely used in the traditional audiology clinic because numerous short sessions, during which time the child is conditioned, are required.

Speech Thresholds

Whereas a speech awareness threshold is often the only response to speech in very young infants, speech recognition thresholds can be evaluated for older infants and children. A child can be conditioned to point to objects (baseball, cowboy, hotdog, etc.) or pictures if the child is too shy to speak or if articulation is unclear. If children are unfamiliar with the objects or pictures that are available, they can be instructed to point to body parts.

Word Intelligibility

Older children can complete word intelligibility testing. Tests that have been developed specifically for use in testing young children include the Northwestern University Children's Perception of Speech (NuCHIPS) (Elliott & Katz, 1980) and the Word Intelligibility by Picture Identification test (WIPI) (Ross & Lerman, 1970). Recommended for testing children as young as 3 years, the NuCHIPS consists of four alternative forced-choice black-and-white pictures in a book (Northern & Downs, 1984). The WIPI is appropriate for use with children from 4 to 5 years of age and has six multicolor foils from which to choose. Word intelligibility in older children with good articulation may be evaluated with the phonetically-balanced kindergarten (PBK-50) word list (Haskins, 1949).

Physiological Tests

Because responses obtained from behavioral tests with infants and children are often not reliable, objective physiological evaluations have gained popularity. Click-evoked ABRs are not frequency specific, and as a result, tone burst protocols are becoming more widely used. Although differences exist between adult and infant ABRs, thresholds can be obtained at similar intensity levels. Differences in ABR and behavioral thresholds are believed to be due to a combination of sensory and nonsensory factors. Nonsensory factors influencing behavioral thresholds include attention, arousal, and motivation. Werner et al (1993) found that sensory factors could account for 25% of the variance between behavioral tests and ABRs at 3 months of age. The remaining variance was attributed to nonsensory factors and possibly central nervous system maturation above the level of the brain stem.

Otoacoustic emissions offer a quick means of verifying the integrity of the inner ear when middle ear function is normal, thereby adding power to the infant and child test battery. Not only can otoacoustic emissions be obtained in newborns, but they are also more robust than in adults (Bonfils et al, 1992; Kok et al, 1993). Distortion-product otoacoustic emissions in newborns are qualitatively similar to those seen in adults with normal-hearing (Lafreniere et al, 1991).

The importance of otoacoustic emissions in assessment of peripheral auditory status has increased the need for effective middle ear measures in infants. Traditionally, immittance measurements in infants have been equivocal. Tympanometry suggesting middle ear fluid (type B) may be of value in infants, but the presence of normal tympanometric results in young infants may be erroneous. Tympanometry with higher frequency probe tones rather than the traditional 226-Hz probe tone may increase the usefulness of tympanometry. Furthermore, evaluation of acoustic reflexes may be included. If the infant has present acoustic reflexes, normal middle ear function can be inferred. Physiological test procedures are discussed more fully in Chapters 17 to 20 and 22.

THE ELDERLY

When assessing elderly patients concomitant sensory and physical problems may affect diagnostic testing. For example, many elderly patients may experience visual impairment, have mobility limitations, or have cognitive impairment, all of which may affect the reliability of test results (Phillips et al, 1993). As individuals age, the rate of information processing decreases. This factor must be considered when structuring the test environment and carrying out test procedures. Audiologists should allow for slower information processing during instruction and explanation of test results and recommendations. Because the capacity of working memory also decreases with age, information presented in short packages will be more readily understood by the elderly patient. Speech comprehension by elderly people improves with exaggeration of stress. In fact, modification of speech in this manner to improve comprehension by elderly patients has been termed *Elderspeak* (Kemper, 1991).

Elderly patients are more conservative in responding to auditory stimuli; thus, because they may wait for a sound to be clearly audible before indicating its presence rather than respond to the softest sound heard (Rees & Botwinick, 1971). For this reason, many elderly patients may need to be (re)instructed to be more aggressive during threshold assessment to ensure that the degree of hearing loss is not overestimated.

Appropriate evaluation of and intervention for possible hearing impairment is important for improving the quality of life in elderly patients. Although hearing loss has been found to have no effect on measures of activities of daily living (Rudberg et al, 1993), hearing loss does have a negative impact on the elderly. These include social isolation and depression (Herbst, 1983; Weinstein & Ventry, 1982), paranoia (Rosch, 1982), and an increased decline in cognitive function when combined with senility and Alzheimer's disease (Herbst & Humphrey, 1980; Uhlmann et al, 1986; Weinstein & Amsell, 1986).

Considerations in Diagnostic Testing

Many elderly patients do not pursue evaluation for hearing impairment. In some cases this is due to denial or the lack of perception of disability, which may be related to the insidious nature of the hearing loss. It is not uncommon for the elderly person to be unaware of how to obtain appropriate audiological testing and habilitation. This often occurs with the infirm or institutionalized elderly. In cases of impaired cognition, senility, or dementia, caregivers may incorrectly interpret the symptoms of hearing loss as manifestations of the cognitive dysfunction.

Because identification of elderly patients at risk for hearing impairment may increase the likelihood of timely connection with appropriate evaluation and habilitation services, screening programs for elderly patients could be very useful. In 1989 the American Speech-Language-Hearing Association drafted guidelines for the Identification of Hearing Impairment/Handicap in Adult/Elderly Persons. The guidelines suggest that the screening include a case history, visual inspection of the external auditory canals, pure tone screening, and a self-assessment of hearing handicap.

The Welch-Allyn Audioscope is used in some nursing homes and physicians offices for identifying elderly patients who should be referred for additional testing. A handheld device that resembles an otoscope, the Audioscope emits pure tones at 40 dB at 500, 1000, 2000, and 4000 Hz. Nurses or physicians instruct patients to respond when they hear the tones, and when the screening is not passed, the patient is referred for diagnostic testing. Studies have found the Audioscope to have a sensitivity of 94% and a specificity of 72 to 90%. Use of the Audioscope in conjunction with a hearing handicap scale, such as the Hearing Handicap Inventory for the Elderly—Screening Version (HHIE-S), has been demonstrated to yield a test accuracy of 83% for noninstitutionalized elderly patients (Lichtenstein et al, 1988). These screening tools are fast—the Audioscope takes approximately 1 to 2 minutes for both ears and the HHIE-S takes approximately 2 minutes to complete (McBride et al, 1994).

Although useful for identifying hearing handicap, self-assessment tools alone may not be appropriate for identifying hearing loss in institutionalized elderly patients. Ciurlia-Guy et al (1993) observed that institutionalized patients in their study tended to deny the presence of hearing loss, which led to a poor correlation between HHIE-S results and audiometric data. The authors suggest that the low priority placed on hearing loss for these patients may be due to concomitant health problems and increased frailty.

PITFALL

Self-assessment scales are very useful for identifying hearing handicap in a wide variety of patient populations. However, they may not be valid in institutionalized elderly populations.

THE MENTALLY/PHYSICALLY CHALLENGED

Developmental Disabilities

Developmental disorders include disabilities evident in childhood such as mental retardation, cerebral palsy, learning difficulties, problems with motor skills, visual impairment, and other physical deficits. Because approximately one-third of hearing-impaired children in special education classes are multiply disabled, the demand for audiologists to have working knowledge of the various developmental disabilities and their impact on diagnostic audiological tests is increased (Karchmer, 1985; Young, 1994). Unfortunately, the various challenges and difficulties experienced when testing patients with multiple handicaps may result in many of the patients having hearing loss being inadequately or improperly diagnosed. This section will focus on patients with developmental disabilities that may have an impact on the audiological evaluation.

Mental Retardation

Mental retardation is defined by diagnostic criteria from DSM-IV (1994) as "significantly sub-average intellectual functioning" (Table 14–4) with "concurrent deficits or impairments in present adaptive functioning" (Table 14–5). To fit the DSM-IV definition, the onset of mental retardation must occur before 18 years of age.

Considerations in Diagnostic Testing

In evaluating patients with mental retardation the developmental age of the patient is factored into selecting appropriate test procedures (Table 14–3). The incidence of cerumen impaction is high in the mentally retarded population so careful otoscopic evaluation should be performed routinely in any audiometric evaluation or hearing screening (Crandell & Roeser, 1993).

Cerebral Palsy

Vining et al (1976) from the Kennedy Institute for Habilitation of the Mentally and Physically Handicapped Child at Johns Hopkins University School of Medicine defined cerebral palsy as "a nonprogressive disorder of motion and posture due to brain insult or injury occurring in the period of early brain growth (generally under 3 years of age)". Some risk factors for cerebral palsy are low birth weight, multiple births, hyperbilirubinemeia, neonatal difficulties (including anoxia, episodes of cyanosis, convulsions, and feeding problems), and a maternal history of complications in pregnancy, including infertility and miscarriages or stillbirths.

In 1897 Sigmund Freud first proposed a classification system for cerebral palsy, including hemiplegia, general cerebral spasticity, paraplegic spasticity, centralized chorea and bilateral athetosis, and bilateral spastic hemiplegia (Vining et al,

TABLE 14–4 Degree of mental retardation based on intellectual functioning (DSM-IV)

Degree of Severity	IQ Level
Mild	50–55 to approximately 70
Moderate	35/40 to 50/55
Severe	20/25 to 35/40
Profound	Less than 20 or 25
Severity unspecified	Strong presumption of MR, but person's IQ is untestable (patient too impaired, uncooperative, or too young)

TABLE 14–5 Indicators of impairments in present adaptive functioning (DSM-IV)

Communication
Self-care
Home living
Social/interpersonal skills
Use of community resources
Self-direction
Functional academic skills
Work
Leisure
Health
Safety

For diagnosis of mental retardation, deficits must be evident in at least two of the areas.

1976). Some types of cerebral palsy are more likely than others to have associated sensorineural hearing loss. Prevalence of hearing loss will depend on the causative factor for the cerebral palsy. For example, patients with choreoathetoid cerebral palsy may have hearing loss as a result of kernicterus, which occurs in some infants with hyperbilirubinemia when unconjugated bilirubin deposits in the brain. This condition leads to various neurological impairments and is a risk factor for both cerebral palsy and sensorineural hearing loss.

Considerations in Diagnostic Testing

Although audiologists do not need to be able to classify the specific type of cerebral palsy, they should be aware that the patient may exhibit some degree of hypertonicity, hyperreflexia, contractures, and extensor plantar reflex (Babinski sign) (Vining et al, 1976). In general, patients with spastic cerebral palsy will move very stiffly and may even exhibit difficulty in moving at all. Involuntary, uncontrolled bodily movements are more characteristic of those with athetoid cerebral palsy. These involuntary body movements often make it difficult to determine whether the patient has responded solely to the presence of the test signal. In addition, these movements may introduce some degree of masking noise, which can affect threshold measurements. Movement artifacts may also make physiological assessments of auditory status, such as OAEs, acoustic reflexes, and ABRs, difficult.

Response modes should vary depending on patient capabilities. One may find that eye movements or eye blinks are the only means for the patient to signal a response. Modified play procedures may be useful with adult patients who understand the process but are physically incapable of responding with traditional response modes. For example, some adult patients may find it easier to release an object that has been placed in their hand when hearing a tone than to raise their hand or push a button. Obtaining as much information as possible about functional capabilities from

<table>
<tr><td>

SPECIAL CONSIDERATON

Many patients with cerebral palsy may have associated visual defects. Before attempting VRA, audiologists should obtain information about the patient's visual status. If uncorrected visual deficits exist, VRA may not be the assessment tool of choice (see section on visual impairment).

</td></tr>
</table>

caregivers and other professionals working with the patient (such as physical therapists, speech-language pathologists, and occupational therapists) is needed in selecting a test procedure that offers the most appropriate response mode.

Down Syndrome

Langdon Down first wrote about the condition now referred to as Down syndrome in 1866 (Diefendorf et al, 1995). Down syndrome is also termed trisomy 21, in reference to its chromosomal abnormality etiology. Patients with Down syndrome have recognizable physical characteristics including upward slanting eyes, epicanthic folds, small noses, low nasal bridges, protruding tongues, broad hands and fingers, and short stature (Gath, 1978). In addition, Down syndrome patients exhibit varying degrees of mental handicap that can affect their ability to participate in age-appropriate audiometric testing.

Because anatomical malformations of the auditory system have been reported from the pinna through the central auditory system, it is estimated that hearing loss occurs in 40 to 70% of Down syndrome patients (Bilgin et al, 1996). Hearing loss may be conductive mixed, or sensorineural. Down syndrome patients have pinnae that are smaller and lower set than in the normal population (Aase et al, 1973). Earcanals are often stenotic and malformations of middle ear structures have been noted (Balkany et al, 1979; Bilgin et al, 1996). As a result, Down syndrome patients have more problems with excessive cerumen and concomitant conductive hearing loss (Maroudias et al, 1994). In addition, ossicular malformations and structural differences in the middle ear, eustachian tube, and nasopharynx have been reported (Sando & Haruo, 1990), which may be partially responsible for the increased incidence of otitis media with effusion in this population (Cunningham & McArthur, 1982; Selikowitz, 1993; Turner et al, 1990).

Although reported inner ear malformations include both the cochlear and the vestibular systems, these structural differences are minor (Bilgin et al, 1996; Harada & Sando, 1981). A greater concern exists with the incidence of early onset sensorineural hearing loss (Keiser et al, 1981) similar to presbyacusis. Walford (1980), in fact, suggested that Down syndrome patients exhibit "accelerated aging," which not only includes the auditory system but also the visual system and cognitive function.

Considerations in Diagnostic Testing

One important consideration in evaluating patients with Down syndrome is the selection of test procedures that are developmentally appropriate. A young Down syndrome child may be best evaluated with VRA, whereas an older Down syndrome patient may be successfully evaluated with CPA even into adulthood. However, caution is called for when interpreting test results because patients with Down syndrome have questionable response validity as a result of excessive false positive responses (Diefendorf et al, 1995).

PEARL

Greenberg et al (1978) suggested the use of the Bayley Scales of Infant Development (BSID) before audiometric assessment of Down syndrome children to determine the mental age equivalent. Their research revealed that Down syndrome patients do not successfully complete VRA until the BSID mental age of 10 to 12 months.

SPECIAL CONSIDERATON

Because of concern about possible conductive hearing loss in children with Down syndrome, it has been recommended that, minimally, a sound-field and bone conduction SRT/SAT be obtained when complete air and bone conduction results are not available (Diefendorf et al, 1995).

Although excessive cerumen and stenotic earcanals may make immittance measurements more difficult in patients with Down syndrome, it is still recommended. It should be recognized that acoustic reflex testing may not be useful with Down syndrome patients because reports have found them to be absent or elevated in many with normal middle ear function and adequate hearing (Schwartz & Schwartz, 1978).

Management of patients with Down syndrome should include careful monitoring of auditory status even after treatment of middle ear pathological conditions. Residual conductive hearing loss requiring additional medical intervention has been reported in many patients even after placement of tympanostomy tubes (Selikowitz, 1993). For children with Down syndrome and chronic hearing loss, appropriate habilitation procedures are needed while the child continues to experience hearing difficulties. Amplification should be considered until the medical condition can be resolved. In some cases the medical intervention may not be successful in alleviating the hearing loss, and in other cases a concomitant sensorineural hearing loss may be present.

Attention Deficit/Hyperactivity Disorder

In delineating the criteria for diagnosis of attention-deficit/hyperactivity disorder (ADHD), the DSM-IV separates the symptoms on the basis of whether they are primarily due to inattention or hyperactivity-impulsivity. To be diagnosed with ADHD, a child must have exhibited a minimum of six of the symptoms of inattention and six of the symptoms for hyperactivity-impulsivity for at least 6 months (Table 14–6). These symptoms must also be evident in more than one setting (e.g., home and school) and to a degree that is considered maladaptive. Furthermore, some of the symptoms must be evident before the age of 7 and cannot be accounted for by another type of mental disorder.

Although attention deficit disorder (ADD) can occur without hyperactivity, for the purpose of this section the two will be considered together. Children with ADD/ADHD have difficulty maintaining attention over a period of time and also exhibit poor impulse control (Keller, 1992; Moss & Sheiffele, 1994; Selikowitz, 1995). They are easily distracted from a task, have difficulty concentrating; and may exhibit poor listening skills, forgetfulness and poor organization skills (Keller, 1992; Moss & Sheiffele, 1994; Selikowitz, 1995). All these characteristics can increase the difficulty in obtaining valid test results in this population.

Sometimes the audiologist or otolaryngologist may be the initial referral for a child with ADD/ADHD. Often, the parents are concerned that a hearing problem may be causing their child to do poorly in school or misbehave. Grundfast et al (1991) listed the following indicators that may suggest that the child should be referred for psychoeducational evaluation:

1. Behavior during office visit
   - Opens cabinet drawers, plays with equipment, and moves around examination room when physician converses with parent
   - Excessively talkative and persistently interrupts conversation between parent and physician
   - Reluctance or seeming inability to hold still for examination
   - Resists examination; generally defiant behavior
   - Spasticity or hypotonia during examination
   - Prolonged crying after completion of examination

2. Audiologic assessment
   - Difficulty sitting still
   - Difficulty following instructions
   - Reluctance to accept earphones, impedance devices, and other procedures readily accepted by age peers
   - Inconsistent auditory thresholds (Grundfast et al, 1991, pp. 72–73)

Considerations in Diagnostic Testing

Because patients with ADD/ADHD are easily distracted and have difficulty remembering, brief instructions should be given so that it is clear about what is expected in the test situation. Distractions in the test environment should be kept to a minimum. For example, toys used for controlling attention in pediatric evaluations may need to be removed from the sound booth when testing an older ADD/ADHD patient. If the test session will be long (as in an evaluation for central auditory processing deficits), frequent breaks are called for and carefully monitoring attentional state throughout testing is needed. Tones and speech should be presented during periods when movement is minimal and the child praised when sitting still to listen.

TABLE 14–6   Symptoms for ADHD (DSM-IV)

Inattention	*Hyperactivity*	Often fails to give close attention to details or makes careless mistakes in schoolwork, work or other activities
		Often has difficulty sustaining attention in tasks or play activities
		Often does not seem to listen when spoken to directly
		Often does not follow through on instructions and fails to finish schoolwork, chores, or duties in the workplace (not due to oppositional behavior or failure to understand instructions)
		Often has difficulty organizing tasks and activities
		Often avoids, dislikes, or is reluctant to engage in tasks that require sustained mental effort (such as schoolwork or homework)
		Often loses things necessary for tasks or activities
		Is often easily distracted by extraneous stimuli
		Is often forgetful in daily activities
Hyperactivity-impulsivity	*Hyperactivity*	Often fidgets with hands or feet or squirms in seat
		Often leaves seat in classroom or in other situations in which remaining seated is expected
		Often runs about or climbs excessively in situations in which it is inappropriate) in adolescents or adults, may be limited to subjective feelings of restlessness)
		Often has difficulty playing or engaging in leisure activities quietly
		Is often "on the go" or often acts as if "driven by a motor"
		Often talks excessively
	Impulsivity	Often blurts out answers before questions have been completed
		Often has difficulty awaiting turn
		Often interrupts or intrudes on others

Autism

Patients with autism are characterized by the symptoms listed in Table 14–7. In addition to these indicators, autism is suspected if a child has delayed social interaction, limited language use in social communication, or symbolic/imaginative play before the age of 3 (DSM-IV, 1994). Because of unresponsiveness to sound, it is not unusual for an audiologist to be the first professional to evaluate a young autistic child. Parents may be confused about their child's inconsistent responses to various sound stimuli. For example, a child with autism may not seem to hear a loud sound such as a train nearby but become distressed at softer, less noticeable sounds. Although these children may seem to be less reactive than normal, they can actually "shut down" with stimulation overload. Unsurprisingly, if an autistic child is not responding in a test environment, the environment/test stimuli may need to be simplified. Some authors have suggested that autistic children do not have a simple sensory deficit but rather an attentional problem (Lovaas et al, 1971). They may have difficulties selectively attending to specific stimuli. In fact, concern about overstimulation or problems with selective attention in autistic children have led to the suggestion that use of ear protectors to reduce auditory stimulation in classroom settings may improve the behavior of some autistic children and their performance on tasks requiring concentration (Fassler & Bryant, 1971).

Considerations in Diagnostic Testing

Sensory integration therapy has been successfully used by speech-language pathologists and occupational therapists in working with autistic patients. Clinicians can use some of the principles found in sensory integration therapy to improve testing autistic children. In general, autistic patients will perform better in an orderly, simple test environment with limited visual distractions (Haack & Haldy, 1996; Quill, 1995). Toys should be stored out of sight and lighting should be soft and subdued. Touching the child unexpectedly during testing should be avoided; when touching is necessary, firm

TABLE 14–7 Criteria for diagnosis of Autistic Disorder (DSM-IV). A total of at least six must be evident for a diagnosis of autism to be made.

Qualitative impairment in social interaction (at least 2)	Marked impairment in the use of multiple nonverbal behaviors such as eye-to-eye gaze, facial expression, body postures, and gestures to regulate social interaction
	Failure to develop peer relationships appropriate to development level
	A lack of spontaneous seeking to share enjoyment, interests, or achievements with other people
	Lack of social or emotional reciprocity
Qualitative impairments in communication (at least 1)	Delay in, or total lack of, the development of spoken language (not accompanied by an attempt to compensate through alternative modes of communication such as gesture or mime)
	In individuals with adequate speech, marked impairment in the ability to initiate or sustain a conversation with others
	Stereotyped and repetitive use of language or idiosyncratic language
	Lack of varied, spontaneous make-believe play or social imitative play appropriate to developmental level
Restricted, repetitive, and stereotyped patterns of behavior, interests, and activities (at least 1)	Encompassing preoccupation with one or more stereotyped and restricted patterns of interest that is abnormal either in intensity or focus
	Apparently inflexible adherence to specific, nonfunctional routines or rituals
	Stereotyped and repetitive motor mannerisms (e.g., hand or finger flapping or twisting, or complex whole-body movements)
	Persistent preoccupation with parts of objects

pressure should be used because light, unexpected touches are known to be overstimulating to autistic children (Haack & Haldy, 1996; Quill, 1995). This factor is important when placing earphones and conducting otoscopy and tympanometry. Slow, rhythmic vestibular stimulation has been found to be calming for autistic children, so one may want to place the child in a rocking chair during testing (Haack & Haldy, 1996; Quill, 1995).

Once environment and interactions with the child have been structured to increase comfort, conditioning the child to auditory stimuli can begin. Unlike normal children who perform better with multisensory cues for play audiometry or VRA conditioning, children with autism may exhibit stimulus overselectivity (Lovaas et al, 1971). As a result, when testing a child with autism, it is best to limit the number of cues.

Patients with Dementia

According to the diagnostic criteria from DSM-IV (1994), dementia can occur as a result of vascular problems, HIV, head trauma, Parkinson's disease, Huntington's disease, Creutzfeldt-Jakob disease, normal-pressure hydrocephalus, hypothyroidism, brain tumor, vitamin B_{12} deficiency, intracranial radiation, substance use (alcohol, drug abuse, or medications), or a combination of these factors. All patients with dementia will exhibit some type of memory impairment that results in difficulty learning new information or recalling information. These patients may also have aphasia, apraxia, agnosias, and problems with various higher level tasks. Two patient populations with dementia commonly seen in audiological practices are those with brain injury and Alzheimer's disease.

Brain Injury

Brain injuries can occur in a variety of ways, such as head trauma or stroke. The type of deficits observed depends on the area of the brain affected. Table 14–8 lists aphasia syndromes produced by strokes within the various areas of the brain. As shown, depending on the area of the lesion, spontaneous speech, comprehension, repetition, naming, reading comprehension, and writing are affected differently. To evaluate patients with brain injury appropriately, it is helpful to

TABLE 14–8   Aphasia syndromes produced by strokes

	Area of Lesion	Spontaneous Speech	Comprehension	Repetition	Naming	Reading Comprehension	Writing
Wernicke's aphasia	Posterior portion of superior temporal gyrus (Wernicke's area)	Fluent	Poor	Poor	Poor	Poor	Poor
Pure word deafness	Both primary auditory cortices, or connection between them and Wernicke's area	Fluent	Poor	Poor	Good	Good	Good
Broca's aphasia	Frontal cortex rostral to base of primary motor cortex (Broca's area)	Nonfluent	Good	Poor*	Poor	Good	Poor
Global aphasia	Broca's area and Wernicke's area	Nonfluent	Poor	Poor	Poor	Poor	Poor
Conduction aphasia	Area of parietal lobe superior to lateral fissure	Fluent	Good	Poor	Good	Good to poor	Good
Anomic aphasia	Various parts of parietal or temporal lobes	Fluent	Good	Good	Poor	Good to poor	Good to poor
Transcortical sensory aphasia	Connections between speech areas and posterior association cortex	Nonfluent or even absent	Poor	Good	Poor	Poor†	Poor
Transcortical motor aphasia	Supplementary motor area	Nonfluent	Good	Good	Poor	Good	Poor

*May be better than spontaneous speech.
†Patient may be able to read words without comprehending them.
Adapted from Carlson (1986).

know which brain functions are impaired and intact, so as to capitalize on the intact capabilities of the patient. For example, if it is known that the patient has a lesion to both primary auditory cortices with pure word deafness, written instructions for pure tone testing can be provided. Patients with Broca's aphasia will not be able to repeat words for word intelligibility testing but comprehension is usually good; therefore a picture pointing task may be a more valid indicator of auditory comprehension.

Alzheimer's Disease

Patients with Alzheimer's disease have progressive memory loss and cognitive dysfunction. In addition, central changes in sensory systems, including those subserving vision, olfaction, and audition, have been documented. Lesions have been documented in patients with Alzheimer's disease in the auditory system at the inferior olivary nucleus (Iseki et al, 1989), the lateral lemniscus (Ishii, 1966), the inferior colliculus, the medial geniculate body, and auditory primary and association cortices (Sinha et al, 1993). Changes have also been noted in the peripheral visual and

olfactory systems of patients with Alzheimer's disease (Blanks et al, 1989; Hinton et al, 1986; Talamo et al, 1989). However, other than those changes that can be attributed to normal aging, the peripheral auditory system does not seem to be similarly affected in these patients (Sinha et al, 1996). The other deficits experienced by patients with Alzheimer's disease contribute to difficulty in obtaining reliable audiological test results.

Considerations in Diagnostic Testing

In general, when evaluating patients with dementia, short, simple instructions should be used. Modeling appropriate behaviors or responses in the test session is especially helpful. For example, for patients with Wernicke's aphasia demonstrating otoscopy and tympanometry rather than describing the procedure is more appropriate. Obviously, a complete case history is the best means to provide information about the patient's lesion and expected deficits. Obtaining information from caregivers about the patient's general behavior and capabilities will aid in making appropriate modifications to test procedures and facilitate obtaining valid test results.

Visual Impairment

Consideration of possible visual deficits in patients being audiologically evaluated is important for selection of appropriate test procedures. The prevalence of visual impairment in patients with hearing loss has been estimated at approximately 38 to 58% (Campbell et al, 1981), with a higher incidence in patients with conditions known to cause hearing and visual impairment, such as congenital rubella, neonatal sepsis, and Rh incompatibility (Woodruff, 1986). Within this group are patients with visual and auditory impairment severe enough to be referred to as "deaf-blind." However, patients labeled as deaf-blind are usually not deaf or blind but exhibit varying degrees of each sensory impairment. Regardless of the degree of visual impairment, the patient's ocular acuity should influence appropriate modification of the test environment and procedures to obtain accurate estimates of auditory sensitivity.

Considerations in Diagnostic Testing

Testing of infants, as previously discussed, often involves the use of visual reinforcement. When evaluating infants with visual impairment, one recommended modification is to use vibrotactile rather than visual reinforcement (Spradlin, 1985). If conditioned play audiometry is considered, selecting items that are tactually interesting and easily discriminated is an important consideration. In addition, equipping the sound room with adjustable lighting and removing the dark Plexiglas covers from the visual reinforcers to increase visibility are important considerations for visually impaired patients (Gustin, 1997). Gustin (1997) also suggests that the visual reinforcers be portable to allow them to be moved closer to the child for testing.

PSEUDOHYPOACUSIS

Pseudohypoacusis was a term originally coined by Carhart (1961) to denote a situation in which a patient exhibits hearing loss inconsistent with audiological test results or medical findings. According to some sources, pseudohypoacusic patients can be divided into two categories (Sohmer et al, 1977). The first category consists of those patients who deliberately, or consciously, feign hearing loss. This category would include patients who expect to receive financial or psychological gain for their hearing loss. Patients who have decreased auditory function caused by an "unconscious, psychogenic process" make up the second category (Spraggs et al, 1994). The term *conversion deafness*, although its existence is controversial (Goldstein, 1966), has been applied to the second group. Conversion disorders can take many forms, including hearing loss, visual impairment, and motor impairments. These nonorganic disorders are attributed by some to be due to "psychologic conflict or need" (Wolf et al, 1993).

Reasons for feigning a hearing loss can be quite complicated. Many patients cannot be neatly categorized as consciously or unconsciously motivated. Some patients may even have a mixture of both. Once a nonorganic hearing loss has been identified, selection of appropriate management depends on accurate determination of type of motivation (i.e., conscious, unconscious, or a mixture).

When evaluating patients with suspected pseudohypoacusis, one must remember that organic causes of hearing loss are more prevalent than nonorganic causes, and thus must first be considered and ruled out. Furthermore, a nonorganic overlay can coexist with some degree of organic hearing impairment, in which case the degree of the true hearing impairment must be determined.

Identification of pseudohypoacusis is extremely important not only to ensure that the patient receives appropriate intervention but also to avoid potentially harmful intervention. Placement of high-power hearing aids on a child who has a functional hearing loss can cause organic damage. More importantly, candidates for invasive management procedures, such as cochlear implants, have also been found to exhibit functional hearing loss or nonorganic overlays (Spraggs et al, 1994).

Children

Pseudohypoacusis in children seems to reach a peak between the ages of 10 and 12 (Andaz et al, 1995; Bowdler & Rogers, 1989) and often is connected to social or academic problems (Bowdler & Rogers, 1989; Yoshida et al, 1989). Children who exhibit nonorganic disabilities are often introverted (Aplin & Rowson, 1986) and may actually be reporting other functional impairments, such as visual problems. Broad (1980) even suggested that children with functional hearing loss may be using malingering as a "psychological self-defense mechanism." In fact, children who are suffering from child abuse have also been reported to exhibit functional hearing loss (Drake et al, 1995).

Some studies suggest that more girls will evidence functional impairments than boys (Andaz et al, 1995; Aplin & Rowson, 1986; Bowdler & Rogers, 1989; Brockman & Hoversten, 1960; Dixon & Newby, 1959; Johnson et al, 1956). Yet, other studies have not found a gender difference in incidence or even suggest the reverse—that there are more male than female pseudohypoacusic patients (Berger, 1965; Rintelmann & Harford, 1963). Many pseudohypoacusic children have a history of middle ear disorders (Aplin & Rowson, 1986; Dixon & Newby, 1959).

Adults

Although some adult patients have been identified with cases of conversion deafness (Monsell & Herzon, 1984; Wolf et al, 1993), most reported cases of pseudohypoacusis in adults are believed to be volitional. Cases of functional hearing loss have been noted in industrial (Harris, 1979) and military (Gold et al, 1991) populations. Feigning hearing loss may be attempted for financial gain, as in many workman's compensation cases, or to avoid work responsibilities. In fact, Gold et al (1991) suggested that the presence of pseudohypoacusis in an enlisted person may indicate that the person was likely to be "prematurely separated from military service."

Diagnostic Testing
Informal Observations and the Basic Audiological Evaluation

In the initial encounter with a new patient, careful attention should be paid to general behavior and communicative competence. Pseudohypoacusic patients may exhibit a variety of almost stereotypical behaviors. For example, a patient may make exaggerated attempts to understand the clinician, such as straining to hear, leaning forward, and making exaggerated motions to lip read. Other patients may have little or no difficulty understanding the clinician in nontest conversation but provide audiometric test results that are inconsistent with the ease observed during informal communication.

In most cases success in obtaining valid test results in patients who exhibit pseudohypoacusis is determined in the first few moments of testing. The most useful information is often that gathered in initial, informal observation by a skilled clinician. For example, in testing children who have presented with sudden moderate-to-severe hearing loss, a clinician may note that they are able to respond appropriately to questions asked in a normal conversational voice when they have their back to the clinician and immittance probes in their ears. In a situation such as this the clinician has a starting point—the clinician will not complete an audiogram indicative of hearing loss of a degree more severe than would be expected with such auditory competence. As testing progresses further without determining valid threshold levels, the more difficult it becomes to encourage an uncooperative patient to provide truthful responses. These simple techniques can provide the audiologist with the basis for modifying test procedures and demanding the patient give more accurate responses.

Once a patient has convinced the clinician, family members, physician, and so forth that the functional hearing loss is organic, the patient often becomes more determined to continue to evidence the hearing loss. Veniar and Salston (1983)

PEARL

An informal technique to use with young or naive pseudohypoacusic patients is to set the audiometer at an intensity significantly below the voluntary SRT, and with monitored live voice ask general questions, such as "How old are you?" "What grade are you in?" and "Where do you go to school?"

---

reported a case in which a 15-year-old child had experienced an ear infection at 8 years of age. After the ear infection was cleared, the child was tested and her physician reported that "all the nerves in the right ear are dead." The child then functioned for the next 7 years as a unilaterally hearing-impaired person. When her hearing was reevaluated at 15 years of age, test results were consistent with normal auditory sensitivity for the left ear and a severe hearing loss in the right. However, results from the Stenger test (described later) suggested that hearing thresholds in the right ear were similar to those in the left. After counseling and a month of "retraining" the right ear to listen, audiological evaluations revealed auditory sensitivity within normal limits for both ears.

During basic audiometry, test-retest reliability, SRT/PTA agreement, ascending/descending threshold agreement and the shadow curve will assist in identifying pseudohypoacusic patients (see Table 14–9).

TABLE 14–9 Tests for pseudohypoacusis

Procedure	Hearing Loss for Test is Applicable	Type of Test
Basic audiometry		
Test-retest threshold reliability	Unilateral/bilateral	Qualitative
SRT/PTA agreement	Unilateral/bilateral	Qualitative
Speech threshold/PTA agreement	Unilateral/bilateral	Qualitative
Failure to demonstrate shadow curve	Unilateral	Qualitative
Tests for pseudohypoacusis		
Stenger (minimum contralateral interference level)	Unilateral	Quantitative
Doerfler-Stewart*	Unilateral/bilateral	Qualitative
Lombard-reflex*	Unilateral/bilateral	Qualitative
Delayed auditory feedback*	Unilateral/bilateral	Qualitative
Swinging story/varying intensity story test (VIST)	Unilateral/bilateral	Qualitative
Immittance measures	Unilateral/bilateral	Quantitative
Otoacoustic emissions	Unilateral/bilateral	Quantitative
Auditory evoked potentials		
Electrocochleography	Unilateral/bilateral	Quantitative
ABR	Unilateral/bilateral	Quantitative
Middle latency response	Unilateral/bilateral	Quantitative
Late components	Unilateral/bilateral	Quantitative

*Historical tests not routinely used in daily audiological practice.
Adapted from Roeser (1987).

Test-Retest Reliability

In conventional audiometric testing the pseudohypoacusic patient will often provide extremely inconsistent responses. Therefore, when it is difficult to obtain a threshold because of inconsistent responding, pseudohypoacusis should be suspected. This inconsistency is also evident in comparing tests obtained at different times.

Expected test-retest reliability for audiometric pure tone and speech tests is ±5- to 10-dB. When tests are administered within close temporal proximity, results should be comparable within this range. Patients who exhibit pseudohypoacusis are often unable to repeat threshold measures within this degree of reliability. Thus whenever thresholds differ more than 10 dB from one test session to the next, the possibility of pseudohypoacusis must be considered. However, some organic conditions of the auditory system can result in threshold variability and clinicians must take this into account before assuming that pseudohypoacusis is present.

Speech Recognition Threshold/Pure Tone Average Agreement

In a standard audiometric evaluation SRT to spondaic words is compared with the pure tone average (PTA) at 500, 1000, and 2000 Hz. If the difference between the SRT and PTA exceeds ±8 dB, pseudohypoacusis should be suspected. When patients attempt to feign hearing loss, a universal finding is that the SRT will be better than the PTA because speech is perceived as being louder than pure tones. As a result, the patient will respond at lower intensities to speech than pure tones. Inconsistent agreement between the SRT and PTA is typically the first indication of pseudohypoacusis during the diagnostic audiological evaluation.

PEARL

Pseudohypoacusic patients will often provide atypical responses on speech threshold test measures. For example, a patient may provide only one syllable of a spondee word or get all of the words right at one time and then miss all of them later.

Ascending-Descending Threshold Agreement

When pseudohypoacusis is considered a possibility for any patient, an ascending approach is advised to establish threshold. The reason is that if a descending approach is used, the patient will be given the opportunity to develop a "loudness yardstick" to be used as a reference.

Use of an ascending approach in conjunction with a descending approach can be an easy method for evaluating patients suspected of being pseudohypoacusic. In cooperative listeners, thresholds derived from ascending tones should be comparable to those derived from descending tones. However, patients with pseudohypoacusis can have thresholds that are 20- to 30-dB better for ascending tones than for descending tones (Harris, 1958). A difference in responses obtained with these two types of presentation is one clinical indicator of pseudohypoacusis.

SPECIAL CONSIDERATION

When establishing pure tone or speech recognition thresholds, an ascending approach is first used whenever pseudohypoacusis is suspected.

Shadow Curve

Many pseudohypoacusic patients feign a unilateral hearing loss. Within the basic audiometric evaluation, clues are available to suggest that the unilateral impairment is not organic. Because of crossover, when a patient has a unilateral loss with significant threshold differences between ears, sounds presented to the impaired ear at 50- to 65-dB above the threshold of the better ear will be heard by the better ear. The patient will respond until masking is presented to the normal ear (see Chapter 12). This unmasked audiometric configuration is called a shadow curve. When a patient is feigning unilateral hearing loss and no responses are obtained with sound to the "impaired" ear, it is clear that a discrepancy is present. The absence of a shadow curve with unilateral hearing loss is indicative of pseudohypoaocusis.

PEARL

The "yes-no" method is helpful in testing young patients thought to demonstrate pseudohypoacusis (Frank, 1976). The patient is instructed to say "yes" whenever the pure tone is heard and "no" when it is not. Patients demonstrating pseudohypoacusis will often respond "no" to stimuli below voluntary threshold.

Tests for Pseudohypoacusis

Special tests have been developed for evaluating patients with pseudohypoacusis. Although many are still in use, some are primarily of historical interest. Many of the tests that are no longer used require specialized equipment or proved to be too difficult. Table 14–8 lists tests for pseudohypoacusis. Note that the asterisks identify those tests that are presented for historical purposes.

Pure Tone and Speech Stenger Tests

When auditory stimuli are presented to both ears simultaneously with the stimulus to one ear being louder than the other, only the louder sound will be perceived by the patient (Newby, 1979). For example, with normal-hearing-listeners, a sound presented to one ear at 50 dB and to the other at 15 dB will be perceived as a monaural sound in one ear only. Responses can be elicited with pure tone or speech stimuli; this is known as the Stenger phenomenon.

The Stenger phenomenon is useful for evaluating patients who exhibit unilateral hearing loss. This task is very difficult for a patient to manipulate. Speech or pure tones are presented 10 dB above threshold in the better ear and 10 dB below the reported threshold in the ear exhibiting hearing loss. Normally, the patient will perceive the stimulus in the better ear because it is 10 dB above threshold. If patients are providing valid responses, they will respond. However, for patients with pseudohypoacusis the sound in the "unilaterally impaired ear" will be louder and they will only hear sound in the "impaired" ear. Therefore they will refuse to respond, and pseudohypoacusis may be inferred.

In this application the Stenger phenomenon is a simple and powerful diagnostic tool for determining pseudohypoacusis in patients exhibiting unilateral hearing loss. However, an additional procedure can be used to glean information about the probable true thresholds in the "impaired" ear. For this additional information, the audiologist must calculate the minimum contralateral interference level (MCIL). After obtaining a positive Stenger test, the intensity of the stimulus to the "impaired" ear is then reduced in 5 dB steps. Eventually, the patient will perceive the stimulus in the better ear and will respond. The level at which the patient responds is the MCIL. True threshold for the "impaired" ear is calculated by subtracting 10- to 15-dB from the level presented to the ear with the nonorganic hearing loss when the patient first responded. This allows quantitative information for the "impaired" ear.

Doerfler-Stewart Test

When feigning hearing loss, patients attempt to use a loudness "yardstick" to decide to which stimuli they will respond. The Doerfler-Stewart test (Doerfler & Stewart, 1946) capitalizes on this behavior by attempting to confuse the patient with removal of this "yardstick." This is accomplished by presenting background noise while obtaining a speech recognition threshold; the presentation of the background noise disrupts the loudness yardstick (Doerfler & Stewart, 1946).

The first step in performing the Doerfler-Stewart test is to obtain a binaural SRT in quiet. Presentation level of the spondaic words is then increased 5 dB SL in each ear, and noise is delivered binaurally at 0 dB SL and then increased in intensity until the patient can no longer repeat the spondaic words. This intensity is the noise interference level (NIL). Next, the clinician increases the level of the noise to 20 dB above the NIL. At this level the SRT is reestablished by gradually decreasing the level of the noise until an additional SRT is obtained in quiet. Finally, the patient's threshold for the noise is obtained, which is termed the noise detection threshold (NDT).

With normative data provided by Martin (1975), the relationships between the three SRTs, the NIL, and the NDT are used to determine whether pseudohypoacusis is present. In general, pseudohypoacusis may be suspected if the SRTs in quiet and noise differ by more than 5 dB, if the noise interferes with speech at a level lower than established norms, if the NDT is better than the SRT, or if the NDT is at a lower level than masking should occur for speech. Because the Doerfler-Stewart Test is performed binaurally, it cannot be used for patients with unilateral hearing loss.

Lombard Reflex

The Lombard reflex is based on the observation that in the presence of background noise, patients will increase the intensity of their speech to be heard (Newby, 1979). If a patient is reading a prepared text and noise is presented at a level too soft for the patient to hear, either because of the very soft level of the noise or the presence of hearing loss, the intensity of the patient's speech should not be affected. If noise is presented at low-to-moderate levels to a patient who is feigning a severe hearing loss, however, the intensity of speech will be modified and the clinician may suspect pseudohypoacusis.

The test is performed by asking the patient to read from a prepared text while wearing earphones. Background noise is presented at a low sensation level and then gradually increased. Pseudohypoacusis may be present if the intensity of speech increases in the presence of noise at lower levels than expected for the reported hearing loss.

Delayed Auditory Feedback

Delayed auditory feedback (DAF) tests are based on the phenomenon that acoustic signals that are fed back to the listener with a delay of about 200 ms disrupt ongoing behavior (Ruhm & Cooper, 1964). For example, if listeners are reading a story with simultaneous feedback, their speech will be unaffected. However, if the feedback is then delayed by 200 ms, vocal production will be affected significantly in most individuals. Similar changes can be seen for other motor activities, such as key tapping. If the acoustic feedback is presented at an intensity below the patient's reported threshold and the patient's behavior is affected, positive evidence of pseudohypoacusis is present.

Although DAF was popular for many years, it proved to be of limited value because many patients were not affected by the delayed auditory input, even though it was above their known threshold. DAF is now used by speech-language pathologists as a treatment for dysfluency.

Swinging Story Test

The Swinging Story Test for unilateral pseudohypoacusis is primarily of historical interest. For this test, a story is presented to a patient with portions presented only to the better ear, portions to both ears, and some only to the poorer ear (Newby, 1979). Although the story information presented to the poorer ear does not contribute to the continuity of the story presented to the good ear, the information does change the meaning. A specially prepared tape recording is necessary for the test so that the presentation may be done in a quick, smooth manner. The information to the poorer ear is presented at a level below the reported speech threshold, and the story presented to the good ear is above the reported threshold. After the patient has heard the story, the clinician asks the patient to repeat the information. Pseudohypoacusis is suspected if the story repeated by the patient contains information presented to the poorer ear.

Martin et al (1998) recommended a variation of the swinging story test for evaluating patients for pseudohypoacusis. Their variation, labeled the Varying Intensity Story Test (VIST) uses three stories, each one paragraph long. The first story is presented above the patient's reported threshold and the second is presented below the patient's threshold. The stories are interleaved and the second story simply modifies the meaning of the first. After the patient listens to the story, 10 questions are given. Five of these questions were designed to identify those patients who heard information below their reported thresholds (using the three frequency PTA for comparison), and five would be answered correctly by patients who only heard information presented above their threshold. This provides a more standardized poststory assessment than the casual retelling of information used with the Swinging Story Test. In addition, this test can be conducted for each ear separately (in the case of patients with unilateral pseudohypoacusis) or binaurally.

Physiological Tests

As with all patients with special needs, many of the physiological assessment tools discussed in other chapters in this book are useful for evaluating patients with suspected pseudohypoacusis. With immittance measures (acoustic reflex) and otoacoustic emissions testing (Chapters 17 and 21), information indicating the expected degree of hearing loss can be obtained. For example, if otoacoustic emissions are present, the patient should not exhibit more than a mild hearing loss (except for in some special cases of patients with auditory neuropathy). Acoustic reflex thresholds alone can provide some indices of auditory function in that reported auditory threshold cannot be poorer than threshold for the acoustic reflex. In addition, evaluation of acoustic reflexes to pure tones in comparison to reflexes to broadband noise, as in the sensitivity predication with acoustic reflexes, can increase the use of acoustic reflex testing with pseudohypoacusic patients (Jerger et al, 1974, 1978).

Finally, in cases in which true thresholds cannot be obtained, electrophysiological evaluations may be needed. Auditory-evoked responses using electrocochleography, ABR, and middle and late components can provide a measure of expected auditory thresholds at various frequencies in patients for whom valid behavioral thresholds cannot be obtained. Material on auditory evoked potentials is covered in Chapters 18 to 20.

HYPERACUSIS

Hyperacusis literally means oversensitive hearing. Patients with hyperacusis manifest severe loudness discomfort to everyday environmental sounds presented at normal intensities. *Hyperacusis dolorosa* has been suggested as a general term for patients having discomfort to moderately loud sound

levels regardless of their hearing sensitivity (Mathisen, 1969). However, Brandy and Lynn (1995) differentiate between two types of hyperacusic patients: *threshold hyperacusis* was suggested for patients with better hearing than age-related hearing sensitivity norms and *suprathreshold hyperacusis* for patients having discomfort to sounds less than 65 dB SPL when hearing sensitivity was normal. Whether hearing sensitivity is within normal levels or not, it is clear that audiologists will, on rare occasions, encounter patients who report extreme hypersensitivity to everyday environmental sounds.

No clear etiological factors have been identified for hyperacusis. Various disorders, such as Bell's palsy, tempromandibular joint problems, central nervous system damage, Meniere's disease, hypothyroidism, and noise exposure, have been associated with this rare disorder. However, a universal relationship does not appear to exist between any one abnormality and hypersensitivity to sound.

Patients with extreme hyperacusis may become incapacitated, with the disorder affecting virtually all aspects of the patient's social and occupational life. Although only limited data support a physiological basis for hyperacusis (Brandy & Lynn, 1995), audiologists should not dismiss the disorder as being purely psychological and do nothing. As part of the treatment program, referral to The Hyperacusis Network (444 Edgedwood Drive, Green Bay, WI 54302) should be considered. Treatments for hyperacusis have included vitamin therapy, antidepressants, tranquilizers, beta-blockers, biofeedback, and counseling. Most recently, desensitization therapy has been successful in treating hyperacusic patients (Jasterboff et al, 1996).

CONCLUSIONS

Providing diagnostic audiological tests for patients with special needs is one of the foremost challenges of the clinical audiologist. This chapter reviews test procedures that have been developed over the years for patients with special needs. Through proper application of available audiological procedures, comprehensive diagnostic audiological data can be successfully obtained from all patients, even those with special needs.

REFERENCES

AASE, J.M., WILSON, A.C., & SMITH, D.W. (1973). Small ears in Down syndrome: A helpful diagnostic aid. *Journal of Pediatrics, 82*;845–847.

AMERICAN NATIONAL STANDARDS INSTITUTE. (1991). *American national standard criteria for permissible ambient noise levels during audiometric testing* (ANSI S3.1-1991). New York: Author.

AMERICAN SPEECH-LANGUAGE-HEARING ASSOCIATION. (1989). Guidelines for the identification of hearing impairment/handicap in adult/elderly persons. (Draft for peer review). *ASHA, 31*;59–60.

ANDAZ, C., HEYWORTH, T., & ROWE, S. (1995). Nonorganic hearing loss in children—a 2-year study. *ORL Journal of Otorhinolaryngology and Related Specialties, 57*(1);33–35.

APLIN, D.Y., & ROWSON, V.J. (1986). Personality and functional hearing loss in children. *British Journal of Clinical Psychology, 25*(Pt 4);313–314.

APUZZO, M., YOSHINAGA-ITANO C. (1995). Early identification of infants with significant hearing loss and the Minnesota Child Development Inventory. *Seminars in Hearing, 16*(2),124–139.

BALKANY, T.J., MISCHKE, R.E., DOWNS, M.P., & JAFEK, B.W. (1979). Ossicular abnormalities in Down syndrome. *Otolaryngology–Head and Neck Surgery, 87*;372–384.

BERGER, K. (1965). Nonorganic hearing loss in children. *Laryngoscope, 75*;447–457.

BILGIN, H., KASEMSUWAN, L., SCHACHERN, P.A., PAPARELLA, M., & LE, C.T. (1996). Temporal bone study of Down syndrome. *Archives of Otolaryngology–Head and Neck Surgery, 122*;271–275.

BLANKS, J.C., HINTON, D.R., SADUN, A.A., & MILLER, C.A. (1989). Retinal ganglion cell degeneration in Alzheimer's disease. *Brain Research, 501*(2);364–372.

BONFILS, P., FRANCOIS, M., AVAN, P., LONDERO, A., TROTOUX, J., & NARCY, P. (1992). Spontaneous and evoked otoacoustic emissions in preterm neonates. *Laryngoscope, 102;* 182–186.

BOWDLER, D.A., & ROGERS, J. (1989). The management of pseudohypoacusis in school-age children. *Clinics in Otolaryngology, 14(3);*211–215.

BRANDY, W.T., & LYNN, J.M. (1995). Audiologic findings in hyperacusis and nonhyperacusis subjects. *American Journal of Audiology, 4(1),* 46–51.

BROAD, R.D. (1980). Developmental and psychodynamic issues related to cases of childhood functional hearing loss. *Child Psychiatry and Human Development, 11(1);*49–58.

BROCKMAN, S.M., & HOVERSTEN, A.S. (1960). Pseudoneural hypacusis in children. *Laryngoscope, 70;* 825–839.

CAMPBELL, C.W., POLOMENO, R.C., ELDER, J.M., MURRAY, J., ALTOSAAR, A. (1981). Importance of an eye examination in identifying the cause of congenital hearing impairment. *Journal of Speech and Hearing Disorders, 46;*258–261.

CARHART, R. (1961). Tests for malingering. *Transactions of the American Academy of Ophthalmology and Otolaryngology, 65;*437.

CARLSON, N.R. (1986). *Physiology of behavior* (3rd ed). Boston, MA: Allyn & Bacon, Inc.

CHENG, L.L. (1993). Asian-American cultures. In: D.E. Battle (Ed.). *Communication disorders in multicultural populations* (pp. 38–77). Boston, MA: Andover Medical Publishers.

CIURLIA-GUY, E., CASHMAN, M., & LEWSEN, B. (1993). Identifying hearing loss and hearing handicap among chronic care elderly people. *The Gerontologist, 33(5);*644–649.

CRANDELL, C., & ROESER, R.J. (1993). Incidence of excessive/impacted cerumen in individuals with mental retardation: a longitudinal investigation. *American Journal of Mental Retardation, 97;*568–574.

CUNNINGHAM, C., & McARTHUR, K. (1982). Hearing loss and treatment in young Down syndrome children. *Child: Care, Health and Development, 7;*357–374.

DENNIS, W. (1973). *Children of the Creche.* Century Psychology Series. New York: Prentice-Hall.

DIAGNOSTIC CRITERIA FROM DSM-IV. (1994). WASHINGTON, DC: American Psychiatric Association.

DIEFENDORF, A.O., BULL, M.J., CASEY-HARVEY, D., MIYAMOTO, R.T., POPE, M.L., RENSHAW, J.J., SCHREINER, R.L., & WAGNER-ESCOBAR, M. (1995). Down syndrome: A multidisciplinary perspective. *Journal of the American Academy of Audiology, 6(1);*39–46.

DIXON, R.F., & NEWBY, H.A. (1959). Children with nonorganic hearing problems. *Archives of Otolaryngology, 70;*619–623.

DOERFLER, L.G., & STEWART, K. (1946). Malingering and psychogenic deafness. *Journal of Speech Disorders, 11;*181–186.

DOWN, J.L. (1866). Observations on ethnic classifications. London Hospital Reports 3;259–262. (As cited by Diefendorf, A.O. et al, [1995]). Down syndrome. *Journal of the American Academy of Audiology, 6;*39–46).

DOWNS, M.P. (1978). Auditory screening. *Otolaryngologic Clinics of North America, 11(3);*611–629.

DRAKE, A.F., MAKIELSKI, K., McDONALD-BELL, C., & ATCHESON, B. (1995). Two new otolaryngologic findings in child abuse. *Archives of Otolaryngology–Head and Neck Surgery, 121(12);*1417–1420.

ELLIOTT, L., & KATZ, D. (1980). *Development of a new children's test of speech discrimination.* St. Louis, MO: Auditec.

FASSLER, J., & BRYANT, N.D. (1971). Disturbed children under reduced auditory input: A pilot study. *Exceptional Child, 38(3);*197–204.

FRANK, T. (1976). Yes-no test for nonorganic hearing loss. *Archives of Otolaryngology, 102;*162–165.

GATH, A. (1978). *Down syndrome and the family.* New York: Academic Press, Inc.

GOLD, S.R., HUNSAKER, D.H., & HASEMAN, E.M. (1991). Pseudohypoacusis in a military population. *Ear Nose Throat Journal, 70(10);*710–712.

GOLDSTEIN, R. (1966). Pseudohypacusis. *Journal of Speech and Hearing Disorders, 31(4);*341–352.

GREENBERG, D.B., WILSON, W.R., MOORE, J.M., & THOMPSON, G. (1978). Visual reinforcement audiometry (VRA) with young Down syndrome children. *Journal of Speech and Hearing Disorders, 43;*448–458.

GREENSTEIN, J.M., GREENSTEIN, B.B., McCONVILLE, K., & STELLINI, L. (1976). *Mother-infant communication and language acquisition in deaf infants.* New York: Lexington School for the Deaf.

GRUNDFAST, K.M., BERKOWITZ, R.G., CONNERS, C.K., & BELMAN, P. (1991). Complete evaluation of the child identified as a poor listener. *International Journal of Pediatric Otorhinolaryngology, 21;*65–78.

GUSTIN, C. (1997). Audiologic testing of children with a visual impairment. *The Hearing Journal, 50(4);*70–75.

HAACK, L., & HALDY, M. (1996). Making it easy—Adapting home and school environments. *OT Practice,* November.

HARADA, T., & SANDO, I. (1981). Temporal bone histopathologic findings in Down syndrome. *Archives of Otolaryngology, 107;*96–103.

HARRIS, D.A. (1958). A rapid and simple technique for the detection of nonorganic hearing loss. *Archives of Otolaryngology, 68;*758–760.

HARRIS, D.A. (1979). Detecting non-valid hearing tests in industry. *Journal of Occupational Medicine, 21(12);*814–820.

HASKINS, H. (1949). A phonetically balanced test of speech discrimination for children, unpublished Master's thesis, 1949. (Cited by J.L. Northern & M.P. Downs. [1984] In *Hearing in Children.* Baltimore, MD: Williams & Wilkins.)

HAYES, D., & NORTHERN, J.L. (1996). *Infants and hearing.* San Diego, CA: Singular Publishing Group, Inc.

HERBST, K.G., & HUMPHREY, C. (1980). Hearing impairment and mental state in the elderly living at home. *British Medical Journal of Clinical Research, 281;*903–905.

HERBST, K.R.G. (1983). Psychosocial consequences of disorders of hearing in the elderly. In: R. Hinchcliffe (Ed.). *Hearing and balance in the elderly* (pp. 174–200). New York: Churchill Livingstone, Inc.

HINTON, D.R., SADUN, A.A., BLANKS, J.C., & MILLER, C.A. (1986). Optic-nerve degeneration in Alzhiemer's disease. *New England Journal of Medicine, 315(8);*485–487.

ISEKI, E., MATSUSHITA, M., KOSAKA, K., KONDO, H., ISHII, T., & AMANO, N. (1989). Distribution and morphology of brain stem plaques in Alzheimer's disease. *Acta Neuropathology, 78(2);*131–136.

ISHII, T. (1966). Distribution of Alzheimer's neurofibrillary changes in the brainstem and hypothalamus of senile dementia. *Acta Neuropathology, 6(2);*181–187.

JASTERBOFF, P.J., GARY, W.C. & GOLD, S.L. (1996). Neurophysiological approach to tinnitus patients. *American Journal of Otology, 17;*236–230.

JERGER, J., BURNEY, P., MAULDIN, L., & CRUMP, B. (1974). Predicting hearing loss from the acoustic reflex. *Journal of Speech and Hearing Disorders, 39;*11–22.

JERGER, J., & HAYES, D. (1976). The cross-check principle in pediatric audiometry. *Archives of Otolaryngology, 102;*614–620.

JERGER, J., HAYES, D., ANTHONY, L., & MAULDIN, L. (1978). Factors influencing prediction of hearing levels from the acoustic reflex. *Monographs in Contemporary Audiology, 1*(1–20).

JOHNSON, K.O., WORK, W.P., & McCOY, G. (1956). Functional deafness. *Annals of Otology, Rhinology, and Laryngology, 65;* 154–170.

KARCHMER, M.A. (1985). A DEMOGRAPHIC PERSPECTIVE. In E. Cherow, N.D. Matkin, & R.J. Trybus (Eds.). *Hearing-impaired children and youth with developmental disabilities* (pp. 36–56). Washington, D.C.: Gallaudet College Press.

KEISER, H., MONTAGUE, J., WOLD, D., MAUNE, S., & PATTISON, D. (1981). Hearing loss of Down syndrome adults. *American Journal of Mental Deficiency, 85*(5);467–472.

KELLER, W.D. (1992). Auditory processing disorder or attention-deficit disorder? In: J. Katz, N.A. Stecker, & D. Henderson (Eds.). *Central auditory processing: A transdisciplinary view* (pp. 107–114). St. Louis, MO: Mosby–Year Book.

KEMPER, S. (1991). Language and aging: Enhancing caregiver's effectiveness with "ELDERSPEAK." *Experimental Aging Research, 17*(2);80.

KOK, M.R., VAN ZANTEN, G.A., & BROCAAR, M.P. (1993). Aspects of spontaneous otoacoustic emissions in healthy newborns. *Hearing Research, 69;*115–123.

LACH, R., LING, D., LING, A.H., & SHIP, N. (1970). Early speech development in deaf infants. *American Annals of the Deaf, 115;*522–526.

LAFRENIERE, D., JUNG, M.D., SMURZYNSKI, J., LEONDARD, G., KIM, D.O., & SASEK, J. (1991). Distortion-product and click-evoked otoacoustic emissions in healthy newborns. *Archives of Otolaryngology–Head and Neck Surgery, 117;*1382–1389.

LEVINE, R.A., CAMPBELL, D.T. (1972). *Ethnocentrism: Theories of conflict, ethnic attitudes, and group behavior.* New York: John Wiley & Sons, Inc.

LICHTENSTEIN, M.J., BESS, F.H., & LOGAN, S.A. (1988). Validation of screening tools for identifying hearing-impaired elderly in primary care. *JAMA, 259*(19);2875–2878.

LING, A.H. (1971). Changes in the abilities of deaf infants with training. *Journal of Communication Disorders, 3;*267–279.

LOVAAS, O.I., SCHREIBMAN, L., KOEGEL, R., & REHM, R. (1971). Selective responding by autistic children to multiple sensory input. *Journal of Abnormal Psychology, 77*(3);211–222.

MAROUDIAS, N., ECONOMIDES, J., CHRISTODOULOU, P., & HELIDONIS, E. (1994). A study on the otoscopical and audiological findings in patients with Down syndrome in Greece. *International Journal of Pediatrics in Otorhinolaryngology, 29;*43–49.

MARTIN, F.N. (1975). *Introduction to audiology.* Englewood Cliffs, NJ: Prentice-Hall.

MARTIN, F.N., CHAMPLIN, C.A., & MARCHBANKS, T.P. (1998). A varying intensity story test for simulated hearing loss. *American Journal of Audiology, 7;*39–44.

MATHISEN, H. (1969). Phonophobia after stapedectomy. *Acta Otolaryngologica, 68;*73–77.

MATKIN, N. (1977). Assessment of hearing sensitivity during the preschool years. In: F. Bess (Ed.). *Childhood deafness.* New York: Grune & Stratton.

McBRIDE, W.S., MULROW, C.D., AGUILAR, C., & TULEY, M.R. (1994). Methods for screening for hearing loss in older adults. *The American Journal of the Medical Sciences, 307*(1); 40–42.

MONSELL, E.M., & HERZON, F.S. (1984). Functional hearing loss presenting as sudden hearing loss: A case report. *American Journal of Otology, 5*(5);407–410.

MOORE, J.M., THOMPSON, G., & FOLSOM, R.C. (1992). Auditory responsiveness of premature infants utilizing visual reinforcement audiometry (VRA). *Ear and Hearing, 13*(3);187–194.

MOORE, J.M., WILSON, W.R. (1978). Visual reinforcement audiometry (VRA) with infants. In: S.E. Gerber, & G.T. Mencher (Eds.). *Early diagnosis of hearing loss* (pp. 177–213). New York: Grune & Stratton.

MOSS, W., & SHEIFFELE, W. (1994). Can we differentially diagnose an attention deficit disorder without hyperactivity from a central auditory processing problem? *Child Psychiatry and Human Development, 25;*85–96.

NATIONAL INSTITUTES OF HEALTH. (1993). Early identification of hearing impairment in infants and young children. NIH Consensus Statement 1993 Mar. 1–3; *11*(1);1–24.

NELLUM-DAVIS, P. (1993). Clinical practice issues. In: D.E. Battle (Ed.). *Communication disorders in multicultural populations* (pp. 306–316). Boston, MA: Andover Medical Publishers.

NEWBY, H. (1979). *Audiology* (4th ed). Englewood Cliffs, NJ: Prentice-Hall.

NORTHERN, J.L., & DOWNS, M.P. (1984). *Hearing in children* (3rd ed.). Baltimore, MD: Williams & Wilkins.

OLSHO, L.W., KOCH, E.G., CARTER, E.A., HALPIN, C.F., & SPETNER, N.B. (1988). Pure tone sensitivity of human infants. *Journal of the Acoustical Society of America, 84;*1316–1324.

OLSHO, L.W., KOCH, E.G., HALPIN, C.F., & CARTER, E.A. (1987). An observer-based psychoacoustic procedure for use with young infants. *Developmental Psychology, 5;*627–640.

PHILLIPS, C.D., CHU, C.W., MORRIS, J.N., & HAWES, C. (1993). Effects of cognitive impairment on the reliability of geriatric assessments in nursing homes. *Journal of the American Geriatrics Society, 41;*136–142.

QUILL, K.A. (1995). *Teaching children with autism: Strategies to enhance communication and socialization.* New York: Delmar Publishers, Inc.

REES, J.N., & BOTWINICK, J. (1971). Detection and decision factors in auditory behavior of the elderly. *Journal of Gerontology, 26*(2);133–136.

RINTELMANN, W., & HARFORD, E. (1963). The detection and assessment of pseudohypoacusis among school-age children. *Journal of Speech and Hearing Disorders, 28;*141–152.

ROBINSHAW, H.M. (1995). Early intervention for hearing impairment: Differences in the timing of communicative and linguistic development. *British Journal of Audiology, 29*(6), 315–334.

ROESER, R.J. (1986). *Diagnostic audiology.* Austin, TX: Pro-Ed.

ROESER, R.J., & NORTHERN, J.L. (1981). Screening for hearing loss and middle ear disorders. In: R.J. Roeser, & M. Downs (Eds.). *Auditory disorders in school children* (pp. 120–150). New York: Thieme Stratton.

ROESER, R.J., & YELLIN, W. (1987). Pure tone test with preschool children. In: F.N. Martin (Ed.). *Hearing disorders in children.* Austin, TX: Pro-Ed.

ROSCH, P.J. (1982). Prepare your practice to keep pace with the aging patient population. *Physical Management, 22;*28–45.

ROSS, M., & LERMAN, J. (1970). A picture identification test for hearing-impaired children. *Journal of Speech and Hearing Research, 13;*44–53.

RUDBERG, M.A., FURNER, S.E., DUNN, J.E., & CASSEL, C.K. (1993). The relationship of visual and hearing impairments to disability: An analysis using the longitudinal study of aging. *Journal of Gerontology, 48(6);*M261–M265.

RUHM, H.B., & COOPER JR., W.A. (1964). Delayed feedback audiometry. *Journal of Speech and Hearing Disorders, 29;*448–455.

SANDO, I., & HARUO, T. (1990). Otitis media in association with various congenital diseases. *Annals of Otology, Rhinology and Laryngology, S148;*13–16.

SCHWARTZ, D.M., & SCHWARTZ, R.H. (1978). Acoustic impedance and otoscopic findings in young children with Down syndrome. *Archives of Otolaryngology, 104;*652–656.

SELIKOWITZ, M. (1993). Short-term efficacy of tympanostomy tubes for secretory otitis media in children with Down syndrome. *Developmental Medicine and Child Neurology, 35;* 511–515.

SELIKOWITZ, M. (1995). *All about ADD: Understanding attention deficit disorder.* Melbourne: Oxford University Press.

SINHA, U.K., HOLLEN, K.M., RODRIGUEZ, R., & MILLER, C.A. (1993). Auditory system degeneration in Alzheimer's disease. *Neurology, 43(4);*779–785.

SINHA, U.K., SAADAT, D., LINTHICUM, F.H., HOLLEN, K.M., & MILLER, C.A. (1996). Temporal bone findings in Alzheimer's disease. *Laryngoscope, 106;*1–5.

SMART, J.F., & SMART, D.W. (1995). The use of translators/interpreters in rehabilitation. *Journal of Rehabilitation, 61(2);* 14–20.

SOHMER, H., FEINMESSER, M., BAUBERGER-TELL, L., & EDELSTEIN, E. (1977). Cochlear, brain stem, and cortical evoked responses in nonorganic hearing loss. *Annals of Otology, Rhinology, and Laryngology, 86(2 Pt. 1);*227–234.

SPRADLIN, J. (1985). Auditory evaluation. In: M. Bullis (Ed.). *Communication development in young children with deafblindness*: Literature review I (pp. 49–61). Monmouth, OR: Teaching Research Publications.

SPRAGGS, P.D., BURTON, M.J., & GRAHAM, J.M. (1994). Nonorganic hearing loss in cochlear implant candidates. *American Journal of Otology, 15(5);*652–657.

TALAMO, B.R., RUDEL, R., KOSIK, K.S., LEE, V.M., NEFF, S., ADELMAN, L., & KAUER, J.S. (1989). Pathological changes in olfactory neurons in patients with Alzheimer's disease. *Nature, 337(6209);*736–739.

THOMPSON, G., & WILSON, W. (1984). Clinical application of visual reinforcement. *Seminars in Hearing, 5;*85–99.

THORNE, B. (1967). Conditioning children for pure tone testing. *Journal of Speech and Hearing Disorders, 27;*84–85.

TURNER, S., SLOPER, P., CUNNINGHAM, C., & KNUSSEN, C. (1990). Health problems in children with Down syndrome. *Child: Care, Health and Development, 16;*83–97.

UHLMANN, R.F., LARSON, E.B., & KOEPSELL, T.D. (1986). Hearing impairment and cognitive decline in senile dementia of the Alzheimer's type. *Journal of the American Geriatric Society, 34;*207–210.

VENIAR, F.A., & SALSTON, R.S. (1983). An approach to the treatment of pseudohypacusis in children. *American Journal of Diseases of Childhood, 137(1);*34–36.

VINING, E.P., ACCARDO, P.J., RUBENSTEIN, J.E., FARRELL, S.E., & ROIZEN, N.J. (1976). Cerebral palsy: A pediatric developmentalist's overview. *American Journal of Diseases of Childhood, 130(6);*643–649.

WALFORD, R.L. (1980). Immunology and aging. *American Journal of Clinical Pathology, 74;*247–253.

WATROUS, B.S., MCCONNELL, F., & SITTON, A.B., et al. (1975). Auditory responses of infants. *Journal of Speech and Hearing Disorders, 40;*357–366.

WEINSTEIN, B.E., & AMSELL, L. (1986). Hearing loss and senile dementia in the institutionalized elderly. *Clinical Gerontologist, 4;*3–15.

WEINSTEIN, B.E., & VENTRY, I.M. (1982). Hearing impairment and social isolation in the elderly. *Journal of Speech and Hearing Research, 25;*593–599.

WERNER, L.A., FOLSOM, R.C., & MANCL, L.R. (1993). The relationship between auditory brain stem response and behavioral thresholds in normal-hearing infants and adults. *Hearing Research, 68;*131–141.

WOLF, M., BIRGER, M., BEN SHOSHAN, J., & KRONENBERG, J. (1993). Conversion deafness. *Annals of Otology, Rhinology, and Laryngology, 102(5);*349–352.

WOODRUFF, M.E. (1986). Differential effects of various causes of deafness on the eyes, refractive errors, and vision of children. *American Journal of Optometry and Physiological Optics, 63(8);*668–675.

YOSHIDA, M., NOGUCHI, A., & UEMURA, T. (1989). Functional hearing loss in children. *International Journal of Pediatric Otorhinolaryngology, 17(3);*287–295.

YOSHINAGA-ITANO, C., SEDEY, A.L., COULTER, D.K., & MEHL, A.L. (1998). Language of early- and later-identified children with hearing loss. *Pediatrics, 102(5);*1161–1171.

YOUNG, C.V. (1994). Developmental disabilities. In: J. Katz (Ed.). *Handbook of clinical audiology* (4th ed.) (pp. 521–533). Philadelphia, PA: Williams & Wilkins.

## Chapter 15

Diagnosing Central Auditory Processing Disorders in Children

Robert W. Keith

The diagnosis and remediation of central auditory processing disorders (CAPDs) in children and adults is one of the more fascinating areas in the audiologist's scope of practice. No other clinical entity presents a more complex set of symptoms to challenge the audiologist. The wide range of intellectual, behavioral, educational, psychological, medical, and social issues associated with CAPD require that the audiologist be widely read in a variety of subjects.

PURPOSES OF THIS CHAPTER

The purposes of this chapter are to introduce students and audiologists to the broad construct of CAPDs, to define various issues related to CAPD, and to discuss the diagnostic approach to children who are thought to be at risk for CAPD. For a better understanding of the diagnosis of central auditory processing disorders the reader is urged to review Chapter 3 on anatomy and physiology of the central auditory system. Diagnostic techniques evolve, sometimes quickly, and some of the tests described here may fall into disuse as others take their place. It is hoped that the background information provided here will be useful in the future as a foundation, despite these changes.

SOME IMPORTANT DEFINITIONS

One of the challenges of central auditory testing is to determine whether an individual is experiencing a primary CAPD, attention deficit disorder, language disorder, or learning disorder. In many cases these problems coexist, and it may not be possible to determine which problem is primary and which is secondary. Nevertheless, it is in the child's best interest to understand the relationships that exist. For clarification, the following definitions of these entities are taken from the *Diagnostic and Statistical Manual of Mental Disorders* (DSM-IV) (American Psychiatric Association, 1994).

Attention-Deficit/Hyperactivity Disorder

The essential feature of attention-deficit/hyperactivity disorder (ADHD) is a persistent pattern of inattention and/or

Audiology: Diagnosis. Edited by Roeser, Valente, and Hosford-Dunn. Thieme Medical Publishers, Inc., New York © 2000

hyperactivity that is more frequent and severe than is typically observed in individuals at a normal level of development. The three subtypes of ADHD are based on the predominant symptom pattern. The subtypes include ADHD combined type, predominantly inattention type, and predominantly hyperactive-impulsive type. The prevalence of ADHD is estimated at 3 to 5% in school-age children. Diagnosis of ADHD is made on the basis of six or more of nine symptoms of inattention or six or more of nine symptoms of hyperactivity. The symptoms, taken from the DSM-IV manual, are listed in Table 15–1.

Learning Disorders

In the DSM-IV learning disorders includes reading, mathematics, and written expression. A diagnosis is made when achievement on individually administered standardized tests in one or more of the areas listed is substantially less than that

expected for age, schooling, and intelligence. Substantially below is usually defined as a discrepancy of more than 2 standard deviations between achievement and IQ. If a sensory deficit is present (e.g., hearing loss), the learning difficulties must be in excess of those usually associated with the deficit.

Associated features of learning disorders include demoralization, low self-esteem, and deficits in social skills. The prevalence of learning disorders range from 2 to 10%, with approximately 5% of students in public schools identified as having a learning disorder.

Communication Disorders

Communication disorders listed in the DSM-IV include expressive language disorder, mixed receptive-expressive language disorder, phonological disorder, stuttering, and communication disorder. Prevalence estimates average around 3% of school-age children for each category. Phonological disorders

TABLE 15–1 Diagnostic criteria for ADHD

A. Either (1) or (2)

  1. Six (or more) of the following symptoms of *inattention* have persisted for at least 6 months to a degree that is maladaptive and inconsistent with developmental level:

  Inattention
    a. Often fails to give close attention to details or makes careless mistakes in schoolwork or other activities
    b. Often has difficulty sustaining attention in tasks or lay activities
    c. Often does not seem to listen when spoken to directly
    d. Often does not follow through on insructions and fails to finish schoolwork, chores, or duties in the workplace (not caused by oppositional behavior or failure to understand instructions)
    e. Often has difficulty organizing tasks and activities
    f. Often avoids, dislikes, or is reluctant to engage in tasks that require sustained mental effort (such as schoolwork or homework)
    g. Often loses things necessary for tasks or activities (e.g., toys, school assignments, pencils, books, or tools)
    h. Often is easily distracted by extraneous stimuli
    i. Often is forgetful in daily activities

  2. Six (or more) of the following symptoms of *hyperactivity-impulsivity* have persisted for at least 6 months to a degree that is maladaptive and inconsistent with developmental level:

  Hyperactivity
    a. Often fidgets with hands or feet or squirms in seat
    b. Often leaves seat in classroom or in other situations in which remaining seated is expected
    c. Often runs about or climbs excessively in situations in which it is inappropriate (in adolescents or adults, may be limited to subjective feelings of restlessness)
    d. Often has difficulty playing or engaging in leisure activities quietly
    e. Often is "on the go" or often acts as if "driven by a motor"
    f. Often talks excessively

  Impulsivity
    g. Often blurts out answers before questions have been completed
    h. Often has difficulty awaiting turn
    i. Often interrupts or intrudes on others (e.g., butts into conversation or games)

B. Some hyperactive-impulsive or inattentive symptoms that caused impairment were present before 7 years of age.
C. Some impairment from the symptoms is present in two or more settings (e.g., at school [or work] and at home).
D. Clear evidence of clinically significant impairment in social, academic, or occupational functioning is present.
E. The symptoms do not occur exclusively during the course of a pervasive developmental disorder, schizophrenia, or other psychotic disorder and are not better accounted for by another mental disorder (e.g., mood disorder, anxiety disorder, dissociative disorder, or a personality disorder).

decrease in prevalence to 0.5% by the age of 17. Linguistic features of an expressive language disorder are many, including limited vocabulary, difficulty in acquiring new words, shortened sentences, simplified grammatical structure, and slow rate of language development. Expressive language disorder may be either acquired or developmental. Both are described as neurologically based, although the acquired type (usually) has a known neurological insult, whereas the neurological insult for the developmental type is not known.

The essential feature of a mixed receptive-expressive language disorder is an impairment in both receptive and expressive language scores. The comprehension deficit is the primary feature that differentiates this from expressive language disorder. The child may intermittently appear not to hear or to be confused or not paying attention when addressed. Deficits in various areas of sensory information processing are common, especially in temporal auditory processing (e.g., processing rate, association of sounds and symbols, sequence of sounds and memory, attention to and discrimination of sounds.) Other associated disorders are ADHD and developmental coordination disorder, among others.

The essential features of a phonological disorder include failure to use developmentally expected sounds that are appropriate for age and dialect. Audiologists may be more familiar with the previous diagnostic term, developmental articulation disorder or phonological disorder.

Central Auditory Processing Disorder

It is instructive to note that DSM-IV does not include a diagnostic category of CAPD. In a discussion of this "problem" that appeared on an Internet ListServe discussion, Watson (1997) (paraphrased here with permission) stated that:

. . . while many audiologists have written a variety of articles and books on CAPD, audiologists should recognize that they are not the only community of clinicians and scientists interested in the origins of learning disabilities, developmental language disorders, and reading disabilities. A review of the literature on those topics finds that very few of the major reviews in recent years have considered auditory (or visual) processing disorders to be major causes of those developmental problems. That is not, by any means, a proof that auditory and visual factors are not important causes of learning difficulties in some children . . . but it does suggest that the auditory and visual research communities have failed to convince many psychologists and educators that they are. The reasons may be partly territorial defense and other political-economic factors, but it is usually the case that those sorts of biases will give way to a large array of rigorously gathered evidence. That research communities have not been so swayed suggests that such evidence is yet to be gathered. . .

Cacace and McFarland (1998) argue that empirical evidence is not sufficient to validate the proposition that CAPD is a modality-specific perceptual dysfunction. Their argument is based on the controversy whether the definition of CAPD is to be inclusive (e.g., see the American Speech-Language-Hearing Association [ASHA] definition) or exclusive of *all* language and attentional processes that service acoustic signal processing.

An ICD-9 (AMA, 1996) diagnosis code has been established for auditory processing disorders (389.14, Central Hearing Loss). However, until CAPD is formally recognized by the DSM guidelines in the same way as ADHD, learning, and communication disorders, it will be difficult for audiologists to obtain reimbursement for testing. Using the DSM-IV guidelines as a model (First et al, 1995) a proposal for differential diagnosis of CAPD is shown in Table 15–2.

Again, *if* the DSM-IV (First et al, 1995) had a diagnostic criteria of CAPD it would read something like the following:

TABLE 15–2   A proposal for differential diagnosis of CAPD

CAPD must be differentiated from . . .	In contrast to **CAPD** the other condition . . .
Normal variations in auditory processing abilities	• Is not substantially below what is expected for a child's age level
Peripheral hearing impairment	• Is characterized by a unilateral or bilateral conductive or sensorineural hearing loss of any degree from mild to severe
Language impairment	• Is characterized by a phonological impairment, limited vocabulary, difficulty in acquiring new words, shortened sentences, simplified grammatical structure, and slow rate of language development
Learning disorder	• Is characterized by an impairment confined to a specific area of academic achievement (i.e., reading, arithmetic, writing skills)
Borderline intellectual functioning	• Is characterized by a degree of intellectual impairment
ADHD	• Is a persistent pattern of inattention and/or hyperactivity that is more frequent and severe than is typically observed in individuals at a normal level of development

1. Behaves as if a peripheral hearing loss was present, despite normal-hearing (Bellis, 1996, p.107)
2. Difficulty with auditory discrimination expressed as diminished ability to discriminate among speech sounds (phonemes)
3. Deficiencies in remembering phonemes and manipulating them (e.g., on tasks such as reading, spelling, and phonics, as well as phonemic synthesis or analysis) (Katz et al, 1992, p. 84)
4. Difficulty understanding speech in the presence of background noise
5. Difficulty with auditory memory, either span or sequence; unable to remember auditory information or follow multiple instructions
6. Demonstrates scatter across subtests with domains assessed by speech-language and psychoeducational tests, with weaknesses in auditory-dependent areas (Bellis, 1996, p. 107)
7. Poor listening skills characterized by decreased attention for auditory information; distractible or restless in listening situations
8. Inconsistent responses to auditory information (sometimes responds appropriately, sometimes not) or inconsistent auditory awareness (one-to-one conversation is better than in a group) (Hall & Mueller, 1997, p. 555)
9. Receptive and/or expressive language disorder; may have a discrepancy between expressive and receptive language skills
10. Difficulty understanding rapid speech or persons with an unfamiliar dialect
11. Poor musical abilities, does not recognize sound patterns or rhythms; poor vocal prosody in speech production

A child must exhibit at least four of these nine symptoms to receive a diagnosis of CAPD. In addition, the symptoms must be present for at least 6 months. Furthermore, the symptoms must deviate from mental age; that is, the behavior is considerably more frequent and intense than that of most children of the same age. If these criteria are met, it would be reasonable to conclude that the child has CAPD.

PEARL

The reader should remember that the proposed models for differential diagnosis of CAPD and diagnostic criteria for CAPD exist in my mind only. The models are proposed in an attempt to demonstrate how things *might* be if CAPD existed in the DSM-IV guidelines.

FURTHER DEFINITION OF CENTRAL AUDITORY PROCESSING DISORDER

In 1995 an ASHA Task Force on Central Auditory Processing Consensus Development met to define central auditory processing and its disorders. A second purpose was to define how the disorders can be identified and ameliorated through intervention.

According to the task force *central auditory processes* are the *auditory system* mechanisms and processes responsible for the following behavioral phenomena:

- Sound localization and lateralization
- Auditory discrimination
- Auditory pattern recognition
- Temporal aspects of audition, including
  Temporal resolution
  Temporal masking
  Temporal integration
  Temporal ordering
- Auditory performance decrements with competing acoustic signals
- Auditory performance decrements with degraded acoustic signals

According to the ASHA statement these mechanisms and processes are presumed to apply to nonverbal and verbal signals and to affect many areas of function, including speech and language. They have neurophysiological and behavioral correlates. Furthermore, many neurocognitive mechanisms and processes are engaged in recognition and discrimination tasks. Some are specifically dedicated to acoustic signals, whereas others (e.g., attentional processes, long-term language representations) are not. With respect to these nondedicated mechanisms and processes, the term *central auditory processes* refers particularly to their deployment in the service of acoustic signal processing.

The ASHA consensus statement defines a CAPD as an observed deficiency in one or more of the behaviors previously listed. For some persons, CAPD is presumed to result from the dysfunction of processes and mechanisms dedicated to audition; for others, CAPD may stem from some more general dysfunction, such as an attention deficit or neural timing deficit, that affects performance across modalities. It is also possible for CAPD to reflect coexisting dysfunctions of both sorts.

THE NEED TO DEVELOP SPECIFIC SUBGROUPS (CATEGORIES) OF CENTRAL AUDITORY DISORDERS

Jerger and Allen (1998) point out that the lack of specificity of central auditory test batteries "can complicate the remediation and management of children diagnosed as having CAPD on the basis of such measures." Their philosophical position is that "our goals should be reoriented toward determining the normalcy/abnormalcy of the component processes involved in spoken word recognition." In practical terms that philosophy translates into determining subtypes of CAPDs in children. Some efforts are being made in that regard at the time of this writing, although more is required. For example, on the basis of the Staggered Spondaic Word Test results, Katz and his colleagues (1992) developed a model that can be used for understanding the CAPD and developing a remediation program. His model includes four categories: phonemic decoding, tolerance-fading memory, integration, and organization. Bellis (1996, p. 193) describes four categories of disorders including auditory decoding

TABLE 15–3 Remediation algorithm based on results of central auditory test

Disorder	Remediation
Disorder of temporal processing	Perceptual training (modify speaker rate, auditory discrimination, phoneme training, computer-assisted remediation [e.g., Fast ForWord])
Disorder of auditory figure ground or other monaural degraded speech test	Reduce noise in environment Classroom management, including preferential seating Use of frequency modulation system or other assistive listening device
Disorders of binaural separation/maturation	Receptive and expressive language remediation usually provided by a speech-language pathologist

deficit, integration deficit, association deficit, and output-organization deficit. Both Katz and Bellis recommend management suggestions on the basis of the CAPD category to which the child is assigned. Similarly, Fallis-Cunningham and Keith (1998) proposed that decisions for remediation should be made on the basis of results of central auditory tests. Table 15–3 provides examples of this model.

These models for categorizing subgroups of CAPDs should be viewed with some caution. It should be clear that the subgroup categories are simplistic, often without clear definition or agreement of what tests or test findings place a child in a certain category. Nevertheless, they represent early efforts to systematize the assessment and remediation of CAPD.

AUDITORY NEUROPATHY

An auditory problem apparently related to, but different from, a typical CAPD is auditory neuropathy. Among audiologists awareness was growing in the 1980s and 1990s of a group of children who fell under a variety of labels including central auditory dysfunction, brain stem auditory processing syndrome, auditory neural synchrony disorder, and finally auditory neuropathy. The basis of this disorder appears to be some combination of problems between the axon terminal of the inner hair cell and dendrite of the spiral ganglion neurons or the axons of the spiral ganglion neuron with the auditory nerve in their course to the brain stem (Stein et al, 1996). Starr et al (1996) provided further information to suggest that auditory neuropathy is an auditory nerve disorder. At this writing the exact cause of auditory neuropathy and its prevalence is unknown. According to Sininger et al (1995) and Hood (1998), the symptoms seen in auditory neuropathy include the following:

- Mild to moderate elevation of auditory thresholds to pure tones by air and bone conduction
- Present otoacoustic emissions (OAEs)
- Absent acoustic reflexes to ipsilateral and contralateral tones
- Absent to severely abnormal auditory brain stem responses in response to high-level stimuli and inability to suppress OAE
- Word recognition ability poorer than expected for pure tone hearing loss configuration

- Absent masking level differences (MLDs)

Sininger states further that one of the characteristics of auditory neuropathy is that intervention appropriate for sensory hearing loss, such as conventional amplification, is not beneficial in these cases. Stein et al (1996) point out the dilemma raised by a failed screening auditory brain stem response and passed OAE when OAEs are used in infant hearing screening programs, as recommended by the NIH Consensus Statement (1993). Those children may be considered to have "normal-hearing" when auditory neuropathy is present. The problems of auditory neuropathy are beyond the scope of this chapter, but the reader should be aware of its existence. Furthermore, Sininger et al (1995) states that auditory neuropathy and CAPD are different entities because "CAPD is characterized by normal-hearing while auditory neuropathy involves the peripheral auditory system and hearing loss." According to Starr et al (1996), auditory neuropathy "could be one etiology for some cases with the disorder known as central auditory processing disorder," especially those in whom pure tone thresholds were elevated. Whether they are different or whether auditory neuropathy is a subset of central auditory processing disorders is still to be determined.

WHEN AND WHO TO REFER AND ON WHAT BASIS

In addition to the diagnostic criteria for CAPD listed previously, some of the following behaviors appear to be characteristic of children with CAPDs:

1. They are often male. According to Arcia and Conners (1998) two theories are proposed to explain this phenomenon. According to one theory girls have a relatively higher threshold to insult than boys. Another is that boys have a relatively more genetic variability. They might be affected more frequently than girls because their relatively slower development results in a longer period than girls have of immaturity and susceptibility to insult.

2. They have normal pure tone hearing thresholds. Some have a significant history of chronic otitis media that has been treated or resolved.

3. They generally respond inconsistently to auditory stimuli. They often respond appropriately, but at other times they seem unable to follow auditory instructions.

4. They may have difficulty with auditory localization skills. This may include an inability to tell how close or far away the source of the sound is and an inability to differentiate soft and loud sounds. There have been frequent reports that these children become frightened and upset when they are exposed to loud noise and often hold their hands over their ears to stop the sound.

5. They may listen attentively but have difficulty following long or complicated verbal commands or instructions.

6. They frequently request that information be repeated.

7. They have poor listening skills. They require a substantial amount of time to answer questions. They have difficulty relating what is heard or to the words seen on paper. They may be unable to appreciate jokes, puns, or other humorous twists of language.

In addition to specific auditory behaviors, many of these children have significant reading problems, are poor spellers, and have poor handwriting. They may have articulation or language disorders. In the classroom they may act out frustrations that result from their perceptual deficits or they may be shy and withdrawn because of the poor self-concept that results from multiple failures.

These examples are only a few of the behaviors that are associated with CAPD. Not every child with an auditory processing problem will exhibit all of the behaviors mentioned. The number of problems experienced by a given child will be an expression of the severity of the CAPD, with symptoms ranging from mild to severe.

The reader will recognize that the behaviors listed above are not unique to children with CAPD. They are common to children with peripheral hearing loss, attention deficit disorders, allergies, and other problems. It should not bother clinicians to find similar behaviors among children with various auditory and language-learning disorders. Children (and adults) are capable of a limited repertoire of responses to the problems of life. However, children with similar behaviors may have very different underlying causes and do not represent a homogenous group. It is the clinician's task to determine the true underlying deficit or deficits among children with similar behaviors and to recommend the appropriate remediation approach for each child.

QUESTIONNAIRES

Checklists of Central Auditory Processing

Several checklists exist to assist school personnel in identifying children who may benefit from central auditory testing. Unfortunately, some have never been validated, including the Fishers (1976) Auditory Problems Checklist and a checklist developed by Willeford and Burleigh (1985). Sanger et al (1985) developed the Checklist of Classroom Observations for Children with Possible Auditory Processing Problems. This 23-item questionnaire was devised for educators to record and rate their observations of children's behavior throughout

a typical day. Teachers rate the behaviors according to the frequency observed. Behaviors addressed include inattentiveness, reading or spelling problems, and recurring ear infections.

One tool useful in reviewing children's behavior is the Children's Auditory Processing Performance Scale (CHAPPS) developed by Smoski et al (1992) to systematically collect and quantify the observed listening behaviors of children. CHAPPS is a questionnaire consisting of 36 items concerning listening behavior in a variety of listening conditions and functions. According to the authors, the clinical applications of this scale are to identify children who should be referred for a CAP evaluation and to prescribe and measure the effects of therapeutic intervention. At this writing CHAPPS is available through the Educational Audiology Association.

A Checklist of Attention and Hyperactivity

The Conners' ADHD/DSM-IV Scales (CADS) (1997) is useful in quantifying parent and teacher perceptions of a child's attention and hyperactivity. This screening tool asks how much caregivers think the child is bothered on 12 questions of restlessness, distractibility, impulsivity, etc. The items are designed to differentiate children with ADHD from normal children. When concern is high, the audiologist may want to determine whether reported behaviors are due to attention deficit disorder or problems with central auditory processing.

HISTORY

The assessment should begin with careful observation of the child, with particular attention to the auditory behavior patterns described previously in this chapter. Care should be taken to identify strengths and weaknesses and to note performance in other modalities, including vision, motor coordination, tactile response, speech, and language.

When possible, an in-depth history from the child's caregiver should be taken. Many years ago Rosenberg (1978) called the case history "the first test" because of the value of the information obtained. He pointed out that a carefully taken history can be extremely useful in differentiating among various problems, can supplement results from auditory tests, and can help in making a decision about the child's educational management.

The case history should be taken systematically to avoid missing important information. The person taking the history should provide an opportunity for the caregiver to state concerns about the child, to describe the child's behaviors, and to express any other related concerns. Specific information that should be requested includes information about: (1) the family; (2) the mother's pregnancy; (3) conditions at birth, the child's growth and development, health, and illnesses; (4) general behavior and socioemotional development; (5) speech and language development; (6) hearing and auditory behavior; and (7) educational progress. The specific questions asked of parents will depend on the setting in which the testing is being done and the purpose of the examination. Areas to be investigated in the history when a CAPD is suspected are given in Table 15–4.

TABLE 15–4 Information model for taking a case history (Keith)

Area	Information Needed
Family history	History of any family member's difficulty in school achievement; the language spoken in the home
Pregnancy and birth	Unusual problems during pregnancy or delivery; abnormalities present in the child at birth
Health and illness	Childhood illnesses, neurological problems, history of seizure, psychological trauma, head trauma or injury, middle ear disease, allergies; drugs or medications prescribed by the physician
General behavior and social-emotional development	Age-appropriate play behavior, social isolation, impulsiveness withdrawal, aggression, tact, sensitivity to others, self-discipline
Speech and language development	Evidence of articulation or receptive/expressive language disorder; ability to communicate ideas verbally; ability to formulate sentences correctly; appropriateness of verbal expression to subject or situation
Hearing and auditory behavior	Ability to localize sounds auditorily; ability to identify the sound with its source; reaction to sudden, unexpected sound; ability to ignore environmental sounds; tolerance to loud sounds; consistency of response to sound; need to have spoken information repeated; ability to follow verbal instructions, listen for appropriate length of time, remember things heard, pay attention to what is said, comprehend words and their meaning, understand multiple meanings of words, understand abstract ideas; discrepancies between auditory and visual behavior
Nonauditory behavior	Motor coordination: gross, fine, and eye-hand; hand dominance; visual perception; spatial orientation; any unusual reaction to touch
Educational history and progress	History of progress in school; reading, math, musical, and art ability

ASSESSMENT: BEFORE CENTRAL AUDITORY TESTING

Testing for Peripheral Hearing Loss Including Conductive and Sensorineural Impairment

Before any attempt is made to diagnose a child as having CAPD, it is necessary to rule out the presence of a peripheral hearing loss of the conductive or sensorineural type. Therefore comprehensive audiometry, including pure tone air and bone conduction threshold tests, middle ear measures, and speech audiometry (see Chapters 11, 13, and 17), should be administered before the central auditory tests. Recent evidence indicates the additional value of obtaining otoacoustic emissions (see Chapter 21) before central auditory processing testing.

In general, central auditory testing is done when hearing is within normal limits, defined as thresholds between 0- and 15-dB Hearing Level for the frequencies 500 through 4000 Hz and within 5 dB for adjacent octave frequencies. When a unilateral hearing loss is present, only monaural sensitized speech tests can be administered. When a sloping hearing loss is present, it may be necessary to identify central auditory tests that can be administered at frequencies of "normal" hearing.

When children have a recent history of otitis media, a single hearing test performed on a child may not be adequate.

> **PITFALL**
>
> Care must be taken to identify any conductive or sensorineural hearing loss before central auditory testing. Unrecognized peripheral hearing loss will contaminate central auditory test results and invalidate findings.

Fluctuating hearing loss associated with allergies or colds makes it unwise to administer central auditory tests based on a previous hearing test. Until recently little information was available on the long-term effects of early and prolonged otitis media with static or fluctuating hearing loss on central auditory abilities. Evidence is growing that otitis media can cause auditory learning problems and is not the innocuous disease that it was once considered to be (Menyuk 1992). The residual effects can be central auditory processing problems that may cause language and learning delays that persist long after the middle ear disease has been resolved (Gravel & Ellis, 1995). Therefore children with histories of frequent colds or chronic middle ear disease should be carefully watched for signs of CAPD.

BEHAVIORAL TESTS OF CENTRAL AUDITORY PROCESSING ABILITIES

Some Background Information on Sensitized Speech Test

Central auditory testing has a rich history going back to the early 1950s. Many of the principles developed at that time are relevant to today's practicing audiologist. Some examples of early work in central auditory testing include Bocca, Calearo, and Antonelli's work on sensitized speech testing in the 1950s (summarized by Calearo & Antonelli, 1973), Matzker's (1959) early work on binaural fusion, Berlin et al (1973) research on dichotic consonant vowel performance, Katz's Staggered Spondee Word Test (1962), Jerger's Distorted Speech Test (1960), the Speech with Alternating Masking Index (1964), and many others. Calearo and Antonelli (1973) summarized a number of principles that explain how auditory messages are handled by the normal central nervous system. They include the following:

- Channel separation: A signal delivered to one ear is kept distinct from a different signal in the other ear.

- Binaural fusion: If a single auditory message is divided into segments and these are delivered biaurally and simultaneously, fusion will take place (at the brain stem level) and the subject will experience one message only.

- Contralateral pathways: Auditory messages from one ear cross at the brain stem level and reach the temporal lobe of the opposite side.

- Hemisphere dominance for language: Although one cerebral hemisphere (usually the left) is verbally dominant, the other hemisphere appears to possess limited verbal abilities. Adding to Bocca and Calearo, we now understand that linguistic information reaching the nondominant hemisphere (the right hemisphere from information presented to the left ear) crosses to the dominant language hemisphere through the densely myelinated fibers in the splenium of the corpus callosum.

Related to the above, some additional principles apply to central auditory assessment. They are as follows:

- Most diseases affecting central hearing pathways produce no loss in threshold sensitivity. Therefore pure tone tests do not generally identify CAPD.

- Undistorted speech audiometry is not sufficiently challenging to the central auditory nervous system to identify the presence of a central auditory lesion/disorder.

- Only tests of reduced acoustic redundancy (distorted speech materials called sensitized speech tests by Teatini [1970]) are sufficiently challenging to the auditory nervous system to identify a central auditory lesion/disorder.

The rationale for sensitized speech testing was further described by Jerger (1960) as the "subtlety principle," in which the subtlety of the auditory manifestation increases as the site of lesion progresses from peripheral to central. More recently Phillips (1995) described these processes in a somewhat different way as "patterns of convergence and divergence in the ascending auditory pathway."

Sensitized speech tests use various means of distortion of the speech stimuli to reduce the intelligibility of the message. Distortion can be accomplished by reducing the range of frequencies in the speech signal, by filtering (filtered speech testing), by reducing the intensity level of speech above a simultaneously presented background noise (auditory figure ground testing), by interrupting the speech at different rates, and by increasing the rate of presentation (time-compressed speech). The basic principle of sensitized speech testing is that a distorted message can be understood by persons with normal-hearing and a normal central auditory system. However, when a central auditory disorder is present, speech intelligibility is poor. The construct of sensitized speech testing is extremely powerful and forms the basis of all behavioral speech tests of central auditory function.

Transition from Site of Lesion to Auditory Learning Disabilities

Most of the distortions of speech used in the diagnosis of the site of the lesion in adults are also used to identify CAPD in children. An excellent example is the Staggered Spondee Word Test (Katz, 1962) that was originally designed to identify cortical lesions in adults. Later the test was successfully applied for identifying CAPD in children. Bornstein and Musiek (1984) stated that "Many of that tasks that were developed to identify site of central auditory nervous system pathology in adults have been used to assess performance of children with various communication problems. Although medically significant pathology affecting the auditory system may be present in children, the primary use of these tasks is to describe the child's performance and how it relates to behavior and communication development. Performance difficulties on these tasks may reflect a dysfunction or a maturational delay of the central auditory nervous system, that precludes adequate perception and therefore optimum speech and language development."

One of the difficulties that occurred in the transition to CAPD testing was the continued use of terms inferring the existence of an auditory "lesion" to describe test findings when no specific lesion existed. The language of central auditory lesion frightened and confused parents. More recently descriptions of auditory performance are based on neuromaturation, hemispheric function, developmental delays, relationships with language impairment and learning disorders, and so on. Also, terminology that describes auditory abilities and disorders is more useful in the design of remediation strategies for affected children.

TEST BATTERY APPROACH TO CENTRAL AUDITORY TESTING

Some attempts have been made to develop algorithms for approaching central auditory assessment in the past (e.g., Bellis, 1996; Hall and Mueller, 1997, Chapter 11, p. 507; Matkin & Hook, 1983; Willeford, 1985, Chapter 14). Because no standard approach to testing existed, audiologists chose from a variety of tests on the basis of their best understanding of the disorder. The disparity of approaches left the professions, and the consumer, confused about CAPDs and remediation.

The 1995 American Speech-Language-Hearing Association (ASHA) report on Central Auditory Processing: Current Status of Research and Implications for Clinical Practice recommended a central auditory test battery on the basis of those mechanisms and processes that are responsible for central auditory processing. The assessment recommended by the panel includes the following:

- History
- Observation of auditory behaviors
- Audiologic test procedures
  - Pure tones, speech recognition, immittance
  - Temporal processes
  - Localization and lateralization
  - Low-redundancy monaural speech
  - Dichotic stimuli
  - Binaural interaction procedures
- Speech-language pathology measures

The panel recommendations provide a framework for a systematic approach to the diagnosis of central processing disorders. That framework standardizes test battery approaches and reduces confusion for consumers and professionals alike. The panel also points out that some measures of auditory function have questionable validity and reliability and have inadequate normative data. The need for understanding the statistical properties of tests that are chosen for central auditory testing cannot be overemphasized. Readers are urged to learn about these concepts and apply them to their clinical practice. Many reasons exist for using well-standardized tests. They include the ability to properly interpret test results and determine with confidence the child's auditory processing abilities. Results from standardized tests can be compared directly with results obtained by other professionals, including speech-language pathologists, psychologists, and others. In addition, parents of affected children can be very sophisticated (through information available on Web sites and other sources) in asking questions about properties of tests being administered to their children. As professionals we need to be able to answer those questions.

SUGGESTED CENTRAL AUDITORY TESTS

Temporal Processes

According to the 1995 ASHA consensus statement, central auditory processes include, among other behavioral phenomena, temporal aspects of audition including temporal resolution, temporal masking, temporal integration, and temporal ordering. The diagnosis of a CAPD is accomplished by use of a variety of indices, including behavioral auditory measures that include... "tests of temporal processes—ordering, discrimination, resolution (e.g., gap detection), and integration."

Many reasons exist for assessing temporal processing during a central auditory test battery. According to Thompson and Abel (1992), the ability to process basic acoustic parameters such as frequency and duration may predict speech intelligibility. Discrimination of a change in frequency is essential for distinguishing place of articulation in stops and manner in stops and glides. The acoustic cue for place in stops is

formant transition (i.e., a rapid change in frequency over a limited time interval). Discrimination of a change in duration likely underlies the recognition of voice contrasts in stops, timing of silent bursts in fricatives, and differentiation of vowel length. Thus deficits in ability to "hear" small differences in timing aspects of ongoing speech create speech discrimination errors, even though hearing thresholds may be normal. According to Bornstein and Musiek (1984), temporal perceptual impairment has negative linguistic implications for children. For example, duration cues play a role in phoneme identification and in providing linguistic cues.

In research conducted over many years, Tallal and her associates (Merzenich et al, 1996; Tallal et al, 1993; Tallal et al, 1996) contend that dysfunction of higher level speech processing, necessary for normal language and reading development, may result from difficulties in the processing of basic sensory information. One component of basic sensory information is the role that temporal processing plays in relation to identification of brief phonetic elements presented in speech contexts (Tallal et al, 1996). Tallal states that ". . . rather than deriving from a primarily linguistic or cognitive impairment, the phonological and language difficulties of language-learning impaired children may result from a basic deficit in processing rapidly changing sensory inputs" (p. 81). She proposes that temporal deficits disrupt normal development of an efficient phonological system and that these phonological processing deficits result in subsequent failure to speak and read normally (Tallal et al, 1993). A brief summary of the work of Tallal and her associates is that processing of rapidly occurring acoustic information is critically involved in the development and maintenance of language. In fact, language-impaired children differ considerably from normally developing children in the rate at which they access sensory information. Tallal's research led to the development of the computerized remediation program called Fast ForWord that is discussed in *Treatment*.

The Auditory Fusion Threshold Test-Revised

The Auditory Fusion Test-Revised (AFT-R) (McCroskey and Keith, 1996) is designed to measure temporal resolution that is one aspect of audition discussed by the ASHA (1995) consensus panel. The method of evaluating temporal resolution in the AFT-R is through determination of the auditory fusion threshold (AFT). The AFT is measured in milliseconds and is obtained by having a listener attend to a series of pure tones presented in pairs. The silent time interval (the interpulse interval) between each pair of tones increases and decreases in duration. As the silent interval changes, the listener reports whether the stimulus pairs are heard as one tone or two tones. The AFT is the average of the points at which the two tones, for the ascending and descending interpulse interval series, are perceptually fused and heard as one. This stimulus protocol is sometimes called "gap detection."

Among the underlying assumptions for this test procedure include the understanding that (1) the acoustic signals that comprise a spoken language have a basis in time, (2) the learning of these temporally bound acoustic signals requires a listening system that can detect the smallest time segment that is part of the spoken language code, and (3) individuals whose auditory systems have varying degrees of temporal processing disorders will exhibit varying kinds of verbal disabilities.

The AFT-R may disclose a temporal processing disorder that can account for language learning problems. The AFT-R is viewed as a test of temporal integrity at the level of the cortex. Even though it is a cortical measure, the test has a low linguistic and cognitive load (e.g., the listener must simply respond by indicating whether one or two tone pulses were heard).

PEARL

Tests using pure tones are thought to reflect nonlinguistic processing.

Duration Patterns Test

The Duration Patterns Test (Musiek et al, 1991) is a sequence of three consecutive 1000 Hz tones, with one differing by being either longer (L), 500 ms, or shorter (S), 200 ms, in duration than the other two tones in the sequence. The tones have a rise/fall time of 10 ms and an interstimulus interval of 300 ms. Six different sequences, LLS, LSL, LSS, SLS, SLL, and SSL, are used in the test. A total of 30 to 50 three-tone sequences are presented monaurally or binaurally at 50 dB re: spondee threshold (ST). Before testing, 5 to 10 practice items are provided to each subject to ensure their understanding of the task (Hurley & Musiek, 1997). The subjects respond to each stimulus presentation with a verbal description of the sequence heard, pointing response, and/or humming. A percent correct score is computed with performance less than 70% considered abnormal by some investigators, although normative data are limited, especially for children at the time of this writing (Hall & Mueller, 1997, p. 535). According to Musiek and his coauthors, the duration patterns test is sensitive to cerebral lesions while remaining unaffected by peripheral hearing loss.

Localization and Lateralization

The ASHA consensus conference recommended inclusion of tests of localization and lateralization in a central auditory test battery on the basis of the relationship between brain stem function and "neural coding of sound time structure" (Phillips, 1995). For example, according to Phillips, determining the location of a sound source requires "temporal processing" in that an acoustic cue underlying the spatial perception is the relative timing of signals arriving at the two ears. Localization refers to the perception of the direction a sound comes from in space for the case of free field stimulation. Lateralization refers to the perceived place a sound seems to occupy within the head, for the case of stimulation using earphones (Watson, 1994). Although these phenomena have been extensively studied by psychoacousticians, little clinical research on abnormalities of localization and lateralization has occurred. Jerger and Harford (1960) described abnormalities of simultaneous median plane localization in patients with brain stem lesions.

Devers et al (1978) studied "dynamic auditory localization" in children who were from regular classrooms and children from self-contained learning disability classrooms. By having the children track a moving sound in a geometric (triangle) pattern, they found significant differences between the two groups of children. Devers et al proposed that results

suggested a difference in binaural integration abilities of the children with learning disabilities. They cautioned against concluding that a causal relationship exists between the poor tracking ability and the learning disability. Nevertheless, this research provided early insights into perceptual problems that may be experienced by children with CAPD.

Recently interest in children with "hyperacusis", a frequent complaint among children with learning disabilities, is growing. Marriage (1996) defines hyperacusis as abnormal loudness discomfort caused by sounds that would be acceptable to most listeners. The symptoms are typically an aversion to loud sound of any kind, with apparent lowering of the loudness discomfort threshold in persons with normal-hearing. I use the term "dysfunctional three-dimensional auditory space" to describe the apparent inability of some children to recognize how near or far away a sound source is and their constant fear of loud sounds. Clearly more research is needed to understand these problems of localization, lateralization, and hyperacusis among children with CAPD.

Low-Redundancy Monaural Speech

The purposes of assessing low-redundancy monaural speech during a central auditory test battery are as follows. Speech in noise testing, commonly called auditory figure ground testing (AFG), has been administered for many years on patients with all types of lesions. Results of testing has found that AFG testing can identify abnormalities in auditory function but cannot precisely determine the site of lesion in the auditory system (Olsen et al, 1975). Similarly, it is generally known that results of low-pass filtered word testing is poorer for the ear contralateral to a temporal lobe lesion compared with the ipsilateral side. However, brain stem lesions may result in decreased performance on the ipsilateral or contralateral ear. Thus as Rintlemann (1985) correctly states, "It is difficult to establish good correlation between test results and the locus of the brain stem pathology. Hence, the primary purpose of these tests is in identifying lesions of the central auditory system rather than localizing them." The same general comment can be made for other degraded speech tests including interrupted and time-compressed speech. A current view of low-redundancy monaural speech testing is to determine *functional disorders of auditory communication,* a term coined by Bergman et al (1987).

One of the most common complaints among children with auditory processing disorders is their inability to communicate when background noise is present. Therefore speech-in-noise testing may be indicated to identify when the child's ability to communicate in the presence of noise is substantially below what is expected for a child's age level. For that reason, it may be beneficial to use different competing signals (e.g., a single speaker versus multitalker speech babble background) at different signal-to-noise ratios (e.g., +8, +4, and zero dB). Research finds that linguistic materials (e.g., multitalker speech babble background noise) are more effective maskers than speech-spectrum noise (SSN), even though the SSN has the same long-term spectrum and amplitude as the meaningful multitalker competing message (Sperry et al, 1997). Other research finds that white noise and narrow band noise are also less effective than speech babble for masking speech. A great deal of variability exists among normal subjects in their ability to discriminate speech in a noise background. As a consequence, when speech-in-noise testing is done to identify central auditory processing disorders, it is important to know the cut off of normal performance for the signal-to-noise ratio and type of noise used in the test.

Few tests of central auditory function are designed to be administered to very young children. One test that includes competing messages that is available for children younger than 6 years is the Pediatric Speech Intelligibility (PSI) test (Jerger, 1987). The PSI consists of monosyllabic word and sentence material with both ipsilateral and contralateral competing messages. Testing is carried out by presenting a sentence or word target and requiring the child to point to the picture corresponding to the sentence or word that was heard. The test is said to be insensitive to developmental differences in cognitive skills and receptive language abilities while being sensitive to the presence of lesions of the central auditory pathways and central auditory processing disorders.

PEARL

Some tests of low-redundancy monaural speech include the following: Pediatric Speech Intelligibility (PSI) test (Jerger, 1987); auditory figure ground and filtered words subtests of SCAN (Keith, 1986) and SCAN-A (Keith, 1994a); high-pass and low-pass filtered speech (VA CD, 1992); and time-compressed speech (VA CD, 1992). Another resource for prerecorded central auditory tests is Auditec (St. Louis, MO).

One proposal for differentiating children with AFG problems and those with ADHD is to administer tests of AFG and auditory vigilance. The rationale for this test approach is that children with CAPD will have difficulty on the AFG but not on tests of auditory vigilance. Children with ADHD will have problems with vigilance but not AFG. When both CAPD and ADHD exist, it may not be possible to separate these co-morbid conditions (Riccio et al 1996). The Auditory Continuous Performance Test (ACPT) (Keith, 1994a) was designed to measure a child's selective attention (indicated by correct responses to specific linguistic cues) and sustained attention (indicated by a child's ability to maintain attention and concentration on a task for an extended period of time). The child listens to a series of familiar monosyllabic words presented at 1/s over 11 continuous minutes. A target word (dog) is presented randomly throughout the test. Errors of omission (misses) and commission (false alarms) are scored. Early validation studies found that the ACPT (Keith, 1994b) correctly identified ADHD 70% of the time. Subsequently, Briggs et al (1998) found that the ACPT correctly identified 86% of children with ADHD.

Another degraded speech task commonly used to identify functional disorders of communication during central auditory testing is the filtered word test. Originally designed to identify temporal lobe tumors in adult patients (Calearo & Antonelli, 1973) low-pass filtered word testing is now used to identify auditory processing disorders in children and adults with CAPD. Obviously, except for telephones and sound systems with poor frequency ranges, filtered speech is seldom encountered in the "real world." The rationale for testing is that individuals with normal-hearing who find it difficult to understand filtered words probably have difficulty understanding degraded speech of many kinds. The inability to resist acoustic distortions in everyday situations provides obstacles to communication for persons so affected.

Low-pass filtered word tests are a category of tests in which speech is degraded by removing part of the frequency spectrum. Some authors consider this a test of auditory closure that is defined as the ability to understand the whole word or message when part is missing. Early research (Willeford, 1976) showed reduced performance on filtered word testing in children who are poor listeners who have central auditory dysfunction. Willeford's early studies have been subsequently verified by other authors (Costello, 1977; Deitrich et al, 1992; Keith & Farrer, 1981). Presumably the child with CAPD is unable to resist acoustic distortions of speech, resulting in poor listening abilities in acoustic environments that are less than optimal.

Filtered word tests are available with different cut-off frequencies and filter slopes (Bornstein et al, 1994; Keith, 1986; Keith, 1994b). Because filtered word test results are particularly vulnerable to high-frequency hearing loss, it is important to rule out peripheral hearing loss before testing. In addition, as with all central auditory testing, it is important to know the mean and range of scores obtained on normal subjects for the filter conditions used.

Dichotic Stimuli

Dichotic speech testing is typically administered to determine hemispheric dominance for language shown by asymmetrical ear responses. A second purpose is to assess neuromaturational development of the auditory system. Dichotic listening tests involve the simultaneous presentation of different acoustic stimuli to the two ears. Commonly used stimuli include digits, consonant-vowel nonsense syllables incorporating the six stop consonants [p, t, k, b, d, g] paired with the vowel /a/, word, spondees, and sentences (Berlin et al, 1993). With the exception of the Staggered Spondee Word Test (SSW), the dichotic signals are recorded with simultaneous alignment of onset and off times. Tests are generally administered at comfortable listening levels with earphones. The listener is required to repeat or write what is heard. Two types of listening instructions are given to subjects, free recall or directed ear testing. Free recall allows the subject to respond to whatever was heard in either ear. Directed ear testing requires the subject to report what is heard in the right or the left ear first. Tests vary whether they require reporting of what was heard in one or both ears. When instructions require the subject to respond to both stimuli, the first ear reported will show better scores and higher reliability than the second ear reported. Because the right ear performance is typically better in young subjects, reflecting the ear to dominant hemisphere relationship, children will usually report what is heard in the right ear first under free recall conditions. Therefore directed ear listening provides better estimates of the true ear score difference and reliability of test scores in the left ear. Directed ear listening provides additional diagnostic information. For example, Obrzut et al (1981) found that children with learning disabilities exhibited a marked switch in ear advantage on directed right and directed left ear first responses. That is, they yielded a right ear advantage when directed to respond from the right ear first and a left ear advantage when directed to respond from the left ear first.

In general, for normal subjects, all dichotic test results show a right ear advantage under free recall and directed ear testing. A right ear advantage is typically present whether the child is right or left handed. For one thing, handedness does not necessarily indicate hemispheric dominance for language (Knox & Roeser, 1980). Furthermore, years ago Satz (1976) reported that a strong right ear advantage is an extremely probable predictor of left hemispheric specialization for speech and language function. However, Satz found that a left ear advantage predicts right hemispheric function for language only rarely. The greater the linguistic content of the signal (going from consonant vowels to words, spondees, and sentences) the larger the right ear advantage (the larger the difference between the right and left ear scores). As the central auditory nervous system matures, the left ear scores improve and the right ear advantage gets progressively smaller. At age 11 or 12 the auditory system is adultlike in terms of performance on dichotic testing. These principles are shown in Figure 15–1, where typical results of a normal 6-year-old child are shown for dichotic consonant-vowel syllables, words from SCAN (Keith, 1986), spondees from the SSW (Katz, 1977), and competing sentences (Willeford, 1977). Typical findings for a normal 11-year-old are shown in Figure 15–2. The figure shows improvement in both left and right ear scores, with narrowing of the ear difference for all but dichotic consonant-vowel test results that remain essentially unchanged from childhood through adulthood.

The interpretation of abnormal dichotic speech tests follows:

1. Poor overall performance
2. Enhanced right ear advantage in the directed-right condition and enhanced left ear advantage in the directed-left condition
3. A marked left ear advantage for both directed-right and directed-left ear conditions

Abnormal performance on dichotic tests indicates delays in auditory maturation, underlying neurological disorganization or damage to auditory pathways. Left ear advantages for all test conditions indicate the possibility of damage to the auditory reception areas of the left hemisphere or failure to develop left hemisphere dominance for language. These abnormalities are related to a wide range of specific learning disabilities, including CAPDs, language, learning, and reading. Longitudinal testing will help the audiologist discern whether maturation is occurring. If repeat testing after an appropriate interval (e.g., a year) shows little change or no change in dichotic test scores, it is likely that the central auditory system is damaged or disordered. The greater the disorder, the more likely that residual deficits will remain in later years.

Binaural Interaction Procedures
Masking Level Differences

The MLD refers to the difference between thresholds obtained under two binaural masking paradigms termed homophasic and antiphasic. According to Wilson et al (1994),

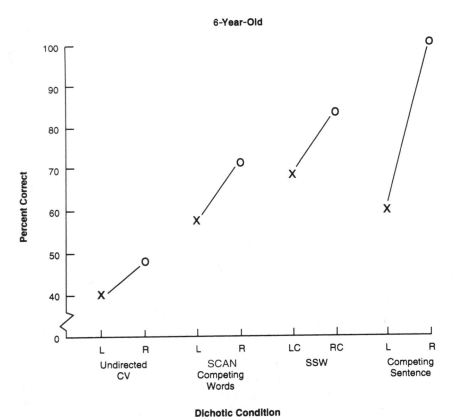

6-Year-Old

Figure 15–1 Typical results of dichotic listening tests expected from a normal 6-year-old. Responses are reported for dichotic consonant-vowel tests for undirected ear listening conditions. The SCAN competing words test, competing conditions of the SSW, and the Competing Sentence Test of the Willeford battery are obtained under directed ear listening conditions. No published data are available for directed ear consonant-vowel testing in 6-year-olds.

a homophasic condition is one in which the signals in two channels are in phase with one another and the noises in two channels are in phase with one another ($S_O N_O$). An antiphasic condition is one in which either the signals or the noises in the two channels are 180 degrees out of phase ($S_O N_\pi$ or $S_\pi N_O$). Masking level differences have been used for many years inpsychoacoustic research and in the clinical evaluation of brain stem function. MLDs are obtained by obtaining binaural masked thresholds for either pure tones or speech under homophasic and antiphasic conditions. The thresholds for the homophasic (e.g., noise in phase at the two ears and signal in phase at the two ears: $S_O N_O$) minus the antiphasic conditions (e.g., noise in phase at the two ears and signal out of phase at the two ears: $S_\pi N_O$) is the MLD. This effect is sometimes called the binaural release from masking. The MLD can be 10- to 15-dB for pure tones and is frequently dependent, with the largest effects in the lower frequencies

(300–600 Hz). The MLD for speech is smaller than for pure tones (Wilson et al, 1994). Subjects must have normal-hearing to maximize the MLD because peripheral hearing loss has a substantial effect on reducing the size of the MLD. Brain stem lesions can reduce or eliminate the MLD (Olsen & Noffsinger, 1976). Early research by Sweetow and Reddell (1978) found reduced MLDs in children with suspected auditory perceptual problems. They found that tonal MLDs were effective in discriminating children with auditory perceptual dysfunction from normal children, but speech MLDs were not. Current interest in the MLD is directed at the fact that it is a nonlinguistic task that may identify dysfunction in the processing of auditory information at brain stem levels. These dysfunctions, when better understood, may underlie certain CAPDs that are related to auditory, language, and learning disorders.

Electrophysiologic Assessment of Central Auditory Function

Some mention should be made of electrophysiologic procedures in central auditory testing. The ASHA task force on central auditory processing (ASHA, 1995) states that

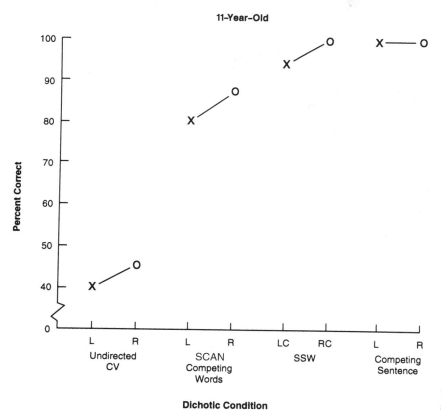

Figure 15–2 Typical results of dichotic listening tests expected from a normal 11-year-old. The tests reported are the same as shown in Figure 15–1.

electrophysiologic procedures "may also be useful" in the diagnosis of CAPD. To quote further from that document, "The auditory brain stem response is well known and applied routinely to detect brain stem lesions. The middle, late, and event-related potentials are still in the development stage, but can be of considerable value in certain clinical situations." For further information the reader is referred to Chapter 20 on late cortical potentials.

LANGUAGE TESTING: WHAT THE AUDIOLOGIST NEEDS TO KNOW

Audiologists who work in the area of CAPD need to know about language and its disorders. The audiologist should become familiar with a range of basic principles. For example, the audiologist must have an understanding of language skill development to formulate meaningful recommendations. They should familiarize themselves with typical language milestones and have a working understanding of approximate age and sequence of emergence. It is essential that the audiologist also have an appreciation for the functional aspects of language that are at the core of communicative competence. The following information comprises a brief outline on aspects of language that will be a helpful reminder for audiologists.

Some of the operative concepts include discrimination, phonology, receptive language, expressive language, prosody, and pragmatics.

Discrimination

Children must have the ability to discriminate fine differences between speech sounds (phonemes) to form the basis for phonemic decoding and ultimate comprehension. Discrimination allows the listener to recognize meaningful segments of language that comprise words and sentences and also allows the listener to tune out distractions and background noise, bringing the relevant information into the foreground. Through this process, information can be selected for comprehension and stored in short-term and long-term memory. Studies have found that infants as young as 3 months demonstrate behaviors that suggest the ability to discriminate between minimally contrasted sound pairs such as "p" and "b." The ability to discriminate between speech sounds is essential to the development of receptive comprehension and expression of speech sounds within the phonology system.

Phonology

The phonological system is comprised of the sound patterns of language, which combine to form meaningful segments of language. Within the age range of 18 to 28 months, children should demonstrate competence in the production of most vowel sounds and the consonant sounds "n," "m," "p," and "h." After the emergence of these speech sounds, children will usually begin to produce "f," "ng," "w," "t," "k," "b," "g," and "d." These sounds generally develop over a longer period of time and require refinement through the ages of 3 to 3½. Other sounds such as "s," "r," "sh," "ch," "zh," "v," "z," and "th" may take several years to develop with mastery occurring as late as 6 to 7 years of age.

Receptive Language

Receptive language is the input system of language that takes in information through the senses. Children typically follow a developmental progression marked by the following milestones: by 1 month, infants should respond to voice and by 2 months they should visually track movement. By 3 months, infants begin to coo in response to a pleasant or familiar voice, and by 4 months they should localize a sound source by head movements. By 5 months, most infants respond to their own name, and by 6 months they should recognize some commonly used words such as daddy, bye-bye, and mama. At 7 months, infants generally show interest in the sounds of objects and by 8 months can recognize the names of some common objects. At 9 months, infants should follow simple directions, and by 10 months they should understand "no" and "stop." By 11 to 12 months, infants begin to understand simple questions and recognize action words, names of objects, people, and pets. Between 13 and 18 months children should understand some new words each week and should be able to identify pictures in a book. They should be able to point to a few body parts and should be able to identify some common objects when they are named. During the 19 to 24 month period, children should recognize many common objects and pictures when they are named, should begin to understand possessive forms, and should follow many simple directions. By 25 to 30 months, children can generally understand prepositions, questions, personal pronouns, and the use of common objects. By 31 to 36 months children should be able to listen to simple stories, follow a two-part direction, and understand turn-taking. It is the progression through these developmental stages that should be emphasized, not a strict or arbitrary adherence to age levels. Ages should serve only as a guide, especially when working with children who have disabilities.

Expressive Language

Although variability exists in individual rate of acquisition, most children follow a developmental sequence that encompasses the following skills. During the first month, infants cry and produce vowel-like sounds. By 2 months, primary caretakers can generally recognize different kinds of cries that signal different needs. By 3 months, infants begin to make "cooing" sounds primarily in the back of the oral cavity and may occasional use consonant sounds such as m, p, and b. By 4 to 6 months, most infants develop greater control over their oral structures and begin to combine consonants and vowels in "babbling" patterns. Between 6 and 11 months, infants continue to babble, repeating sequences of sounds in reduplicated patterns. First words should emerge between 12 and 18 months, and most children begin combining words into two-word combinations between the ages of 2 and 2½. Beyond this stage, language skills should expand rapidly toward sentence use by the age of 3 to 3½.

Prosody

Speech is shaped by the prosodic features of stress, duration, and loudness. These features are important for early discrimination of speech and nonspeech sounds. Prosodic features complement the linguistic signal and aid the listener in his or her interpretation of grammatical and semantic functions, as well as emotional intent and social cues. Early prosodic development can be seen in infants' differentiated cries, with later evidence appearing in intonated babbling patterns. As children approach first word usage, it is often possible to detect inflection patterns of "jargon" that approximate the prosodic features of adult speech.

Pragmatics

Interaction is the key in language development and usage. The area of pragmatics addresses the functional, communicative parameters that govern language usage within an interactive context. The development of social or pragmatic skills begins long before the emergence of first words. Eye contact should begin within the first month, closely followed by early turn-taking during face-to-face interaction. This provides a foundation for later turn-taking during conversation. Young children should also be able to focus jointly, with a communicative partner, on a topic or object of interest. Communicative or pragmatic function of language is also illustrated by the child's use of language to signal a variety of functions. These social/semantic functions include requesting an object, requesting an action, protesting, requesting a social routine, requesting comfort, greeting, requesting permission, commenting, requesting information, and providing information. It is the child's ability to develop language as a social and interactive tool (taking precedence over phonological and syntactic development) that forms the basis of communicative competence.

LANGUAGE TESTING

Language tests are designed to assess areas of strength and weakness for aspects of language described earlier. Nonstandardized language sampling and standardized language measures are both used by speech-language pathologists for assessment. That information is used in the development of remediation programs for children with central auditory processing and language disorders. The ASHA (1995) consensus statement on CAPD points out that clinicians should be cautious in attributing language/learning difficulties to CAPD in any simple fashion. Clinicians should not infer the existence of CAPD solely from evidence of learning disability or language impairment or vice versa.

INTERPRETING TEST RESULTS

In the preceding pages definitions of central auditory processing and related attention, language, and learning disorders have been provided. The purpose of providing this information is to assist the audiologist in understanding what is a CAPD and what is not. A brief review of the ASHA consensus statement finds that careful examination of the child's history, observation of auditory behaviors, and results of audiologic procedures are used to identify deficits in auditory processing. Audiologic test results should be reviewed to develop an auditory profile. Does the child have difficulty listening under conditions of degraded speech as shown by tests of time-compressed speech or filtered words? Is there difficulty understanding speech in the presence of background noise? If so, what kind of noise, and what signal-to-noise ratio is necessary for adequate understanding? Are there apparent problems in the neurologic pathways, as indicated by difficulty in localization or lateralization, or tests of MLDs? Is there indication of delays in maturation or damage to the auditory nervous system shown by poor performance or abnormal ear advantages on dichotic tests? Does the child have problems of auditory discrimination because of a temporal processing disorder? Does the temporal processing disorder compromise understanding speech presented at rapid rates?

PEARL

Examples of cognitive factors that may affect central auditory test results include low intelligence, poor short-term memory, speed of mental processing, attention, reaction time, and communication strategies.

Audiologic findings are viewed in conjunction with results of speech-language pathology, psychology, learning disabilities, and other specialties. Only when findings are integrated can meaningful remediation programs be designed. The combination of test results will be used to determine whether the child will benefit from direct perceptual training, compensation for auditory deficits, or cognitive training. A discussion of remediation of children and adults with CAPDs is presented in *Treatment*.

ACKNOWLEDGMENTS

Appreciation is expressed to my speech-language pathologist colleague Melinda Chalfonte-Evans, who assisted in writing comments on what audiologists should know about language.

REFERENCES

American Medical Association. (1996). *AMA international classification of diseases* (9th Revision Clinical Modification). Chicago, IL: The Association.

American Psychiatric Association. (1994). *Diagnostic and statistical manual of mental disorders: DSM-IV.* (4th Ed.). Washington, DC: The Association.

American Speech-Language-Hearing Association. (1995). *Task force on central auditory processing consensus development,* Washington, DC: The Association.

Arcia, E., & Conners, C.K. (1998). Gender differences in ADHD? *Developmental and Behavioral Pediatrics, 19*(2),77–83.

Bellis, T.J. (1996). *Assessment and management of central auditory processing disorders in the educational setting.* San Diego, CA: Singular Publishing Group.

Bergman, M., Hirsch, S., Solzi, P., & Mankowitz, Z. (1987). The threshold-of-interference test: A new test of interhemispheric suppression in brain injury. *Ear and Hearing, 8*(3),147–150.

Berlin, C.E., Hughes, L.F., Lowe-Bell, S.S., & Berlin, H.L. (1973). Dichotic right ear advantage in children 5 to 13. *Cortex, 3*(9),394–402.

Bornstein, S.P., & Musiek, F.E. (1984). Implications of temporal processing for children with learning and language problems. In: D.S. Beasley (Ed.), *Methods of Study. Audition in childhood.* San Diego, CA: College Hill Press.

Bornstein, S.P., Wilson, R.H., & Cambron, N.K. (1994). Low- and high-pass filtered Northwestern University auditory test No. 6 for monaural and binaural evaluation. *Journal of the American Audiology Association, 5,*259–264.

Briggs, S.R., House, J., Keith, R.W., & Weiler, E. (1998) *The Auditory Continuous Performance Test as part of an attention deficit-hyperactivity disorder test battery.* M.A. Thesis, University of Cincinnati.

Cacace, A.T., & McFarland, D.J. (1988). Central auditory processing disorder in school-aged children: A critical review. *Journal of Speech and Hearing Research, 41,*355–373.

Calearo, C., & Antonelli, A.R. (1973). Disorders of the central auditory nervous system. In: M. Paparella, & D.A. Shumrick (Eds.), *Otolaryngology:* Philadelphia, PA: Saunders.

Conners, C.K. (1997). *Conners' rating scales-revised.* North Tonawanda, NY: Multi-Health Systems Inc.

Costello, M.R. (1977). Evaluation of auditory behavior of children using the Flowers-Costello test of central auditory abilities. In: R.W. Keith (Ed.), *Central auditory dysfunction.* New York: Grune & Stratton.

Deitrich, K.N., Succop, P.A., Berger, O.G., & Keith, R.W. (1992). Lead exposure and the central auditory processing abilities and cognitive development of urban children: The Cincinnati lead study cohort at age 5 years. *Neurotoxicology and Teratology, 14,*51–56.

Devers, J.S., Hoyer, E.A., & McCroskey, R.L. (1978). Dynamic auditory localization by normal and learning disability children. *Journal of the American Auditory Society, 3,*172–178.

Fallis-Cunningham, R., & Keith, R.W. (1998). *Auditory testing for temporal processing disorders.* Presentation to the annual meeting of the American Auditory Society, Los Angeles, CA.

First, M.B., Frances, A., & Pincus, H.A. (1995). *DSM-IV handbook of differential diagnosis.* Washington, DC: American Psychiatric Press.

Fisher, L.I. (1976). *Auditory problems checklist.* Bemidji, MN: Life Products.

Gravel, J., & Ellis, M.A. (1995). The auditory consequences of otitis media with effusion: The audiogram and beyond. *Seminars in Hearing, 16,*(1),44–58.

Hall, J.W., & Mueller, H.G. (1997). *Audiologists' desk reference.* (Vol. 1) (p. 507). San Diego, CA: Singular Publishing Group.

Hood, L.J. (1998). Auditory neuropathy: What is it and what can we do about it? *The Hearing Journal, 51*(8),10–18.

Hurley, R.M., & Museik, F.M. (1997). Effectiveness of three central auditory processing (CAP) tests in identifying cerebral lesions. *Journal of the American Academy of Audiology, 8,*257–262.

Jerger, J. (1960). Observations on auditory behavior in lesions of the central auditory pathways *Archives of Otolaryngology, 71,*797–806.

Jerger, J. (1964). Auditory tests for disorders of the central auditory mechanisms. In: W.S. Fields & B.R. Alford (Eds.), *Neurological aspects of auditory and vestibular disorders.* Springfield, IL: Charles C. Thomas.

Jerger, J., & Harford, E. (1960). Alternate and simultaneous binaural balancing of pure tones. *Journal of Speech and Hearing Research, 3,*15–30

Jerger, S. (1987). Validation of the Pediatric Speech Intelligibility Test in children with central nervous system lesions. *Audiology, 26,*298–311.

Jerger, S., & Allen, J.S. (1998). How behavioral tests of central auditory processing may complicate management. In: F. Bess (Ed.), *Proceedings from the fourth international symposium on childhood deafness.* Nashville, TN: Bill Wilkerson Center Press.

Katz (1962). The use of staggered spondaic words for assessing the integrity of the central auditory nervous system. *Journal of Audiology Research, 2,*327–337.

Katz, J. (1977). The Staggered Spondaic Word Test. In: R.W. Keith (Ed.), *Central auditory dysfunction.* New York: Grune & Stratton.

Katz, J., Stecker, N., & Henderson, D. (1992). *Central auditory processing: A transdisciplinary view.* St. Louis, MO: Mosby–Year Book.

Keith, R.W. (1986). *SCAN: Screening test for auditory processing disorders in children.* San Antonio, TX: The Psychological Corporation.

Keith, R.W. (1994a). *SCAN-A: Test of auditory processing abilities for use with adolescents and adults.* San Antonio, TX: The Psychological Corporation.

Keith, R.W. (1994b). *Auditory Continuous Performance Test.* San Antonio, TX: The Psychological Corporation.

Keith, R.W. (1999). *SCAN-C: Test of auditory processing disorders in children–revised.* San Antonio, TX: The Psychological Corporation.

Keith, R.W., & Farrer, S. (1981). Filtered word testing in the assessment of children with central auditory disorders. *Ear and Hearing, 12,*267–289.

Knox, C., & Roeser, R.J. (1980). Cerebral dominance in normal and dyslexic children. In: R.W. Keith (Ed.), *Seminars in Speech, Language, and Hearing, 1,*181–194.

Marriage, J. (1996). *Hyperacusis in Williams syndrome.* Unpublished Ph.D. Dissertation, University of Manchester, England.

Matkin, N.D., & Hook, P.E. (1983). A multidisciplinary approach to central auditory evaluations. In: E.Z. Lasky & J. Katz (Eds.), *Central Auditory Processing Disorders.* Baltimore, MD: University Park Press.

Matzker, J. (1959). Two new methods for the assessment of central auditory functions in cases of brain disease. *Annals of Otology, 68,*1185–1190.

McCroskey, R.L., & Keith, R.W. (1996). *The Auditory Fusion Test-Revised.* St. Louis, MO: AUDiTEC.

Menyuk, P. (1992). Relationship of otitis media to speech processing and language development. In: J. Katz, N. Stecker, & D. Henderson (Eds.), *Central auditory processing: A transdisciplinary view.* St. Louis, MO: Mosby–Year Book.

Musiek, F.E., Baran, J.A., & Pinheiro, M.L. (1991). Duration pattern recognition in normal subjects and patients with cerebral and cochlear lesions. *Audiology, 29,*304–313.

Musiek, F.E., Gollegly, K.M., Kibbe, K.S., & Verkest-Lenz, S.B. (1991). Proposed screening test for central auditory disorders: Follow-up on the Dichotic Digits Test. *American Journal of Otology, 12,*109–113.

NIH Consensus Statement. (1993). Early identification of hearing impairment in infants and young children. *11,*1–24.

Obrzut, J.E., Hynd, G.W., Obrzut, A., & Pirozzolo, F.J. (1981). Effect of directed attention on cerebral asymmetries in normal and learning-disabled children. *Developmental Psychology, 17*(1),118–125.

Olsen, W.O., & Noffsinger, D. (1976). Masking level differences for cochlear and brain stem lesions. *Annals of Otolaryngology Rhinology and Laryngology, 86,*820–825.

Olsen, W.O., Noffsinger, D., & Kurdziel, S. (1975). Speech discrimination testing in quiet and in white noise by patients with peripheral and central lesions. *Acta Otolaryngologica, 80,*375–382.

Phillips, D.P. (1995). Central auditory processing and its disorders: A view from neuroscience. *The American Journal of Otology, 19*(3),338–351.

Riccio, C., Cohen, G., Hynd, G., & Keith, R.W. (1996). Validity of the Auditory Continuous Performance Test in differentiating central auditory processing disorders with and without ADHD. *Journal of Learning Disabilities, 29*(5), 561–566.

Rintelmann, W.F. (1985). Monaural speech tests in the detection of central auditory disorders. In: M.L. Pinheiro & F.E. Musiek (Eds.), *Assessment of central auditory dysfunction.* Baltimore, MD: Williams & Williams.

Rosenberg, P.E. (1978). Case history: The first test. In: J. Katz, *Handbook of clinical audiology.* (2nd ed.). Baltimore: Williams & Wilkins.

Sanger, D.D., Freed, J.M., & Decker, T.N. (1985). Behavioral profile of preschool children suspected of auditory language processing problems. *The Hearing Journal, 38*(10),17–20.

Satz, P. (1976). Cerebral dominance and reading disability: An old problem revisited. In: R.M. Knights & D.J. Bakker (Eds.), *The neuropsychology of learning disorders: Theoretical approaches,* Baltimore, MD: University Park Press.

Sininger, Y., Hood, L.H., Starr, A., Berlin, C.I., & Picton, R.W. (1995). Hearing loss due to auditory neuropathy. *Audiology Today, 7*(2),10–13.

Smoski, W.J., Brunt, M.A., & Tannahill, J.C. (1992). Listening characteristics of children with central auditory processing disorders. *Language, Speech, and Hearing Services, 23,*145–152.

Sperry, J.L., Wiley, T.L., & Chial, M.R. (1997). Word recognition performance in various background competitors. *Journal of American Academy of Audiology Association, 8,* 71–80.

Starr, A., Picton, T.W., Sininger, Y., Hook, L.J., & Berlin, C.I. (1996). Auditory neuropathy. *Brain, 119,*741–753.

Stein, L., Tremblay, K., Pasterak, J., Banerjee, S., Lindermann, K., & Kraus, N. (1996). Brainstem abnormalities in neonates with normal otoacoustic emissions. *Seminars in Hearing, 17*(2),197–213.

Sweetow, R.W., & Reddell, R.D. (1978). The use of masking level differences in the identification of children with perceptual problems. *Journal of the American Academy of Audiology, 4,*52–56.

Teatini, G.P. (1970). *Sensitized speech tests: Results in normal subjects.* II Danavox Symposium, Odense, Denmark.

Thompson, M.E., & Abel, S.M. (1992). Indices of hearing in patients with central auditory pathology. *Scandinavian Audiology,* (Suppl.) 35, 3–15.

VA CD. (1992). *Tonal and speech materials for auditory perceptual assessment.* Long Beach, CA: Research and Development Service, Veterans Administration Central Office.

Watson, C.S. (1994). *How does basic science show that central auditory processing is critical to audition? The view from psychoacoustics.* Presentation to the ASHA consensus development conference, March 11–13. Albuquerque, NM.

Watson, C.S. (1997). Personal communication, paraphrased here with permission.

Willeford, J. (1976). Central auditory function in children with learning disabilities. *Audiology and Hearing Education, 2*(2),12–20.

Willeford, J. (1977). Assessing central auditory behavior in children: A test battery approach. In: Keith, RW. (Ed.), *Central auditory dysfunction.* New York: Grune & Stratton.

Willeford, J. (1985). Assessment of central auditory disorders in children. In: M.L. Pinheiro, & F.E. Musiek (Eds.), *Assessment of central auditory dysfunction: Foundations and clinical correlations.* Baltimore, MD: Williams and Wilkins.

Willeford, J., & Burleigh, J. (1985). *Handbook of central auditory processing disorders in children.* Orlando, FL: Grune & Stratton.

Wilson, R.H., Zizz, C.A., & Sperry, J.L. (1994). Masking level difference for spondaic words in 2000-msec bursts of broadband noise. *Journal of the American Academy of Audiology Association, 5,*236–242.

## Chapter 16

Diagnosing Central Auditory Processing Disorders in Adults

Brad A. Stach

Outline

The central auditory nervous system is a highly complex network that analyzes and processes neural information from both ears and transmits the processed information to the auditory cortex and other areas within the nervous system. Auditory processing ability is usually defined as the capacity with which the central auditory nervous system transfers information from the eighth nerve to the auditory cortex. Central auditory processing disorder (CAPD) is an impairment in this function of the central auditory nervous system.

Much of our knowledge of the way in which the brain processes sound has been gained from studying normally functioning systems. The central auditory nervous system plays an important role in comparing sound at the two ears for the purpose of sound localization. The central auditory nervous system also plays a major role in extracting a signal of interest from a background of noise. Although signals at the cochlea are analyzed exquisitely in the frequency, amplitude, and temporal domains, it is in the central auditory nervous system where those fundamental analyses are eventually perceived as speech or some other meaningful nonspeech sound.

We have also gained substantial knowledge by studying central auditory systems that are impaired because of neurological disorders. For example, we have learned that the peripheral portion of the auditory system serves as a bottleneck for information transfer. Disorders at this level can have a dramatic impact on hearing ability. At more central levels, the effects of the disorder are more subtle and more challenging to measure.

The ability of the central auditory nervous system to process sound was evaluated historically for diagnostic purposes to identify specific lesions or disease processes of the nervous system. Numerous measures of auditory nervous system function were scrutinized for what they could reveal about the presence of such neurological disorders. These diagnostic site-of-lesion efforts formed a basis for the assessment of central auditory disorders today, which is much more focused on describing communication disorder than on diagnosing specific neurological disorders.

If the role of audiological evaluation is defined as the assessment of hearing in a broad sense, it is easy to understand why many clinicians and researchers embrace the importance of evaluating more than just the sensitivity of the ears to faint sounds and the ability of the ear to detect single-syllable words presented in quiet. Although both measures provide important information to the audiological assessment, they stop short of offering a complete picture of an individual's auditory ability. Certainly, knowledge of the complexity of auditory perception, as evidenced by the ability to follow a conversation in a noisy room or the effortless ability to localize sound, leads to an understanding that the rudimentary assessment of hearing sensitivity and speech recognition do not adequately characterize what it takes to hear. Neither do they adequately describe the possible disorders that a person might have. As a result, it is becoming increasingly common for assessment of central auditory ability to be included as a routine component of the basic audiological evaluation.

Audiology: Diagnosis. Edited by Roeser, Valente, and Hosford-Dunn. Thieme Medical Publishers, Inc., New York © 2000

Over the past two decades, techniques that were once used to assist in the diagnosis of neurological disease have been adapted for use in the assessment of communication impairment that occurs as a result of CAPD. Speech audiometric measures that are sensitized in certain ways, along with other psychophysical measures designed to challenge the auditory nervous system, are now commonly used to evaluate auditory processing ability. A typical battery of tests might include the assessment of speech recognition across a range of signal intensities, the assessment of speech recognition in the presence of competing speech signals, the measurement of dichotic listening, and an assessment of temporal processing capacity. Results of such an assessment provide an estimate of central auditory processing ability and a more complete profile of a patient's auditory abilities and handicap (Chmiel & Jerger, 1996; Jerger et al, 1990b). Such information is often useful in providing guidance regarding appropriate amplification strategies or other rehabilitation approaches (Chmiel et al, 1997; Stach et al, 1985, 1991). The value of this information has led many clinicians to choose to evaluate central auditory ability as a routine component of any thorough assessment of hearing.

Auditory evoked potentials and other electrophysiological measures have also proven to be useful in the diagnosis of central auditory processing disorders. These techniques are described in later chapters of this textbook. This chapter will describe behavioral tests that have been developed over the years for the assessment of central auditory processing.

PURPOSES OF ASSESSING CENTRAL AUDITORY PROCESSING

The aim of central auditory processing assessment is to evaluate the ability of the central auditory nervous system to process acoustic signals. Advanced speech audiometric and other behavioral measures can be used to measure central auditory nervous system function, often referred to as central auditory processing ability. At least two important reasons exist for doing so: (1) to assist the medical profession in identifying specific lesions of the auditory system, and (2) to describe a communication disorder.

Identification of a Specific Lesion

It was in the 1950s that speech audiometric measures were first used successfully to identify lesions of the central auditory nervous system (Bocca et al, 1954). Speech recognition measures, including monotically presented words sensitized by low-pass filtering and dichotic testing, were found to be effective in identifying patients with temporal lobe lesions and other neurological disorders. From those beginnings, speech audiometric measures, along with other behavioral techniques, were designed and evaluated for their effectiveness in identifying lesions of the auditory nervous system.

Refinement of these behavioral measures ensued throughout the 1960s and 1970s, bringing with it an enhanced understanding of the function of the auditory nervous system and the impact of neurological disorder on that function. Much of the design of our approach today is a direct result of concepts that were formulated during these early efforts.

During the 1980s, the importance of the diagnostic, site-of-lesion role of central auditory testing began to diminish with the advent of radiological imaging techniques and the refinement of auditory evoked potential assessment. As ever smaller lesions were being detected by the progressively increasing accuracy of these imaging and evoked-potential measures, the sensitivity of central auditory processing tests diminished accordingly. As a result, the role of central auditory assessment in the identification of specific lesions changed from one of diagnosis to one of screening.

Although measures of central auditory processing ability remain useful diagnostically in helping to identify the presence of neurological disorders, particularly in a screening role, they are used more often now to assess the functional impact of such a disorder and to monitor the course of the disease process.

PEARL

The real value of measures of CAPD lie not in their ability to screen for medical problems but in their ability to quantify the impact of neurological disorders on communication ability.

Description of a Communication Disorder

As measures of central auditory processing ability were being refined for diagnostic, site-of-lesion purposes, many researchers and clinicians began to understand their value in providing insight into a patient's auditory abilities beyond the level of cochlear processing. It became readily apparent that these behavioral measures designed to identify lesions could be used to assess and quantify hearing disorder, resulting from an impaired central auditory nervous system. That is, their value in quantifying functional deficits became apparent as they were being applied in an effort to identify structural deficits. These functional deficits, referred to collectively as central auditory processing disorders, were found to be readily quantifiable with the same strategies used for diagnostic purposes.

Today, assessment of central auditory processing ability is used for several purposes. It serves as a screener for retrocochlear neurological disorder, and it is useful in quantifying the consequences of such a neurological disorder. In addition, the measurement of central auditory processing serves as a metric of suprathreshold hearing ability, which permits a more complete understanding of communication function. As a result, it is valuable in quantifying hearing impairment resulting from functional deficits in the auditory nervous system. Finally, it assists in defining how a patient will hear after a peripheral hearing sensitivity loss has been corrected with hearing aids.

THE NATURE OF CENTRAL AUDITORY PROCESSING DISORDERS

Although a tendency exists to think of hearing impairment as the sensitivity loss that can be measured on an audiogram,

> ## PEARL
>
> Central auditory processing (1) screens for retro-cochlear disorder, (2) measures suprathreshold hearing, and (3) helps define communication ability after the peripheral loss has been corrected with hearing aids

other types of hearing impairment may or may not be accompanied by sensitivity loss. These other impairments result from disease, damage, or degradation of the central auditory nervous system in adults or delayed or disordered auditory nervous system development in children.

A disordered auditory nervous system, regardless of cause, will have functional consequences that can vary from subclinical to a substantial, easily measurable auditory deficit. Auditory nervous system impairments tend to be divided into two groups, depending on the nature of the underlying disorder, even though the functional consequences may be similar. When an impairment is caused by an active, measurable disease process, such as a tumor or other space-occupying lesion, or from damage caused by trauma or stroke, it is often referred to as a retrocochlear disorder. That is, retrocochlear disorders result from structural lesions of the nervous system. When an impairment is due to a developmental disorder or delay or from diffuse changes such as the aging process, it is often referred to as a CAPD. That is, CAPDs result from "functional lesions" of the nervous system. The term CAPD is also used to describe the functional consequence of a retrocochlear disorder.

The consequences of both types of disorder can be remarkably similar from a hearing perspective, but the disorders tend to be treated differently because of the consequences of diagnosis and the likelihood of a significant residual communication disorder. Retrocochlear disorders are those that are often addressed first by medical management. Residual communication disorder is often a secondary consideration because of the immediate health threat of most retrocochlear disease, which must be treated first. CAPDs often are seen as communication disorders and are either the residual consequence of a retrocochlear disorder or the consequence of diffuse changes or disorders that are not amenable to medical management. That both types of disorder may present similar audiological findings can be challenging clinically, but their treatment as a communication disorder is not likely to differ because the functional deficit to the patient will be similar regardless of the underlying cause.

Symptoms

Some adults with CAPDs will have normal-hearing sensitivity. Others, especially those who are elderly, will have some degree of peripheral hearing sensitivity loss on which the central auditory disorder is imposed. In the former group, the most common symptom is that of a hearing disorder in the presence of normal-hearing sensitivity. Such patients will describe difficulty hearing in certain listening situations despite their ability to detect faint sounds. In the latter group the most common symptom will be a hearing disorder that seems to be disproportionate to the degree of hearing sensitivity loss. Regardless of category, adults with CAPDs share common difficulties along a continuum of severity.

The most common symptom of CAPD is difficulty extracting a signal of interest from a background of noise. Patients with central auditory disorders will simply have difficulty hearing in noise. Typical environments in which difficulties occur include parties, restaurants, and in the car. Another common symptom is difficulty localizing a sound source, especially in the presence of background noise. Perhaps as a consequence of these symptoms, patients and their families are also likely to describe behaviors such as inattentiveness and distractibility.

These symptoms, of course, are not unlike those of patients with peripheral hearing sensitivity loss. It should be no surprise that an auditory disorder, regardless of its locus, would result in similar perceived difficulties.

> ## PEARL
>
> A distinguishing feature of CAPD is the inability to extract sounds of interest in noisy environments despite an ability to perceive the sounds with adequate loudness.

Signs

Not surprisingly, clinical findings in patients with CAPDs reflect impairments in those functions attributable to the central auditory nervous system. That is, tests of central auditory processing have been designed to try to assess those functions uniquely attributable to the auditory nervous system rather than to the cochlea. Indeed, one important clinical challenge is to rule out or control the influences of the cochlea or cochlear hearing loss. A list of common clinical signs is shown in Table 16–1.

TABLE 16–1 Clinical signs of central auditory processing disorder

Categories of Reduced Function
Recognition of frequency-altered speech
Recognition of speech in competition
Recognition of speech at high-intensity levels
Temporal processing
Localization
Lateralization
Dichotic listening
Binaural processing
Acquired suprathreshold asymmetry

Following is a description of many of the diverse clinical signs of CAPD. Although the clinical signs attributable to a central disorder may provide insight into the basis and locus of the underlying disorder, the symptoms related to the various signs seem to be reasonably similar across patients. That is, whether a disorder is identified as a problem in temporal processing, dichotic listening, or localization, the functional consequence to the patient tends to be difficulty hearing in adverse listening environments. Indeed, development of these various measures did not evolve from a systematic plan to assess the central auditory mechanism, rather it evolved from efforts to challenge the integrity of the central nervous system by measuring functions that are attributable to it.

Subtlety and Bottleneck Principles

As a general rule, the more peripheral a lesion, the greater its impact will be on auditory function (the bottleneck principle). Conversely, the more central the lesion, the more subtle its impact will be (the subtlety principle). One might conceptualize this by thinking of the nervous system as a large oak tree. If one of its many branches was damaged, overall growth of the tree would be affected only subtly. Damage to its trunk, however, could have a significant impact on the entire tree. A well-placed lesion on the auditory nerve can have a substantial impact on hearing, whereas a lesion in the midbrain is likely to have more subtle effects.

PEARL

The bottleneck principle holds that the more peripheral a lesion, the greater its impact on auditory function, and the subtlety principle holds that the more central the lesion, the more subtle its impact.

Perhaps the best illustration of the bottleneck principle comes from reports of cases with lesions that effectively disconnect the cochlea from the brain stem. These cases demonstrate the presence of severe or profound hearing loss and very poor speech recognition despite normal cochlear function, as indicated by normal otoacoustic emissions or eighth nerve action potentials. In cases involving lesions of the cerebellopontine angle resulting from tumor (Cacace et al, 1994), multiple sclerosis (Stach & Delgado-Vilches, 1993), and miliary tuberculosis (Stach et al, 1998), results have shown how a strategically placed lesion at the bottleneck can substantially affect hearing ability. The bottleneck in the case of the auditory system is, of course, the eighth nerve as it enters the auditory brain stem.

One specific type of auditory nervous system disorder identified recently is auditory neuropathy (Starr et al, 1996, 1998), a term used to describe a condition in which cochlear function is normal and eighth nerve function is abnormal. It is distinguishable from disorders caused by space-occupying lesions in that imaging results of the nerve and brain stem are normal. Nevertheless, auditory neuropathy is a disorder that

exemplifies the consequences of a disorder at the level of the bottleneck.

If the bottleneck is unaffected, lesions at higher levels will have effects on auditory processing ability that are more subtle. These effects tend to become increasingly subtle as the lesions are located more centrally in the system. For example, whereas a lesion at the bottleneck can cause a substantial hearing sensitivity loss, a brain stem lesion often results in only a mild low-frequency sensitivity loss (Jerger & Jerger, 1980), and a temporal lobe lesion is unlikely to affect hearing sensitivity at all. Similarly speech recognition of words presented in quiet can be very poor in the case of a lesion at the periphery but will be unaffected by a lesion at the level of the temporal lobe.

Reduced Recognition of Frequency-Altered Speech

One hallmark sign of CAPD is a reduction in recognition of speech materials that have been altered in the frequency domain. It has been known for more than 40 years that reducing the informational content, or redundancy, of speech targets by low-pass filtering creates a challenge to an impaired auditory nervous system that is not present in an intact system (Boca et al, 1954). As a result, patients with auditory processing disorder are likely to perform more poorly on a low-pass filtered speech test than those with normal-hearing ability.

Reduced Recognition of Speech in Competition

As stated earlier, one of the most important consequences of CAPD is an inability to extract signals of interest from a background of noise. This can be measured directly with a number of different speech audiometric techniques. Results show that patients with auditory processing disorders have significant difficulty identifying speech in the presence of competition. In general, the more meaningful or speechlike the competition, the more interfering will be its influence on perception (Sperry et al, 1997; Stuart & Phillips, 1996).

Much of the early work in this area focused on monaural perception of speech targets in a background of competition presented to the same ear. Other results have shown deficits in patients with CAPDs when competition is presented to the opposite ear or when both targets and competition are presented to both ears in a sound field.

Reduced Speech Recognition at High Intensity Levels

In cases of normal auditory processing ability, speech recognition performance increases systematically as speech intensity is increased to an asymptomatic level representing the best speech understanding that can be achieved in that ear. In some cases, however, a paradoxical *rollover* effect exists, in which performance declines substantially as speech intensity increases beyond the level producing the maximal performance score. In other words, as speech intensity increases, performance rises to a maximum level, then declines or "rolls over" sharply as intensity continues to increase. This rollover effect is commonly observed when the site of the hearing loss is retrocochlear, in the auditory nerve or the auditory pathways in the brain stem (Dirks et al, 1977; Jerger & Jerger, 1971).

Reduced Temporal Processing

Impairment in processing in the time domain is also a common sign in central auditory disorders. Temporal processing deficits have been identified on the basis of a number of measures, including time compression of speech, duration pattern discrimination, duration difference limens, gap detection, and so on. Some researchers believe that deficits in temporal processing are the underlying cause of and primary contributors to many of the other measurable deficits associated with CAPDs.

Disordered Localization and Lateralization

The ability to localize acoustic stimuli generally requires auditory system integration of sound from both ears. Some patients with central auditory disorders have difficulty locating the directional source of a sound. Disorders of the central auditory nervous system have been associated with deficits in the ability to localize the source of a sound in a sound field or to lateralize the perception of a sound within the head.

Deficits in Dichotic Listening

Most people with intact auditory nervous systems are able to identify different signals presented simultaneously to both ears. If the signals are linguistic in nature, most individuals will experience a slight right ear advantage in dichotic listening ability. CAPDs, particularly those caused by impairment of the corpus callosum and auditory cortex, often result in dichotic deficits characterized by substantial reduction in left ear performance.

Other Deficits in Binaural Processing

The binaural auditory system is an exquisite detector of differences in timing of sound reaching the two ears. This helps in localizing low-frequency sounds, which reach the ears at different points in time. One way of assessing how sensitive the ears are to these timing, or phase, cues is by measuring binaural release from masking. When identical low-frequency tones are presented in phase to both ears, these tones will be substantially less audible than when the phase of one of the tones is reversed. If noise is introduced so that the in-phase tones are just masked, changing the phase of one of the tones will make them audible again despite the masking noise. This is referred to as *binaural release from masking,* and it occurs as a result of processing in the brain stem at the level of the superior olivary complex. Abnormal binaural release from masking is a common sign of auditory processing disorder that occurs as a result of impairment in the lower auditory brain stem.

A different kind of deficit in binaural processing is referred to as *binaural interference.* Under normal circumstances, binaural hearing provides an advantage over monaural hearing.

This so called binaural advantage has been noted in loudness judgments, speech recognition, and evoked potential amplitudes. In contrast, in cases of binaural interference, binaural performance is actually poorer than the best monaural performance. In such cases, performance on a perceptual task with both ears can actually be poorer than performance on the better ear in cases of asymmetrical perceptual ability. It appears that the poorer ear reduces binaural performance below the better monaural performance. Binaural interference has been reported in elderly individuals (Jerger et al, 1993) and in patients with multiple sclerosis (Silman, 1995). The functional consequence of binaural interference may be to reduce the potential benefit of binaural hearing aids when hearing with both ears is poorer than hearing with one ear.

Acquired Suprathreshold Asymmetry

Emerging evidence suggests that asymmetry in peripheral hearing sensitivity can have a disproportionate effect on processing by the poorer hearing, or deprived, ear. Results are intriguing in that they point to changes in central auditory function as a consequence of the asymmetry. Some asymmetry occurs naturally as a result of greater cochlear disorder in one ear than the other. In such cases, evidence is mounting that processing by the poorer ear is adversely affected beyond that which might be expected if the loss were symmetrical (Moore et al, 1997; Silverman & Emmer, 1993).

PITFALL

The detrimental effects of asymmetry on the central auditory nervous system can be created by fitting a hearing aid to one ear of a person with symmetrical hearing loss.

Asymmetry can also occur by fitting a hearing aid on one ear only. The concept of late-onset auditory deprivation as a result of unilateral hearing aid fitting has emerged over the past several years (Neuman, 1996; Silman et al, 1984, 1992; Silverman & Silman, 1990). Late-onset auditory deprivation refers to an apparent asymmetrical decline in speech-recognition ability in the unaided ear of a person who was fitted with only one hearing aid. That is, in a patient fitted with one hearing aid, speech recognition ability in that ear remains constant over time while the same ability in the unaided ear begins to show signs of deterioration. As long as hearing is symmetrical in both ears, this decline is not apparent. However, once a hearing aid is fitted in one ear, resulting in asymmetrical hearing, ability appears to decline in the disadvantaged ear. Although this reduction may be reversible if the unaided ear is aided within a reasonable time frame, in some patients the decline in speech understanding may not recover (Gelfand, 1995). As a result, a binaural interference phenomenon may occur, wherein binaural ability is actually poorer than the better monaural ability.

CAUSES OF CENTRAL AUDITORY PROCESSING DISORDERS

There are two primary causes of CAPDs in adults. One is neuropathology of the peripheral and central auditory nervous systems, resulting from tumors or other space-occupying lesions or from damage caused by trauma or stroke. The other is from diffuse changes in brain function, usually related to the aging process. A list of potential causes of CAPD is shown in Table 16–2.

TABLE 16–2 Causes of central auditory processing disorder

Locus of Disorder	Pathology
Eighth Nerve	Cochleovestibular schwannoma
	Neurofibromatosis (NF-2)
	Lipoma
	Meningioma
	Neuritis
	Diabetic neuropathy
Brain stem	Infarct
	Glioma
	Multiple sclerosis
Cortex	Cerebrovascular accident
	Tumor
	Trauma
Diffuse	Meningitis
	Toxicity
	Deprivational effects of peripheral pathological conditions
	Degenerative effects of biological aging

Disorders Resulting from Neuropathology

A retrocochlear disorder is caused by a change in neural structure of some component of the peripheral or central auditory nervous system. The effect that this structural change will have on function depends primarily on lesion size, location, and impact. For example, a retrocochlear lesion may or may not affect auditory sensitivity. A tumor on the eighth cranial nerve can cause a substantial sensorineural hearing loss, depending on how much pressure it places on the nerve, the damage that it causes to the nerve, or the extent to which it interrupts blood supply to the cochlea. A tumor in the temporal lobe, however, is quite unlikely to result in any change in hearing sensitivity, although it may result in a more subtle hearing disorder as noted in measures of suprathreshold function such as speech recognition ability.

Retrocochlear neuropathological conditions can occur at any level in the peripheral and central auditory nervous system pathway. The likely causes and consequence of retrocochlear disorders are delineated below.

Eighth Nerve Disorders

The most common neoplastic growth affecting the auditory nerve is called a cochleovestibular schwannoma. The more generic terms acoustic tumor or acoustic neuroma typically refer to a cochleovestibular schwannoma. Other terms used to describe this tumor are acoustic neurinoma and acoustic neurilemoma.

A cochleovestibular schwannoma is a benign, encapsulated tumor composed of Schwann cells that arises from the eighth cranial nerve. Schwann cells serve to produce and maintain the myelin that ensheathes the axons of the eighth nerve. This tumor arising from the proliferation of Schwann cells is benign in that it is slow growing; is encapsulated, thereby avoiding local invasion of tissue; and does not disseminate to other parts of the nervous system. Acoustic tumors are unilateral and most often arise from the vestibular branch of the eighth nerve. Thus they are sometimes referred to as vestibular schwannomas.

The effects of a cochleovestibular schwannoma depend on its size, location, and the extent of the pressure it places on the eighth nerve and brain stem. Auditory symptoms may include tinnitus, hearing loss, and unsteadiness. Depending on the extent of the tumor's impact, it may cause headache, motor incoordination from cerebellar involvement, and involvement of adjacent cranial nerves. For example, involvement of the fifth cranial nerve can cause facial numbness, involvement of the seventh cranial nerve can cause facial weakness, and involvement of the fourth cranial nerve can cause diplopia.

Among the most common symptoms of cochleovestibular schwannoma are unilateral tinnitus and unilateral hearing loss. The hearing disorder varies in degree, depending on the location and size of the tumor. Hearing sensitivity can range from normal to a profound hearing loss. Speech recognition ability typically is disproportionately poor for the degree of hearing loss. If the tumor is affecting function of the eighth nerve, its effects are unlikely to be subtle because of the bottleneck principle.

One other important form of schwannoma is neurofibromatosis. This tumor disorder has two distinct types. Neurofibromatosis-1 (NF-1), also known as von Recklinghausen's disease, is an autosomal dominant disease characterized by café-au-lait spots and multiple cutaneous tumors, with associated optic gliomas, peripheral and spinal neurofibromas, and, rarely, acoustic neuromas. In contrast, neurofibromatosis-2 (NF-2) is characterized by bilateral cochleovestibular schwannomas. The schwannomas are faster growing and more virulent than the unilateral type. This is also an autosomal dominant disease and is associated with other intracranial tumors. Hearing loss in NF-2 is not particularly different from a unilateral type of schwannoma, except that it is bilateral and often progresses more rapidly.

In addition to cochleovestibular schwannoma a number of other types of tumors, cysts, and aneurysms can affect the eighth nerve and the cerebellopontine angle where the eighth nerve enters the brain stem. These other neoplastic growths, such as lipoma and meningioma, occur more rarely than cochleovestibular schwannoma. The effect of these various forms of tumor on hearing is often indistinguishable.

In addition to acoustic tumors other disease processes can affect the function of the eighth nerve. Two important neural disorders are cochlear neuritis and diabetic cranial neuropathy.

Not unlike any cranial nerve, the eighth nerve can develop neuritis or inflammation of the nerve. Although rare, acute cochlear neuritis can occur as a result of a direct viral attack on the cochlear portion of the nerve. This results in degeneration of the cochlear neurons in the ear. Hearing loss is sensorineural and often sudden and severe. It is accompanied by poorer speech understanding than would be expected from the degree of hearing loss. One specific form of this disease occurs as a result of syphilis. Meningoneurolabyrinthitis is an inflammation of the membranous labyrinth and eighth nerve that occurs as a predominant lesion in early congenital syphilis or in acute attacks of secondary and tertiary syphilis.

Diabetes mellitus is a metabolic disorder caused by a deficiency of insulin, with chronic complications including neuropathy and generalized degenerative changes in blood vessels. Neuropathies can involve the central, peripheral, and autonomic nervous systems. When neuropathy from diabetes affects the auditory system, it usually results in a vestibular disorder and hearing loss consistent with retrocochlear disorder.

Brain Stem Disorders

Brain stem disorders that affect the auditory system include infarcts, gliomas, and multiple sclerosis. Brain stem infarcts are localized areas of ischemia produced by interruption of the blood supply. Auditory disorder varies depending on the site and extent of the disorder. Two syndromes related to vascular lesions that include hearing loss are inferior pontine syndrome and lateral inferior pontine syndrome. Inferior pontine syndrome results from a vascular lesion of the pons involving several cranial nerves. Symptoms include ipsilateral facial palsy, ipsilateral sensorineural hearing loss, loss of taste from the anterior two thirds of the tongue, and paralysis of lateral conjugate gaze movement of the eyes. Lateral inferior pontine syndrome results from a vascular lesion of the inferior pons, with symptoms that include facial palsy, loss of taste from the anterior two thirds of the tongue, analgesia of the face, paralysis of lateral conjugate gaze movements, and sensorineural hearing loss.

Gliomas are tumors composed of neuroglia, or supporting cells of the brain. They develop in various forms, depending on the types of cells involved, including astrocytomas, ependymomas, glioblastomas, and medulloblastomas. Any of these can affect the auditory pathways of the brain stem, resulting in various forms of retrocochlear hearing disorder, including hearing sensitivity loss and speech perception deficits.

Multiple sclerosis is a demyelinating disease. It is caused by an autoimmune reaction of the nervous system that results in small scattered areas of demyelination and the development of demyelinated plaques. During the disease process, local swelling of tissue exacerbates symptoms and is followed by periods of remission. If the demyelination process affects structures of the auditory nervous system, hearing disorder can result. No characteristic hearing sensitivity loss emerges as a consequence of the disorder, although all possible configurations have been described. Speech perception deficits are not uncommon in patients with multiple sclerosis (Stach et al, 1990a).

CAPDs associated with brain stem lesions will vary, depending on level at which they occur in the brain stem and the extent of the lesion's influence. Generally, the higher in the brain stem, the more subtle are the effects of the lesion. In lower brain stem lesions, performance on difficult monotic tasks is typically poor in the ear ipsilateral to the disorder. In addition, abnormalities are often found in measures of binaural release from masking. In higher brain stem lesions, performance on difficult monotic tasks can be abnormal in both the ipsilateral and contralateral ear. Brain stem lesions have also been associated with reduction in localization, lateralization, and temporal processing abilities.

Cortical Disorders

One of the more common cortical pathological conditions is caused by cerebrovascular accident, or stroke, which results from an interruption of blood supply to the brain as a result of aneurysm, embolism, or clot. This in turn causes a sudden loss of function related to the affected portion of the brain. Any other disease processes, lesions, or trauma that affect the central nervous system can affect the central auditory nervous system as well. When the temporal lobe is involved, audition may be affected, although more typically receptive language processing is affected, whereas hearing perception is relatively spared.

Central auditory processing disorders associated with temporal lobe lesions include poor dichotic performance, some reduction in performance on difficult monotic tasks typically in the ear opposite to the lesion, impaired localization ability, and reduced temporal processing ability.

Bilateral temporal lobe lesions are an exception to the subtlety principle. In such cases "cortical deafness" can occur, resulting in symptoms that resemble auditory agnosia or profound hearing sensitivity loss (Hood et al, 1994; Jerger et al, 1969; 1972).

Functional Disorders of Aging

Changes in structure and function occur throughout the peripheral and central auditory nervous systems as a result of the aging process. Structural degeneration occurs in the cochlea and in the central auditory nervous system pathways. Evidence of neural degeneration has been found in the auditory nerve, brain stem, and cortex.

Anatomical and physiological aging of the auditory system results from at least two processes (Willott, 1996). One is the central effects of peripheral pathological conditions or those that are a result of the deprivational effects of cochlear hearing loss. The other is the central effects of biological aging of the nervous system structures themselves. As with all other structures of the body, the brain undergoes changes related to the aging process. These central effects of biological aging include a loss of neuronal tissue; loss of dendritic branches, reducing the number of synaptic contacts; changes in excitatory and inhibitory neurotransmitter systems; and other degenerative changes.

Whereas the effect of structural change in the auditory periphery is to attenuate and distort incoming sounds, the major effect of structural change in the central auditory nervous system is the degradation of auditory processing. Hearing impairment in the elderly, then, can be quite complex, consisting of attenuation of acoustic information, distortion of that information, and/or disordered processing of neural information. In its simplest form, this complex disorder can be thought of as a combination of peripheral cochlear effects (attenuation and distortion) and central nervous system effects (auditory processing disorder). The consequences of peripheral sensitivity loss in the elderly are similar to those of younger hearing-impaired individuals. The functional consequence of structural changes in the central auditory nervous system is CAPD.

Auditory processing ability is usually defined operationally on the basis of behavioral measures of speech understanding. Degradation in auditory processing has been demonstrated most convincingly by the use of "sensitized" speech audiometric measures (Antonelli, 1970; Bergman, 1971; Bergman et al, 1976; Bosatra & Russolo, 1982; Hinchcliffe, 1962). Age-related changes have been found on degraded speech tests that use both frequency (Bocca, 1958) and temporal alteration (Konkle et al, 1977; Letowski & Poch, 1996; Lutterman et al, 1966; McCroskey & Kasten, 1982; Price & Simon, 1984; Sticht & Gray, 1969). Tests of dichotic performance have also been found to be adversely affected by aging (Arnst, 1982; Fifer et al, 1983; Gelfand et al, 1980; Jerger et al, 1990c; 1995). In addition, aging listeners do not perform as well as younger listeners on tasks that involve the understanding of speech in the presence of background noise (Goetzinger et al, 1961; Helfer & Wilber, 1990; Jerger, 1973; Jerger & Hayes, 1977; Konig, 1969; Orchik & Burgess, 1977; Pestalozza & Shore, 1955; Shirinian & Arnst, 1982; Wiley et al, 1998). Some aging patients also experience binaural interference (Jerger et al, 1993).

In addition to reduced performance on speech audiometric measures, temporal processing deficits (Fitzgibbons & Gordon-Salant, 1996; Grose, 1996) have been described on measures of precedence (Cranford & Romereim, 1992), duration difference limens (Fitzgibbons & Gordon-Salant, 1996), duration discrimination (Phillips et al, 1994), and gap detection (Lutman, 1991; Moore et al, 1992; Schneider et al, 1994).

PEARL

The functional consequences of cochlear hearing loss in patients who are elderly appear to be similar to those of younger individuals. The functional consequences of structural changes in the central auditory nervous system with aging is CAPD.

FACTORS INFLUENCING DIAGNOSTIC ASSESSMENT

The measurement of central auditory processing ability in adults is typically carried out with a test battery approach that assesses absolute speech recognition ability, speech recognition in competition, dichotic listening, and temporal processing ability. Within each of these categories, substantial variation exists in test use across clinical sites. In addition, new developments in testing strategies hold promise to enhance the ability to quantify central auditory function.

Regardless of test or test battery used in the assessment of auditory processing ability, some factors influence both the selection of testing tools and approaches and the success with which they are likely to be implemented. One of the most important factors in speech audiometric testing is the way in which information content of the test materials is manipulated. Other factors that are critical are those related to hearing sensitivity loss and cognitive ability of the patients being tested.

Informational Content

As neural impulses travel from the cochlea through the eighth nerve to the auditory brain stem and cortex, the number and complexity of neural pathways expand progressively. The system, in its vastness of pathways, includes a certain level of redundancy or excess capacity of processing ability. Such redundancy serves many useful purposes, but it also makes the function of the central auditory nervous system somewhat impervious to our efforts to examine it. For example, a patient can have a rather substantial lesion of the auditory brain stem or cortex and still have normal-hearing and normal word-recognition ability. To be able to assess the impact of such a lesion, the speech audiometric measures must be sensitized in some way before we can adequately examine the brain and understand its function and disorder.

PEARL

Intrinsic and extrinsic redundancy combine to make the function of the central auditory nervous system somewhat impervious to our efforts to examine it. Nevertheless, if a neurological system with reduced intrinsic redundancy is presented with speech materials with reduced extrinsic redundancy, the abnormal processing caused by the neurological disorder will be revealed.

Redundancy in Hearing

A great deal of redundancy is associated with our ability to hear and process speech communication. Intrinsically, the central auditory nervous system has a rich system of anatomical, physiological, and biochemical overlap. Among other functions, such *intrinsic redundancy* permits multisensory processing and simultaneous processing of different auditory signals. Another aspect of intrinsic redundancy is that the nervous system can be altered substantially by neurological disorder and still maintain its ability to process information.

Extrinsically, speech signals contain a wealth of information related to phonological, syntactical, and semantic content and rules. Such *extrinsic redundancy* allows a listener to hear only part of a speech segment and still understand what is being said. For example, consonants can be perceived from the coarticulatory effects of vowels even when the acoustic segments of the consonants are not heard. An entire sentence can be perceived from hearing only a few words that are embedded into a semantic context.

Extrinsic redundancy increases as the content of the speech signal increases. Thus nonsense syllables are least redundant; continuous discourse is most redundant. The immunity of speech perception to the effects of hearing sensitivity loss varies directly with the amount of redundancy of the signal. The more redundancy inherent in the signal, the more immune that signal is to the effects of hearing loss. Stated another way, perception of speech that has lower redundancy is more likely to be affected by the presence of hearing loss than is perception of speech with greater redundancy.

Extrinsic and Intrinsic Redundancy Relationship

The issue of redundancy plays a role in the selection of speech materials. In assessing the effects of a cochlear hearing impairment on speech perception, signals that have reduced redundancy can be used. Nonsense syllables or monosyllable words are sensitive to peripheral hearing impairment and are useful in quantifying its effect. Sentential approximations and sentences, on the other hand, are not. Redundancy in these materials is simply too great to be affected by most degrees of hearing impairment.

In assessing the effects of a disorder of the central auditory nervous system on speech perception, however, the situation becomes more difficult. Speech signals of all levels of redundancy provide too much information to a central auditory nervous system that, itself, has a great deal of redundancy. Even if the intrinsic redundancy is reduced by a neurological disorder, the extrinsic redundancy of speech may be sufficient to permit normal processing. The solution to assessing central auditory nervous system disorders is to reduce the extrinsic redundancy of the speech information enough to reveal the reduced intrinsic redundancy caused by a neurological disorder. This concept is shown in Table 16–3.

TABLE 16–3 The relationship of intrinsic and extrinsic redundancy to speech recognition ability

Intrinsic		Extrinsic		Speech Recognition
Normal	+	Normal	=	Normal
Normal	+	Reduced	=	Normal
Reduced	+	Normal	=	Normal
Reduced	+	Reduced	=	Abnormal

Normal intrinsic redundancy and normal extrinsic redundancy result in normal processing. Reducing the extrinsic redundancy, within limits, will have little effect on a system with normal intrinsic redundancy. Similarly, a neurological disorder that reduces intrinsic redundancy will have little impact on perception of speech with normal extrinsic redundancy. However, if a system with reduced intrinsic redundancy is presented with speech materials that have reduced extrinsic

redundancy, the abnormal processing caused by the neurological disorder will be revealed.

Methods of Reducing Extrinsic Redundancy

To reduce extrinsic redundancy, speech signals must be *sensitized* in some way. Table 16–4 shows some methods for sensitizing test signals. In the frequency domain, speech can be

TABLE 16–4 Methods for sensitizing speech audiometric measures

Domain	Technique
Frequency	Low-pass filtering
Time	Time compression
Intensity	High-level testing
Competition	Speech in noise
Binaural	Dichotic measures

sensitized by removing high frequencies, or low-pass filtering, thus limiting the phonetic content of the speech targets. Speech can also be sensitized in the time domain by time-compression, a technique that removes segments of speech and compresses the remaining segments to increase speech rate. In the intensity domain, speech can be presented at sufficiently high levels at which disordered systems cannot seem to process effectively. Another very effective way to reduce redundancy of a signal is to present it in a background of competition. Yet another way to challenge the central auditory system is to present different but similar signals to both ears simultaneously in a dichotic paradigm.

Patient Factors

One of the most limiting factors in the selection of test measures of CAPD is the influence of hearing sensitivity loss on the ability to interpret test outcome. Another is the influence of cognitive competence on the complexity of the task that can be administered.

Hearing Sensitivity Loss

A significant confounding variable in the measurement of central auditory processing ability is the presence of cochlear hearing impairment. In cases in which hearing loss is present, signals that have enhanced redundancy need to be used so that hearing sensitivity loss does not interfere with interpretation of the measures. That is, materials should be used that are not affected by peripheral hearing impairment so that assessment can be made of processing at higher levels of the system. The issue is usually one of interpretation of test scores. For example, nonsense-syllable perception is usually altered by peripheral hearing impairment, and any effects of central nervous system disorder might not be revealed because they are difficult or impossible to separate from the effects of the hearing sensitivity loss. Use of sentences would likely overcome the peripheral hearing impairment, but their redundancy would be too great to challenge nervous-system processing, even if it is disordered.

In some cases the presence of hearing sensitivity loss simply precludes test interpretation, and testing cannot be carried out effectively. For example, the consonant-vowel (CV) nonsense syllables used in the dichotic CV test are notoriously influenced by even a slight amount of cochlear hearing loss. If the test is used in a patient with hearing sensitivity loss, poor performance cannot be interpreted as a dichotic deficit because the performance level could also be attributed to the cochlear hearing loss. As another example, the masking level difference (MLD) test of binaural release from masking is an excellent test of lower brain stem function. However, the same performance abnormality attributable to a brain stem disorder can be obtained in a patient with a mild degree of low-frequency hearing loss. Thus interpretation of the test is equivocal in the presence of hearing sensitivity loss.

In other cases, however, the influence of cochlear hearing loss on the speech measure is known, which may allow adequate interpretation. For example, absolute performance on one speech-in-competition measure, the synthetic sentence identification (SSI) test, can be compared with normative data on the basis of degree of hearing loss (Yellin et al, 1989). In this way a patient's performance can be compared with expectations for someone with a cochlear hearing loss of the same degree. If performance is within the expected range, auditory processing ability is classified as normal. If performance falls below the expected range, performance on the test is considered abnormal, consistent with an auditory processing disorder. As another example, expectations of performance on a dichotic measure, the dichotic digits test, can be adjusted to more accurately assess central auditory ability in the presence of hearing loss (Musiek, 1983a). Without knowing the expected influence of hearing sensitivity loss, performance on these tests could not be interpreted accurately.

The easiest solution to the issue of cochlear hearing loss is to use highly redundant speech signals to overcome the hearing sensitivity loss and then to sensitize those materials enough to challenge central auditory processing ability. The targets can be sensitized by adding background competition, testing at high intensity levels, and so on.

The issue of hearing sensitivity loss and its influence on measuring central auditory processing ability is particularly challenging in the aging population. Much of the reduction in speech recognition ability, particularly in quiet, that is attributable to the aging process can actually be explained by degree of hearing sensitivity loss. That being said, reduction in central auditory processing ability, as measured with speech recognition in competition, can be attributed to central auditory aging when hearing sensitivity loss is adequately controlled during test interpretation.

For example, several studies have addressed the role of peripheral sensitivity loss in declining speech understanding with age. One study attempted to estimate the prevalence of auditory processing disorder in a clinical population (Stach et al, 1990b) and to assess the possibility that increased peripheral sensitivity loss was, in fact, the cause of increased speech audiometric abnormalities. Seven-hundred patient files, 100 patients from each of seven half-decades, were evaluated. Auditory processing disorder was operationally defined on the basis of speech audiometric test results. Absolute test scores were compared against empirically established norms (Yellin et al, 1989) for hearing loss and test performance and helped to ensure against the potential bias caused by the inevitable increase in peripheral hearing loss that occurs with age. Hearing loss was then matched across age groups. Despite equivalent peripheral sensitivity loss across groups, the prevalence of auditory processing disorder increased systematically with age. These results serve to emphasize that auditory processing disorder cannot be explained simply as an artifact of peripheral sensitivity loss.

In another study (Jerger et al, 1991a) a battery of speech audiometric tests and a battery of neuropsychological measures were administered to 200 elderly individuals with varying degrees of sensitivity loss. Although results showed a predictable influence of hearing sensitivity loss on most measures, a significant amount of the total variance in SSI performance was attributable to knowledge of subject age.

As a final example, another study (Jerger, 1992) analyzed speech audiometric scores from 137 aged subjects across four age groups that were matched for degree of pure tone sensitivity loss. Results showed a statistically significant decline in SSI score as a function of age that could not be explained on the basis of hearing sensitivity loss.

These examples serve to illustrate that auditory processing disorder can be assessed in patients with hearing sensitivity loss, but that great care must be taken in doing so if the influences of peripheral and central effects are to be isolated.

Absolute Speech Recognition

The need to control for or at least understand absolute speech recognition is much the same concept as the influence of hearing sensitivity loss. Absolute speech recognition in quiet will have some influence on speech recognition in noise, and interpretation of the latter cannot be made without adequate assessment of the former. This concept is perhaps easiest to illustrate in cases of asymmetry. Suppose, for example, that absolute speech recognition scores for sentence materials were 100% and 70% for the right and left ears, respectively. A competing sentence dichotic measure is then carried out and shows an asymmetry in dichotic performance, with the left ear score being poorer than the right. Is this a dichotic deficit or simply a reflection of the monotic asymmetry? Similarly, speech in noise scores should not be compared with normative data if speech in quiet scores are not known or somehow anchored to expected levels.

SPECIAL CONSIDERATION

Absolute speech recognition in quiet will have some influence on speech recognition in noise, and interpretation of the latter cannot be made without adequate assessment of the former.

Cognitive Competence

Can the patient perform the perceptual task? It seems like such an easy question. Not unlike the issue of hearing sensitivity loss, this question often arises when assessing the aging population. Are these changes in speech recognition ability attributable to true auditory processing disorder or are they simply a reflection of reduced capacity to perform the task brought on by senescent changes in cognition? The answer seems to be that for most of the perceptual tasks in the central auditory processing test battery, task-related demands are low enough to not be influenced by reductions in memory or cognition (Jerger et al, 1990a). In others, however, evidence exists that reduced scores can be related to the task rather than to an auditory problem.

What, then, is the role of cognitive ability in declining speech understanding with age? Jerger and colleagues (1989b) suggested that speech audiometric tests of central function were not necessarily related to cognitive disability. Audiological data were analyzed from 23 patients with a neuropsychological diagnosis of dementia. Among the cognitive deficits found in these patients were those of memory, tolerance of distraction, mental tracking and sequencing, and cognitive flexibility. Despite such deficits, 12 of the 23 subjects (52%) yielded speech audiometric results consistent with normal auditory processing ability. Although the auditory processing disorder found in the remaining 11 subjects could be related to cognitive deficits, it might also be the case that results on the neuropsychological evaluation were confounded by the effects of auditory processing disorder. That is, in these 11 subjects, the relative contribution of auditory and cognitive deficits could not be separated. In any event the fact that some patients with dementia could perform well on behavioral speech audiometric tests argues against the explanation that auditory processing disorders can be explained as easily by subtle cognitive decline as by an auditory deficit.

In another study Jerger and colleagues (1989a) measured both auditory and cognitive status in 130 aged subjects. They found that auditory processing ability and cognitive function were congruent in only 64% of subjects, indicating that the two measures are relatively independent. That is, auditory processing disorders can occur in those individuals with normal cognitive status, and cognitive decline can occur in those with normal auditory processing ability.

PEARL

Disorders of cognitive ability and disorders of central auditory processing are independent entities, yet each may influence interpretation of measures of the other.

These results suggest that, in general, speech audiometric measures are independent of significant cognitive decline. However, the story is not quite that simple. In another study of the aging process, this time using dichotic measures, some performance deficits were found to be task related (Jerger et al, 1990c). These results suggest that dichotic results could be overinterpreted as deficits if care was not taken to limit these nonauditory influences. Patients were asked to perform a dichotic measure in two ways. One was a free-recall mode, in which the patient's task was to identify both sentences in either order. The other was a focused-recall task, in which the patient was asked to identify only those sentences perceived in the right ear. The task was then repeated for the left ear. Results showed that a number of elderly patients had difficulty on the free-recall task but improved when the task was simplified. It appears that short-term memory problems were influencing the results on this dichotic measure. When the task was simplified, some patients still showed deficits, but they appeared to be truly auditory in nature. Care must be taken when selecting tests for clinical populations that include older individuals to ensure that task-related performance issues are well understood and controlled.

PITFALL

Memory and other nonauditory cognitive factors can cause task-related deficits that are not reflective of auditory ability, especially on measures of dichotic listening.

Influence of Medication and Other Drugs

Performance on any behavioral measure, and particularly on those that are designed to stress the auditory system, can be adversely influenced by some medications and intoxicants. Performance can be reduced temporarily from acute drug use or intoxication, or it can be reduced permanently from chronic exposure to toxins. As an example of the former, patients who have ingested alcohol before the evaluation can perform poorly on measures of central auditory processing ability. As an example of the latter, workers who are exposed to industrial toxins for a number of years will show permanent changes in auditory processing ability.

Procedural Factors

Procedural factors can certainly influence the successful implementation of a central auditory processing test battery. Most commercially available tests have been designed to control many of these factors. Nevertheless, applicability of certain tests and test materials can be limited, especially in older patients.

Speech versus Nonspeech Stimuli

Merits and controversies are related to the use of speech and nonspeech targets and competition. Regarding targets, the more speechlike the signal, the more redundant the informational content. This helps in overcoming hearing loss but requires sensitizing to challenge the central auditory system. The less speechlike the targets, the easier they are to control, but the more distant they are from being readily generalized to communication ability.

Regarding competition, the issue is related to how interfering the competitor can be. White noise or multitalker babble tends to act like a masker without much interference other than that which is achieved acoustically. The more speechlike and meaningful the competition, the more interfering it is likely to be and the more effective it will be in challenging the auditory processing system (Sperry et al, 1997; Stuart & Phillips, 1996). For this reason, competition consisting of single-talkers, double-talkers, or even noise that has been temporally altered to resemble speech has been used effectively to provide interference with the perceptual task.

SPECIAL CONSIDERATION

The more speechlike the competition, the more interfering it will be in perceiving speech in noise, and the more valuable it will be as a competitor in CAPD assessment.

Response Modes

Another procedural factor that can influence outcomes is whether the measure is open-set or closed-set in nature. This issue relates primarily to speech audiometric measures. At least two advantages exist to closed-set measures. First, the use of closed-set responses generally allows the "anchoring" of performance at a known level. For example, if performance on a measure in quiet is 100% on a closed-set measure, it is readily assured that the patient has the language, cognition, memory, and attention to perform the particular task. Once competition is added or some other sensitizing is done to the targets, the tester is assured that the patient has the capacity to perform the task. A second advantage can be achieved when testing is being carried out on adults with limited language ability, such as those with aphasia. In such cases, picture-pointing tasks can be used, wherein the patient has a limited number of foils from which to choose the correct answer, and the language level may be low enough to overcome the effects of aphasia (S. Jerger et al, 1990).

Monaural versus Binaural versus Dichotic

Assessing all three conditions, monaural speech recognition, binaural ability, and dichotic listening, is probably meritorious. Each has the potential to provide insight about the presence

and nature of a CAPD. In isolation, each reveals only a portion of the system's ability to process information.

Task Complexity

Complexity of the perceptual or response tasks tends to add a variable that can be difficult to control. As learned in the example of elderly listeners' difficulty with free recall of dichotically presented sentences, if a task is to be applicable to all ages of adults, it must take into considerations task-related limitations of aging patients. Tasks that require perceptual judgments, adaptive psychophysical procedures, and measures that tax memory can all add confounding variables to the assessment of CAPD in older adults.

SOME DIAGNOSTIC MEASURES OF CENTRAL AUDITORY PROCESSING DISORDER

Following are descriptions of some available measures of central auditory processing ability. Although not exhaustive, those described are among the measures that have stood the test of time or that hold promise as effective measures for clinical testing.

Monaural Measures

Monaural measures of central auditory processing ability are typically speech audiometric measures that are in some way sensitized in an effort to challenge the central auditory mechanisms. Monaural speech audiometric measures include high-level word-recognition testing, time-compressed speech, low-pass filtered speech, and speech in competition. Other monaural measures include nonspeech assessment of temporal processing ability.

Word Sentence Recognition in Quiet

Interpretation of word-recognition measures is based on the predictable relation of maximum word-recognition scores to degree of hearing loss. If the maximum score falls within a given range for a given degree of hearing loss, the results are considered to be within expectation for a cochlear hearing loss. If the score is poorer than expected, word-recognition ability is considered to be abnormal for the degree of hearing loss and consistent with retrocochlear disorder.

One modification of this original word-recognition paradigm has been the exploration of speech understanding across the patient's entire dynamic range of hearing rather than at just a single suprathreshold level. The goal here is to determine a maximum score regardless of test level. To obtain a maximum score, lists of words or sentences are presented at three to five different intensity levels, extending from just above the speech threshold to the upper level of comfortable listening. In this way, a *performance versus intensity* or PI function is generated for each ear. In most cases the PI function rises systematically as speech intensity is increased to an asymptomatic level representing the best speech understanding that can be achieved in the test ear. In some cases, however, a paradoxical *rollover* effect occurs, in which the function declines substantially as speech intensity increases beyond the level producing the maximal performance score. In other words as speech intensity increases, performance rises to a maximum level, then declines or "rolls over" sharply as intensity continues to increase. This rollover effect is commonly observed when the site of the hearing loss is retrocochlear, in the auditory nerve or the auditory pathways in the brain stem (Dirks et al, 1977; Jerger & Jerger, 1971).

PEARL

The use of high-level speech-recognition testing is a way of sensitizing speech audiometric measures by challenging the auditory system at high intensity levels. Reduced performance at high intensity levels is not uncommon in disordered central auditory nervous systems.

The use of PI functions is a way of sensitizing speech by challenging the auditory system at high intensity levels. Because of its ease of administration, many audiologists use it routinely as a screening measure for retrocochlear disorders.

Sensitized Speech

One of the first measures of central auditory processing ability was the low-pass filtered speech test. In this test, single-syllable words are low-pass filtered below 500 Hz to eliminate higher frequency information and the redundancy it provides. Most listeners with normal-hearing sensitivity and normal auditory nervous systems can perceive these targets accurately, despite the severity of filtering. However, patients with auditory processing disorders require more redundancy and tend to perform poorly on these measures. Results in patients with temporal lobe lesions showed poorer scores in the ear contralateral to the lesion (Boca et al, 1954; Jerger, 1960; Lynn & Gilroy, 1977) and patients with brain stem lesions showed ipsilateral, contralateral, and bilateral ear effects (Calearo & Antonelli, 1968; Lynn & Gilroy, 1977).

Time compression of speech targets is another way to reduce the redundancy. Time compression effectively speeds up speech by eliminating segments of the speech signal and compressing the remaining speech into a smaller time window. This results in rapid speech that is unaltered in the frequency and amplitude domains. Processing of time-compressed speech has been shown to be abnormal in patients with brain stem lesions (Calearo & Antonelli, 1968), cortical disorder (Calearo & Lazzaroni, 1957; Kurdziel et al, 1976), and in aging populations (Konkle et al, 1977; Letowski & Poch, 1996; Sticht & Gray, 1969).

Although redundancy can be reduced by low-pass filtering or time compression, these methods have clinical limitations because of their susceptibility to the effects of cochlear hearing loss. That is, hearing sensitivity loss of cochlear origin may affect scores on these measures in a manner that does not permit the interpretation of central auditory system integrity. As a result, test results are generally only interpretable on individuals who have normal-hearing sensitivity, which does not give these measures widespread clinical applicability in adult populations.

Perhaps the most successfully used sensitized speech measures are those in which competition is presented as a means of stressing the auditory system. Two examples of speech-in-competition measures are the speech-perception-in-noise (SPIN) test and the synthetic sentence identification (SSI) test (Jerger et al, 1968). The SPIN test (Kalikow et al, 1977) has as its target a single word that is the last in a sentence. In half the sentences the word is predictable from the context of the sentence. These signals are presented in a background of multitalker competition. Although useful in assessing speech-recognition in competition, the influence of cochlear hearing loss does not always allow accurate interpretation.

The SSI test (Jerger et al, 1968) also uses sentence materials presented in competition. The SSI uses sentential approximations that are presented in a closed-set format. The patient is asked to identify the sentence from a list of 10. Sentences are presented in the presence of single-talker competition. Testing typically is carried out with the signal and the competition at the same intensity level, a message/competition ratio of 0 dB. The SSI has some advantages inherent in its design. First, because it uses sentence materials, it is relatively immune to hearing loss. Said another way, the influence of mild degrees of hearing loss on identification of these sentences is minimal, and the effect of more severe hearing loss on absolute scores is known. Second, it uses a closed-set response, thereby permitting practice that reduces learning effects and ensures that a patient's performance deficits are not task related. Third, the single-talker competition, which has no influence on recognition scores of those with normal auditory ability, can be quite interfering to sentence perception in those with central auditory processing ability. Reduced performance on the SSI has been reported in patients with brain stem disorders (Jerger & Hayes, 1977; Jerger & Jerger, 1975; Jerger & Jerger, 1983; Russolo & Poli, 1983) and in the aging population.

Temporal Processing

Various measures of temporal processing have been used to assess central auditory ability. One measure is known as the auditory duration patterns test (ADPT) (Musiek et al, 1990). The ADPT is a sequence of three 1000 Hz tones, one of which varies from the others in duration. The duration of a tone is either longer (500 ms) or shorter (200 ms). The patient's task is to identify the pattern of tones as long-long-short, long-short-long, short-short-long, and so on. Practice items can be given before testing to eliminate learning effects. Abnormal performance has been reported in patients with temporal lobe disorder (Musiek et al, 1990; Hurley & Musiek, 1997).

Other measures of temporal processing have shown changes related to the aging process (Fitzgibbons & Gordon-Salant, 1996). These measures include assessment of temporal resolution by gap detection or modulation detection and assessment of duration discrimination by duration difference limen determination. Although these psychophysical measures are not generally applicable clinically, results from the aging population show the potential for their usefulness in assessing central auditory processing ability in the time domain.

Binaural Measures

One important aspect of auditory processing ability is the manner in which both ears work together to integrate and separate information. Measures of binaural ability include assessment of the manner in which the ears process phase cues, integrate information, lateralize and localize the source of sound, and extract signals of interest from background competition.

Masking Level Difference

One behavioral diagnostic measure that has stood the test of time is a measure of lower brain stem function known as the masking level difference (MLD). The MLD measures binaural release from masking caused by interaural phase relationships. As described earlier, the binaural auditory system is an exquisite detector of differences in timing of sound reaching the two ears. This helps in localizing low-frequency sounds, which reach the ears at different points in time. As described earlier, the concept of binaural release from masking reveals how sensitive the ears are to these timing, or phase, cues.

The MLD test is the clinical strategy designed to measure binaural release from masking. To carry out the MLD, a 500 Hz interrupted tone is split and presented in phase to both ears. Narrowband noise is also presented at a fixed level of 60 dB HL. Using the Bekesy tracking procedure, threshold for the in-phase tones is determined in the presence of the noise. Then the phase of one of the tones is reversed, and threshold is tracked again. The MLD is the difference in threshold between the in-phase and the out-of-phase conditions. For a 500 Hz tone, the MLD should be greater than 7 dB and is usually around 12 dB.

Abnormal performance on the MLD is consistent with brain stem disorder (Hannley et al, 1983; Hendler et al, 1990; Lynn et al, 1981; Noffsinger et al, 1975; Olsen & Noffsinger, 1976; Quaranta & Cervellera, 1977). Care must be taken in interpreting MLD results in the presence of hearing loss because the MLD shift is reduced with reduced hearing thresholds (Jerger et al, 1984).

SPECIAL CONSIDERATION

Care must be taken in interpreting MLD results in the presence of hearing loss, especially when losses occur at 500 Hz or thresholds at 500 Hz are asymmetric.

Binaural Integration

Efforts have been made to assess how the two ears can work together to integrate partial information from each into a binaural perception of the whole. Two such efforts include the measures of binaural fusion and binaural resynthesis.

Binaural fusion is a measure in which words, usually monosyllables, are pass-band filtered into a low-pass band and a high-pass band. In the original description of the binaural fusion test, the low-pass band was from 500 to 800 Hz and the high-pass band from 1815 to 2500 Hz (Matzker, 1959). The low-pass band is presented to one ear and the high-pass band to the other. Recognition of either band in isolation is generally poor. However, normal listeners are capable of fusing the two pass-bands when they are presented binaurally and recognizing the words with a high level of accuracy. Abnormally poor binaural fusion scores have been reported

in some patients with brain stem disorder (Palva & Jokinen, 1975; Smith & Resnick, 1972) and in some patients with temporal lobe disorder (Lynn & Gilroy, 1972).

Another test of binaural integration, often referred to as binaural resynthesis, is the rapidly alternating speech perception (RASP) test (Bocca & Calearo, 1963; Lynn & Gilroy, 1977; Willeford, 1977), wherein a sentence stimulus is alternated between the ears every 300 ms. The segments presented to one ear are minimally intelligible under normal conditions. The segments from both ears fuse together into an easily recognizable message under normal circumstances. Abnormal performance on the RASP test has been associated with disorders at the level of the lower brain stem (Lynn & Gilroy, 1977; Musiek & Geurkink, 1982).

Precedence

The precedence effect in sound localization is measured by presenting identical clicks from two speakers on opposite sides of the subject's head. The onset of clicks from one speaker is presented earlier than that from the other speaker. With proper delays, normal subjects perceive a fused image originating from the leading speaker. The precedence effect has been shown to be abnormal in elderly individuals (Cranford & Romereim, 1992) and in patients with multiple sclerosis (Cranford et al, 1990).

Localization

Localization ability is usually measured in a sound field and expressed as the accuracy of identifying a signal source. Numerous strategies for measuring localization ability have been implemented over the years, but few have proven to be practical clinically. Nevertheless, poor localization ability has been associated with auditory nervous system disorders at the level of the brain stem (Hausler et al, 1983; Stephens, 1976) and cortex (Sanchez-Longo & Forster, 1958; Stephens, 1976).

One of the more promising strategies for assessment of localization ability is the three-dimensional (3-D) auditory test of localization (Koehnke & Besing, 1997). By use of virtual reality techniques and digital signal processing technology, 3-D assessment of sound-source localization can be made under earphones, with the source being externalized to various spatial locations outside of the head. This new technique promises to bring the measurement of localization ability under control to an extent that it can be implemented clinically for assessment of this important aspect of auditory processing ability.

Cued Discourse

Another promising strategy for the assessment of binaural hearing is the cued discourse technique (Jerger et al, 1991b). Identical ongoing speech signals are presented from speakers opposite the right and left ear. The speech signal is a single talker reading a story written in the first person. The same story is presented from both speakers with a delay of 1 minute in one of the speakers. The patient's task is to count the number of times that the personal pronoun "I" is perceived from the speaker that is being cued. The number of errors is counted, and the opposite speaker is cued. After completion, multi-talker babble is introduced from an overhead speaker, and the process is repeated over a range of signal-to-noise ratios. Results of the cued discourse measure have shown significant asymmetries in patients with CAPDs (Jerger et al, 1991b) and in the aging population (Jerger & Jordan, 1992). The listening situation is a challenging one, and the technique seems likely to assist in quantifying disorders in those patients with obscure and difficult-to-measure auditory complaints.

Dichotic Measures

Another effective approach to assessing central auditory processing ability is the use of dichotic tests. In the dichotic paradigm two different speech targets are presented simultaneously to the two ears. The patient's task is usually either to repeat back both targets in either order or to report only the target heard in the precued ear. In this latter case the right ear is precued on half the trials and the left on the other half. Two scores are determined, one for targets correctly identified from the right ear, the other for targets correctly identified from the left ear. The patterns of results can reveal auditory processing deficits, especially those caused by disorders of the temporal lobe and corpus callosum. Dichotic tests have been constructed using nonsense syllables, monosyllabic words, spondaic words, sentences, and synthetic sentences.

Dichotic Consonant Vowels

CV nonsense syllables have been used as dichotic stimuli (Berlin et al, 1972), presented either simultaneously or in a manner that staggers the presentation from 30 to 90 ms. Simultaneous presentation yields normal scores of approximately 60 to 70% correct identification. In the staggered condition, scores are better for the lagging ear than for the leading ear. Regardless of method, abnormal results on the dichotic CV test have been reported in patients with temporal lobe lesions (Collard et al, 1986; Olsen, 1983), temporal lobectomy (Berlin et al, 1972), and hemispherectomy.

Dichotic Digits

Dichotic listening has been assessed for many years with a paradigm that uses digits as stimuli (Broadbent, 1954; Kimura, 1961). More recent efforts (Musiek, 1983a) have rekindled interest in use of the digits test to assess dichotic performance. In its current version the dichotic digits test consists of 40 pairs of digits delivered simultaneously to both ears. The patients' task is to identify the digits in a free-recall mode (i.e., in any order). One advantage of the dichotic digits test is its relative resistance to the effects of peripheral hearing loss. Abnormal performance on the dichotic digits test has been reported in patients with brain stem lesions (Musiek 1983b), temporal lobe lesions (Hurley & Musiek, 1997; Kimura, 1961; Musiek, 1983b; Sparks et al, 1970), and as a result of the aging process (Wilson & Jaffe, 1996). Although the predominant findings have shown contralateral ear effects, many patients with brain stem and temporal lobe lesions will also show abnormal ipsilateral performance.

Staggered Spondaic Word Test

The staggered spondaic word (SSW) test (Katz, 1962) is one in which a different spondaic word is presented to each ear, with the second syllable of the word presented to the leading ear overlapping in time with the first syllable of the word presented to the lagging ear. Thus the leading hear is presented with one syllable in isolation (noncompeting), followed by one syllable in a dichotic mode (competing). The lagging ear begins with the first syllable presented in the dichotic mode and finishes with the second syllable presented in isolation. The right ear serves as the leading ear for half of the test presentations. Error scores are calculated for each ear in both the competing and noncompeting modes. A correction can be applied to account for hearing sensitivity loss. Abnormal SSW performance has been reported in patients with brain stem (Musiek, 1983b), corpus callosum (Baran et al, 1986), and temporal lobe lesions (Lynn & Gilroy, 1977; Olsen, 1983; Winkelaar & Lewis, 1977).

Competing Sentence Test

The competing sentence test (Willeford, 1977) uses short natural sentences that average six to seven words in length. The sentence presented to the target ear is generally set at an intensity level 15 dB below the level of the sentence presented to the nontarget ear. Sentences are generally scored as correct if the meaning and content of the sentence was identified appropriately. Abnormal competing sentence test performance has been reported in patients with temporal lobe lesions (Lynn & Gilroy, 1977; Musiek, 1983b), predominantly on the ear contralateral to the lesion.

Dichotic Sentence Identification Test

The dichotic sentence identification (DSI) test (Fifer et al, 1983) uses synthetic sentences from the SSI test aligned for presentation in the dichotic mode. The response is closed-set, and the subject's task is to identify the sentences from among a list on a response card. The DSI was designed in an effort to overcome the influence of hearing sensitivity loss on test interpretation and was found to be applicable for use in ears with a pure tone average of up to 50 dB and asymmetry of up to 40 dB. Abnormal DSI results have been reported in aging patients (Jerger et al, 1990c, 1994).

TOWARD A COGENT CLINICAL STRATEGY

With such a wide array of diagnostic options, the challenge of deciding which to use for clinical assessment can be a daunting one. A number of test batteries have been applied over the years (e.g., Keith, 1995; Musiek et al, 1994; Willeford, 1977) with varying degrees of success.

A test battery will be described briefly here in an effort to illustrate one approach to the diagnosis of CAPD that has proven successful clinically (Jerger & Hayes, 1977; Stach et al, 1990b). The approach that is used to diagnose CAPD is based on the assumptions that (1) CAPD is an auditory perceptual problem, not a cognitive or linguistic problem; (2) that it can be operationally defined on the basis of speech audiometric measures; and (3) that tests can be administered in a manner that limits the influences of cochlear hearing loss, language, and cognition on interpretation of results. Although it is by no means the only strategy that exists, it is successful for several reasons. First, the measures have been validated in populations of patients with confirmed neurological disease processes, making them useful for diagnostic screening purposes and applicable for describing CAPD as a communication disorder (Jerger & Jerger, 1975; Jerger & Jerger, 1983). Second, the measures can be used with most patients in a manner that is clinically efficient. Third, the approach has a reasonable degree of specificity in that factors unrelated to central auditory disorders seldom result in poor performance on the measures used. Fourth, to the extent possible, the approach is effective in controlling the influences of cochlear hearing loss on test interpretation. In addition, the measures can be applied in a manner that controls the cognitive influences of factors such as memory, thereby isolating auditory disorder from nonauditory influences on test interpretation.

PEARL

The key factors in any successful test battery approach are the efficient and effective controls over cochlear sensitivity loss, absolute speech recognition ability, and nonauditory influences.

Applying such a clinical strategy to any of a number of existing tests of CAPD would likely enhance their usefulness in a test battery as well. The key factors are the efficient and effective controls over cochlear sensitivity loss, absolute speech recognition ability, and nonauditory influences.

A Test Battery Approach

The test battery described here includes word-recognition testing in quiet, the SSI test (Jerger et al, 1968) with ipsilateral competing message, and the DSI test (Fifer et al, 1983). CAPD is operationally defined on the basis of patterns of speech audiometric scores.

Word-recognition testing is carried out in quiet across a range of intensity levels, providing a PI function. The maximum word recognition score is compared with empirically derived normative scores on the basis of the degree of hearing sensitivity loss. These normative scores are based on the performance of a large number of patients with cochlear hearing loss and no evidence of retrocochlear disorder. If performance equals or exceeds the lower limits of normal, the score is considered appropriate for that degree of hearing loss and consistent with normal-hearing, conductive hearing loss, or sensorineural hearing loss of cochlear origin. If performance is less than the lower limits of normal, the score is considered abnormal for that degree of hearing loss consistent with retrocochlear disorder. A PI function is obtained to look for rollover. A small amount of rollover (<20%) can be attributable to cochlear hearing loss. A more significant rollover is consistent with retrocochlear disorder.

The SSI test is administered monaurally, with ipsilateral competition at a message-to-competition ratio of 0 dB. This test is also administered across a range of intensity levels to determine a PI function. Interpretation is based on maximum score compared with established norms on the basis of degree of hearing loss, the amount of rollover, and the discrepancy between speech recognition of words in quiet and the sentences in competition. Excessive reduction in sentence recognition in competition compared with word-recognition scores obtained in quiet is a finding that is often consistent with retrocochlear disorder.

The DSI test is generally presented at a single intensity level. If hearing sensitivity is normal, sentences are delivered at 50 dB HL to both ears. If a hearing loss exists, the level is increased in both ears. Testing is always carried out at equal HL in both ears. Over the past few years, dichotic performance has been evaluated under two task conditions, free recall and focused recall. In the free-recall condition, the patient is asked to identify both sentences regardless of the ear in which they are heard. In the focused-recall condition, the patient is asked to identify only those sentences identified in a specified ear, and then the other ear is tested. Results are consistent with a dichotic deficit when scores on the focused-recall condition show significant asymmetry or reduced scores in both ears.

In terms of screening for retrocochlear disorder, general patterns have emerged as being consistent with lesions at certain levels within the auditory system. These patterns are summarized in Table 16–5. When a hearing loss is cochlear, word-recognition and SSI scores will be consistent with the degree of loss, and little if any rollover will occur on the PI function. DSI scores will be normal.

When a hearing loss is sensorineural because of an eighth nerve lesion, suprathreshold word recognition ability is likely to be substantially affected. Maximum scores are likely to be

TABLE 16–5 Expected patterns of abnormality related to central auditory processing disorder on a battery of tests, including maximum word-recognition scores presented in quiet (WRS max), performance intensity function of word-recognition scores in quiet (WRS PI), maximum synthetic sentence identification scores (SSI max), performance intensity function of SSI scores (SSI PI), and scores on the dichotic sentence identification (DSI) test. Predicted performance on these measures would be: (-) normal or predictable from the degree of hearing sensitivity loss; (±) sometimes abnormal, depending on the site, size, and extent of influence of the lesion; or (+) abnormal.

Site	WRS max	WRS PI	SSI max	SSI PI	DSI
Cochlea	−	−	−	−	−
Eighth nerve	+	+	+	+	−
Brain stem	−	±	+	+	−
Temporal lobe	−	−	±	±	+

poorer than predicted from the degree of hearing loss, and rollover of the PI function is likely to occur. SSI scores are also likely to be depressed. Abnormal results will occur in the ear ipsilateral to the lesion. Dichotic measures will be normal.

When a hearing disorder occurs as a result of a brain stem lesion, suprathreshold word-recognition ability is likely to be affected. Word-recognition scores in quiet may be normal, or they may be depressed or show rollover. SSI scores are likely to be depressed or show rollover in the ear ipsilateral to the lesion. Dichotic measures will likely be normal.

When a hearing disorder occurs as the result of a temporal lobe lesion, hearing sensitivity is unlikely to be affected, and word-recognition scores are likely to be normal. SSI scores may or may not be abnormal in the ear contralateral to the lesion. DSI scores are most likely to show a deficit caused by the temporal lobe lesion, usually characterized by a substantial left ear deficit.

In patients with CAPD and no identifiable neuropathological condition, patterns of results are similar to those of patients with brain stem and/or temporal lobe lesions. In an elderly patient, for example, it is not uncommon to observe reduced SSI maximum scores with rollover and reduced dichotic performance.

Controlling for Hearing Sensitivity Loss

One of the benefits of this type of test battery approach is that it can be used in patients with a wide range of hearing sensitivity loss. That is, scores can be interpreted in the presence of a hearing loss because the influence of the loss on speech-recognition scores is known or controllable.

The influence of hearing sensitivity loss is controlled in several ways. First, as stated previously, maximum scores can be compared with normative data on the basis of degree of hearing loss. This can be done for both word-recognition and SSI scores. An example of the normative data for the SSI test is shown in Table 16–6. Thus, if a patient with a pure tone average of 35 dB HL has a maximum SSI score of 70%, the result is consistent with what could be expected from a hearing loss of that magnitude. However, if the maximum score was 30%, performance would be interpreted as poorer than that which would be attributable to the hearing loss alone, implicating a retrocochlear disorder as a contributor to the performance deficit.

A second way of controlling the influence of hearing sensitivity loss is by establishing a performance-intensity function. If maximum scores approach 100%, the hearing loss is not influencing absolute word-recognition ability. Should rollover occur at higher intensity, the reduced performance could not be attributable to any influence of sensitivity loss on absolute performance.

Another way of managing hearing loss influence is by testing at more than one message/competition ratio. For example, one strategy used with the SSI test is to begin testing at a favorable ratio of +10 dB. If a patient scores 100%, the hearing sensitivity loss is not interfering with perception of the sentence. A reduced score at a reduced message/competition ratio, then, is more appropriately attributable to a problem in auditory processing ability. A similar strategy can be used in dichotic testing. Each ear can be assessed in isolation to deter-

TABLE 16–6 Lower limits of maximum SSI scores (SSI max) for different degrees of cochlear hearing sensitivity loss as quantified by the pure tone average (PTA) of thresholds at 500, 1000, and 2000 Hz

PTA (dB)	SSI max (%)
0	86
5	81
10	76
15	71
20	66
25	61
30	56
35	51
40	46
45	41
50	36
55	31
60	26
65	21
70	16
75	11
80	6
85	0

After Yellin et al (1989), with permission.

mine absolute sentence-recognition ability. Any reduction in scores with dichotic presentation can then be attributed to a dichotic deficit rather than any peripheral influences.

Controlling Nonauditory Influences on Test Interpretation

Nonauditory influences are controlled in much the same way as the influence of cochlear sensitivity loss. Good performance at one intensity level and poorer performance at a higher intensity level is difficult to explain on the basis of a cognitive or language deficit. Similarly, good performance at one message/competition ratio and poorer performance at another is difficult to attribute to these nonauditory influences. Often performance will be asymmetrical as well, forcing the unlikely argument necessary to explain ear asymmetry on the basis of a cognitive or language deficit. That is, can there be a left ear cognitive deficit? Can there be a left ear language deficit? Obviously, the likelihood of asymmetry resulting from a cognitive or language deficit is small. An argument would also have to be made to explain the rollover of the PI function. Could it be that a patient might somehow be cognitively more impaired at higher intensity levels than at lower intensity levels? An intensity-level specific cognitive deficit would be a very difficult one to explain.

By use of this type of test battery approach, with words and sentences presented at various intensity levels and message/competition ratios, it is possible to ensure that the patient is cognitively capable of carrying out the task, linguistically capable of carrying out the task, and has the attentional ability to carry out the task. Any deficit, then, could be attributable to an auditory processing disorder.

Thus use of PI functions, various message/competition ratios, and word-versus-sentence comparisons permits the assessment of auditory processing ability in a manner that reduces the likelihood of nonauditory factors influencing the interpretation of test results. Clinical experience with this diagnostic strategy has been encouraging. In conjunction with thorough immittance, otoacoustic emission, and auditory evoked potential measurements, the use of well-controlled speech audiometric measures has proven to be quite powerful in defining the presence or absence of an auditory processing disorder.

ILLUSTRATIVE CASES

The following cases illustrate results from two patients, one with retrocochlear disorder resulting from brain stem lesions and the other with CAPD resulting from auditory nervous system aging.

Central Auditory Processing Disorder in Neuropathological Conditions

Patient 1 has auditory complaints as a result of multiple sclerosis. The patient is a 34-year-old woman. Two years before her evaluation, she experienced an episode of diplopia, accompanied by a tingling sensation and weakness in her left leg. These symptoms gradually subsided and reappeared in slightly more severe form a year later. Ultimately, she was diagnosed with multiple sclerosis. Among various other symptoms, she had vague hearing complaints, particularly in the presence of background noise.

Immittance audiometry, as shown in Figure 16–1A is consistent with normal middle ear function, characterized by a type A tympanogram, normal static immittance, and normal right and left uncrossed reflex thresholds. However, crossed reflexes are absent bilaterally. This unusual pattern of results is consistent with a central pathway disorder of the lower brain stem.

Pure tone audiometric results are shown in Figure 16–1B. The patient has a mild low-frequency sensorineural hearing loss bilaterally, a finding that is not uncommon in brain stem disorder (Jerger & Jerger, 1980; Stach et al, 1990a).

Suprathreshold speech-recognition performance is abnormal in both ears. Although word-recognition scores are normal when presented in quiet, scores on sentence-recognition in the presence of competition are abnormal, as shown in Figure 16–1C. Dichotic scores were normal.

auditory evoked potentials are also consistent with abnormality of brain stem function. On the left no waves were identifiable beyond component wave II, and on the right none were identifiable beyond wave III.

Multiple sclerosis is a disease that involves the formation of demyelinating plaques within the white matter of the brain stem. When the plaques occur in or near the auditory pathways, function can be disrupted. In this case the speech audiometric results showed a classic pattern of brain stem disorder. Recognition of words in quiet was normal. The measure was not sensitized, and the signals contained too much redundancy to challenge the impaired nervous system. Had the lesions been more peripheral at the juncture of the eighth nerve and brain stem, these scores may well have been significantly reduced. Because neural information coursed through the bottleneck without disruption, perception of undistorted speech remained normal. In contrast, sentence recognition in competition was reduced bilaterally. This is likely due to bilateral lesions, with the ipsilateral ear affected on both sides. Dichotic performance remains normal because the temporal lobes and corpus callosum remain intact. Once again, these undistorted signals are perceived clearly at the level of the temporal lobe because of the redundancy of the signal.

One other characteristic of multiple sclerosis is that it goes through periods of exacerbation and remission. Results in Figure 16–1C were obtained during a period of exacerbation of the disease process. Results in Figure 16–1D were obtained 3 months later during a period of remission. SSI scores returned to near-normal levels as function of the brain stem improved.

Central Auditory Processing Disorder in Aging

Patient 2 has a long-standing sensorineural hearing loss. The patient is a 78-year-old woman with bilateral sensorineural hearing loss that has progressed slowly over the past 15 years. She has worn hearing aids for the past 10 years and has an annual audiological re-evaluation each year. Her major complaints are in communicating with her grandchildren and trying to hear in noisy restaurants. Although her hearing aids worked well for her at the beginning, she is not receiving the benefit from them that she did 10 years ago.

Immittance audiometry, a shown in Figure 16–2A is consistent with normal middle ear function, characterized by a type A tympanogram, normal static immittance, and normal crossed and uncrossed reflex thresholds bilaterally.

Pure tone audiometric results are shown in Figure 16–2B. The patient has a moderate, bilateral, symmetrical, sensorineural hearing loss. Hearing sensitivity is slightly better in the low frequencies than in the high frequencies.

Speech audiometric results are consistent with those found in older patients. Word-recognition scores are reduced, but not below a level predictable from the degree of hearing sensitivity loss. However, speech recognition in the presence of competition is substantially reduced, as shown in Figure 16–2C, consistent with the patient's age. Performance on the SSI at +10 dB message/competition ratio was 100% bilaterally.

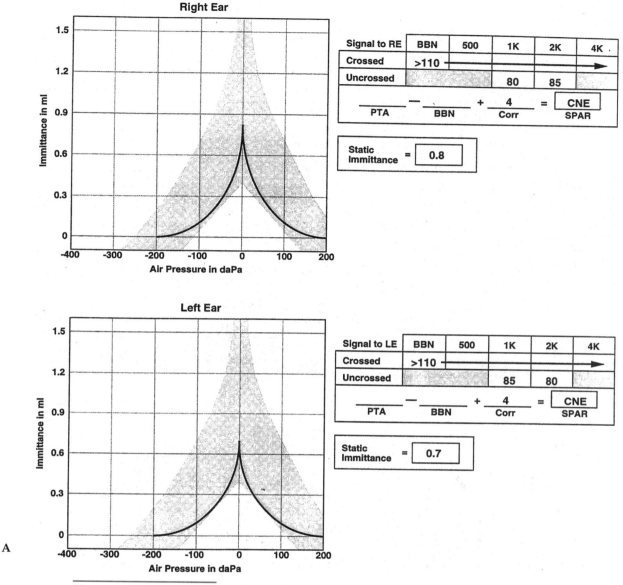

Figure 16–1 Hearing consultation results in a 34-year-old woman with multiple sclerosis. Immittance measures **(A)** are consistent with normal middle ear function. However, left-crossed and right crossed reflexes are absent, consistent with brain stem disorder. (*Figure continued next page.*)

However, at a 0 dB ratio, performance was substantially reduced. In addition to these monotic deficits, she also shows evidence of a dichotic deficit, with reduced performance in the left ear. Results are shown in Figure 16–2D. Performance on a free-recall task were reduced, with performance reduced even further on the focused-recall task.

Results of a hearing handicap assessment show that she has communication problems a significant proportion of the time in most listening environments, especially those involving background noise.

These results are not uncommon in many aging patients with hearing disorders. Word recognition in quiet is consistent with the degree of hearing loss. Speech perception in the

presence of competition is reduced beyond what might be expected from the hearing sensitivity loss. In addition, dichotic performance is abnormal in the left ear.

CONCLUSIONS

- Auditory processing ability is usually defined as the capacity with which the central auditory nervous system transfers information from the eighth nerve to the auditory cortex. CAPD is an impairment in this function of the central auditory nervous system.

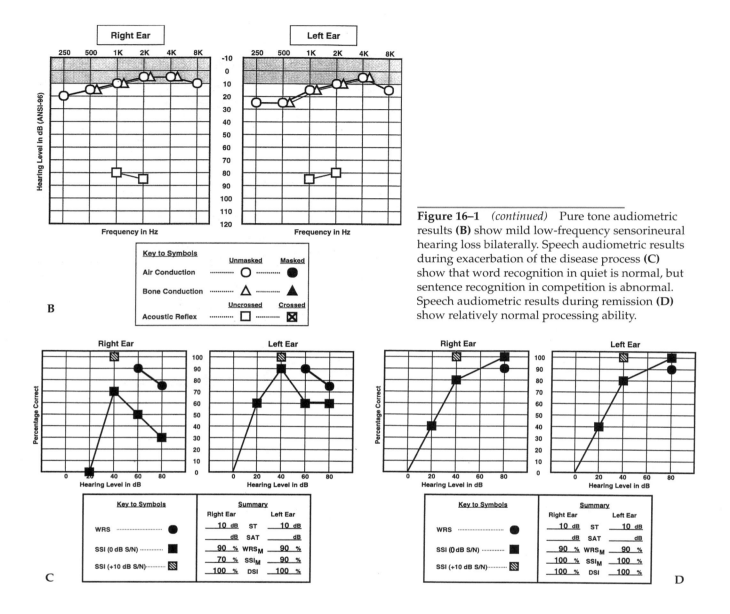

Figure 16–1 *(continued)* Pure tone audiometric results **(B)** show mild low-frequency sensorineural hearing loss bilaterally. Speech audiometric results during exacerbation of the disease process **(C)** show that word recognition in quiet is normal, but sentence recognition in competition is abnormal. Speech audiometric results during remission **(D)** show relatively normal processing ability.

- The aim of central auditory processing assessment is to evaluate the ability of the central auditory nervous system to process acoustic signals. Advanced speech audiometric and other behavioral measures can be used to measure central auditory nervous system function to assist in the screening of specific lesions of the auditory system and to describe a communication disorder.

- A disordered auditory nervous system, regardless of cause, will have functional consequences that can vary from subclinical to a substantial, easily measurable auditory deficit.

- A distinguishing feature of CAPD is the inability to extract sounds of interest in noisy environments despite an ability to perceive the sounds with adequate loudness.

- Two primary causes of CAPDs exist in adults. One is neuropathological conditions of the peripheral and central auditory nervous systems resulting from tumors or other space-occupying lesions or from damage caused by trauma

or stroke. The other is from diffuse changes in brain function usually related to the aging process.

- The measurement of central auditory processing ability in adults is typically carried out with a test battery approach that assesses absolute speech recognition ability, speech recognition in competition, dichotic listening, and temporal processing ability.

- Several factors influence the selection of testing tools and approaches and the success with which they are likely to be implemented. One of the most important factors in speech audiometric testing is the way in which information content of the test materials is manipulated. Other factors that are critical are those related to hearing sensitivity loss and cognitive ability of the patients being tested.

- Monaural speech audiometric measures include high-level word-recognition testing, time-compressed speech, low-pass filtered speech, and speech in competition. Other

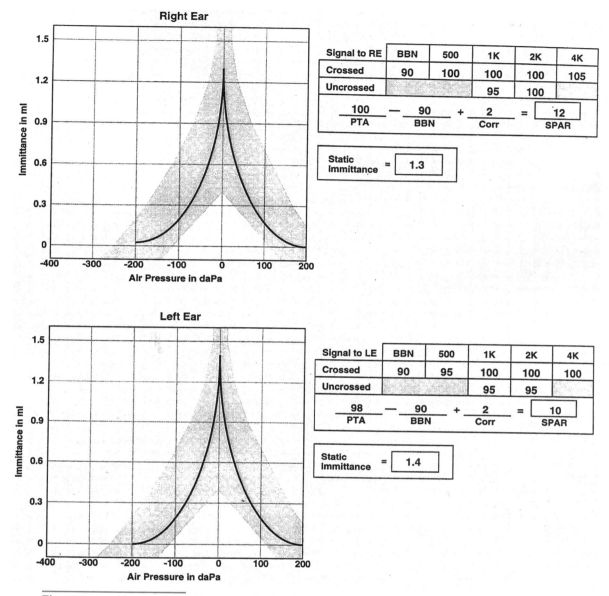

Figure 16–2 Hearing consultation results in a 78-year-old woman with long-standing, progressive hearing loss. Immittance measures **(A)** are consistent with normal middle ear function. (*Figure continued next page.*)

monaural measures include nonspeech assessment of temporal processing ability.

- Measures of binaural ability include assessment of the manner in which the ears process phase cues, integrate information, lateralize and localize the source of sound, and extract signals of interest from background competition.
- Another effective approach to assessing central auditory processing ability is the use of dichotic tests.
- A number of test batteries have been applied over the years with varying degrees of success. With such a wide array of diagnostic options, the challenge of deciding which to use for clinical assessment can be a daunting one.
- The key factors in any successful test battery approach are the efficient and effective controls over cochlear sensitivity loss, absolute speech recognition ability, and nonauditory influences.
- The use of performance-intensity functions, various message/competition ratios, and word-versus-sentence comparisons permits the assessment of auditory processing ability in a manner that reduces the likelihood of cochlear hearing loss and nonauditory factors influencing the interpretation of test results.
- In conjunction with thorough immittance, otoacoustic emission, and auditory evoked potential measurements, the use of well-controlled speech audiometric measures has proven to be quite powerful in defining the presence or absence of an auditory processing disorder.

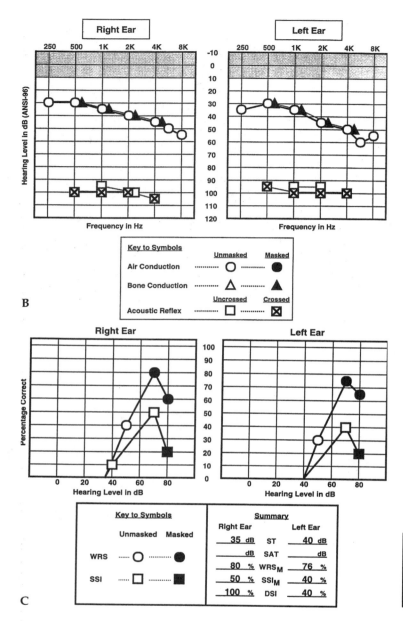

Figure 16–2 *(continued)*   Pure tone audiometric results **(B)** show bilateral, symmetrical, moderate, sensorineural hearing loss. Speech audiometric results **(C)** show reduced word recognition in quiet, consistent with the degree and configuration of cochlear hearing loss. Sentence recognition in competition is substantially reduced. Dichotic performance **(D)** is reduced in the left ear, regardless of task complexity.

	Right Ear	Left Ear
Free Recall	100	60
Focused Recall	100	40

D

REFERENCES

ANTONELLI, A. (1970). Sensitized speech tests in aged people. In: C. Rojskjaer (Ed.), *Speech audiometry.* Second Danavox Symposium. Odense, Denmark: Danavox.

ARNST, D. (1982). Staggered spondaic word test performance in a group of older adults. A preliminary report. *Ear and Hearing, 3;*118–123.

BARAN, J.A., MUSIEK, F.E., & REEVES, AG. (1986). Central auditory function following anterior sectioning of the corpus callosum. *Ear and Hearing, 7;*359–362.

BERGMAN, M. (1971). Hearing and aging. *Audiology, 10;* 164–171.

BERGMAN, M., BLUMFIELD, B., CASCARDO, D., DASH, B., LEVITT, H., & MARGUILES, M. (1976). Age-related decrement in hearing for speech: Sampling and longitudinal studies. *Journal of Gerontology, 31;*533–538.

BERLIN, C.I., LOWE-BELL, S.S., JANNETTA, P.J., & KLINE, D.G. (1972). Central auditory deficits of temporal lobectomy. *Archives of Otolaryngology, 96;*4–10.

BOCCA, E. (1958). Clinical aspects of cortical deafness. *Laryngoscope, 68;*301–309.

BOCCA, E., & CALEARO, C. (1963). Central hearing processes. In: J. Jerger (Ed.), *Modern developments in audiology* (pp. 337– 370.) New York: Academic Press.

BOCCA, E., CALEARO, C., & CASSINARI, V. (1954). A new method for testing hearing in temporal lobe tumours. *Acta Oto-laryngologica, 44;*219–221.

BOSATRA, A., & RUSSOLO, M. (1982). Comparison between central tonal tests and central speech tests in elderly subjects. *Audiology, 21*;334–341.

BROADBENT, D.E. (1954). The role of auditory localization of attention and memory span. *Journal of Experimental Psychology, 47*;191–196.

CACACE, A.T., PARNES, S.M., LOVELY, T.J., & KALATHIA, A. (1994). The disconnected ear: Phenomenological effects of a large acoustic tumor. *Ear and Hearing, 15*;287–298.

CALEARO, C., & ANTONELLI, A.R. (1968). Audiometric findings in brain stem lesions. *Acta Otolaryngologica, 66*;305–319.

CALEARO, C., & LAZZARONI, A. (1957). Speech intelligibility in relation to the speed of the message. *Laryngoscope, 67*; 410–419.

CHMIEL, R., & JERGER, J. (1996). Hearing aid use, central auditory disorder, and hearing handicap in elderly persons. *Journal of the American Academy of Audiology, 7*;190–202.

CHMIEL, R., JERGER, J., MURPHY, E., PIROZZOLO, F., & TOOLEY-YOUNG, C. (1997). Unsuccessful use of binaural amplification by an elderly person. *Journal of the American Academy of Audiology, 8*;1–0.

COLLARD, M.E., LESSER, R.P., LÜDERS, H., DINNER, D.S., MORRIS, H.H., HAHN, J.F., & ROTHNER, A.D. (1986). Four dichotic speech tests before and after temporal lobectomy. *Ear and Hearing, 7*;363–369.

CRANFORD, J.L., BOOSE, M., & MOORE, CA. (1990). Tests of precedence effect in sound localization reveal abnormalities in multiple sclerosis. *Ear and Hearing, 11*;282–288.

CRANFORD, J.L., & ROMEREIM, B. (1992). Precedence effect and speech understanding in elderly listeners. *Journal of the American Academy of Audiology, 3*;405–409.

DIRKS, D.D., KAMM, C., BOWER, D., & BETSWORTH, A. (1977). Use of performance-intensity functions for diagnosis. *Journal of Speech and Hearing Disorders, 42*;408–415.

FIFER, R.C., JERGER, J.F., BERLIN, C.I., TOBEY, E.A., & CAMPBELL, J.C. (1983). Development of a dichotic sentence identification test for hearing-impaired adults. *Ear and Hearing, 4*;300–305.

FITZGIBBONS, P.J., & GORDON-SALANT, S. (1996). Auditory temporal processing in elderly listeners. *Journal of the American Academy of Audiology, 7*;183–189.

GELFAND, S.A. (1995). Long-term recovery and no recovery from the auditory deprivation effect with binaural amplification: Six cases. *Journal of the American Academy of Audiology, 6*;141–149.

GELFAND, S.A., HOFFMAN, S., WALTZMAN, S.B., & PIPER, N. (1980). Dichotic CV recognition at various interaural temporal onset asynchronies: Effect of age. *Journal of the Acoustical Society of America, 68*;1258–1261.

GOETZINGER, C., PROUD, G., DIRKS, D., & EMBREY, J. (1961). A study of hearing in advanced age. *Archives of Otolaryngology, 73*;662–674.

GROSE , J.H. (1996). Binaural performance and aging. *Journal of the American Academy of Audiology, 7*;168–174.

HANNLEY, M., JERGER, J.F., & RIVERA, V.M. (1983). Relationships among auditory brain stem responses, masking level differences and the acoustic reflex in multiple sclerosis. *Audiology, 22*;20–33.

HAUSLER, R., COLBURN, S., & MARR, E. (1983). Sound localization in subjects with impaired hearing: Spacial-discrimination and interaural-discrimination tests. *Acta Oto-Laryngologica Supplement, 400*;1–62.

HELFER, K.S., & WILBER, L.A. (1990). Hearing loss, aging, and speech perception in reverberation and noise. *Journal of Speech and Hearing Research, 33*;149–155.

HENDLER, T., SQUIRES, N.K., & EMMERICH, D.S. (1990). Psychophysical measures of central auditory dysfunction in multiple sclerosis: Neurophysiological and neuroanatomical correlates. *Ear and Hearing, 11*;403–416.

HINCHCLIFFE, R. (1962). The anatomical locus of presbycusis. *Journal of Speech and Hearing Disorders, 27*;301–310.

HOOD, L.J., BERLIN, C.I., & ALLEN, P. (1994). Cortical deafness: A longitudinal study. *Journal of the American Academy of Audiology, 5*;330–342.

HURLEY, R., & MUSIEK, F.E. (1997). Effectiveness of three central auditory processing (CAP) tests in identifying cerebral lesions. *Journal of the American Academy of Audiology, 8*;257–262.

JERGER, J. (1960). Observations on auditory behavior in lesions of the central auditory pathways. *Archives of Otolaryngology, 71*;797–806.

JERGER, J. (1973). Audiological findings in aging. *Advances in Oto-Rhino-Laryngology, 20*;115–124.

JERGER, J. (1992). Can age-related decline in speech understanding be explained by peripheral hearing loss? *Journal of the American Academy of Audiology, 3*;33–38.

JERGER, J., ALFORD, B., LEW, H., RIVERA, V., & CHMIEL, R. (1995). Dichotic listening, event-related potentials, and interhemispheric transfer in the elderly. *Ear and Hearing, 16*;482–498.

JERGER, J., BROWN, D., & SMITH, S. (1984). Effect of peripheral hearing loss on masking level difference. *Archives of Otolaryngology, 110*;290–296.

JERGER, J., CHMIEL, R., ALLEN, J., & WILSON, A. (1994). Effects of age and gender on dichotic sentence identification. *Ear and Hearing, 15*;274–286.

JERGER, J., & HAYES, D. (1977). Diagnostic speech audiometry. *Archives of Otolaryngology, 103*;216–222.

JERGER, J., & JERGER, S. (1971). Diagnostic significance of PB word functions. *Archives of Otolaryngology, 93*;573–580.

JERGER, J., & JERGER, S. (1975). Clinical validity of central auditory tests. *Scandinavian Audiology, 4*;147–163.

JERGER, J., JERGER, S., OLIVER, T., & PIROZZOLO, F. (1989a). Speech understanding in the elderly. *Ear and Hearing, 10*;79–89.

JERGER, J., JERGER, S., & PIROZZOLO, F. (1991a). Correlational analysis of speech audiometric scores, hearing loss, age, and cognitive abilities in the elderly. *Ear and Hearing, 12*;102–109.

JERGER, J., JOHNSON, K., JERGER, S., COKER, N., PIROZZOLO, F., & GRAY, L. (1991b). Central auditory processing disorder: A case study. *Journal of the American Academy of Audiology, 2*;36–54.

JERGER, J., & JORDAN, C. (1992). Age-related asymmetry on a cued-listening task. *Ear and Hearing, 4*;272–277.

JERGER, J., LOVERING, L., & WERTZ, M. (1972). Auditory disorder following bilateral temporal lobe insult: Report of a case. *Journal of Speech and Hearing Disorders, 37*;523–535.

JERGER, J., MAHURIN, R., & PIROZZOLO, F. (1990a). The separability of central auditory and cognitive deficits: Implications for the elderly. *Journal of the American Academy of Audiology, 1*;116–119.

JERGER, J., OLIVER, T.A., & PIROZZOLO, F. (1990b). Impact of central auditory processing disorder and cognitive deficit on the self-assessment of hearing handicap in the elderly. *Journal of the American Academy of Audiology, 1*;75–80.

Jerger, J., Silman, S., Lew, H.L., & Chmiel, R. (1993). Case studies in binaural interference: Converging evidence from behavioral and electrophysiologic measures. *Journal of the American Academy of Audiology, 4;*122–131.

Jerger, J., Speaks, C., & Trammel, J.L. (1968). A new approach to speech audiometry. *Journal of Speech and Hearing Disorders, 33;*319–328.

Jerger, J., Stach, B.A., Johnson, K., Loiselle, L.H., & Jerger, S. (1990c). Patterns of abnormality in dichotic listening in the elderly. In: J.H. Jensen (Ed.), *Proceedings of the 14th Danavox Symposium on Presbyacusis and Other Age Related Aspects* (pp. 143–150). Odense, Denmark: Danavox.

Jerger, J., Stach, B., Pruitt, J., Harper, R., & Kirby, H. (1989b). Comments on speech understanding and aging. *Journal of the Acoustical Society of America, 85;*1352–1354.

Jerger, J., Weikers, N., Sharbrough, F., & Jerger, S. (1969). Bilateral lesions of the temporal lobe: A case study. *Acta Otolaryngalogica Supplement,* 258.

Jerger, S., & Jerger, J. (1980). Low-frequency hearing loss in central auditory disorders. *American Journal of Otology, 2;*1–4.

Jerger, S., & Jerger, J. (1983). Neuroaudiologic findings in patients with central auditory disorder. *Seminars in Hearing, 4;*133–159.

Jerger, S., Oliver, T.A., & Martin, R.C. (1990). Evaluation of adult aphasics with the pediatric speech intelligibility test. *Journal of the American Academy of Audiology, 1;*89–100.

Kalikow, D.N., Stevens, K.N., & Elliott, L.L. (1977). Development of a test of speech intelligibility in noise using sentence materials with controlled word predictability. *Journal of the Acoustical Society of America, 61;*1337–1351.

Katz, J. (1962). The use of staggered spondaic words for assessing the integrity of the central auditory system. *Journal of Audiological Research, 2;*327–337.

Keith, R.W. (1995). Development and standardization of SCAN-A: Test of auditory processing disorders in adolescents and adults. *Journal of the American Academy of Audiology, 6;*286–292.

Kimura, D. (1961). Some effects of temporal lobe damage on auditory perception. *Canadian Journal of Psychology, 15;*157–165.

Koehnke, J., & Besing, J. (1997). Clinical application of 3-D auditory tests. *Seminars in Hearing, 18;*345–354.

Konig, E. (1969). Audiological tests in presbycusis. *International Audiologist, 8;*240–259.

Konkle, D., Beasley, D., & Bess, F. (1977). Intelligibility of time-altered speech in relation to chronological aging. *Journal of Speech and Hearing Research, 20;*108–115.

Kurdziel, S., Noffsinger, D., & Olsen, W. (1976). Performance by cortical lesion patients on 40 and 60% time-compressed materials. *Journal of the American Audiological Society, 2;*3–7.

Letowski, T., & Poch, N. (1996). Comprehension of time-compressed speech: Effects of age and speech complexity. *Journal of the American Academy of Audiology, 7;*447–457.

Lutman, M.E. (1991). Degradations in frequency and temporal resolution with age and their impact on speech identification. *Acta Otolaryngalogica Supplement, 476;*120–126.

Lutterman, D., Welsh, O., & Melrose, J. (1966). Responses of aged males to time altered speech stimuli. *Journal of Speech and Hearing Research, 9;*226–230.

Lynn, G.W., & Gilroy, J. (1972). Neuro-audiological abnor-

malities in patients with temporal lobe tumors. *Journal of Neurological Science, 17;*167–184.

Lynn, G.W., & Gilroy, J. (1977). Evaluation of central auditory dysfunction in patients with neurological disorders. In: R.W. Keith (Ed.), *Central auditory dysfunction* (pp. 177–222). New York: Grune & Stratton.

Lynn, G.E., Gilroy, J., Taylor, P.C., & Leiser, RP. (1981). Binaural masking-level differences in neurological disorders. *Archives of Otolaryngologica, 107;*357–362.

Matzker, J. (1959). Two methods for the assessment of central auditory function in cases of brain disease. *Annals of Otology, Rhinology, and Otolaryngology, 68;*115–119.

McCroskey, R., & Kasten, R. (1982). Temporal factors and the aging auditory system. *Ear and Hearing, 3;*124–127.

Moore, B.C.J., Peters, R.W., & Glasberg, B.R. (1992). Detection of temporal gaps in sinusoids by elderly subjects with and without hearing loss. *Journal of the Acoustical Society of America, 92;*1923–1932.

Moore, B.C.J., Vickers, D.A., Glasberg, B.R., & Baer, T. (1997). Comparison of real and simulated hearing impairment in subjects with unilateral and bilateral cochlear hearing loss. *British Journal of Audiology, 31;*227–245.

Musiek, F.E. (1983a). Assessment of central auditory dysfunction: The dichotic digit test revisited. *Ear and Hearing, 4;*79–83.

Musiek, F.E. (1983b). Results of three dichotic speech tests on subjects with intracranial lesions. *Ear and Hearing, 4;*318–323.

Musiek, F.E., Baran, J.A., & Pinheiro, M.L. (1990). Duration pattern recognition in normal subjects and patients with cerebral and cochlear lesions. *Audiology, 29;*304–313.

Musiek, F.E., Baran, J.A., & Pinheiro, M.L. (1994). *Neuroaudiology case studies.* San Diego, CA: Singular Publishing Group.

Musiek, F.E., & Geurkink, N.A. (1982). Auditory brain stem response and central auditory test findings for patients with brain stem lesions: A preliminary report. *Laryngoscope, 92;*891–900.

Neuman, A.C. (1996). Late-onset auditory deprivation: A review of past research and an assessment of future research needs. *Ear and Hearing Supplement, 17;*3S–13S.

Noffsinger, D., Kurdziel, S., & Applebaum, E.L. (1975). Value of special auditory tests in the latero-medial inferior pontine syndrome. *Annals of Otology, 84;*384–390.

Olsen, W.O. (1983). Dichotic test results for normal subjects and for temporal lobectomy patients. *Ear and Hearing, 4;*324–330.

Olsen, W.O., & Noffsinger, D. (1976). Masking level differences for cochlear and brain stem lesions. *Annals of Otology, 85;*820–825.

Orchik, D., & Burgess, J. (1977). Synthetic sentence identification as a function of age of the listener. *Journal of the American Audiological Society, 3;*42–46.

Palva, A., & Jokinen, K. (1975). The role of the binaural test in filtered speech audiometry. *Acta Otolaryngologica, 79;*310–314.

Pestalozza, G., & Shore, I. (1955). Clinical evaluation of presbycusis on the basis of different tests of auditory function. *Laryngoscope, 65;*1136–1163.

Phillips, S.L., Gordon-Salant, S., Fitzgibbons, P.J., & Yeni-Komshian, G.H. (1994). Auditory duration discrimination in young and elderly listeners with normal-hearing. *Journal of the American Academy of Audiology, 5;*210–215.

Price, P.J., & Simon, H.J. (1984). Perception of temporal differences in speech by "normal-hearing" adults: Effect of age and intensity. *Journal of the Acoustical Society of America, 76*;405–410.

Quaranta, A., & Cervellera, G. (1977). Masking level differences in central nervous system diseases. *Archives of Otolaryngology, 103*;482–484.

Russolo, M., & Poli, P. (1983). Lateralization, impedance, auditory brain stem response and synthetic sentence audiometry in brain stem disorders. *Audiology, 22*;50–62.

Sanchez-Longo, L.P., & Forster, F.M. (1958). Clinical significance of impairment of sound localization. *Neurology, 8*;119–125.

Schneider, B.A., Pichora-Fuller, M.K., Kowalchuk, D., & Lamb, M. (1994). Gap detection and the precedence effect in young and old adults. *Journal of the Acoustical Society of America, 95*;980–991.

Shirinian, M., & Arnst, D. (1982). Patterns in performance intensity functions for phonetically balanced word lists and synthetic sentences in aged listeners. *Archives of Otolaryngology, 108*;15–20.

Silman, S. (1995). Binaural interference in multiple sclerosis: Case study. *Journal of the American Academy of Audiology, 6*;193–196.

Silman, S., Gelfand, S.A., & Silverman, C.A. (1984). Effects of monaural versus binaural hearing aids. *Journal of the Acoustical Society of America, 76*;1357–1362.

Silman, S., Silverman, C.A., Emmer, M.B., & Gelfand, S.A. (1992). Adult-onset auditory deprivation. *Journal of the American Academy of Audiology, 3*;390–396.

Silverman, C.A., & Emmer, MB. (1993). Auditory deprivation from and recovery in adults with asymmetric sensorineural hearing impairments. *Journal of the American Academy of Audiology, 4*;338–346.

Silverman, C.A., & Silman, S. (1990). Apparent auditory deprivation from monaural amplification and recovery with binaural amplification: Two case studies. *Journal of the American Academy of Audiology, 1*;175–180.

Smith, B.B., & Resnick, D.M. (1972). An auditory test for assessing brain stem integrity: Preliminary report. *Laryngoscope, 82*;414–424.

Sparks, R., Goodglass, H., & Nickel, B. (1970). Ipsilateral versus contralateral extinction in dichotic listening resulting from hemisphere lesions. *Cortex, 6*;249–260.

Sperry, J.L., Wiley, T.L., & Chial, M.R. (1997). Word recognition performance in various background competitors. *Journal of the American Academy of Audiology, 8*;71–80.

Stach, B.A., & Delgado-Vilches, G. (1993). Sudden hearing loss in multiple sclerosis: Case report. *Journal of the American Academy of Audiology, 4*;370–375.

Stach, B.A., Delgado-Vilches, G., & Smith-Farach, S. (1990a). Hearing loss in multiple sclerosis. *Seminars in Hearing, 11*;221–230.

Stach, B.A., Jerger, J.F., & Fleming, KA. (1985). Central presbyacusis: A longitudinal case study. *Ear and Hearing, 6*;304–306.

Stach, B.A., Loiselle, L.H., & Jerger, J.F. (1991). Special hearing aid considerations in elderly patients with auditory processing disorders. *Ear and Hearing Supplement, 12*; 131S–138S.

Stach, B.A., Spretnjak, M.L., & Jerger, J. (1990b). The prevalence of central presbyacusis in a clinical population. *Journal of the American Academy of Audiology, 1*;109–115.

Stach, B.A., Westerberg, B.D., & Roberson, J.B. (1998). Auditory disorder in central nervous system miliary tuberculosis: A case report. *Journal of the American Academy of Audiology, 9*;305–310.

Starr, A., Picton, T.W., Sininger, Y., Hood, L.J., & Berlin, C.I. (1996). Auditory neuropathy. *Brain, 119*;741–753.

Starr, A., Sininger, Y., Winter, M., Derebery, M.J., Oba, S., & Michalewski H.J. (1998). Transient deafness due to temperature-sensitive auditory neuropathy. *Ear and Hearing, 19*;169–179.

Stephens, S.D.G. (1976). Auditory temporal summation in patients with central nervous system lesions. In: S.D.G. Stephens (Ed.), *Disorders of auditory function* (pp. 243–252). London: Academic Press.

Sticht, T., & Gray, B. (1969). The intelligibility of time-compressed words as a function of age and hearing loss. *Journal of Speech and Hearing Research, 12*;443–448.

Stuart, A, & Phillips, D.P. (1996). Word recognition in continuous and interrupted broadband noise by young normal-hearing, older normal-hearing, and presbyacusic listeners. *Ear and Hearing, 17*;478–489.

Wiley, T.L., Cruickshanks, K.J., Nondahl, D.M., Tweed, T.S., Klein, R., & Klein, B.E.K. (1998). Aging and word recognition in competing message. *Journal of the American Academy of Audiology, 9*;191–198.

Willeford, J. (1977). Assessing central auditory behavior in children: A test battery approach. In: R.W. Keith (Ed.), *Central auditory dysfunction* (pp. 43–72). New York: Grune & Stratton.

Willott, JF. (1996). Anatomic and physiologic aging: A behavioral neuroscience perspective. *Journal of the American Academy of Audiology, 7*;141–151.

Wilson, R.H., & Jaffe, M.S. (1996). Interactions of age, ear, and stimulus complexity on dichotic digit recognition. *Journal of the American Academy of Audiology, 7*;358–364.

Winkelaar, R.G., & Lewis, T.K. (1977). Audiological tests for evaluation of central auditory disorders. *Journal of Otolaryngology, 6*;127–134.

Yellin, M.W., Jerger, J., & Fifer, RC. (1989). Norms for disproportionate loss of speech intelligibility. *Ear and Hearing, 10*;231–234.

## Chapter 17

Acoustic Immittance Measurements

Robert H. Margolis and Lisa L. Hunter

Outline

*See also Margolis (1981); Van Camp (1986); and Wiley (1997).

INTRODUCTION AND HISTORY

Tympanometry is unique among audiological procedures. Although most audiological tests are rather logical applications of methods that were developed for behavioral or physiological assessment—audiometry from auditory psychophysics, auditory brain stem response from electrophysiology—the roots of acoustic immittance measurements are as diverse as the principles governing transoceanic transmission lines, research on early telephone transducers, and observations of the effects of air pressure on hearing. An understanding of the clinical application of acoustic immittance measurements does not come naturally from knowledge of the anatomy, physiology, and pathology of the middle ear. A different set of underlying principles is required—one that is usually better understood by physicists and acoustic engineers than by clinicians concerned with ear disease. In this chapter the physical principles of aural acoustic immittance measurement are reviewed and applied to the clinical test called tympanometry.

The history of the development of tympanometry, reviewed elsewhere (Shallop, 1976; Van Camp et al, 1986), might begin with informal observations of the effects of air pressure on hearing published early in the nineteenth century in England by William Hyde Wollaston and Sir Charles Wheatstone. Although these papers described some perceptive observations and predate any real research in the area, they are not the tightly controlled research papers found in our contemporary journals. In fact, it is hard to imagine that anything like them would be published by any present-day scientific journal. However, the observation that air pressure on either side of the tympanic membrane (TM) alters the function of the ear would be applied to clinical problems as early as the latter half of the nineteenth century by the pioneers of otology, Toynbee and Politzer.

At about the same time, Wheatstone's uncle, Oliver Heaviside (1850–1925), working out of his parent's home because he was unemployed from the time he was 24 until his death at age 75, wrote prolifically on a variety of electrical engineering topics (Fig. 17–1). Heaviside was hearing-impaired; perhaps this was the reason for his reclusive lifestyle (Nahin, 1988). An important issue of the day was the problem of transmitting electrical signals across transoceanic cables. In the process of defining the characteristics of long transmission lines, Heaviside coined the term *impedance*, wrote its defining equations for electrical circuits, and originated the

Audiology: Diagnosis. Edited by Roeser, Valente, and Hosford-Dunn. Thieme Medical Publishers, Inc., New York © 2000

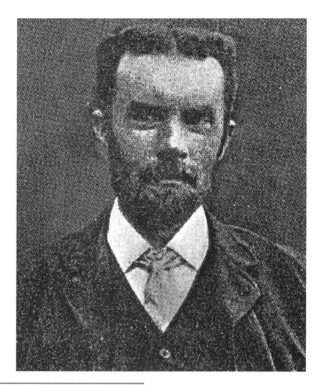

Figure 17–1 Oliver Heaviside (1850–1925).

use of vectors for circuit analysis. Precisely the same principles would be applied to acoustic systems by the early telephone engineers in this century (West, 1928), and a powerful tool, acoustic impedance measurement, was born. That tool would be used to design loudspeakers for acoustic systems as large as a sports stadium and as small as the space in front of a completely-in-the-canal hearing aid. It would form the basis for the clinical test we call tympanometry.

PEARL

Oliver Heaviside's hearing loss may have contributed to his reclusive lifestyle, his ostracism from mainstream science, and his germinal contribution to the development of the impedance concepts on which tympanometry is based.

The clinical application of acoustic impedance measurement was born in the *Rigshospitalet* (State Hospital) in Copenhagen, Denmark, in the 1940s. There Otto Metz produced his landmark work on the acoustic impedance of normal and pathological ears (Metz, 1946). By use of an ingenious, pre-electric device, Metz developed the theory of acoustic impedance of the ear and tested a large number of normal subjects and patients with ear disease. He was also the first to study the acoustic stapedius reflex in patients with ear disease.

The method that Metz developed would be further refined by several of his colleagues at the same hospital. Acoustic impedance measurement would not be useful for routine clinical evaluation until an additional dimension, earcanal air

pressure, was added to the measurement. By measuring impedance as a function of earcanal pressure, it was possible to estimate the impedance of the middle ear without the contaminating influence of the earcanal. In addition, the tympanometric patterns that were observed in normal and abnormal ears were quickly found to have diagnostic significance. Although several investigators contributed to this refinement, it was Terkildsen (Terkildsen & Nielsen, 1960; Terkildsen & Thomsen, 1959) who developed the method that would be incorporated in the first commercially produced clinical instrument.

The advent of clinical instruments in the 1960s and 1970s led to many observations of the effects of specific pathological conditions on tympanograms. A variety of tympanometric patterns were described for patients of different ages, for different probe frequencies, and for different ear diseases. The wide variety of patterns was not well understood until a group of physicists at the University of Antwerp took an interest in understanding the relations between tympanometric patterns and the physics of the middle ear. The result was the *Vanhuyse model* (pronounced van-EYES-uh), perhaps the most important single contribution to understanding tympanograms (Vanhuyse et al, 1975). The model provides a basis for understanding the effects of frequency, pathological conditions, and middle ear development on tympanometric patterns. It is the basis for clinical interpretation of tympanograms and a tool for experimental studies of pathological conditions on middle ear function.

There are other significant characters in the story (von Bekesy, Zwislocki, Jerger, Colletti, and Van Camp). Although much has been learned about the acoustic immittance characteristics of normal and pathological ears, the usual clinical approach to tympanometry is not substantially different than that used by the clinicians who first used this tool in the late 1960s and early 1970s. Although that approach is adequate for most patients, a more systematic and quantitative approach, based on an understanding of the underlying physical principles, can enhance the usefulness of the technique and make us better clinicians.

PHYSICAL PRINCIPLES OF AURAL ACOUSTIC IMMITTANCE

The middle ear is a transducer that converts acoustic energy into mechanical energy. It is so efficient that eardrum vibrations for sounds that are near threshold cannot be detected by the most sensitive instruments. Yet it responds with almost unmeasurable distortion to sound pressures that are a million times greater than the sound pressure at threshold. This remarkable system achieves its sensitivity and dynamic range by a delicate mechanical balance of anatomical structures that exist in an equally delicate physiological environment. It is not surprising that pathological disturbances of the middle ear produce changes in its mechanical properties. With ingenious electroacoustic devices and an understanding of some basic physical principles, pathological changes in middle ear function can be measured, and these measurements can be used to diagnose ear disease and understand the effect of disease on middle ear function.

The direct approach to the evaluation of a mechanical system is to observe the effect that a known force has on the system.

With a procedure as simple and direct as deforming the basilar membrane with a hair, von Bekesy determined some of the mechanical characteristics of the cochlear partition. If we could use a similar direct approach to examine the response of the middle ear, we could probably improve our ability to evaluate middle ear function. Because it is not feasible to directly probe the eardrum or ossicles, an indirect method has been developed on the basis of measurements of the *acoustic immittance* in the earcanal. The acoustic immittance measured in the earcanal is a result of the combined effects of the air volume in the canal and the characteristics of the middle ear. If we know the effect of the earcanal, we can evaluate the middle ear. Studies of the acoustic immittance of normal ears form a basis for determining abnormal middle ear conditions.

Acoustic immittance is a generic term that refers to *acoustic impedance* and *acoustic admittance* and all of their components. Acoustic immittance measurement is a method for analyzing the responses of acoustic systems to sound. Other kinds of systems (e.g., mechanical and electrical systems) can be analyzed with similar techniques. Because mechanical systems are simpler and more familiar, the concept of *mechanical immittance* will be developed in this chapter, and then the same principles will be applied to acoustic systems, specifically, the ear. The immittance of a mechanical system is determined by exerting a force on the system and observing its response. We will begin with the concept of *force*.

Force

An action that is capable of moving a body or changing the motion of a body is a *force*. In the international unit system (*Systéme Internationale*, SI)* the unit of force is the Newton (N). One N is the force required to change the velocity of a mass of 1 kg by 1 m/s in 1 second. For example, if a 1-kg mass at rest is set into motion accelerating to a velocity of 1 m/s in 1 second, the force was 1 N.

Force can be static (constant) or dynamic (changing with time). Of course an infinite number of ways exist that a force could change in time. The simplest time-varying pattern is one that changes sinusoidally, illustrated in Figure 17–2. A sinusoidally changing force can be described mathematically by

$$F(t) = A \sin (2\pi ft) \qquad (1)$$

where $F(t)$ is the force at any instant in time, A is the peak amplitude, f is the frequency of the sinusoidal change, and t is the time at which the measurement is made. The period of a sinusoidal waveform, denoted T, is the time elapsed during one cycle. It is convenient to express a sinusoidally changing force with one number that expresses its magnitude. This is typically done by calculating the root mean square (rms) value of the sinusoidally changing force. That is, each instantaneous force is squared, the squared values are averaged, and the square root of the average is the rms force. We commonly use this rms method to express the sound pressure of an acoustic signal.

Mechanical Immittance

When a force is applied to an object, the object moves with a velocity that is proportional to the applied force. The relationship

*See Van Camp et al (1986) for a discussion of units and unit systems.

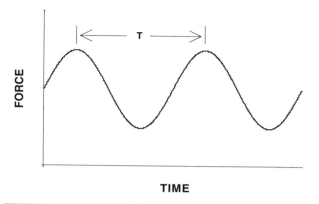

Figure 17–2 Sinusoidally varying force with period T.

between the velocity and the applied force provides the basis for quantitative analysis of the mechanical characteristics of the system. This relationship can be expressed in a number of ways. Recall that *immittance* is a generic term that includes a number of quantities with different units of measurement. The two approaches to immittance measurement are *impedance* and *admittance*.

Mechanical Impedance

Mechanical impedance is the opposition offered by an object to the flow of energy. In simple terms the mechanical impedance of an object is an expression of how difficult it is to move. If the same force moves one object faster than another, the first object has a lower mechanical impedance than the second. Stated more formally, mechanical impedance, Z_m, is the ratio of the applied force, F, to the resulting velocity, V:

$$Z_m = F/V \angle \emptyset_z \qquad (2)$$

Because the unit of force is the Newton, and the unit of velocity is meters per second, mechanical impedance has units N/m/s, or more simply, N • s/m. One N • s/m is a mechanical ohm.

The force may be static or dynamic. A dynamic force is usually expressed as an rms value. In a linear system a sinusoidal force results in a sinusoidally changing velocity, also expressed as an rms value. The frequency of the sinusoidally changing velocity is identical to that of the force. $\angle \emptyset_z$ is the impedance phase angle and represents the time relationship between F and V. The phase angle gives important information about the characteristics of *mass*, *compliance*, and *friction* that contribute to the impedance of the system.

The mass, compliance, and friction of a mechanical system determine its impedance. *Ideal* mass, compliance, and friction elements are those that possess only one of these characteristics. Ideal elements do not exist in the real world, but they are useful concepts. The three types of ideal elements respond in a unique manner when acted on by a force.

When a force is applied to an ideal mass, it moves in the direction of the applied force until another force stops it. In the real world it does not move indefinitely because it encounters friction, which eventually stops the motion. The impedance offered by a mass is its *mass reactance*, X_m.

A compliant element is a spring. Compliance is the ability of the spring to be compressed, the inverse of stiffness. When a force is applied to an ideal spring, it is compressed and returns to its original position when the applied force is removed. The impedance offered by a spring is its *compliant reactance*, X_c.

The *total reactance* of a system is the combination of all the component mass and spring elements. That is:

$$X_{total} = X_m + X_c \qquad (3)$$

A system that has both mass and spring elements can be characterized as a mass *or* a spring, depending on which type of reactance is greater. Because values of X_c are negative, a negative total reactance indicates that the system is dominated by spring elements, and a positive total reactance indicates that the system is dominated by mass elements.

The impedance that results from friction is called *resistance*, R. Friction causes energy loss through dissipation as heat. Thus mass and spring elements (*reactive* elements) store energy and friction dissipates energy.

The total impedance of a mechanical system composed of mass, spring, and friction elements is:

$$Z_m = R + jX_{total} \qquad (4)$$

The j mathematically represents $\sqrt{-1}$ in complex number notation and indicates that resistance and reactance cannot be combined by simple arithmetic.*

Eqs. 2 and 4 represent two ways to define the mechanical impedance of a system. Eq. 2 defines impedance as a force/velocity ratio with a specific time relationship between the force and velocity. Eq. 4 expresses impedance as the combined contributions of mass and spring elements (X_{total}) and friction (R). Because Eq. 2 can be represented by a vector with a specific length and angle, it is referred to as *polar notation*. Eq. 4 represents the vector in terms of its rectangular components (R and X_{total}) and is referred to as *rectangular notation*.

Vector Analysis

The relations expressed in Eqs. 2 and 4 indicate that impedance is a *vector*, a two-dimensional quantity that can be analyzed into polar or rectangular components.

Vector analysis is a useful way to understand the concept of *complex impedance*. A complete description of the impedance of a system requires two numbers, either magnitude and phase (Eq. 2) or resistance and reactance (Eq. 4). A graphic representation of a vector plot shows how these representations are related. Consider the complex mechanical system schematized in Figure 17–3. To move the system, a mass has to be set into motion, a spring has to be compressed, and friction is encountered when the components move. Similar processes need to occur to set the middle ear into vibration. This system, then, has compliant reactance associated with the spring, mass reactance associated with the mass, and resistance resulting from friction. In the vector system illustrated in

*See Nahin (1988, Tech Note 1, p. 204) for the mathematical basis for $\sqrt{-1}$ in vector analysis.

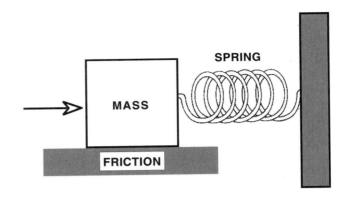

Figure 17–3 A complex mechanical system composed of a mass and spring. Friction is encountered when the mass and spring move. The impedance of the system is the vector sum of the effects of the mass, spring, and friction.

Figure 17–4A, compliant reactance X_c is shown as a negative value on the y-axis, mass reactance, X_m, is shown as a positive value on the y-axis, and resistance, R, is shown as a positive value on the x-axis. Total reactance, X_{total}, is the sum of X_c and X_m. X_{total} and R can be thought of as vectors that produce a resultant vector, impedance, Z, with a phase angle, $\emptyset_z$. From Eq. 2 it is evident that $|Z| = F/V$. (When the impedance magnitude is given without the phase angle, it is placed in absolute value signs.)

Mechanical Admittance

For reasons that will be discussed later, it is convenient to characterize the immittance of the ear as an admittance rather than impedance. The mechanical admittance Y of a system is the reciprocal of impedance:

$$Y = V/F \angle \emptyset_Y \qquad (5)$$

Just as impedance has components representing mass, compliance, and friction, admittance can be analyzed into similar components. The admittance associated with a mass is *mass susceptance*, B_m. The admittance associated with spring elements is *compliant susceptance*, B_c. The admittance resulting from friction is *conductance*, G. The total susceptance, B_{total}, is the sum of the mass and compliant susceptances:

$$B_{total} = B_m + B_c \qquad (6)$$

Admittance can be stated in terms of susceptance and conductance:

$$Y = G + jB_{total} \qquad (7)$$

Eqs. 5 and 7 represent the polar and rectangular forms of admittance. Just as impedance can be graphically represented as a vector system, admittance can also be represented as a pair of vectors representing conductance on the x-axis and susceptance on the y-axis. Figure 17–4B illustrates the vector representation of admittance.

Table 17–1 presents a summary of immittance quantities, their definitions, and their units. Table 17–2 presents the formulas defining the relationships among immittance quantities. For further discussion of immittance quantities,

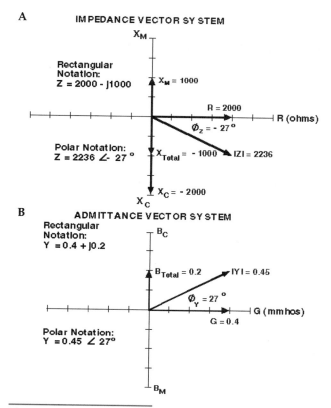

A

IMPEDANCE VECTOR SYSTEM

Rectangular
Notation:
Z = 2000 - j1000

Polar Notation:
Z = 2236 ∠- 27 °

B

ADMITTANCE VECTOR SYSTEM

Rectangular
Notation:
Y = 0.4 + j0.2

Polar Notation:
Y = 0.45 ∠ 27°

Figure 17–4 Impedance and admittance vector systems. **(A)** The impedance vector system is composed of mass reactance (X_m) and compliant reactance (X_c), which sum to total reactance (X_{total}), and resistance (R). X_t and R combine to form Z, the impedance magnitude that has a phase angle Ø. **(B)** The admittance vector system is calculated from the impedance vector values by the conversion equations given in Table 17–2.

their relationships, and their units, see American National Standards Institute (1987) and Van Camp et al (1986).

Acoustic Immittance

The principles governing mechanical systems can be applied to acoustic systems. Like mechanical systems, the acoustic immittance of a system is determined by its mass, compliance, and friction. An acoustic mass is a volume of air that moves as a unit without compression, such as the air in an open tube. An acoustic spring (compliance) is a volume of air that is alternately compressed and expanded, such as a rigidly enclosed volume of air. Friction occurs as a result of collisions of molecules in the medium (such as air) and between the medium and surrounding structures.

Acoustic impedance, Z_a, can be defined by modifying Eq. 2. *Sound pressure*, P, is substituted for force and *volume velocity*, U is substituted for velocity:

$$Z_a = P/U \ \angle \emptyset_z \tag{8}$$

Eq. 8 is the polar form of acoustic impedance. In rectangular form,

$$Z_a = R_a + jX_a \tag{9}$$

X_a (or X_{total}) is the sum of the compliant reactance and mass reactance. When X_a has a positive value, the reactance associated with mass elements is greater than the reactance associated with spring elements and the system is said to be mass controlled. When X_a is negative, the system is stiffness controlled or compliance controlled.

Acoustic admittance is the reciprocal of acoustic impedance. From Eq. 8,

$$Y_a = U/P \ \angle \emptyset_Y \tag{10}$$

or in rectangular form

$$Y_a = G_a + jB_a \tag{11}$$

When B_a is positive, the system is compliance controlled or stiffness controlled. A negative B_a indicates a mass-controlled system.

Measurements of acoustic immittance in the earcanal are influenced by both mechanical and acoustic elements. Because the middle ear is a transducer, converting acoustic energy to mechanical energy, both acoustic and mechanical structures comprise the system. The enclosed volumes of air on both sides of the TM act as acoustic compliance elements (acoustic springs). At high frequencies significant acoustic-mass effects are associated with these air volumes. The eardrum, ligaments, tendons, and muscles of the middle ear act as mechanical springs that return to their original position when stretched and released. The ossicles are mechanical masses. Although tympanometry is based on the measurement of acoustic impedance in the earcanal, it is really the *mechanoacoustic* middle ear system that we are evaluating.

Acoustic Immittance Units

From Eq. 8 we can determine the units for acoustic impedance. Sound pressure, P, is force per unit area and has units N/m^2. One N/m^2 is a Pascal (Pa). Volume velocity is the rate at which a volume of air moves past an imaginary plane and has units m^3/s. Acoustic impedance, then, has units $N/m^2/m^3/s$, or $Pa/m^3/s$, or more simply, $Pa \cdot s/m^3$. One $Pa \cdot s/m^3$ is one acoustic ohm in the mks unit system. It has become conventional in tympanometry to use the cgs unit system. One cgs ohm is equal to 10,000 mks ohms. One cgs ohm, then, is $10^5 \ Pa \cdot s/m^3$.

The unit of admittance is the mho, the inverse of the ohm. One mks mho is $1 \ m^3/Pa \cdot s$, and 1 cgs mho is $1 \ m^3/10^5 Pa \cdot s$ or $10^{-5} m^3/Pa \cdot s$. Because the admittance of the ear is a fraction of an mho, it is convenient to use the millimho (mmho), which is 1000 of an mho. One cgs mmho is $10^{-8} m^3/Pa \cdot s$.

Frequency Dependence of Acoustic Immittance

Virtually every measure of auditory function depends on the frequency of the stimulus. Audiometric thresholds are typically measured over a five-octave range because hearing sensitivity in normal and impaired ears is frequency dependent. One of the sources of the frequency dependence of auditory

TABLE 17–1   Immitance quantities

Quantity	Symbol	Unit	Definition
Force	F	Newton (N)	An action that is capable of moving a body or changing the motion of a body.
Pressure	P	Pascal (Pa)	Force per unit area (1 Pa = 1 N/m²).
Volume velocity	U	m³/s	Volume of a medium (e.g., air) that moves past an imaginary plane per unit time.
Acoustic mass	M_a	Pa • s²/m³	Ratio of sound pressure to the resulting change in volume velocity. An acoustic mass element is a volume of air that moves as a unit in response to sound, such as the air in an open tube.
Acoustic stiffness	K_a	Pa/m³	Ratio of change in sound pressure to the resulting change in volume displacement. An acoustic stiffness element is a volume of air that is alternately compressed and expanded by sound, such as the air in rigid enclosure.
Acoustic compliance	C_a	m³/Pa	The inverse of acoustic stiffness.
Acoustic immittance	None	None	A generic term referring to acoustic impedance, acoustic admittance, and all of their rectangular and polar components.
Acoustic impedance	Z_a	Acoustic ohm	Opposition offered by a system to the flow of acoustic energy; the reciprocal of acoustic admittance.
Acoustic reactance	X_a	Acoustic ohm	The impedance offered by acoustic mass and acoustic compliance elements.
Compliant (stiffness) reactance	X_c	Acoustic ohm	The impedance offered by acoustic compliance elements.
Mass reactance	X_m	Acoustic ohm	The impedance offered by mass elements.
Acoustic resistance	R_a	Acoustic ohm	The impedance resulting from friction.
Acoustic admittance	Y_a	Acoustic millimho (mmho)	The ease with which energy flows through an acoustic system; the reciprocal of acoustic impedance.
Acoustic susceptance	B_a	Acoustic millimho (mmho)	The admittance offered by acoustic compliance and acoustic mass elements.
Compliant susceptance	B_c	Acoustic millimho (mmho)	The admittance offered by acoustic compliance elements.
Mass susceptance	B_m	Acoustic millimho (mmho)	The admittance offered by acoustic mass elements.
Acoustic conductance	G_a	Acoustic millimho (mmho)	The admittance associated with friction in an acoustic system.

sensitivity is the frequency dependence of the transmission of sound through the middle ear.

Of the three types of mechanical and acoustic elements, one (acoustic resistance) is independent of frequency. The immittance associated with springs and masses, however, strongly depends on frequency. This is evident in the next two equations:

$$X_m = 2\pi f M \qquad (12)$$

$$X_c = \frac{-\rho c^2}{2\pi f V} \qquad (13)$$

where M is mass, ρ is the density of the medium (usually air), c is the velocity of sound, and V is the volume of an enclosed quantity of air (an acoustic spring). Eq. 12 expresses the relationship between mass reactance (X_m), mass (M), and frequency (f). The reactance of a mass increases in direct proportion to frequency. Mass elements, then, have a low

TABLE 17–2 Relations among acoustic immittance quantities

Defining equations

$$Z_a = P/U \angle \varnothing_z \qquad Y_a = U/P \angle \varnothing_Y$$

$$Z_a = R_a + jX_a \qquad Y_a = G_a + jB_a$$

Computational equations

$$|Z_a| = \sqrt{R_a^2 + X_a^2} \qquad R_a = \frac{G_a}{G_a^2 = B_a^2}$$

$$\varnothing_Z = \arctan (X_a/R_a) \qquad \varnothing_Y = \arctan (B_a/G_a)$$

Conversion equations

$$R_a = \frac{G_a}{G_a^2 = B_a^2} \qquad G_a = \frac{R_a}{R_a^2 = X_a^2}$$

$$X_a = \frac{-B_a}{G_a^2 = B_a^2} \qquad B_a = \frac{-X_a}{R_a^2 = X_a^2}$$

$$\varnothing_Z = -\varnothing_Y \qquad \varnothing_Y = -\varnothing_Z$$

reactance at low frequencies and a high reactance at high frequencies. In contrast, Eq. 13 shows that the reactance of a spring is inversely proportional to frequency so that spring elements have a high reactance at low frequencies and a low reactance at high frequencies.

Because mass reactance increases with frequency, adding mass to a system will have a greater effect at high frequencies than at low frequencies. A mass on the TM causes a downward sloping hearing loss (mass tilt). Because stiffness reactance decreases with frequency, adding stiffness to a system has a greater effect at low frequencies. Conditions that stiffen the middle ear, such as ossicular adhesion or negative middle ear pressure, cause an upward sloping hearing loss (stiffness tilt).

If the reactance of spring elements decreases with frequency and the reactance of mass elements increases with frequency, then a system composed of a combination of mass and spring elements will be maximally efficient at one frequency at which the compliant and mass suspectance are in balance. This is called the *resonant frequency*. At the resonant frequency $X_{total} = 0$ and $Z = R$. That is, the reactances associated with the masses and springs cancel and the impedance of the system consists solely of the resistive component.

Acoustic Immittance of Complex Systems

Complex systems are those comprised of a combination of mass, compliance, and resistive elements. The middle ear system has been modeled as a complex network of elements representing the various anatomical structures of the ear (Goode et al, 1994; Kringlebotn, 1988; Zwislocki, 1962). These models predict the input and output characteristics of the middle ear and can be used to predict the effects of a pathological condition on middle ear function. The Zwislocki model is shown in Figure 17–5.

The Zwislocki model represents the transmission pathway from the earcanal to the cochlea and is composed of series elements (components 1, 3, 5, and 7) and parallel, or shunt, elements (components 2, 4, and 6). For sound to reach the cochlea it must travel through the series elements. Sound that passes through the shunt elements does not reach the cochlea and represents energy that does not contribute to hearing. Note that the middle ear cavities are shown as the first element (component 1), preceding the eardrum (components 2 and 3). This seems counterintuitive because we know that anatomically the eardrum precedes the middle ear cavities. However, for the eardrum to move, the air in the middle ear must expand or contract. Functionally, then, the middle ear cavities represent a series element at the input to the system.

The eardrum appears in two locations, as a shunt element (component 2) and as a series element (component 3). This indicates that some of the vibration of the eardrum is coupled to the ossicular chain and some of its vibration is energy that is not transmitted through the middle ear.

The incus-malleus joint (component 4) and the incus-stapes joint (component 6) are shown as shunt elements because some energy loss occurs at the joints.

The model helps us understand why the relationship between tympanometry and hearing is complex. Because

ZWISLOCKI MIDDLE EAR MODEL

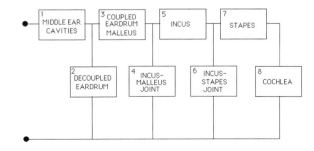

Figure 17–5 Zwislocki middle ear model.

tympanometry is a measure of the *input immittance* of the system, it is influenced by both shunt and series elements. Sound that is heard is transmitted through only the series elements. The components that most influence the input immittance are those series and shunt elements that are closest to the input. Thus the tympanogram is dominated by the middle ear cavities, the eardrum, and the malleus. A substantial change at the output of a complex system can have a small or negligible effect on the input immittance. An example of this is otosclerosis in which the impedance of the stapes becomes virtually infinite, but it has little effect on the tympanogram (Shahnaz & Polka, 1999).

The goal of tympanometry is to determine the input characteristics of the middle ear, independent of the earcanal. The earcanal and middle ear can be modeled as a system with two impedances that may be either in series or in parallel. Network representations of series and parallel systems are shown in Figure 17–6.

The input impedance of the series system shown in Figure 17–6 is:

$$Z_i = Z_1 + Z_2 \qquad (14)$$

The input impedance of the parallel system shown in Figure 17–6 is given by:

$$\frac{1}{Z_i} = \frac{1}{Z_1} + \frac{1}{Z_2} \qquad (15)$$

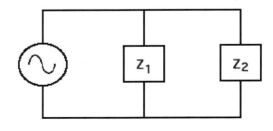

PARALLEL SYSTEM

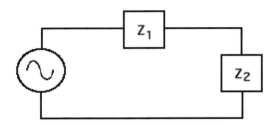

SERIES SYSTEM

Figure 17–6 Parallel and series systems. *Top panel*, A parallel circuit composed of a sinusoidal source of energy and two impedances (Z_1 *and* Z_2) configured in parallel. *Bottom panel*, A series circuit composed of a sinusoidal source of energy and two impedances (Z_1 *and* Z_2) configured in series.

Solving for Z_i

$$Z_i = \frac{Z_1 Z_2}{Z_1 + Z_2} \qquad (16)$$

Because admittance is the reciprocal of impedance, Eq. 15 can be rewritten as follows:

$$Y_i = Y_1 + Y_2 \qquad (17)$$

Eqs. 14 and 17 reveal two simple rules governing the immittance of series and parallel systems. The input impedance of a series system is the sum of the impedances of its components. The input admittance of a parallel system is the sum of the admittances of its components.

By viewing the ear as a system consisting of two components, the interaction between the earcanal and the middle ear can be analyzed. Anatomically, the earcanal and middle ear appear to be in series. However, acoustically, they behave as parallel elements.

From Eq. 14 we see that the input impedance, Z_i, of a series system is greater than the impedance of either component. Not so obviously, Eqs. 15 and 16 indicate that the input impedance of a parallel system is less than either component. Acoustic impedance measurements have shown that the input impedance at the entrance to the earcanal is less than the impedance of either the earcanal volume or the middle ear measured separately. This suggests that the earcanal and middle ear are configured as a parallel acoustic system. Another characteristic of a parallel acoustic system is that the sound pressure delivered to each element is the same. At the low frequencies typically used for aural acoustic impedance measurements, the sound pressure at the entrance to the eardrum and the sound pressure at the TM are virtually identical. This again suggests that the earcanal and middle ear can be represented as a parallel acoustic system.

If we let Z_1 represent the earcanal and Z_2 represent the middle ear, we can solve Eq. 16 for the middle ear impedance. Denoting the earcanal impedance as Z_{ec}, the middle ear impedance as Z_{me}, and the measured impedance at the lateral end of the earcanal as Z, we can rewrite Eq. 16 as follows:

$$Z = \frac{Z_{ec} Z_{me}}{Z_{ec} + Z_{me}} \qquad (18)$$

Solving for Z_{me}

$$Z_{me} = \frac{Z_{ec} Z}{Z_{ec} - Z} \qquad (19)$$

Alternately, the input admittance can be determined from Eq. 16. First let us rewrite Eq. 16 in terms of the admittance of the earcanal Y_{ec}, the admittance of the middle ear Y_{me}, and the admittance at the lateral end of the earcanal Y.

$$Y = Y_{ec} + Y_{me} \qquad (20)$$

Solving for Y_{me}

$$Y_{me} = Y - Y_{ec} \qquad (21)$$

The point of this exercise is to demonstrate that the admittance measured at the lateral end of the earcanal is more easily corrected for earcanal volume than the impedance. Eq. 19 is a complex relationship, whereas Eq. 21 is a simple one. Eq. 21 tells us that a simple subtraction of the admittance associated with earcanal volume from the measured admittance will yield the admittance of the middle ear. The simpler relationship expressed in Eq. 21 compared with Eq. 19 is the reason that tympanometric measurements are made in admittance rather than impedance.

PEARL

Tympanometric measurements are commonly made in admittance rather than impedance because the effect of earcanal volume on admittance is simple and the effect of earcanal volume on impedance is complex.

Determining the Admittance of the Earcanal

Eq. 21 provides a method for determining the admittance of the middle ear from the measured admittance Y and the admittance of the earcanal Y_{ec}. How can we estimate Y_{ec}? If we know the earcanal volume, V, we can calculate Y_{ec}. Because the susceptance of a volume of air is the reciprocal of its reactance, we can rewrite Eq. 13 in terms of compliant susceptance B_c and volume V:

$$B_c = \frac{2\pi f V}{\rho c^2} \tag{22}$$

where the unit of B_c is the mho (the inverse of an ohm) and volume, V, is in cc. At 226 Hz, $2\pi f/\rho c_2 = 0.001$, so we can write Eq. 22 as follows:

$$B_c = 0.001\ V \tag{23}$$

Converting to mmhos,

$$B_c\ (in\ mmhos) = V \tag{24}$$

That is, at 226 Hz, the susceptance (in mmho) of an enclosed volume of air that conforms to certain constraints on its geometry is numerically equal to its volume (in cc). So the susceptance of a volume of air of 1 cc is 1 mmho. This is a convenient relationship that simplifies the calibration of instruments that use a 226-Hz probe frequency. In fact, that is precisely why the 226-Hz probe frequency was selected.

Now we can calculate the susceptance of the earcanal if we know its volume. Because an enclosed volume of air has no resistive (or conductance) component, we also know its admittance. The G term in Eq. 11 is zero, so at 226 Hz, $Y_{ec} = B = V$.

How is the volume of the earcanal determined? The first commercially available instrument for measurement of aural acoustic immittance, the Zwislocki acoustic impedance bridge, manufactured by Grason-Stadler, Inc., obtained an estimate of the earcanal volume by pouring alcohol into the earcanal from a calibrated syringe (Zwislocki, 1963). This approach produces a good measurement of earcanal volume but is not practical in the clinic. An alternative approach was suggested by Terkildsen and Thomsen (Terkildsen & Thomsen, 1959) in the very first article on tympanometry. By pressurizing the earcanal, the middle ear could be stiffened to the point that the middle ear admittance becomes nearly zero. From Eq. 21 it is evident that the measured admittance in that condition becomes the admittance of the earcanal. This acoustic method provides a reasonably accurate measure of

the earcanal volume (Shanks & Lilly, 1981) and provides the basis for measurement of the middle ear impedance from tympanometry. This method has been shown to produce estimates of middle ear impedance that are comparable to those obtained by laboratory methods (Margolis et al, 1985).

Calculating the Admittance of the Middle Ear

Using Eq. 21, the admittance of the middle ear can be calculated by subtracting the admittance of the earcanal from the measured admittance. The measured admittance that we are most interested in is the one corresponding to the peak of the tympanogram. The admittance of the earcanal is taken from the positive or negative tail of the tympanogram. The negative tail provides the more accurate estimate of earcanal volume (Shanks & Lilly, 1981). Many instruments, however, use the positive tail value. From the tympanogram in Figure 17–7, the admittance of the middle ear is 0.52 mmho using the negative tail and 0.45 using the positive tail. Because of the asymmetry of tympanograms, the middle ear admittance using the negative tail value is almost always greater than that obtained using the positive tail (Margolis & Smith, 1977). It is necessary, therefore, to use different norms for admittance calculated using the positive tail and that obtained using the negative tail.

The admittance calculated in this manner is referred to as the *peak compensated static acoustic admittance* (American National Standards Institute, 1987) or more concisely, the *static admittance*.

The static admittance can be accurately determined from the admittance tympanogram only if no significant phase shifts occur when the ear is pressurized. In fact, the admittance phase changes during pressurization, becoming larger at the tails of the tympanogram than at the peak. At 226 Hz, these phase shifts are usually small enough that the error is negligible. At higher frequencies it is necessary to calculate compensated conductance and susceptance separately. From the compensated conductance and susceptance, the compensated admittance can be determined. The compensated conductance G_{tm} and susceptance B_{tm} are:

$$G_{tm} = G_{peak} - G_{tail} \tag{25}$$

$$B_{tm} = B_{peak} - B_{tail} \tag{26}$$

Compensated admittance is calculated from compensated conductance and susceptance with the computational equation in Table 17–2:

$$Y_{tm} = \sqrt{G_{tm^2} + B_{tm^2}} \tag{27}$$

INSTRUMENTATION

Design Principles of Clinical Acoustic Immittance Instruments

The earliest devices for evaluation of middle ear function were acoustic instruments that presented a sound to the ear and evaluated the sound energy that was developed in the earcanal. Eq. 8 indicates that if a sound (probe tone) with a certain volume velocity is presented to a system, the impedance of the system is proportional to the sound pressure. A

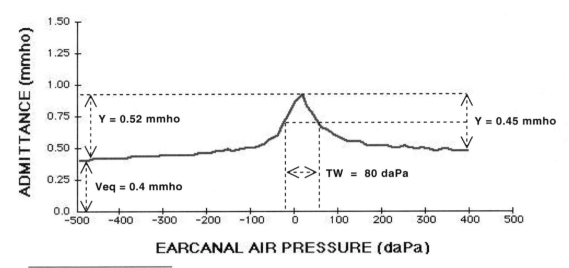

Figure 17–7 Single-component, single-frequency (226-Hz) tympanogram. This tympanogram, from a normal adult ear, has a compensated static admittance *(Y)* of 0.45 mmho compensated from the positive tail, 0.52 mmho compensated from the negative tail, tympanometric width *(TW)* of 80 daPa calculated from the positive tail, and an equivalent volume *(V^{eq})* of 0.4 mmho calculated from the negative tail.

probe tone presented to a system with high impedance has a high sound pressure; if the impedance is low, the probe tone sound pressure will be low. This is a convenient method for measuring the impedance of a system. A constant volume velocity probe tone is presented to the ear and the sound pressure is measured in the earcanal. A calibration procedure provides a conversion from sound pressure to impedance.

Alternately, the probe tone sound pressure could be held constant and the volume velocity could be measured. This approach has been adopted by most commercially produced acoustic immittance systems.

Figure 17–8 illustrates the design of a typical probe used for acoustic immittance measurement. A tube is used to couple an air pump and manometer to the probe to pressurize the earcanal. A miniature loudspeaker delivers the probe tone to the ear. A microphone picks up the acoustic signal in the earcanal and converts it to an electrical signal that is used to measure the acoustic immittance. Some systems have a second transducer for delivering a stimulus for ipsilateral acoustic reflex measurement.

Figure 17–9 shows a block diagram of an admittance meter. A sinusoidal electrical signal is generated, amplified, and delivered to the miniature loudspeaker housed in the probe. The microphone picks up the probe tone in the earcanal and converts it to an electrical signal. An automatic gain control (AGC) keeps the probe tone at a constant sound pressure by controlling the gain of the probe tone amplifier. The voltage that is required to keep the probe tone at a fixed level is proportional to the admittance of the ear. The electrical signal that drives the probe tone transducer is also delivered to a comparator along with the amplified output of the microphone. The comparator provides a measurement of the magnitude of the probe tone signal and the phase of the microphone signal. Once the system is calibrated, the magnitude and phase are identical to |Y| and $\emptyset_Y$, the polar components of acoustic admittance.

The first electroacoustic admittance meters were analog electrical systems similar to that depicted in Figure 17–9. Current instruments use microprocessors that perform the same functions by digital signal processing. Many of the functions of the components in Figure 17–9 are accomplished in software. The block diagram in Figure 17–9, however, is a good representation of the functions designed into these digital acoustic immittance systems.

ANSI Standard for Acoustic Immittance Instruments

The American National Standards Institute (ANSI) published a standard in 1987 describing the desirable characteristics of clinical acoustic immittance systems (American National Standards Institute, 1987). Manufacturers of these systems generally design their instruments to comply with the standard. The goal of the standard is to ensure that aural acoustic immittance measurements, using a 226-Hz probe tone, are equivalent when measured with any instrument that meets the specifications of the standard. In addition, the standard helps to promote uniform terminology and plotting formats. However,

TO PUMP AND MANOMETER

MICROPHONE OUTPUT

PROBE TONE

IPSILATERAL REFLEX

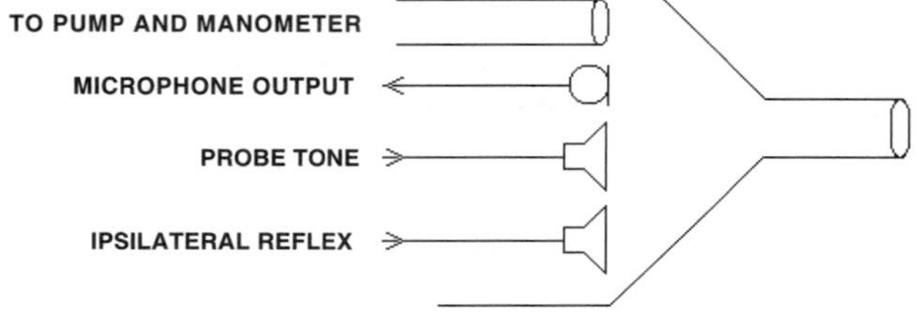

Figure 17–8 Components of a tympanometric probe.

TWO-COMPONENT ADMITTANCE METER

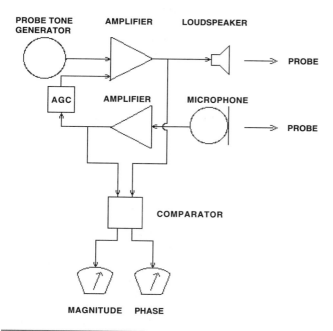

Figure 17–9 Block diagram of an acoustic immittance measurement system. The probe tone is produced by the signal generator, amplified, and delivered to the miniature loudspeaker in the probe (Fig. 17–7). The acoustic signal in the earcanal is picked up by the microphone, converted to an electrical signal, and amplified. The automatic gain control (*AGC*) dynamically adjusts the gain of the probe tone amplifier to keep the sound pressure in the earcanal constant. The comparator compares the amplified microphone signal and the probe signal to determine the relative amplitude and phase in the earcanal. The calibration process allows the amplitude and phase to be converted to admittance units.

compliance with a standard is entirely voluntary, unless a stipulation in statute requires conformity to a standard.

Measurement Units and Terminology

The ANSI standard recommends the use of the international units system. The SI unit of pressure is the dekapascal (daPa). Another pressure unit that has been commonly used for tympanometry is the mm H_2O. These units are related in the following manner:

$$1 \text{ mm } H_2O = 0.98 \text{ daPa}$$

$$1 \text{ daPa} = 1.02 \text{ mm } H_2O$$

For practical purposes, the two units can be considered to be equivalent.

Because clinical acoustic immittance measurement was widely used before the existence of the standard, inconsistent, and sometimes confusing terminology has been used.

The standard provides the following definitions of terms, many of which are frequently misused by manufacturers and in published reports.

Acoustic immittance refers collectively to acoustic impedance, acoustic admittance, and all of their components.

Acoustic compliance, the reciprocal of acoustic stiffness, is the ratio of a change in volume displacement to a change in sound pressure. Compliance is a characteristic of a spring. This term has been improperly used for measurements that are actually admittance magnitude values. A variety of units have been used in conjunction with incorrectly reported "compliance" values, including "arbitrary units" and cubic centimeters. Because most instruments are actually admittance meters, the correct unit is the millimho (mmho).

Compensated static acoustic immittance is the immittance that has been compensated (or corrected) for the acoustic immittance of the earcanal. This value represents the acoustic immittance of the middle ear at the TM.

Peak compensated static acoustic immittance is the static immittance obtained with the earcanal air pressure adjusted to produce a peak in the measured immittance. This is frequently referred to as the static admittance or the peak admittance.

Measurement-plane tympanometry is a measurement of acoustic immittance at the probe tip and represents the combined acoustic immittance of the earcanal and middle ear.

Compensated tympanometry is a measurement of acoustic immittance that has been compensated (or corrected) for the acoustic immittance of the earcanal.

Plotting Format

The appearance of a tympanogram is affected by the scale proportions (aspect ratio) of the plot. Just as the audiometer standard (American National Standards Institute, 1996) describes the specifications for an audiogram, the acoustic immittance standard provides a standard format for plotting 226-Hz tympanograms. The standard recommends an aspect ratio of 300 daPa to 1 mmho. Note in Figure 17–7 that a distance corresponding to 300 daPa on the *x*-axis is equivalent to the distance corresponding to 1 mmho on the *y*-axis.

The standard also recommends the following axis labels. The *y*-axis should be labeled with one of the following:

Acoustic admittance (10^{-8} m³/Pa • s [acoustic mmho])
Acoustic admittance of an equivalent volume of air (cm³)
Acoustic impedance (10^8 Pa • s/m³ [Acoustic kohm])

The *x*-axis should be labeled as follows:

Air pressure (daPa) (1 daPa = 1.02 mm H_2O)

These rather cumbersome labels were recommended because of the confusion that existed resulting from inconsistent use of terminology and units. The ANSI working group wanted to be as specific as possible so that there would be no ambiguity in the quantities that are represented on tympanograms. Perhaps because the recommended labels are quite cumbersome, they have not been used consistently. We recommend the following axis labels for tympanograms.

These are adequately specific but not as unwieldy as those recommended by ANSI.

y-axis: Acoustic admittance (mmho)
x-axis: Earcanal air pressure (daPa)

Calibration

Many features of an acoustic immittance instrument must be calibrated. These include the probe tone, the admittance measurement system, the air pressure measurement system, and the ipsilateral and contralateral reflex stimuli. All these features should be calibrated on a regular basis.

Probe Tone

The standard is applicable to instruments that use a 226-Hz probe tone. Although that frequency is not necessarily the one that is best for clinical diagnosis, it has been widely used, and more is known about tympanograms obtained at that frequency than other frequencies. It is a convenient frequency because of the simple relationship between acoustic admittance and the volume of air-filled calibration cavities.

The standard specifies that the actual frequency of the probe tone should be within 3% of the nominal frequency. That is, the actual frequency of the 226-Hz probe tone must be between 219 and 233 Hz. The sound pressure level must be ≤90 dB measured in a 2-cc (HA-1) coupler.

Admittance Measurement System

The admittance measurement section of the acoustic immittance instruments are calibrated by placing the probe into a known acoustic admittance. An enclosed volume of air can be used as the known admittance because its admittance can be calculated from the volume of the enclosure. At 226 Hz, the admittance of an air-filled enclosure is equal to its volume. That is, the admittance of a 1 cc volume is 1 mmho. This simple relationship holds if the cavity dimensions are within certain limits (the length cannot be much greater than the diameter) and the atmospheric conditions (temperature and pressure) are not extreme.

Because the admittance of a volume of air depends on atmospheric conditions, it may be necessary to adjust the calibration in cities where the altitude is significantly different from sea level. At an elevation of 1 mile (e.g., Denver), the admittance of a volume of air is 22% higher than at sea level. This requires a correction in the calibration, which is usually incorporated into the software calibration routine that is built into the instrument.

The standard specifies that the acoustic immittance measurement system should be calibrated in three calibration cavities with volumes of 0.5, 2.0, and 5.0 cc. The admittance magnitude and phase indicators (Figure 17–9) are adjusted to read 0.5, 2.0, and 5.0 mmho with phase angles of 90 degrees for all three cavities. The 90-degree phase angle results from the fact that an enclosed cavity is nearly an ideal compliant element. That is, the admittance is composed of a positive (compliant) susceptance value that is equal to the volume and a conductance of 0 mmho.

For instruments that measure admittance at other frequencies, the calibration method is similar. Instead of the

admittance being equal to the volume, the admittance is determined from the following formula:

$$Y = V \frac{f_p}{226} < 90°$$

where V is the volume of the calibration cavity and f_p is the probe frequency. Eq. 28 tells us that the admittance of an enclosed volume increases in proportion to the frequency and the phase angle remains 90 degrees.

CLINICAL APPLICATIONS OF TYMPANOMETRY

The Vanhuyse Model

As clinical experience with tympanometry accumulated in the 1970s, a variety of tympanometric patterns was observed. A few investigators, experimenting with higher frequency probe tones, observed that tympanometric patterns are more complex at higher frequencies (Alberti & Jerger, 1974; Colletti, 1976; Liden et al, 1974a, 1974b, 1977; Margolis & Popelka, 1977; Van Camp et al, 1976). The first studies of tympanometry in neonates revealed that newborns have complex tympanometric shapes even at low frequencies (Bennett, 1975; Keith, 1973, 1975). Although certain patterns appeared to be associated with certain ear conditions, it was the model developed at the University of Antwerp that would provide a framework for understanding the variety of tympanometric shapes (Vanhuyse et al, 1975).

The Vanhuyse model is based on assumptions of the shapes of resistance and reactance tympanograms. Because admittance, conductance, and susceptance tympanograms are simply mathematical transformations of impedance components (resistance and reactance) (see Table 17–2), impedance can be manipulated and the effects on admittance, conductance, and susceptance can be observed. The reason that this approach is informative is that simple changes in impedance quantities produce complex changes in admittance quantities.

The Vanhuyse model is represented graphically in Figure 17–10. On the basis of acoustic impedance measurements that had been made in the cat (Moller, 1965a), the resistance tympanogram was assumed to be a monotonically decreasing function of air pressure, with a higher resistance for negative pressure than for positive pressure, and reactance is a single-peaked function that is symmetrical around ambient earcanal pressure (upper left panel of Fig. 17–10A). The reactance values are negative because at low frequencies the ear is stiffness controlled. The absolute values of reactance are greater than resistance at all pressures. (Compare the reactance X tympanogram with the dashed line in Fig. 17–10A.)

As the reactance tympanogram shifts from negative to positive values, four tympanometric patterns occur (see Fig. 17–10). These were named by Vanhuyse et al (1975) according to the number of positive and negative peaks (extrema) in the susceptance and conductance patterns.

1B1G

In the 1B1G pattern both susceptance B and conductance G are single peaked. The admittance Y tympanogram is also single peaked. This pattern occurs when acoustic reactance is

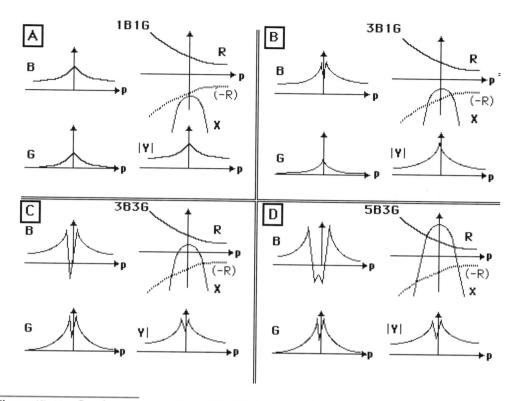

Figure 17–10 Graphic representation of the Vanhuyse model (Vanhuyse et al, 1975). The model determines the shapes of susceptance *(B)* and conductance *(G)* tympanograms from assumptions of the shapes and locations of reactance *(X)* and resistance *(R)* tympanograms using the conversion equations shown in Table 17–2. The upper right corner of each panel shows the reactance and resistance tympanograms. The resistance tympanogram is also shown as negative values *(−R)* to compare its magnitude with the reactance tympanogram. The corresponding susceptance *(B)*, conductance *(G)*, and admittance *(Y)* tympanograms are also shown in each panel. **(A)** The 1B1G pattern occurs when reactance is negative (stiffness controlled) and its absolute value is greater than resistance at all pressures. **(B)** The 3B1G pattern occurs when the reactance is negative and its absolute value is less than resistance at low pressures but greater than resistance at high pressures. **(C)** The 3B3G pattern occurs when reactance is positive (mass controlled) and less than resistance at low pressures and negative at high pressures. **(D)** The 5B3G pattern occurs when reactance is positive and greater than resistance at low pressures and negative at high pressures.

negative at all earcanal pressures and greater in absolute value than resistance (Fig. 17–10A). That is, $X < 0$ and $|X| > R$.

3B1G

In the 3B1G tympanogram, conductance G is single peaked and there is a central notch in susceptance B, resulting in three extrema. This occurs when the reactance tympanogram is shifted toward zero so that at low pressures the absolute value of reactance is less than resistance ($X < 0$ and $|X| < R$) and at high pressures the absolute value of reactance is greater than resistance ($X < 0$ and $|X| > R$). The model predicts that the admittance Y tympanogram is single peaked. In some cases, however, admittance can be notched in the 3B1G pattern (Margolis et al, 1985).

3B3G

In the 3B3G pattern conductance G and susceptance B are both notched. This occurs when reactance at low pressure becomes positive but remains less than resistance ($0 < X < R$). That is, the ear becomes mass controlled. When the ear is pressurized, the system is stiffened and reactance is negative. The susceptance B notch dips below the tail values, resulting in a negative compensated susceptance indicating a mass-controlled ear. The admittance Y tympanogram is also notched.

5B3G

In the 5B3G pattern, the conductance G tympanogram is notched and the susceptance B tympanogram has five extrema. This occurs when the reactance X tympanogram shifts further into positive values so that at low pressures reactance is positive and greater than reactance ($X > R$). Pressurizing the ear has a stiffening effect, and at high pressures the reactance is negative (stiffness controlled).

Resonant Frequency

The resonant frequency is the frequency at which the total reactance is 0. At that frequency, the stiffness reactance and mass reactance are equal but of opposite sign so the total is zero. According to the Vanhuyse model, the resonant frequency of the middle ear is the transition frequency from 3B1G to 3B3G. Another way to identify the resonant frequency is to locate the frequency at which the compensated susceptance is zero. A number of methods for estimating resonant frequencies have been compared (Hanks & Rose, 1993; Margolis & Goycoolea, 1993). The method that appears to be optimal is the frequency at which the minimum susceptance (in the notch) is equal to the positive tail value.

The model provides an understanding of the greater complexity of tympanometric patterns as frequency increases. We know that the reactance of the ear shifts from large negative values toward zero with increasing frequency. The effect of probe frequency on tympanometric shapes can be predicted by shifting the reactance tympanogram accordingly. Shifting the reactance tympanogram from large negative values to positive values results in a sequence beginning with 1B1G and progressing through 5B3G. This is the sequence that occurs in a typical normal adult ear (Margolis & Goycoolea, 1993; Margolis et al, 1985).

The effects of some pathological conditions can also be predicted. A stiffening of the middle ear is expected to shift the reactance tympanogram toward larger negative values while an ossicular discontinuity would have the opposite effect. This approach has been found to account for the effects of frequency and many pathological conditions on tympanometric shapes.

The Vanhuyse model is useful for interpreting tympanometric shapes at any frequency. However, because more complex shapes occur at higher frequencies, the model is most useful for interpreting multifrequency tympanograms.

Single-Frequency (226-Hz) Tympanometry
Tympanometric Features

A number of features of the 226-Hz tympanogram have been used for qualitative and quantitative analysis in the evaluation of middle ear function. These include tympanometric shape, static acoustic admittance, tympanometric width (gradient), tympanometric peak pressure, and equivalent earcanal volume.

Tympanometric Shapes

Two approaches have been taken to the interpretation of 226-Hz tympanograms—qualitative and quantitative. Many of the early instruments that were used for tympanometry were uncalibrated and presented tympanometric results as "arbitrary compliance units." Because it was not appropriate to quantitatively measure tympanometric characteristics from

such data, qualitative methods were used based on judgments of the shapes of tympanograms. The most popular of these methods was the classification scheme originally described by Liden (1969), Liden et al (1974a), and Jerger (1970). Tympanograms are classified according to the height and location of the tympanometric peak. A type A tympanogram has a normal peak height and location on the pressure axis. A type B tympanogram is flat. A type C tympanogram has a peak that is displaced toward negative pressure. Liden also described a type D pattern characterized by a double peak. Later, subtypes A_d and A_s were added (Feldman, 1976), indicating a high-peaked and a low-peaked type A pattern, respectively. Although this approach is useful for identifying abnormal tympanometric features, its lack of precision leads to occasional errors and misinterpretations. For example, without quantitative criteria, no rule for distinguishing types A, A_s, and A_d exists. Even the type B and type A designations are not always agreed on when small peaks occur.

After the publication of the ANSI standard, manufacturers began to conform with the requirement that the immittance indicator must be calibrated in physical units. Virtually all clinical instruments produced since then have been admittance meters. Although some have labeled the y-axis cm^3, the units are equivalent to the millimho. With the current calibrated instruments, it is possible to present results quantitatively and determine pass-fail criteria for tympanometric features. Four features are useful to consider in the clinical interpretation of 226-Hz tympanograms.

Static Admittance

The peak compensated static acoustic admittance, or static admittance, is perhaps the most important feature of the 226-Hz tympanogram. Static admittance is sensitive to many middle ear conditions, including otitis media with effusion, some chronic otitis media sequelae such as cholesteatoma and ossicular adhesions, space-occupying lesions of the middle ear that are in contact with the eardrum or ossicular chain such as glomus tumor, ossicular discontinuity, eardrum perforation, and earcanal occlusion. Table 17–3 includes normative values for children and adults.

Tympanometric Width

A number of studies demonstrated that the sharpness of the tympanometric peak is an indicator of middle ear pathology (Fiellau-Nikolajsen, 1983; Haughton, 1977; Nozza et al, 1992a; Nozza et al, 1994; Paradise et al, 1976). Brooks (1968) introduced the term *gradient* for this tympanometric characteristic. Methods for quantifying the gradient were proposed by Brooks (1968), Paradise et al (1976), and Liden et al (1970). Two studies have compared gradient measures obtained with the various techniques in normal children and adults (de Jonge, 1986; Koebsell & Margolis, 1986). These studies concluded that the preferred method is the tympanometric width. Figure 17–7 illustrates the calculation of this measure. The distance from the peak to the positive tail of the tympanogram is bisected. The width of the tympanogram at that point is determined in dekapascals. Although it has been suggested that abnormally narrow width may indicate stapes fixation (Ivey, 1975), this has not been confirmed. Only abnormally wide tympanometric width should be considered an indication of middle ear dysfunction. Normative data for

TABLE 17–3 Norms for static admittance (Y), tympanometric width (TW), equivalent earcanal volume (V$_{ea}$), and resonant frequency (Res F) determined from sweep frequency (SF) and sweep pressure (SP) methods

Age group		Y (mmho)	TW (daPa)	V$_{ea}$ (cm^3)	Res F SF (Hz)	Res F SP (Hz)
Children (3–10 y)	Mean	0.52[*a]	114[a]	0.58[d]	1153[a]	1041[a]
	90% Range	(0.25–1.05)[*a]	(80–159)[a]	(0.3–0.9)[d]	(850–1525)[a]	(755–1425)[a]
	Fail	≤0.2[*]	≥160	≥1.0	<850 Hz	<755 Hz
	Criteria	≤0.3[†]			>1525 Hz	>1425 Hz
Adults (≥18 y)	Mean	0.79[*b]	77[c]	1.36[e]	1135[b]	990[b]
	90% Range	(0.30–1.70)[b]	(51–114)[c]	(0.9–2.0)[e]	(800–2000)[b]	(630–1400)[b]
	Fail	≤0.3[*]	≥115	≥2.0	<800 Hz	<630 Hz
	Criteria	≤0.4[†]			>2000 Hz	>1400 Hz

[*] +200 daPa compensation.
[†] Negative tail compensation.
[a] Hunter (1993); [b]Margolis and Goycoolea (1993); [c]Margolis and Heller (1987); [d]Shanks et al (1992); [e]Wiley et al (1996).

tympanometric width are presented in Table 17–3. Figure 17–11 shows a tympanogram from a patient with otitis media in which static admittance is normal but tympanometric width is abnormal.

Tympanometric Peak Pressure

The earcanal air pressure at which the peak of the tympanogram occurs is the *tympanometric peak pressure* (TPP). TPP is an indicator of the pressure in the middle ear space. Although TPP overestimates the actual middle ear pressure, sometimes by as much as 100% (Elner et al, 1971; Renvall & Holmquist, 1976), it is an indicator of the status of the middle ear pressure. A TPP of −300 daPa, for example, indicates a significant negative middle ear pressure, but the actual middle ear pressure may be quite different in two ears having the same TPP.

TPP has been widely used to evaluate middle ear pressure. In fact, the first tympanometry article was subtitled "A Method for Objective Determination of the Middle-ear Pressure" (Terkildsen & Thomsen, 1959). Since then, it has been used in the classification of tympanometric shapes (Jerger, 1970; Liden, 1969; Paradise et al, 1976), as a pass-fail criterion for screening for middle ear disease (American Speech-Language-Hearing Association, 1979) and as a diagnostic indicator for otitis media (Renvall et al, 1975).

The clinical use of TPP has been based on the *ex vacuo* theory of middle ear function. (See Magnuson [1983] for a review.) The theory holds that the absorption of gases by the middle ear mucosa results in negative middle ear pressure that accumulates until the eustachian tube opens, restoring the middle ear pressure to ambient. If the eustachian tube fails to open, the negative pressure continues to build, resulting in the large negative pressures that are frequently observed in children.

Recent observations indicate that the gas exchange mechanism for the middle ear is more complex than previously thought (Ostfeld & Silberberg, 1992). The diffusion of gases depends on many factors related to gas concentrations in the middle ear, mucosa, and blood. Diffusion is bidirectional and,

under certain circumstances, can produce positive middle ear pressures (Hergils & Magnuson, 1985, 1987). Experimental evidence has failed to verify that chronic closure of the eustachian tube leads to large negative middle ear pressures (Cantekin et al, 1980b; Proud et al, 1971).

Other mechanisms may be responsible for the large negative pressures observed in patients. The ciliary action of the eustachian tube may lower the middle ear pressure as it moves fluid through the closed tube (Hilding, 1944; Murphy, 1979). Alteration of middle ear gas composition may also contribute to negative middle ear pressure (Cantekin et al, 1980b; Yee & Cantekin, 1986). In some patients, particularly in children, sniffing may produce large negative middle ear pressures (Falk, 1981, 1983; Magnuson, 1981). The negative pressure that occurs in the nasopharynx during sniffing can cause evacuation of air through the eustachian tube. Rather than indicating chronic closure of the eustachian tube, negative pressure caused by sniffing may result from an abnormally compliant tube that is too easily opened by the rush of air in the nasopharynx.

> ## PITFALL
>
> **Negative middle ear pressure does not always indicate an obstructed eustachian tube. In children, negative pressure often results from evacuation of the middle ear, resulting from sniffing. This indicates a eustachian tube that opens easily as air moves through the nasopharynx.**

Perhaps because of the multiple mechanisms that produce middle ear pressure, TPP is not a reliable indicator of medically significant middle ear disease. Several studies have revealed that TPP is not a good predictor of middle ear effusion (Fiellau-Nikolajsen, 1983; Haughton, 1977; Nozza et al,

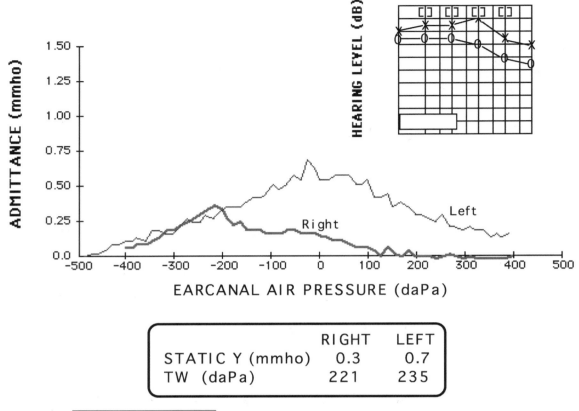

	RIGHT	LEFT
STATIC Y (mmho)	0.3	0.7
TW (daPa)	221	235

Figure 17–11 Tympanogram from a child with bilateral otitis media. The static admittance is normal but tympanometric widths are abnormal in both ears.

1994; Paradise et al, 1976). In the absence of other tympanometric, audiometric, or otoscopic abnormality, negative middle ear pressure probably does not indicate a significant middle ear disorder.

PITFALL

Tympanometric peak pressure is not a reliable indicator of medically significant middle ear disease.

Positive middle ear pressure has been reported in patients with acute otitis media (Margolis & Nelson, 1992; Ostergard & Carter, 1981). Although only a few cases have been reported in the literature, positive TPP (>50 daPa) should raise a suspicion of acute otitis media, and should be followed with a careful history, otoscopic examination, audiometric evaluation, and, if appropriate, medical referral.

PEARL

Positive middle ear pressure may be an indication of acute otitis media.

Equivalent Earcanal Volume

In the presence of a flat tympanogram, an estimate of the volume of air in front of the probe can be useful for detecting eardrum perforations and evaluating the patency of tympanostomy tubes. Although a normal equivalent volume (V_{ea}) does not rule out a perforation, a flat tympanogram with a large volume is evidence of an opening in the TM.

Acoustic immittance measurements using a 226-Hz probe tone are useful for estimating the volume of air in front of the probe (Lindeman & Holmquist, 1982; Shanks et al, 1992). In normal ears the admittance at high positive or negative pressure is primarily determined by the earcanal volume. However, because the eardrum and earcanal walls are not perfectly rigid when the ear is pressurized, the admittance at 226 Hz, expressed as an equivalent volume, overestimates the actual earcanal volume by about 25% in adults (Shanks & Lilly, 1981). The average tympanometrically measured equivalent earcanal volume is about 0.3 cc in 4-month infants (Holte et al, 1991), 0.75 cc in preschool-aged children (Margolis & Heller, 1987), and 1.0 to 1.4 cc in adults (Margolis & Heller, 1987; Wiley et al, 1996). An opening in the TM adds the volume of the middle ear space and contiguous mastoid air cells to the volume of the earcanal. Estimates of the size of the middle ear and mastoid vary considerably among studies. Estimates of 2.0 and 4.7 cc have been reported for 1-year-old infants (Palva & Palva, 1966; Rubensohn, 1965); 6.5, 8.6, and 12.0 cc for adults (Diamant et al, 1958; Moller, 1965b; Zwislocki, 1962). Within studies, a wide range of volumes have been reported, with a range of 2 to 22 cc in one study of adults (Molvaer et al, 1978).

On the basis of these measurements, it should be possible to distinguish between ears with intact eardrums and those with perforations without difficulty. However, ears with past or present middle ear disease have smaller middle ear/mastoid volumes than normal ears for several reasons. First, an ear with active disease may contain fluid, inflammation, granulation, fibrosis, and cholesteatoma, which displace air volume, reducing the middle ear/mastoid volume. Second, ears with active disease may have obstructions of the mastoid air cell system, reducing the total mastoid volume. Third, when chronic disease occurs in infancy, an interruption of the pneumatization process occurs, resulting in a smaller air-filled space (Palva & Palva, 1966). Fourth, chronic disease is more prevalent in ears with poorly pneumatized mastoids (Diamant et al, 1958).

Shanks demonstrated that ears with perforations that are otherwise free of disease have abnormally large volumes (Shanks, 1985). However, when perforations occurred in the presence of active disease, V_{ea} was often normal. The data from Shanks (1985) are shown in Figure 17–12. The subjects were older male adults so the volumes are larger than would be obtained from the general population. A criterion of 6 cc

results in a specificity of 95%. That is, 95% of the normal subjects had equivalent volume $\leq$ 6 cc. For subjects with eardrum perforations who were free of active middle ear disease, equivalent volume exceeded 6 cc in 92% of the cases. That is, the sensitivity was 92%. For subjects with perforations and active middle ear disease, the sensitivity dropped to 50%. Thus a normal volume in the presence of a flat tympanogram may indicate an intact eardrum or a perforation with active middle ear disease. An abnormally large volume suggests a perforation and a normal middle ear/mastoid air space. The Shanks study demonstrates a very important point; a normal volume does not rule out an eardrum perforation.

PITFALL

Although a large equivalent volume suggests a tympanic membrane perforation or patent tympanostomy tube, a normal volume can occur in the presence of a perforation, especially when active middle ear disease is present.

Shanks et al (1992) recommended an abnormal criterion of 1.0 cc for children. For adults, a value of 2.0 cc appears to effectively separate ears with intact eardrums from those with perforations but without active disease (Margolis & Heller, 1987; Wiley et al, 1996).

Another useful clinical application for equivalent volume is to monitor the course of middle ear disease after the insertion of tympanostomy tubes. It has been shown that equivalent volume correlates highly with indices of disease severity (Hunter et al, 1992) and with recurrence otitis media (Takasaka et al, 1996). A progressively larger equivalent volume after tube insertion is an indication of recovery from otitis media. When the equivalent volume remains small, it is an indication of persistent disease. In a study of 157 children aged 6 months to 8 years, treated with tympanostomy tubes for chronic otitis media with effusion (OME), Hunter et al (1992) found that ears with postoperative equivalent volumes of less than 1.5 cc had recurrences of otitis media on average 9.5 months after surgery, whereas ears with equivalent volumes of 3.0 cc or more were otitis free twice as long after surgery (17.5 months on average). This difference was highly significant. Therefore it appears that equivalent volume can be a useful predictor of postoperative recovery and that ears with equivalent volumes of 1.5 cc or less should be followed more closely for recurrence of otitis media.

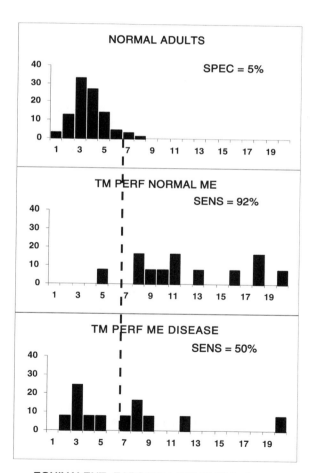

EQUIVALENT EARCANAL VOLUME (cc)

Figure 17–12 Equivalent volume measures for three groups of adult male patients. *Top panel*, Normal middle ear, intact TM. *Middle panel*, TM perforation with otherwise normal middle ear. *Bottom panel*, TM perforation with middle ear inflammation. (Data from Shanks [1985], with permission.)

Sensitivity and Specificity of Tympanometry and Otoscopy

To gauge the clinical usefulness of any diagnostic test, a complete understanding must be developed of the test's performance in various populations at high and low risk for the disease of interest. Tympanometry is no different in this regard. Tympanometry is one of the most highly used diagnostic tests for diagnosing a specific disease in audiological practice. However, we have had adequate information about sensitivity and specificity of tympanometry obtained with calibrated instruments for well-described populations only within the past few years.

Pneumatic otoscopy requires skill, experience, and the proper equipment. With the proper equipment and a highly trained, experienced otoscopist, pneumatic otoscopy is about 94% sensitive and 78% specific, using myringotomy as the "gold standard" (Gates et al, 1986a). Tympanometry is generally less sensitive, but more specific than otoscopy. This fact makes tympanometry a good adjunct to pneumatic otoscopy. It is important for the audiologist and physician to understand that the two procedures will not always agree and that the combination in this case is stronger than either procedure alone.

In most studies before 1990, tympanometry was measured with arbitrary units and therefore qualitative types were compared with otoscopic examination or surgery. For example, Bluestone et al (1973) correlated tympanogram types with the presence of OME at surgery in ears at high risk for OME (all had surgery because of suspected fluid). Flattened or extremely rounded tympanograms were associated with OME in 82% of ears, whereas normal, sharply peaked tympanograms were associated with absence of fluid in 100% of ears. Paradise et al (1976) expanded the familiar Liden-Jerger classification of tympanogram types into 14 types on the basis of arbitrary "compliance" units and gradient. They studied 280 subjects aged 10 days to 5 years, 11 months. These infants and children were from two groups; 107 were scheduled to receive myringotomy and tubes, and 173 were selected from various outpatient clinics. Tympanometry and otoscopy were completed within 1 hour and within 2 hours of myringotomy for the surgical group. Overall, agreement between otoscopy and surgery was 86%. Sensitivity of otoscopy for presence of OME was 91%, and specificity was 75%. Percentage of ears with OME varied by type of tympanogram, with the highest prevalence of fluid (89%) found in the flat or rounded tympanogram. Normal tympanograms were associated with no OME in 95% of ears. In tympanograms with pressure peaks at or less than -100 daPa, presence of OME depended highly on the gradient or width of the tympanogram. If gradient alone was considered, then sensitivity was 95% and specificity was 76% for presence of OME, similar to the test performance of otoscopy. Cantekin et al (1980a) combined otoscopy and tympanometry into an algorithm and found that tympanometry in combination with otoscopy resulted in better test performance than either test alone. The combined sensitivity of otoscopy and tympanometry was 97%, and specificity was 90%. Gates et al (1986a) used the 14 tympanogram types suggested by Paradise et al (1976). Five of these types were found to be associated with a low prevalence of OME (8% of ears with these tympanogram types had OME at surgery). Three types were highly associated with OME with a prevalence of 88%. The other six types were intermediate, with prevalences varying from 20 to 54%.

Because otitis media is a continuum of middle ear conditions with tympanometric results also varying along a continuum, it is highly unlikely that any criterion, no matter how carefully selected, will identify all affected ears. This fact was demonstrated by Le and colleagues in two studies of tympanometry in ears before and after intubation (Le et al, 1992; 1994).

As in the Le studies, more recent investigators have used calibrated equipment that allows static admittance and tympanometric width to be quantified and compared among groups of individuals. Silman et al (1992) investigated several protocols for sensitivity and specificity of detection of middle ear OME in children. Children were identified with OME on the basis of pneumatic otoscopy by an experienced otolaryngologist. Sensitivity and specificity of four combinations of immittance variables were estimated. Variables included static admittance, tympanometric width, tympanometric peak pressure, and ipsilateral acoustic reflex. The sensitivity of the various combinations ranged from 76 to 95%.

Performance of two screening procedures was also assessed by Roush et al (1992) in 374 ears of 3- to 4-year-old children in a preschool program. A "traditional" procedure, based on TPP < -200 daPa or absent ipsilateral acoustic reflex was compared with the interim norms published in the 1990 ASHA Guidelines (American Speech-Language-Hearing Association, 1990). The "gold standard" was pneumatic otoscopy performed by an experienced, validated otoscopist. The "traditional" procedure had high sensitivity (95%) but low specificity (65%). Although the negative predictive value was high (99%), the positive predictive value was low (27%). The ASHA interim norms had high sensitivity (84%) and specificity (95%), with a positive predictive value of 69% and a negative predictive value of 98%. The guidelines will perform differently in different populations, and other variables, such as the time interval between screening and medical examination, personnel used for screening, and use of case history and visual inspection, will all affect the performance of the screening protocol.

Nozza and colleagues (1992b) have made important contributions in their studies of acoustic immittance in various populations of children (Nozza et al, 1992b, 1994). In the first study two groups of children were evaluated. One group ($n = 61$, aged 1 to 8 years) received myringotomy and intubation and thus was at high risk for OME. Tympanometry was performed no more than 30 minutes before surgery. The surgeon was unaware of the results of tympanometry. Six different protocols were evaluated; three of these included ipsilateral acoustic reflexes. Sensitivity, specificity, positive and negative predictive values were all measured. Positive and negative predictive values are influenced by the prevalence of the disease in the population, which was very high in this sample (73%). Sensitivity (90%) and specificity (86%) were highest for gradient combined with acoustic reflexes. Gradient combined with static admittance also produced relatively high sensitivity (83%) and specificity (87%). A second group of children ($n = 77$, aged 3 to 16 years) who attended an allergy clinic and were unselected with regard to otitis media history were also studied and reported in the same paper (Nozza et al, 1992b). The same six immittance protocols were compared against a validated otoscopist. In this sample sensitivity was 78% for all protocols except ipsilateral reflex alone (sensitivity = 88%) and gradient or static admittance < 0.1 mmho (sensitivity = 67%). Gradient + ipsilateral reflex and gradient + static admittance performed equally well for specificity (99%). Positive predictive value was higher for gradient + static admittance (88%) than it was for gradient + ipsilateral reflex (78%).

In a subsequent study (Nozza et al, 1994), a group of children ($n = 171$, aged 1 to 12 years) with recurrent or chronic OME, who were scheduled for myringotomy and tubes, received otoscopy by a validated otoscopist and tympanometry by a certified audiologist. The prevalence of OME in this group was 55%. Eleven criteria, with various cut-points for each criterion were evaluated. As expected, there was a trade-off so that as sensitivity increased with changes in cut-point,

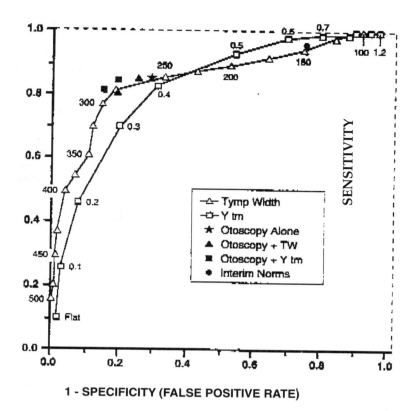

1 - SPECIFICITY (FALSE POSITIVE RATE)

Figure 17–13 ROC for tympanometric measures alone and in combination with otoscopy. (From Nozza et al [1994], with permission.)

specificity decreased. Sensitivity and specificity for various criteria are depicted on a receiver-operator curve in Figure 17–13. Sensitivity is depicted on the *y*-axis and the false positive rate (1–specificity) is depicted on the *x*-axis. Points that fall closest to the upper left corner show best test performance (high sensitivity and low false positive rate). It can be seen that tympanometric width >275 daPa performs best as a single criterion, but width combined with otoscopy performs slightly better. The study also evaluated tympanometric criteria against otoscopy findings based on the child rather than the ear. TW of >250 daPa performed better than cutoffs of 150 or 200 when judged against otoscopy.

These studies demonstrate that the choice of cutoff criteria affects test performance greatly. It appears that combinations of criteria, such as otoscopy and TW, perform better than single criteria. Static admittance alone has low sensitivity but good specificity. Use of either ipsilateral reflex or tympanometric width combined with static admittance provides good test performance, as does otoscopy combined with width. However, all studies have used highly experienced, validated otoscopists, and results may be very different with less experienced or knowledgeable personnel. Prevalence of the disease in the population will affect negative and positive predictive values. With lower prevalence, the positive predictive value goes down; that is, fewer referrals will turn out to have real problems. As the positive predictive value decreases, the number of unnecessary referrals increases. Cutoff criteria may need to be more stringent when prevalence is lower and more lax when prevalence or risk of the disease is greater. Therefore it is very helpful to estimate the prevalence of the disease in the population of interest when choosing pass/fail criteria.

The results of these studies indicate that both tympanometry and pneumatic otoscopy are good tests for identifying OME. It is important to remember that highly skilled otoscopists were used in the evaluation of otoscopy and that most clinicians who examine ears are probably not as skilled as those used in the studies. Most patients with middle ear disease are initially evaluated by primary care physicians who are less experienced in ear examination and in cleaning the earcanal to perform an adequate evaluation of the ear. In view of the fact that otoscopy and tympanometry are both effective screening tests, tympanometry would appear to be a very useful adjunct to otoscopy for evaluation of the ear by primary care physicians and by audiologists.

Screening Tympanometry

Tympanometry has been widely used in screening programs, primarily for identifying middle ear disease in pediatric populations. (See Holte & Margolis [1987] and Roush [1990] for discussions.) The value of mass screening programs for identifying middle ear disease has been controversial (American Academy of Audiology, 1997b; Bluestone et al, 1986). Although various conferences, organizations, and agencies have been hesitant to recommend large-scale screening programs, many programs for preschool and school-age children have incorporated tympanometric screening into the protocol. Most programs combine audiometric screening with tympanometric screening to detect both sensorineural hearing loss and middle ear disorders (American Speech-Language-Hearing Association, 1990; American Academy of Audiology, 1997a).

Margolis and Heller (1987) developed a screening protocol that was later incorporated into the 1990 ASHA Guideline.

PEARL

Tympanometry, performed carefully by experienced audiologists, and pneumatic otoscopy, performed by highly skilled otoscopists, are equally effective for detecting OME.

That protocol, shown in a flowchart format in Figure 17–14, uses case history information, visual inspection of the ear, audiometric screening, and tympanometry to identify significant hearing loss and middle ear disorders requiring medical referral.

Case History

In a screening program, time is not sufficient to take a complete history. However, certain information warrants a medical referral without the need to perform any tests. This includes a recent history of otalgia (ear pain) or otorrhea (ear discharge).

Visual Inspection

Personnel who administer screening tests vary widely in their skills for examining the ear. Some may be quite experienced otoscopists, whereas others may not be able to visualize the TM and reliably evaluate its appearance. However, every screening program should include an inspection of the ear to identify obvious signs of active disease. The visual inspection should include examination of the head and neck and otoscopic inspection of the earcanal and TM. Conditions that warrant additional testing or medical referral include developmental defects; earcanal occlusion or inflammation; and TM abnormalities associated with ear disease, including inflammation, perforation, and abnormal landmarks or color.

Audiometric Screening

Guidelines for audiometric screening have been recommended by various professional associations (American Speech-Language-Hearing Association, 1990; American Academy of Audiology, 1997a). Typically these involve a three-frequency screen at a fixed hearing level, such as 20 dB HL at 1, 2, and 4 kHz. Failure to respond to one or more frequencies in either ear constitutes a fail and results in further testing, audiological evaluation, or medical referral.

Tympanometry

Variables that have been used in screening programs include qualitative assessment of tympanometric shapes, static admittance, tympanometric width, tympanometric peak pressure, and equivalent volume. Because tympanometric peak pressure has been shown to be weakly related to significant middle ear disease, it has been largely abandoned as a screening indicator. Early studies indicated that tympanometric screening resulted in an unacceptably high rate of referrals (Roush & Tait, 1985). More recent protocols have incorporated a rescreening requirement to reduce the number of false positive failures (Margolis & Heller, 1987). Adequate normative data are available to set reasonable fail criteria for static admittance, tympanometric width, and equivalent earcanal volume. Table 17–3 includes fail criteria for these variables for children and adults.

The flowchart illustrated in Figure 17–14 illustrates the logic used to determine the need for an audiological or medical referral, not necessarily the order in which the tests are performed. A positive history or visual inspection results in an immediate referral, most likely to a physician. The audiometric screen requires a second test before a referral is made. The second test can be performed on the same day as the screen or at a later date. Failure of both audiometric screening tests is required to result in a referral. The tympanometric portion of the protocol uses equivalent earcanal volume, static admittance, and tympanometric width. A flat tympanogram with a large volume is an indication of a perforation and warrants an immediate referral if the patient is not already under the care of a physician. Patent tympanostomy tubes, for example, do not require a referral because the patient is obviously in medical treatment. Failure on static admittance or tympanometric width requires a second screening 4 to 6 weeks after the first screen. Failure on both occasions is required for a referral.

The nature of the referral will depend on the circumstances of the screening program. In some cases, patients may be referred to an audiologist for complete audiological evaluation, the outcome of which will determine the need for medical referral. Those referred for medical evaluation may be referred to a primary care physician or to an otolaryngologist. This is determined by the available resources, the requirements of the healthcare provider, and the relationships between the screening program and other clinical facilities.

Multifrequency Tympanometry
High Impedance Pathological Conditions

High impedance pathological conditions are conditions that increase the impedance of the middle ear, ranging from simple middle ear effusion to invasive neoplasms. OME increases the impedance of the middle ear space in direct proportion to the quantity of fluid occupying the normally air-filled space. With large quantities of fluid, varying the earcanal air pressure does not change the impedance at the eardrum, so the tympanogram is flat. A typical 226-Hz admittance tympanogram in an ear with OME is shown in Figure 17–15A. Because the tympanogram is flat, tympanometric width and tympanometric peak pressure are not measurable. Equivalent volume is within the normal range, indicating that the probe tip is not obstructed by the earcanal wall. A flat tympanogram at low frequencies is strong evidence for OME, but some high impedance pathological conditions may be evident only at higher frequencies. In various stages of OME, impedance may be altered by increased mass caused by thick effusion in contact with the ossicles or decreased compliance caused by reduction of the air volume of the mastoid and middle ear space. In these stages the 226-Hz tympanogram may not be flat, but it likely will be more rounded and broader than normal. Tympanometric width is more sensitive than static admittance for some of these conditions. However, even width can be normal in some cases of OME. Examination of the higher frequencies may be necessary to reveal impedance changes in some stages of OME. A 226-Hz tympanogram from a patient with chronic OME is shown in Figure 17–15B.

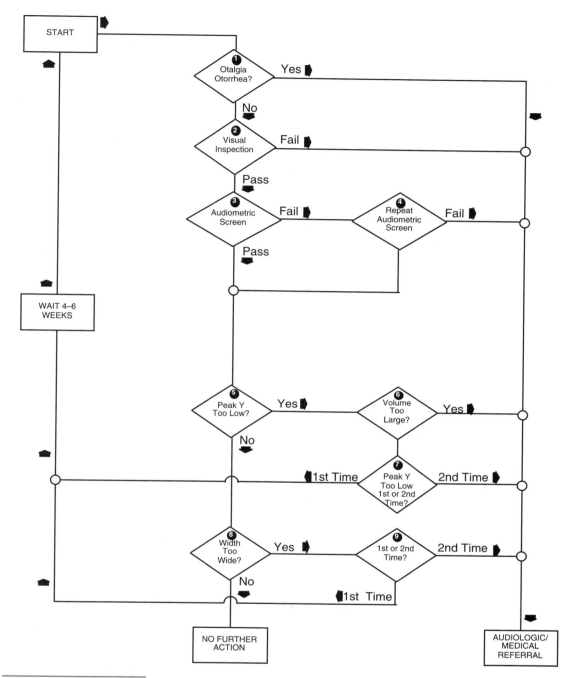

Figure 17–14 Flowchart for screening for hearing loss and middle ear disease. (From Margolis & Heller [1987], with permission.)

The TM was retracted and thickened with reduced mobility on pneumatic otoscopy. She had been treated for acute otitis media 3 months earlier. Static admittance is within normal limits, but the tympanogram is abnormally wide. Multifrequency tympanograms for the same patient are shown in Figure 17–16. At all frequencies greater than 226 Hz, tympanograms are nearly flat and do not progress through the normal Vanhuyse sequence.

As with other sequelae of otitis media, TM retraction occurs on a continuum (Maw & Bawden, 1994; Sade & Berco,

1976), ranging from slight retraction of pars tensa without atrophy to collapse of the eardrum onto the ossicles and promontory of the middle ear. Figure 17–15C shows a 226-Hz tympanogram from an ear with retraction caused by negative middle ear pressure. Multifrequency tympanograms for the same patient are shown in Figure 17–17. The patterns are normal Vanhuyse patterns with a tympanometric peak pressure of −277 daPa and a resonant frequency of 1250 Hz. Retraction by itself results only in a shift of the tympanogram on the pressure axis. When retraction occurs with atrophy,

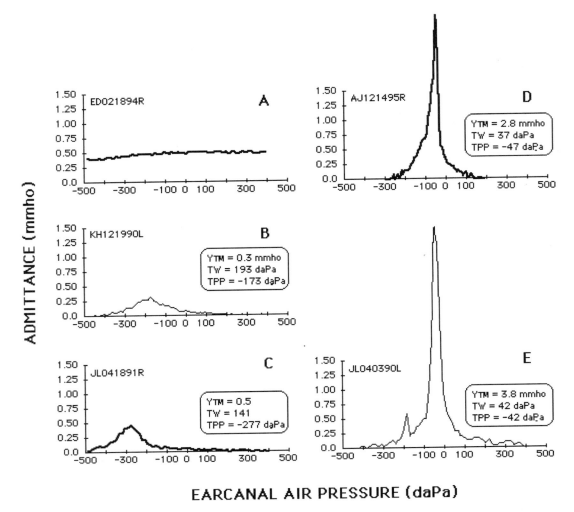

Figure 17–15 226-Hz admittance tympanograms from two patients with chronic otitis media with effusion **(A,B)**, patient with TM retraction **(C)**, patient with TM atrophy **(D)**, and patient with an ossicular discontinuity **(E)**.

tympanosclerosis, or other middle ear sequelae, other tympanometric abnormalities may be present.

Another high-impedance pathological condition, cholesteatoma (keratoma), is a collection of epithelial debris that usually originates in the lateral epithelial layer of the eardrum and migrates into the middle ear. In severe cases cholesteatoma can result in destruction of ossicles and invasion of the mastoid air cell system (Proctor, 1991). In a study of acquired cholesteatoma in 1024 children and adults, Sheehy and colleagues (1977) found that most occurred in the attic or the posterosuperior quadrant (73%), whereas 18% had a complete marginal perforation, 6% had a partial, central perforation, and only 3% had an intact TM. Cholesteatomas are rare, even among people with histories of chronic OME. In children treated with tympanostomy tubes, prevalence of cholesteatoma 6 to 20 years later is approximately 1% (Daly et al, 1997). A case study of a patient with cholesteatoma is presented in the last section of this chapter.

Otosclerosis is a high-impedance pathological condition that has defied attempts to develop a definitive diagnostic test. Although 226-Hz tympanograms tend to show low static admittance in otosclerotic ears, the overlap between normals and otosclerotics has prevented this measure from being an effective diagnostic test (Alberti & Jerger, 1974; Jerger, 1970; Jerger et al, 1974). In a study of experimentally produced stapes fixation in cats (Margolis et al, 1978), there was a clear separation of static impedance at 220 and 660 Hz between cats with stapes fixation and normals. This clear separation is not apparent between otosclerotic patients and normal subjects. Because the site of the lesion is at the stapes footplate, where the input impedance to the cochlea is very high, increasing the impedance at that point has little effect on the impedance at the TM. In addition, the wide normal variability among human individuals makes it more difficult to detect small impedance changes in clinical populations than in a controlled experiment.

Multifrequency tympanometry does not appear to increase the sensitivity of tympanometry for otosclerosis (Colletti, 1976; Shahnaz & Polka, 1999). Shahnaz and Polka (1999) compared static admittance, tympanometric width, resonant

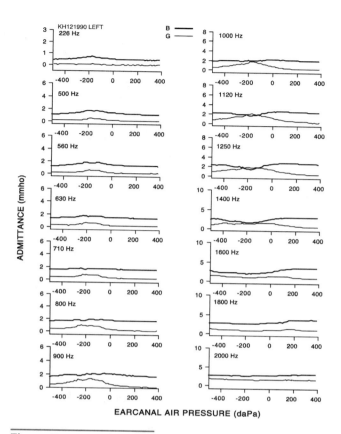

Figure 17–16 Multifrequency tympanograms from a patient with chronic otitis media with effusion. The 226-Hz admittance tympanogram is shown in Figure 17–15B.

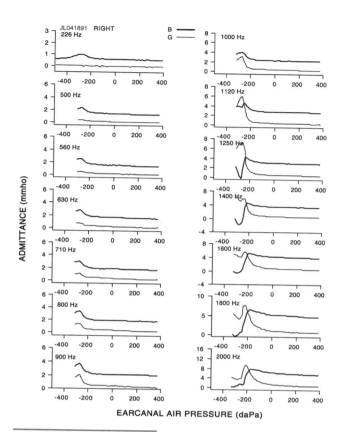

Figure 17–17 Multifrequency tympanograms from a patient with TM retraction caused by negative middle ear pressure. The 226-Hz admittance tympanogram is shown in Figure 17–15C.

frequency, and the frequency corresponding to an admittance phase angle of 45 degrees in 36 normal-hearing adults and 14 patients diagnosed with otosclerosis. Results showed no statistically significant difference in static admittance or width between normal and otosclerotic ears. A significant difference existed between normal and otosclerotic ears for resonant frequency, and for the frequency corresponding to an admittance phase angle of 45 degrees. However, the sensitivity was only 79% and the specificity was 71%. Thus multifrequency tympanometry does not perform particularly well as a diagnostic test for otosclerosis. The combination of absent acoustic reflexes, conductive hearing loss, relatively normal 226-Hz tympanogram, and normal eardrum appearance in an adult with an otherwise unremarkable history for ear disease remains the best indication of otosclerosis.

Low-Impedance Pathological Conditions

Low-impedance pathological conditions are those that decrease the impedance at the eardrum. Tympanometry is very effective for identifying these pathological conditions because they cause a large impedance change at the TM. However, clinically significant low-impedance pathological conditions are more rare than high-impedance pathological conditions. The most common low-impedance pathological condition is TM atrophy, often called a monomeric or dimeric membrane. Thinning or destruction of the middle fibrous layer (lamina

propria) of the TM resulting from otitis media, traumatic perforation, or surgical placement of tympanostomy tubes results in decreased stiffness and hypermobility. Atrophy can occur in small, focal areas, often at a previous myringotomy site, or may be more generalized across the eardrum. Atrophy may lead to atelectasis (collapse of the eardrum into the ossicles and middle ear promontory) when combined with eustachian tube dysfunction and otitis media, resulting in a clinically significant pathological condition. TM atrophy is associated with increased static admittance, narrow tympanometric width, and decreased resonant frequency. Atrophy does not, however, appear to be associated with conductive hearing loss unless it is also accompanied by retraction of the TM or ossicular erosion. Figure 17–15D shows a 226-Hz tympanogram from a patient with a history of otitis media and generalized TM atrophy. Note the high-static admittance (2.8 mmho) and narrow width (37 daPa). Figure 17–18 shows multifrequency tympanograms for the same patient. The resonant frequency is abnormally low (<500 Hz). Tympanometric patterns are normal Vanhuyse patterns through 1400 Hz. The transitions from one Vanhuyse pattern to the next are all shifted toward lower frequencies. The 3B1G pattern at 500 Hz, 3B3G pattern at 710 Hz, and 5B3G pattern at 900 Hz are not observed in normal ears at those low frequencies. This indicates a decreased stiffness, resulting in a decreased resonant frequency. At the highest frequencies (>1400 Hz) the

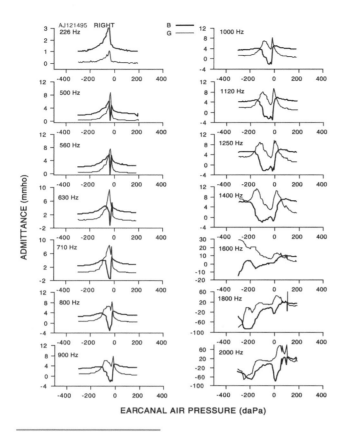

Figure 17–18 Multifrequency tympanograms from a patient with an atrophic TM. The 226-Hz admittance tympanogram is shown in Figure 17–15D.

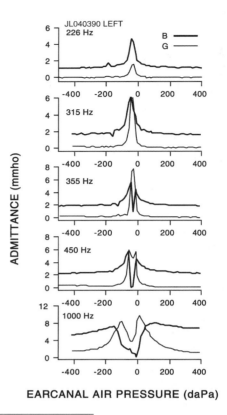

Figure 17–19 Multifrequency tympanograms from a patient with a complete disarticulation of the ossicular chain. The 226-Hz admittance tympanogram is shown in Figure 17–15E.

patterns become very high amplitude and irregular, probably indicating that the measurement system is not capable of measuring such high admittance values. Because hearing is normal, it can be surmised that the changes are due to TM atrophy and not to ossicular disarticulation, which would result in conductive hearing loss.

The effect of ossicular erosion and disarticulation is similar to atrophy, although the effects can be more marked. Typically, complete disarticulation results in extremely high static admittance at 226 Hz and extremely low resonant frequency. Figure 17–15E shows the 226-Hz tympanogram from a patient with surgically confirmed traumatic disarticulation. Like the patient with tympanometric atrophy, the static admittance is high (3.8 mmho) and the tympanometric width is narrow (42 daPa). Figure 17–19 shows multifrequency tympanograms for the same patient. At 355 Hz the pattern is 3B1G and the depth of the susceptance notch indicates that the ear is beyond the resonant frequency. This is an extremely low-resonant frequency and an unusually low frequency for a 3B1G pattern. 3B3G and 5B3G patterns occur at 450 and 1000 Hz, respectively, again, very low frequencies for these complex patterns.

A careful otologic examination is required to discover the cause of the hearing loss, when present, and the tympanometric abnormalities. Multiple pathological conditions can coexist, obscuring the true cause of hearing loss. For example, when otosclerosis coexists with atrophy of the TM, the more lateral, and less significant, pathological condition dominates the tympanogram. Thus an ear with both otosclerosis and atrophy may be confused with ossicular discontinuity.

Tympanometry in Infants

Tympanograms recorded from normal ears of newborn infants are very different from those obtained from older infants, children, and adults. In neonate ears with confirmed middle ear disease, 226-Hz tympanograms are not reliably different from those obtained from normal ears. For these reasons, the 226-Hz tympanometry is not an effective test for middle ear disease in newborns.

The earliest tympanometric recordings from neonate ears were made with single-component instruments that used a 220-Hz probe tone and expressed the results as "arbitrary compliance units" (Bennett, 1975; Keith, 1973, 1975; Poulsen & Tos, 1978). These studies reported a frequent occurrence of double-peaked tympanograms, indicating that the newborn ear is very different from the adult ear. Recall from the Vanhuyse model that double-peaked admittance tympanograms occur in 3B1G, 3B3G, or 5B3G patterns, that is, when the absolute value of reactance is less than resistance or when reactance becomes positive (mass controlled). This never occurs in the normal adult ear at 220 or 226 Hz because at low frequencies reactance is a large negative value indicating a stiffness-controlled system.

Later studies recorded two-component tympanograms at two probe frequencies, 220 and 660 Hz (Himelfarb et al, 1979;

Sprague et al, 1985). These two-component recordings permit an analysis of the components of immittance. These studies indicated that at low frequencies, the newborn ear is characterized by a large resistive component and a very low reactance. The low reactance suggests a significant mass effect that offsets the stiffness of the middle ear system. The patterns, particularly at 660 Hz, were generally not consistent with the Vanhuyse model.

Holte recorded multifrequency tympanograms (226 to 900 Hz) from newborns and, from the same babies, at several ages up to 4 months (Holte et al, 1991). Tympanometric patterns were classified by shape using the four categories of the Vanhuyse model and "other" for patterns that do not conform to any of the Vanhuyse categories. For newborns (1 to 7 days) at 226 Hz, all tympanograms conformed to the Vanhuyse categories, approximately equally distributed among the four patterns. Recall that adult ears are all 1B1G at that frequency. As frequency increases from 226 Hz to 900 Hz, the proportion of "other" patterns increases, reaching 100% at 900 Hz. With increasing age, the proportion of "other" patterns decreases and the tympanograms conform more consistently to the Vanhuyse model. By 3 to 4 months, most patterns conformed to the Vanhuyse model with 100% 1B1G patterns at 226 Hz and 82% either 1B1G or 3B1G at 900 Hz. The results of that study indicated that tympanograms of newborns do not progress in an orderly sequence with changes in probe frequency and are apparently influenced by mass and resistive elements that are not present in older subjects. By 4 months of age tympanometric patterns behave in a manner that is consistent with the Vanhuyse model, although developmental changes are not yet complete.

PEARL

By 4 months of age, multifrequency tympanograms of normal infant ears behave in an orderly fashion, similar to those of older children and adults.

Figure 17–20 shows multifrequency tympanograms from a 2-day-old infant and from the same infant at age 4 months. At 2 days, the 226-Hz tympanogram is a 1B1G pattern but the peak susceptance is lower than conductance, a reversal of the relationship seen in older infants and adults. At higher frequencies, the patterns are irregular and do not conform to the Vanhuyse model. At 4 months, the patterns are regular 1B1G patterns up to 900 Hz where a 3B1G pattern is observed. These patterns are very similar to those seen in older children and indicates a rapid maturation of the external and/or middle ear.

The reasons for the disorganized behavior of tympanograms in newborns are not clear. Because the osseous portion of the earcanal wall of the newborn is not rigid as it is in adults, it has been suggested that movement of the canal wall influences tympanometric recordings (Keefe et al, 1993; Paradise et al, 1976). There is evidence for and against this hypothesis. Holte et al (1990) found no relationship between canal wall movement of neonates measured with video otomicroscopy and tympanometric patterns. Hsu et al (1996) found similarly chaotic tympanometric patterns in newborn chinchillas despite the fact that the canal wall appeared to be

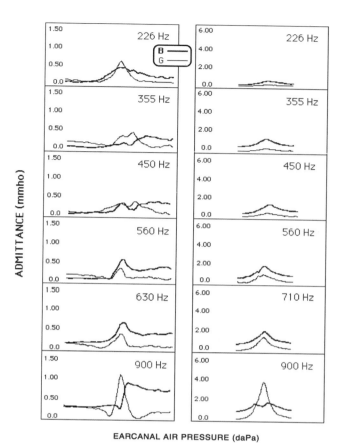

Figure 17–20 Tympanogram from a full-term 1-day-old infant and from the same infant at age 133 days.

fully ossified on histological analysis. On the other hand, Keefe et al (1993) measured complex impedance in infants at various ages and found a mass effect that appeared to be similar to the acoustic properties of soft tissue elsewhere in the body. Because this effect dominates at low frequencies, they argued that probe tones less than 1000 Hz would probably not be effective for evaluating middle ear function in newborns. Although a mass component of earcanal wall vibration in newborns is certainly a possibility, it does not account for the irregular (non-Vanhuyse patterns that are prevalent in that age group).

Another possible source of the differences between infants and older subjects is the presence of material in the middle ear. Mesenchyme (unresorbed fetal tissue), amniotic fluid, and other cellular debris have been observed in the middle ears of infant temporal bones (Eavey, 1993; Paparella et al, 1980). Abnormal tissue that is in contact with the ossicles and eardrum has been shown to produce irregular tympanometric patterns in chinchillas (Margolis et al, 1998). On the other hand the middle ears of newborn chinchillas with irregular tympanometric patterns were free of debris and appeared mature in structure (Hsu et al, 1996).

Although the reasons for the chaotic nature of tympanometric patterns in newborns are not clear, it is evident that low-frequency tympanometry is not effective for detecting middle ear pathological conditions in the neonate. Balkany

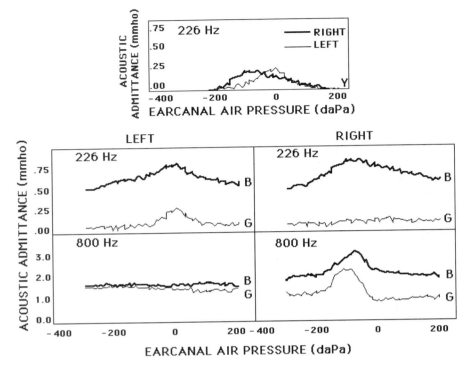

Figure 17–21 Tympanograms from a 2-week-old infant with acute otitis media in the left ear. The 226-Hz tympanograms appear to be normal and bilaterally similar. The 800-Hz tympanogram is flat in the involved ear and normal in the uninvolved ear.

et al (1978) reported that 30% of 125 consecutively examined neonatal intensive care unit infants had middle ear effusion (MEE), based on otoscopy and/or tympanocentesis. All were judged to have normal 226-Hz tympanograms. Others also have reported normal 226-Hz tympanograms in the presence of confirmed MEE in neonates (Hunter & Margolis, 1992; Paradise et al, 1976). Figure 17–21 shows tympanograms from a newborn intensive care nursery patient with confirmed acute otitis media with effusion. The 226-Hz tympanogram appeared to be normal and similar to that of the unaffected ear. Using a higher probe tone frequency, however, the tympanogram was clearly abnormal. Evidence is mounting that tympanograms obtained with probe tone frequencies that are higher than the conventional 226 Hz are more sensitive to middle ear disease in newborns than conventional tympanometry (Marchant et al, 1986; Rhodes et al, 1998).

Wideband Reflectance

A new technique has been used recently to evaluate middle ear function. *Energy reflectance* is the ratio of energy reflected from a surface to the energy that strikes the surface (incident energy). This is a useful concept for evaluating middle ear function because it tells us how much energy is reflected from the eardrum and how much is absorbed by the middle ear. Recall that because of the complexity of the middle ear system, the amount of energy absorbed by the middle ear is not the same as the energy delivered to the cochlea. Consequently, although energy reflectance indicates how much energy is transmitted into the middle ear, it may not always correlate with hearing sensitivity.

Measurement systems used to measure energy reflectance are calibrated differently than those used for multifrequency tympanometry. Whereas multifrequency tympanometry is

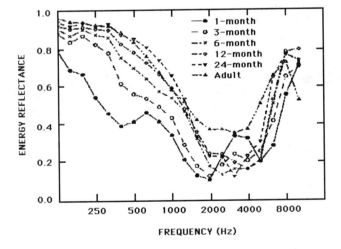

Figure 17–22 Energy reflectance for normal subjects aged 1 month to adult. (From Keefe et al [1993], with permission.)

restricted to frequencies less than 2 kHz, energy reflectance systems can measure over a much wider frequency range. Because energy reflectance is mathematically related to impedance and admittance, it is possible to derive any immittance quantity from measures of reflectance.

Keefe and colleagues (1993) measured energy reflectance from normal subjects aged 1 month to adult. The results are shown in Figure 17–22. In normal adult ears more than 90% of low-frequency energy is reflected, accounting for our relatively poor auditory sensitivity below 500 Hz. As frequency increases above 500 Hz, reflectance decreases, forming a broad minimum near 3000 Hz. It is in this range that energy is most efficiently transmitted into the middle ear. Infants show roughly the same pattern. The youngest infants in the study (1 month) show an additional dip near 400 Hz, possibly an effect of the incomplete development of the earcanal wall. A compliant earcanal wall would absorb energy, decreasing the reflectance of the ear. Keefe et al suggested that the 400-Hz frequency is the expected location of a reflectance dip because of the vibration of soft tissue in the earcanal.

Keefe and Levi (1996) introduced the concept of the reflectance tympanogram. Using a multifrequency tympanometry instrument they calculated reflectance from admittance and plotted it against earcanal air pressure. Margolis et al (1999) recorded reflectance tympanograms from normal adult subjects. Figure 17–23 shows the average reflectance for varying earcanal pressures. Pressurizing the earcanal changes the reflectance pattern in several ways. At low frequencies reflectance is increased. The broad minimum that occurs around 3 kHz becomes narrower, deepens, and shifts up in frequency, forming a narrow minimum around 5000 Hz. At

this frequency, pressurizing the ear *increases* the sound absorption by the middle ear. This would be expected to *improve* hearing in a narrow, high-frequency region. This is consistent with observations made as early as 1820 (Wollaston, 1820) that middle ear pressure significantly decreases the loudness of low-frequency sounds with little effect on higher frequencies.

Figure 17–24 shows mean reflectance tympanograms from 20 normal adult subjects for frequencies ranging from 250 to 11,000 Hz. As frequency increases, reflectance tympanograms progress through a sequence of three patterns. At low frequencies where reflectance is increased by positive and negative pressure, the reflectance tympanogram shows a single minimum near ambient pressure. At higher frequencies, where reflectance decreases with pressure, the pattern is inverted with a single maximum. At the highest frequencies the pattern is nearly flat, indicating that pressure has little effect on reflectance. This sequence of patterns may form the

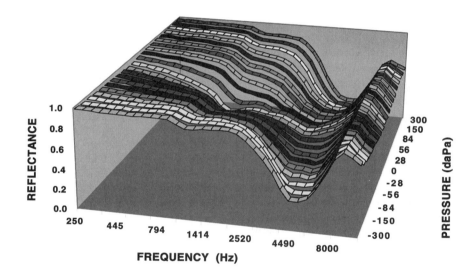

Figure 17–23 Energy reflectance for normal subjects at various earcanal air pressures. *(See Color Plate 19.)*

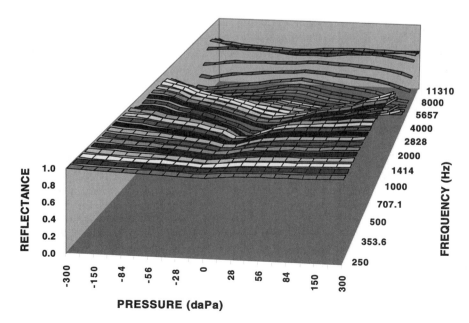

Figure 17–24 Average reflectance tympanograms for 20 normal adult subjects. As the test frequency progresses from low to high, tympanometric patterns progress from V-shaped, to inverted V, to flat. *(See Color Plate 20.)*

basis for evaluating ears with middle ear pathological conditions, much the same as the Vanhuyse model is used for multifrequency tympanometry.

Identification of Patulous Eustachian Tube

Clinical acoustic immittance instruments are useful for identifying the chronically patulous eustachian tube, a condition that is often characterized by symptoms of aural fullness and autophony (abnormal sensation of one's own voice). It can be unilateral or bilateral, chronic, transient, or intermittent. The condition has been linked to rapid weight loss (O'Connor & Shea, 1981) and to pregnancy (Plate et al, 1979) but is also seen in isolation. The symptoms can be quite troublesome to some patients, whereas other patients with the condition are not bothered by it and, in some cases, were not aware of the condition. A variety of surgical procedures have been used to correct the condition with limited success. Identifying the condition and distinguishing it from otitis media can be helpful to the patient and the physician, even if it cannot be successfully treated. See Henry and DiBartolomeo (1993) for a review.

A variety of methods have been used to identify the condition. One that is readily performed with many clinical acoustic immittance instruments is the recording of breathing-related changes in the apparent admittance of the ear. Because of the patent eustachian tube, nasopharyngeal pressure changes are transmitted to the middle ear, producing changes in middle ear admittance similar to those produced by earcanal pressure changes in tympanometry. These are readily detected by the immittance instrument and quite distinct from the normal ear.

The test is performed by setting the instrument to the acoustic reflex mode without presentation of a reflex-eliciting stimulus. Recordings can be made with the patient (1) breathing normally, (2) breathing deeply, and (3) holding the breath. The case presented later in this chapter illustrates the use of this test.

THE ACOUSTIC STAPEDIUS REFLEX

A Short History

The first observations of the acoustically evoked contraction of the middle ear muscles were made by Hensen (1878), who observed the responses of both the tensor tympani and stapedius muscles of dogs to sound stimulation. Other investigators described similar responses in cat and rabbit. (See Hallpike [1935] for a review.) As early as 1913, Kato (1913) observed that only the stapedius muscle, and not the tensor tympani, responded to acoustic stimulation in monkeys. Nevertheless, the role of the tensor tympani in the acoustic reflex in humans would not be understood until the latter half of the century.

Lüscher (1929) was the first of several investigators to report direct observations of the acoustic stapedius reflex in humans. By observing the movement of the stapedius tendon through a perforated TM, Lüscher was able to study stimulus-response relationships of the reflex. Kobrak (1948) tried, with limited success, to observe the acoustic-stapedius reflex

through the intact TM by treating it with a mixture of water, glycerine, and potassium iodide to induce transparency. The clinical usefulness of acoustic reflex measurement required the development of electroacoustic instruments that measure the change in the acoustic admittance of the middle ear produced by contraction of one or both middle ear muscles.

The first electroacoustic device used for clinical acoustic reflex measurement was the Metz bridge (Metz, 1946). Metz recorded acoustic reflexes from a wide variety of patients with ear disease, including patients with unilateral otosclerosis and facial nerve paralysis. The absence of an acoustic reflex in these patients is strong evidence that the tensor tympani, innervated by cranial nerve V, is not active during the acoustic reflex. Jepsen (1955) working with the same device, made similar observations and concluded that only the stapedius muscle in humans is acoustically activated and referred to the response and the *acoustic-stapedius reflex*. Although the issue was debated as late as 1957 by Terkildsen (1957) who was a colleague of Metz and Jepsen at Rigshospitalet in Copenhagen, it is now widely accepted that the acoustic reflex in humans results from stapedius, and not tensor tympani, contraction. Nevertheless, acoustically evoked activity of the tensor tympani has been demonstrated in some subjects under certain conditions (Stach et al, 1984).

The availability of commercial acoustic-immittance instruments beginning in the early 1960s gave rise to many clinical studies on various groups of patients with ear disease. Observations of acoustic-reflex adaptation (decay) (Anderson et al, 1970) provided another dimension for the clinical usefulness of the acoustic reflex.

Anatomy of the Human Middle Ear Muscles

The middle ear muscles are penniform; that is, they converge on a central tendon. Both the tensor tympani and the stapedius are almost entirely encased in bony canals. They are largely striated with some fat surrounding the muscle tissue.

The tensor tympani is 2 cm long and lies in a curved, bony channel, the semicanal, next to the eustachian tube. The muscle originates from the eustachian tube wall and the greater wing of the sphenoid bone. Its tendon emerges from the cochleariform process, a projection from the anterior-medial wall of the middle ear, and attaches to the neck of the malleus on its anterior and medial surface. Like the other muscles of the eustachian tube (tensor veli palatini, levator veli palatini, and salpingopharyngeus), the tensor tympani is innervated by the trigeminal nerve (cranial nerve V). Contraction of the tensor tympani medializes the manubrium of the malleus and the TM.

The stapedius muscle is the smallest muscle of the body and it inserts on the smallest bone of the body, the stapes. It lies just beneath and parallel to the medial wall of the fallopian canal, which houses the vertical segment of the facial nerve, lateral to the vestibule, and posterior to the middle ear. At its superior end it turns anteriorly and its tendon emerges from the bony canal through the pyramidal eminence. The tendon attaches to the stapes just medial to the capitulum on its posterior surface. The stapedial branch of the facial nerve (cranial nerve VII) arises just superior to the chorda tympani and exits through a foramen in the medial wall of the fallopian canal to innervate the stapedius muscle. Contraction of

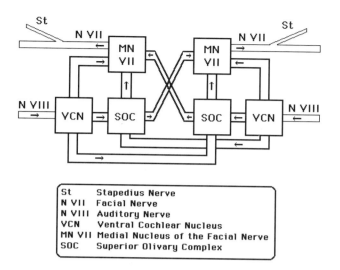

St	Stapedius Nerve
N VII	Facial Nerve
N VIII	Auditory Nerve
VCN	Ventral Cochlear Nucleus
MN VII	Medial Nucleus of the Facial Nerve
SOC	Superior Olivary Complex

Figure 17–25 Acoustic-stapedius reflex pathways.

the stapedius causes the stapes footplate to rock in the oval window, the anterior portion of the footplate being displaced laterally while the posterior portion is medialized. Occasionally, the stapedius muscle is malformed or absent, resulting in an absent acoustic reflex (Wright & Etholm, 1973).

The Acoustic-Stapedius Reflex Arc

Information on the acoustic-reflex pathways comes entirely from animal studies. The block diagram in Figure 17–25 is a representation of the acoustic-reflex pathways in rabbits suggested from the work of Borg (1973). The afferent portion of the reflex arc consists of the eighth cranial nerve fibers that synapse with dendrites in the ventral cochlear nucleus (VCN). Three separate reflex pathways emerge from the VCN: a projection to the ipsilateral superior olivary complex (SOC); a projection to the contralateral SOC; and a projection to the ipsilateral medial nucleus of the seventh cranial nerve (MN VII). The SOC sends projections to the ipsilateral and contralateral MN VII. The seventh cranial (facial) nerve contains the axons of the stapedius motoneurons that branch off of the main trunk to form the stapedial branch of the seventh nerve.

The neural network depicted in Figure 17–25 produces a bilateral contraction of the stapedius muscle to monaural stimulation. The contraction of the stapedius muscle in the ear that receives the eliciting stimulus is referred to as the ipsilateral reflex. The contraction in the opposite ear is the contralateral reflex.

Subsequent work has explained the organization of the pathway that Borg described, without substantially altering the representation in Figure 17–25. Several investigators found that the origin of the stapedius motor neurons is a region near, but not in, MN VII (Joseph et al, 1985). These motoneurons are organized into highly specialized groups that respond differentially to stimulus characteristics. For example, clusters of motoneurons have been identified that

respond exclusively to ipsilateral stimulation, others to contralateral stimulation, and still others to bilateral stimulation. Another group responds to both ipsilateral and contralateral stimulation and another may exist that is not acoustically activated.

The effect of stapedius contraction is a frequency-dependent attenuation of sound that is transmitted through the middle ear. The maximum attenuation produced by the contralateral reflex is about 10 dB at 600 Hz, decreases with increasing frequency, and reaches 0 dB at 2000 Hz (Rabinowitz, 1977). Experiments on cats suggest that attenuation may be substantially greater in the ear ipsilateral to the stimulus than in the contralateral ear (Guinan & McCue, 1987).

Characteristics of the Acoustic-Stapedius Reflex

Although several methods have been used for measurement of the acoustic-stapedius reflex, the most widely used method is measurement of the changes in the acoustic admittance of the ear caused by stapedius contraction. Figure 17–26 presents a series of ipsilateral reflex recordings from a normal-hearing subject. As the stimulus level decreases, the magnitude of the acoustic admittance change decreases monotonically until no response is observed. The lowest stimulus level that produces a change in acoustic admittance is the acoustic reflex *threshold*. In the example shown the reflex threshold is 80 dB HL. Several studies have shown that the threshold of both the ipsilateral and contralateral acoustic reflex for tonal stimuli is 80- to 85-dB HL for frequencies ranging from 500 to 4000 Hz. The acoustic-reflex threshold for broadband noise stimuli is 10- to 20-dB lower than for tonal stimuli. (See Wilson & Margolis, 1990, for a review.)

A decrease in the strength of stapedius contraction during continuous stimulation is referred to as acoustic-reflex adaptation or acoustic-reflex decay. In normal-hearing individuals adaptation is frequency dependent with the greatest adaptation occurring for high-frequency tones, less for low-frequency tones, and very little for broadband noise (Wilson et al, 1978).

A common method for quantifying acoustic-reflex adaptation is the *half-life*. The half-life is the time required for reflex magnitude to diminish to one half of its maximum value during a continuous stimulus. The most commonly used clinical method for measuring acoustic-reflex adaptation is to present the stimulus for 10 s and determine whether the half-life occurs in that interval. A half-life of ≤ 10 s at 500 or 1000 Hz is abnormal. At higher frequencies, the measure is less useful because of the presence of adaptation in normal subjects. Abnormal acoustic-reflex adaptation has been shown to be related to retrocochlear pathology (Anderson et al, 1970) and to pressure on the auditory nerve (Lusk et al, 1990a).

Clinical Applications of Acoustic-Stapedius Reflex Measurements

Acoustic-reflex measures are helpful in the differential diagnosis of ear disease. They can help to (a) confirm a questionable diagnosis of middle ear pathological conditions, (b)

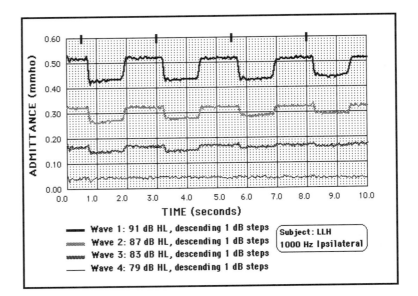

Figure 17–26 Ipsilateral acoustic reflex recordings from a normal adult ear.

TABLE 17–4 Typical ipsilateral (ipsi) and contralateral (contra) acoustic-reflex results in patients with unilateral ear disease

Site of Lesion/Ear	Ipsi/Right	Mode/Probe Ear Contra/Right	Ipsi/Left	Contra/Left
Middle ear/right	A	A	N	A
Middle ear/left	N	A	A	A
Cochlea/right	E, A	N	N	E, A
Cochlea/left	N	E, A	E, A	N
Eighth N/right	E, A, Ad	N	N	E, A, Ad
Eighth N/left	N	E, A, Ad	E, A, Ad	N
Seventh N/right*	A	A	N	N
Seventh N/left*	N	N	A	A
Brain stem/right	A	A	N	A
Brain stem/left	N	A	A	A
Brain stem/midline	N	A	N	A

N, Normal; *E*, elevated threshold; *A*, absent; *Ad*, abnormal adaptation.
* Proximal to the stapedial branch.

distinguish between cochlear and retrocochlear pathological conditions, (c) identify patients at risk for eighth nerve tumors and other retrocochlear pathological conditions, (d) identify the site of a facial nerve lesion, and (e) identify pseudohypacusis in patients with apparently severe hearing losses.

Acoustic-reflex findings in patients with various sites of disease are summarized in Table 17–4. The table presents typical ipsilateral and contralateral acoustic-reflex results for patients with unilateral disease. Bilateral disease would be characterized by the combination of results of unilateral disease on each side.

Middle Ear Disease

The acoustic reflex is usually absent in patients with middle ear disease. Two mechanisms produce this result. First, a conductive hearing loss in the stimulated ear reduces the effectiveness of the eliciting stimulus. Because the normal reflex threshold is 80- to 85-dB HL, a conductive loss as small as 20 dB may be sufficient to elevate the reflex threshold beyond the range of the acoustic-immittance measurement system. Second, the middle ear pathological condition may decrease the acoustic admittance of the ear to the extent that the effect of stapedial contraction cannot be detected. When the tympanogram is flat, for example, the stapedius is incapable of changing the middle ear admittance sufficiently to be detected by the measuring equipment. Patients with otosclerosis typically have normal tympanograms and absent acoustic reflexes. This is because the stapes fixation has little effect on the input impedance at the eardrum, but the stapedius contraction is not capable of altering the impedance of the ossicular chain.

Inner Ear Disease

The effects of cochlear hearing loss on acoustic-reflex thresholds is quite variable. In general, mild cochlear hearing loss has little effect on acoustic-reflex thresholds for tonal stimuli. As the hearing loss increases beyond about 40 dB, acoustic-reflex thresholds increase approximately linearly. For patients with hearing losses exceeding 70 dB, reflexes are typically absent. The effect of cochlear hearing loss on the acoustic-reflex threshold for broadband noise is different from tonal thresholds. Mild hearing losses cause significant elevations in the acoustic-reflex threshold for noise. The differential effect of hearing loss on tonal and noise thresholds reflects a reduction in the effect of stimulus bandwidth on acoustic-reflex threshold. The effects of cochlear hearing loss on acoustic-reflex thresholds has been exploited to provide a nonbehavioral screening test for sensorineural hearing loss. (See Popelka [1981] for a review.)

Disease of the Auditory Pathway

Many reports have documented the effects of tumors in the internal auditory canal and cerebellopontine angle (CPA) on acoustic reflex characteristics. Experimental evidence exists that pressure on the auditory nerve causes both a reduction in amplitude and an increased rate of adaptation (decay) of the stapedius response (Lusk et al, 1990b). Before the widespread availability of ABR and magnetic resonance imaging (MRI) techniques, acoustic reflex measures were among the most sensitive tests for eighth nerve pathological conditions. At present, ABR is thought to be the most sensitive physiological test for retrocochlear disease. Because most eighth nerve pathological conditions are space-occupying lesions of which vestibular schwannomas (acoustic neuromas) are the most common, imaging studies have long been used to detect these lesions. Gadolinium-enhanced MRI is thought to have a nearly perfect sensitivity to CPA tumors measuring 3 mm in diameter or greater. Although MRI is superior to all auditory tests for diagnosis of space-occupying lesions of the CPA, acoustic-reflex measurements are still useful in the audiological test battery for evaluation of the auditory pathway. Because of the expense of MRI, the acoustic reflex and other audiological tests can be useful for selecting patients to be referred for imaging studies.

Disease of the eighth cranial nerve has complex effects on the acoustic-stapedius reflex (see Table 17–4). Intracanalicular vestibular schwannomas may abolish the reflex or they may

---

> ### PEARL
>
> **Although gadolinium-enhanced MRI is the most accurate diagnostic test for CPA tumors, acoustic reflex, ABR, and other audiological tests can be helpful for selecting patients for referral for imaging studies.**

have more subtle effects. The acoustic-reflex threshold may be elevated or normal. An elevated acoustic-reflex threshold or absent reflex in the presence of normal-hearing or mild sensorineural hearing loss and a normal tympanogram suggests a retrocochlear pathological condition. Abnormal acoustic-reflex adaptation is also a strong indicator of retrocochlear disease. Reflex decay recordings from a patient with an eighth nerve tumor are shown in Figure 17–27.

Although acoustic-reflex measurements were shown to be sensitive to eighth nerve lesions before the advent of MRI, this needs to be re-evaluated now that tumors are routinely diagnosed at an earlier (and smaller) stage. It is generally true that any test for a space-occupying lesion is more sensitive to large masses than to small masses. So just how sensitive are acoustic reflex measures to small acoustic neuromas? This question was investigated in a recent study of patients with acoustic neuromas (Lynn et al, 1996). They separated their patients with acoustic neuroma into two groups—those with asymmetrical hearing loss and those with normal-hearing or symmetrical hearing loss. In general, the latter group had smaller tumors. Although this way of grouping patients does not separate them into nonoverlapping groups in terms of tumor size, it is a useful way to divide the subjects because those with asymmetrical hearing loss are likely to be tested by ABR or MRI. Those with normal-hearing or symmetrical hearing loss are more likely to be undiagnosed. A group of patients with normal-hearing who were seen for vestibular testing served as the control group. In patients with normal or symmetrical hearing loss with vestibular schwannomas, 66% had abnormal reflexes (defined as elevated thresholds, abnormal reflex decay, or absent responses). Only 4% of normal-hearing patients seen for vestibular evaluation had abnormal reflexes. Other studies have also reported a high prevalence of abnormal reflexes in normal-hearing patients with eighth nerve tumors (Morrison & Sterkers, 1996; Prasher & Cohen, 1993; Valente et al, 1995). These studies suggest that abnormal reflexes in the absence of asymmetrical hearing loss should be considered a risk factor for eighth nerve disease with appropriate follow-up testing, either ABR or MRI.

Another recent study evaluated both safety and test efficiency for 1000-Hz ipsilateral acoustic reflexes. Hunter et al (In press) studied receiver-operator characteristics (ROC) for the ipsilateral acoustic reflex and interaural pure tone threshold difference for detection of acoustic neuroma. The acoustic neuroma group consisted of 56 patients. The control group consisted of 108 patients without acoustic neuroma who are representative of the general clinical population of the Fairview University Medical Center Audiology Clinic. These patients had audiograms ranging from normal-hearing to profound hearing loss that was either cochlear or mixed.

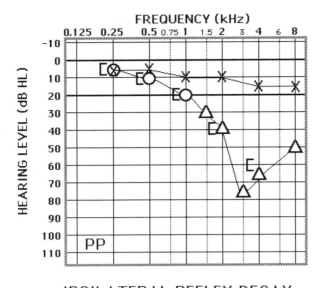

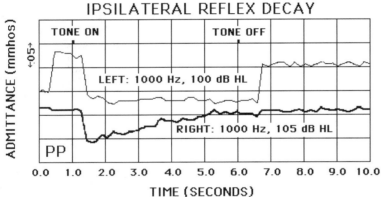

Figure 17–27 Audiogram and acoustic-reflex decay recordings from a patient with a right vestibular schwannoma (acoustic neuroma).

Presence or absence of acoustic neuroma was confirmed by MRI, usually with gadolinium contrast. Acoustic-reflex sensitivity and specificity was evaluated for all subjects and also for various groups subdivided on the basis of degree of hearing loss and type of hearing loss. Receiver-operator analyses showed that acoustic-reflex thresholds at 1000 Hz did not perform well at any criterion used (cutoff for abnormal set between 85 dB HL and 105 dB HL). For all ears with sensorineural hearing loss, the hit rate using the optimal criterion (>95 dB HL) was only 54%, and the false alarm rate was 32%. Exclusion of ears with hearing loss >50 dB HL improved the hit rate slightly to 62%, but the false alarm rate was still high (34%). The presence of a conductive component tended to increase the false alarm rate with no effect on the hit rate. The pure tone threshold difference between ears (averaged at 1.0, 2.0, 4.0, and 8.0 kHz) was also evaluated. When all hearing loss degrees and types were included, the highest hit rate (86%) and lowest false alarm rate (23%) was obtained with a 15 dB criterion. The ROC curve analysis clearly showed that the pure tone threshold difference performs better than the ipsilateral acoustic-reflex threshold, at least at 1000 Hz.

Taken together, the results of the Lynn et al study and the Hunter et al study suggest that acoustic-reflex threshold measures probably do not contribute significantly to the identification of acoustic neuromas when asymmetrical hearing loss exists. The 86% hit rate for hearing loss asymmetry would

probably be judged sufficiently high to justify an MRI evaluation in most centers. However, when normal-hearing or symmetrical hearing loss exists, unilaterally abnormal acoustic reflexes should raise a concern about the possibility of an acoustic neuroma. MRI evaluation in these cases can lead to the detection of acoustic neuromas that would not be identified on the basis of the audiogram.

Safety of the acoustic-reflex threshold and decay tests was also addressed in the Hunter et al study. Several cases of permanent threshold shift after reflex decay testing at levels exceeding 115 dB SPL have been reported in the literature. On the basis of safety and test performance considerations, a maximum stimulus level of 115 dB SPL is recommended. Converting to hearing level and allowing for intersubject variation in earcanal sound pressure, a maximum of 105 dB HL would be prudent. When reflex thresholds are above this level, no added diagnostic benefit exists to determining the reflex threshold. Because it is the patients with symmetrical or normal-hearing for whom acoustic-reflex testing is most useful, this restriction on stimulus level would not limit the value of reflex testing.

Brain stem lesions may abolish the reflex without affecting the pure tone audiogram (Griesen & Rasmussen, 1970) or they may differentially affect the contralateral and ipsilateral responses. Cases have been reported in which ipsilateral reflexes are normal while contralateral reflexes are abnormal

(Jerger & Jerger, 1977; Wilson & Margolis, 1990), presumably because of a midline lesion of the brain stem, affecting only the decussating reflex pathways.

Pseudohypoacusis

For mild and moderate hearing losses, acoustic reflexes elicited by tonal stimuli are usually within normal limits (Popelka, 1981). In those cases the presence of a reflex does not help to evaluate the validity of the pure tone audiogram (Gelfand, 1994). However, in severe losses the presence of a reflex may indicate that the hearing loss is not as great as the audiogram suggests. The presence of a reflex in those cases may indicate pseudohypoacusis. A case is presented later in this chapter that illustrates the usefulness of acoustic reflex measures in a patient with an apparently severe hearing loss that may have been of hysterical origin. Another case was described in a previous chapter on this topic (Margolis & Levine, 1991).

CASE STUDIES

Recurrent Otitis Media

SR is a 10-year-old boy who has been followed since early childhood. He had frequent episodes of otitis media in his first 2 years and had bilateral myringotomy with tympanostomy tubes at age 2 and again at age 3. After the second surgery, he responded well and his hearing was normal. At ages 6 and 7 he had several episodes of acute otitis media, which were treated with antibiotics. Although his 226-Hz tympanograms returned to normal, the hearing in the left ear continued to show a mid-frequency conductive hearing loss, which has persisted to age 10. At his 10-year study visit the audiogram (Fig. 17–28) showed a 35 dB conductive loss on the left in the mid-frequencies (0.5 to 2.0 kHz). The eardrum on the left was retracted and showed areas of atrophy

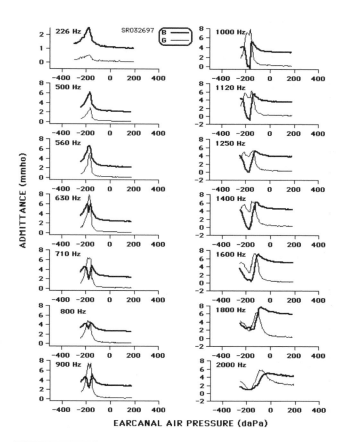

Figure 17–29 Multifrequency tympanograms for the left ear of patient SR with recurrent otitis media. The patterns are 1B1G for frequencies ≤ 560 Hz, 3B1G at 630 Hz, and 3B3G at frequencies above 630 Hz.

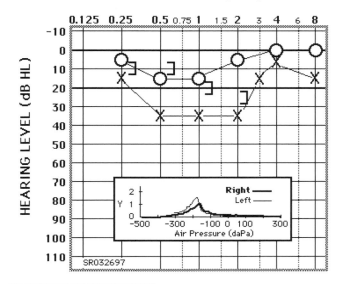

Figure 17–28 Audiogram and 226-Hz tympanograms from patient SR with recurrent otitis media.

and fibrosis, but there was no evidence of inflammation or effusion.

The 226-Hz tympanograms for the left ear, shown in Figure 17–28, showed negative tympanometric peak pressure (−170 daPa), indicating negative middle ear pressure and high static admittance, probably caused by the atrophic areas on the eardrum. Multifrequency tympanograms (Fig. 17–29) were characterized by regular, Vanhuyse patterns, shifted toward negative pressure. The resonant frequency was low-normal (710 Hz) with 3B3G and 5B3G patterns occurring at unusually low frequencies (900 and 1000 Hz, respectively). Above 1000 Hz, the patterns were 3B3G.

Wideband reflectance is shown in Figure 17–30. The measurements were made with the earcanal air pressure set to compensate for the middle ear pressure (i.e., at tympanometric peak pressure). Two frequency regions exist in which reflectance is abnormal. Below 1500 Hz, reflectance is abnormally high. Below 1200 Hz reflectance is nearly 1.0, indicating that almost all the energy is reflected. This region of abnormality corresponds roughly to the region of hearing loss. Between 5 and 8 kHz, reflectance is abnormally low, indicating more than the normal sound absorption, perhaps because of the atrophic eardrum.

Reflectance tympanograms are shown in Figure 17–31. The patterns appear to be quite disorganized compared with

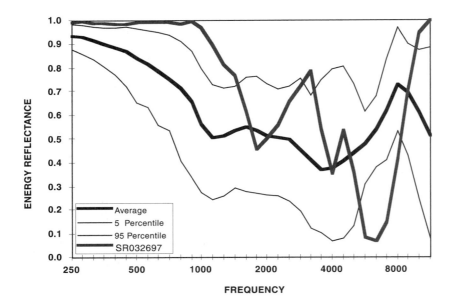

Figure 17–30 Wideband reflectance for patient SR with recurrent otitis media and conductive hearing loss. The mean, 5th, and 95th percentiles are shown for 20 normal adult subjects. The patient has a region of abnormal reflectance from 250 to 1500 Hz and a region of abnormally low reflectance from about 5 to 7 kHz.

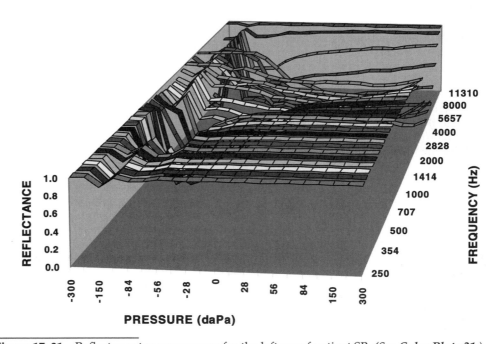

Figure 17–31 Reflectance tympanograms for the left ear of patient SR. *(See Color Plate 21.)*

normal subject data in Figure 17–24. In this case reflectance tympanograms seem to more clearly identify the middle ear pathological condition than either the 226-Hz tympanograms or multifrequency tympanograms. The data shown in tympanogram format (Fig. 17–31) appear more clearly abnormal than the same data displayed as reflectance plotted against frequency (Fig. 17–30).

This case illustrates the complex relationship between acoustic admittance as measured by multifrequency tympanometry and energy reflectance. Multifrequency tympanograms indicate a high admittance system that has reduced stiffness, resulting in a low resonant frequency and the occurrence of 3B3G and 5B3G patterns at relatively low

frequencies. The reflectance results, however, indicate an abnormally high reflectance at frequencies roughly corresponding to the frequency range of the hearing loss (Fig. 17–30) and a rather disorganized response to earcanal air pressure (Fig. 17–31).

The hearing loss is greater than expected from the otoscopic features of retraction, atrophy, and fibrosis. Many ears with those pathological conditions have normal-hearing. It is likely that middle ear adhesions have been formed as a result of recurrent otitis media. (See Margolis et al [1998] for an example.) The multifrequency tympanograms show the expected effects of the atrophic eardrum. The correspondence of the frequency region of high reflectance and the hearing loss suggests that reflectance may be a useful diagnostic indicator for this type of pathological condition. More cases like this are required to determine the relative value of multifrequency tympanometry and wideband reflectance for detecting middle ear pathological conditions.

Cholesteatoma

SP had bilateral myringotomy and tubes when he was 18 months old. On the preoperative examination, the right ear was thick and immobile and the left ear had a retraction pocket. No fluid was present at the time of surgery. At the 7-year study visit, video-otomicroscopy indicated two areas of crusted debris on the right eardrum (Fig. 17–32). The otologist

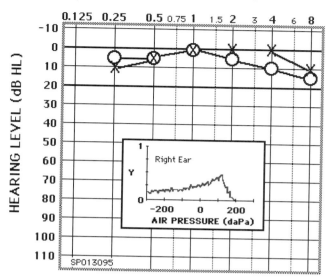

Figure 17–33 Audiogram and 226-Hz tympanogram *(right ear)* for patient SP with a cholesteatoma originating from the TM and invading the middle ear.

attempted to remove them by suction without success. Two weeks later the patient underwent exploratory surgery of the right ear and a cholesteatoma, adherent to one of the areas of debris on the eardrum, was removed from the middle ear.

The audiogram indicated normal-hearing (Fig. 17–33). The 226-Hz tympanogram (Fig. 17–33 *inset*) had a distinct peak with static admittance in the normal range, although the morphology was unusual. Multifrequency tympanograms were clearly abnormal at every frequency (Fig. 17–34).

The case illustrates the superiority of multifrequency tympanometry over 226-Hz tympanometry for detecting some middle ear pathological conditions. Although the 226-Hz tympanogram was a bit odd, the static admittance was normal, and it probably would be categorized as a type A with positive pressure. Multifrequency tympanograms were unambiguous in suggesting abnormal middle ear function.

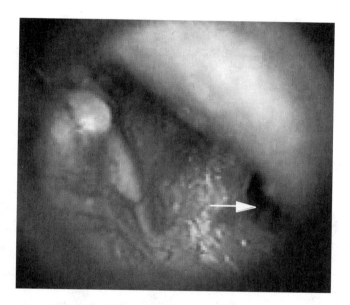

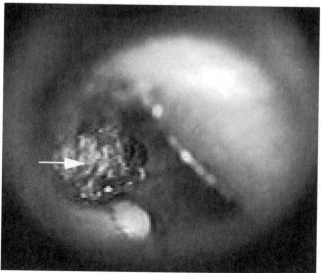

Figure 17–32 Otomicroscopic image of the right TM of patient SP. The image shows two areas of squamous debris, one on pars tensa and one on pars flaccida. A cholesteatoma in the middle ear originated from the squamous debris on pars tensa. *(See Color Plate 22.)*

PEARL

Multifrequency tympanometry detects middle ear pathological conditions in some patients with normal 226-Hz tympanograms.

Chronic Otitis Media

JT was 10 months old when he had his first surgery and had a second set of tubes inserted at age 27 months. After each surgery, he responded well but then developed recurrent episodes of otitis media. After the second surgery, the tube in the right ear extruded within the first postoperative month. Otitis media developed in that ear by the fifth postoperative month and frequent episodes occurred over the next 22 months. On subsequent examinations, the right eardrum

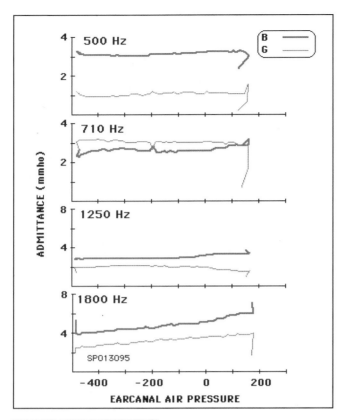

Figure 17–34 Multifrequency tympanograms from patient SP with a cholesteatoma. At approximately 200 daPa the values went out of range of the measurement instrument.

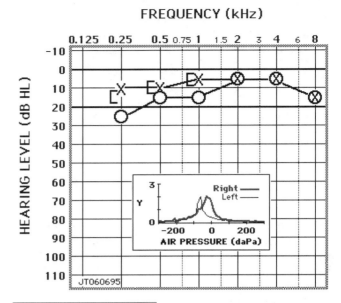

Figure 17–35 Audiogram and 226-Hz tympanograms from patient JT with chronic otitis media.

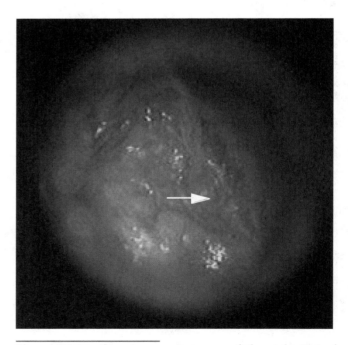

Figure 17–36 Otomicroscopic image of the right TM of patient JT. Identifiable landmarks were completely absent. A deep retraction pocket was present anteriorly and a tympanosclerotic region was present in the anterosuperior region. Most of the drum was retracted against the promontory of the middle ear and was immobile on pneumatic stimulation. Only a small portion of the drum was mobile. (*See Color Plate 23.*)

appeared progressively retracted without active disease. At his 7-year study visit he had normal-hearing and no indication of recent symptoms. His audiogram and 226-Hz tympanograms were normal (Fig. 17–35).

The otomicroscopic examination showed a complete absence of identifiable landmarks on the right eardrum (Fig. 17–36). A deep retraction pocket was present anteriorly and a tympanosclerotic region was present in the anterosuperior region. Most of the drum was retracted against the promontory of the middle ear and was immobile on pneumatic stimulation. Only a small portion of the drum was mobile (identified by the arrow in Fig. 17–36).

Multifrequency tympanograms (Fig. 17–37) show an abnormally low resonant frequency (500 Hz) and broad, flat patterns at high frequencies. 3B3G patterns occur at abnormally low frequencies (≥560 Hz).

Considering the severity of the pathological condition, it is surprising that abnormalities did not appear on the audiogram and 226-Hz tympanograms. The normal-hearing and 226-Hz tympanogram are particularly unexpected. Only the multifrequency tympanograms indicated the presence of middle ear pathological conditions. This type of middle ear pathological condition frequently leads to chronic sequelae like atelectasis, cholesteatoma, ossicular erosion, and con-

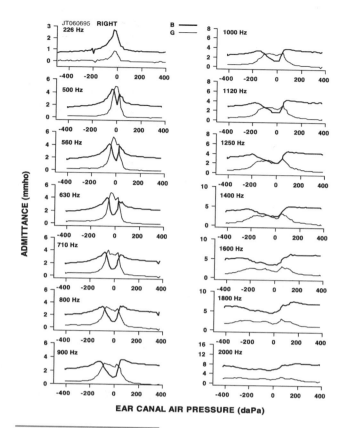

Figure 17–37 Multifrequency tympanograms from patient JT with chronic otitis media. The 226-Hz tympanograms are normal. At 500 Hz the pattern is 1B1G and the susceptance notch reaches the positive tail, indicating resonance at that frequency. The 3B3G pattern occurs at an abnormally low-frequency (560 Hz) and the high-frequency patterns are abnormally flattened.

ductive hearing loss. It is important to identify this condition and make the appropriate referral for otologic management. In this case audiometry and single-frequency tympanometry did not reveal the middle ear pathology.

Patulous Eustachian Tube

LF is a 29-year-old woman with severe progressive scleroderma, a degenerative disease that causes atrophy of the epidermis and other organ involvement. Her body weight was about 80 lb at the time of the evaluation, but there was no significant recent weight loss. She had essentially normal-hearing, although she had consistently shown small air-bone gaps bilaterally (see Fig. 17–38 *inset*); 226-Hz and multifrequency tympanograms were normal, and otoscopic evidence of middle ear disease was absent.

The patient complained of the sound of her own voice, which she described as "Darth Vader," and the sound of her breathing, a symptom referred to as *autophony*. She found this to be very annoying and sought an ENT evaluation and treatment for the condition.

Figure 17–38 shows recordings made with a clinical acoustic immittance instrument in the acoustic-reflex mode. The reflex eliciting stimulus was set to 40 dB HL (the minimum allowed by the instrument) to prevent acoustic-reflex activation. Recordings were made during normal breathing, deep breathing, and holding the breath. Recordings are shown for the left ear of patient LF and for a normal subject.

In the normal breathing and deep breathing conditions the patient had a distinct vascular pulse on the recording. This is not unusual, but when it occurs (especially unilaterally) the patient should be evaluated for middle ear abnormalities such as glomus tumors. Vascular pulses can be identified by their rate, which coincides with the pulse rate (usually about 1/s). In the deep breathing condition large pulsations are seen with a much slower rate than the vascular pulse. These correspond to the breathing cycle. In this case they are about 2 seconds apart. The recordings made from a normal subject, shown at the bottom of Figure 17–38, are distinctly different with no breathing-related admittance change. The apparently large changes in admittance are caused by transmission of pressure (either sound pressure or static air pressure) from the nasopharynx to the middle ear through the patent eustachian tube.

The patient was counseled by the otolaryngologist on the limited success of surgical treatment for patulous eustachian tube. As O'Connor and Shea (1981) pointed out, many patients are able to tolerate the symptoms when they have been counseled on the cause and the limited success of surgical procedures. This patient has not opted for surgery.

Pseudohypoacusis

LW is a 29-year-old woman who had a history of hearing loss since childhood. Attempts to obtain medical and school history information were not successful because the patient could not provide the names of previous physicians or schools. Her speech had a distinct "deaf" quality, and she appeared to communicate by speechreading. Her husband accompanied her to visits with the health professional and served as an oral interpreter. She had no response at audiometric limits to pure tones. The absence of vibrotactile responses and the presence of acoustic reflexes (see Fig. 17–39) led to a suspicion of pseudohypoacusis. Otoacoustic emissions and ABRs were normal. When it was explained to her that these results indicate normal function of the cochlea and auditory pathways, she responded tearfully, "Then why can't I hear?" The patient was referred to a psychologist for counseling. After a period of counseling, a repeat audiogram indicated responses in one ear in the 100- to 110-dB range at 500 to 8000 Hz, an improvement over previous audiograms. The patient will be followed to determine whether the apparent hearing improvement continues. It is possible that this patient has a true hysterical deafness. This case illustrates that acoustic-reflex measures can provide a warning of the possibility of pseudohypoacusis.

ACKNOWLEDGMENT

This work was supported by grant no. P50 DC03093 from the NIH National Institute of Deafness and Other Communication Disorders. Portions of this chapter were published previously in Margolis and Hunter (1999), and are used by permission of the publisher.

PEARL

Acoustic-reflex measures can provide a warning of the possibility of pseudohypoacusis.

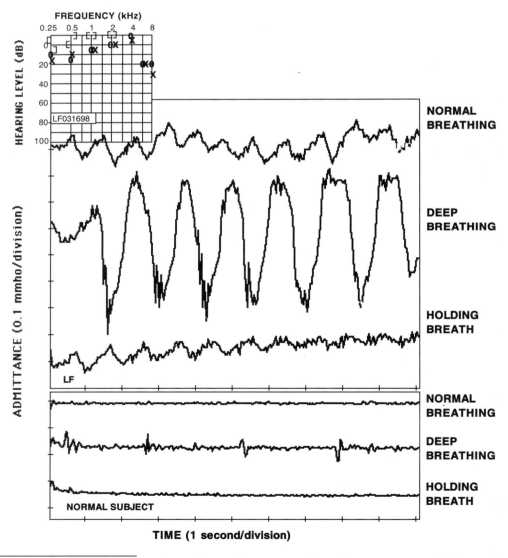

Figure 17–38 Audiogram and eustachian tube test recordings from a patient with bilaterally patulous eustachian tubes.

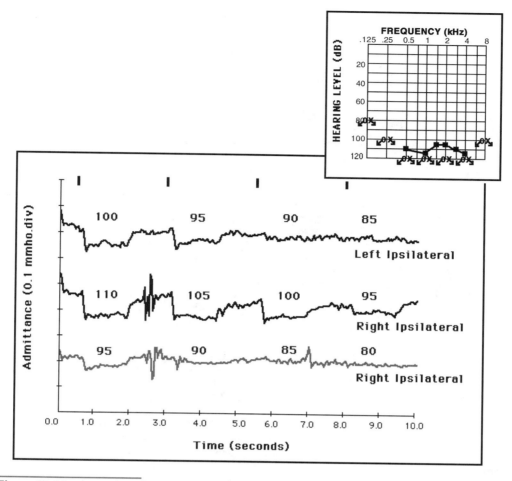

Figure 17–39 Acoustic-reflex recordings from patient LW showing normal ipsilateral responses bilaterally. The audiogram showed no response on the first two visits. After a period of psychological counseling, the patient responded at high levels *(squares)*.

REFERENCES

ALBERTI, P.W., & JERGER, J.F. (1974). Probetone frequency and the diagnostic value of tympanometry. *Archives of Otolaryngology, 99,*206–10.

AMERICAN ACADEMY OF AUDIOLOGY. (1997a). Identification of hearing loss and middle ear dysfunction in children. *Audiology Today, 9*(3),18–20.

AMERICAN ACADEMY OF AUDIOLOGY. (1997b). Identification of hearing loss and middle-ear dysfunction in preschool and school-age children. *Audiology Today, 9*(3),21–23.

AMERICAN NATIONAL STANDARDS INSTITUTE. (1987). American National Standard Specifications for instruments to measure aural acoustic impedance and admittance (ANSI S3.39-1987). New York: American National Standards Institute.

AMERICAN NATIONAL STANDARDS INSTITUTE. (1996). American National Standard Specification for Audiometers (ANSI S3.6-1989). New York: American National Standards Institute.

AMERICAN SPEECH-LANGUAGE-HEARING ASSOCIATION. (1979). Guidelines for acoustic immittance screening for middle-ear function. *ASHA, 21,* 283–8.

AMERICAN SPEECH-LANGUAGE-HEARING ASSOCIATION. (1990). Guidelines for screening for hearing impairment and middle-ear disorders. *ASHA, 32*(Suppl. 2),17–24.

ANDERSON, H., BARR, B., & WEDENBERG, E. (1970). Early diagnosis of VIIIth-nerve tumours. *Acta Otolaryngologica (Stockholm), 262,*232–237.

BALKANY, T.J., BERMAN, S.A., SIMMONS, M.A., & JAFEK, B.W. (1978). Middle ear effusion in neonates. *Laryngoscope, 88,*398–405.

BENNETT, M. (1975). Acoustic impedance bridge measurements with the neonate. *British Journal of Audiology*, 9,117–124.

BLUESTONE, C.D., BEERY, Q.C., & PARADISE, J.L. (1973). Audiometry and tympanometry in relation to middle ear effusions in children. *Laryngoscope, 83*,594–604.

BLUESTONE, C.D., FRIA, T.J., ARJONA, S.K., CASSELBRANT, M.L., SCHWARTZ, D.M., RUBEN, R.J., GATES, G.A., DOWNS, M.P., NORTHERN, J.L., JERGER, J.F., et al. (1986). Controversies in screening for middle ear disease and hearing loss in children. *Pediatrics, 77*(1),57–70.

BORG, E. (1973). On the neuronal organization of the acoustic middle ear reflex. A physiological and anatomical study. *Brain Research, 49*,101–123.

BROOKS, D.N. (1968). An objective method of determining fluid in the middle ear. *International Journal of Audiology, 7*, 280–286.

CANTEKIN, E.I., BLUESTONE, C.D., FRIA, T J., STOOL, S.E., BEERY, Q.C., & SABO, D.L. (1980a). Identification of otitis media with effusion in children. *Annals of Otology, Rhinology, and Laryngology, 89*(Suppl. 68),190–195.

CANTEKIN, E.I., DOYLE, W.J., PHILLIPS, D.C., & BLUESTONE, C.D. (1980b). Gas absorption in the middle ear. *Annals of Otology, Rhinology, and Laryngology, 89*(Suppl. 68),71–75.

COLLETTI, V. (1976). Tympanometry from 200 to 2000 Hz probe tone. *Audiology, 15*,106–119.

DALY, K.A., L.L., H., LEVINE, S.C., LINDGREN, B. R., & GIEBINK, G. S. (1997). Sequelae of otitis media from childhood through young adulthood. In *Abstracts of the Midwinter Meeting of the Association for Research in Otolaryngology*. St. Petersburg Beach, FL.

DE JONGE, R. R. (1986). Normal tympanometric gradient: A comparison of three methods. *Audiology, 25*,299–308.

DIAMANT, M., RUBENSOHN, G., & WALANDER, A. (1958). Otosalpingitis and mastoid pneumatization. *Acta Otolaryngologica, 49*,381–388.

EAVEY, R.D. (1993). Abnormalities of the neonatal ear: Otoscopic observations, histologic observations, and a model for contamination of the middle ear by cellular contents of amniotic fluid. *Laryngoscope, 103*(Suppl. 58),1–31.

ELNER, A., INGELSTEDT, S., & IVARSSON, A. (1971). The elastic properties of the tympanic membrane. *Acta Otolaryngologica, 72*,397–403.

FALK, B. (1981). Negative pressure induced by sniffing, a tympanometric study in healthy ears. *Journal of Otolaryngology, 10*,299–305.

FALK, B. (1983). Variability in the tympanogram due to eustachian tube closing failure. *Scandinavian Audiology, (Suppl. 17)*,11–17.

FELDMAN, A.S. (1976). Tympanometry—Procedures, interpretations, and variables. In: A.S. Feldman, & L.A. Wilber (Eds.), *Acoustic impedance and admittance—The measurement of middle ear function.* (pp. 103–155). Baltimore, MD: Williams & Wilkins.

FIELLAU-NIKOLAJSEN, M. (1983). Tympanometry and secretory otitis media. Observations on diagnosis, epidemiology, treatment, and prevention in prospective cohort studies of three-year-old children. *Acta Otolaryngolica, (Suppl. 394)*,1–73.

GATES, G. A., AVERY, C., COOPER, J. C., HEARNE, E. M., & HOLT, G.R. (1986a). Predictive value of tympanometry in middle ear effusion. *Annals of Otology, Rhinology, and Laryngology, 95*,46–50.

GELFAND, S.A. (1994). Acoustic reflex threshold tenth percentiles and functional hearing impairment. *Journal of the American Academy of Audiology, 5*,10–16.

GOODE, R.L., KILLION, M., NAKAMURA, K., & NISHIHARA, S. (1994). New knowledge about the function of the human middle ear: development of an improved analog model. *American Journal of Otology, 15*,145–154.

GRIESEN, O., & RASMUSSEN, P.E. (1970). Stapedius muscle reflexes and otoneurological examinations in brainstem tumors. *Acta Otolaryngologica (Stockholm), 70*,366–370.

GUINAN, J.J., & MCCUE, M.P. (1987). Asymmetries in the acoustic reflexes of the cat stapedius muscle. *Hearing Research, 26*,1–10.

HALLPIKE, C.S. (1935). On the function of the tympanic muscles. *Journal of Laryngology and Otology, 50*,362–366.

HANKS, W.D., & ROSE, K.J. (1993).2 Middle ear resonance and acoustic immittance measures in children. *Journal of Speech and Hearing Research, 36*(1),218–21.

HAUGHTON, P. M. (1977). Validity of tympanometry for middle ear effusions. *Archives of Otorhinolaryngology, 103*,505–513.

HENRY, D.F., & DIBARTOLOMEO, J.R. (1993). Patulous eustachian tube identification using tympanometry. *Journal of the American Academy of Audiology, 4*,53–57.

HENSEN, V. (1878). Beobachtungen uber die Trommelfell-spanners bei hund und katze. *Archiv fur Anatomie und Physiologie (physiologische Abtheilung), 2*,312.

HERGILS, L., & MAGNUSON, B. (1985). Morning pressure in the middle ear. *Archives of Otolaryngology, 111*,86–89.

HERGILS, L., & MAGNUSON, B. (1987). Middle-ear pressure under basal conditions. *Archives of Otolaryngology–Head and Neck Surgery, 113*,829–832.

HILDING, A.C. (1944). Role of ciliary action in production of pulmonary atelectasis, vacuum in paranasal sinuses, and in otitis media. *Transactions of the American Academy of Ophthalmology and Otolaryngology*, 367–378.

HIMELFARB, M.Z., POPELKA, G.R., & SHANON, E. (1979). Tympanometry in normal neonates. *Journal of Speech and Hearing Research, 22*,179–191.

HOLTE, L.A., CAVANAGH, R.M., & MARGOLIS, R. H. (1990). Earcanal wall mobility and tympanometric shape in young infants. *Journal of Pediatrics, 117*,77–80.

HOLTE, L.A., & MARGOLIS, R.H. (1987). Screening tympanometry. *Seminars in Hearing, 8*,329–338.

HOLTE, L.A., MARGOLIS, R.H., & CAVANAUGH, R.M. (1991). Developmental changes in multifrequency tympanograms. *Audiology, 30*,1–24.

HSU, G.S., MARGOLIS, R.H., SCHACHERN, P.L., SUTHERLAND, C., & JAVEL, E. (1996). The development of hearing and middle ear function in neonatal chinchillas. In *Abstracts of the Midwinter Meeting of the Association for Research in Otolaryngology*. St. Petersburg Beach, FL.

HUNTER, L.L., & MARGOLIS, R.H. (1992). Multifrequency tympanometry: Current clinical application. *American Journal of Audiology, 1*,33–43.

HUNTER, L.L., MARGOLIS, R.H., DALY, K.A., & GIEBINK, G.S. (1992). Relationship of tympanometric estimates of middle ear volume to middle ear status at surgery. In *Abstracts of the Midwinter Research Meeting of the Association for Research in Otolaryngology*. St. Petersburg Beach, FL.

HUNTER, L.L., RIES, D., SCHLAUCH, R.S., LEVINE, S.C., & WARD, W.D. (In press). Safety and clinical performance of acoustic reflex tests. *Ear and Hearing.*

IVEY, R. (1975). Tympanometric curves and otosclerosis. *Journal of Speech and Hearing Research, 18,*554–558.

JEPSON, O. (1995). *Studies on the acoustic stapedius reflex in man. Measurements of the acoustic impedance of the tympanic membrane in normal individuals and in patients with peripheral facial palsy.* Unpublished doctoral thesis. University of Aarhus, Denmark.

JERGER, J. (1970). Clinical experience with impedance audiometry. *Archives of Otolaryngology, 92,*311–324.

JERGER, J., & JERGER, S.J. (1977). Diagnostic value of crossed vs uncrossed acoustic reflexes. *Archives of Otolaryngology, 103,* 445–453.

JERGER, J., JERGER, S., MAUDLIN, L., & SEGAL, P. (1974). Studies in impedance audiometry: II. Children less than six years old. *Archives of Otolaryngology, 99,*1–9.

JOSEPH, M.P., GUINAN, J.J., FULLERTON, B.C., NORRIS, B.E., & KIANG, N.Y.S. (1985). Number and distribution of stapedius motoneurons in cats. *Journal of Comparative Neurology, 232,*43–54.

KATO, T. (1913). Zur physiologie der binnenmuskeln des ohres. *Pfluegers Archiv fur die gesamte physiologie des menschen und der tiere, 150,*569.

KEEFE, D.H., BULEN, J.C., AREHART, K.H., & BURNS, E.M. (1993). Earcanal impedance and reflection coefficient in human infants and adults. *Journal of the Acoustical Society of America, 94*(5),2617–2638.

KEEFE, D.H., & LEVI, E. (1996). Maturation of the middle and external ears: Acoustic power-based responses and reflectance tympanometry. *Ear and Hearing, 17,*361–373.

KEITH, R.W. (1973). Impedance audiometry with neonates. *Archives of Otolaryngology, 97,*465–476.

KEITH, R.W. (1975). Middle ear function in neonates. *Archives of Otolaryngology, 101,*376–379.

KOBRAK, H.G. (1948). Present status of objective hearing tests. *Annals of Otology, Rhinology, and Laryngology, 57,*1018–1026.

KOEBSELL, K.A., & MARGOLIS, R. H. (1986). Tympanometric gradient measured from normal preschool children. *Audiology, 25,*149–157.

KRINGLEBOTN, M. (1988). Network model for the human middle ear. *Scandinavian Audiology, 17,*75–85.

LE, C.T., DALY, K.A., MARGOLIS, R.H., LINDGREN, B.R., & GIEBINK, G.S. (1992). A clinical profile of otitis media. *Archhives of Otolaryngology–Head and Neck Surgery, 118,* 1225–1228.

LE, C.T., HUNTER, L.L., MARGOLIS, R.H., DALY, K.A., LINDGREN, B.R., & GIEBINK, G.S. (1994). A clinical profile of otitis media without an intact tympanic membrane. *Archives of Otolaryngology–Head and Neck Surgery, 120,*513–516.

LIDEN, G. (1969). The scope and application of current audiometric tests. *Journal of Laryngology and Otology, 83,*507–520.

LIDEN, G., BJORKMAN, G., NYMAN, H., & KUNOV, H. (1977). Tympanometry and acoustic impedance. *Acta Otolaryngologica, 83,*140–145.

LIDEN, G., HARFORD, E., & HALLEN, O. (1974b). Automatic tympanometry in clinical practice. *Audiology, 13,*126–39.

LIDEN, G., HARFORD, E., & HALLEN, O. (1974a). Tympanometry for the diagnosis of ossicular disruption. *Archives of Otolaryngology, 99,*23–9.

LIDEN, G., PETERSON, J., & BJORKMAN, G. (1970). Tympanometry. *Archives of Otolaryngology, 92,*248–57.

LINDEMAN, P., & HOLMQUIST, J. (1982). Volume measurement of middle ear and mastoid air cell system with impedance audiometry on patients with eardrum perforations. *Acta Otolaryngologica, 386(Suppl.),*70–73.

LUSCHER, E. (1929). Die funktion des musculus stapedius bein menschen. *Z Hals-Nasen-Ohrenheilkunde, 23,*105–132.

LUSK, R.P., LILLY, D.J., & LENTH, R.V. (1990a). Pressure-induced modifications of the acoustic nerve. Part I. The acoustic reflex. *American Journal of Otolaryngology, 11,*398–406.

LUSK, R.P., LILLY, D.J., & LENTH, R.V. (1990b). Pressure-induced modifications of the acoustic nerve. Part I. The acoustic reflex. *American Journal of Otolaryngology, 11,*398–406.

LYNN, S., FABRY, D., & HARNER, S. (1996). *Acoustic reflex remains sensitive in normal-hearing acoustic neuroma patients.* Presentation to the Annual Convention of the American Academy of Audiology, Salt Lake City, UT.

MAGNUSON, B. (1981). On the origin of the high negative pressure in the middle ear space. *American Journal of Otolaryngology, 2,*1–12.

MAGNUSON, B. (1983). Eustachian tube pathophysiology. *American Journal of Otolaryngology, 4,*123–130.

MARCHANT, C.D., MCMILLAN, P M., SHURIN, P.A., JOHNSON, C.E., TURCZYK, V.A., FEINSTEIN, J.C., & PANEK, D.M. (1986). Objective diagnosis of otitis media in early infancy by tympanometry and ipsilateral acoustic reflex thresholds. *Journal of Pediatrics, 109*(4),590–595.

MARGOLIS, R.H., (1981). Fundamentals of acoustic immitance. In: G.R. Popelka (Ed.), *Hearing assessment with the acoustic reflex* (pp. 117–144). New York: Grune & Stratton.

MARGOLIS, R.H., & GOYCOOLEA, H.G. (1993). Multifrequency tympanometry in normal adults. *Ear and Hearing, 14,* 408–413.

MARGOLIS, R.H., & HELLER, J.W. (1987). Screening tympanometry: Criteria for medical referral. *Audiology, 26,*197–208.

MARGOLIS, R.H., & HUNTER, L.L. (1999). Tympanometry: Basic principles and clinical applications. In: W.F. Rintelmann, & F. Musiek (Eds.), *Contemporary perspectives on hearing assessment* (pp. 89–130). Boston, MA: Allyn & Bacon.

MARGOLIS, R.H., & LEVINE, S.C. (1991). Acoustic reflex measures in audiologic evaluation. *Otolaryngology Clinics of North America, 24,*329–347.

MARGOLIS, R.H., & NELSON, D.A. (1992). Acute otitis media with transient sensorineural hearing loss: A case study. *Archives of Otolaryngology–Head and Neck Surgery, 119,*682–686.

MARGOLIS, R.H., OSGUTHORPE, J.D., & POPELKA, G.R. (1978). The effects of experimentally-produced middle ear lesions on tympanometry in cats. *Acta Otolaryngologica, 86,*428–436.

MARGOLIS, R.H., & POPELKA, G.R. (1977). Interactions among tympanometric variables. *Journal of Speech and Hearing Research, 20,*4474–62.

MARGOLIS, R.H., SALY, G.L., & KEEFE, D.H. (1999). Wideband reflectance tympanometry in normal adults. *Journal of the Acoustical Society of America, 106,*265–280.

MARGOLIS, R.H., SCHACHERN, P.L., & FULTON, S. (1998). Multifrequency tympanometry and histopathology in chinchillas with experimentally-produced middle-ear pathologies. *Acta Otolaryngologica, 118,*216–225.

MARGOLIS, R.H., & SMITH, P. (1977). Tympanometric asymmetry. *Journal of Speech and Hearing Research, 20,*437–446.

Margolis, R.H., Van Camp, K.J., Wilson, R.H., & Creten, W.L. (1985). Multifrequency tympanometry in normal ears. *Audiology, 24,*44–53.

Maw, A.R., & Bawden, R. (1994). Tympanic membrane atrophy, scarring, atelectasis and attic retraction in persistent untreated otitis media with effusion and ventilation tube insertion. *International Journal of Pediatric Otorhinolaryngology, 30,*189–204.

Metz, O. (1946). The acoustical impedance measured on normal and pathological ears. *Acta Otolaryngologica (Stockholm), 63(Suppl.),*3–254.

Moller, A. (1965a). An experimental study of the acoustic impedance of the middle ear and its transmission properties. *Acta Otolaryngologica (Stockholm), 60,*129–149.

Moller, A.R. (1965b). Network model of the middle ear. *Journal of the Acoustical Society of America, 33,*168–176.

Molvaer, O., Vallersnes, F., & Kringlebotn, M. (1978). The size of the middle ear and the mastoid air cell. *Acta Otolaryngologica, 85,*24–32.

Morrison, G.A., & Sterkers, J.M. (1996). Unusual presentations of acoustic tumors. *Clinics in Otolaryngology, 21,*80–83.

Murphy, D. (1979). Negative pressure in the middle ear by ciliary propulsion of mucus through the eustachian tube. *Laryngoscope, 89,*954–961.

Nahin, P.J. (1988). *Oliver Heaviside: Sage in solitude.* New York: IEEE Press.

Nozza, R.J., Bluestone, C.D., & Kardatze, D. (1992a). Sensitivity, specificity, and predictive value of immittance measures in the identification of middle-ear effusion. In: F. H. Bess, & J.W. Hall (Eds.), *Screening children for auditory function.* Nashville, TN: Bill Wilkerson Center Press.

Nozza, R.J., Bluestone, C.D., Kardatze, D., & Bachman, R. (1992b). Towards the validation of aural acoustic immittance measures for diagnosis of middle ear effusion in children. *Ear and Hearing, 13,*442–453.

Nozza, R.J., Bluestone, C.D., Kardatze, D., & Bachman, R. (1994). Identification of middle ear effusion by aural acoustic admittance and otoscopy. *Ear and Hearing, 15,*310–323.

O'Connor, A.F., & Shea, J.J. (1981). Autophony and the patulous eustachian tube. *Laryngoscope, 91,*1427–1435.

Ostergard, C.A., & Carter, D.R. (1981). Positive middle ear pressure shown by tympanometry. *Archives of Otolaryngology, 107,*353–356.

Ostfeld, E.J., & Silberberg, A. (1992). Theoretic analysis of middle ear gas composition under conditions of nonphysiologic ventilation. *Annals of Otology, Rhinology, and Laryngology, 101,*445–51.

Palva, T., & Palva, A. (1966). Size of the human mastoid air cell system. *Acta Otolaryngologica, 62,*237–251.

Paparella, M.M., Shea, D., Meyerhoff, W.L., & Goycoolea, M.V. (1980). Silent otitis media. *Laryngoscope, 90,*1089–1098.

Paradise, J.L., Smith, G.C., & Bluestone, C.D. (1976). Tympanometric detection of middle ear effusion in infants and children. *Pediatrics, 58,*198–210.

Plate, S., Johnsen, N.J., Nodskov Pedersen, S., & Thomsen, K.A. (1979). The frequency of patulous Eustachian tubes in pregnancy. *Clinics in Otolaryngology, 4,*393–400.

Popelka, G.R. (1981). *Hearing assessment with the acoustic reflex.* New York: Grune & Stratton.

Poulsen, G., & Tos, M. (1978). Screening tympanometry in newborn infants and during the first six months of life. *Scandinavian Audiology, 7,*159–166.

Prasher, D., & Cohen, M. (1993). Effectiveness of acoustic reflex threshold criteria in the diagnosis of retrocochlear pathology. *Scandinavian Audiology, 22,*11–18.

Proctor, B. (1991). Chronic otitis media and mastoiditis. In: M.M. Paparella, D.A. Shumrick, J.L. Gluckman, & W.L. Meyerhoff (Eds.), *Otolaryngology* (pp. 1349–1376). Philadelphia, PA: W.B. Saunders.

Proud, G.O., Odoi, H., & Toledo, P.S. (1971). Bullar pressure changes in eustachian tube dysfunction. *Annals of Otology, Rhinology, and Laryngology, 80,*835–837.

Rabinowitz, W.M. (1977). *Acoustic-reflex effects on the input admittance and transfer characteristics of the human middle ear.* Unpublished Ph.D. thesis, Cambridge, MA: Massachusetts Institute of Technology.

Renvall, U., & Holmquist, J. (1976). Tympanometry revealing middle ear pathology. *Annals of Otology, Rhinology, and Laryngology, 85(Supplement 25),*209–215.

Renvall, U., Liden, G., Jungert, S., & Nilsson, E. (1975). Impedance audiometry in the detection of secretory otitis media. *Scandinavian Audiology, 4,*119–124.

Rhodes, M.C., Margolis, R.H., Hirsch, J.E., & Napp, A.P. (1998). Hearing screening in the newborn intensive care nursery: A comparison of methods. *Otolaryngology–Head and Neck Surgery.*

Roush, J. (1990). Identification of hearing loss and middle ear disease in preschool and school-age children. *Seminars in Hearing, 11,*357–371.

Roush, J., Drake, A., & Sexton, J.E. (1992). Identification of middle ear dysfunction in young children: A comparison of tympanometric screening procedures. *Ear and Hearing, 13(2),*63–69.

Roush, J., & Tait, C.A. (1985). Puretone and acoustic immittance screening of preschool-aged children: An examination of referral criteria. *Ear and Hearing, 6,*245–249.

Rubensohn, G. (1965). Mastoid pneumatization in children at various ages. *Acta Otolaryngologica, 60,*11–14.

Sade, J., & Berco, E. (1976). Atelectasis and secretory otitis media. *Annals of Otology, Rhinology, and Laryngology, 85(Suppl. 25),*66–72.

Shahnaz, N., & Polka, L. (1999). Standard and multifrequency tympanometry in normal and otosclerotic ears. *Ear and Hearing.*

Shallop, J.K. (1976). The historical development of the study of middle ear function. In: A.S. Feldman & L.A. Wilber (Eds.), *Acoustic impedance and admittance—The measurement of middle ear function* (pp. 8–48). Baltimore, MD: Williams & Wilkins.

Shanks, J.E. (1985). Tympanometric volume estimates in patients with intact and perforated eardrums. *ASHA, 27,*78.

Shanks, J.E., & Lilly, D.J. (1981). An evaluation of tympanometric estimates of earcanal volume. *Journal of Speech and Hearing Research, 24,*557–566.

Shanks, J.E., Stelmachowicz, P.G., Beauchaine, K.L., & Schulte, L. (1992). Equivalent earcanal volumes in children pre- and post-tympanostomy tube insertion. *Journal of Speech and Hearing Research, 35,*936–941.

Sheehy, J., Brachmann, D., & Graham, M. (1977). Complications of cholesteatoma: A report on 1024 cases. In: B. McCabe, J. Sade, & M. Abramson (Eds.), *Cholesteatoma: First international conference* (pp. 420–429). Birmingham, AL: Aesculapius Publishing Co.

Silman, S., Siverman, C.A., & Arick, D.S. (1992). Acoustic immittance screening for detection of middle-ear effusion in children. *Journal of the American Academy of Audiology, 3,*262–268.

Sprague, B.H., Wiley, T.L., & Goldstein, R. (1985). Tympanometric and acoustic reflex studies in neonates. *Journal of Speech and Hearing Research, 28,*265–272.

Stach, B.A., Jerger, J.F., & Jenkins, J.A. (1984). The human acoustic tensor tympani reflex. *Scandinavian Audiology, 13,*93–99.

Takasaka, T., Hozawa, K., Shoji, F., Takahashi, Y., Jingu, K., Adachi, M., & Kobayashi, T. (1996). Tympanostomy tube treatment in recurrent otitis media with effusion. In: D.J. Lim, C.D. Bluestone, M. Casselbrant, J.O. Klein, & P.L. Ogra (Eds.), *Recent advances in otitis media* (pp. 197–199). Hamilton, Ontario: B.C. Decker, Inc.

Terkildsen K. (1957). Movements of the eardrum following inter-aural muscle reflexes. *Archives of Otolaryngology, 66,*484.

Terkildsen, K., & Nielsen, S. (1960). An electroacoustic impedance measuring bridge for clinical use. *Archives of Otolaryngology, 72,* 339–346.

Terkildsen, K., & Thomsen, K.A. (1959). The influence of pressure variations on the impedance of the human ear drum. *Journal of Laryngology and Otology, 73,*409–418.

Valente, M., Peterein, J., Goebel, J., & Neely, J.G. (1995). Four cases of acoustic neuromas with normal-hearing. *Journal of the American Academy of Audiology, 6,*203–210.

Van Camp, K.J., Margolis, R.H., Wilson, R.H., Creten, W.L., & Shanks, J.E (1986). Principles of tympanometry. *ASHA Monographs* (24),1–88.

Van Camp, K.J., Raman, E.R., & Creten, W.L. (1976). Two-component versus admittance tympanometry. *Audiology, 15,*120–127.

Vanhuyse, V.J., Creten, W.L., & Van Camp, K.J. (1975). On the W-notching of tympanograms. *Scandinavian Audiology, 4,*45–50.

West, W. (1928). Measurements of the acoustical impedances of human ears. *Post Office Elect Engin, 21,*293–300.

Wiley, T.L., Cruikshanks, K.J., Nondahl, D.M., Tweed, T.S., Klein, R., & Klein, B.E.K. (1996). Tympanometric measures in older adults. *Journal of the American Academy of Audiology, 7,*260–268.

Wilson, R.H., & Margolis, R.H. (1999). Acoustic-reflex measurements. In: M.E. Musiek, & W.F. Rintelmann (Eds.), *Contemporary perspectives in hearing assessment* (pp. 131–166) Boston, MA: Allyn and Bacon.

Wilson, R.H., Steckler, J.F., Jones, H.C., & Margolis, R.H. (1978). Adaptation of the acoustic reflex. *Journal of the Acoustical Society of American, 64,*782–791.

Wollaston, W.H. (1820). On sounds inaudible to certain ears. *Philosophical Transactions of the Royal Society of London, 110,*306–314.

Wright, J.L., & Etholm, B. (1973). Abnormalities of the middle ear muscles. *Journal of Laryngology and Otology, 87,*281–288.

Yee, A.L., & Cantekin, E.I. (1986). Effect of changes in systemic oxygen tension on middle ear gas exchange. *Annals of Otology, Rhinology, and Laryngology, 95,*369–372.

Zwislocki, J. (1962). Analysis of the middle-ear function. I. Input impedance. *Journal of the Acoustical Society of America, 34,* 1514–1523.

Zwislocki, J.J. (1963). An acoustic method for clinical examination of the ear. *Journal of Speech and Hearing Research, 6,*303–314.

Electrocochleography

John A. Ferraro

Outline

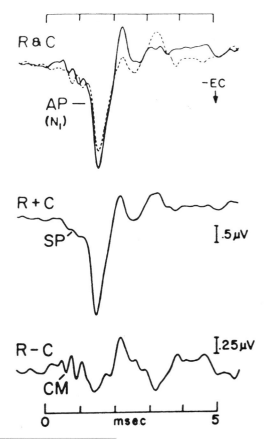

Figure 18–1 Components of the human electrocochleogram evoked by click stimuli. Top tracings show responses to rarefaction (*R*) and condensation (*C*) polarity clicks. Adding separate R and C responses (*middle tracing*) enhances the cochlear summating potential (*SP*) and auditory nerve action potential (*AP*), which are not phase-locked to the stimulus. Subtracting R and C responses (*bottom tracing*), enhances the cochlear microphonic (*CM*) (From ASHA [1988], p. 9, based on data from Coats [1981].)

The transduction of acoustic energy in the auditory periphery involves the generation of stimulus-related, electrical potentials in the cochlea. As the term implies, *electrocochleography* (ECochG) is a method for recording these potentials. The clinical application of ECochG, however, often includes measurement of the whole nerve or compound action potential (AP) of the auditory nerve. Thus we can add the term *ECochG* to our list of auditory evoked potentials (AEPs) that comprise components from the auditory nerve but fail to indicate this by their most popular name or acronym. Chief among these terms, of course, is *auditory brain stem response* (ABR) or any of the more than 10 terms or acronyms commonly used for this particular AEP.

The product of ECochG is referred to as an electrocochleogram (ECochGm). As shown in Figure 18–1 (from ASHA [1988] based on data from Coats, [1981]), the ECochGm comprises the cochlear microphonic (CM), cochlear summating potential (SP), and auditory nerve AP. These three

425

components may be recorded independently or in various combinations.

Historically, attempts to record the CM (also referred to as the cochlear potential) from humans date back almost to the time of its discovery in the cat by Wever and Bray (1930) (e.g., Andreev et al, 1939; Fromm et al, 1935; Lempert et al, 1947; Lempert et al, 1950; Perlman & Case, 1941). Although the SP was described in animals in 1950 (Davis et al, 1950; von Bekesy, 1950), its recording in humans received little to no attention until the mid-to-late 1970s (e.g., Eggermont, 1976; Gibson, 1978; Gibson et al, 1977). The first recordings of human auditory nerve APs are credited to Ruben et al (1960).

Although available to the hearing scientist/clinician for more than half a century, ECochG's emergence as a clinical tool did not begin until the 1970s. Renewed and increased attention to all AEPs during this period was due in part to the discovery and application of the ABR. Another important factor, which has facilitated the recent clinical popularity of ECochG in particular, is the development and refinement of noninvasive recording techniques. Ruben and coworkers, for example, performed their AP measurements on patients undergoing middle ear surgery. Within a few years, nonsurgical techniques that involved passing a needle electrode through the tympanic membrane (TM) to rest on the cochlear promontory were introduced (e.g., Aran & LeBert, 1968; Yoshie et al, 1967). This *transtympanic* (TT) approach to ECochG is still used widely in Europe. However, invasive recording methods have not been well accepted in the United States for a variety of reasons to be discussed later. Fortunately, the components that constitute an ECochGm can also be measured noninvasively from *extratympanic* (ET) sites such as the earcanal or the lateral surface of the TM. Pioneering work in this area was performed by Sohmer and Feinmesser (1967), Coats and Dickey (1970), and Cullen et al (1972), among others. A more thorough discussion and description of ECochG recording approaches is presented in the "Recording Techniques" section of this chapter.

The technical capability to record cochlear and auditory nerve potentials in humans has led to a variety of clinical applications for ECochG, including the following:

- Diagnosis/assessment/monitoring of Meniere's disease/ endolymphatic hydrops (MD/ELH) and the assessment/ monitoring of treatment strategies for these disorders
- Enhancement of wave I of the ABR in the presence of hearing loss or less than optimal recording conditions
- Measurement and monitoring of cochlear and auditory nerve function during surgery involving the auditory periphery (Ferraro and Krishnan, 1997; Ruth et al, 1988).

Although other uses for ECochG have been described, the above three applications continue to be the most popular and will therefore receive the most attention in this chapter. Our intention is to provide background information and reference material for the practitioner who currently uses ECochG in the laboratory, clinic, and/or operating room or is interested in doing so. The material has been organized to include reviews and descriptions under the general headings of salient features of the CM, SP, and AP; recording techniques; preparing for an examination; interpretation of the ECochGm; and clinical applications.

SALIENT FEATURES OF THE COCHLEAR MICROPHONIC, COCHLEAR SUMMATING POTENTIAL, AND ACTION POTENTIAL

Detailed descriptions of the CM, SP, and AP are abundant in the hearing science literature and beyond the scope of this chapter. The reader is encouraged to review this literature to gain a better understanding and appreciation of the specific features of these potentials and their relevance to hearing function. Indeed, this knowledge is essential to the clinical application of ECochG. The following section summarizes the salient features of the CM, SP, and AP, especially as related to their recording in humans.

Cochlear Microphonic

At least in animals, the CM is perhaps the most thoroughly investigated inner ear potential. However, as a clinical tool in humans, the SP and AP have received considerably more attention than the CM. The historical popularity of the CM in the laboratory has been facilitated by the relative ease with which it can be recorded and its considerable magnitude compared with other electrical phenomena associated with hearing. This is not necessarily the case in humans, however, in part because of the CM's characteristics. For example, the CM is an alternating current (AC) voltage that reflects an instantaneous displacement pattern of point sources on the cochlear partition (Berlin, 1986). Because of this feature, the CM waveform tends to mirror that of the acoustic stimulus, which makes it difficult to separate from stimulus artifact in clinical, noninvasive recordings. In addition, the effectiveness of the CM in the differential diagnosis of inner ear/auditory nerve disorders has yet to be established. Although reductions in CM magnitude and distorted waveform structure have been reported for various disorders such as MD and acoustic neuromas (Gerhardt et al, 1985; Gibson and Beagley, 1976; Kumagami et al, 1982; Moriuchi and Kumagami, 1979; Morrison et al, 1980), these characteristics tend to reflect general as opposed to specific cochlear pathological conditions.

The current inadequacy of the CM as a clinical tool may be more attributable to our incomplete understanding of its specific features than to the features themselves. For example, it has recently been observed that the spectral and temporal characteristics of CM recorded from the round window are strikingly similar to those of evoked otoacoustic emissions (EOAEs) measured from the earcanal (Norton et al, 1989). These findings suggest that both CM and EOAEs may have a common, place-specific generator. For a time, the CM was considered to be primarily a by-product of cochlear processing. Recent evidence, however, indicates that the CM may provide the input to the motor activity of the organ of Corti's outer hair cells (Evans & Dallos, 1993). Current attention to inner hair cell CM has focused on its role as a generator potential for the auditory nerve (Dallos, 1997).

New knowledge about the CM may expand its usefulness in the clinic. For example, Bian and Chertoff (1998) derived indices of mechanical to electrical transduction from the CM. Some of the indices were able to distinguish between cochlear pathological conditions, even though auditory thresholds were similar. These findings suggest that new analytic approaches to quantifying the CM may prove useful in the differential diagnosis of inner ear pathology. In addition, it has long been known that measurement of cochlear potentials at the round window (the most dominant component of which is the CM) in animals is sensitive to changes in middle ear transmission characteristics (Galambos & Rupert, 1959; Gerhardt et al, 1979; Guinan & Peake, 1967). This characteristic may prove useful for intraoperative monitoring and predicting outcome for patients undergoing middle ear surgery.

The mysteries of cochlear transduction processes are being unraveled at a rapid pace. In addition, the noninvasive techniques for recording the electrical events associated with these processes are becoming more sensitive. As new knowledge and technology in this area are applied to humans, the CM will most assuredly assume a more prominent role in clinical ECochG.

Summating Potential

The SP is a complex response that comprises several components. Like the CM, the SP is stimulus-related and generated by the hair cells of the organ of Corti. Also like the CM, the SP is a reflection of the displacement-time pattern of the cochlear partition. However, whereas the CM reflects the stimulus waveform, the SP displays a rectified, direct current (DC) version of this pattern more representative of the stimulus envelope (Dallos, 1973). The SP manifests itself as a shift in the CM baseline, the direction (or polarity) of which is dictated by an interactive effect between stimulus parameters (i.e., frequency and intensity) and the location of the recording electrode. The relationship between the CM and SP waveforms is illustrated in Figure 18–2 (Durrant, 1981). When recorded extratympanically (i.e., from the TM or earcanal), the SP is often seen as a downward (negative) deflection that persists for the duration of the acoustic stimulus.

Because of its complexity, the SP is probably the least understood cochlear potential, and its role in hearing function remains unclear. However, as a DC response to AC

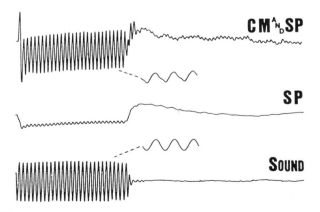

Figure 18–2 Relationship among the waveforms of the acoustic stimulus (*Sound*), and resultant cochlear microphonic (*CM*) and summating potential (*SP*). Insets show details of the CM and Sound tracings via an expanded timebase (from Durrant [1981], p. 23).

stimuli, at least some of the components of the SP are thought to represent the sum of various nonlinearities associated with transduction processes in the cochlea (Dallos et al, 1972; Davis, 1968; Engebretson & Eldridge, 1968; Gulick et al, 1989; Ruth, 1994; Tasaki et al, 1954; Whitfield & Ross, 1965). Thus the magnitude of the SP may be a reflection of the amount of distortion that accompanies or is produced by these processes. This characteristic has made the SP useful for certain clinical conditions. In particular, it is now well documented that the ECochGms of patients with MD/ELH often display SPs that are enlarged compared with the SPs of normally hearing subjects or patients with cochlear disorders other than MD/ELH (e.g., Coats, 1981, 1986; Dauman et al, 1988; Ferraro et al, 1983; Ferraro et al, 1985; Ferraro & Krishnan, 1997; Gibson et al, 1977; Gibson, 1978; Goin et al, 1982; Kitahara et al, 1981; Kumagami et al, 1982; Moriuchi & Kumagami, 1979; Morrison et al, 1980; Ruth et al, 1988; Schmidt et al, 1974; Staller, 1986). Conventional rationale for this finding is that an increase in endolymph volume creates additional distortion within the system, which is reflected in the SP. Whether the nature of this increased distortion is mechanical (Gibson et al, 1977) and/or electrical (Durrant & Dallos, 1972, 1974; Durrant & Gans, 1977) has not been resolved, and other factors such as biochemical and/or vascular changes may also be responsible for an enlarged SP in MD/ELH (Goin et al, 1982; Staller, 1986). Regardless of the specific pathophysiology, measurement of the SP to help diagnose, assess, and monitor MD/ELH has emerged as a primary application for modern-day ECochG.

Action Potential

The AP recorded by ECochG represents the summed response of several thousand auditory nerve fibers that have fired in synchrony. When evoked by click stimuli, the term *whole nerve AP* is sometimes applied because, theoretically, the *"square"* waveform of the click has a flat spectrum that contains all frequencies and therefore stimulates the entire basilar membrane. A stimulus with a narrower bandwidth, such as a tone burst, excites a more limited segment of the membrane to produce a "compound AP" (Gibson, 1978). In reality, although both of the above adjectives for the AP can be misleading, "whole nerve," in particular is a true misnomer. This is because the spectrum of the acoustic click that reaches the cochlea is far from flat and substantially narrower in bandwidth than the spectrum of the electrical pulse driving the transducer. Furthermore, synchronicity of neural firings is essential to producing a well-defined AP. Maximum synchrony, in turn, occurs at the onset of the stimulus, even for tone bursts. If this onset is abrupt, the response will be dominated by neural contributions from the basal, high-frequency end of the normal cochlea (Kiang, 1965). Thus the whole nerve is not excited in response to click stimuli, nor is the segment of the basilar membrane excited by tonal stimuli necessarily limited to that which codes for the signal's frequency.

The AP, like the CM (or unlike the SP), is an AC voltage. However, unlike either of the cochlear potentials whose waveforms reflect the displacement-time pattern of the cochlear partition, the AP waveform is characterized by a series of brief, predominantly negative peaks representative of the pattern of resultant neural firings. At suprathreshold stimulus levels, the first and largest of these peaks is referred to as N_1. N_1 is virtually the same component as wave I of the ABR and, as such, arises from the distal portion of the auditory nerve (Moller & Janetta, 1983). AP peaks beyond N_1 (such as N_2 and N_3) are analogous to corresponding ABR components (i.e., waves II and III) but have received little, if any, clinical attention in ECochG.

For clinical purposes the most useful features of the AP relate to its magnitude and latency. The former is a reflection of the number of nerve fibers firing. However, because the afferent fibers of the auditory nerve primarily innervate the inner hair cells (Spoendlin, 1966), AP magnitude also can be viewed as a reflection of inner hair cell output. AP latency represents the time between stimulus onset and the peak of N_1. This measure is analogous to the "absolute latency" for ABR components and incorporates stimulus travel time from the output of the transducer to the inner ear, traveling wave propagation time along the basilar membrane, and the time associated with the synchronization of neural impulses that produces the AP peaks. As with all waves of the ABR, reductions in signal intensity at suprathreshold levels for the AP are accompanied by changes in the N_1, including magnitude reduction leading to eventual disappearance into the electrical noise floor, and latency prolongation.

Since its initial recording in humans in 1960, the AP has been the most widely studied component of the ECochGm. Early interest in the AP, however, was directed toward the development of an electrophysiological index of hearing status in children (Cullen et al, 1972). This effort was overshadowed by the advent of the ABR for such purposes, primarily because wave V of the ABR appeared to be more sensitive and easier to measure than the AP-N_1. As AEP applications and technology have evolved over the years, the use of the AP to assess and monitor cochlear and auditory nerve function has received renewed attention, especially in surgical settings. In addition, the use of a combined AP-ABR approach for assessing retrocochlear status in hard-of-hearing subjects is gaining popularity. At present, perhaps the most popular application of the AP involves the measurement of its magnitude compared with that of the SP in patients suspected of having MD/ELH. As described earlier, an enlarged SP often characterizes the

ECochGms of patients with MD/ELH. The clinical consistency of this finding, however, improves considerably when the SP amplitude is compared with the amplitude of N_1 to form the SP/AP amplitude ratio (Coats, 1981; Coats, 1986; Eggermont, 1976). It is now widely accepted that an enlarged SP/AP amplitude ratio to click stimuli is a positive finding for ELH.

RECORDING TECHNIQUES

Transtympanic versus Extratympanic ECochG

As mentioned previously, there are two general approaches for recording ECochG: transtympanic (TT) and extratympanic (ET). TT ECochG is an invasive procedure that involves passing a needle electrode through the TM to rest on the cochlear promontory. During surgeries that expose the middle ear space, TT recordings can also be made with a ball electrode on the round window through the surgical field. Photographs of needle and ball electrodes used for TT ECochG are shown in Figure 18–3. ET recordings are performed with an electrode resting against the skin of the earcanal or surface of the TM. For the latter recording site, the procedure is also referred to as "tympanic (or TM) ECochG" (Ferraro & Ferguson, 1989), even though this approach is still considered to be ET. Although ET ECochG can be performed with a needle electrode in the skin of the earcanal, this option is rarely, if ever, chosen. Therefore virtually all ET recordings tend to be noninvasive. Examples of currently popular ET electrodes are shown in Figure 18–4.

Both TT and ET approaches to ECochG have advantages and disadvantages. The primary advantage of the TT approach is the proximity of the recording electrode to the response generators. This "near field" situation produces large components with relatively little signal averaging.

The greatest advantage associated with ET approaches is that they can be performed in nonmedical settings with minimal discomfort to the patient. This latter condition also obviates the need for sedation/local anesthesia. By virtue of these advantages, ET ECochG is becoming increasingly popular among audiologists, and even physicians, who perform AEP

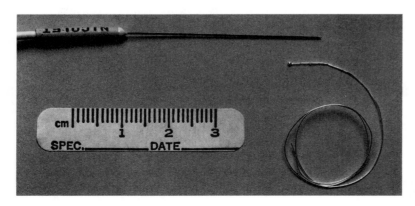

Figure 18–3 Photographs of needle (promontory placement) and ball-tipped (round window placement) electrodes used for transtympanic ECochG.

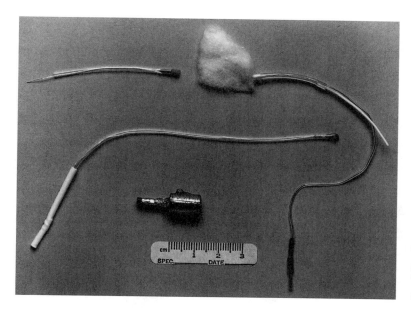

Figure 18–4 Photographs of electrodes used for extratympanic ECochG: Modified (and home-made) version of Stypulkowski-Staller Tymptrode (*top left*), Lilly wick electrode (*top right*), and Bio-Logic EcochGtrode (*middle*) are placed at the surface of the tympanic membrane. Gold-foil TIPtrode (*bottom*) rests in the outer portion of the earcanal.

PITFALL

The major limitations of TT ECochG relate to its invasiveness. Such procedures require the assistance of a physician and are therefore limited to a medical setting. In addition, penetrating the TM with a needle is not accomplished without some degree of pain/discomfort to the patient, even when local anesthetics are used. These disadvantages certainly have limited the use of TT ECochG in the United States. By comparison, ECochG responses recorded from ET sites require more signal averaging and tend to be smaller in amplitude than their counterparts measured from the promontory or round window.

CONTROVERSIAL POINT

Should I perform TT or ET ECochG? Given the advantages and disadvantages of both approaches, the decision to perform ET or TT ECochG often depends on the traditional practices, personnel, and attitudes of the clinic.

---

testing. Another factor that has contributed to the growing popularity of ET ECochG relates to advances in electrode design (discussed in following section) and the practice of using the TM as a recording site. The TM offers a practical compromise between earcanal and TT placements with respect to component magnitudes and signal averaging time (Ferraro, Blackwell et al, 1994; Ferraro, Thedinger et al, 1994; Ruth et al, 1988; Schoonhoven et al, 1995). Perhaps most importantly for clinical purposes, however, the waveform patterns that lead to the interpretation of the TT ECochGm tend to be preserved in TM recordings (Ferraro, Thedinger et al, 1994).

Obviously, TT recordings depend on the availability of a physician who has the time and interest to perform the examination. Although a physician is not needed for ET ECochG, placing an electrode on the TM is certainly a more delicate maneuver than attaching surface electrodes to the scalp or resting them in the earcanal. With proper instruction and materials, however, this procedure is easily learned and well within the scope of professional practice for audiologists.

Recording Parameters

Selection of recording parameters for ECochG will vary according to the components of interest. Because these components generally occur within a latency epoch of 5 ms after stimulus onset, they can be considered to be in the family of "early- or "short-latency" AEPs (Picton et al, 1974). They are, in fact, the earliest (shortest) members of this family. As relatives, ECochG components and the ABR can be recorded with similar parameters. A notable exception occurs in the selection of the bandpass of the preamplifier for ECochG when the SP is of interest. That is, the high-pass setting of the filter must be low enough to accommodate a DC component. Other differences between ECochG and ABR recording parameters involve the electrode array and the number of samples to be averaged. For ECochG, the latter depends on the choice of recording approaches, with TT requiring considerably fewer repetitions than ET. Table 18–1 illustrates suitable parameters for recording the SP and AP together, which are the components of interest when ECochG is used in the diagnosis of MD/ELH.

TABLE 18–1 ECochG recording parameters

Electrode Array	
Primary (+)	Earcanal/Tympanic Membrane/Promontory/Round Window
Secondary (−)	Contralateral Earlobe/Mastoid Process/Earcanal
Common	Nasion/Ipsilateral Earlobe
Signal Averaging Settings	
Timebase	5–10 milliseconds
Amplification Factor	50,000X–100,000X (Extratympanic–ET) 5,000X–25,000X (Transtympanic–TT)
Filter Bandpass	5 Hz–3,000 Hz
Repetitions	1,000–1,500 (ET) 100–200 (TT)
Stimuli	
Type	Broadband Clicks (BBC), Tone bursts (TB)
Duration (BBC)	100 microsecond electrical pulse
Envelope (TB)	2 millisecond linear rise/fall, 5–10 millisecond plateau
Polarity	Rarefaction and Condensation (BBC), Alternating (TB)
Repetition Rate	11.3/second
Level	85 dB HL (115 dB pe SPL)

A description of these parameters with rationale is provided in the following.

Electrode Array

Many clinicians/researchers use an electrode array that displays the AP as a downward (negative) deflection. To accomplish this, the primary electrode (i.e., the electrode connected to the +/noninverted input of the differential preamplifier) should rest in the earcanal or on the TM, promontory, or round window (depending on the choice of ET or TT recording approaches). Sites for the secondary (−/inverted) electrode include the vertex of the scalp, high forehead, or contralateral earlobe or mastoid process.

Choices for "ground" or "common" sites include the nasion and ipsilateral earlobe or mastoid process. Reversing the + and − inputs to the preamplifier shifts the polarity of the ECochGm by 180 degrees. This array would display the AP-N_1 as a positive peak, which might be preferable when compared with conventional ABR recordings.

It often is the case that the test battery for a given patient includes both ECochG and measurement of the ABR. These recordings can be accomplished with five electrodes: a TM electrode (because our choice is TM ECochG) and surface electrodes attached to both earlobes (or mastoid processes), the high forehead (or vertex), and nasion. A common electrode configuration for this approach is TM (+)-to-contralateral earlobe (−) for ECochG, and high forehead or vertex (+)-to-ipsilateral earlobe (−) for ABR, with ground at the nasion for both arrays.

Timebase

As indicated previously, ECochG components represent the earliest voltage changes to occur in the ear in response to acoustic stimulation. For brief transient stimuli (such as clicks), the timebase (or signal averaging window) must therefore be set to capture the electrophsyiological activity occurring within the first few milliseconds after stimulus onset. For click stimuli, a timebase of 10 ms allows for visualization ABR

PEARL

We prefer the earlobe or mastoid process as the secondary (−) electrode site for ECochG simply because electrodes tend to be easier to attach and secure to these sites. An array that uses the ipsilateral earlobe or mastoid process as the secondary site produces ECochG components with smaller amplitudes than those obtained with a contralateral reference.

components that follow N_1. For longer duration stimuli (such as tone bursts) the timebase should extend beyond the duration of the stimulus envelope so that the entire response is observable within the averaging window (remember that both the SP and CM persist for the duration of the stimulus). For example, a 20 ms window could be used if the stimulus were a 1000 Hz tone burst with a two-cycle rise/fall time, and a 10 cycle plateau (i.e., a 14 ms envelope).

Amplification Factor

Preamplifier amplification factor is selected to maximize the signal-to-noise ratio for a given recording condition. The amount of amplification needed for suitable recordings of the SP and/or AP for ET measurements generally ranges between 50,000 and 100,000 times, whereas the factor for TT recordings can be 5 to 10 times smaller. In part, selection of this parameter is made on the basis of the level of the electrical noise floor, which incorporates several elements (e.g., myogenic and electroencephalographic activity, electrical artifact from the equipment, and/or testing environment). The sensitivity setting of the signal averager's analog-to-digital converter also must be taken into account. Thus amplification/sensitivity settings may vary from laboratory to laboratory and also among evoked potential units from different manufacturers. However, the manipulation of these variables to provide settings appropriate to recording conditions is easily accomplished in most commercial instruments.

Filter Bandpass

As mentioned earlier, when the SP is of interest, the bandpass of the preamplifier filter must be wide enough to allow for the amplification of a DC component. To record the SP-AP complex, the bandpass must also include the fundamental frequency of the AP, which is approximately 1000 Hz.

PITFALL

Recording the SP and AP together presents a dilemma in that the amplification systems generally used for ECochG are not designed for DC signals. Thus the selection of a bandpass to accommodate both the SP and AP represents a compromise that introduces some degree of distortion to both components.

When such a wide bandpass is used, the DC (SP) component is frequency filtered, and recording of the AC (AP) component may be distorted by the presence of low-frequency noise.

Repetitions

In general, the number of stimulus repetitions needed to evoke a well-defined ECochGm will vary with recording conditions and the subject's degree of hearing loss. The former depends on the recording approach, with TT ECochG requiring considerably fewer averages than ET ECochG. For subjects with hearing loss in the 1000 to 4000 Hz range, more

---

PEARL

Practically speaking, the click-evoked SP is tolerable of a certain degree of filtering because it is a transient of brief duration and therefore not a true DC component (Durrant & Ferraro, 1991).

SPECIAL CONSIDERATION

When sensorineural hearing loss in the mid-to-high frequencies exceeds 50- to 60-dB hearing level (HL), the use of ECochG to help diagnose or assess MD/ELH is questionable. The basis for this statement is that losses of this magnitude generally involve (i.e., reduce the output of) the population of outer hair cells that produce the SP. On the other hand, when hearing loss of similar or greater magnitude precludes the identification of wave I in the presence of wave V in the conventionally recorded ABR, ECochG can be very useful. Ferraro and Ferguson (1989), for example, have shown that the AP-N_1 is usually recordable under such conditions, and can be substituted for ABR wave I to determine the I to V interwave interval.

---

repetitions may be necessary than are usually needed for normally hearing subjects or those with low-frequency losses.

Stimuli

As mentioned earlier, the broadband click tends to be the most popular stimulus for short-latency AEPs because it excites synchronous discharges from a large population of neurons to produce well-defined peaks. In addition, 100 μs is a popular choice for the duration of the driving rectangular pulse because the first spectral null for a click of this duration occurs at 10,000 Hz. (i.e., 1/100 μs). Thus the signal theoretically contains equal energy at all frequencies less than this value. In reality, the frequency range of the transducer is usually lower than 10,000 Hz and the outer and middle ears filter the acoustic signal further. Thus, as described earlier in this chapter, the spectrum of the acoustic signal reaching the cochlea is not flat or as wide as 10,000 Hz.

PITFALL

Unfortunately, the brevity of the click makes it a less-than-ideal stimulus for studying cochlear potentials.

Because the duration of both the CM and SP are stimulus dependent, both components appear only as brief deflections when evoked by clicks (see Fig. 18–1). Despite this limitation, the use of clicks has proven to be very effective in evoking the SP-AP complex for certain ECochG applications, even though the duration of the SP is abbreviated under these conditions (Durrant & Ferraro, 1991).

Although the click continues to remain popular, several recent studies have also advocated the use of tonal stimuli for ECochG (Ferraro, Blackwell et al, 1994; Ferraro, Thedinger et al, 1994; Koyuncu et al, 1994; Levine et al, 1992; Margolis et al, 1995; Orchik et al, 1993). Tonal stimuli generally provide for a higher degree of response frequency specificity than clicks. This feature can be useful for monitoring cochlear status in progressive disorders (such as MD/ELH), where hearing is usually not affected at all frequencies during the initial stages. In addition, the use of extended-duration stimuli such as tone bursts allows for better visualization of the SP and CM than can be achieved with clicks (Durrant & Ferraro, 1991).

PITFALL

A problem related to the use of tonal stimuli for ECochG (and other AEPs) is the lack of standardization regarding stimulus parameters.

Most studies use tone bursts of only one or two frequencies, stimulus envelopes are different, and the approach to defining stimulus intensity is not standardized. These inconsistencies make it difficult to compare data across laboratories/clinics. For tone bursts, we prefer an envelope with a linear rise-fall time of 2 ms and a 10 ms plateau. Shorter plateaus (e.g., 5 ms) can sometimes be used to avoid interference by ABR components (Levine et al, 1992).

Stimulus polarity relates to the initial deflection of the transducer diaphragm and is an important factor for ECochG. Presenting clicks or tone bursts in alternating polarity inhibits the presence of recorded signals that are phase locked to the stimulus, such as stimulus artifact and CM. The former can sometimes be large enough to obscure early ECochG components, and the latter generally overshadows both the SP and AP. Thus the use of alternating-polarity stimuli is preferable if the SP amplitude and SP/AP amplitude ratio are measurements of interest (such as when ECochG is used in the diagnosis of MD/ELH). On the other hand, several studies have now shown that recording separate responses to condensation and rarefaction clicks may provide useful clinical information. In particular, certain subjects with MD/ELH display abnormal latency differences between AP-N_1 latencies to condensation versus rarefaction clicks (Levine et al, 1992; Margolis & Lilly, 1989; Margolis et al, 1992; Margolis et al, 1995; Orchik et al, 1997; Sass et al, 1997).

For ECochG, as with most signal-averaged AEPs, it is important that the cochlear/neural response to one stimulus be complete before the next stimulus is presented. For click-evoked, short-latency AEPs, this requirement allows for considerable latitude in the selection of stimulus repetition rate. For ECochG, however, increasing this rate beyond 10 to 30/s may cause some adaptation of the AP (Suzuki & Yamane, 1982). Rates on the order of 100/s cause maximal suppression of the AP while leaving the SP relatively unaffected.

CONTROVERSIAL POINT

What is the appropriate polarity for delivering click stimuli? In deference to recent studies, measurement of separate responses to condensation and rarefaction clicks should be used to assess the AP-N_1 latency difference. These responses can be added together off-line (which is analogous to using alternating clicks) to derive the SP amplitude and SP/AP amplitude ratio.

Gibson et al (1977) and Coats (1981) applied this approach to maximize visualization of the SP. Unfortunately, the use of very fast stimulus repetition rates has not proven to be very successful in the clinic, in part because the AP contribution is not completely eliminated and the SP may also be reduced (Durrant, 1986). In addition, rapid clicks presented at loud levels tend to be obnoxious for patients.

When ECochG is performed to help diagnose MD/ELH, the signal should be intense enough to evoke a well-defined SP-AP complex. Thus for this application stimulus presentation should begin at a level near the maximum output of the stimulus generator. Unfortunately, as mentioned earlier, a lack of standardization exists for AEP stimuli regarding signal calibration and decibel reference. Common references include decibel HL (or hearing threshold level [HTL] or normal-hearing level [nHL]), decibel sensation level (SL), and decibel peak equivalent sound pressure level (pe SPL). As in conventional audiometry, decibel HL is based on the mean behavioral threshold of a group of normally hearing subjects, whereas decibel SL is the number of decibels above an individual threshold. Decibel pe SPL is determined by matching the SPL of a transient signal to that of a continuous sinusoid, and therefore represents the only physical measure of intensity of the three common references. It may be necessary to calibrate ECochG signals in both HL and pe SPL. Zero decibel HL represents the average behavioral threshold of a group of normally hearing subjects to the various stimuli used for ECochG (e.g., clicks and tone bursts). For decibel pe SPL, an oscilloscope is used to match the level of the click to that of a 1000 Hz continuous sinusoid. Consistent with the findings of Stapells et al (1982), 0 decibel HL for clicks corresponds to approximately 30 dB pe SPL.

PEARL

Masking of the contralateral ear is not a concern for conventional ECochG because the magnitude of any electrophysiological response from the nontest ear is very small. In addition, ECochG components are generated before crossover of the auditory pathway.

A final note regarding stimuli relates to stimulus artifact, which can be quite large for ECochG because of the nature of

ET (especially TM) electrodes. These wire devices also serve as antennae that are very receptive to electromagnetic radiation from the transducer and other electrical sources in the environment. The following suggestions are offered to help to reduce stimulus artifact:

- Use a tubal insert transducer
- Separate the transducer from the electrode cables as much as possible
- Braid the electrode cables
- Test subjects in a shielded sound booth with the examiner and AEP unit located outside of the booth
- Plug the AEP unit into an isolated socket equipped with a true-earth ground
- Use a grounded cable for the primary electrode (such cables are commercially available)
- Turn off the lights in the testing room and *unplug* unnecessary electronic equipment (it also may be necessary to turn off the lights in the examiner room)
- Consider encasing the transducer in grounded mu metal shielding.

PREPARING FOR AN EXAMINATION

Selection of Recording Approach

As described in the previous section of this chapter, the selection of recording approaches to ECochG generally depends on reasons related to the traditional practices and attitudes of the clinic and the availability of qualified personnel to perform the examination.

PITFALL

Unfortunately, a factor that usually is not considered in the selection of ET versus TT approaches is the attitude of the patient.

Given an informed choice (i.e., an explanation of options with advantages and disadvantages of each), most patients will select ET ECochG for obvious reasons. Taking all the above into account, the approach to ECochG in many clinics is limited exclusively to ET methods even though personnel and resources may be available to perform TT recordings.

PEARL

Virtually all ET recordings in the author's clinic/laboratory are made from the TM because of the advantages this site offers over other ET locations (i.e., along the earcanal).

The benefits TM ECochG offers over other ET approaches include increased component amplitudes, more stable/repeatable responses, and reduced testing time because less

signal averaging is needed (Arsenault & Benitez, 1991; Ferraro & Ferguson, 1989; Ruth, 1990; Ruth & Lambert, 1988; Ruth et al, 1988; Stypulkowski & Staller, 1987). Given our preference for TM ECochG, the following information emphasizes this particular approach.

Instructions to the Patient

Most patients are unfamiliar with ECochG and therefore confused as to what it is, why they need it, and how it will be performed. The lengthiness of the term *electrocochleography* sometimes adds to this confusion. Instructions to the patient can begin on the way to the testing room with an assurance that the examination is noninvasive and painless, that the test will take approximately 1 hour, and they can sleep through it if they wish. Engaging patients in conversation at this point and watching them walk also provides some insight regarding their hearing and balance status. Once in the sound booth, the patient lies in a supine position on an examining bed, which can be adjusted to maximize comfort of the head, neck, and upper back. Eyeglasses and/or earrings are removed (usually by the patient), and food/chewing gum/candy/and so forth must be swallowed or discarded. When the patient is comfortable and attentive, ECochG is described as a method for recording the electrical responses of the inner ear to click-type sounds. It also helps to explain that their doctor has requested this examination to assess whether too much fluid in the inner ear is the basis for their symptoms. The patient should then be informed that surface electrodes will be attached to the scalp, a small, sponge-tipped electrode will be inserted along the earcanal to rest on their TM, and an earplug will be used to hold the electrode in place and deliver the clicks.

SPECIAL CONSIDERATION

Patients should be cautioned that the TM electrode might feel strange and may even be a little uncomfortable, but that it should not be particularly painful.

The procedures for preparing the skin and placing the surface electrodes are described while performing these tasks (for more detailed instructions on how to prepare the skin for surface electrodes see Ferraro, 1997). After the surface electrodes are attached (or beforehand for that matter), otoscopy is performed to assess the patency of the earcanal and normalcy of the TM. Cerumen removal may be necessary to visualize the TM and clear a pathway along the earcanal large enough for the electrode. Once the surface electrodes have been placed and otoscopy performed, the TM electrode can be constructed and placed.

SPECIAL CONSIDERATION

If either the earcanal or TM appear abnormal or damaged, ECochG is not advisable.

Construction and Placement of the TM Electrode (Tymptrode)

The photograph of ET electrodes in Figure 18–4 includes the Tymptrode (originally described by Stypulkowski and Staller [1987] and modified by Ferraro and Ferguson [1989]), the Lilly wick electrode (Lilly & Black, 1989), and the TM-ECochGtrode manufactured by Bio-Logic. The latter two electrodes are commercially available. The Tymptrode can be fabricated using "store-bought" materials such as those listed in the following (see Ferraro [1992] and Ferraro [1997]):

- Medical grade silicon (Silastic) tubing (0.058" ID, 0.077" OD)
- Teflon-insulated silver wire (0.008" bare diameter, 0.011" insulated diameter)
- Tight-celled, but soft, rubber foam
- Electrode gel (not paste or cream)
- Fine, needle-nosed forceps
- 1-ml disposable tuberculin syringe with needle
- Copper microalligator clip soldered to the end of an electrode cable

The procedure for constructing the Tymptrode involves cutting the wire and tubing into segments a few centimeters longer than the earcanal, with the wire approximately 2 cm longer than the tubing. Fine forceps are used to scrape the insulation off both ends of the wire (a crucial step), which is then threaded through the tubing. One end of the wire protruding from the tubing remains bare, and the other end is hooked to the end of a small plug (approximately 2 mm × 3 mm) of the rubber foam. Once again using the fine forceps, that portion of the plug hooked to the wire is tucked into the end of the tubing to leave only a small portion of the plug extending beyond the tubing. Figure 18–5 is a labeled drawing of a Tymptrode constructed as described earlier. Tymptrodes, at this stage, can be made and stockpiled for indefinite periods of time. Immediately before use, the foam tip of the Tymptrode must be impregnated with electrode gel. This step is accomplished by filling the tuberculin syringe with gel and injecting the entire piece of foam until it is thoroughly saturated (including that portion of the foam within the tubing attached to the wire). Attach the microalligator clip of the electrode cable to the other (bare) end of the wire, and the Tymptrode is ready for insertion.

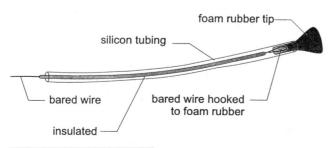

Figure 18–5   Construction of the Tymptrode.

> ### PEARL
> Both ears should tested, even if unilateral disease is suspected. Comparison between affected and unaffected sides can provide important diagnostic information. The affected side should be tested first in case the patient becomes restless as the examination progresses.

Inserting the Tymptrode

To gain the assistance of gravity when placing the Tymptrode, the patient is instructed to gently roll over onto his or her side so that the test ear is facing up. The Tymptrode is then inserted into the entrance of the earcanal and gently advanced (by hand or using the fine forceps) until the tip makes contact with the TM. The latter is confirmed with ototscopic observation and electrophysiological monitoring. It also helps to ask the patient when they feel the electrode touching the TM. The use of an immittance probe tip to insert the Tymptrode "blindly" into the canal until the patient acknowledges contact with the TM has been reported (Ferraro & Ferguson, 1991; Storms et al, 1996). Durrant (1990) used the port of a vented earmold in similar fashion. Recent research, however, indicates that achieving proper contact with the TM is more successful when the Tymptrode is placed visually by use of an otoscope or operating microscope rather than blindly by means of a probe tip (Lopez et al, 1993).

> ### PITFALL
> Even with an otoscope, it sometimes is difficult to actually see the point of contact between the Tymptrode tip and TM.

> ### PEARL
> Monitoring the electrophysiological noise floor during electrode placement helps to achieve proper contact with the TM.

As the electrode is being advanced into the earcanal, the raw EEG/noise floor is displayed on-screen. Large, spurious and cyclic or peak-clipped voltages (i.e., an open-line situation) characterize this electrical activity. When proper contact of the Tymptrode tip with the TM is achieved, the noise floor drops dramatically and becomes more stable. Both visual and electrophysiological monitoring provide the best opportunity for achieving proper contact with the TM on the "first try."

Once the Tymptrode is in contact with the TM, the foam tip of the sound delivery tube is compressed and inserted into the earcanal alongside the Tymptrode tubing.

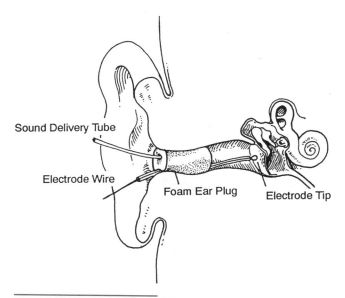

Figure 18–6 Illustration of the Tymptrode in position and held in place by the foam ear tip of the sound delivery tube (Ferraro [1992], p. 28).

Only a portion of the transducer earplug needs to be inserted into the canal to achieve proper stimulation for evoking the ECochGm. Figure 18–6 is a schematic representation of the Tymptrode and sound delivery tube in the earcanal (Ferraro, 1992). With the Tymptrode and other electrodes attached to the preamplifier and the sound tube in place and the patient comfortable, relaxed, and still, the signal averaging process can begin.

INTERPRETATION OF THE ELECTROCOCHLEOGRAM

As with most AEPs, measures of component amplitude and latency form the bases for interpreting the ECochGm. Figure 18–7 depicts a normal ECochGm to click stimuli recorded from the TM. Stimulus level was 80 dB HL, and click polarity was alternated to favor the SP and AP at the expense of inhibiting the CM. Component amplitudes can be measured from peak-to-peak (*left panel*) or using a baseline reference (*right panel*).

SPECIAL CONSIDERATION
Care must be taken during this stage not to push the electrode further against the TM when inserting the earplug, because this can cause some discomfort to the patient. However, the materials that comprise the Tymptrode are relatively soft and flexible, which allows the tip to compress or bend at the TM rather than penetrate the membrane.

CONTROVERSIAL POINT
Should SP and AP amplitudes be measured from peak to peak or with a baseline reference? The method of choice in our laboratory for TM and other ET approaches is peak to peak because of the considerable lability of the baseline amplitude for ET recordings.

By use of peak-to-peak values from our laboratory, normal SP amplitudes measured from the TM to 80 dB HL clicks

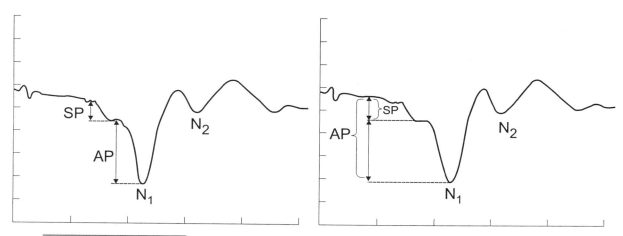

Figure 18–7 Normal ECochGm from the tympanic membrane to clicks presented in alternating polarity at 80 dB HL. The amplitudes of the summating potential (*SP*) and action potential (*AP*) can be measured from peak-to-trough (*left panel*), or with reference to a baseline value (*right panel*). Amplitude/time scale is 1.25 microvolts/1 millisecond per gradation. Insert phone delay is 0.90 milliseconds.

generally range from 0.1 to 1.0 μV, with a mean of 0.4 μV. AP amplitudes can be as large as 5.0 μV, although our mean value is approximately 2.0 μV. AP-N_1 latency is measured from stimulus onset to the peak of N_1 and, as mentioned earlier in this chapter, should be identical to the latency of ABR wave I. At 80 dB HL, normal N_1 latencies generally range from 1.3 to 1.7 ms, with a mean of approximately 1.5 ms. These values have been corrected for the 0.9 ms delay

opposed to click-evoked responses, where the SP appears as a small shoulder preceding the AP, the SP to tone bursts persists as long as the stimulus. The AP and its N_1, in turn, are seen at the onset of the response. SP amplitude is measured at the midpoint of the waveform to minimize the influence of the AP and with reference to baseline amplitude. Thus the polarity of the SP depends on whether the voltage at midpoint is greater than (positive SP) or less than (negative SP)

TABLE 18–2   Mean SP/AP amplitude ratios to click stimuli from recent studies

	SP/AP Ratio (SD)	Recording Approach	N
Campbell et al (1992)	0.27 (0.15)	TM*	17
Levine et al (1992)	0.31 (0.11)	TM	13
Margolis et al (1995)	0.26 (0.09)	TM	53
Koyuncu et al (1994)	0.24 (0.20)	Earcanal	20
Roland et al (1993)	0.21 (0.09)	Earcanal	17
Densert et al (1994)	0.16 (0.06)	TT†	17
Aso et al (1991)	0.24 (0.05)	TT	29

*TM = Tympanic membrane
†TT = Transtympanic

attributable to stimulus travel time through the sound tube of the tubal insert transducer. Although labeled in Figure 18–7, N_2 has received little interest for ECochG applications.

Also as shown in Figure 18–7, SP and AP amplitudes are made from the leading edge of both components. The resultant values are used to derive the SP/AP amplitude ratio, which is a key measure when ECochG is used to help diagnose and monitor MD/ELH. Table 18–2 (Ferraro & Krishnan, 1997) compares mean SP/AP amplitude ratios to click stimuli from several recent studies. These values occur within a relatively small range (i.e., 0.16 to 0.31) despite the use of different recording approaches.

Figure 18–8 (Ferraro, Blackwell et al, 1994) depicts a normal electrocochleogram evoked by an 80 dB HL, 2000 Hz tone burst (2 ms rise/fall, 10 ms plateau, alternating polarity). As

the baseline voltage. Figure 18–9 (Ferraro, Blackwell et al, 1994) illustrates tone burst SPs at several frequencies recorded from both the TM and promontory (TT) of the same normally hearing subject. Note that for both recording approaches, the polarities of the SPs at 500 and 8000 Hz are slightly positive, whereas negative SPs are seen at 1000, 2000, and 4000 Hz. This feature tends to vary across frequencies, recording approaches and within and across subjects.

Another noteworthy aspect of Figure 18–9 is that although the magnitudes of the TM responses are approximately one-quarter that of the promontory responses (note amplitude scales), the corresponding patterns of the TM and TT recordings at each frequency are virtually identical.

In Figure 18–10 (Ferraro, Blackwell et al, 1994, p. 21), mean SP amplitudes recorded from the TMs of 20 normally

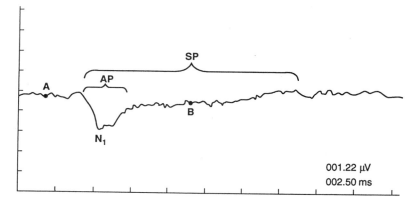

001.22 μV
002.50 ms

Figure 18–8   Normal ECochGm from the tympanic membrane to a 2000 Hz tone burst presented in alternating polarity at 80 dB HL. Action potential (*AP*) and its first negative peak (*N_1*) are seen at the onset of the response. Summating potential (*SP*) persists as long as the stimulus. SP amplitude is measured at midpoint of response (*point B*), with reference to a baseline value (*point A*). Amplitude (microvolts)/time (milli-seconds) scale at lower right (Ferraro, Blackwell et al [1994], p. 19).

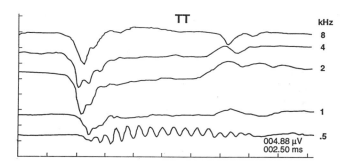

TT

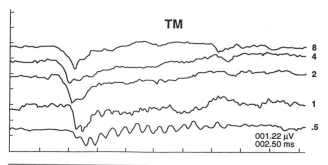

TM

Figure 18–9 ECochGms evoked by tone bursts of different frequencies presented at 80 dB HL. Stimulus frequency in kHz indicated at the right of each waveform. Amplitude (microvolts)/time (milliseconds) scale at lower right (Ferraro, Blackwell et al [1994], p. 20).

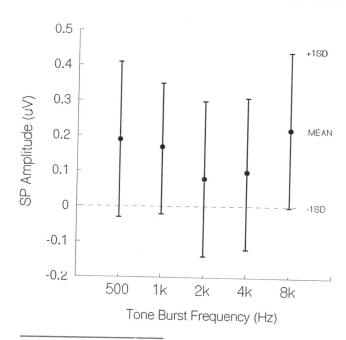

Figure 18–10 Mean summating potential (*SP*) amplitudes measured from the tympanic membrane of 20 normal ears as a function of tone burst frequency. Bars represent ± 1 standard deviation (*SD*). Stimulus level was 80 dB HL (Ferraro, Blackwell et al [1994], p. 21).

hearing subjects are plotted as a function of tone burst frequency. All mean values are slightly positive and range between 0.10 and 0.22 μV. Standard deviations (indicated by the bars) are comparatively large and range from 0.18 to 0.22 across frequencies.

CLINICAL APPLICATIONS

Meniere's Disease/Endolymphatic Hydrops

Although much has been learned about MD (or idiopathic ELH) since its initial description in the literature more than 135 years ago (Meniere, 1861), the true pathophysiology of this disorder(s) continues to elude us. As a result, neither a cure nor an effective treatment strategy that works for all patients has been developed. The symptoms on which the diagnosis of MD/ELH is based include recurrent, spontaneous vertigo, hearing loss, aural fullness, and tinnitus (Committee on Hearing and Equilibrium, 1995). However, the presence and severity of these symptoms tend to vary over time both among and within patients. The capricious nature of this disorder makes it difficult to diagnose and evaluate with a high degree of specificity and/or sensitivity.

As mentioned earlier in this chapter, ECochG has emerged as one of the more powerful tools in the diagnosis, assessment, and monitoring of MD/ELH, primarily through the measurement of the SP and AP. Examples of this application are shown in Figures 18–11 and 18–12 (Ferraro, Thedinger et al, 1994) and Figure 18–13 (Ferraro, 1993). The upper tracings in both Figures 18–11 (click-evoked ECochGms) and 18–12 (tone burst-evoked ECochGms) were measured from the promontory (TT), whereas the lower waveforms represent TM recordings. Figure 18–13 displays TM tracings to tone bursts from the right (affected) and left (unaffected) sides of an MD/ELH patient. For the click-evoked ECochGms in Figure 18–11, the SP/AP amplitude ratios (on the basis of

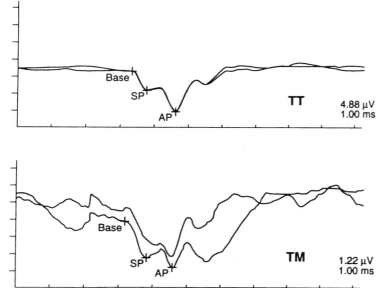

Figure 18–11 Abnormal responses to clicks recorded from the promontory (*TT*) and tympanic membrane (*TM*) of the affected ear of the same patient. Both TT and TM responses display an enlarged summating potential (*SP*)/action potential (*AP*) amplitude ratio, which is a positive finding for endolymphatic hydrops. "Base" indicates reference for SP and AP amplitude measurements. Amplitude (microvolts)/ time (milliseconds) scale at lower right. Stimulus onset delayed by approximately 2 ms (Ferraro, Thedinger et al [1994], p. 27).

absolute SP and AP amplitudes) were approximately 1.0 and 2.0 for the TT and TM recordings, respectively. Both values are enlarged beyond the normal limits. Thus despite different recording approaches that led to different values for the SP/AP amplitude ratio, both TT and TM ECochGms were positive for MD/ELH. Also notable in Figure 18–11 is the instability of the TM waveforms' baseline voltages compared with those of the TT recordings. As mentioned previously, this instability is the reason some clinicians prefer to measure absolute as opposed to baseline-referenced component amplitudes. Had the SP and AP amplitudes been measured with respect to a baseline voltage, SP/AP amplitude ratios would have been approximately 0.50 (TT) and 0.75 (TM).

As mentioned earlier in this chapter, the SP/AP amplitude ratio is a more consistent feature across and within subjects than the individual amplitudes of either component (Eggermont, 1976). Coats (1986), however, noted that this ratio does not represent a simple linear relationship. In normal patients, for example, fourfold increases in AP amplitude may be accompanied by twofold decreases in SP amplitude. This relationship is illustrated in Figure 18–14 (Coats, 1986), wherein SP amplitudes have been normalized to AP amplitudes to derive the 95% confidence interval of normal values (dashed line). Any SP/AP amplitude ratio above the confidence interval is considered to be abnormal.

SP amplitudes for the tone burst ECochGms in Figure 18–12 vary slightly across frequencies. However, a pronounced SP trough is seen at all frequencies and in all tracings, once again regardless of recording approach. It also should be noted for tone burst responses that the measurement of interest is the magnitude of the SP trough rather than the SP/AP amplitude ratio. Indeed, the AP component to tone bursts may not even be visible in the face of an abnormally enlarged SP. As shown in Figure 18–13, enlargement of the SP trough can be even more dramatic when the affected and unaffected sides are displayed together.

The reported incidence of an enlarged SP and SP/AP amplitude ratio in the general population with Meniere's disease is only approximately 60% to 65% (Coats, 1981; Gibson et al,

1977; Kitahara et al, 1981; Kumagami et al, 1982). This situation makes the diagnostic usefulness of ECochG somewhat questionable, particularly for patients whose symptoms are not "classic" and for whom the clinical profile is unclear (Campbell et al, 1992). Thus, researchers continue to seek ways to improve the sensitivity of ECochG (i.e., the percentage of patients with MD/ELH who display ECochGms that are positive for this disorder).

One way to make ECochG more sensitive is to test patients when they are experiencing symptoms of MD/ELH. Ferraro et al (1985) found positive ECochGms in more than 90% of patients who were symptomatic at the time of testing and whose symptoms included aural fullness and hearing loss. Unfortunately, the practicality of testing patients when they are symptomatic is questionable given the fluctuating nature of the disorder, especially in its early stages. In addition, many patients are unwilling or unable to complete an examination during a vertiginous attack.

Other approaches to increasing the sensitivity of ECochG have been directed toward the parameters associated with recording and interpreting the ECochGm. An example of such a method involves measuring the AP-N_1 latency difference between responses to condensation versus rarefaction clicks (as described earlier in this chapter). Figure 18–15 from Margolis et al (1995) exemplifies this procedure. The AP-N_1 latency difference (LD) between clicks of opposite polarity for this patient with MD/ELH was 0.75 ms. The upper limit of the LD in normal subjects from this study was 0.38 ms. The basis for comparing AP-N_1 latencies to clicks of opposite polarity relates to changes in the velocity of the traveling wave in an endolymph-loaded cochlea. That is, the up and down movement of the cochlear partition under such conditions may be abnormally restricted (or enhanced) in one direction over the other. If this condition occurs, the velocity of the traveling wave (on which the AP-N_1 latency is dependent) will differ if the initial movement of the cochlear partition is upward (as with rarefaction clicks) versus downward (as with condensation clicks).

Another interesting feature in Figure 18–15 is that the AP-N_1 latency difference is obscured when responses to rarefaction

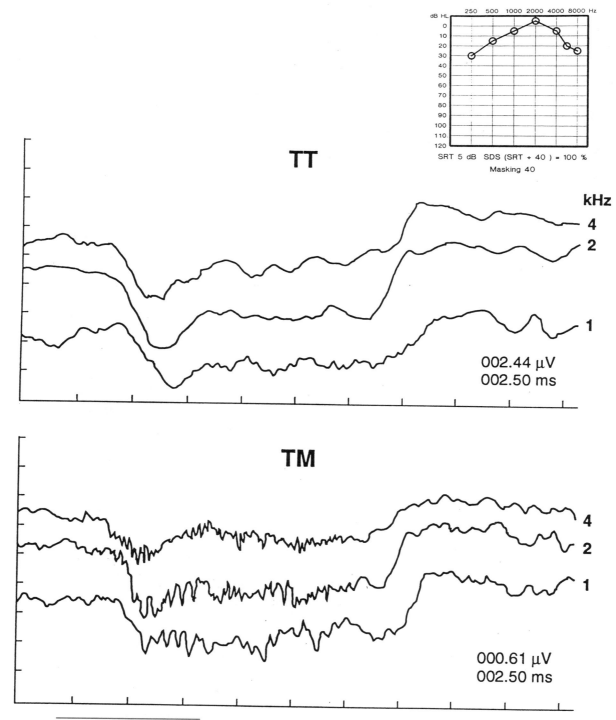

Figure 18–12   Abnormal responses to tone bursts recorded from the promontory (*TT*) and tympanic membrane (*TM*) of the affected ear of the same patient. All tracings show an enlarged summating potential trough which is a positive finding for endolymphatic hydrops. Tone burst frequency in kHz indicated at the right of each tracing. Amplitude (microvolts)/time (milliseconds) scale at lower right. Pure tone audiogram at upper right (Ferraro, Thedinger et al [1994], p. 26).

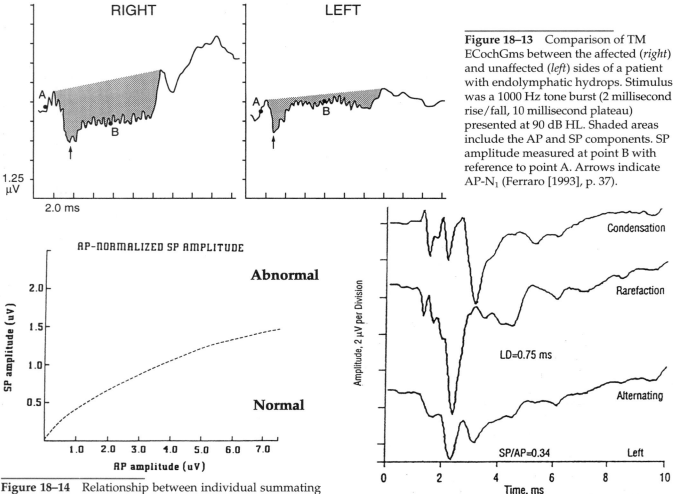

Figure 18–13 Comparison of TM ECochGms between the affected (*right*) and unaffected (*left*) sides of a patient with endolymphatic hydrops. Stimulus was a 1000 Hz tone burst (2 millisecond rise/fall, 10 millisecond plateau) presented at 90 dB HL. Shaded areas include the AP and SP components. SP amplitude measured at point B with reference to point A. Arrows indicate AP-N$_1$ (Ferraro [1993], p. 37).

Figure 18–14 Relationship between individual summating potential (*SP*) and action potential (*AP*) amplitudes to click stimuli. Dashed line represents 95% confidence limit for normal SP/AP amplitude ratio (Ferraro & Ruth [1994], p. 112, adapted from Coats [1986]).

Figure 18–15 ECochGm from a Meniere's patient evoked with condensation (*top tracing*) and rarefaction (*middle tracing*) polarity clicks. The latency difference of 0.75 ms between AP-N$_1$ components is a positive finding for endolymphatic hydrops since it is greater than 0.38 ms. This feature is obscured if the condensation and rarefaction tracings are combined to derive the response to alternating clicks (*bottom tracing*) (Margolis et al [1995], p. 52).

and condensation clicks are combined (lowest tracing), which is analogous to presenting clicks in alternating polarity. What appears instead is an SP-AP complex that looks to be abnormally wide or prolonged. This latter finding is not new, in that Morrison et al (1980) reported a widening of the SP-AP duration in patients with Meniere's disease almost 20 years ago. Prolongation of the complex was attributed to an "after-ringing" of the CM caused by ELH. In light of more recent studies, however, it may be more likely that differences in AP-N$_1$ latency to condensation versus rarefaction clicks produced what appeared to be a widened SP-AP complex to the alternating clicks used by Morrison et al (1990).

Even though the underlying mechanisms may be unclear, the preceding studies suggest that the duration of the SP-AP complex may be important to consider in the interpretation of the ECochGm. Ferraro and Tibbils (1997) explored this notion by combining both amplitude and duration features of the response to measure the "areas" of the SP and AP.

Figure 18–16 displays representative tracings from this study. The waveforms in the left panel are from a normal subject, whereas the right tracings are from a patient suspected of having MD/ ELH. The shaded portions of the top tracings in both panels represent the SP area, which was defined by the onset of the SP (baseline) and that point in the tracing where the waveform returned to the baseline amplitude. It should be noted that despite the label this measurement included the areas of components other than the SP (such as the AP-N$_1$, and often -N$_2$). The shaded portions of the lower tracings represent the area of the AP-N$_1$. The results from this study revealed that patients with MD/ELH with enlarged SP/AP amplitude ratios also have enlarged SP/AP area ratios. However, enlarged area ratios also were seen in several patients suspected of having MD/ELH, but whose SP/AP amplitude

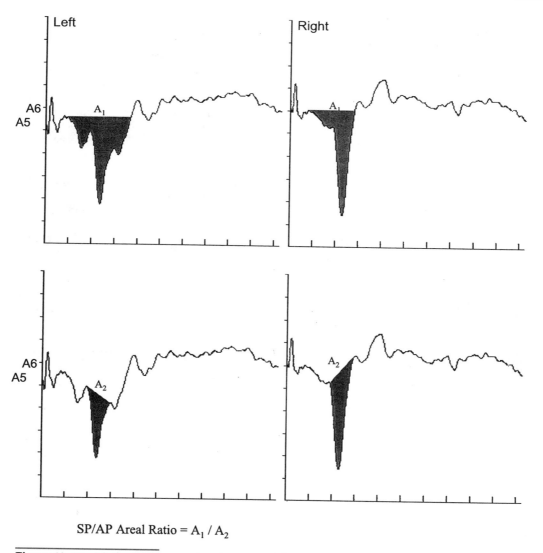

SP/AP Areal Ratio = A_1 / A_2

Figure 18–16   Method for measuring the areas of the summating potential (*SP*) and action potential (*AP*) to click stimuli to derive the SP/AP area ratio. Shaded portions represent the area of each component. ECochGm in the left panel is from a normal subject. ECochGm in the right panel is from a patient suspected of having Meniere's disease and displays an enlarged SP area (and SP/AP area ratio).

ratio was within normal limits. These findings suggest that use of the SP/AP area ratio may improve the sensitivity of ECochG. Additional research using larger clinical populations and outcome measures is needed to verify this possibility and to assess whether any of the other approaches described (such as measurement of the AP-N_1 latency difference to clicks of opposite polarity) actually improve the diagnostic sensitivity of ECochG.

An important aspect regarding the use of ECochG in the evaluation of MD/ELH is the association between the results of an examination and the subsequent diagnosis and treatment of the patient. An outcome study was recently completed to examine this aspect (Murphy et al, 1997). Chi-square analysis was applied to a database established from 103 patients referred for ECochG to help diagnose or rule out MD/ELH. As shown in Table 18–3, 50 patients from this study had negative

TABLE 18–3   ECochG outcome vs. diagnosis of MD/ELH for 103 patients

	Negative Diagnosis	Positive Diagnosis	Total
Negative ECochGm:	26	24	50
Positive ECochGm:	2	51	53
Total:	28	75	103

ECochGms, but only 26 of these individuals received a negative diagnosis for MD/ELH. The remaining 24 patients received positive diagnoses despite the ECochGm. This finding translates to a sensitivity factor (or true positive rate) for ECochG of 68%. On the other hand, 51 of the 53 patients who had positive ECochGms received positive diagnoses for MD/ELH. The specificity factor (true negative rate) derived from this finding is approximately 93%. The results from this outcome study simply help to confirm empirical observations from several other studies. Namely, ECochG is a fairly sensitive, yet highly specific, tool in the evaluation of MD/ELH.

PEARL

Enlarged SP/AP amplitude ratios also have been reported for perilymphatic fistulas (Ackley et al, 1994; Kobayashi et al, 1993). Thus the fluid pressure of the scala media may be the underlying feature to which ECochG is specific. Overpressure in the scala media, in turn, may be caused by ELH or underpressure in the scalae vestibuli and/or tympani (as in a fistula).

Enhancement of Wave I

Identification of waves I, III, and V and the subsequent measurement of the I to III, I to V and III to V interwave intervals (IWIs) are crucial to the interpretation of the ABR, especially in the diagnosis of retrocochlear disorders. However, when the ABR is recorded conventionally with surface electrodes on the scalp and earlobes (or mastoid processes), wave I is among the first components to disappear as stimulus intensity is lowered from suprathreshold levels (Fria, 1980; Schwartz & Berry, 1985). In hard of hearing subjects, including those with acoustic tumors, wave I may be reduced, distorted, or absent, despite the presence of an identifiable wave V (Cashman & Rossman, 1983; Hyde & Blair, 1981). This situation significantly reduces the diagnostic usefulness of the ABR because the I to V and III to V IWIs are immeasurable. Under all the preceding and other "less than optimal" recording conditions (e.g., noisy electrical and/or acoustical environment, restless subject), simultaneous recording of the AP-N_1 through ECochG and the ABR has been shown to be very beneficial (Ferraro & Ferguson, 1989; Ferraro & Ruth, 1994). Specifically, the amplitude of the AP-N_1 (or wave I) recorded from the TM is larger across intensities than corresponding amplitudes measured from the mastoid process or earcanal Figure 18–17 (Ferraro & Ferguson, 1989) displays TM-ECochG (left panel) and ABR (right panel) recordings from a normally hearing individual. The electrode array for ECochG is vertex (+)-to-TM (−), which displays the AP-N_1 as a positive peak in accordance with the conventional display of the ABR. The filter bandpass for ECochG also is conventional to the ABR (i.e., 100 to 3000 Hz) because the SP is not of interest. Corresponding amplitude scales highlight the disparity in magnitudes between ECochG and ABR components. Of particular importance, however, is that the visual detection thresholds of N_1 and wave V are the same (16 dB nHL), whereas wave I in the ABR becomes poorly defined at 46 dB nHL, and is absent at 26 dB nHL. Figure 18–18 from the same study applies the combined

ECochG-ABR approach to a clinical situation. Wave I is absent in the presence of wave V in the conventionally recorded ABR for this hard of hearing patient (top tracings). However, when the ABR is recorded with a vertex (+)-to-TM (−) electrode array (bottom tracings), N_1 is identifiable, permitting the measurement of the N_1 to V IWI. The mean value for the conventionally-recorded I to V IWI in our laboratory is 4.0 ms, and our normal range extends from 3.5 to 4.5 ms. In the face of high-frequency hearing loss, however, we have observed slightly shorter I to V IWIs because the absolute latency of wave I appears to be more delayed than the wave V latency as a result of the loss. In addition, the second component of N_1 (which is analogous to N_2 or wave II) becomes dominant at low stimulus levels. These observations indicate that the upper limit of the I to V IWI established from normal listeners may not apply to patients with significant hearing loss, including those with retrocochlear lesions. These individuals are the very ones for whom the combined ECochG-ABR approach would be applicable. Additional research using the combined approach in hard of hearing patients with and without retrocochlear lesions is needed to address this issue.

Intraoperative Monitoring

Intraoperative monitoring of inner ear and auditory nerve status during surgeries that involve the peripheral auditory system has become an important application for ECochG. Such monitoring usually is done to help the surgeon avoid potential trauma to the ear/nerve in an effort to preserve hearing (Ferraro & Ruth, 1994; Lambert & Ruth, 1988). In addition, intraoperative ECochG recordings may be helpful in the identification of anatomical landmarks (such as the endolymphatic sac) (Gibson & Arenberg, 1991). Finally, ECochG monitoring has been examined as a method to help predict postoperative outcome, especially for patients undergoing endolymphatic decompression/shunt surgery for the treatment of MD/ELH (Arenberg et al, 1993; Gibson & Arenberg, 1991; Gibson et al, 1988; Mishler et al, 1994; Wazen, 1994). Examples of the preceding applications for intraoperative ECochG monitoring are presented in the following.

Hearing Preservation

Figure 18–19 (Musiek et al, 1994) illustrates a series of intraoperative ECochGms recorded from a patient undergoing vestibular neurectomy for treatment of intractable vertigo. These responses were measured from the promontory and also include ABR components. The presence of the AP throughout the surgery indicates that hearing was preserved during the procedure, which was verified postoperatively. Combining both ECochG and ABR measures also allows for monitoring auditory brain stem status in addition to cochlear/auditory nerve function.

Figure 18–20 (Gibson & Arenberg, 1991) displays serial tracings from an ear in which a cochleostomy was performed, also for treatment of intractable vertigo. In this example the AP disappeared when the cochlear duct was opened, which was predictive of the patient's total loss of hearing greater than 2 to 3 kHz after surgery.

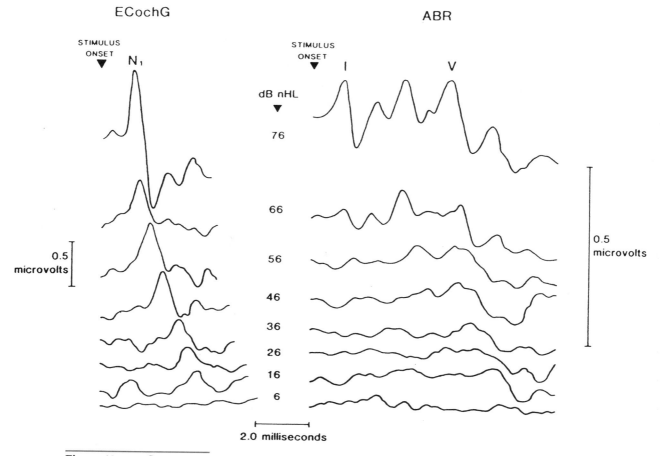

Figure 18–17 Comparison between AP-N$_1$ recorded from the TM (*left tracings*) and conventional ABR (*right tracings*) in a normally hearing subject. Note the disparity between ECochG and ABR amplitude scales which illustrates how much larger the TM recordings were. Threshold of N$_1$ and wave V are the same (between 16- and 6-dB nHL). Wave I in the conventional ABR disappears between 36- and 26-dB nHL (Ferraro & Ferguson [1989], p. 163).

On the basis of a review of recent literature, three important questions should be considered regarding the use of ECochG (and other AEP) intraoperative monitoring for the purpose of preserving hearing. First, will trauma to the ear be reflected in the ECochGm? Evidence from several studies (including the example in Figure 18–20) is ample that the answer to this question is yes. Second, are changes in the ECochGm that reflect trauma to the ear reversible? That is, if the ear is damaged as indicated by the ECochGm, can the surgical approach be altered in time to correct or at least mitigate the problem? The answer to this question is "not always" because the auditory nerve is very unforgiving. It is not unusual to lose the AP (and hearing) very rapidly, especially when the surgical field includes the cochlear blood supply (such as during the removal of an acoustic neuroma). Animal studies have shown that cessation of cochlear blood flow completely abolishes the AP within 30- to 45-seconds (Perlman et al, 1959). When this situation occurs, ECochG monitoring to preserve hearing is akin to locking the gate after the horse has left the corral Because time is of the essence in such situations, direct nerve opposed to far field, signal-averaged monitoring should be applied.

The third question to consider regarding intraoperative monitoring to preserve hearing is whether the surgical approach can be altered at all if the ECochGm indicates trauma to the ear. The answer to this question is once again "not always." During acoustic tumor removal, for example, it may be that complete resection of the tumor is not possible without compromising the nerve. Thus hearing may be lost regardless of monitoring.

The preceding questions are not posed to discourage the use of intraoperative ECochG monitoring to preserve/protect hearing. Rather, they are presented merely as issues to consider when applying the procedure.

Identification of Anatomical Landmarks

Although controversial in its own right, decompression or shunting of the endolymphatic sac is an option for patients who have nonsurgical approaches for treatment of MD/ELH fail. During such surgeries, instantaneous measurements of the mechanoelectrical processes of the inner ear can be achieved by means of ECochG. As described above, these measurements can alert the surgeon to imminent damage to the

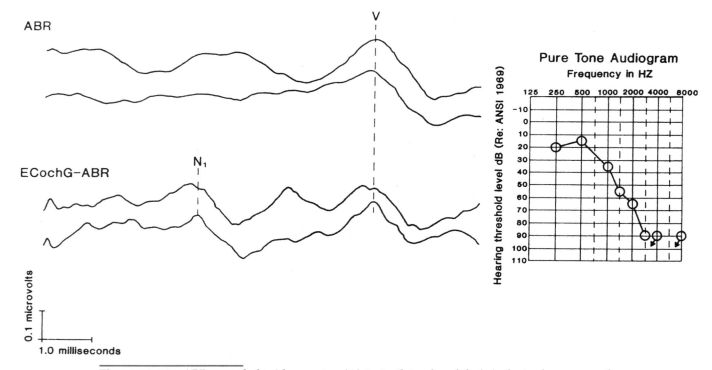

Figure 18–18 ABR recorded with a vertex (+)-to-ipsilateral earlobe(−) electrode array, and ECochG-ABR recorded with a vertex(+)-to-ipsilateral tympanic membrane(−) electrode array from a patient with hearing loss (*audiogram at right*). Wave I is absent in the conventional ABR tracings, whereas N_1 is recordable with the ECochG-ABR approach (Ferraro & Ferguson [1989], p. 165).

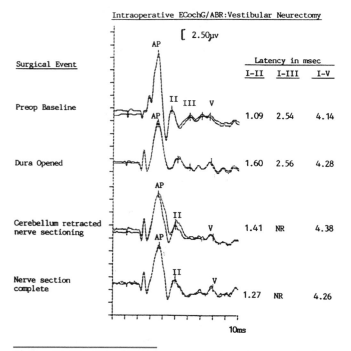

Figure 18–19 ECochGms measured at various events during vestibular neurectomy surgery. ABR components also are visible. Preservation of all components throughout surgery indicates preservation of the cochlear nerve (Musiek et al [1994], p. 369).

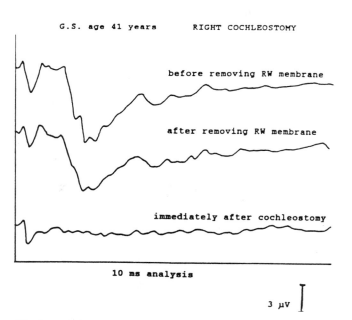

Figure 18–20 ECochGms measured during cochleostomy surgery involving removal of the round window (*RW*) membrane. All components disappeared immediately after puncturing the cochlear duct (Gibson & Arenberg [1993], pg. 299).

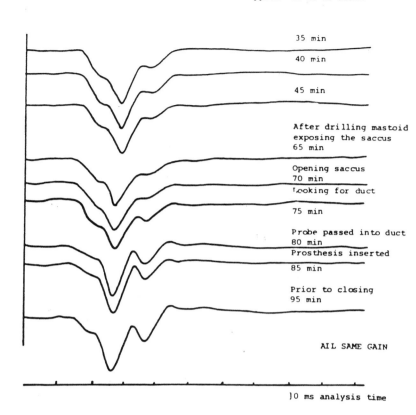

A.T.   Approx 80 dB HL Click

35 min

40 min

45 min

After drilling mastoid
exposing the saccus
65 min

Opening saccus
70 min

Looking for duct

75 min

Probe passed into duct
80 min

Prosthesis inserted

85 min

Prior to closing
95 min

ALL SAME GAIN

]0 ms analysis time

Figure 18–21   ECochGms measured at various events during endolymphatic sac surgery. "Probe passed into duct" tracing shows a reduction in the summating potential. This alteration helped to differentiate the location of the endolymphatic duct from surrounding tissue (Gibson & Arenberg [1993], p. 300).

cochlea. However, identifying the endolymphatic sac with certainty is not an easy task, especially in MD when congenital abnormalities and unusual anatomical variations may be present (Arenberg, 1980). As indicated in Figure 18–21 (Gibson & Arenberg, 1991), ECochG may be helpful in these situations. The uppermost tracings display an enlarged SP and SP/AP amplitude ratio. However, the SP becomes smaller and remains that way after a metal probe is passed into the endolymphatic duct (bottom three tracings). Probing of surrounding tissue did not alter the ECochGm.

SPECIAL CONSIDERATION

Both reduction and abolition of ECochG and ABR components can occur during surgical retraction of the nerve/brain stem/cerebellum that recovers when the retractor(s) is repositioned or removed. Thus disappearance of the AP may not always be indicative of hearing loss.

Prediction of Postoperative Outcome

As indicated, several recent studies have shown that intraoperative monitoring of ECochG may be helpful in predicting the postoperative status of patients. Figures 18–19 and 18–20 represent examples of this application. That is, maintenance of the AP during surgery is predictive of postoperative preservation of hearing, whereas disappearance of the AP indicates that some, if not all, hearing may be lost. This latter occurrence should be interpreted very cautiously.

Another feature of the ECochGm that has been used to predict postoperative outcome is changes in the SP/AP amplitude ratio during endolymphatic sac surgery. Reductions in the ratio when the sac is open or shunted are interpreted as predictive of successful outcome (i.e, improvement in symptoms including hearing status). However, the long-term predictive value of intraoperative ECochG (or ECochG in general) remains questionable. Figure 18–22 displays selected tracings measured from a patient undergoing endolymphatic shunt decompression surgery. A noticeable reduction in the SP/AP amplitude ratio to click stimuli and the SP amplitude to tone bursts were observed when the sac was decompressed. Likewise, this patient reported an improvement in symptoms after surgery. Figure 18–23 displays the intraoperative ECochGm from another patient. In this example, the SP amplitude and SP/AP amplitude ratio remained enlarged throughout surgery. Yet this patient, too, reported considerable improvement in symptoms after surgery.

Many of the statements found in the literature regarding the predictive value of intraoperative ECochG monitoring are based on anecdotal observations. Long-term studies that include a comparison of preoperative, perioperative, and postoperative data (ECochG and other tests) are needed to fully assess this application.

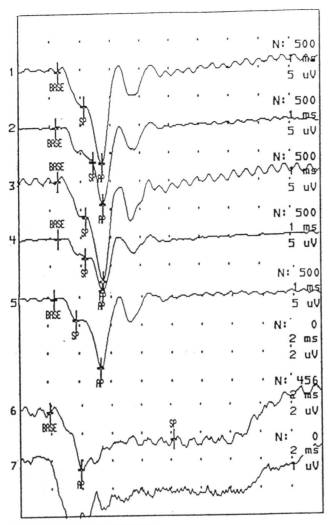

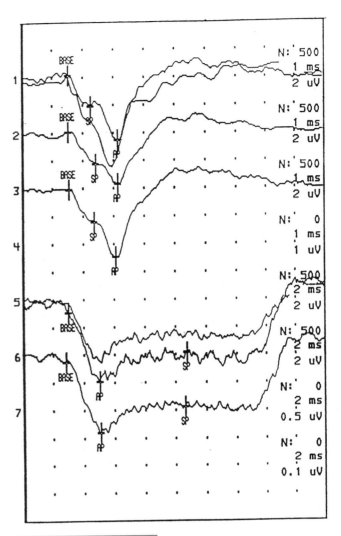

Figure 18–22 ECochGms recorded during endolymphatic shunt surgery. Baseline tracing (*1*), drilling on mastoid (*2*), probing for endolymphatic duct (*3*), inserting prosthesis (*4*), closing (*5*). Tracing 5 shows a reduction in the summating potential (*SP*)/action potential (*AP*) amplitude ratio compared to tracing 1. Tracings 1 to 5 are in response to clicks, whereas tracings 6 to 7 were recorded to tone bursts at the onset of surgery. This patient reported improvement in symptoms following surgery.

Figure 18–23 ECochGms recorded to clicks (*tracings 1 to 4*), and 2000 Hz tone bursts (*5 to 7*) during endolymphatic shunt surgery. Summating potential (*SP*)/action potential (*AP*) amplitude ratio remained enlarged throughout surgery, yet this patient also reported improvement in symptoms post-operatively.

CONTROVERSIAL POINT

Can intraoperative ECochG monitoring be used to predict patient outcome after surgery? In my experience, ECochG is more analogous to a "thermometer" than a "barometer" of inner ear function. That is, ECochG reflects the acute status of the ear at the time of testing but is not necessarily predictive of long-term cochlear/auditory nerve function.

Other Applications

As indicated in the introductory section of this chapter, the three most popular applications for ECochG are evaluation of MD/ELH, identification of wave I, and intraoperative monitoring. However, other uses, such as estimation of hearing thresholds, have been reported. Laureano et al (1995), for example, found significant correlation between AP and behavioral thresholds to mid- to high-frequency tone bursts. As described earlier, Ferraro and Ferguson (1989) found no differences between TM-recorded AP and conventionally recorded wave V thresholds in normally hearing individuals. Wave V threshold, of course, often is used to estimate hearing sensitivity in infants and other difficult-to-test populations.

Despite the studies mentioned previously, it is unlikely that ECochG will emerge as a "tool of choice" for estimating hearing sensitivity. In most cases other electrophysiological and behavioral approaches that tend to be more accurate, less time-consuming, and easier to administer are available. This is not to say, however, that the relationship between ECochG and hearing status should not continue to be studied. Lilly (Personal communication, 1997), for example, has reported on the usefulness of ECochG for estimating hearing reserve in cochlear implant candidates. Schoonhoven et al (1995) found a relationship between the slopes of AP input-output functions measured from the TM and cochlear recruitment. Keith et al (1992) used ECochG to assess the integrity of the inner ear before stapedectomy surgery in a patient who was unable to be tested behaviorally.

CONCLUSIONS

In summary the evaluation of inner ear and auditory nerve function by means of ECochG continues to be useful for a variety of clinical applications. This basic premise persists in the face of continued controversy regarding how ECochG is recorded, interpreted, and applied. Increased attention to resolving these controversies and to expanding current applications is apparent in the recent literature, and these efforts bode well for the future of ECochG. It truly is the case that ECochG provides a window through which the physiology and pathophysiology of the human auditory periphery can be studied in the laboratory, clinic, and operating room. We may not yet fully understand what we are seeing through this window or even how or where to look. However, the key to unlocking these mysteries most certainly involves our ability to make the window larger and our resolve to continue looking through it.

REFERENCES

ACKLEY, R.S., FERRARO, J.A., & ARENBERG, I.K. (1994). Diagnosis of patients with perilymphatic fistula. *Seminars in Hearing, 15;*37–41.

AMERICAN SPEECH-LANGUAGE-HEARING ASSOCIATION. (1988). The short latency auditory evoked potentials: A tutorial paper by the Working Group on Auditory Evoked Potential Measurements of the Committee on Audiologic Evaluation.

ANDREEV, A.M., AROPOVA, A.A., & GERSUNI, S.V. (1939). On electrical properties in the human cochlea. *Journal of Physiology USSR, 22;*206–212.

ARAN, J.M., & LEBERT, G. (1968). Les responses nerveuse cochleaires chex l'homme, image du fonctionnement de l'oreille et nouveau test d'audiometrie objectif. *Revue de Laryngologie, Otologie, Rhinologie (Bordeaux), 89;*361–365.

ARENBERG, I.K. (1980). Abnormalities, congenital abnormalities and unusual anatomic variations of the endolymphatic sac and vestibular aqueduct: Clinical, surgical and radiographic correlations. *American Journal of Otology, 2;*118–149.

ARENBERG, I.K., GIBSON, W.P.R., & BOHLEN, H.K.H. (1993). Improvements in audiometric and electrophysiologic parameters following nondestructive inner ear surgery utilizing a valved shunt for hydrops and Meniere's disease. *Proceedings of the Sixth Annual Workshops on Electrocochleography and Otoacoustic Emissions* (pp. 545–561). International Meniere's Disease Research Institute.

ARSENAULT, M.D., & BENITEZ, J.T. (1991). Electrocochleography: A method for making the Stypulkowski-Staller electrode and testing technique. *Ear and Hearing, 12;*358–360.

ASO, S., WATANABE, Y., & MIZUKOSHI, K. (1991). A clinical study of electrocochleography in Meniere's disease. *Acta Otolaryngologica (Stockholm), 111;*44–52.

BERLIN, C.I. (1986). Electrocochleography: An historical overview. *Seminars in Hearing, 7;*241–246.

BIAN, L., & CHERTOFF, M. (1998). Similar hearing loss, different physiology: Characterizing cochlear transduction in pure tone or salicylate damaged ears. *Abstracts of the Twenty-First Midwinter Research Meeting of the Association for Research in Otolaryngology,* p. 84 (A #334).

CAMPBELL, K.C.M., HARKER, L.A., & ABBAS, P.J. (1992). Interpretation of electrocochleography in Meniere's disease and normal subjects. *Annals of Otology, Rhinology, and Laryngology, 101;*496–500.

CASHMAN, M., & ROSSMAN, R. (1983). Diagnostic features of the auditory brain stem response in identifying cerebellopontine angle tumors. *Scandinavian Audiology, 12;*35–41.

COATS, A.C. (1981). The summating potential and Meniere's disease. *Archives of Otolaryngology, 104;*199–208.

COATS, A.C. (1986). Electrocochleography: Recording technique and clinical applications. *Seminars in Hearing, 7;*247–266.

COATS, A.C., & DICKEY, J.R. (1970). Non-surgical recording of human auditory nerve action potentials and cochlear microphonics. *Annals of Otology, Rhinology, and Laryngology, 29;*844–851.

COMMITTEE ON HEARING AND EQUILIBRIUM. (1995). Committee on Hearing and Equilibrium guidelines for the diagnosis and evaluation of therapy in Meniere's disease. *Otolaryngology–Head and Neck Surgery, 113;*181–185.

CULLEN, J.K., ELLIS, M.S., BERLIN, C.I., & LOUSTEAU, R.J. (1972). Human acoustic nerve action potential recordings from the tympanic membrane without anesthesia. *Acta Otolaryngologica, 74;*15–22.

DALLOS, P. (1973). *The auditory periphery: Biophysics and physiology* (pp. 218–381). New York: Academic Press.

DALLOS, P. (1997). Outer hair cells: The inside story. *American Academy of Audiology 9th Annual Convention Program,* p. 70 (A).

DALLOS, P., SCHOENY, Z.G., & CHEATHAM, M.A. (1972). Cochlear summating potentials: Descriptive aspects. *Acta Otolaryngologica, 301*(Suppl.),1–46.

DAUMAN, R., ARAN, J.M., SAUVAGE, R.C., & PORTMANN, M. (1988). Clinical significance of the summating potential in Meniere's disease. *American Journal of Otology, 9;*31–38.

DAVIS, H. (1968). Mechanisms of the inner ear. *Annals of Otology, Rhinology, and Laryngology, 77;*644–656.

DAVIS, H., FERNANDEZ, C., & MCAULIFFE, D.R. (1950). The excitatory process in the cochlea. *Proceedings of the National Academy of Science, 36;*580–587.

Densert, B., Arlinger, S., & Herglis, L. (1994). Reproducibility of the electric response components in clinical electrocochleography. *Laryngoscope, 33;*254–263.

Durrant, J.D. (1981). Auditory physiology and an auditory physiologist's view of tinnitus. *Journal of Laryngology and Otology, 4*(Suppl.),21–28.

Durrant, J.D. (1986). Combined ECochG-ABR versus conventional ABR recordings. *Seminars in Hearing, 7;*289–305.

Durrant, J.D. (1990). Extratympanic electrode support via vented earmold. *Ear and Hearing, 11;*468–469.

Durrant, J.D., & Dallos, P. (1972). Influence of direct current polarization of the cochlear partition on the summating potential. *Journal of the Acoustical Society of America, 52;*542–552.

Durrant, J.D., & Ferraro, J.A. (1991). Analog model of human click-elicited SP and effects of high-pass filtering. *Ear and Hearing, 12;*144–148.

Durrant, J.D., & Gans, D. (1977). Biasing of the summating potentials. *Acta Otolaryngologica, 80;*13–18.

Eggermont, J.J. (1976). Summating potentials in electrocochleography: Relation to hearing disorders. In: R.J. Ruben, C. Elberling, & G. Salomon (Eds.). *Electrocochleography* (pp. 67–87). Baltimore, MD:University Park Press.

Engebretson, A.M., & Eldridge, D.H. (1968). Model for the nonlinear characteristics of cochlear potentials. *Journal of the Acoustical Society of America, 44;*548–554.

Evans, B., & Dallos, P. (1993). Sterocilia displacement induced somatic motility of cochlear outer hair cells. *Proceedings of the National Academy of Science (USA), 90;*8347–8351.

Ferraro, J.A. (1992). Electrocochleography: How, Part I. *Audiology Today, 4;*26–28.

Ferraro, J.A. (1993). Electrocochleography: Clinical applications. *Audiology Today, 5;*36–38.

Ferraro, J.A. (1997). *Laboratory exercises in auditory evoked potentials.* San Diego, CA: Singular Publishing Group, Inc.

Ferraro, J.A., Arenberg, I.K., & Hassanein, R.S. (1985) Electrocochleography and symptoms of inner ear dysfunction. *Archives of Otolaryngology, 111;*71–74.

Ferraro, J.A., Best, L.G., & Arenberg, I.K. (1983). The use of electrocochleography in the diagnosis, assessment and monitoring of endolymphatic hydrops. *Otolaryngology Clinics of North America, 16;*69–82.

Ferraro, J.A., Blackwell, W., Mediavilla, S.J., & Thedinger, B. (1994). Normal summating potential to tone bursts recorded from the tympanic membrane in humans. *Journal of the American Academy of Audiology, 5;*17–23.

Ferraro, J.A., & Ferguson, R. (1989). Tympanic ECochG and conventional ABR: A combined approach for the identification of wave I and the I–V interwave interval. *Ear and Hearing, 3;*161–166.

Ferraro, J.A., & Ferguson, R. (1991). A new TM electrode design. In: I.K. Arenberg (Ed.). *Proceedings of the Third International Symposium and Workshops on the Surgery of the Inner Ear* (pp. 253–256). Amsterdam: Kugler Publications.

Ferraro, J.A., & Krishnan, G. (1997). Cochlear potentials in clinical audiology. *Audiology and Neuro-Otology, 2;*241–256.

Ferraro, J.A., & Ruth, R.A. (1994). Electrocochleography. In: J.T. Jacobson (Ed.). *Auditory evoked potentials: Overview and basic principles.* (pp. 101–122). Boston, MA: Allyn & Bacon.

Ferraro, J.A., Thedinger, B., Mediavilla, S.J., & Blackwell, W. (1994). Human summating potential to tone bursts: Observations on TM versus promontory recordings in the same patient. *Journal of the American Academy of Audiology, 6;*217–224.

Ferraro, J.A., & Tibbils, R. (1997). SP/AP area ratio in the diagnosis of Meniere's disease. *Abstracts of the XV Biennial Symposium of the International Evoked Response Audiometry Study Group,* p. 13(A).

Fria, T. (1980). The auditory brain stem response: Background and clinical applications. *Monographs in Contemporary Audiology, 2;*1–44.

Fromm, B., Bylen, C.O., & Zotterman, Y. (1935). Studies in the mechanisms of Wever and Bray effect. *Acta Otolaryngologica, 22;*477–483.

Galambos, R., Rupert, A. (1959). Action of the middle ear muscles in normal cats. *Journal of the Acoustical Society of America, 31;*349–355.

Gerhardt, H.J., Wagner, H., & Werbs, M. (1985). Electrocochleography (ECochG) and brain stem evoked response recordings (BSER) in the diagnosis of acoustic neuromas. *Acta Otolaryngologica, 99;*384–386.

Gerhardt, K.J., Melnick, W., Ferraro, J.A. (1979). Reflex threshold shift in chinchillas following a prolonged exposure to noise. *Journal of Speech and Hearing Research, 22;*63–72.

Gibson, W.P.R. (1978). *Essentials of electric response audiometry.* New York: Churchill and Livingstone.

Gibson, W.P.R., & Arenberg, I.K. (1991). The scope of intraoperative electrocochleography. In: I.K. Arenberg (Ed.). *Proceedings of the Third International Symposium and Workshops on the Surgery of the Inner Ear* (pp. 295–303). Amsterdam: Kugler Publications.

Gibson, W.P.R., Arenberg, I.K., & Best, L.G. (1988). Intraoperative electrocochleographic parameters following nondestructive inner ear surgery utilizing a valved shunt for hydrops and Meniere's disease. In: J.G. Nadol (Ed.). *Proceedings of the Second International Symposium on Meniere's Disease* (pp. 170–171). Amsterdam: Kugler and Ghedini Publications.

Gibson, W.P.R., & Beagley, M.A. (1976). Transtympanic electrocochleography in the investigation of retrocochlear disorders. *Revue Laryngology, 97*(Suppl.),507–516.

Gibson, W.P.R., Moffat, D.A., & Ramsden, R.T. (1977). Clinical electrocochleography in the diagnosis and management of Meniere's disorder. *Audiology, 16;*389–401.

Goin, D.W., Staller, S.J., Asher, D.L., & Mischke, R.E. (1982). Summating potential in Meniere's disease. *Laryngoscope, 92;*1381–1389.

Guinan, J., & Peake, W. (1967). Middle-ear characteristics of anesthetized cats. *Journal of the Acoustical Society of America, 41;*1237–1261.

Gulick, W.L., Gescheider, G.A., & Frisina, R.D. (1989). *Hearing: Physiological acoustics, neural coding, and psychoacoustics.* New York: Oxford University Press.

Hyde, M.L., & Blair, R.L. (1981). The auditory brain stem response in neuro-otology: Perspectives and problems. *Journal of Otolaryngology, 10;*117–125.

Keith, R.W., Kereiakes, T.J., Willging, J.P., & Devine, J. (1992). Evaluation of cochlear function in a patient with 'far-advanced' otosclerosis. *American Journal of Otology, 13;*347–349.

KIANG, N.S. (1965). Discharge patterns of single nerve fibers in the cat's auditory nerve. *Research Monograph 35*. Cambridge, MA: MIT Press.

KITAHARA, M., TAKEDA, T., & YAZAMA, T. (1981). Electrocochleography in the diagnosis of Meniere's disease. In: K.H. Volsteen (Ed.). *Meniere's disease: Pathogenesis, diagnosis and treatment* (pp. 163–169). New York: Thieme-Stratton.

KOBAYASHI, H, ARENBERG, I.K., FERRARO, J.A., & VAN DER ARK, G. (1993). Delayed endolymphatic hydrops following acoustic tumor removal with intraoperative and postoperative auditory brain stem response improvements. *Acta Otolaryngologica (Stockholm)*, 504(Suppl.),74–78.

KOYUNCU, M., MASON, S.M., & SHINKWIN, C. (1994). Effect of hearing loss in electrocochleographic investigation of endolymphatic hydrops using tone-pip and click stimuli. *Journal of Laryngology and Otology*, 108;125–130.

KUMAGAMI, H., NISHIDA, H., & MASAAKI, B. (1982). Electrocochleographic study of Meniere's disease. *Archives of Otology*, 108;284–288.

LAMBERT, P., & RUTH, R.A. (1988). Simultaneous recording of noninvasive ECoG and ABR for use in intraoperative monitoring. *Otolaryngology–Head and Neck Surgery*, 98;575–580.

LAUREANO, A.N., MURRAY, D., McGRADY, M.D., & CAMPBELL, K.C.M. (1995). Comparison of tympanic membrane-recorded electrocochleography and the auditory brain stem response in threshold determination. *American Journal of Otology*, 16;209–215.

LEMPERT, J., MELTZER, P.E., WEVER, E.G., & LAWRENCE, M. (1950). The cochleogram and its clinical applications: Concluding observations. *Archives of Otolaryngology*, 51;307–311.

LEMPERT, J., WEVER, E.G., & LAWRENCE, M. (1947). The cochleogram and its clinical applications: A preliminary report. *Archives of Otolaryngology*, 45;61–67.

LEVINE, S.M., MARGOLIS, R.H., FOURNIER, E.M., & WINZENBURG, S.M. (1992). Tympanic electrocochleography for evaluation of endolymphatic hydrops. *Laryngoscope*, 102;614–622.

LILLY, D.J., & BLACK, F.O. (1989). Electrocochleography in the diagnosis of Meniere's disease. In: J.B. Nadol (Ed.). *Meniere's disease* (pp. 369–373). Berkeley, CA: Kugler and Ghedini.

LOPEZ, W., FERRARO, J.A., & CHERTOFF. M. (1993). Comparison between blind and visual electrode placement in tympanic electrocochleography. *ASHA*, 35;183(A).

MARCHBANKS, R. (1997). Why monitor perilymphatic pressure in Meniere's disease? *Acta Otolaryngologica (Stockholm)*, 526(Suppl.);27–29.

MARGOLIS, R.H., LEVINE, S.M., FOURNIER, M.A., HUNTER, L.L., SMITH, L.L., & LILLY, D.J. (1992). Tympanic electrocochleography: Normal and abnormal patterns of response. *Audiology*, 31;18–24.

MARGOLIS, R.H., & LILLY, D.J. (1989). Extratympanic electrocochleography: Stimulus considerations. *ASHA*, 31;183(A).

MARGOLIS, R.H., RIEKS, D., FOURNIER, M., & LEVINE, S.M. (1995). Tympanic electrocochleography for diagnosis of Meniere's disease. *Archives of Otolaryngology–Head and Neck Surgery*, 121;44–55.

MENIERE, P. (1861). Pathologic auriculaire. Memoire sur les lesions de l'oreille interne donnant lieu a des symptomes de congestion cerebrale applectiforme. *Gazzette Medicine*, 16;88–89.

MISHLER, E.T., LOOSMORE, J.L., HERZOG, J.A., SMITH, P.G., & KLETZKER, G.K. (1994). The efficacy of electrocochleography in monitoring endolymphatic shunt procedures. *Annual Meeting of the American Neuro-Otology Society*, p. 45(A).

MOLLER, A., & JANETTA, P. (1983). Monitoring auditory functions during cranial nerve microvascular decompression operations by direct monitoring from the eighth nerve. *Journal of Neurosurgery*, 59;493–499.

MORIUCHI, H., & KUMAGAMI, H. (1979). Changes of AP, SP and CM in experimental endolymphatic hydrops. *Audiology*, 22;258–260.

MORRISON, A.W., MOFFAT, D.A., & O'CONNOR, A.F. (1980). Clinical usefulness of electrocochleography in Meniere's disease: An analysis of dehydrating agents. *Otolaryngologic Clinics of North America*, 11;703–721.

MURPHY, L.A., FERRARO, J.A., CHERTOFF, M., McCALL, S., & PARK, D. (1997). Issues in auditory evoked potentials. *American Academy of Audiology Convention Program*, p. 64(A).

MUSIEK, F.E., BORENSTEIN, S.P., HALL, J.W. III, & SCHWABER, M.K. (1994). Auditory brain stem response: Neurodiagnostic and intraoperative applications. In: J. Katz (Ed.). *Handbook of clinical audiology* (4th ed.) (pp. 351–374). Baltimore, MD: Williams & Wilkins.

NORTON, S.J., FERGUSON, R., & MASCHER, K. (1989). Evoked otoacoustic emissions and extratympanic cochlear microphonics recorded from human ears. *Abstracts of the Twelfth Midwinter Research Meeting of the Association for Research in Otolaryngology*, p. 227(A).

ORCHIK, J.G., GE, X., & SHEA, J.J. (1997). Action potential latency shift by rarefaction and condensation clicks in Meniere's disease. *American Journal of Otology*, 14;290–294.

ORCKIK, D.J., SHEA, J.J. JR., & GE, X. (1993). Transtympanic electrocochleography in Meniere's disease using clicks and tone bursts. *American Journal of Otology*, 14;290–294.

PERLMAN, M.B., & CASE, T.J. (1941). Electrical phenomena of the cochlea in man. *Archives of Otolaryngology*, 34;710–718.

PERLMAN, M.B., KIMURA, R., & FERNANDEZ, C. (1959). Experiments on temporary obstruction of the internal auditory artery. *Laryngoscope*, 69;591–613.

PICTON, T.W., HILLYARD, S.H., FRAUZ, H.J., & GALAMBOS, R. (1974). Human auditory evoked potentials. *Electroencephalography and Clinical Neurophysiology*, 36;191–200.

ROLAND, P.S., ROSENBLOOM, J., YELLIN, W., & MEYERHOFF, W.I. (1993). Intrasubject test-retest variability in clinical electrocochleography. *Laryngoscope*, 103;963–966.

RUBEN, R., SEKULA, J., & BORDELY, J.E. (1960). Human cochlear responses to sound stimuli. *Annals of Otorhinolaryngology*, 69;459–476.

RUTH, R.A. (1990). Trends in electrocochleography. *Journal of the American Academy of Audiology*, 1;134–137.

RUTH, R.A. (1994). Electrocochleography. In: J. Katz (Ed.). *Handbook of clinical audiology* (4th ed.). (pp. 339–350). Baltimore: Williams & Wilkins.

RUTH, R.A., LAMBERT, P.R., & FERRARO, J.A. (1988). Electrocochleography: Methods and clinical applications. *American Journal of Otology*, 9;1–11.

SASS, K., DENSERT, B., & ARLINGER, S. (1997). Recording techniques for transtympanic electrocochleography in clinical practice. *Acta Otolaryngologica (Stockholm)*, 118;17–25.

SCHMIDT, P., EGGERMONT, J., & ODENTHAL, D. (1974). Study of Meniere's disease by electrocochleography. *Acta Otolaryngologica, 316*(Suppl.);75–84.

SCHOONHOVEN, R., FABIUS, M.A.W., & GROTE, J.J. (1995). Input/output curves to tone bursts and clicks in extratympanic and transtympanic electrocochleography. *Ear and Hearing, 16*;619–630.

SCHWARTZ, D.M., & BERRY, G.A. (1985). Normative aspects of the ABR. In: J.T. Jacobson (Ed.). *The auditory brain stem response* (pp. 65–97). San Diego, CA: College Hill Press.

SOHMER, H., & FEINMESSER, M. (1967). Cochlear action potentials recorded from the external canal in man. *Annals of Otology, Rhinology, and Otolaryngology, 76*;427–435.

SPOENDLIN, H. (1966). Organization of the cochlear receptor. *Advances in Otorhinolaryngology, 13*;1–227.

STALLER, S.J. (1986). Electrocochleography in the diagnosis and management of Meniere's disease. *Seminars in Hearing, 7*;267–278.

STAPELLS, D., PICTON, T.W., & SMITH, A.D. (1982). Normal-hearing thresholds for clicks. *Journal of the Acoustical Society of America, 72*;74–79.

STORMS, R.F., FERRARO, J.A., & THEDINGER, B. (1996). Electrocochleographic effects of earcanal pressure change in subjects with Meniere's disease. *American Journal of Otology, 17*;874–882.

STYPULKOWSKI, P.H., & STALLER, S.J. (1987). Clinical evaluation of a new ECoG recording electrode. *Ear and Hearing, 8*;304–310.

SUZUKI, J.F., & YAMANE, H. (1982). The choice of stimulus in the auditory brain stem response test for neurological and audiological examinations. *Annals of the New York Academy of Science, 388*;731–736.

TASAKI, I., DAVIS, H., & ELDRIDGE, D.H. (1954). Exploration of cochlear potentials in guinea pig with a microelectrode. *Journal of the Acoustical Society of America, 26*;765–773.

VON BEKESY, G. (1950). DC potentials and energy balance of the cochlear partition. *Journal of the Acoustical Society of America, 22*;576–582.

WAZEN, J.J. (1994). Intraoperative monitoring of auditory function: Experimental observation, and new applications. *Laryngoscope, 104*;446–455.

WEVER, E.G., & BRAY, C. (1930). Action currents in the auditory nerve response to acoustic stimulation. *Proceedings of the National Academy of Science, 16*;344–350.

WHITFIELD, I.C., & ROSS, H.F. (1965). Cochlear microphonic and summating potentials and the outputs of individual hair cell generators. *Journal of the Acoustical Society of America, 38*;126–131.

YOSHIE, N., OHASHI, T., & SUZUKI, T. (1967). Non-surgical recording of auditory nerve action potentials in man. *Laryngoscope, 77*;76–85.

## Chapter 19

The Auditory Brain Stem Response

Sally A. Arnold

The auditory brain stem response (ABR) is one component of the auditory evoked potentials (AEPs), which also include electrocochleography, the auditory middle latency response, and the auditory late response. The term *auditory evoked potential* refers to electrical activity of the auditory system that occurs in response to an appropriate acoustic stimulus. One way to classify the AEPs is according to their time of occurrence (latency) after onset of the eliciting stimulus. The ABR is the group of potentials occurring within the first 10 ms after the stimulus. The ABR has also been called the brain stem–evoked response (BSER), brain stem–auditory evoked potential (BAEP), and brain stem–auditory evoked response (BAER).

The existence of the ABR was first reported in 1967 (Sohmer & Feinmesser, 1967) and later explored in greater detail and attributed to the brain stem by Jewett and his colleagues in the early 1970s (Jewett & Williston, 1971; Jewett et al, 1970). Since that time, a tremendous amount of both basic and clinical research has been done concerning the ABR, and it has become a standard and valuable component of the audiological test battery.

GENERAL DESCRIPTION OF THE ABR

The ABR Waveform

The ABR consists of a series of seven positive-to-negative going waves, occurring within about 10 ms after stimulus onset. Several systems of nomenclature have been devised for labeling the individual waveform peaks of the ABR, but the most popular convention in the United States is to label the positive peaks with Roman numerals: waves I to VII. Wave I occurs about 1.5–2 ms after onset of the eliciting stimulus, depending on stimulus intensity, with the successive waves following at about 1- to 2-ms intervals. Figure 19–1 shows the ABR waveform recorded from a normal subject, using a high-intensity click stimulus (*click* is defined in a later section). Positive polarity is plotted in an upward direction. Two waveforms obtained under identical stimulus and recording conditions are shown. Note that the amplitude of the peaks are extremely small—<1μV. A desirable characteristic of the ABR is the high degree of repeatability between repetitions, as shown in this figure. The large negative deflection at the beginning of the waveform between 0–1 ms is stimulus artifact. This artifact can occur, particularly at high stimulus levels, because the earphones radiate electrical energy that may be picked up by the recording electrodes.

451

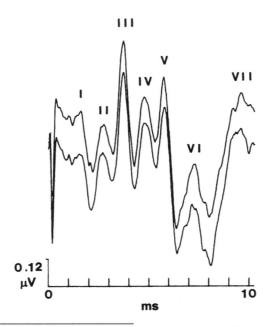

Figure 19–1   Two ABR waveforms, obtained from an adult subject using 80 dB nHL clicks. The individual waves of the ABR are labeled with Roman numbers I to VII.

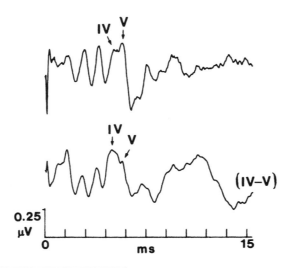

Figure 19–2   Examples of the "wave IV–V complex." In the top waveform, wave IV occurs as a shoulder on the wave V peak. In the bottom waveform, wave V appears as a shoulder on wave IV. Stimulus was 80 dB nHL clicks for both recordings.

The full complement of seven waves shown in Figure 19–1 is not always present in the ABR waveform. A normal variant is for waves II, VI, and especially VII to be absent. Also, the structure of waves IV and V varies considerably. These waves may occur separately as two distinct peaks (as in Fig. 19–1), they may be merged into a single peak, or they may occur together as the *IV–V complex,* in which one wave occurs in the form of a shoulder on the other wave (see Fig. 19–2).

Again, these variations in waveform structure are considered normal (Chiappa et al, 1979).

Origins of the Auditory Brain Stem Response

A great deal of research has been done with both humans and animals concerning the origins of the various ABR waves. In humans with confirmed pathological conditions of the auditory pathway, abnormalities in the ABR have been related to lesion site (Sohmer, et al, 1974; Starr & Hamilton, 1976; Stockard & Rossiter, 1977). This strategy has also been used in animals with experimentally induced lesions (Achor & Starr, 1980b; Buchwald & Huang, 1975). Another technique used in animal studies is to examine the temporal correspondence between the ABR components recorded from the scalp and recordings made with electrodes placed within individual structures along the auditory pathway (Achor & Starr, 1980a; Huang & Buchwald, 1977).

It is generally agreed that the ABR is generated by the auditory nerve and subsequent fiber tracts and nuclei within the auditory brain stem pathways; however, controversy exists regarding the precise generators of the various waves. For many years, it was widely believed that the primary generator sites for the ABR were as follows: wave I—auditory nerve, wave II—cochlear nucleus, wave III—superior olivary complex, wave IV—lateral lemniscus, and wave V—inferior colliculus. Waves VI and VII were not extensively studied. Later, a series of experiments by Moller and Jannetta and their colleagues (Moller & Jannetta, 1985) shed new light on the generators of the ABR. In human patients undergoing various neurosurgical procedures, the authors simultaneously measured electrical activity from exposed locations along the auditory brain stem pathway and the ABR recorded from the scalp in the standard manner. They were able to examine the temporal correspondence between the responses from these various intracranial sites and particular waves of the ABR. They concluded that *both* waves I and II arise from the auditory nerve—wave I from the distal portion of the nerve in the cochlea and wave II from the proximal portion of the auditory nerve as it enters the brain stem. They believe that subsequent waves are generated at lower levels of the brain stem than previously assumed: wave III—cochlear nucleus, wave IV—superior olivary complex, wave V—lateral lemniscus as it terminates in the inferior colliculus. The large, slow, negative deflection after wave V, as well as waves VI and VII, is presumably generated mainly in the inferior colliculus. Similar experiments, also using intracranial recordings from humans (Hashimoto et al, 1981), are in basic agreement with these conclusions, which are now widely accepted. The contradictions with the earlier research are believed to be related in part to species differences.

It is important to note that the above-mentioned sites should be viewed as primary but not exclusive generators because it is overly simplistic to assume that each ABR component is derived from only a single structure. More likely, activity from lower structures interacts with activity in higher structures to generate the successive ABR potentials (Jewett & Williston, 1971; Moller & Jannetta, 1985; Picton et al, 1974). The exception is wave I, which because of its short latency undoubtedly represents activity solely from the auditory nerve.

RECORDING PROCEDURES

Electrodes

The ABR is recorded from electrodes attached to various positions on the head. Typical electrodes are small metal cups or disks, coated with various materials such as silver, silver-chloride, gold, tin, or platinum. Other electrode styles, such as self-adhesive disposables, ear clips, and earcanal electrodes are also available. The electrodes are attached to insulated lead wires and connector pins that insert into electrode jacks.

The ABR is actually recorded by measuring the difference in electrical activity between two electrodes, a technique known as *differential recording.* One of the electrodes (the non-inverting electrode) is usually placed on the vertex (on top of the head, at the center) or on the middle of the forehead just below the hairline. Another electrode (the inverting electrode) is usually placed on the earlobe or mastoid process of the ipsilateral ear (i.e., the ear receiving the stimulus). A third electrode, typically placed on the contralateral earlobe, contralateral mastoid, forehead, or nape of the neck, serves as the ground electrode.

Before attaching the electrodes, the skin must be thoroughly cleaned to remove excess oil, dead skin, and dirt to obtain a good contact between the skin and the electrode. Commercial cleansing preparations are available for this task. Once the electrodes have been applied, the adequacy of contact with the skin is assessed by measuring the electrical impedance between each electrode pair. For high-quality recordings, interelectrode impedances ≤6kΩ are generally considered acceptable; impedances also should be fairly equal between electrode pairs. Low and balanced impedances will help reduce unwanted interference such as electrical noise and muscle artifact that can make waveform interpretation difficult.

PEARL

If the impedance of one or more electrodes is discovered to be high, it can often be lowered by pressing on the electrode(s) for a few moments. If this is unsuccessful, the skin in the area of electrode placement may need to be rescrubbed to lower the impedance. This may be impractical in the case of an infant or young child who is already sleeping. Acceptable ABR recordings can often be obtained in these circumstances with much higher impedances, on the order of 10 to 12 kΩ, provided that the impedances are fairly balanced between electrode pairs and the recording environment is favorable.

Analysis Time Period

When recording the ABR, electrical activity from the electrodes is collected and analyzed over a certain time period, beginning at the onset of the stimulus and continuing long enough to encompass all the response of interest. Although the entire ABR waveform occurs within the first 10 ms after stimulus onset for high-level clicks, the response will be considerably delayed at lower stimulus levels, for low-frequency stimuli, and when testing infants. To encompass the entire ABR under all these various conditions, it is recommended that a longer time window of either 15 or 20 ms be used.

Processing of Electrical Activity

Electrical activity picked up by the recording electrodes within the specified time window must be processed through several stages to visualize the ABR waveform. This is because the ABR peaks are of extremely low voltage ($< 1 \mu V$) and are buried in a background of interference (termed *noise*), which includes ongoing EEG activity, muscle potentials caused by movement or tension, and 60 Hz power line radiation. The stages of processing include amplification, filtering, and signal averaging.

Amplification and Filtering

Because of the small size to the ABR peaks, amplification is necessary to increase the magnitude of the electrical activity picked up by the electrodes. An amplifier gain of 10^5 is typically used.

The problem of interference obscuring the ABR can be diminished partially by filtering the electrical activity coming from the electrodes. Band-pass filters are used to accept energy only within the particular frequency band of interest and reject energy in other frequency ranges. For ABR recording, band-pass filter settings of 100 to 3000 Hz or 30 to 3000 Hz are commonly used. A filter setting of 30 to 3000 Hz is recommended to enhance the ABR when testing infants or when using low-frequency tone bursts or bone conduction stimuli (see details later).

Filtering can only eliminate a portion of the interfering noise because of overlap between the frequency content of the ABR and the frequency of the interference. Therefore another technique, called *signal averaging,* must be used to further reduce unwanted interference.

Signal Averaging

The ABR is very small and, even with filtering, is buried in a background of noise. Signal averaging helps to reduce this noise so that the signal, in this case the ABR, can be detected. Signal averaging is possible because the ABR is *time locked* to stimulus onset, whereas the noise interference occurs randomly. That is, the signal occurs at the same points in time after onset of the eliciting stimulus, but the noise has no regular pattern. In signal averaging a large number of stimuli are presented, and the responses to each of the individual stimulus presentations (termed *sweeps*) are averaged together to obtain a final averaged waveform. By averaging, the random noise tends to cancel out, whereas the evoked potential is retained because it is basically the same in each sweep. The greater the number of stimulus presentations used, the greater the improvement in signal-to-noise ratio and the more clearly the ABR can be visualized in the final averaged waveform. For ABR recording, between 1000 and 2000 sweeps are typically used. However, for efficient use of test time, averaging may be terminated before the specified number of sweeps is reached as soon as a clear waveform is visualized in the averaged response.

Even with signal averaging, the patient must be reclining or lying in a relaxed state without moving, or interference from muscle activity will make identification of the ABR difficult. For infants and young children, this generally requires that they be tested while asleep. A sedative such as chloral hydrate is often used to induce sleep.

STIMULUS PARAMETERS

Stimulus Types

Clicks

The ABR is an *onset response,* meaning that it is generated by the onset of an auditory stimulus. The stimulus onset or rise time must be rapid to synchronize all the neurons contributing to the ABR. The ideal stimulus for eliciting the ABR is a *click,* which is a brief rectangular pulse of 50–200 μs duration, with an instantaneous onset. The rapid onset of the click provides good neural synchrony, thereby eliciting a clearly defined ABR.

PITFALL

A drawback to the use of click stimuli exists. Because of the reciprocal relationship between time and frequency of acoustic signals, a click is a broad-spectrum signal, containing energy across a wide range of frequencies. Because of this frequency spread, clicks cannot be used to assess sensitivity in specific frequency regions but rather to provide a gross estimate of hearing sensitivity.

Brief Tone Bursts

When assessing hearing sensitivity, it is desirable to take separate measurements within different frequency regions. To do this, one must use *frequency-specific* stimuli or stimuli containing energy within a discrete band of frequencies. The pure tone stimuli used for traditional audiometry, with long rise/fall times, are inappropriate for ABR because they are too slow to generate an onset response.

A stimulus used for ABR that represents a compromise between the desired frequency specificity and the required temporal brevity is the short-duration tone burst (also termed *tone pip*). These stimuli are brief tones with rise/fall times of only a few milliseconds (generally <5 ms) and brief or no plateau duration. Tone burst stimuli are more confined in their frequency range than clicks but still have considerable spectral splatter (i.e., sidebands of energy above and below the nominal frequency of the stimulus). Spectral splatter can be reduced by appropriate shaping or *windowing* of the rise/fall time (i.e., the manner in which the stimulus waveform goes from 0 to maximum amplitude). The stimulus may rise linearly or may be

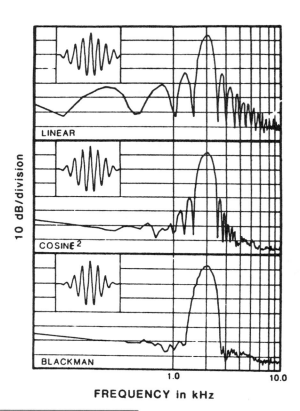

Figure 19–3 Examples of spectra of 2000 Hz tone bursts, shaped with linear, cosine squared, and Blackman windows. Each tone burst has a 2 ms rise/fall time with no plateau. The insets show the time waveform for each stimulus. (From Gorga & Thornton [1989], with permission.)

shaped by use of a mathematical formula of some sort. The preferred shaping for reducing spectral splatter is the Blackman window. Figure 19–3 (Gorga & Thornton, 1989) shows the amplitude spectra and time waveforms (*inset*) of 2000 Hz tone bursts having 2 ms rise/fall times and no plateau. Three gating functions are shown: a linear window (*top*), a cosine-squared or Hanning window (*middle*), and a Blackman window (*bottom*). Notice that the Blackman window reduces the amplitude of the sidebands compared with the other two.

Stimulus Polarity

Clicks

Most commercial evoked potential instruments allow a choice of rarefaction, condensation, or alternating rarefaction and condensation phase for the click onset. At present no consensus has been reached regarding which polarity is the best to use; however, most researchers recommend using either rarefaction or alternating phase. Rarefaction is the phase that stimulates the afferent dendrites of the auditory nerve and has been shown to produce shorter latencies and larger amplitudes of the major ABR waveform components (Schwartz & Morris, 1990). Alternating phase is useful in reducing stimulus artifact, which may interfere with identification of wave I. The stimulus artifact follows the phase of the stimulus and therefore cancels out when opposite polarities are added together.

Alternating phase, however, may degrade the clarity of the waveform, especially in the case of high-frequency hearing loss (Coats & Martin, 1977).

Tone Bursts

The difference between rarefaction and condensation phase is less important for tone bursts than clicks because the stimulus rise time will include excursions of both polarities. Alternating phase can be used to cancel out the cochlear microphonic and stimulus artifact; however, for low-frequency tone bursts, alternating phase will broaden the ABR peaks and may degrade clarity.

Stimulus Rate

During signal averaging, the stimulus must be presented at a specified rate, which must be slow enough to prevent the overlapping of responses that will occur if a new stimulus is presented before the response to the previous stimulus has been completed. For example, for a 10 ms time window, a rate of 100/s would be the fastest rate possible. The choice of stimulus rate is a compromise between response clarity and test efficiency. A slower stimulus rate produces the most clearly defined waveform but increases the amount of time required to obtain a single average. A higher stimulus rate reduces test time but decreases the amplitude of the ABR, particularly the early components of the waveform (Jewett & Williston, 1971; Pratt & Sohmer, 1976). Stimulus rates of 17 to 20/s are typically used clinically. Another clinical strategy is to use a slow rate (<20/s) when clear definition of all waveform components is required, as for otoneurological assessment (see following), and to use a higher rate (e.g., >60/s) when measuring wave V latency-intensity functions for threshold estimation (see following) because wave V is most resistant to the effects of a high stimulus rate.

PEARL

An important factor to consider when choosing a stimulus rate is that the value should not be evenly divisible into 60 to avoid time locking onto any 60 Hz electrical interference that may be in the test environment. For maximum cancellation of a 60 Hz artifact, an odd stimulus rate (e.g., 21.1/s, 27.7/s) is typically used.

Calibration of Stimulus Intensity

Unlike pure tone audiometry, no standards for intensity calibration exist for the stimuli used in ABR measurement because of their short duration. A typical method of specifying intensity for both clicks and tone bursts is to find the average behavioral threshold for the stimulus in a group of normal adults. The average threshold is termed 0 dB *normalized hearing level* or 0 dB nHL. All intensities are then expressed in decibels of normalized hearing level relative to this previously determined zero point.

A physical measurement that is used to express intensity of clicks is the *peak equivalent SPL (peSPL)*. To measure this, the click is routed to an oscilloscope, and the peak amplitude or peak-to-peak amplitude is measured. Then, a sine wave is routed through the ABR earphone to the oscilloscope, and its amplitude is adjusted to equal that of the click. The SPL of the sine wave is measured with a sound level meter. The amplitude of the click can then be expressed as dB peSPL re: frequency of the comparison sinusoid (Gorga et al, 1985a). Generally, average behavioral threshold (0 dB nHL) will be about 30 dB peSPL.

A sound level meter can be used to obtain a physical measurement of tone burst intensity by increasing the duration of the burst so that it is long relative to the response time of the meter. The intensity can then be measured and expressed in terms of decibels of sound pressure level re: 20 μPa (Gorga et al, 1985a).

CLINICAL USEFULNESS OF THE AUDITORY BRAIN STEM RESPONSE

The ABR is used clinically both in the estimation of auditory sensitivity and in otoneurological assessment (i.e., to detect lesions along the auditory nerve and brain stem pathways). It is by far the most widely used AEP in audiology. The popularity of the ABR stems from the fact that its characteristics are quite similar between people, making the response fairly easy to identify under most circumstances. It is also highly stable (i.e., it is unaffected by subject state). Characteristics of the response do not vary between wakefulness and sleep and are not affected by most medications. This means that children may be tested reliably during natural or sedation-induced sleep.

AUDITORY BRAIN STEM RESPONSE IN ESTIMATION OF AUDITORY SENSITIVITY

ABR is an important tool for the evaluation of auditory sensitivity in those individuals who are not readily testable by conventional behavioral audiometric procedures. Such persons include infants, developmentally delayed children, multiply handicapped children and adults, autistic individuals, and persons suspected of pseudohypoacusis.

Click Stimuli

In using the ABR for threshold estimation, the click is the most commonly used stimulus because it yields the clearest ABR response. The following discussion of ABR in estimation of auditory sensitivity will pertain to click stimuli. The use of frequency-specific stimuli will be described in a subsequent section.

In assessing hearing sensitivity, wave V of the ABR is used because it is the most robust of the waves and the one best

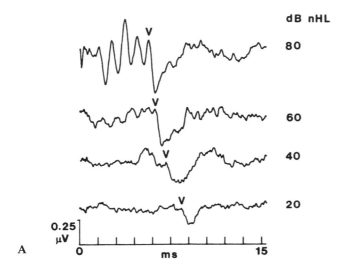

dB nHL

80

60

40

20

0.25
μV

A

0   ms   15

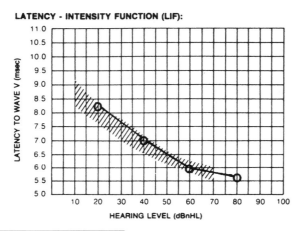

LATENCY - INTENSITY FUNCTION (LIF):

B

Figure 19–4 **(A)** ABR intensity series, obtained from a normal subject, at click levels of 80- to 20-dB nHL. Wave V latency ranges from 5.64 ms at 80 dB to 8.28 ms at 20 dB nHL. **(B)** Wave V latency-intensity function, plotted from the ABR intensity series shown in **A**.

correlated with behavioral audiometric threshold. The full complement of ABR waves is seen only at intense click levels. As the intensity of the click decreases, most of the ABR waves disappear, except wave V, which generally can be elicited at intensity levels within 10- to 20-dB of behavioral threshold for the click. This can be seen in Figure 19–4A, which shows a series of ABRs collected in a normal-hearing adult at click levels from 80- to 20-dB nHL. Notice that as stimulus intensity decreases, the amplitude of wave V decreases and its latency increases.

To estimate auditory sensitivity, ABR waveforms are obtained at a series of click intensity levels, beginning at a moderate to high intensity (e.g., 60 dB nHL) and continuing down to lower levels until wave V is no longer seen. If no response occurs at the starting level, intensity must of course be increased. Wave V threshold is usually found to the nearest 5- to 10-dB. If wave V is present at 20 dB nHL, this is

considered normal, and testing at lower stimulus levels is not needed. It is good clinical practice to obtain two waveforms at each stimulus level so that the repeatability of the waveform can be examined. This aids in determining whether wave V is present at a particular stimulus level.

Once the intensity series is obtained, the latency of wave V is measured at each stimulus level where present and plotted on a graph known as a *latency-intensity function* (LIF). Figure 19–4B shows the wave V LIF for the intensity series of Figure 19–4A. The shaded area on the graph represents the adult normative wave V latency values (mean latency ± 2 SD). A characteristic of wave V latency is its between-subject consistency. This can be seen by the narrow width of the shaded normal region in Figure 19–4B.

PEARL

Even though between-subject variability in wave V latency is small, it is vital that each test facility establish its own normative data. Because latency can be affected by stimulus and recording parameters, by equipment characteristics, and by the test environment, normative values will vary between facilities (see the "Establishment of Clinical Norms" section later in this chapter).

After the wave V intensity series is obtained, two factors are used in hearing estimation: wave V threshold and the LIF.

Wave V Threshold

The lowest click level at which Wave V can be elicited provides information about the degree of hearing loss. It is well accepted that click threshold will be determined by auditory sensitivity within the mid-frequency to high-frequency range, although disagreement exists regarding the particular frequencies involved. Click threshold reportedly correlates best with hearing sensitivity between 2 and 4 kHz (Gorga et al, 1985b; Picton et al, 1981), or between 1 and 4 kHz (Hyde, 1985; Jerger & Mauldin, 1978; Picton et al, 1994).

In normal individuals and those with conductive hearing loss, click threshold will generally be about 10- to 20-dB higher than the best audiometric threshold within the mid-frequency to high-frequency range. For cochlear losses, the difference between click threshold and audiometric thresholds is often reduced, and click threshold may be as close as 5 dB above best behavioral threshold. For convenience in the clinical setting, the behavioral threshold may be predicted to be a constant value (e.g., 10 dB) below click threshold. Because of individual variability, however, a constant correction factor will not be accurate in all cases.

The value of wave V threshold will range along a continuum, from ≤20 dB nHL (considered normal) to wave V absent at equipment limits. Because maximum output for clicks is limited to about 90- to 100-dB nHL (recall that 0 dB nHL ≅30 dB peSPL), one will not be able to differentiate between severe and profound losses.

PITFALL

Because of limitations in maximum output, the absence of wave V to clicks does not imply the absence of hearing. Rather, it suggests a severe or profound degree of hearing loss within the mid-frequency to high-frequency range. In one study (Rance et al, 1998), 25% of children with no click ABR at 100 dB nHL had useful residual hearing at all frequencies through 4 kHz.

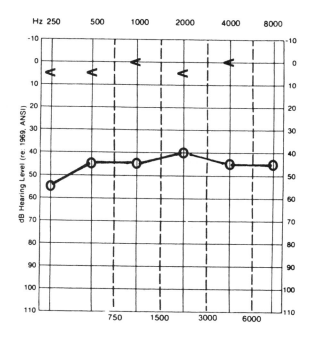

Wave V Latency-Intensity Function

The slope of the LIF for click stimuli and the position of the curve relative to normal can be used to provide information concerning the type of hearing loss and the audiometric configuration. Slope is defined as the amount of change in latency per decibel change of intensity measured in microseconds per decibel. Slope is computed by finding the difference in wave V latency at threshold and at the highest intensity measured and then dividing by the total change in intensity. Using the LIF in Figure 19–4B as an example, the latency at 20 dB nHL is 8.28 ms, whereas the latency at 80 dB nHL is 5.64 ms. This is a total change in latency of 2.64 ms over a range of 60 dB, for a slope of 0.044 ms/dB or 44 μs/dB. Normal slope is typically about 40 ms/dB on the average (Don et al, 1977; Picton et al, 1981; Stapells et al, 1985), but normal values as low as 20 μs/dB (Picton et al, 1981) and as high as 63 μs/dB (Gorga et al, 1985b) have been reported.

Several characteristic LIF types have come to be associated with certain audiometric patterns, as explained in the following:

Conductive Hearing Loss

In conductive hearing loss the slope of the LIF typically is normal. However, the latency of wave V at each intensity will be prolonged, resulting in an LIF that runs parallel to the normal curve but is shifted to the right. This occurs because conductive pathological conditions primarily cause an attenuation of sound reaching the cochlea, thereby causing latency shifts as would be seen with lower stimulus intensities. Figure 19–5 shows the audiogram and LIF for the right ear of a patient with a conductive hearing loss. The wave V threshold of 50 dB nHL is 10 dB above the best pure tone threshold in the 1 to 4 kHz range (i.e., 40 dB at 2 kHz). At each stimulus level, wave V latency is quite prolonged re: normal value. The slope of the LIF (46.7 μs/dB) is normal.

Flat Cochlear Loss

A normal slope to the LIF is also seen with cochlear losses having a flat audiometric configuration. In this case the wave V latencies may fall within the normal range or may be somewhat prolonged. The prolongation will generally be less than for conductive losses. It should be noted, however, that no definitive value of latency shift will consistently differentiate between cochlear and conductive losses. Figure 19–6 shows the audiogram and corresponding LIF for a patient with a right flat cochlear loss. Here again, the wave V threshold is 50 dB nHL, which is 5 dB above the best threshold within the 1 to 4 kHz range (i.e., 45 dB at 4 kHz). The slope of the LIF,

LATENCY - INTENSITY FUNCTION (LIF):

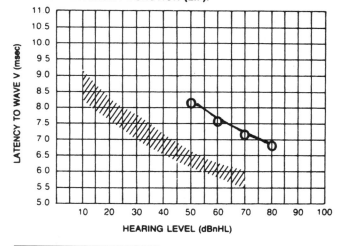

Figure 19–5 Pure tone audiogram *(top)* and wave V LIF *(bottom)* for a person with a right conductive hearing loss. Wave V latency ranges from 6.80 ms at 80 dB nHL to 8.20 ms at 50 dB nHL, resulting in a slope of 46.7 μs/dB.

computed between 50- and 80-dB, is 48.7 μs/dB. Notice that the wave V latencies show less prolongation from normal than the conductive loss in the previous example.

Sloping High-Frequency Cochlear Loss

In high-frequency cochlear hearing losses, the slope of the LIF is typically steeper than normal. A steep slope occurs when wave V latency is prolonged at and near threshold but is normal or nearly normal at higher intensity levels. Although originally attributed to loudness recruitment (Stapells et al, 1985), the steep slope is now believed to be related to the configuration of the pure tone audiogram (Gorga et al, 1985b). Because wave V latency is determined in part by the region of

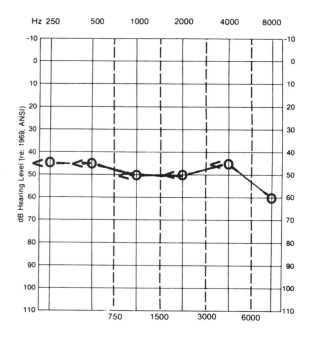

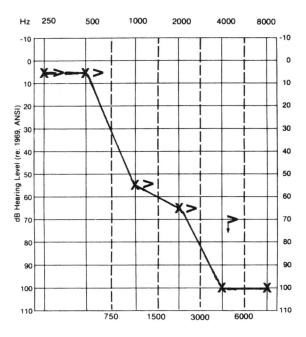

LATENCY - INTENSITY FUNCTION (LIF):

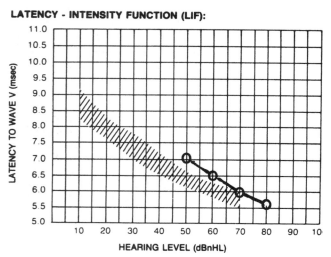

LATENCY - INTENSITY FUNCTION (LIF):

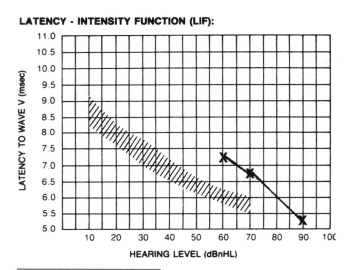

Figure 19–6 Pure tone audiogram *(top)* and wave V LIF *(bottom)* for a person with a right flat sensorineural hearing loss of cochlear origin. Wave V latency ranges from 5.66 ms at 80 dB nHL to 7.12 ms at 50 dB nHL, for a slope of 48.7 μs/dB.

Figure 19–7 Pure tone audiogram *(top)* and wave V LIF *(bottom)* for a person with a left steeply sloping high-frequency sensorineural hearing loss of cochlear origin. Wave V latency ranges from 5.26 ms at 90 dB nHL to 7.24 ms at 60 dB nHL, for a slope of 66 μs/dB.

the cochlea where the response is initiated, latency will be shorter when high-frequency fibers in the basal region are stimulated and longer when lower frequency fibers toward the apical region are stimulated. In sloping high-frequency losses the basal portions of the cochlea contribute to the ABR only at high intensities, provided the stimulus exceeds the threshold for high-frequency fibers, whereas more apical regions contribute to the response for lower intensities. Figure 19–7 shows an audiogram from the left ear of a patient with a high-frequency sensorineural hearing loss, along with the wave V LIF for that ear. Note that wave V threshold was determined to be 60 dB nHL, which is 5 dB above the best threshold within the 1–4 kHz range (i.e., 55 dB at 1000 Hz).

The slope of the LIF, computed between 60- to 90-dB nHL, is 66 μs/dB, which is steeper than normal, consistent with a high-frequency loss.

In summary, ABR testing with click stimuli can predict auditory sensitivity within the 1 to 4 kHz range to within 5- to 20-dB. By providing a measure of sensitivity within the critical speech frequencies, click ABR testing is a valuable tool for detecting hearing loss in difficult-to-test populations. The slope of the wave V LIF can be somewhat helpful in ascertaining the type and configuration of the hearing loss. However, because of between-subject variability, not all individuals will show the slope expected for their hearing loss.

The LIF can only *suggest* audiometric patterns, which may not apply in individual cases.

A major limitation of click stimuli is that they are not frequency specific and therefore cannot provide information regarding the entire audiogram. Notice how, for the steeply sloping high-frequency loss shown in Figure 19–7, the click threshold did not adequately describe the entire audiometric configuration. In addition, because click threshold gives an estimate of hearing within the mid-frequency to high-frequency range, it is possible to have a normal ABR and still have significant hearing loss. Specifically, click ABR will not be sensitive to hearing loss below 1 kHz or above 4 kHz.

PITFALL

A normal click ABR threshold does not necessarily imply normal-hearing. Rather, it implies an area of normal sensitivity between 1 and 4 kHz. Many patterns of hearing loss (e.g., low-frequency rising, high-frequency notch, "island" of normal-hearing) can yield normal click thresholds.

Frequency-Specific Stimuli

In attempting to approximate the behavioral pure tone audiogram, it has become fairly common to include brief tone bursts as part of the test protocol. As previously stated, these stimuli have narrower frequency spectra than clicks but are substantially broader than the pure tone stimuli used for conventional audiometry because of the brief rise/fall time. Brief tone bursts, especially with linear ramps, contain sidebands of energy at frequencies above and below the predominant energy peak. Because the sidebands are less intense than the peak of energy, the frequency spread is more of a problem at high levels of stimulation. With steeply sloping audiograms, this spread of stimulation may cause hearing loss in the frequency region under test to be underestimated because neighboring frequency regions with better sensitivity will be stimulated, generating a response at a lower stimulus level. This frequency spread has been shown to be more of a problem for low-frequency tone pips than for mid-frequency to high-frequency tone pips (Kileny, 1981; Stapells & Picton, 1981).

Enhancement of Frequency Specificity

As previously stated, a way to improve frequency specificity in ABR testing is to use tone bursts that are shaped with a Blackman function, which reduces the sidebands of energy. Such stimuli are now widely available on commercial ABR instrumentation. At high stimulus intensities, however, stimulation can still spread to adjacent frequency areas with better hearing because of basilar membrane mechanics.

An alternative way to ensure frequency specificity of the ABR is to combine the tone pips with *notched noise masking* presented to the same ear (Picton et al, 1979; Picton et al, 1981; Stapells et al, 1995). Notched noise is similar to wide band noise, containing energy across the frequency spectrum, except within a certain narrow range of frequencies (the *notch*). The frequency at which the notch occurs corresponds

to the frequency of the tone pip being used. Thus the sidebands of energy present in the tone pip are masked out, restricting the area of stimulation to the nominal frequency of the tone pip. This ensures that the ABR is generated by neurons sensitive only to the test frequency. The notched noise masking procedure requires more sophisticated instrumentation than is currently available on most commercial ABR instrumentation, a factor that has limited widespread implementation of this procedure.

Waveform Morphology

The structure of the ABR waveform elicited with high-frequency tone pips is similar to that obtained using clicks. However, for tone pip frequencies of 1000 Hz and less, the early waveform components are not clearly seen, and wave V is broader than normal. This is related to the loss of neural synchrony in the apical, low-frequency region of the cochlea. The broad structure and poor repeatability of the ABR to low-frequency stimuli can make wave V difficult to identify (Gorga et al, 1988; Stapells et al, 1995), especially at low intensities, and considerable experience is necessary to accurately evaluate low-frequency ABR thresholds in the clinical setting. Figure 19–8, from Stapells and colleagues (Stapells et al, 1995), shows examples of ABR waveforms obtained to 500, 2000, and 4000 Hz tone bursts in notched noise from a 21-month-old girl with normal-hearing. The arrows pinpoint the location of wave V when it is present in a particular waveform. Wave V threshold for all frequencies is 20 dB nHL, which

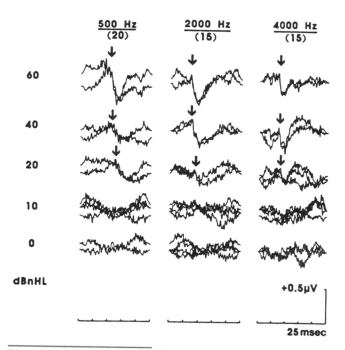

Figure 19–8 ABRs recorded with 500, 2000, and 4000 Hz tone bursts in notched noise from a 21-month-old girl with normal-hearing. The arrows above each waveform indicate the location of wave V, whereas the numbers below the tone burst frequency indicate the behavioral pure tone thresholds, obtained at 24 months of age. (From Stapells et al [1995], with permission.)

agrees with the behavioral pure tone thresholds noted at the top of the figure. Note the broad structure of wave V for the 500 Hz stimuli.

Accuracy of Threshold Prediction

The validity with which tone burst ABR can predict behavioral thresholds has been studied extensively. For mid-frequency to high-frequency tone pips, wave V can be elicited within about 10- to 25-dB of behavioral threshold (Kodera et al, 1977; Munnerley et al, 1991; Stapells, 1989; Stapells et al, 1995; Suzuki et al, 1977; Weber & Folsom, 1977). The threshold correspondence for low-frequency stimuli was originally thought to be poor (Davis & Hirsh, 1976; Gerken, 1978; Gorga et al, 1988). However, it is now known that the response filter setting is a critical factor when recording low-frequency ABRs. Because of the broadening of the ABR waveform with low-frequency stimuli, the low-frequency cut-off (high-pass filter setting) must be set low enough to encompass the low-frequency portion of the ABR spectrum. It has been shown (Stapells & Picton, 1981; Suzuki et al, 1977) that the amplitude of wave V for 500 Hz stimuli is attenuated as the low-frequency cut-off of the response filter is increased. A filter setting of 30 to 3000 Hz (rather than the typical 100 to 3000 Hz) is recommended when recording low-frequency ABRs to enhance wave V amplitude. Using this filter setting, fairly good correspondence is seen between ABR threshold and behavioral threshold for low frequencies.

The predictive accuracy of tone burst ABR has been studied extensively by Stapells and colleagues (Stapells et al, 1995; Stapells et al, 1990) in populations of normal and hearing-impaired infants, children, and adults. They used tone bursts with linear rise/fall times, at frequencies between 500–4000 Hz, presented with notched noise to enhance frequency specificity. The authors found similar results for all age groups. About 98% of ABR thresholds were within 30 dB of pure tone behavioral thresholds, 91 to 93% were within 20 dB, and 66 to 69% within 10 dB. The average ABR threshold was about 10 dB higher for 500 Hz tone bursts than for higher frequencies.

Suggested Test Protocol Using Clicks and Tone Bursts

The duration of an ABR test session for infants and young children is determined by the amount of time they will remain sleeping. Because this time is often quite limited (as short as 30 minutes), the clinician must collect ABR data in an efficient, judicious manner.

A suggested protocol for maximizing the usefulness of information obtained is as follows: First, measure the click threshold and LIF in both ears. To accomplish this, begin at a moderately high stimulus level (e.g., 60 dB nHL) and use bracketing to find wave V threshold in as few steps as possible. With experience, the clinician can learn to select test levels wisely on the basis of the appearance of the response at the current intensity level, to zero in on threshold in as few steps as possible. For example, in individuals with normal-hearing, one can obtain the LIF by using only 60- and 20-dB nHL test levels. The click data provide a gross estimate of hearing sensitivity in the mid- to high-frequency range, as well as some insight into the type and configuration of hearing

loss. In addition, analysis of the waveform at high click levels can be used to assess integrity of the auditory brain stem (see section on Otoneurological Assessment later in the chapter). Second, obtain wave V threshold to 500 Hz tone bursts in both ears. (The LIF is typically not analyzed for tone bursts, only the threshold.) The 500 Hz and click threshold data together provide a two-point approximation of the audiometric configuration. Third, if test time remains, find threshold for a high-frequency burst (e.g., 3000 or 4000 Hz) in both ears to obtain more detail regarding the audiometric configuration.

Bone Conduction Auditory Brain Stem Response Testing

Several investigators have shown that it is feasible to do ABR testing with bone conduction (BC) stimulation, using both clicks (Cone-Wesson & Ramirez, 1997; Mauldin & Jerger, 1979; Stuart et al, 1994; Yang et al, 1987) and tone bursts (Cone-Wesson & Ramirez, 1997; Nousak & Stapells, 1992). As in pure tone audiometry, BC ABR testing is administered to estimate cochlear reserve in an attempt to define the type of hearing loss. Bone conduction ABR testing is especially useful for infants with earcanal atresia or other structural malformations of the external and/or middle ear, when knowledge of cochlear status is crucial for planning habilitation. The clinical procedure involves comparing ABR wave V thresholds for air conduction (AC) and BC stimulation using clicks and/or tone bursts.

Characteristics of the Auditory Brain Stem Response to Bone Conduction Stimulation

When BC stimulation is used to elicit the ABR, wave V is the predominant component. The earlier waves, especially wave I, are often obscured by a large stimulus artifact. In adults, wave V latencies for BC clicks are about 0.5 ms longer than latencies for AC clicks at the same sensation level (Mauldin & Jerger, 1979), a difference that has been attributed to differences in the amplitude spectra of clicks for AC and BC (Mauldin & Jerger, 1979). In infants, on the other hand, wave V latencies are shorter for BC clicks than AC clicks (Yang et al, 1987). Also, wave V thresholds for BC are lower in infants than adults for both click and 500 Hz stimuli, with no difference seen for 4000 Hz stimuli (Cone-Wesson & Ramirez, 1997). Both the shorter latencies and lower thresholds for BC in infants have been attributed to differences in skull characteristics between infants and adults (Yang et al, 1987) and to greater SPL values developed in the infant earcanal during BC stimulation (Cone-Wesson & Ramirez, 1997).

Procedure for Recording the Auditory Brain Stem Response with Bone Conduction Stimulation

Details of recommended stimulus and recording parameters for BC ABR testing have been reviewed by Cone-Wesson (1995). A basic description follows.

An oscillator placement on the temporal bone in the superoposterior auricular position (Yang et al, 1987) is recommended because it yields the lowest ABR threshold, particularly in infants. Yang and colleagues (Yang et al, 1987) showed that wave V threshold was 30 to 40 dB higher in neonates using a forehead placement and 15- to 25-dB higher using an occipital bone placement compared with a temporal bone placement. These differences were attributed to the fact that in infants the skull sutures are not fused and therefore the BC stimulation is not efficiently conducted to the ear from the more remote locations. In adults use of a forehead placement is not recommended because the behavioral threshold for BC clicks in this location is about 10 dB higher than for a temporal bone placement, thereby reducing the maximum output available from the bone oscillator.

The oscillator may be held in place with a Velcro band placed around the head (Yang et al, 1987). To ensure consistency of placement between patients, the vibrator-to-head coupling force should be measured with a spring scale and maintained between 400 and 450 g (Stuart et al, 1994).

In recording BC ABR, the inverting electrode should be placed at some distance from the oscillator to minimize stimulus artifact. Locations used include an inferior postauricular location, on the ear lobe, in the earcanal, or low on the nape of the neck.

Both click and tone burst stimuli may be used for BC ABR as for AC ABR. It is important to calibrate the BC stimuli in terms of dB nHL. This is accomplished by finding the average behavioral threshold (0 dB nHL) for the BC stimuli in a group of normal listeners, using the same oscillator placement as will be used for ABR testing. The 0 dB nHL value will be about 40 dB higher for BC than AC. This correction factor must then be applied to the intensity levels specified on the ABR instrumentation.

Normative data for threshold and wave V latency must be established for all BC stimuli to be used. Because of the observed differences between infants and adults (Cone-Wesson & Ramirez, 1997; Yang et al, 1987), it is crucial to establish norms for the ages to be tested.

The clinical test protocol involves comparing the threshold of AC and BC stimuli to estimate the amount of air-bone gap. As for pure tone audiometry, it is important to use masking in the contralateral ear when indicated.

Automated Auditory Brain Stem Response Screening

In recent years, *automated* ABR instruments have been developed for screening newborns in a hospital setting. The need for such instrumentation arose because traditional ABR testing proved to be too expensive and time-consuming for the mass screening of large numbers of infants.

The first automated ABR screener to be developed and the most widely used at present is the ALGO, currently manufactured by Natus Medical Inc. (Hall et al, 1988; Kileny, 1987; Peters, 1986). The ALGO uses a single, low-level click stimulus at 35 dB nHL to elicit the ABR. A computerized detection algorithm is used to decide whether a response is present by comparing incoming data to a template of a normal waveform stored in memory. The result of this comparison yields a decision of either "pass" or "refer," depending on whether a response is detected. It is important to remember that because a single click level is used, one cannot determine the degree of any existing hearing loss; rather the test merely indicates which babies are in need of follow-up.

PITFALL

Several problems related to BC ABR testing should be noted. At the higher stimulus levels, stimulus artifact from the oscillator can interfere with visualization of the ABR response, especially for tone burst stimuli. Stimulus artifact can be minimized by placing the oscillator high on the temporal bone and by using an ear lobe, earcanal, or nape of neck location for the inverting electrode. The use of alternating-phase stimuli will also minimize stimulus artifact, although this may substantially broaden the ABR response, especially for low-frequency tone bursts. Another problem is that the maximum output of the BC vibrator is only about 45- to 55-dB nHL. This limits the ability to distinguish between mixed and sensorineural losses when AC thresholds are elevated beyond the moderate loss range.

Because very little technical expertise is required to screen infants with the ALGO, the device can be used by nonprofessionals such as technicians or volunteers. This contributes to the cost-effectiveness of the device and reduces personnel costs for universal hearing screening programs. Large-scale, multicenter clinical trials have confirmed the accuracy and clinical feasibility of the ALGO (Hall, 1992; Herrmann et al, 1995).

At present, two more automated ABR screeners are on the market—the Clarity System by SonaMed Corp. and the Smart Screener by Intelligent Hearing Systems. It is likely that more will be developed in the future because of increasing support for the concept of universal hearing screening.

AUDITORY BRAIN STEM RESPONSE IN OTONEUROLOGICAL ASSESSMENT

The ABR is not only useful in assessing auditory threshold sensitivity. It is also used for detection of *retrocochlear* lesions (i.e., abnormalities along the auditory pathway beyond the cochlea), including the auditory nerve and various structures of the auditory brain stem.

Common examples of retrocochlear lesions are tumors of various types (Musiek et al, 1986; Selters & Brackmann, 1977; Starr & Achor,1975; Starr & Hamilton, 1976; Stockard & Rossiter, 1977; Stockard et al, 1977; Stockard et al, 1980; Terkildsen et al, 1977), which may occur on the auditory nerve, within the auditory brain stem itself (*intra-axial*), or outside the brain stem (*extra-axial*). Extra-axial tumors affect the auditory system when they grow large enough to exert pressure on the auditory brain stem pathways (Stockard et al, 1980). A second type of retrocochlear lesion is demyelinating disease, most notably multiple sclerosis (MS) (Robinson & Rudge, 1975; Starr & Achor, 1975; Stockard et al, 1977; Stockard et al, 1980), but also including central pontine myelinolysis seen in chronic alcoholics (Begleitter et al, 1981; Stockard et al, 1976) and multifocal leukoencephalopathy (Stockard &

Rossiter, 1977). The ABR has also proven useful in the detection of vascular lesions of the brain stem, including hemorrhage from a ruptured blood vessel or interruption of blood flow because of occlusion of a blood vessel (Starr & Hamilton, 1976; Stockard & Rossiter, 1977; Stockard et al, 1980). The ABR has been used in the differential diagnosis of comatose patients. The ABR will typically not be affected if coma is due to metabolic or toxic causes (e.g., drug overdose) but will show changes if coma is due to a structural lesion (Starr & Achor, 1975; Stockard et al, 1980). ABR testing can help to determine the extent of brain damage in head trauma victims (Starr & Hamilton, 1976) or infants suffering from lack of oxygen because of birth complications and is used in the determination of brain death (Starr & Achor, 1975; Stockard & Rossiter, 1977).

In otoneurological applications, the ABR is useful in assessing the status of the auditory nerve and brain stem pathways because damage to these areas can alter the ABR in characteristic ways. The location of the lesion will affect the ear in which ABR abnormalities are manifested. In general, a lesion of the auditory nerve will affect the ABR generated by stimulation of the ear ipsilateral to the lesion. In cases of large tumors located at the cerebellopontine angle, contralateral effects may also be seen due to compression of the brain stem. Lesions of the brain stem may cause ipsilateral, contralateral, or bilateral abnormalities of the ABR.

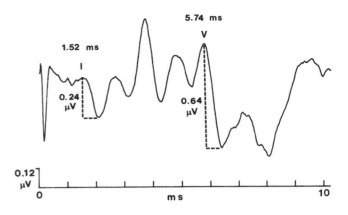

I – V   IPL = 5.74 – 1.52 = 4.22 ms

V/I amp. ratio = 0.64 ÷ 0.24 = 2.67

Figure 19–9   ABR waveform from Figure 19–1, showing calculation of the wave I to V interpeak latency and the wave V/I amplitude ratio. The absolute latencies and amplitudes of waves I and V are labeled on the waveform. Calculation of interpeak latency and amplitude ratio are shown under the tracings.

> ## PITFALL
>
> **It is not possible to diagnose the type of pathological condition causing the ABR abnormality (e.g., tumor vs. vascular lesion). Abnormal findings merely indicate the possibility of a retrocochlear lesion, not the type of lesion.**

In using ABR to assess the integrity of the central auditory pathways, click stimuli are generally used because they elicit the clearest waveform. Because information regarding auditory sensitivity is not of primary interest here, it is not necessary to find wave V threshold. Rather, the ABR is elicited at an intense stimulus level (typically between 60- and 90-dB nHL) and various parameters of the ABR waveform are examined. These parameters are described in the following.

Interpeak Latencies

The wave I to V interpeak latency (IPL) is the difference between the latency of wave I and the latency of wave V in a given waveform (see Fig. 19–9). This IPL is often termed *central conduction time* or *brain stem transmission time*. Because wave I is generated by the auditory nerve at the periphery of the auditory system and wave V is presumably generated by lateral lemniscus fibers as they enter the inferior colliculus, the difference in latency between these waves is the time required for neural impulses to be conducted through the auditory brain stem. The normal wave I to V IPL is about 4.0 ms (Stockard et al, 1980). Retrocochlear lesions (e.g., a tumor causing pressure on the auditory nerve or brain stem) may slow neural conduction velocity and therefore increase the time between the ABR peaks. The IPL is usually considered

abnormal if it is greater than 2 or 2.5 standard deviations above the mean.

Figure 19–10, from Stockard et al (1977) shows the ABR obtained from a 48-year-old man with a brain stem tumor compared with that of a normal adult. Note that the wave V peak is prolonged for the tumor patient, increasing the wave I to V IPL by 0.89 ms.

A further refinement of the IPL measure is to obtain the wave I to III and wave III to V IPLs as well. These measures are made in an attempt to more precisely pinpoint the location of the abnormality within the auditory pathway (Stockard & Rossiter, 1977; Stockard et al, 1980).

In addition to comparing the IPLs to normative data, the IPLs may also be compared between ears in a given patient for greater sensitivity. With retrocochlear pathological conditions, the IPL may remain within normal limits but may be longer in the affected ear compared with the other side.

> ## SPECIAL CONSIDERATION
>
> **It is important for the clinician to note that the wave I to V IPL can be influenced by the audiometric configuration. Specifically, high-frequency hearing loss of cochlear origin may prolong wave I more than wave V, resulting in a shortening of the wave I to V IPL (Coats & Martin, 1977). Thus high-frequency cochlear loss can counteract the lengthening effect of retrocochlear pathological conditions on the wave I to V IPL, resulting in a false-negative outcome.**

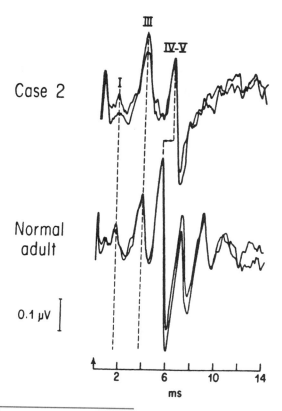

Figure 19–10 Example of an ABR obtained from a 48-year-old man with a tumor arising from the floor of the fourth ventricle, presumably exerting pressure on the auditory brain stem (*upper trace*). An ABR from a normal adult is shown for comparison (*lower trace*). Stimuli for both recordings were 75 dB nHL clicks. The wave I–V interpeak latency is prolonged in the tumor patient. (From Stockard et al [1977], with permission.)

Absolute Latency of Wave V

Measurement of interpeak latencies depends on obtaining wave I, which usually appears in the ABR waveform only at moderate to high stimulus intensity levels. With significant hearing loss, it may not be possible to elicit wave I at the maximum stimulus level available, making calculation of the wave I to V IPL impossible. However, because a prolongation of the wave I to V IPL will also result in a prolongation of the wave V latency itself, some have used the wave V absolute latency in evaluating patients for retrocochlear lesions (Coats & Martin, 1977; Robinson & Rudge, 1975). A problem with using absolute latency is that hearing loss, both conductive and sensorineural of cochlear origin, can cause some delay in wave V latency. Because many patients seen for otoneurological assessment will have associated hearing loss, this causes problems of interpretation and raises the possibility of excessive false positive results.

Interaural Wave V Latency Difference

The interaural wave V latency difference is the difference in wave V latency obtained at the same stimulus level between the two ears. This measure is also useful when inability to elicit wave I makes measurement of IPLs impossible. The interaural wave V latency difference may be more sensitive than the absolute wave V latency because wave V may be prolonged in one ear relative to the other ear but still not fall outside the normal range for latency. A latency difference greater than 0.3 to 0.4 ms between ears is generally considered abnormal (Bauch & Olsen, 1989; Clemis & McGree, 1979; Josey et al, 1988; Selters & Brackmann, 1977). As with the wave V absolute latency measure, a problem exists with false positive results when using the interaural latency comparison if hearing loss is present. If a unilateral or asymmetrical hearing loss exists, wave V latency may be significantly prolonged in one ear simply because of the hearing loss and not because of retrocochlear pathology. Various correction factors have been proposed to compensate for the effects of hearing loss (Hyde et al, 1981; Selters & Brackmann, 1977), but none has gained universal acceptance. Another problem occurs when a retrocochlear lesion results in a bilateral prolongation of wave V. In this case, no difference may be found in wave V latency between ears, and the retrocochlear pathological condition will be missed.

Wave V/I Amplitude Ratio

Measures of *absolute* amplitude of the ABR waves have not proven to be useful clinically because amplitude is highly variable both within and between subjects and varies considerably with levels of physiological noise, electrode impedance, and electrode location. However, a *relative* amplitude measure, the wave V/I amplitude ratio, has proven to be useful in assessing brain stem integrity (Starr & Achor, 1975; Stockard et al., 1977). To obtain this measure, the peak-to-peak amplitudes of waves I and V are measured (from the maximum positive peak to the following negative trough) and compared in the form of a ratio, as demonstrated in Figure 19–9. In normal adults wave V is larger than wave I, resulting in an amplitude ratio of >1.0. Retrocochlear pathology may cause a decrease in wave V amplitude, resulting in a ratio of <1.0.

Figure 19–11, from Stockard et al (1977) shows the ABR obtained from the left and right ears of a patient with MS. Notice that, for right ear stimulation, wave V amplitude is less than wave I amplitude and results in an abnormal V/I amplitude ratio of >1.0. The amplitude ratio for left ear stimulation is normal (>1.0).

Shift in Wave V Latency at High Stimulus Rates

Another measure for otoneurological diagnosis involves comparing wave V latency obtained using a slow stimulus rate (20/s or less) and a fast stimulus rate (50/s or greater). There will be some increase in wave V latency at the high stimulus rate for normal subjects (Don et al, 1977; Pratt & Sohmer, 1976; Zollner et al, 1976) caused by adaptation. However, those with damaged auditory systems caused by retrocochlear lesions may show a latency shift beyond the range expected for normal individuals (Fowler & Noffsinger, 1983; Musiek & Gollegly, 1985; Stockard & Rossiter, 1977). Before this measure can be used with confidence, it is necessary to establish criteria for abnormality for the stimulus rates that are to be used.

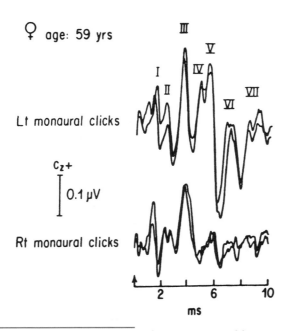

Figure 19–11 ABRs obtained from a 59-year-old patient with multiple sclerosis for left *(top)* and right *(bottom)* ear stimulation. Stimuli were 60 dB nHL clicks. It can easily be seen that the wave V/I amplitude ratio is abnormally small for right ear stimulation. The latency of wave V is also slightly prolonged in the right ear relative to the left ear. (From Stockard et al [1977], with permission.)

Absent Waveform Components

Retrocochlear pathological conditions may be severe enough to disrupt the generation of components of the ABR entirely, resulting in absent waves. The presence of a lesion at a given location can eliminate waves generated at the lesion site and rostral to the lesion (Musiek et al, 1986; Starr & Hamilton, 1976). For example, with a tumor of the auditory nerve, wave I may be present because it is generated peripherally to the site of the tumor, whereas all the remaining waves may be absent. It is important to note that the absence of waves VI or VII is not diagnostically significant because the presence of these waves is highly variable, even in normal individuals. An example of missing ABR waves for a patient with an extensive brain stem tumor is shown in Figure 19–12 from Starr and Hamilton (1976). Note that for both right and left ear stimulation, only waves I to III are clearly present.

Reproducibility

In normal individuals ABR waveforms obtained under identical stimulus conditions are usually highly repeatable. Poor reproducibility has been reported in patients with MS (Prasher & Gibson, 1980; Robinson & Rudge, 1980), presumably as a result of loss of neural synchrony caused by the demyelination process. This measure is not widely used in otoneurological diagnosis, however, because fluctuating levels of physiological noise may also affect the degree to which waves replicate. Also, the judgment of reproducibility can be quite subjective, unless a mathematical procedure such as correlation is used.

SUBJECT FACTORS AFFECTING THE AUDITORY BRAIN STEM RESPONSE

The ABR is not affected by changes in the mental state of the subject, such as level of arousal or degree of attention paid to the eliciting stimulus. Also no difference exists between waking and sleeping state or with stages of sleep. For clinical use, the stability of the ABR across changes in mental state is an important advantage of the ABR over the later components of the AEPs. However, several subject factors do influence characteristics of the ABR that the clinician needs to be aware of, including the following.

Young Age

The age of the patient must be considered in interpreting ABR results. In neonates and young children, ABR waveform structure, peak latencies, and peak amplitudes differ from adults.

The ABR waveform in neonates consists primarily of three component peaks, corresponding to waves I, III, and V in the adult ABR (Jacobson et al, 1982; Salamy et al, 1975). During the first 18 months of life, the other component peaks of the ABR emerge until the waveform assumes an adult structure. The change in ABR waveform between newborn and adults is shown in Figure 19–13 from Jacobson & Hall (1994).

Wave I amplitude in newborns is larger than in adults (Salamy & McKean, 1976; Salamy et al, 1975; Stockard et al, 1978), possibly because the recording electrode is closer to the

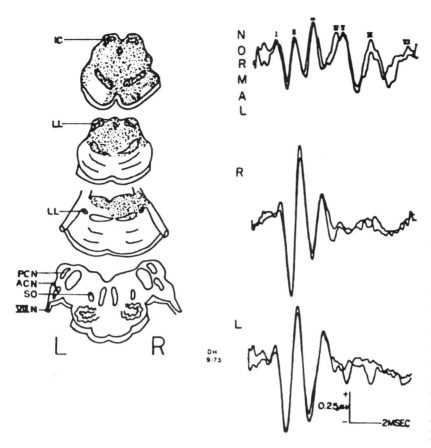

Figure 19–12 ABR waveforms obtained for right and left ear stimulation from an 18-year-old man with a large intra-axial brain stem tumor, with a normal ABR waveform at the top for comparison. For the tumor patient, only waves I to III are clearly seen (although a hint of the wave IV–V complex is seen in the right ear tracing). The extent of the lesion is indicated by the stippled area to the left. IC, Inferior colliculus; LL, lateral lemniscus; PCN, posterior cochlear nucleus; ACN, anterior cochlear nucleus; SO, superior olivary nucleus; VIII N, auditory nerve. (From Starr et al [1976], with permission.)

cochlea because of the smaller head size of infants. On the other hand, wave V amplitude is smaller in infants than in adults. Therefore the wave V/I amplitude ratio will be reduced for infants, often having a value less than 1.0 (Jacobson et al, 1982).

The latencies of the ABR waveform components are longer in neonates compared with adults and decrease progressively throughout the neonatal period because of maturation of the cochlea and brain stem. Wave I matures most rapidly, assuming an adult latency value by about 2 to 3 months of age (Jacobson et al, 1982; Salamy et al, 1982). Various reports show wave V assuming an adult value either by 12 or 18 months (Finitzo-Hieber, 1982; Hecox & Galambos, 1974) by slightly more than 2 years (Gorga et al, 1989) or as late as 2.5 years of age (Salamy et al, 1975). This differential maturation of waves I and V means that the wave I to V IPL progressively shortens as the infant grows. The wave I to V IPL decreases from approximately 5.0 ms at term to the adult value of about 4.0 ms by 12 to 18 months of age (Salamy et al, 1982). The time course of wave III maturation follows that of wave V.

The infant ABR is more vulnerable to the effects of increasing stimulus repetition rate. Consequently, slower rates of stimulus presentation may need to be used to maximize waveform clarity. In one study, for example, for infants less than 6 weeks of age, waveform clarity improved when stimulus rate was lowered from 15/s to 5/s (Salamy et al, 1975). The amount of wave V latency shift with increasing stimulus repetition rate is greater in infants than adults (Fujikawa & Weber,

1977; Salamy, 1984). This must be kept in mind when using the repetition rate shift as an indicator of brain stem integrity.

When testing infants from birth to about 18 to 24 months of age, it is important to use normative data appropriate for age rather than adult values (see "Establishment of Clinical Norms" in this chapter).

In premature infants the ABR can be recorded as early as 27 to 30 weeks' gestational age (Starr et al, 1977; Stockard & Westmoreland, 1981), although only at high stimulus intensity levels. As might be expected because of immaturity of the auditory system, latencies of waves I and V, and the I to V IPL are prolonged re: full term infants and decrease rapidly week by week until they reach full-term neonatal values at abut 39 to 40 weeks' gestation (Roberts et al, 1982; Starr et al, 1977). When testing premature infants, compensation must be made for the prematurity. The normative data used must be appropriate for *conceptual age*, which is the gestational age at birth plus the postnatal age. If premature infants are to be tested before they reach a conceptual age of 38 to 40 weeks (equivalent to full-term), norms must be established for various ages within the preterm period.

Advanced Age

Some investigators have reported that the absolute latency of wave V increases systematically with increasing age (Jerger & Hall, 1980; Jerger & Johnson, 1988; Rowe, 1978). However,

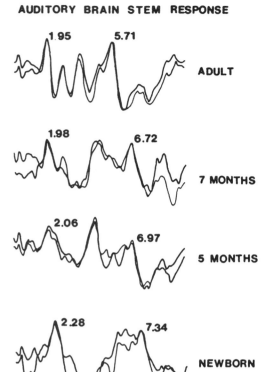

AUDITORY BRAIN STEM RESPONSE

ADULT — 1.95 5.71

7 MONTHS — 1.98 6.72

5 MONTHS — 2.06 6.97

NEWBORN — 2.28 7.34

0.2μV

3 MSEC

Figure 19–13 ABR waveforms showing maturation of the response from newborn to adult. In each example, the latencies of waves I and V are indicated. Over time, the progressive emergence of waveform components, decrease in latencies, and change in amplitude ratio can be observed. (From Jacobson & Hall [1994], with permission.)

others have not found this effect of aging (Beagley & Sheldrake, 1978; Rosenhamer et al, 1980; Schwartz et al, 1994).

CONTROVERSIAL POINT

The issue of whether it is necessary to establish separate normative data for elderly adults remains unresolved at this time.

Gender

A gender difference in ABR latencies and amplitude is well documented (Jerger & Hall, 1980; McClelland & McCrea, 1979; Stockard et al, 1978). Beginning at adolescence, females have slightly shorter wave III and V latencies than males. This difference is greatest for wave V, resulting in a wave I–V

interpeak latency about 0.1 to 0.2 ms shorter in females (Stockard et al, 1979). Females also show larger amplitudes for the later waves than males. Although the cause of this gender effect is not known for certain, the difference has been attributed to smaller head size and brain dimensions on the average in women (Stockard et al, 1978). Shorter distance between generators would result in shorter latencies, whereas smaller head size would cause the recording electrodes to be closer to the generators, resulting in larger amplitude.

CONTROVERSIAL POINT

Many clinicians recommend establishing separate normative data for male and female adults to compensate for the gender difference. Others disagree (Schwartz et al, 1994), believing that although a statistical effect of gender may be present, the differences are not clinically significant.

Pharmacological Agents

Most sedatives, general anesthetics, and neuromuscular blocking agents have no effect on the ABR. This means that patients may be validly tested under sedation or anesthesia, a factor that makes the ABR particularly suited for clinical use. An exception is the general anesthetic enflurane (Stockard et al, 1980), which causes increased IPLs.

Other drugs that have been shown to increase IPLs of the ABR are phenytoin, an anticonvulsant, and lidocaine, a local anesthetic that is used to treat cardiac dysrhythmias. Alcohol intoxication has also been noted to increase IPLs (Squires et al, 1978), but some of this effect may be related to a concomitant decrease in body temperature (Jones et al, 1980) (see effect of body temperature in the following).

Body Temperature

A decrease in body temperature below normal causes an increase in ABR IPLs (Stockard et al, 1980). This effect is thought to be due to slowed neural conduction velocity and synaptic transmission speed in hypothermia (Picton et al, 1981). Because low-birth-weight infants and comatose patients are prone to hypothermia, temperature should be measured before an ABR evaluation in these patients. One investigator (Hall, 1992) has published correction factors for the I to V IPL to compensate for the effects of hypothermia.

ESTABLISHMENT OF CLINICAL NORMS

When using ABR for threshold estimation and/or otoneurological assessment, it is vital to have appropriate normative values against which to compare patient data. Many of the ABR indices used clinically are highly dependent on a host of stimulus and recording parameters, such as stimulus transducer type, stimulus intensity, stimulus polarity, stimulus presentation rate, tone burst frequency, tone burst rise/fall time, response filter settings, electrode locations, and ambient noise level in the test environment. Therefore it is important to use norms that were obtained under conditions that are identical to the clinical protocol in use.

Because many ABR characteristics also vary with age and gender, normative values must be established for all populations to be evaluated. When gathering norms, subjects are grouped by age intervals, which should be smallest where the expected rate of change in ABR parameters is largest. For example, if infants and young children are to be tested, an age grouping might be as follows: birth to 6 weeks, 7 weeks to 3 months, 4 to 6 months, 7 to 9 months, 10 to 12 months, and so forth. If premature infants are to be tested before term, smaller age intervals should be used (e.g., 31 to 32 weeks, 33 to 34 weeks, 35 to 36 weeks, 37 to 38 weeks) because of rapid maturation during this period. If separate norms are to be established for the elderly, the age groupings can be larger (e.g., 5-year or 10-year intervals) because the rate of change in the ABR is much slower. In addition to age-related norms, separate norms are sometimes established for male and female adults because of gender differences in the ABR.

Normative values should be established for the following ABR parameters: absolute latencies (waves I, III, and V), interpeak latencies (I to V, I to III, and III to V), the V/I amplitude ratio, wave V interaural latency difference, shift in wave V latency at a high stimulus rate, wave V LIF for clicks, wave V threshold for bone-conducted stimuli, and wave V threshold for tone burst stimuli.

The process of establishing normative data involves recording the ABR data of interest in a number of normal subjects, grouped within the pre-established age and gender categories. For each group, the mean and standard deviation of each ABR parameter is computed. The criterion for normality is typically considered to be within 2.0 or 2.5 standard deviations from the mean. The number of subjects required per group is not universally agreed on. Many clinicians arbitrarily use 10 subjects per group, although no statistical basis exists for this practice. A better method has been described (Sklare, 1987) in which subjects are added to each group until the standard error of measurement is less than the time resolution of the response waveform. Using this approach, the number of subjects required per group will depend on the variability in the data.

Gathering normative data can be a lengthy process. As an alternative, many sets of published norms are available (Cox, 1985; Gorga et al, 1989; Gorga et al, 1987; Musiek et al, 1984).

LIMITATIONS OF THE AUDITORY BRAIN STEM RESPONSE

Although ABR has proven to be a valuable clinical tool for auditory assessment, it does have limitations that must be kept in mind. First, because the ABR is generated subcortically, it does not truly measure "hearing." Rather, it assesses the integrity of the peripheral auditory system and auditory brain stem pathways before sound is received by the cortex. Consequently, persons with cortical damage interfering

---

> ### PITFALL
>
> The clinician must be extremely cautious before using norms established at another facility. One needs to be certain that stimulus and recording parameters and population characteristics for the published normative database are identical to the clinical protocol in use. If not, serious errors in interpretation of clinical ABR data may arise.

with auditory reception may have perfectly normal ABR results. For example, Ozdmar and colleagues (Ozdamar et al, 1982) reported on a patient who was deaf as a result of bilateral temporal lobe lesions but who had a normal ABR. Fortunately, such cases of cortical deafness are quite rare.

Conversely, ABR may also *overestimate* the degree of hearing loss. Many paradoxical cases have been reported of patients who showed no ABR at maximum stimulus levels, who later were found by behavioral testing to have normal-hearing or no more than a moderate sensorineural hearing loss (Kraus et al, 1984; Rance et al, 1998; Worthington & Peters, 1980). Recently, with the widespread clinical use of otoacoustic emissions (OAEs), many similar cases have been reported of patients who show normal OAEs and absent ABR (Berlin et al, 1998; Sininger et al, 1995). Absence of the ABR in the presence of normal OAEs and normal or near-normal behavioral thresholds has been termed *auditory neuropathy* and is speculated to be caused by damage to the auditory nerve or brain stem that disrupts the neural synchrony necessary for ABR generation, yet leaves hearing relatively intact. Significantly, many of the reported patients have histories of birth complications including prematurity, respiratory distress, and hyperbilirubinemia, placing them at risk for neurological damage (Berlin et al, 1998; Kraus et al, 1984). These paradoxical case reports highlight the importance of using a test battery approach, including ABR, OAEs, and behavioral audiological testing if and when it becomes feasible, especially for individuals identified with significant hearing loss for whom amplification is contemplated.

CONCLUSIONS

ABR testing is an important clinical tool for estimating hearing sensitivity and assessing the integrity of the auditory nerve and auditory brain stem pathways. This chapter has provided an overview of the ABR, including normative aspects of the waveform, recording procedures, and clinical protocols and interpretation. Numerous factors affecting the ABR, including stimulus and recording parameters, and pathological and nonpathological subject characteristics, have been described. It is vitally important for the audiologist to be aware of these factors for accurate interpretation of ABR data in the clinical setting.

REFERENCES

ACHOR, L., & STARR, A. (1980a). Auditory brain stem responses in the cat. I. Intracranial and extracranial recordings. *Electroencephalography and Clinical Neurophysiology, 48*,154–173.

ACHOR, L., & STARR, A. (1980b). Auditory brain stem responses in the cat. II. Effects of lesions. *Electroencephalography and Clinical Neurophysiology, 48*,174–190.

BAUCH, C.D., & OLSEN, W.O. (1989). Wave V interaural latency differences as a function of asymmetry in 2000-4000 Hz hearing sensitivity. *American Journal of Otology, 10*,389–392.

BEAGLEY, H., & SHELDRAKE, J. (1978). Differences in brain stem response latency with age and sex. *British Journal of Audiology, 12*,69–77.

BEGLEITTER, J., PORJESZ, B., & CHOU, C.L. (1981). Auditory brain stem potentials in chronic alcoholics. *Science, 211* (6),1064–1066.

BERLIN, C.I., BORDELON, J., ST. JOHN, P., WILENSKY, D., HURLEY, A., KLUKA, E., & HOOD, L.J. (1998). Reversing click polarity may uncover auditory neuropathy in infants. *Ear and Hearing, 19*(1),37–47.

BUCHWALD, J.S., & HUANG, C.-M. (1975). Far-field acoustic response: Origins in the cat. *Science, 189*,382–384.

CHIAPPA, K.H., GLADSTONE, K.J., & YOUNG, R.R. (1979). Brain stem auditory-evoked responses: Studies of waveform variations in 50 normal human subjects. *Archives of Neurology, 36*,81–87.

CLEMIS, J.D., & McGEE, T. (1979). Brain stem electric response audiometry in the differential diagnosis of acoustic tumors. *Laryngoscope,* (89),31–42.

COATS, A.C., & MARTIN, J.L. (1977). Human auditory nerve action potentials and brain stem evoked responses. Effects of audiogram shape and lesion location. *Archives of Otolaryngology, 103*,605–622.

CONE-WESSON, B. (1995). Bone-conduction ABR tests. *American Journal of Audiology, 4*(3),14–19.

CONE-WESSON, B., & RAMIREZ, G.M. (1997). Hearing sensitivity in newborns estimated from ABRs to bone-conducted sounds. *Journal of the American Academy of Audiology, 8*(5), 299–307.

COX, L.C. (1985). Infant assessment: developmental and age-related considerations. In J.T. Jacobson (Ed.). *The auditory brain stem response.* (pp. 297–316). San Diego, CA: College Hill Press.

DAVIS, H., & HIRSH, S.K. (1976). The audiometric utility of brain stem responses to low-frequency sounds. *Audiology, 15*,181–195.

DON, M., ALLEN, A., & STARR, A. (1977). Effect of click rate on the latency of auditory brain stem responses in humans. *Annals of Otology, Rhinology and Laryngology, 86*(2), 186–196.

FINITZO-HIEBER, T. (1982). Auditory brain stem response: its place in infant audiological evaluations. *Seminars in Speech, Language and Hearing, 3*(1),76–87.

FOWLER, C.G., & NOFFSINGER, D. (1983). Effects of stimulus repetition rate and frequency on the auditory brain stem response in normal, cochlear-impaired, and VIII nerve/ brain stem-impaired subjects. *Journal of Speech and Hearing Research, 26*,560–567.

FUJIKAWA, S., & WEBER, B. (1977). Effects of increased stimulus rate on brain stem electric response (BER) audiometry as a function of age. *Journal of the American Audiology Society, 3*,147–150.

GERKEN, G.M. (1978). Brain stem evoked potentials and auditory analysis of single cycle transients. In R.F. Naunton & C. Fernandez (Eds.). *Evoked electrical activity in the auditory nervous system.* New York: Academic Press.

GORGA, M.P., ABBAS, P.J., & WORTHINGTON, D.W. (1985a). Stimulus calibration in ABR measurements. In J.T. Jacobson (Ed.). *The auditory brain stem response.* San Diego, CA: College-Hill Press, Inc.

GORGA, M.P., KAMINSKI, J.R., BEAUCHAINE, K.A., & JESTEADT, W. (1988). Auditory brain stem responses to tone bursts in normally hearing subjects. *Journal of Speech and Hearing Research, 31*(1),87–97.

GORGA, M.P., KAMINSKI, K.A., BEAUCHAINE, W., JESTEADT, W., & NEELY, S.T. (1989). Auditory brain stem responses from children three months to three years of age: normal patterns of response II. *Journal of Speech and Hearing Research, 32*,281–288.

GORGA, M.P., REILAND, J.K., BEAUCHAINE, K.A., WORTHINGTON, D. W., & JESTEADT, W. (1987). Auditory brain stem responses from graduates of an intensive care nursery: Normal patterns of response. *Journal of Speech and Hearing Research, 30*,311–318.

GORGA, M.P., & THORNTON, A R. (1989). The choice of stimuli for ABR measurements. *Ear and Hearing, 10*,217–230.

GORGA, M.P., WORTHINGTON, D.W., REILAND, J.K., BEAUCHAINE, K.A., & GOLDGAR, D.E. (1985b). Some comparisons between auditory brain stem response thresholds, latencies and the pure-tone audiogram. *Ear and Hearing, 6*(2),105–112.

HALL, J.W.I. (1992). *Handbook of auditory evoked responses.* Boston, MA: Allyn and Bacon.

HALL, J.W.I., KRIPAL, J.P., & HEPP, T. (1988). Newborn hearing screening with auditory brain stem response: Measurement problems and solutions. *Seminars in Hearing, 9*(1), 15–33.

HASHIMOTO, I., ISHIYAMA, Y., YOSHIMOTO, T., & NEMOTO, S. (1981). Brain stem auditory-evoked potentials recorded directly from human brain stem and thalamus. *Brain, 104*(4),841–859.

HECOX, K., & GALAMBOS, R. (1974). Brain stem auditory evoked responses in human infants and adults. *Archives of Otolaryngology, 99*,30–33.

HERRMANN, B.S., THORNTON, A.R., & JOSEPH, J. (1995). Automated infant hearing screening using the ABR: Development and validation. *American Journal of Audiology, 4*, 6–14.

HUANG, C., & BUCHWALD, J. (1977). Interpretation of the vertex short-latency acoustic response: A study of single neurons in the brain. *Brain Research, 137*,291–303.

HYDE, M.L. (1985). The effect of cochlear lesions on the ABR. In J.T. Jacobson (Ed.). *The auditory brain stem response* (pp. 133–146). San Diego, CA: College-Hill Press.

HYDE, M.L. &. BLAIR, R.L. (1981). The auditory brain stem response in neuro-otology: Prospective and problems. *Journal of Otolaryngology, 10*,117–125.

JACOBSON, J., MOREHOUSE, C.R., & JOHNSON, J. (1982). Strategies of infant auditory brain stem response assessment. *Ear and Hearing, 3*,263–269.

JACOBSON, J.T., & HALL, J.W.I. (1994). Newborn and infant auditory brain stem response applications. In J.T. Jacobson (Ed.). *Principles and applications in auditory evoked potentials.* (pp. 313–344). Boston, MA: Allyn and Bacon.

JERGER, J., & HALL, J.W., III. (1980). Effects of age and sex on auditory brain stem response (ABR). *Archives of Otolaryngology, 106,*387–391.

JERGER, J., & JOHNSON, K. (1988). Interactions of age, gender, and sensorineural hearing loss on ABR latency. *Ear and Hearing, 9,*168–175.

JERGER, J., & MAULDIN, L. (1978). Prediction of sensorineural hearing level from the brain stem evoked response. *Archives of Otolaryngology, 104,*456–461.

JEWETT, D.L., ROMANO, M.N., & WILLISTON, J.S. (1970). Human auditory evoked potentials: possible brain stem components detected on the scalp. *Science, 167,*1517–1518.

JEWETT, D. L., & WILLISTON, J. S. (1971). Auditory-evoked far fields averaged from the scalp of humans. *Brain, 94,*681–696.

JONES, T.A., STOCKARD, J.J., & WEIDNER, W.J. (1980). The effects of temperature and acute alcohol intoxication on brain stem auditory evoked potentials in the cat. *Electroencephalography and Clinical Neurophysiology, 49,*23–30.

JOSEY, A.F., GLASSCOCK, M.E., II, & MUSIEK, F.E. (1988). Correlation of ABR and medical imaging in patients with cerebello-pontine angle tumors. *American Journal of Otology, 9,*12–16.

KILENY, P. (1981). The frequency specificity of tone-pip evoked auditory brain stem responses. *Ear and Hearing, 2,*270–275.

KILENY, P. (1987). ALGO-1 automated infant hearing screener: Preliminary results. *Seminars in Hearing, 8,*125–131.

KODERA, K., YAMANE, H., YAMADA, O., & SUZUKI, J.-I. (1977). Brain stem response audiometry at speech frequencies. *Audiology, 31,*61–71.

KRAUS, N., OZDAMAR, O., STEIN, L., & REED, N. (1984). Absent auditory brain stem response: peripheral hearing loss or brain stem dysfunction? *Laryngoscope, 94* (March),400–406.

MAULDIN, L., & JERGER, J. (1979). Auditory brain stem evoked responses to bone-conducted signals. *Archives of Otolaryngology, 105,*656–661.

MCCLELLAND, R.J., & MCCREA, R.S. (1979). Intersubject variability of the auditory-evoked brain stem potentials. *Audiology, 18,*462-471.

MOLLER, A.R., & JANNETTA, P.J. (1985). Neural generators of the auditory brain stem response. In J. T. Jacobson (Ed.), *The auditory brain stem response.* San Diego, CA: College-Hill Press, Inc.

MUNNERLEY, G.M., GREVILLE, K.A., PURDY, S.C., & KEITH, W.J. (1991). Frequency-specific auditory brain stem responses relationship to behavioural thresholds in cochlear-impaired adults. *Audiology, 30,*25–32.

MUSIEK, F.E., & GOLLEGLY, K.M. (1985). ABR in Eight Nerve and Low Brain stem Lesions. In J.T. Jacobson (Ed.). *The auditory brain stem response* (pp. 181–202). San Diego, CA: College-Hill Press, Inc.

MUSIEK, F.E., KIBBE, K., RACKLIFFE, L., & WEIDER, D.J. (1984). The auditory brain stem response I-V amplitude ratio in normal, cochlear, and retrocochlear ears. *Ear and Hearing, 5,*52–55.

MUSIEK, F. E., KIBBE-MICHAL, K., GEURKINK, N. A., & JOSEY, A. F. (1986). ABR results in patients with posterior fossa tumors and normal pure-tone hearing. *Otolaryngology—Head and Neck Surgery, 94*(5),568–573.

NOUSAK, J.K., & STAPELLS, D.R. (1992). Frequency specificity of the auditory brain stem response to bone-conducted tones in infants and adults. *Ear and Hearing, 13,*87–95.

OZDAMAR, O., KRAUS, N., & CURRY, F. (1982). Auditory brain stem and middle latency responses in a patient with cortical deafness. *Electroencephalography and Clinical Neurophysiology, 53,*224–230.

PETERS, J.G. (1986). An automated infant screener using advanced evoked response technology. *The Hearing Journal, 39*(September),25–30.

PICTON, T.W., DURIEUX-SMITH, A., & MORAN, L.M. (1994). Recording auditory brain stem responses from infants. *International Journal of Pediatric Otorhinolaryngology, 28,*93–110.

PICTON, T.W., HILLYARD, S.A., KRAUSZ, H.I., & GALAMBOS, R. (1974). Human auditory evoked potentials. I. Evaluation of components. *Electroencephalography and Clinical Neurophysiology, 36,*179–190.

PICTON, T.W., OUELLETTE, J., HAMEL, G., & SMITH, A.D. (1979). Brain stem evoked potentials to tonepips in notched noise. *The Journal of Otolaryngology, 8*(4),289–314.

PICTON, T.W., STAPELLS, D.R., & CAMPBELL, K.B. (1981). Auditory evoked potentials from the human cochlea and brain stem. *The Journal of Otolaryngology, 10,*(Suppl. 9),1–41.

PRASHER, D.K., & GIBSON, W.P.R. (1980). Brain stem auditory evoked potentials: A comparative study of monaural vs. binaural stimulation in the detection of multiple sclerosis. *Electroencephalography and Clinical Neurophysiology, 50,* 247–253.

PRATT, H., & SOHMER, H. (1976). Intensity and rate functions of cochlear and brain stem evoked responses to click stimuli in man. *Archives of Oto-Rhino-Laryngology, 212,*85–92.

RANCE, G., DOWELL, R.C., RICKARDS, F.W., BEER, D.E., & CLARK, G.M. (1998). Steady-state evoked potential and behavioral hearing thresholds in a group of children with absent click-evoked auditory brain stem responses. *Ear and Hearing, 19*(1),48–61.

ROBERTS, J.L., DAVIS, H., PHON, G.L., REICHERT, T.J., STURTEVANT, E.M., & MARSHALL, R.E. (1982). Auditory brain stem responses in preterm neonates: maturation and follow-up. *The Journal of Pediatrics, 101*(2),257–263.

ROBINSON, K., & RUDGE, P. (1975). Auditory evoked responses in multiple sclerosis. *Lancet, 1,*1164–1166.

ROBINSON, K.H., & RUDGE, P. (1980). The use of the auditory evoked potential in the diagnosis of multiple sclerosis. *Journal of Neurological Science, 45,*235–244.

ROSENHAMER, H.J., LINDSTROM, B., & LUNDBORG, J. (1980). On the use of click-evoked electric brain stem responses in audiological diagnosis. II. The infuence of sex and age upon the normal response. *Scandinavian Audiology, 9,*93–100.

ROWE, M.I. (1978). Normal variability of the brain stem auditory evoked response in young and old adult subjects. *Electroencephalography and Clinical Neurophysiology, 44,*459–470.

SALAMY, A. (1984). Maturation of the auditory brain stem response from birth through early childhood. *Journal of Clinical Neurophysiology, 1,*293–329.

SALAMY, A., & MCKEAN, C.M. (1976). Postnatal development of human brain stem potentials during the first year of life. *Electroencephalography and Clinical Neurophysiology, 41,*418–426.

SALAMY, A., MCKEAN, C.M., & BUDA, F.B. (1975). Maturational changes in auditory transmission as reflected in human brain stem potentials. *Brain Research, 96,*361–366.

SALAMY, A., MENDELSON, T., & TOOLEY, W.H. (1982). Developmental profiles for the brain stem auditory evoked potential. *Early Human Development, 6,*331–339.

SCHWARTZ, D.M, MORRIS, M.D., SPYDELL, J.D., BRINK, C.T., GRIM, M.A., & SCHWARTZ, J.A. (1990). Influence of click polarity on the auditory brain stem response (BAER) revisited. *Electroencephalography and Clinical Neurophysiology, 77*,445–457.

SCHWARTZ, D.M., MORRIS, M.D., & JACOBSON, J.T. (1994). The normal auditory brain stem response and its variants. In J.T. Jacobson (Ed.). *Principles and applications in auditory evoked potentials* (pp. 123–153). Boston, MA: Allyn and Bacon.

SELTERS, W.A., & BRACKMANN, D.E. (1977). Acoustic tumor detection with brain stem electric response audiometry. *Archives of Otolaryngology, 103*(April),181–187.

SININGER, Y.S., HOOD, L.J., STARR, A., & BERLIN, C.I. (1995). Hearing loss due to auditory neuropathy. *Audiology Today, 7*(2),10–13.

SKLARE, D.A. (1987). Auditory brain stem response laboratory norms: When is the data base sufficient? *Ear and Hearing, 8,* 56–57.

SOHMER, H., & FEINMESSER, M. (1967). Cochlear action potentials recorded from the external ear in man. *Annals of Otology, Rhinology, and Laryngology, 76*,427–436.

SOHMER, H., FEINMESSER, M., & SZABO, G. (1974). Sources of electrocochleographic responses as studied in patients with brain damage. *Electroencephalography and Clinical Neurophysiology, 37*,663–669.

SQUIRES, K.C., CHU, N.S., & STARR, A. (1978). Auditory brain stem potentials with alcohol. *Electroencephalography and Clinical Neurophysiology, 45*,577–584.

STAPELLS, D.R. (1989). Auditory brain stem response assessment of infants and children. *Seminars in Hearing, 10,* 229–251.

STAPELLS, D.R., GRAVEL, J.S., & MARTIN, B.A. (1995). Thresholds for auditory brain stem responses to tones in notched noise from infants and young children with normal-hearing or sensorineural hearing loss. *Ear and Hearing, 16*(4),361–371.

STAPELLS, D.R., & PICTON, T.W. (1981). Technical aspects of brain stem evoked potential audiometry using tones. *Ear and Hearing, 2*(1),20–29.

STAPELLS, D.R., PICTON, T.W., DURIEUX-SMITH, A., EDWARDS, C.G., & MORAN, L.M. (1990). Thresholds for short-latency auditory-evoked potentials to tones in notched noise in normal-hearing and hearing-impaired subjects. *Audiology, 29*,262–274.

STAPELLS, D.R., PICTON, T.W., PEREZ-ABALO, M., READ, D., & SMITH, A. (1985). Frequency specificity in evoked potential audiometry. In J.T. Jacobson (Ed.). *The auditory brain stem response* (pp. 147–177). San Diego, CA: College-Hill Press.

STARR, A., & ACHOR, L.J. (1975). Auditory brain stem responses in neurological disease. *Archives of Neurology, 32*(November), 761–768.

STARR, A., AMLIE, R., MARTIN, W.H., & SANDERS, S. (1977). Development of auditory function in newborn infants revealed by auditory brain stem potential. *Pediatrics, 60,* 831–839.

STARR, A., & HAMILTON, A.E. (1976). Correlation between confirmed sites of neurological lesions and abnormalities of far-field auditory brain stem responses. *Electroencephalography and Clinical Neurophysiology, 41*,595–608.

STOCKARD, J.E., STOCKARD, J.J., WESTMORELAND, B.F., & CORFITS, J.L. (1979). Brain stem auditory-evoked responses. Normal variation as a function of stimulus and subject characteristics. *Archives of Neurology, 36*(13),823–831.

STOCKARD, J.E., & WESTMORELAND, B.F. (1981). Technical considerations in the recording and interpretation of the brain stem auditory evoked potential for neonatal neurologic diagnosis. *American Journal of EEG Technology, 21*,31–54.

STOCKARD, J.J., & ROSSITER, V.S. (1977). Clinical and pathological correlates of brain stem auditory response abnormalities. *Neurology, 27*(4),316–325.

STOCKARD, J.J., ROSSITER, V.S., WIEDERHOLT, W.C., & KOBAYASHI, R.M. (1976). Brain stem auditory-evoked responses in suspected central pontine myelinolysis. *Archives of Neurology, 33*(October),726–728.

STOCKARD, J.J., STOCKARD, J.E., & SHARBROUGH, F.W. (1977). Detection and localization of occult lesions with brain stem auditory responses. *Mayo Cinic Proceedings, 52*(December), 761–769.

STOCKARD, J.J., STOCKARD, J.E., & SHARBROUGH, F.W. (1978). Nonpathological factors influencing brain stem auditory evoked potentials. *American Journal of EEG Technology, 18,* 177–209.

STOCKARD, J.J., STOCKARD, J.E., & SHARBROUGH, F.W. (1980). Brain stem auditory evoked potentials in neurology: methodology, interpretation, clinical application. In M.J. Aminoff (Ed.). *Electrodiagnosis in clinical neurology* (pp. 370–413). New York: Churchill Livingstone.

STUART, A., YANG, E.Y., & GREEN, W.B. (1994). Neonatal auditory brain stem response thresholds to air- and bone-conducted clicks: 0 to 96 hours postpartum. *Journal of the American Academy of Audiology, 5*(3),163–172.

SUZUKI, T., HIRAI, Y., & HORIUCHI, K. (1977). Auditory brain stem responses to pure tone stimuli. *Scandinavian Audiology, 6*,51–56.

TERKILDSEN, K., HUIS IN'T VELD, F., & OSTERHAMMEL, P. (1977). Auditory brain stem responses in the diagnosis of cerebellopontine angle tumours. *Scandinavian Audiolgy, 6,* 43–47.

WEBER, B.A., & FOLSOM, R.C. (1977). Brain stem wave V latencies to tone pip stimuli. *Journal of the American Academy of Audiology, 2*,182–184.

WORTHINGTON, D.W., & PETERS, J.F. (1980). Quantifiable hearing and no ABR: paradox or error? *Ear and Hearing, 1,* 281–285.

YANG, E.Y., RUPERT, A.L., & MOUSHEGIAN, G. (1987). A developmental study of bone conduction auditory brain stem response in infants. *Ear and Hearing, 8,*244–251.

ZOLLNER, C., KARNAHL, T., & STANGE, G. (1976). Input-output function and adaptation behavior of the five early potentials registered with he earlobe-vertex pick-up. *Archives of Oto-Rhino-Laryngology, 212,*23-33.

## Chapter 20

Middle and Long Latency Auditory Evoked Potentials

David L. McPherson and Bopanna Ballachanda

Outline

HISTORICAL PERSPECTIVE OF AUDITORY EVOKED POTENTIALS

The development of auditory evoked potentials (AEPs) closely follows advances in electronic technology. The earliest recording of a human AEP was accomplished by Vladimirovich Pravdich-Neminsky, a Russian scientist, in 1913 (Brazier, 1984). These recordings consisted of dim tracings on a cathode tube oscilloscope. Later a camera would be used to take photographs of the cathode tube and the waveforms that "overlayed" would become dark because of the repetitive exposure of the cathode tube tracings on the film. The storage oscilloscope (i.e., the ability of an oscilloscope to "store" a recording without overwriting the previous tracing) coupled with a camera permitted an easier more reliable means of reading the evoked potential recording.

During this same time the recording oscilloscope, or what is more commonly called the strip-chart recorder, replaced the use of photographic film. However, it was the advent of the computer that brought AEPs out of the research laboratory and into the clinic. Allsion Laboratories was a pioneer in this area and manufactured the first commercial clinical evoked potential unit. Unfortunately, it was very expensive and short lived. Interestingly, the demise of the early clinical use of AEPs was because its use in establishing auditory thresholds was controversial and poorly defined. The discovery of auditory brain stem evoked potentials (ABR) by Don Jewett in 1971 (Jewett & Williston, 1971) rekindled interest in the use of AEPs for estimating hearing sensitivity. The purpose of this chapter is to present material on the clinical use of the middle and long latency AEPs.

GENERAL CONSIDERATIONS

Some conventions used in this chapter need to be clarified. For example, the designation of polarity (positivity/negativity) may appear as positive up, negative down or negative

Audiology: Diagnosis. Edited by Roeser, Valente, and Hosford-Dunn. Thieme Medical Publishers, Inc., New York © 2000

up, positive down. These differences have a long history. In this chapter the more conventional designation of positive up and negative down is used. However, in reading the literature it is always important to refer to the figure designators and confirm the polarity of the waveforms.

Ferraro et al (1996) proposed a standard for presenting and specifying parameters in AEP testing and reporting. The tables in this chapter conform to those recommendations. Throughout this chapter, the designation dB nHL is used as a reference to average behavioral threshold in normal subjects according to stimulus specifications.

Figure 20–1 illustrates an overview of the morphological features of the AEPs discussed in this chapter. These were recorded from normal young adults (18 to 26 years of age) without respect to gender. Table 20–1 gives an overview of the description of the middle (MLAEP) and long latency auditory potentials (LAEP) discussed in this chapter. The reader is encouraged to use this chapter as a basis for further study and exploration into AEPs.

Electrodes

Electrodes consist of a metal alloy, the most common being tin, gold, silver, and silver-sliver chloride (Ag-AgCl). For recording of responses whose frequencies are greater than about 100 Hz, the metal alloy is not particularly significant, especially for recording the brain stem AEP (ABR). Tin electrodes are frequently used in the clinical recording of the ABR unless extended recording times, beyond about 1 hour, are used. In such cases both silver and gold electrodes have been found to be more stable. Low-frequency recordings, less than about 50 Hz, require stability as to changes in the surface potential between the electrode and the scalp. Gold electrodes tend to hold a potential and become polarized. Ag-AgCl electrodes are more stable, thus allowing long-term recordings of DC potentials.

Because infection is always a possibility when abrading the skin as needed for electrode preparation, it is strongly recommended that disposable electrodes be used. In addition, skin preparation and electrode application should be carried out with examining gloves.

It is common practice to use the linked earlobe, or linked mastoid, as a reference electrode site when recording many of the LAEPs. This is particularly true for the P300 event–related potential. However, all electrode sites across the scalp are active. Therefore one can expect electrical interactions of neural sites to bias the recordings obtained from other electrodes. This poses a particular problem in recordings, whereby the precise nature of the response across the scalp is desired, or in single channel recordings, where hemispheric specificity is of interest. Consequently, our preferred reference site is C7, a noncephalic electrode position.

Electrode Montage

In referring to electrode montages, the 10 to 20 international system will be used (Jasper, 1958). The exception to this is when referring to mastoid placement of an electrode. Mastoid electrode placement will be abbreviated as M1 (left mastoid) and M2 (right mastoid). Also, Mi and Mc are used to designate ipsilateral mastoid (signal and electrode placement on the same side) and contralateral mastoid (electrode placement on the mastoid opposite the signal). Unless specifically stated as an exception, earlobe placement of an electrode (A1, A2) and mastoid placement of an electrode (M1, M2) are used interchangeably. That is, one may be substituted for the other. However, the nonstandard use of a frontal placement for the noninverting electrode instead of the vertex (Cz) electrode for

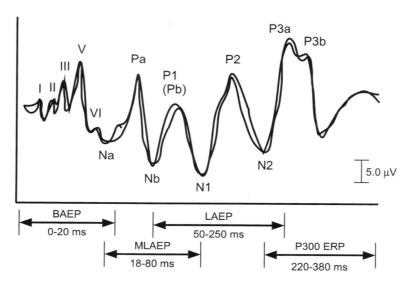

Figure 20–1 General morphological features of the AEP and the ERP. The ABR occurs between 1 and 20 ms poststimulus; the MLAEP occurs between 18 and 80 ms poststimulus, the LAEP occurs between 50 and 250 ms poststimulus, and the auditory ERP occurs between 220 and 380 ms poststimulus.

TABLE 20–1   Description of the MLAEP and LAEP

Component	Classification	Latency (ms)	Amplitude (μU)	Response Features
Na	MLAEP Exogenous	18–25	5–7	a. May be present even when the Pa is absent.
Pa	MLAEP Exogenous	24–36	8–12	
Nb	MLAEP Exogenous	34–47	8–12	a. Not always fully developed until 8–10 y of age.
Pb	MLAEP* Exogenous	55–80	5–7	a. Sensitive to changes in stimulus parameters (i.e., frequency, intensity, "on" and "off" effects). b. Amplitude changes with sleep state.
P50 gating response	MLAEP Exogenous/ gating response	40–70	3–8 (S1) 0–6 (S2)	a. S2 amplitude is 60% or less of the S1 amplitude in normal individuals. b. Absent in ADHD and schizophrenia.
P1	LAEP[†] Exogenous	55–80	5–7	a. Sensitive to changes in stimulus parameters (i.e., frequency, intensity, "on" and "off" effects). b. Amplitude changes with sleep state.
N1	LAEP Exogenous	80–150	5–10	a. Sensitive to changes in the acoustic features of the stimulus (i.e., spectrum). b. Amplitude changes with sleep state and attention. c. Sensitive to changes in the acoustic features of the stimulus (i.e., spectrum).
P2	LAEP Exogenous	145–180	3–6	a. Amplitude changes with sleep state and attention.
N2	LAEP endogenous	180–250	3–6	a. Sensitive to change in the acoustic features of the stimulus. b. Amplitude significantly affected by attention and sleep state.
MMN	Exogenous	200–300	30–50	a. Not affected by attention. b. Subject sleep state will vary both amplitude and latency.
P300, P300a, P300b	Endogenous cognitive	220–380	12	a. The P300a is related to stimulus novelty. b. The P300b is related to task response. c. The amplitude is affected by attention and sleep state.
N400	Endogenous linguistic	390–510	−10	a. Sensitive to linguistic content. b. Amplitude changes with low versus high predictability sentences.

*Designated as a MLAEP when labeled Pb. If labeled P1, then it is associated with the LAEP.
[†]Designated as a LAEP when labeled P1. If labeled Pb, then it is associated with the MLAEP.

ABRs, MLAEPs, and LAEPs is not acceptable. This common, but technically incorrect practice, even in ABR recordings, is discouraged.

All electrode sites across the scalp should be considered neural active sites. Wolpaw and Wood (1982) have clearly shown that the nasion, ear, and mastoid, as well as other cephalic locations, are in the auditory evoked field potential. Referential locations on or below the inferior neck provide the best and most accurate reference location. One of the most common locations is C7 located at the nape of the neck (McPherson & Starr, 1993).

Amplifiers

Considerable confusion exists over the use of amplifier and channel designations in evoked potentials. Much of the confusion is created at the manufacture level. The terms "noninverting" and "inverting" should be used in describing the amplifier inputs, and this convention has been used throughout this chapter. In general, the following are equated: (1) noninverting, positive, +, active; and (2) inverting, negative, −, reference. It is beyond the scope of this chapter to engage in a discussion of the technicalities of these terms. For a good discussion, readers are referred to Hall (1992) and McPherson (1996).

Many books and reference materials give gain specifications for the various AEPs. These are starting points, but what is important is not so much the actual gain, but what permits a strong enough signal that meets the input requirements to the signal averager. It is also important to have a signal that does not overdrive the artifact reject. The best method to determine proper gain is to make an initial adjustment and then, while viewing the raw unaveraged signal on the monitor, adjust the gain so that muscle movement will cause a reject. When the patient is quiet, the ongoing tracing will be relatively stable. Generally, a good starting for all AEPs is a gain setting somewhere between 10K and 20K. Some manufacturers specify gain in terms of voltage per division. If a visual (i.e., screen) adjustment of gain is completed, as recommended earlier, it is a matter of adjusting the artifact to about three-quarters total screen excursion. Specifics need to be addressed on a manufacturer-by-manufacturer basis.

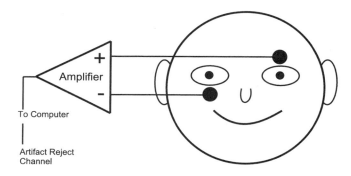

> ## PEARL
>
> Having the patient gently clench the teeth or lightly close the eyes is a good way to check the artifact reject setting.

Figure 20–2 Placement of eye monitoring electrodes for eye muscle artifact. One electrode is placed above the orbit and the second electrode is placed below the orbit of the opposite eye. This permits both eye blinks and eye movement to be monitored and rejected from the recordings.

Monitoring Eye Movement Artifact

Eye movement is a known major contaminant in the recording of AEPs, especially for activity that is occurring beyond about 50 ms. This problem has two basic considerations. First, the amplitude and latency are such that not only may they obscure the desired response but they may actually be mistaken for the response (Barrett, 1993; McPherson, 1996). Second, the eye blink is an easily conditioned response and may become synchronized with the auditory stimuli and has a latency of about 250 ms.

An oblique electrode placement (Fig. 20–2) will permit the monitoring of both eye movement (i.e., electro-oculography) and eye blinks. The preferred situation is when the eye movement or blinks activate the artifact rejection during eye monitoring. An alternate procedure is to affix the electrode superior and lateral to the orbit of one eye and reference it to the contralateral mastoid (or earlobe). The bandpass of the amplifier should be approximately .1 to 30 Hz.

Postauricular Muscle Reflex

The postauricular muscle reflex (PAM) is a muscle innervated by the posterior auricular branch of the facial nerve (seventh nerve). The PAM contracts in response to moderately loud sounds and may become a conditioned reflex. Because of its timing, about 18 to 30 ms, it may contaminate the MLAEP and be mistaken for a neural response within the MLAEP. The

main feature in recognizing the PAM is that it is a very large response whose amplitude is not within the range of a known MLAEP. The PAM may easily be avoided by routinely using earlobe electrodes (A1, A2) instead of mastoid electrodes (M1, M2). If mastoid electrodes are used, placing the electrode on the head of the bony prominence will significantly reduce the probability of the PAM being recorded.

Repetition Rate and Interstimulus Interval

In most instances the repetition rate (number of presentations per second) is the reciprocal of the interstimulus interval (ISI) (the time between each individual stimulus presentations). However, in some instances this is not the case, especially in paradigms that use paired or multiple stimuli. The ISI must be long enough to capture the entire desired response before the occurrence of the next trial.

Prestimulus Recording

We strongly recommend that all recordings include a prestimulus sample. That is, a sample that is approximately 10% of the sample window is obtained before the presentation of the acoustic event. This provides a better estimate of the baseline of the response and some indication of the noise present in the recording.

> ## PEARL
>
> A good way to obtain an estimate of the noise level is to make a set of replicated averages with the stimulus off.

Subject State

The subject should be placed in a comfortable position with the neck at rest such that the muscles of the face and neck are in a relaxed position. The room should be sound isolated with no visual or other sensory distractions. A low light level is best. The person being tested should be told to be alert but not active.

Attention

The effects of attention vary across components. In cochlear recordings and the ABR, it is not a significant factor. In the MLAEP, there is some indication that active attention may enhance the later components (Pb), but to a very small degree. However, in the LAEP and in auditory event–related potentials (ERPs) the effect becomes significant, especially for responses occurring beyond about 150 ms.

Attention includes *selective* attention, whereby attention is maintained through an active discrimination task (i.e., same-difference task); *active* attention, whereby the observer is asked to respond to the stimuli (i.e., button push); *passive* attention, whereby the individual being tested is to be in an awake alert state but not necessarily attending to the stimuli; and an *ignore* condition, whereby the individual is being distracted from the stimuli. The effect of these various states of attention on the component varies with the component being measured.

Special Considerations

In the original paper on auditory neuropathy (Starr et al, 1991) it was noted that conditions exist whereby time-locked AEPs, such as in the ABR as seen in auditory neuropathy, may be absent and cognitive AEPs may be present. This poses an interesting perspective on the interpretation of AEPs. It would appear that if the ABR is absent, one must ascertain whether the individual being tested fits this profile. Specifically, an auditory neuropathy is suspected when a percept of the auditory stimulus is present, but an absence of the ABR in the presence of the cochlear microphonic and otoacoustic emissions. If such is the case, then this significantly changes the interpretation of the AEPs. For example, if one is looking at a particular component of the MLAEP or LAEP and the components are absent, or significantly abnormal, it becomes necessary to examine earlier components, especially wave I of the ABR. We strongly recommend the practice of preceding any AEP evaluation with both acoustic immittance measures, including tympanometry, and measures of otoacoustic emissions.

The use of the ABR for hearing screening and threshold estimation has been well established for almost two decades. It is primarily predicated on the observation that as intensity increases or decreases, latency demonstrates an inverse relationship. Wave V of the ABR is primarily used in this technique because it is very robust, stable, and repeatable (McPherson & Starr, 1993). Historically, the LAEPs have not been used for hearing threshold assessment because latencies of these components generally do not show the same trend nor have they been considered as robust (McPherson, 1996). Over the early years of developing the ABR as a measure of hearing amplitude, measures have been criticized as being unstable, especially across individuals. However, today these issues have changed, primarily because of changes in technology and a better understanding of factors affecting these measures. It has clearly been established that the amplitude of the predominant AEP components are stable within the individual and that the changes seen in the amplitude with stimulus changes are consistent across individuals, although the amplitude values across individuals may vary somewhat (McPherson, 1996).

Although the amount of enhancement varies with each component, in general it is important to realize that the greater a target signal is attended, the more robust the component is, with large effects of attention seen for the P300 and later responses (i.e., P300a, P300b, N400).

Calibration and Normal Values

Issues of stimulus calibration and specification are significant when recording and reporting AEPs, especially those discussed in this chapter. Significant differences exist between specifying a stimulus in dB HL, dB nHL, dB SPL, dB SPLpe, and dB SL. In some instances, the components will be more sensitive to threshold levels and sensation levels than to the actual sound pressure levels. The reader is referred to Hall (1992), McPherson (1996), and Gorga and Neely (1994) for a more complete discussion on calibrating AEPs.

Peak latencies are fairly stable and robust in the major components of AEPs. Consequently, latency values may generally be used across studies and laboratories. This is not necessarily true for amplitude values. Electrode placement, filter settings, biological noise, stimulus specification, and subject state affect amplitude to a much greater extent than these factors affect latency. Although it is possible to use amplitude values from other studies and laboratories, it is absolutely necessary to maintain the exact stimulus and recording parameters as those that were used to obtain the normative data (Table 20–2). Even minor changes can affect the waveform. One of the greatest violations that occurs in AEPs, and especially those using ABR, is to adjust filter settings and other parameters to obtain "better" waveforms. Indeed, such poor and naïve techniques not only result in abuses of the procedure but also give the tester a false sense of obtaining reliable and meaningful test results. Unless one understands exactly what the consequences are of changing a particular parameter, exact protocols should be followed. Clinicians should avoid using the term "In my clinical experience. . . ." This phrase is commonly used as an excuse for the lack of rigor and understanding as related to established and proven procedures. The best procedure is to develop one's own normative data on the basis of the protocols chosen and keep within those protocols. Second, and one that works quite well, is to adopt published data while maintaining the identical techniques that were used to collect the normative information.

MIDDLE LATENCY AUDITORY EVOKED POTENTIALS (MLAEPs)

Introduction

The MLAEPs consist a of biphasic waveform (Fig. 20–3) with a negative wave occurring at about 20 ms (Na), a positive wave

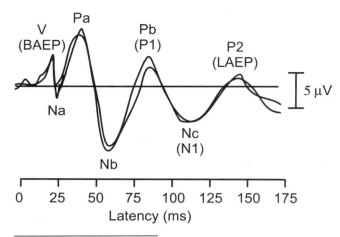

Figure 20–3   MLAEPs to a 2000 Hz pip presented at 70 dB nHL. The components Pb and Nc are often considered part of the LAEPs. Wave V of the ABR and the P2 component of the LAEP are also shown to illustrate the distribution of the MLAEP.

occurring at about 30 ms (Pa), a second negative wave occurring at about 40 ms (Nb), and a second positive wave occurring at about 50 ms (Pb). The Pb component of the MLAEP is oftentimes identified as the P1 component of the LAEP. However, because of the stimulus response nature of the Pb, we prefer to classify it as a MLAEP. Further separation of these components is seen because the Na-Pa wave has been identified as abnormal in temporal lobe lesions of the auditory system, and Pb has been reported as abnormal in schizophrenia, autism, stuttering, and attention disorder hyperactive disorder (ADHD). Buchwald and others have stated that the Pb component of the MLAEP is related to activity of the reticular activating system and is responsible for the modulation of sensory stimuli (Buchwald et al, 1981; Erwin et al, 1991; Freedman et al, 1987; Hillyard & Kutas, 1983).

TABLE 20–2   Summary of AEP recording parameters

Component	Montage*,†	Time base (ms)	No. Averages	Filter (Hz)	Stimuli (type)	Level	Rate	ISI
MLAEP	Cz-Ai	80–100	500–1000	3–1500	Brief tones	75–80 dB nHL	5–11/s	90–200 ms (adult) 300–500 ms (young children)
P50	Cz-C7 or Ai	80	250–500	1–3000	Brief tone	70–75 dB nHL for both pairs	(see ISI)	S1–S2 interval, 500 ms S2–S1 interval, 10 s
LAEP	Cz-Ai	300	200–250	1–300	Tone burst	75–80 dB HL	0.9–2.9/s	300 ms–1.1 s
MMN	Fpz, F4, Fz, F3, C4, Cz, C3, Oz to Tip of nose or C7	400	50–100	0.1–100	Oddball paradigm	75–80 dB HL	1/s	1000 ms
P300	Cz'-C7	500	200–250	.05–50 Hz	Oddball paradigm	75–80 dB HL	0.9/s or less	1.1s or longer
N400	Cz-C7	100 (before) 750 (after)	100	.05–50	Speech	75–80 dB HL	(see ISI)	1–2 s from end of sentence

*Montages are noted with the noninverting electrode stated first and the inverting electrode stated last (i.e., Cz-Mi, or Fpz, Cz to C7).
†A (earlobe) and M (mastoid) electrode designations are used interchangeably.

The MLAEPs represent primarily exogenous responses (i.e., those responses primarily generated by the physical characteristics of the stimulus) of the auditory system. The study of the generators of the MLAEP have given strong support for thalamocortical projections to primary and secondary auditory cortices (Kraus et al, 1994a; McPherson & Starr, 1993; Parving et al, 1980; Shi Di & Barth, 1992; Wolpaw & Wood, 1982; Wood & Wolpaw, 1982). However, clear evidence also exists that overlapping sources are present (Kraus et al, 1994a; McPherson & Davies, 1995; Wood & Wolpaw, 1982). Kraus and McGee (1995) suggest that the MLAEP pathways are sensory specific to the auditory stimulus, demonstrating a high degree of frequency specificity and temporal sequencing. Early portions of the MLAEP pathway are from the ventral portion of the medial geniculate with radiations into the primary auditory cortex. The MLAEP as recorded over the vertex is a mixture of both primary and secondary afferents, with the secondary afferents showing some state dependency; especially for sleep (Kraus & McGee, 1995).

Studies on the development of the middle latency response have yielded a variety of results and recommendations. The most important recommendation is that made by McGee and Kraus (1996) showing that to obtain reliable recordings of the middle latency response in infants it is necessary to control and maintain sleep state. Specifically, these authors recommend that a constant state of light sleep or awakefulness be maintained throughout the testing. It is likewise necessary that this same state be maintained across subjects to develop and compare an individual recording to a set of age-matched norms.

PEARL

Light periodic fanning of a sleeping infant is enough to help keep the infant in a relatively stable and moderate state of sleep.

Filter settings are critical in the MLAEP, and incorrect filtering may provide false information, especially when using the MLAEP for maturation studies. Scherg (1982) has observed waveform distortion in infants when filtering was narrowed, thus creating "phantom" peaks occurring within the middle latency segment. Tucker and Ruth (1996) have shown that latency decreases and amplitude increases for the Pa component from birth (i.e., 24 hours postpartum) to adulthood. Most researchers agree that the MLAEP reaches adult values in the early teens.

McGee and Kraus (1996) have suggested that the middle latency response has a long developmental time course that is complete just after the first 10 years of life. The developmental aspects of the middle latency response appear to be related not only to amplitude and latency but also to the stability of the response and the effects of subject state. They attribute these factors to multiple generators of the MLAEP that may have different developmental sequences. Developmental studies by McPherson et al (1989) and Buchwald (1990b) have also shown that changes in morphology occur during development and that responses up to the Pb are usually present in

the normal newborn period. The Na response is seen fairly consistently after the age of 8.

Technical Specifications

The MLAEP is obtained with an 80 to 100 ms window. Between 500 and 1000 averages should be sufficient to collect replicable waveforms. A high-pass filter between 3 and 10 Hz and a low-pass filter between 1500 and 2000 Hz may be used (author preference is a bandpass of 3 to 1500 Hz). A presentation rate of about 5/s will generally give good Na-Pa responses in adults; however, if the Na-Pa is not present or young children or infants are being tested, it may be necessary to decrease the rate to 2 to 3/s (Table 20–3). Unlike the Pa component that is present and is part of the primary auditory pathway, the later response, Pb, is part of the nonspecific auditory pathway and reticular activating system; thus its presence and variation may depend on subject state.

Electrodes

The electrode type (i.e., Ag-AgCl, silver, or gold) is not critical, except tin is not recommended. The MLAEP does not require long time constants to record the response. Single-channel recordings are most common in the MLAEP. The MLAEP is maximally recorded over the vertex at Cz and referenced to the ipsilateral earlobe or mastoid. However, this gives a single vertex response (Cz) and does not provide information about interhemispheric responses. A more useful technique is to use three channels with electrodes located at Cz, T3, and T4 (noninverting) with a noncephalic electrode located at C7 or linked mastoids (A1 + A2). A ground, in either situation, is located at Fpz. Similar montages have been consistently reported in the literature for use in measures of the middle latency auditory pathway function (Kraus et al, 1982, 1994a; McPherson & Starr, 1993).

Although the MLAEP does not have problems with eye movement contamination, it may become contaminated with activity of the PAM. This is no trivial matter and was the cause of extreme controversy in the early stages of evoked potential use. Contamination from the PAM may easily be resolved by using earlobe electrodes instead of mastoid electrodes (Fig. 20–4).

Recording Parameters

A 10-ms preanalysis baseline is obtained with an 80-ms poststimulus recording. The signal is bandpass filtered between 3 and 1500 Hz, and 500 averages are obtained for each condition. An artifact reject is set to 75% maximum sampling amplitude to exclude the PAM reflex.

Stimulus

Oates and Stapells (1997a,b) demonstrated that the Na-Pa response of the MLAEPs, when using a derived band center frequency technique, showed good frequency specificity to brief tones. This would suggest that frequency specificity may be obtained in the MLAEP using brief tones with a linear 2-1-2 cycle window tone pip or a Blackman 5-cycle window tone pip. Both result in excellent frequency specificity for the MLAEPs.

Nelson et al (1997) showed that the variability of the Pb component of the MLAEP was reduced by using low-

TABLE 20–3   MLAEP recording parameters

Parameter	Note
Electrodes	
Type:	Ag-AgCl, silver, gold
Montage:	*Single channel:*
	Cz (noninverting).
	Ai (inverting).
	FpZ (ground).
	Multichannel (see text):
	Cz, T3, and T4 (noninverting).
	C7–noncephalic (inverting).
	FpZ (ground).
Recording Parameters	
Channels:	One channel is standard.
	Two or more channels for hemispheric specificity.
Timebase:	80–100 ms with a 10 ms preanalysis.
# Averages:	500–1000.
Filter (bandpass):	3–1500 Hz.
Artifact Rejection:	3/4 maximum sampling amplitude.
Stimuli	
Type:	100 µs acoustic clicks may be used, but are not preferred.
	Brief tone with a 2-1-2 cycle.
	Blackman 5-cycle brieftone.
Transducer:	Tubal insert phones.
	Calibrated earphones (i.e., TDH-39, etc.).
	Sound field speakers.
Polarity:	Rarefaction.
	NOTE: in children sometimes it is necessary to reverse the polarity for better morphology.
Level:	75–80 dB nHL for a robust response showing all of the subcomponents.
	Brief tones may be used to estimate hearing sensitivity and the actual level would vary.
Rate:	Up to 11/s, but lower rates are preferable (5/s).
	In young children rates as low as 2–3/s yield best results.
ISI:	90–200 ms with the longer ISI preferred.
	300–500 ms in young children.

frequency (500 Hz) stimulation with a duration not less than about 60 ms and a repetition rate of 1.1/s. The response was recorded optimally at Fz (inverting electrode) when a noncephalic reference (noninverting electrode) was used. They also reported that Pb had a larger amplitude and longer latency in children than adults. It should be realized, however, that a Cz placement is more common than Fz.

A rise/fall time of at least 2 ms is recommended to reduce spectral splatter and appears to maximize frequency specificity. Rise/fall times of greater than 4 ms appear to significantly reduce the amplitude of the Na-Pa response. That is, the amplitude of the Na-Pa response increases for rise/fall times up to about 2 ms, asymptotes, and then shows a reduction in amplitude for rise/fall times greater than 2 ms. A rise/fall time of four cycles and a plateau time of two cycles is believed to be a good compromise in estimating a MLAEP threshold (Xu et al, 1997).

The stimulus may be presented either in the sound field, through earphones, or through tubal insert phones. The intensity, except for threshold estimation, is usually at a moderately comfortable level (75- to 80-dB nHL). In adults a rate of 5/s gives the best results, but in young children and infants a slower rate, between 2 to 3/s, is necessary for reliable recordings.

Hearing threshold may be estimated by completing an intensity series beginning at 80 dB nHL and decreasing in either 10- or 15-dB steps. Threshold is estimated as the lowest level in which the Na-Pa response may be identified and is repeatable. Threshold estimation is completed by evaluating the changes in amplitude with intensity. Little or no latency change occurs with changes in the intensity of the acoustic stimulus.

The use of the MLAEP as a means of threshold estimate is extremely limited because of the necessity of controlling for sleep state, muscle contamination, and suppression of the

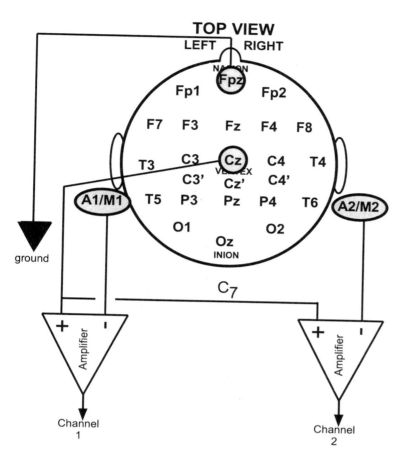

Figure 20–4 Electrode montage for the MLAEP (Cz-A1 and Cz-A2).

MLAEP with sleep-enhancing drugs (i.e., chloral hydrate, barbiturates). The advantage, however, has been in the ability to obtain frequency-specific information, especially for the low frequencies where the use of click stimuli to obtain the ABR results in primarily mid- to high-frequency recordings. On the other hand, use of frequency-specific ABR techniques has greatly overcome this limitation in ABR (Oates & Stapells, 1997a,b).

Subject State and Variables

Kraus and McGee (1996) have shown that the MLAEP may be recorded in infants, however, it is necessary to control for sleep state. A classic article by Kraus et al (1989) showed that the MLAEP is most consistent in the awake, stage 1, and REM sleep conditions, but extremely variable in stage 4 sleep. That is, changes occur in the morphology and detectability of the MLAEP as a function of sleep state. Consequently, it is necessary that a laboratory or clinic, when making these measurements in infants and very young children, be consistent in subject state. This necessitates the development of normative measures, group measures (e.g., age related), and repeated measures to be obtained in the same sleep state. It may be necessary to develop several sets of normative tables.

Litscher (1995) has shown that the amplitude of the Na-Pa component of the MLAEP decreases as body temperature decreases (similar to the amplitude and latency changes seen in the ABR). The author also demonstrated that increases in latencies and decreases in amplitudes of the MLAEP occurred during sedation of comatose patients. Although body temperature

does not need to be monitored routinely, certain situations, such as coma or intraoperative monitoring of the MLAEP, exist where this must be taken into account.

The MLAEP is suppressed with the patient under general anesthesia with the use of halothane, enflurane, isoflurane, and desflurane (Schwender et al, 1996). The amount of suppression is dose dependent and hence makes an excellent means of monitoring the depth of the anesthesia. Studies that have compared the electroencephalograph and the MLAEP during anesthesia have reported that the MLAEP is more sensitive to changes in the level of anesthesia (Plourde et al, 1997; Tatsumi et al, 1995).

Clinical Applications

Cottrell and Gans (1995) have reported significant differences in infants and children with multiple handicaps. Although no specific discriminant analysis or categorical profile was identified, the authors characterized the responses from these individuals as being "depressed" with "substantial waveform variability."

Arehole et al (1995) recorded the MLAEP over the vertex and referenced the recordings to both the contralateral and ipsilateral mastoid in an attempt to obtain some hemispheric information on the MLAEP in a group of children classified as learning disabled. These authors reported abnormal recordings that varied with recording condition. The deviation from normal was varied and no consistent trend was identified other than the MLAEP was abnormal, mostly for latency. Such inconsistencies are not surprising when one considers the observation that AEPs are not disorder specific but appear to represent function.

Dietrich et al (1995) completed a study on 10 male stutterers and found that the latency of the Pb component of the MLAEP was significantly shorter than those of age-matched and gender-matched controls, suggesting that some subcortical functional differences may be present in individuals who stutter.

The Pa component of the MLAEP has been used successfully in the establishment of threshold information and audiogram reconstruction. Although clicks have been used by some

to obtain threshold estimates in the absence of ABRs (Kraus & McGee, 1990), tone pips provide a means to better assess the frequency response of the ear (Oats & Stapells, 1997a,b).

For example, the top panel of Figure 20–5 shows the morphological changes in the Pa-Nb waves for three frequencies as intensity is decreased. In the left panel responses are seen at the lowest test level, 15 dB nHL; in the right panel Pa-Nb is present at 15 dB nHL for the 500 Hz tone, 25 dB nHL for the 1000 Hz tone, and 45 dB nHL for the 4000 Hz tone. These have then been plotted as an amplitude-intensity function in the center panel. The bottom panel shows both the pure tone

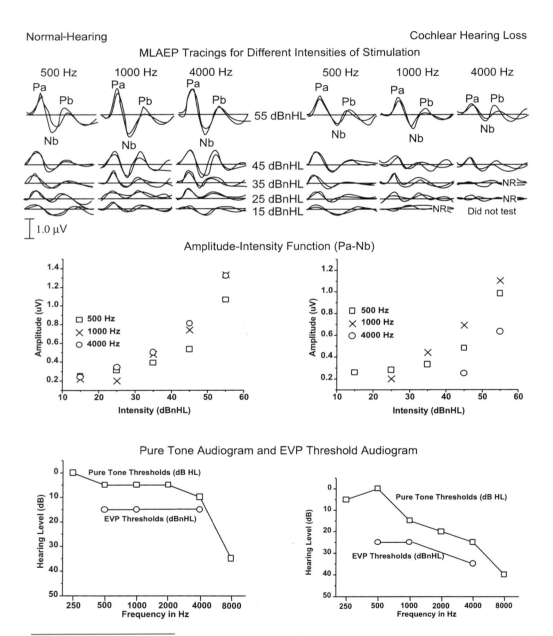

Figure 20–5   MLAEPs in a normal ear (*left side of figure*) and in a cochlear hearing loss (*right side of the figure*) for 500-, 1000-, and 4000-Hz tone pips. The top panel shows the averaged tracings for the Pa, Nb, and Pb components. The middle panel shows the amplitude-latency plots of the Pa-Nb components. The bottom panel shows both the pure tone threshold audiogram and the reconstructed audiogram using the information obtain from the MLAEP.

audiogram and the evoked visual potential (EVP) thresholds plotted on a more traditional looking audiogram (remember a difference in calibration does exist). The EVP thresholds over-estimate the audiometric threshold by about 10 dB. Although this may seem excessive at first, it is better than no informa-tion and provides some frequency specificity. In using this information clinically one takes into account the "average" difference.

Others have reported either absent or "abnormal" MLAEPs in central auditory processing disorders (CAPDs). These include Fifer and Sierra-Irizarry (1988), Özdamar and Kraus (1983), McPherson and Davies (1995), and also in development by McGee and Kraus (1996).

P50 GATING RESPONSE

Introduction

Two of the greatest challenges in audiology are the assessment of auditory thresholds in individuals in whom behavioral audiometric testing is either unreliable or not possible, or when the auditory disorder is not one of sensitivity but related to the processing of auditory information by the central ner-vous system. Sensory gating, which occurs in the MLAEP at about 50 ms after stimulus, has been found to be related to central auditory disorders, especially auditory attention.

Sensory gating in the auditory system is represented by a diminished response for repeated stimulation and appears to be necessary for targeted attention (Waldo et al, 1992). Auditory sensory gating uses a paired stimuli paradigm whereby two identical signals are separated by a short ISI (i.e., 500 ms), and the presentation of the pair has a much longer ISI (i.e., 10 s). The two stimuli presentations in the pair are averaged separately, and in the normal individual the amplitude of the second paired stimulus will have a smaller amplitude, usually by about 40% (Nagamoto et al, 1989; Waldo et al, 1992).

The latency of the P50 auditory gating response occurs between 40 and 70 ms, suggesting a time window consistent with thalamic activity. Erwin et al (1991), in a study using a population of schizophrenic patients, stated that a sensory gating deficit is suggestive of subcortical dysfunction in the thalamus. However, Nagamoto et al (1989) believed that because gating depends on the interval between the paired stimuli and because responses in schizophrenic patients var-ied, multiple mechanisms were involved in sensory gating with various CNS pathways contributing to neuronal inhibi-tion. Other areas such as the temporal cortex and hippocam-pus have been proposed, but the thalamic origin appears most likely at this time.

Technical Specifications

Electrodes

Because a relatively long time constant is used in the record-ing of the P50, it is recommended that Ag-AgCl electrodes be used. Other metals used in making electrodes tend to cause a shift in the DC potential gradient, thus giving rise to possible contamination from low-frequency artifact. A single channel Cz- C7 (preferred) or Cz- Mi configuration is sufficient to record this response. A ground electrode may be placed at

Fpz. In addition, eye movement must be monitored because the P50 response is in the general latency region of eye blinks that may become time locked to an acoustic event (Fig. 20–6). The signal is bandpassed between 1 and 3000 Hz (3 dB down, 6 dB/octave).

> ### PEARL
>
> If excessive eye movement occurs, the use of cotton balls taped gently to the closed eyelid will provide enough light pressure to suppress involuntary eye movement.

Recording Parameters

Although a single channel is used to record the P50 gating response to a paired stimuli paradigm, each stimulus (S1 and S2) must be averaged in separate buffers. Most commercial equipment allows for a P300 paradigm. The P50 protocol may be established by setting the P300 paradigm to identical stim-uli, probability at 50%, nonrandom sequence, S1-S2 interval at 500 ms, and the ISI, or repeat cycle interval, at 10 s. This will permit the recording of the P50 on commercial equipment.

Each stimulus response, S1 and S2, is collected using an 80-ms sample window with a 10 ms preanalysis baseline. The signal is bandpassed between 1 and 3000 Hz and an artifact reject set on the eye blink channel.

Stimuli

Matched pairs of tone pips (i.e., stimulus 1, S1; and stimulus 2, S2) with a two-cycle rise time, one-cycle plateau time, and two-cycle decay time (2-1-2 cycle) are commonly used for these recordings (Table 20–4). Both S1 and S2 must be identi-cal in frequency, intensity, temporal characteristics, and mode of presentation. That is, nothing can be different or novel between S1 and S2. Tubal insert phones or calibrated ear-phones, either a monaural or binaural (the latter being the most common), may be used and the stimulus should be pre-sented at a moderate intensity, 70- to 75-dB nHL. A 500 ms ISI exists between S1 and S2 and a 10 s interval between the pairs. The 10-s interval is needed for the CNS to "forget" about the stimulus, whereas the shorter interval between S1 and S2 does not give the nervous system enough time to con-sider S2 a novel stimulus.

> ### PITFALL
>
> Differences between S1 and S2 produce a mismatch negativity and will be evaluated by the nervous system as two different stimuli, thus suppressing the gating response.

Subject State and Variables

No thorough and consistent studies have been done showing the effect of subject state on the response. However, active attention to the paired stimuli produces more consistent responses but does not account for the amount or frequency of suppression. Because this is a middle latency response, it

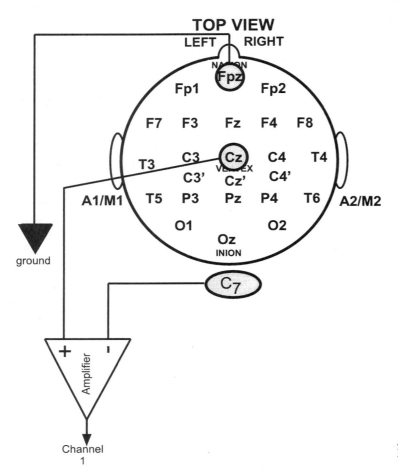

Figure 20–6   Electrode montage for the P50 (Cz-C7).

must be assumed that, to a large extent, subject state considerations are similar for both types of responses.

Some aging effects appear on sensory gating. Freedman et al (1987) reported that in subjects younger than 18, the gating effect was more varied and perhaps absent before adolescence.

Other factors, such as attention (Jerger et al, 1992) and mood (Waldo & Freedman, 1986), do not affect sensory gating; however, anxiety, anger-hostility, and extreme tension tend to suppress the gating response.

Clinical Applications

It has been reported that in normal subjects the P50 amplitude of the second paired stimulus (S2) is about 5% of the P50 amplitude for the first paired stimulus (S1). The P50 may be completely absent in about 40 to 50% of those with normal auditory gating.

In our laboratory for a vertex electrode recording the upper limit for normal for the S2/S1 ratio is .68. For example, Boutros et al (1991) reported that the P50 to S2 will be completely absent (i.e., S2/S1 ratio of 0) in approximately 40% of the normal population. This is in contrast to schizophrenic patients who will exhibit poorer suppression ratios on the order of magnitude of 95% or greater (Nagamoto et al 1989), resulting in little or no suppression (Fig. 20–7). Similar findings are seen in adolescent males with ADHD.

Some have suggested that abnormal gating responses may be a genetic marker in schizophrenia. Siegel et al (1984) reported that approximately 50% of first-degree relatives of schizophrenic patients showed abnormalities in the gating response.

In addition to schizophrenia, the gating response has been found to change in manic depressive persons. Baker et al (1990) found that as depression increased, the ratio of the P50 auditory response increased (i.e., the amplitude of the P50 to S2 became larger). This type of graded response has not been observed in schizophrenic patients.

SPECIAL CONSIDERATION

A neuropsychiatric history should be obtained before using this procedure.

LONG LATENCY AUDITORY EVOKED POTENTIALS (LAEPs)

Introduction

The LAEPs traditionally have four components (Fig. 20–8): P1, occurring between 55 and 80 ms; N1, occurring between

TABLE 20–4 P50 recording parameters

Parameter	Note

Electrodes

Type: Ag-AgCl

Montage: *Single channel:*
Cz (noninverting).
A1+A2, linked mastoid electrodes (inverting).
FpZ (ground).

Single channel:
Cz (noninverting).
C7–noncephalic (inverting).
FpZ (ground).

Eye movement (see text):
Superior orbit of one eye to the inferior orbit of the opposite eye (polarity not specified).

Recording Parameters

Channels: One channel is standard.
S1 and S2 must be averaged with equal trials, but separately. Most equipment allows this by using a P300 paradigm with a probability of 50%.

Timebase: 80 ms with a 10 ms preanalysis.

\# Averages: 250–500.

Filter (bandpass): 1–3000 Hz.

Artifact Rejection: 3/4 maximum sampling amplitude.

Stimuli

Type: Brief tone with a 2-1-2 cycle.
Blackman 5-cycle brieftone.
Both S1 and S2 are matched identically.

Transducer: Tubal insert phones.
Calibrated earphones (i.e., TDH-39, etc.).

Polarity: Rarefaction.
NOTE: in children sometimes it is necessary to reverse the polarity for better morphology.

Level: 70–75 dB nHL for both pairs.
Brief tones may be used to estimate hearing sensitivity and the actual level would vary.

Rate: See ISI for details.

ISI: S1–S2 interval, 500 ms.
S2–S1 interval, 10 s.

90 and 110 ms; P2, occurring between 145 and 180 ms; and N2, occurring between 180 and 250 ms (McPherson, 1996). In some instances the P1 of the LAEP is also considered to be the Pb in the MLAEP.

The P1 response is primarily an exogenous potential occurring at about 60 ms. It is thought to represent late thalamic projections into the early auditory cortex and is part of the specific sensory system (Velasco et al, 1989). The P1 response appears to be strongly related to stimulus parameters. The N1 is primarily an exogenous potential, occurring at about 100 ms and is associated with activity of the nonspecific polysensory system within the contralateral supratemporal auditory cortex (Knight et al, 1988). The P2

occurs at about 160 ms and is primarily an exogenous potential of the nonspecific polysensory system demonstrating activity in the lateral-frontal supratemporal auditory cortex (Scherg et al, 1989). The N2 is the first of the primarily endogenous potentials occurring at about 200 ms and is part of the nonspecific polysensory system in the supratemporal auditory cortex (Velasco et al, 1989). The term *endogenous* refers to an ERP that is produced after internal processing of the stimulus. The N2 is highly related to attention as is the entire N1-P2-N2 response, being related to the acoustic features of audition. The P1 differs greatly from the N1, P2, N2 components of the LAEP and consequently is considered, in general, to be part of the MLAEP.

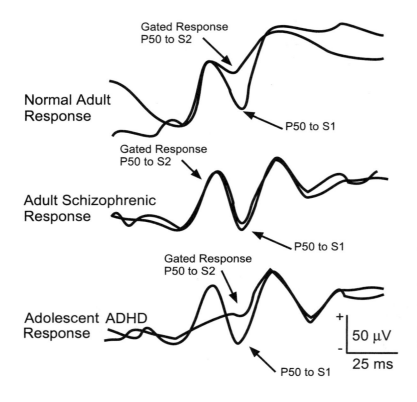

Gated Response
P50 to S2

Normal Adult
Response

P50 to S1

Gated Response
P50 to S2

Adult Schizophrenic
Response

P50 to S1

Gated Response
P50 to S2

Adolescent ADHD
Response

P50 to S1

50 μV

25 ms

Figure 20–7 The P50 auditory gating response in a normal young adult male, a young adult female with schizophrenia, and a teenage male with ADHD. Notice on the top tracing that the S2 response is gated (i.e., a small amplitude negative wave) compared with the S1 response. Also, as noted in the bottom tracing, only partial gating has occurred to S2 illustrating the phenomena that the amount of gating varies.

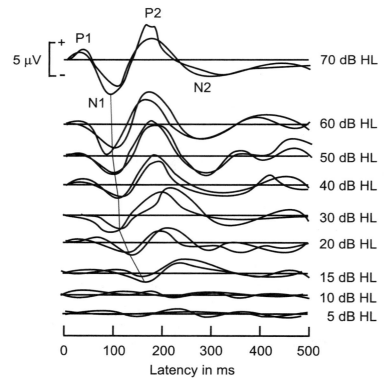

5 μV

P1

P2

70 dB HL

N2

N1

60 dB HL

50 dB HL

40 dB HL

30 dB HL

20 dB HL

15 dB HL

10 dB HL

5 dB HL

0   100   200   300   400   500
Latency in ms

Figure 20–8 The LAEP to different intensities. Notice that the latency of the response shows little variation at high to moderate levels and then quickly increases near threshold. In contrast, the amplitude shows a graded response with intensity.

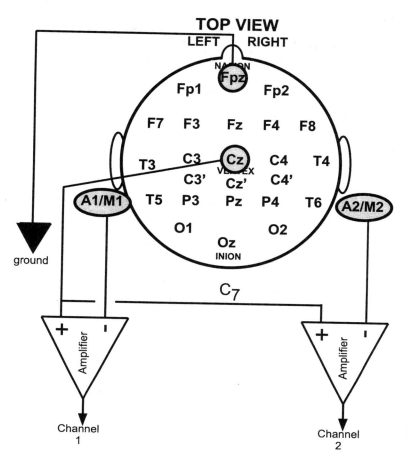

Figure 20–9 Electrode montage for the LAEP (Cz-A1 and Cz to A2).

Technical Specifications

Electrodes

The LAEP is maximal when recorded over the vertex at Cz. The typical recording is to record from Cz (noninverting electrode) to C7 (preferred) or the ispsilateral earlobe or mastoid (Ai) (inverting electrode). Hemispheric asymmetry measures may be obtained by using two channels, Cz-Ai and Cz-Ac (Fig. 20–9). Because the LAEP may become contaminated with eye movement, it is highly recommended that eye movement be monitored by placing electrodes lateral to the orbit of one eye and superior to the orbit of the opposite eye. This will permit the simultaneous monitoring of vertical and horizontal eye movement and eye blinks (see the discussion at the beginning of this chapter).

Recording Parameters

The most common type of recording is completed using a single channel. However, more useful information is obtained by the use of two or more channels, thus providing some information on hemispheric specificity. The recording should include a 50-ms preanalysis sample followed by a 300-ms poststimulus sample (Table 20–5). A series of 200 to 250 artifact-free samples is obtained for each average with a bandpass filter of 1 to 300 Hz.

Stimulus

The LAEP is best recorded using tone bursts, speech, or speech-like stimuli. The response of the LAEP is primarily to the acoustic features of audition, especially to the transition features. The most common, albeit the most simplistic, is a tone burst consisting of a rise and fall time between 5 and 10 ms and a plateau time between 25 and 50 ms. Speech material needs to have a total duration not greater than about 50 to 60 ms or minimally less than the first component of interest. Longer stimulus times will result in the recording of a sustained potential that may include stimulus artifact. For tonal stimulation, a rarefaction tone burst should be used and in cases of poor morphological features, such as often seen in very young children, the polarity should be reversed between trials. The stimuli are presented at a rate between 0.9 and 2.9/s, with the faster rates showing a reduction in the N1 amplitude.

Subject State and Variables

Both attention and subject state affect the LAEPs. Attention appears to have its greatest effect on the N2 response, although the effects of subject and attention on the N2 are similar. This results in a decreased amplitude of the N2 response when attention wanes. Subjects should be awake and attentive but not necessarily active in the task itself.

TABLE 20–5   LAEP recording parameters

Parameter	Note
Electrodes	
Type:	Ag-AgCl
Montage:	*Single channel:*
	Cz (noninverting).
	Ai (inverting).
	FpZ (ground).
	Multichannel (see text):
	Cz (noninverting).
	A1 (inverting).
	A2 (inverting).
	FpZ (ground).
	Eye movement (see text):
	Superior orbit of one eye to the inferior orbit of the opposite eye (polarity not specified).
Recording Parameters	
Channels:	One channel is standard.
	Two or more channels for hemispheric specificity.
Timebase:	300 ms with a 50 ms preanalysis.
# Averages:	200–250.
Filter (bandpass):	1–300 Hz.
Artifact Rejection:	3/4 maximum sampling amplitude.
Stimuli	
Type:	Tone bursts with a 5–10 ms rise/fill time and a 25–50 ms plateau time.
	Brief duration speech material (i.e., CVC) may be used.
Transducer:	Tubal insert phones.
	Calibrated earphones (i.e., TDH-39, etc.).
	Sound field speakers.
Polarity:	Rarefaction.
	NOTE: in children sometimes it is necessary to reverse the polarity for better morphology.
Level:	75–80 dB nHL for a robust response showing all of the subcomponents.
	Tone bursts may be used to estimate hearing sensitivity and the actual level would vary.
Rate:	0.9–2.9/s (we prefer the lower rate of about 0.9–1.3/s).
ISI:	300 ms–1.1 s with the longer ISI preferred.

Drugs that produce a central suppression of brain activity such as barbiturates will significantly influence and usually diminish the LAEP.

> **PEARL**
>
> **A simple motivational technique for young children is to periodically award the child with tokens that may be exchanged for various rewards, such as toys, depending on the number of tokens accumulated throughout the test session.**

Clinical Applications

The P1 was discussed under the MLAEP Pb component because its characteristics are more representative of responses in that time domain. In clinical situations, the LAEP is usually seen as two distinct components: (1) the N1-P2 component, and (2) the P2-N2 or N2 component. We would like to suggest, however, that our preference for measurement is from baseline to the particular peak of the component (i.e., baseline-N1, baseline-P2, etc.). Because this is not a common convention in the clinical literature in the field of communicative disorders, we have chosen to use the more common method of amplitude measurement (i.e., peak-to-

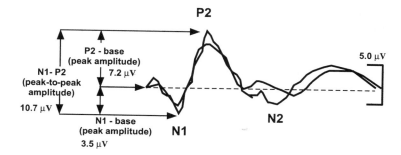

Figure 20–10 LAEP showing the measurement of the N1 peak amplitude, the P2 peak amplitude, and the N1-P2 peak-to-peak amplitude. Note the asymmetry in the amplitudes between the peak amplitudes of the N1 and P2.

peak). The difficulty with peak-to-peak measures of the LAEP components is that the amplitudes of the positive and negative peaks are not symmetrical, and each individual peak (i.e., positive peak, negative peak) varies. Figure 20–10 shows the N1-P2-N2 complex of the LAEPs. Measurements include the N1-P2 peak-to-peak amplitude (10.7 μ V), the P2 peak amplitude (7.2 μ V), and the N1 peak amplitude (3.5 μ V). As noted, the peaks are not symmetrical, with the positive peak having a greater amplitude. Because the generators and the stimulus response patterns are different between the individual peaks, using peak-to-peak measurements would reduce the value of the measurement.

N1-P2 (N1) Component

Both the latency and amplitude of the N1-P2 response should be obtained. If one is interested in hemispheric asymmetries, the dominance (i.e., handedness) of the subject should be noted.

Because the latency of the N1-P2 is relatively stable within a variety of stimulus conditions or pathological conditions, this measure may provide mean latencies within age groups. In children older than 5 and adults, we would expect to see this response out to approximately 195 ms. This would provide the following possibilities for the interpretation of latency: (1) normal (within age group); (2) maturational delay (below age group, but older than 5); (3) prolonged latency (i.e., abnormal); and (4) absent.

Amplitude, unlike latency, varies considerably with both stimulus condition and pathological condition. Amplitude may also be expected to vary within the effect of age (i.e., increase with age to some extent). Stimulus intensity changes are also reflected in amplitude changes. As with the ABR, as the intensity of the stimulus decreases, the amplitude of the N1-P2 complex also decreases. However, latency remains stable except at and less than approximately 20 dB SL. Also, as the intensity becomes within about 10- to 15-dB of threshold, the P2 is no longer seen and the N1 becomes the lowest observable response. This makes the N1-P2 a reasonable response for frequency-specific threshold information using an evoked potential paradigm. However, unlike the ABR, sedation cannot be used in recording the N1-P2 and may limit its use in obtaining frequency-specific threshold information.

The N1-P2 reflects the acoustic characteristics of the acoustic stimulus. That is, it reflects changes in timing, the sequence of the event, and other physical dimensions such as frequency and intensity. As a result, acoustic clicks, such as those used in the ABR, are poor stimuli.

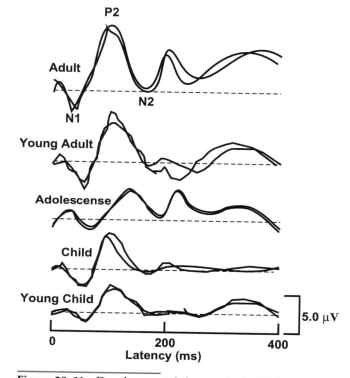

Figure 20–11 Developmental changes in the P2 from young child (approximately 3 years in age), to adult (approximately 42 years of age).

P2-N2 (N2) Component

Similar to the N1-P2 component, both the latency and amplitude should be obtained for this response along with information about dominance (i.e., handedness). Unlike the N1-P2 that is primarily exogenous, the N2 shows a greater influence of endogenous factors on the response than does the earlier N1-P2 component. In addition, the P2 shows a developmental sequence (Fig. 20–11). The P2 peaks becomes larger with maturation and develops a sharper peak (McPherson, 1996).

Intensity changes have little effect on the N2 for either latency or amplitude. However, significant changes are seen in the amplitude of the N2 for attention. Although the subject does not need to be actively attending to the task itself, the subject does need to be awake and alert (i.e., not drowsy, etc.). Active attention will slightly enhance the response.

The N2 first appears at about 3 years of age, with a latency between 200 and 280 ms, and reaches adult values by about 12 years of age, with a range from 185 to 235 ms. Because the changes in latency are not particularly outstanding with age, it is probably not a good measure of sensory maturation, although certainly the absence of the response in individuals older than 5 must be considered abnormal, particularly in light of the presence of earlier LAEP components.

Similar to the latency of the N2, the amplitude is relatively stable and does not particularly vary with stimulus parameters. However, significant effects of amplitude have been seen in individuals with attention disorders. Specifically, the amplitude of the N2 shows approximately a 50% reduction of the N1/N2 ratio in these individuals.

The N2 is best obtained using a discrimination task of the acoustic aspects of the auditory event or a task requiring semantic discrimination. Hence, it may be used to evaluate such functions.

These measures have been used to study auditory function in cochlear implant patients. For example, Jordon et al (1997) studied the N1 and P300 in a group of cochlear implant patients. Findings revealed a general shortening of the latency of the N100 in the implant patients that began to approximate normal-hearing subjects. A two-tone perceptual task was used (i.e., detection of a 400 Hz versus 1450 Hz tone). Scalp distribution across the skull was broader for the implant patients than for the normal-hearing subjects. In addition, Micco et al (1995) reported, in a group of Nucleus 22 cochlear implant patients, no significant differences in the latency of the N1 and P2 when using the phonemes /dα/ and /di/ as a stimulus.

One of the more interesting studies is that of Eggermont et al (1997) who used the P1 latency to study maturation of the auditory system in children with cochlear implants. These authors observed a graded maturation of the auditory system, as measured by changes in P1 with age. The normal-hearing group demonstrated a mature P1 by about age 15 years; whereas, the children with cochlear implants showed a P1 delay in maturation about equal to the duration of the deafness. In earlier reports (Ponton et al, 1996a,b) they were able to demonstrate that the regression line for development, as measured by P1, was interrupted in the deaf children but began after implant and eventually reached maturation.

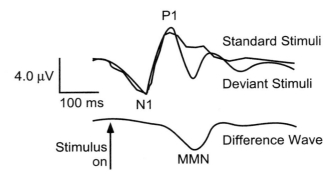

Figure 20–12   The MMN to the phonemes /bα/ (standard stimulus) and /dα/ (deviant stimulus). The bottom tracing shows the MMN as a difference wave, however, the MMN is clearly seen when the two waveforms (standard and deviant) are overlayed as seen in the top tracing.

subject is not involved in the auditory task, such as while reading and performing visual discrimination. A typical response recorded from one subject is shown in Figure 20–12. Responses to the deviant stimuli, that is, the infrequent and physically different stimuli, and for the sequence of the homogeneous standard stimuli are illustrated. The bottom trace labeled as MMN is derived by subtracting the responses to standard stimuli from that to the deviant stimuli. The derived waveform (MMN) shows a clear negative deflection beginning at the N1 wave latency (about 100 ms) and peaking later between 200 and 300 ms.

Amplitude and latency of the MMN are the most commonly measured parameters. Amplitude typically is measured between the positive peak and the following negative trough. The latency is measured from the time of stimulus onset to the initial peak of MMN waveform. In addition to these two measures, several researchers have used other analysis techniques to reflect additional changes in the waveform. Most common is multiplying the peak amplitude of the MMN with its duration (Groenen et al, 1996). It is believed that this is a better indicator of the total amount of processing occurring in the MMN.

Studies investigating the scalp distribution of the MMN (Giard et al, 1990; Scherg et al, 1989), magnetic encephalography studies (Alho, 1995; Alho et al, 1994; Hari et al, 1984; Näätänen, 1992), intracranial studies in humans and animals (Csepe et al, 1987; Javit et al, 1992; Kraus et al, 1994b), and studies involving brain lesions in humans (Woods et al, 1993) have been used to identify the neural structures responsible for the generation of MMN. These studies indicate that the underlying neural structures contributing to the generation of the MMN are believed to originate in auditory cortex. However, the exact location of MMN appears to change, depending on what aspect of the stimulus condition is varied (i.e., frequency, duration, intensity, etc.) and the complexity of the sounds (i.e., speech vs. nonspeech sounds). In addition to auditory cortex, strong indications show that frontal cortex activity contributes to the MMN, most probably related to automatic switching of attention from standard signal to

MISMATCH NEGATVITY

Introduction

Mismatch negativity (MMN) is a recent introduction to the family of LAEPs (Näätänen et al, 1978). The MMN is elicited by a physically deviant stimulus in a sequence of homogeneous "standard" stimuli. The term *mismatch negativity* refers to the central nervous system's ability to compare a deviant stimulus from a previous standard set stored in short-term memory. It is assumed that MMN reflects an automatic mismatch process between the sensory inflow created by the deviant stimuli and the memory trace of the standard stimuli. These responses are automatic, not confounded by attention and cognitive factors and can be observed even when the deviant stimuli. Animal studies suggest MMN subcomponents may be generated in the thalamus and hippocampus.

Technical Specifications
Electrodes

The most common electrode montage, recording parameters, and stimuli for MMN acquisition are listed in Table 20–6. Disk electrodes are used for MMN recordings and Ag-AgCl electrodes are preferred compared with tin or gold-coated electrodes. No set montages, but good recordings, can be obtained by electrodes placed over the vertex (Cz), frontal area (Fz), parietal area (Pz), and, in some situations, over the occipital (Oz) and prefrontal (Fpz) areas. A single channel recording may be obtaining by using an Fz electrode placement (Fig. 20–13). Electrodes placed at A1 or A2 produce a polarity reversal (Sandridge & Boothroyd, 1996), indicating variations in current density caused by dipole orientation. Electrode placements on the vertex and frontal cortex provide the best recordings sites. The best recording site for the noninverting electrode is the tip of the nose. However, C7 as a noncephalic site is acceptable. The ground electrode can be placed on the forehead.

Recording

The number of electrodes can vary from three to seven, with three electrode recordings providing adequate information. In addition to the scalp electrodes, two electro-oculogram electrodes should be used for monitoring eye movements. The time base of the recording window is usually set from 0 to 400 ms. A prestimulus baseline is recorded. Maturational studies require a wider recording window (Table 20–6).

Given that the MMN is part of the late-evoked potentials, the amplitude values are considerably high. As a result, the number of averages can be as low as 50 or as high as 100. In addition, because the MMN contains very low-frequency signals the filters should be set between 0.1 and 100 Hz.

Stimuli

The stimulus condition applied to the recording of the MMN is a typical oddball paradigm using a probability for the deviant, or oddball, stimulus between .15 and .20 and the standard stimulus having a probability of $1 - p$ (deviant). For example, given a deviant stimulus probability of .20, the standard stimulus probability would be .80. The MMN has been elicited by changes in stimulus parameters such as frequency

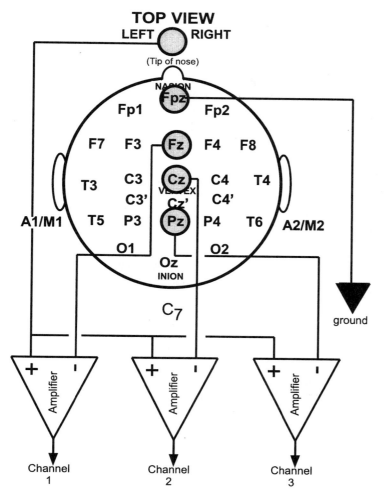

Figure 20–13 Electrode montage for the MMN (Fz, Cz, Pz—tip of nose).

TABLE 20–6   MMN recording parameters

Parameter	Note
Electrodes	
Type:	Ag-AgCl
Montage:	Fpz, F4, Fz, F3, C4, C3, Oz (inverting).
	A1, A2, or tip of nose (noninverting).
Recording Parameters	
Channels:	3–7.
Timebase:	400 ms.
# Averages:	50–100.
Filter (bandpass):	0.1–100 Hz.
Artifact Rejection	
Stimuli	
Type:	Oddball paradigm
Transducer:	Tubal insert phones.
	Calibrated earphones.
Polarity:	Not applicable.
Level:	75–80 dB HL.
Rate:	1/s.
ISI:	1000 ms.

(Sams et al, 1985), duration (Kaukoranta et al, 1989), intensity (Näätänen et al, 1987), and location (Paavilainen et al, 1989; Schroger, 1996). Sams et al (1985) presented a 1.0 kHz standard signal and a slightly higher frequency (1.008 kHz) deviant stimulus. MMN changes have also been observed for intensity (Näätänen, 1992). Other factors affecting the MMN include stimulus duration and ISIs. For example, the shorter the ISI, the larger the MMN amplitude (Näätänen 1992). However, the MMN appears to be a suprathreshold phenomenon and to elicit a robust MMN, stimuli must be presented at suprathreshold levels.

In addition to the tonal signals and their elementary variations, speech sounds have served to evaluate the discrimination abilities between categorical boundaries (Kraus et al, 1992, 1995), although they do not recognize categorical boundaries per se and have been used in newborns to determine simple discrimination abilities (Cheour-Luhtanen et al, 1995).

Subject State and Variables

Unlike the late endogenous potentials, the MMN is not affected by subject state such as attention. Variations occur in individual MMN amplitudes and latencies across subjects and within subjects. However, the amplitude variations seem to be greater than latency changes. Therefore latency rather than amplitude appears to be a better indicator of the MMN response. The MMN amplitude and latency changes with sleep level. When subjects are drowsy, amplitude and latency increase. For deep sleep, amplitude decreases and the latency increases. Consequently, it is important for the subject to maintain alertness during the testing. Studies have also shown a positive relationship between MMN and drugs, with changes in waveforms noted with drugs, such as barbiturates, that have a general activating or deactivating effect on the central nervous system (Näätänen, 1992).

Clinical Applications

The MMN shows promise as a clinical tool in evaluating feature-specific testing of auditory functions in various hearing disorders. It can also be used to measure auditory analysis, storing, and discrimination abilities. One of the advantages of the MMN is that it does not depend on attention and is a good technique to evaluate preattentive auditory discrimination processes and sensory memory.

Most of the clinical application is in the area of perceptual or processing abilities related to the psychophysical features of sound perception. The MMN has been used to examine the central auditory processing accuracy in patients with cochlear implant compared with normal-hearing subjects (Kraus et al, 1993a; Ponton & Don, 1995). In both of these studies MMN findings suggest that the MMN can be used as an evaluation tool during rehabilitation.

Kraus et al (1992, 1993b, 1994c) using a passive oddball paradigm and speech stimuli to obtain the MMN were able to demonstrate that the MMN to speech stimuli provided a stable and reliable measure in school-age children and adults. They suggested that the MMN is a good tool for the study of central auditory function. In a subsequent study (Kraus et al, 1993c) they reported on an adult with severely abnormal ABR in the presence of normal-hearing. The MLAEPs, N1, P2, and P300 of the LAEPs were normal. However, the MMN was normal for speech stimuli in which the individual had relative good speech perception, but poor in other areas consistent with her behavioral discrimination abilities. The case study points out the usefulness of the MMN and other AEPs in understanding auditory processing deficits. Other uses for the MMN have been in the study of voice onset time and central auditory plasticity (Tremblay et al, 1997), categorization of speech sounds (Sharma et al, 1993), and evaluation of speech in cochlear implant users (Kraus et al, 1993d). The latter study showed, using /da/ and /ta/ as paired stimuli, that the cochlear implant users were processing the speech stimuli the same as the normal-hearing individuals in the study. That is, essentially no difference was present in the MMN. The authors concluded that the MMN has potential as being an objective measure of cochlear implant function.

The N1, P2, N2, P3, and MMN were studied to both speech and tonal stimuli in children with cochlear implants (Kileny et al, 1997). Intensity contrasts (1500 Hz for 75- vs. 90-dB SPL), tonal contrasts (80 dB SLP for 1500 Hz vs. 3000 Hz), and speech contrasts consisting of the words "heed" versus "who'd" were used. Each of the components were identified, and correlations were found between speech recognition and cognitive evoked potential latencies. It was believed that evoked potentials are useful in the assessment of cochlear implant function in children.

The MMN was used to study discrimination in patients with cochlear implants. Ponton and Don (1995) showed that the MMN is a good tool for evaluating both duration and pitch in cochlear implant users and suggest that it may be a good technique to study discriminability in children with cochlear implants and assist in the rehabilitative process.

The MMN may provide an objective measure of speech perception in patients with cochlear implants. For example, both Ponton and Don (1995) and Groenen et al (1996) have shown that the MMN is a reliable tool for studying pitch and duration and that differences are seen in length of use of implant and difference in implant effectiveness.

The MMN has also been shown to be useful in evaluating patients who are comatose, the aging population, those with Alzhemiers disease-dementia, those with Parkinsons disease, and in patients with central nervous system processing problems (for a review see Csepe & Molnar, 1997).

P300 COGNITIVE AUDITORY EVOKED POTENTIAL

Introduction

The P300 is a cognitive auditory ERP. The P300 occurs in internal higher level brain processing associated with stimulus recognition and novelty. The P300 is classified as an endogenous auditory ERP and is nonsensory specific (i.e., it occurs to both unimodality and multimodality sensory stimulation). The P300 occurs between about 220 ms and 380 ms. In some instances it will be a bimodal peak with a P300a and P300b component (Fig. 20–14). The P300 is used in the study of memory disorder, information processing, and decision making.

The P300 has its maximum amplitude over the centroparietal areas at the midline. The generation sites of the P300 are complex, having multiple overlapping sites that appear to be simultaneously activated, especially in the frontal and temporal cortex. Activity is also seen in the temporoparietal association cortex. Other areas have included the primary auditory cortex and the polysensory association cortex (Buchwald, 1990a,b).

Technical Specifications
Electrodes

The P300 may be recorded from an electrode placed between Cz and Pz, often referred as Cz', for the noninverting electrode, and between C_7 for the inverting electrode (Fig. 20–15). The ground may be placed at FpZ. A slight normal variation appears in the maximum amplitude of the P300 from individual to individual between Cz and Pz. It is highly recommended that a three-channel system be used and all three noninverting electrode positions be used (i.e., Fz, Cz, and Pz).

Eye movement can produce an artifact in the recording of the P300. The latency of this artifact is about the same as the P300. Therefore protocol dictates that eye movement be monitored and that any such activity cause the sample to be discarded.

Recording Parameters

Although frequently used, single-channel recordings of the P300 are not recommended. This is primarily due to the normal variation of the response characteristics of the P300 along the midline. In the normal individual the maximum may occur from Cz to Pz. The targets (rare stimuli) are averaged separately from the nontarget (standard or common stimuli) (Table 20–7).

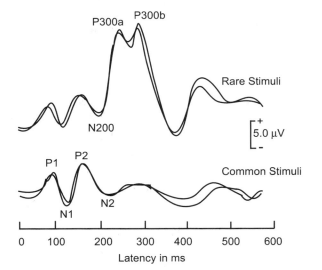

Figure 20–14 The P300 event-related auditory potential in response to the phoneme /bɑ/ (rare or oddball stimulus) and /dɑ/ (common or frequent stimulus). The rare stimulus was presented with a probability of .20 and presentation of the stimulus did not occur in two consecutive trials.

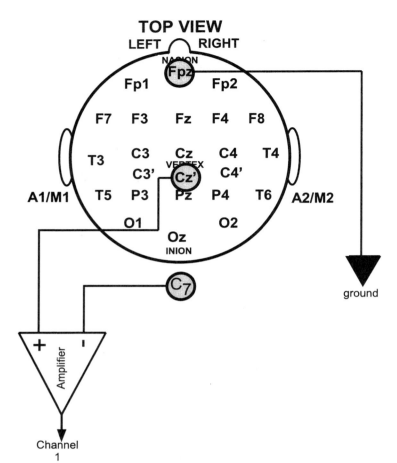

Figure 20–15   Electrode montage for the MMN (Cz-C7).

ing the subject to actively attend to the rare stimulus. The two most common activities are to either have the subject count the rare stimuli, or to push a button each time the rare stimulus occurs. Figure 20–14 is an example of a P300 recording.

Stimuli

Tone bursts are the most common stimuli having a rise/fall time of 10 ms and a plateau of 25 to 50 ms. Because stimulus novelty is paramount in obtaining a P300 response, two distinct tones should be used as the stimuli. This is referred to as an "oddball" paradigm, whereby one tone is the standard, common, or frequent, and the second tone is the deviant, oddball, or rare. Research has shown that the rare tone should randomly occur with a probability not greater than .20 and should not occur twice in succession (McPherson, 1996). The response is not particularly affected by intensity, but differences in intensities between the two stimuli will affect the P300 response. Again, it is important to remember that it is the occurrence and recognition of stimulus differences that are the basis of the P300. An intensity level of 70- to 75-dB HL is sufficient to evoke a robust response.

Subject State and Variables

The significance, or *task relevancy,* is a key feature in the elicitation of the P300. Likewise the occurrence of the rare, or target, stimulus must be uncertain. The more uncertainty or

---

SPECIAL CONSIDERATION

During active tasks, such a button press, a premovement or premotor response may occur. The is called the *Bereitschaftspotential* or "readiness" potential. This is a slow negative potential that occurs up to 1 s before the onset of movement. In addition two other potentials have been identified to occur just before motor movement. The characteristics of these potentials are such that they may both contaminate ERPs or be mistaken for an auditory neural response. The effect of these potentials becomes greater in conditioned-response paradigms or where the subject has developed a sense predictability in responding. Consequently, the more random and lower the probability of the oddball stimulus, the less these influences are observed in the recordings (a .20 probability of occurrence is optimum).

A 500 ms to 800 ms epoch is recorded with a filter bandpass between .05 and 50 Hz. Two hundred (200) artifact free samples are collected consisting of 160 common samples and 40 rare samples. The amplitude of the P300 is enhanced by requir-

TABLE 20–7   P300 recording parameters

Parameter	Note
Electrodes	
Type:	Ag-AgCl, gold (not preferred)
Montage:	*Single channel* (not preferred)
	Cz' (noninverting).
	C7 (inverting).
	FpZ (ground).
	Multichannel (see text):
	Fz (noninverting).
	Cz (noninverting).
	Pz (noninverting).
	C7 (inverting).
	FpZ (ground).
	Eye movement (see text):
	Superior orbit of one eye to the inferior orbit of the opposite eye (polarity not specified).
Recording Parameters	
Channels:	One channel (not recommended)
	Three channels for best localization of the response.
	The target, or oddball (rare), stimuli are averaged in one buffer, and the common or frequent stimuli are averaged in a second buffer.
Timebase:	500 ms with a 100 ms preanalysis.
# Averages:	200–250.
Filter (bandpass):	.05–50 Hz.
Artifact rejection:	3/4 maximum sampling amplitude.
Stimuli	
Type:	Tone bursts with 10 ms rise/fall time and a 25–50 ms plateau time.
	Brief duration speech material (i.e., CVC) may be used.
	The target, or oddball (rare) stimuli, should occur not more than 20% (.20) of the time, randomly presented and not occurring in succession.
Transducer:	Tubal insert phones.
	Calibrated earphones (i.e., TDH-39, etc.).
	Sound field speakers.
Polarity:	Not specified.
Level:	75–80 dB nHL for a robust response showing all of the subcomponents.
Rate:	0.9/s or less depending on the stimulus length.
ISI:	1.1 s or longer depending on the stimulus length.

surprise (Donchin, 1981), the larger the amplitude of the P300. The P300 may be bimodal having both an "a" and "b" component, depending on the particular paradigm being used. The "a" peak is present regardless of subject participation, whereas the "b" peak occurs when the subject is actively involved in the detection of the target stimuli, such as stimuli counting or button pushing (Michalewski et al, 1986). The amplitude of the P300 is primarily determined by two properties of the acoustic stimulus: (1) the probability of occurrence; and (2) the meaning (i.e., perceived meaning) of the acoustic stimulus. Both of these factors need to be viewed relative to the subject's response. That is, *subjective probability* and *subjective meaning*. It is the subjectiveness of these factors that makes the P300 so interesting and clinically useful.

Picton and Hillyard (1974) have shown that the scalp distribution of the P300 shifts from a more frontal distribution to a more parietal distribution across the scalp as the task changes from active participation to passive participation. Consequently, a shift in the generators of the P300 is correlated with a shift in attention.

SPECIAL CONSIDERATION

The use of tonal stimuli in a P300 paradigm is a simplistic type of task and is not as sensitive as using other stimuli, such as phonemes, that require more complex processing.

Clinical Applications

The clinical application of auditory P300 testing must begin with the fact that the P300 is *task revelant*. Because of this, the P300 may be considered an index of stimulus processing and has great potential for studying higher level processing skills (McPherson, 1996).

In using an auditory continuous task paradigm, Salamat and McPherson (1999) found that the amplitude of the P300 in both a normal and adult (ADHD) population decreased as ISI decreased. However, the decrement of the P300 amplitude was greater in the ADHD adult population, suggesting that although the cognitive processes that are available in a normal population are present in an ADHD population, the degree of availability or quality of processes relevant to cognition is affected in the ADHD population. The use of P300 in trying to identify patients having ADHD versus ADHD type of behavior is useful in planning intervention schemes; especially because auditory attention disorders are generally present in ADHD populations, and treatment of auditory disorders with and without ADHD would vary.

The latency of the P300 is more variable and longer in school-age children with confirmed ADHD than in age-matched normal children when task difficulty was held constant and equal for both groups. It was concluded that P300 abnormalities in ADHD reflect processing differences as opposed to discrimination differences.

Kileny (1991) has reported on the use of the P300 in the assessment of cochlear implant users as a means of determining cognition and discrimination. Likewise, others have shown its use in auditory discrimination tasks including intensity (Hillyard et al, 1971), frequency, and duration (Polich, 1989b; Polich et al, 1985). In general, changes in frequency, intensity, and duration may be seen in changes in P300 latency. Frequency also affects amplitude of the P300.

Hurley and Musiek (1997) studied the the effectiveness of central auditory processing tests in the identification of cerebral lesions in adults (from 22 to 73 years old). The P300 was recorded using an oddball paradigm with a 1000 Hz tone used as the frequent stimulus and a 2000 Hz tone used as the oddball stimulus. The P300, using this paradigm, had a hit rate of approximately 59%. They also reported a 98% probability of a patient not having a central auditory nervous system disorder when the P300 was normal.

The auditory P300 has been used to study auditory deprivation. Hutchinson and McGill (1997) looked at 17 children with profound bilateral deafness between the ages of 9 and 18 years that had been fitted with monaural hearing aids. An oddball paradigm using tonal stimulation revealed asymmetry in P300 results between years and between an age-matched group of children with normal-hearing. Although the purpose of the study was to show the importance of binaural amplification, the study illustrates the use of the P300 in the assessment of auditory function.

The use of P300 recordings in patients with cochlear implants has shown changes in the P300 consistent with behavioral performance in an oddball task. That is, patients that could behaviorally identify the oddball presentation showed a clear P300. In a few patients with cochlear implants that could behaviorally perform the oddball task, the P300 was not absent (Jordon et al, 1997).

Micco et al (1995), using an oddball paradigm to synthesized phonemes of /dɑ/ and /di/, reported that in the patients implanted with the Nucleus 22 device essentially no differences were seen in the P300 between the implant users and normal-hearing individuals. It was concluded that the P300 possibly may be a useful tool in evaluating cognitive function in cochlear implant users.

The P300 has been of greatest use in the study and diagnosis of dementia and Alzheimer's disease. The latency of the P300 is significantly increased for adjusted age level in dementia and shows both a decrease in amplitude and increase in latency of the P300 in Alzheimer's disease. These differences, along with other clinical signs, help to distinguish Alzheimer's disease from dementia and other neuropsychiatric diseases such as Korsakoff psychosis (Barrett, 1993; Michaelewski et al, 1986; Polich 1989a; St Clair et al, 1988).

The amplitude and latency of the P300 is abnormal in several types of neuropsychiatric and behavioral disorders. The P300 has been found to demonstrate reduced amplitudes in autism and schizophrenia. An increase in the latency of the P300a and P300b, along with a decrease in the amplitude of the P300b, has been observed in ADHD. A decreased amplitude and increased latency of the P300 has been reported in children with CAPDs (Allred et al, 1994; Goodin, 1990; Jirsa, 1992; Kraiuhin et al, 1990; Marsh et al, 1990; Martineau et al, 1989, 1992; McPherson & Davies, 1995; Muir et al, 1988; Polich, 1989a; Polich et al, 1990; Satterfield et al, 1990; St Clair et al, 1988).

N400 SEMANTIC EVOKED POTENTIAL

Introduction

AEPs occurring between 300 and 500 ms after stimulus onset are sensitive to lexical aspects of speech (Kutas & Hillyard, 1980). The N400 is an ERP that may be elicited after a semantically incorrect sentence, specifically one in which the ending is unexpected (Fig. 20–16). For example, "The dog bit the *cat*" has high contextual constraints and the ending a high probability of occurrence. This would be contrasted by "the dog bit the *moon*" whose ending would have a low probability of occurrence. The latter sentence would produce an N400. Terminal words in spoken sentences with varying degrees of contextual constraint and probability will produce different amplitudes in the N400. Ending words with a high degree of expectation produce a low-amplitude N400, whereas ending words with a low degree of expectation produce a high-amplitude N400 (Connolly et al, 1990).

The latency of the N400 shifts with the complexity of the task (Connolly et al, 1992), whereas the amplitude of the N400 shifts inversely with the expectancy of the terminal word (Kutas & Hillyard, 1984). As can be understood from this brief discussion, the occurrence of an N400 requires a high level of linguistic processing, thus providing a mechanism of assessing brain processing of language.

The N400 demonstrates a centroparietal distribution in scalp topography (Connolly et al, 1990; Kutas & Hillyard, 1980, 1982). Similar to the P300, undoubtedly multiple, simultaneous overlapping generators exist.

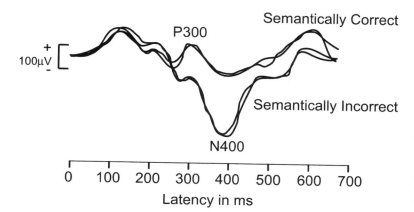

Figure 20–16   The N400 ERP to a semantically correct sentence ("the dog chewed the bone") and to a semantically incorrect sentence ("the dog chewed the green"). The N400 appears to the semantically incorrect sentence.

Technical Specifications

Electrodes are placed at Cz (noninverting) and referenced to C_7 (Fig. 20–17). The signal is bandpassed filtered between DC and 300 Hz. A 750 ms poststimulus sample is acquired. Eye movement must be monitored.

Because the response diminishes rather quickly as a result of semantic adaptation, a total of 100 samples is obtained by collecting 50 trials of high-constraint, high-predictable sentences and 50 trials of low-constraint, low-predictable

sentences (Table 20–8). The sentence presentations should be pseudorandomized. The sentences are presented at a comfortable level, approximately 70 dB HL in the binaural condition. A 1500 ms ISI is used. The subjects are merely instructed to listen carefully to the sentences. A good source for sentences is the SPIN test (Bilger et al, 1984). A subset of the sentences that have been found appropriate for first graders and above are as follows.

High-contextual constraint high-predictability sentences:

1. The dog chewed on a bone.
2. Football is a dangerous sport.
3. A bicycle has two wheels.

Low-contextual constraint low-predictability sentences:

1. Betty knew about the nap.
2. Jane has a problem with the coin.
3. They knew about the fur.

Subject State and Variables

The subjects must be awake and alert. They should attend by "listening carefully" to the sentences. Because eye movement may contaminate the results, they must be monitored. Because of the necessity of using a relatively small number of averages, eye movement artifact must be reduced and not just "rejected" by the averaging process.

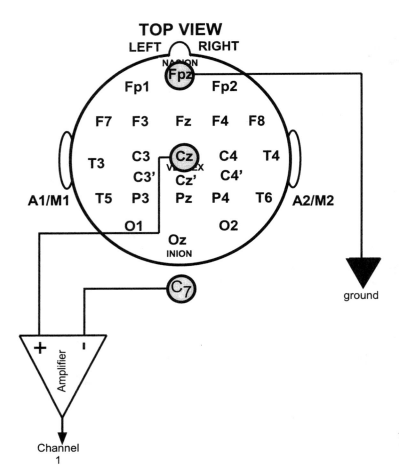

Figure 20–17 Electrode montage for the N400 (Cz-C7).

Clinical Applications

Kutas and Hillyard (1984) have shown that semantic "unexpectancy" results in the N400 and not a semantic "unrelatedeness." Likewise, grammatical incongruities do not produce an N400 and consequently the two, grammatical incongruities and semantic incongruities, are not produced in the same manner.

The N400 does not appear to be part of the stimulus discrimination process associated with the N200. For example, in a phonological masking paradigm, Connolly et al (1992) showed the N400 latency increased for a phonologically correct masker. No changes were noted in the N2. Connolly et al (1992) concluded that their findings support a cognitive, semantic processing of the sentence.

The presence of an N400 depends on the complexity of the processing task, which shifts the latency of the N400, and the degree of expectancy of the terminal word, which is inversely related to the amplitude of the N400. In other words, amplitude shifts give information as to the ability to predict word usage from contextual cues, and latency shifts indicate the ability to process complex linguistic information.

Kutas and Hillyard (1983) reported in a series of school-age children that the N400 was present to semantic processing but was not present in sentences containing grammatical errors, thus concluding that grammatical errors are processed in a different manner than semantic incongruities.

Phonologically correct masking (i.e., 12 talker babble) was studied by Connolly et al (1992) using both the N200 and

N400 ERPs. The N400 was affected by the presence of the phonological correct masking; whereas the N200 showed no effects, suggesting that the N400 responds to linguistic processing, and the N200 responds to the acoustic processing of the sentence. Because both potentials may be observed in the same recording, it is apparent that the N200 and N400 represent two distinct ERPS.

Other levels of language activity have also been studied. For example, syntactic anomalies such as subcategorization, agreement violations, and tense violations have been found to elicit a negative wave occurring between 300 and 500 ms, similar to the N400, but with a maximal amplitude over the frontal region of the scalp as opposed to centroparietal distribution of the N400 (Connolly et al, 1990; Friederici, Pfeifer et al, 1993; Kutas & Hillyard, 1980, 1982, 1983).

CONCLUSIONS

The purpose of this chapter is to introduce practitioners to MLAEPs and long LAEPs. These potentials are not considered as mainstream electrophysiological tests in routine audiology practice. However, they promise to be a valuable tool in diagnosing various auditory processing problems. Therefore the contents and orientation of this chapter are toward clinical applications relevant to audiology practice. It is anticipated that future developments in auditory electrophysiology will prove the value of late auditory evoked responses in clinical applications.

TABLE 20–8   N400 recording parameters

Parameter	Note
Electrodes	
Type:	Ag-AgCl
Montage:	*Single channel:* Cz (noninverting). C7 (inverting). FpZ (ground). *Eye movement* (see text): Superior orbit of one eye to the inferior orbit of the opposite eye (polarity not specified).
Recording Parameters	
Channels:	Single-channel response. Each of the two stimuli, highly predictable and less predictable, are averaged in separate buffers.
Timebase:	100 ms prestimulus. 750 ms poststimulus.
# Averages:	200 (100 for each stimulus). Presentations greater than 100/stimulus set will cause a diminished N400 (similar to habituation).
Filter (bandpass):	.05–50.
Artifact Rejection:	3/4 maximum sampling amplitude.
Stimuli	
Type:	Speech stimuli where S1 is a highly constrained and predictable sentence, and S2 is a less constrained and less predictable sentence. The sentences are pseudorandomized.
Transducer:	Tubal insert phones. Calibrated earphones (i.e., TDH-39, etc.). Sound field speakers.
Polarity:	Not specified.
Level:	75–80 dB nHL for a robust response showing all of the subcomponents.
Rate:	See ISI.
ISI:	1–2 s from end of sentence.

ACKNOWLEDGMENTS

Appreciation is expressed to Herbert Gould, Ph.D., Associate Professor, School of Audiology & Speech-Language Pathology, University of Memphis for his review of this manuscript. Partial funding for this work was provided by a grant from the David O. McKay School of Education, Brigham Young University.

REFERENCES

ALHO, K. (1995). Cerebral generators of mismatch negativity (MMN) and its magnetic counterpart (MMN) elicited by sound changes. *Ear and Hearing, 16*(1);38–51.

ALHO, K., WOODS, D.L., ALGAZI, A., KNIGHT, R.T., & NÄÄTÄNEN, R. (1994). Lesions of frontal cortex diminish the auditory mismatch negativity. *Electroencephalography and Clinical Neurophysiology, 91*(5);353–362.

ALLRED, C., MCPHERSON, D.L., & BARTHOLOMEW, K. (1994). *Auditory training in a patient with severe dysfunction in auditory memory and figure ground.* Presented at the Annual Meeting of the Academy of Rehabilitative Audiology. Salt Lake City, Utah.

AREHOLE, S., AUGUSTINE, L.E., & SIMHADRI, R. (1995). Middle latency response in children with learning disabilities: Preliminary findings. *Journal of Communication Disorders, 28*(1);21–38.

BAKER, N.J., STAUNTON, M., ADLER, L.E., GERHARDT, G.E., DREBING, C., WALDO, M., NAGAMOTO, H., & FREEDMAN, R.

(1990). Sensory gating deficits in psychiatric inpatients: Relation to catecholamine metabolites in different diagnostic groups. *Biological Psychiatry, 27;*519–528.

BARRETT, G. (1993). Clinical applications of event-related potentials. In A.M. Halliday (Ed.). *Evoked potentials in clinical testing.* (pp. 589–633). London: Churchill Livingstone.

BILGER, R.C., NUETZEL, J.M., RABINOWITZ, W.M., & RZECZKOWSKI, C. (1984). Standardization of a test of speech perception in noise. *Journal of Speech and Hearing Research, 27;* 32–48.

BILLINGS, R.J. (1989). The origin of the initial negative component of the averaged lambda potential recorded from midline electrodes. *Electroencephalography and Clinical Neurophysiology, 72*(2);114–117.

BOUTROS, N., ZOURIDAKIS, G., & OVERALL, J. (1991). Replicating and extension of P50 findings in schizophrenia. *Electroencephalography and Clinical Neurophysiology, 22;*40–45.

BRAZIER, M.A.B. (1984). Pioneers in the discovery of evoked potentials. *Electroencephalography and Clinical Neurophysiology, 59;*2–8.

BUCHWALD, J.S. (1990a). Animal models of event-related potentials. In: J. Rohrbaugh, R. Parasuraman, & R. Johnson (Eds.). *Event-related potentials of the brain* (pp. 57–75). New York: Oxford Press.

BUCHWALD, J.S. (1990b). Comparison of plasticity in sensory and cognitive processing systems. *Clinical Perinatology, 17*(1);57–66.

BUCHWALD, J.S., HINMAN, C., NORMAN, R., HUANG, C., & BROWN, K. (1981). Middle and long latency auditory evoked responses recorded from the vertex of normal and chronically lesioned cats. *Brain Research, 205*(1);91–109.

CHATRIAN, C.E. (1976) The lambda waves. In: A. Remond (Ed.). *Handbook of electroencephalography and clinical neurophysiology* (Vol. 6a) (pp. 123–149). Amsterdam: Elsevier.

CHEOUR-LUHTANEN, M., ALHO, K., KUJALA, T., SAINIO, K., REINIKAINEN, K., RENLUND, M., AALTONEN, O., EEROLA, O., & NÄÄTÄNEN, R. (1995). Mismatch negativity indicates vowel discrimination in newborns. *Hearing Research, 82*(1);53–58.

CONNOLLY, J.F., PHILLIPS, N.A., & STEWART, S.H. (1990). The effects of processing requirements on a neurophysiological responses to spoken sentences. *Brain and Language, 39;*302–318.

CONNOLLY, J.F., PHILLIPS, N.A., STEWART, S.H., & BRAKE, W.G. (1992). Event-related potential sensitivity to acoustic and semantic properties of terminal words in sentences. *Brain and Language, 43;*1–18.

COTTRELL, G., & GANS, D. (1995). Auditory evoked response morphology in profoundly-involved multi-handicapped children: comparisons with normal infants and children. *Audiology, 34*(4);189–206.

CSEPE ,V., KARMOS, G., & MOLNAR, M. (1987). Evoked potential correlates of stimulus deviance during wakefulness, and sleep in the cat—Animal model of mismatched negativity. *Electroencephalography and Clinical Neurophysiology, 66;*571–578.

CSEPE, V., & MOLNAR, M. (1997). Towards the possible clinical application of the mismatch negativity component of event-related potentials. *Audiology and Neurootology, 2*(5);354–369.

DIETRICH, S., BARRY, S., & PARKER, D. (1995). Middle latency auditory responses in males who stutter. *Journal of Speech and Hearing Research, 38;*5–17.

DONCHIN, E. (1981) Surprise! . . . Surprise? *Psychophysiology, 18;*493–513.

EGGERMONT, J.J., PONTON, C.W., DON, M., WARING, M.D., & KWONG, B. (1997). Maturational delays in cortical evoked potentials in cochlear implant users. *Acta Otolaryngologian (Stockholm), 117*(2);161–3.

ERWIN, R.J., MAWHINNEY-HEE, M., GUR, R.C., & GUR, R.E. (1991). Midlatency auditory evoked responses in schizophrenics. *Biological Psychiatry, 30;*430–442.

FERRARO, J.A., DURRANT, J.D., SINIGER, Y.S., & CAMPBELL, K. (1996). Recommended guidelines for reporting AEP specifications. *American Journal of Audiology, 5;*35–37.

FIFER, R.C., & SIERRA-IRIZARRY, B. (1988). Clinical applications of the auditory middle latency response. *American Journal of Otology, 9;*47–56.

FREEDMAN, R., ADLER, L.E., & WALDO, M. (1987). Gating of the auditory evoked potential in children and adults. *Psychophysiology, 24;*223–227.

FRIEDERICI, A.D., PFEIFER, E., et al. (1993). Event-related brain potentials during natural speech processing: Effects of semantic, morphological and syntactic violations. *Brain Research and Cognitive Brain Research, 1*(3);183–92.

GIARD, M.H., PERRIN, F., PERNIER, J., & BOUCHET, P. (1990). Brain generators implicated in processing of auditory stimulus deviance: A topographic event-related potential study. *Psychophysiology, 27;*627–640.

GOODIN, D.S. (1990). Clinical utility of long latency 'cognitive' event-related potentials (P3): The pros. *Electroencephalography and Clinical Neurophysiology, 76*(1);2–5.

GORGA, M., & NEELY, S.T. (1994). Stimulus calibration in auditory evoked potential measurements. In J.T. Jacobson (Ed.). *Principles and applications in auditory evoked potentials.* (pp. 85–98). New York: Allyn & Bacon.

GROENEN, P., SNIK, A., & VAN DEN BROEK, P. (1996). On the clinical relevance of mismatch negativity: Results from subjects with normal-hearing and cochlear implant users. *Audiology and Neurootology, 1*(2);112–124.

HALL, J.W. (1992). *Handbook of auditory evoked potentials.* Boston, MA: Allyn & Bacon.

HARI, R., HAMALAINEN, M., ILMONIEMI, R., KAUKORANTA, E., REINIKAINEN, K., SALMINEN, J., ALHO, K., NÄÄTÄNEN, R., & SAMS, M. (1984). Responses of the primary auditory cortex to pitch changes in a sequence of tone pips: Neuromagnetic recordings in man. *Neuroscience Letters, 50;*127–132.

HILLYARD, S.A., & KUTAS, M. (1983). Electrophysiology of cognitive processing. *Annual Review of Psychology, 34;*33–61.

HILLYARD, S.A., SQUIRES, K.C., BAUER, J.W., & LINDSAY, P.H. (1971). Evoked potential correlates of auditory signal detection. *Science, 172;*1357–1360.

HURLEY, R.M., & MUSIEK, F.E. (1997). Effectiveness of three central auditory processing (CAP) tests in identifying cerebral lesions. *Journal of the American Academy of Audiology, 8*(4);257–262.

HUTCHINSON, K.M., & McGILL, D.J. (1997). The efficacy of utilizing the P300 as a measure of auditory deprivation in monaurally aided profoundly hearing-impaired children. *Scandinavian Audiology, 26*(3);177–185.

JASPER, H.H. (1958). Report on Committee on Methods of Clinical Examination in Clinical Electroencephalography. *Electroencephalography and Clinical Neurophysiology, 10;*370–375.

Javit, D.C., Schroeder, C.E., Steinschneider, M., Arezzo, J.C., & Vaughan Jr, H.G. (1992). Demonstration of mismatch negativity in the monkey. *Electroencephalography and Clinical Neurophysiology, 83;*87–90.

Jerger, K., Biggins, C., & Fein, G. (1992). P50 suppression is not affected by attentional manipulations. *Biology and Psychology, 31;*365–377.

Jewett, D.L., & Williston, J.S. (1971). Auditory evoked far fields recorded from scalp of humans. *Brain, 94;*681–696.

Jirsa, R.E. (1992). The clinical utility of the P3 AERP in children with auditory processing disorders. *Journal of Speech and Hearing Research, 35*(4);903–912.

Jordan, K., Schmidt, A., Plotz, K., von Specht, H., Begall, K., Roth, N., & Scheich, H. (1997). Auditory event-related potentials in post- and prelingually deaf cochlear implant recipients. *American Journal of Otology, 18*(6 Supp.);116–117.

Kileny, P.R. (1991). Use of electrophysiologic measures in the management of children with cochlear implants: Brain stem, middle latency, and cognitive (P300) responses. *American Journal of Otology, 12*(Supp.);37–42.

Kileny, P.R., Boerst, A., & Zwolan, T. (1997). Cognitive evoked potentials to speech and tonal stimuli in children with implants. *Otolaryngology–Head and Neck Surgery, 117*(3 Pt. 1);161–169.

Knight, R.T., Scabini, D., Woods, D.L., & Clayworth, C. (1988). The effects of lesions of superior temporal gyrus and inferior parietal lobe on temporal and vertex components of the human AEP. *Electroencephalography and Clinical Neurophysiology, 70*(6);499–509.

Kraiuhin, C., Gordon, E., Coyle, S., Sara, G., Rennie, C., Howson, A., Landau, P., & Meares, R. (1990). Normal latency of the P300 event-related potential in mild-to-moderate Alzheimer's disease and depression. *Biological Psychiatry, 28*(5);372–386.

Kraus, N., & McGee, T. (1990). Clinical applications of the middle latency response. *Journal of the Acoustical Society of America, 1;*130–133.

Kraus, N., & McGee, T. (1995). The middle latency response generating system. *Electroencephalography and Clinical Neurophysiology Supplement, 44;*76–92.

Kraus, N., & McGee, T. (1996). Auditory development reflected by middle latency response. *Ear and Hearing, 17*(5);419–429.

Kraus, N., McGee, T., Carrell, T., King, C., Littman, T., & Nicol, T. (1994c). Discrimination of speech-like contrasts in the auditory thalamus and cortex. *Journal of the Acoustical Society of America, 96*(5 Pt. 1); 2758–2768.

Kraus, N., McGee, T., Carrell, T., Sharma, A., Micco, A., & Nicol, T. (1993b). Speech evoked cortical potentials in children. *Journal of the American Academy of Audiology, 4*(4);238–248.

Kraus, N., McGee, T., Carrell, T., Sharma, A., & Nicol, T. (1995). Mismatch negativity to speech stimuli in school-age children. *Electroencephalography and Clinical Neurophysiology Supplement, 44;*211–217.

Kraus, N., & McGee, T. & Comperatore, C. (1989). MLRs in children are consistently present during wakefulness, stage 1, and REM sleep. *Ear and Hearing, 10*(6);339–345.

Kraus, N., McGee, T., Ferre, J., Hoeppner, J.A., Carrell, T., Sharma, A., & Nicol, T. (1993c). Mismatch negativity in the neurophysiologic/behavioral evaluation of auditory processing deficits: A case study. *Ear and Hearing, 14*(4);223–234.

Kraus, N., McGee, T., Litman, T., Nicol, T., & King, C. (1994b). Non-primary auditory thalamic representation of acoustic change. *Journal of Neurophysiology, 72;*1270–1277.

Kraus, N., McGee, T., Sharma, A., Carrell, T., & Nicol, T. (1992). Mismatch negativity event-related potential elicited by speech stimuli. *Ear and Hearing, 13*(3);158–164.

Kraus, N., McGee, T., & Stein, L. (1994a). The auditory middle latency response: Clinical uses, development, and generating system. In: J.T. Jacobson (Ed.). *Principles and applications in auditory evoked potentials* (pp. 155–178). Needham Heights: Simon & Schuster.

Kraus, N., Micco, A.G., Koch, D.B., McGee, T., Carrell, T., Sharma, A., Wiet, R.J., & Weingarten, CZ. (1993d). The mismatch negativity cortical evoked potential elicited by speech in cochlear-implant users. *Hearing Research, 65* (1–2),118–124.

Kraus, N., Özdamar, Ö., Hier, D., & Stein, L. (1982). Auditory middle latency responses (MLRs) in patients with cortical lesions *Electroencephalography and Clinical Neurophysiology, 54;*275–287.

Kutas, M., & Hillyard, S.A. (1980). Reading senseless sentences: Brain potentials reflect semantic incongruity. *Science, 207;*203–205.

Kutas, M., & Hillyard, S.A. (1982). The lateral distribution of event-related potentials during sentence processing. *Neuropsychologia, 20*(5);579–590.

Kutas, M., & Hillyard, S.A. (1983). Event-related brain potentials to grammatical errors and semantic anomalies. *Memory and Cognition, 11*(5);539–550.

Kutas, M., & Hillyard, S.A. (1984). Brain potentials during reading reflect word expectancy and semantic association. *Nature, 307;*161–163.

McPherson, D.L. (1996). *Late potentials of the auditory system.* San Diego, CA: Singular Publishing Group Inc.

McPherson, D.L., & Davies, K. (1995). Binaural interaction in school age-children with attention deficit hyperactivity disorder. *Journal of Human Physiology, 21*(1);47–53.

McPherson, D.L., & Starr, A. (1993). Auditory evoked potentials in the clinic. In: A.M. Halliday (Ed.). *Evoked potentials in clinical testing* (pp. 359–381). New York: Churchill Livingstone.

McPherson, D.L., Tures, C., & Starr, A. (1989). Binaural interaction of the auditory brain stem potentials and middle latency auditory evoked potentials in infants and adults. *Electroencephalography and Clinical Neurophysiology, 74;* 124–130.

Micco, A.G., Kraus, N., Koch, D.B., McGee, T.J., Carrell, T.D., Sharma, A., Nicol, T., & Wiet, J. (1995). Speech-evoked cognitive P300 potentials in cochlear implant recipients. *American Journal of Otology, 16*(4);514–520.

Michalewski, H.J., Rosenberg, C., & Starr, A. (1986). Event-related potentials in dementia. In: R.Q. Cracco, I. Bodis-Wollner (Eds.). *Evoked potentials* (pp. 521–528). New York: Alan R. Liss.

Muir, W.J., Squire, I., Blackwood, D.H., Speight, M.D., St Clair, D., Oliver, C., & Dickens, P. (1988). Auditory P300 response in the assessment of Alzheimer's disease in Down's syndrome: A 2-year follow-up study. *Journal of Mental Deficiency Research, 32;*455–463.

NÄÄTÄNEN, R. (1992). *Attention and brain function.* Hillsdale, NJ: Earlbaum.

NÄÄTÄNEN, R., GAILLARD, A.W.K., & MANTYSALO, S. (1978). Early selective attention effect on evoked potential reinterpreted. *Acta Psychologica,42*;313–329.

NÄÄTÄNEN, R., PAAVILAINEN, P., ALHO, K., REINIKAINEN, K., & SAMS, M. (1987). The mismatch negativity to intensity changes in an auditory stimulus sequence. *Electroencephalography and Clinical Neurophysiology Supplement, 40;* 125–131.

NAGAMOTO, H.T., ADLER, L.E., WALDO, M.C., & FREEDMAN, R. (1989). Sensory gating in schizophrenics and normal controls: Effects of changing stimulation interval. *Biological Psychiatry, 25*;549–561.

NELSON, M.D., JACOBSON, J.T., HALL, J.W., ET AL. (1997). Factors affecting the recordability of auditory evoked response component Pb (P1). *Journal of the American Academy of Audiology, 8*(2);89–99.

NIEDERMEYER, E. (1987). The normal EEG in the waking adult. In: E. Niedermeyer, & F. Lopes da Silva (Eds.). *Electroencephalography* (pp. 110–112). Munich: Urban & Schwarzenberg.

OATES, P., & STAPELLS, D. (1997a). Frequency specificity of the human auditory brain stem and middle latency responses to brief tones. I. High-pass noise masking. *Journal of the Acoustical Society of America, 102*(2);3597–3608.

OATES, P., & STAPELLS, D. (1997b). Frequency specificity of the human auditory brain stem and middle latency responses to brief tones. II. Derived responses. *Journal of the Acoustical Society of America, 102*(2);3609–3619.

ÖZDAMAR, Ö., & KRAUS, N. (1983). Auditory middle latency responses in humans. *Audiology, 22*;34–49.

PAAVILAINEN, P., KARLSSON, M.L., REINIKAINEN, K., & NÄÄTÄNEN, R. (1989). Mismatch negativity to change in spatial location of an auditory stimulus. *Electroencephalography and Clinical Neurophysiology, 73*(2);129–141.

PARVING, A., SALOMON, G., ELBERLING, C., LARSEN, B., & LASSAN, N.A. (1980). Middle components of the auditory evoked response in bilateral temporal lobe lesions. *Scandinavian Audiology (Copenhagen), 9*;161–167.

PERZ-BORJA, C., CHATRIAN, G.E., TYCE, F.A., & RIVERS, M.H. (1962) Electrographic patterns of the occipital lobes in man: A topographic study based on use of implanted electrodes. *Electroencephalography and Clinical Neurophysiology, 14*;171–182.

PICTON, T.W., & HILLYARD, S.A. (1974). Human auditory evoked potentials. II: Effects of attention. *Electroencephalography and Clinical Neurophysiology, 36*;191–199.

PLOURDE, G., BARIBEAU, J., & BONHOMME, V. (1997). Ketamine increases the amplitude of the 40-Hz auditory steady-state response in humans. *British Journal of Anaesthesiology, 78*(5);524–529.

POLICH, J. (1989a). P300 and Alzheimer's disease. *Biomedical Pharmacotherapy, 43*(7);493–499.

POLICH, J. (1989b). Frequency, intensity, and duration as determinants of P300 from auditory stimuli. *Electroencephalography and Clinical Neurophysiology, 6*;277–286.

POLICH, J., HOWARD, L., & STARR, A. (1985) Stimulus frequency and masking as dereminants of P300 latency in event-related potentials from auditory stimuli. *Biologic Psychiatry, 21*;309–318.

POLICH, J., LADISH, C., & BLOOM, F.E. (1990). P300 assessment of early Alzheimer's disease. *Electroencephalography and Clinical Neurophysiology, 77*(3);179–189.

PONTON, C.W., & DON, M. (1995). The mismatch negativity in cochlear implant users. *Ear and Hearing, 16*(1);131–146.

PONTON, C.W., DON, M., EGGERMONT, J.J., WARING, M.D., KWONG, B., & MASUDA, A. (1996a). Auditory system plasticity in children after long periods of complete deafness. *Neuroreport, 8*(1);61–65.

PONTON, C.W., DON, M., EGGERMONT, J.J., WARING, M.D., & MASUDA, A. (1996b). Maturation of human cortical auditory function: differences between normal-hearing children and children with cochlear implants. *Ear and Hearing, 17*(5);430–437.

SALAMAT, M., & MCPHERSON, D.L. (1999). Interactions among variables in the P300 response to a continuous performance task. *Journal of the American Academy of Audiology, 10*;379–387.

SALLINEN, M., & LYYTINEN, H. (1997). Mismatch negativity during objective and subjective sleepiness. *Psychophysiology, 34*(6);694–702.

SANDRIDGE, S.A., & BOOTHROYD, A. (1996). Using naturally produced speech to elicit the mismatch negativity. *Journal of the American Academy of Audiology, 7*(2);105–112.

SATTERFIELD, J.H., SCHELL, A.M., NICHOLAS, T.W., SATTERFIELD, B.T., & FREESE, T.E. (1990). Ontogeny of selective attention effects on event-related potentials in attention-deficit hyperactivity disorder and normal boys. *Biological Psychiatry, 28*(10);879–903.

SCHERG, M. (1982). Distortion of middle latency auditory response produced by analog filtering. *Scandinavian Audiology, 11*;57–60.

SCHERG, M., VAJSAR, J., & PICTON, T. (1989). A source analysis of the late human auditory evoked potentials. *Journal of Cognitive Neuroscience, 1*(4);3336–3355.

SCHWENDER, D., KLASING, S., CONZEN, P., FINSTERER, U., POPPEL, E., & PETER, K. (1996). Midlatency auditory evoked potentials during anesthesia with increasing endexpiratory concentrations of desflurane. *Acta Anaesthesiology Scandinavia, 40*(2);171–176.

SHARMA, A., KRAUS, N., MCGEE, T., CARRELL, T., & NICOL, T. (1993). Acoustic versus phonetic representation of speech as reflected by the mismatch negativity event-related potential. *Electroencephalography and Clinical Neurophysiology, 88*(1);64–71.

SHI DI, & BARTH, S. (1992). The functional anatomy of middle-latency auditory evoked potentials: Thalamocortical connections. *Journal of Neurophysiology, 68*;425–431.

SHIH, J.J., & THOMPSON, S.W. (1998). Lambda waves: Incidence and relationship to photic driving. *Brain Topography, 10*(4);265–272.

SIEGEL, C., WALDO, M., MIZNER, G., ADLER, L.E., & FREEDMAN, R. (1984). Deficits in sensory gating in schizophrenic patients and their relatives: Evidence obtained with auditory evoked responses. *Archives of General Psychiatry, 41;*607–612.

ST CLAIR, D., BLACKBURN, I., BLACKWOOD, D., & TYRER, G. (1988). Measuring the course of Alzheimer's disease. A longitudinal study of neuropsychological function and changes in P3 event-related potential. *British Journal of Psychiatry, 152*(48);48–54.

Starr, A., McPherson, D., Patterson, J., Don, M., Luxford, W., Shannon, R., Sininger, Y., Tonakawa, L., & Waring, M. (1991). Absence of both auditory evoked potentials and auditory percepts dependent on timing cues. *Brain, 114*;1157–1180.

Tatsumi, K., Hirai, K., Furuya, H., & Okuda, T. (1995). Effects of sevoflurane on the middle latency auditory evoked response and the electroencephalographic power spectrum. *Anesthesiology Analgesics, 80*(5); 940–943.

Tremblay, K., Kraus, N., Carrell, T., & McGee, T. (1997). Central auditory system plasticity: Generalization to novel stimuli following listening training. *Journal of the Acoustical Society of America, 102*(6);3762–3773.

Tucker, D., & Ruth, R. (1996). Effects of age, signal level, and signal rate on the auditory middle latency response. *Journal of the American Academy of Audiology, 7*;83–91.

Velasco, M., Eelasco, F., & Velasco, A.L. (1989). Intracranial studies on potential generators of some vertex auditory evoked potentials in man. *Stereotactic and Functional Neurosurgery, 53*(1);49–73.

Waldo, M.C., & Freedman, R. (1986). Gating of auditory evoked responses in normal college students. *Psychiatric Research, 19*(3);233–239.

Waldo, M., Gerhardt, G., Baker, N., Drebing, C., Adler, L., & Freedman, R. (1992). Auditory sensory gating and catecholamine metabolism in schizophrenic and normal subjects. *Psychiatric Research, 44*;21–32.

Wolpaw, J.R., & Wood, C.C. (1982). Scalp distribution of human auditory evoked potentials: I. Evaluation of reference electrode sites. *Electroencephalography and Clinical Neurophysiology, 54*;15–24.

Wood, C.C., & Wolpaw, J.R. (1982). Scalp distribution of human auditory evoked potentials. II. Evidence for overlapping sources and involvement of auditory cortex. *Electroencephalography and Clinical Neurophysiology, 54*; 25–38.

Woods, D.L., Knight, R.T., & Scabini, D. (1993). Anatomical substrates of auditory selective attention: Behavioral and electrophysiological effects of posterior association cortex lesions. *Brain Research Cognitive Brain Research, 1*; 227–240.

Xu, Z.M., Cawenberge, K., Vinck, D., & De Vel, E. (1997). Choice of a tone-pip envelope for frequency-specific threshold evaluations by means of the middle-latency response: Normally hearing subjects and slope of sensorineural hearing loss. *Auris Nasus Larynx, 24*(4); 333–340.

PREFERRED PRACTICE GUIDELINES

Professionals Who Perform the Procedure(s)

▼ Audiologists
▼ Neurophysiologists
▼ Neurologists
▼ Otologists

Expected Outcomes

▼ Auditory evoked potentials will provide frequency and sensitivity information about hearing.
▼ Auditory evoked potentials will provide information about the integrity of the auditory system.
▼ Auditory evoked potentials will provide information about specific and non-specific auditory processing.
▼ Auditory evoked potentials to speech stimuli will provide information about speech processing, cognitive processing of speech, and linguistic processing of speech depending upon the type of stimulus.

Clinical Indications

▼ Auditory evoked potentials may be conducted on individuals that are difficult to test using behavioral protocols.
▼ Auditory evoked potentials may be conducted on individuals with central auditory processing disorders and other types of perceptual and cognitive disorders.

▼ Auditory evoked potentials may be conducted on individuals with language processing disorders.

Clinical Process

▼ Electrophysiological evaluation of the auditory system.
▼ Adjunct procedure in obtaining information about auditory sensitivity.
▼ Adjunct procedure to obtaining information about auditory processing.
▼ Adjunct to planning of intervention programs.
▼ Adjunct to monitoring status of the disorder.

Documentation

▼ Documentation contains pertinent background about the suspected disorder and any behavioral auditory evaluations.
▼ Documentation should include information about the status of the patient in educational and social settings.
▼ Documentation includes specific information about the electrophysiological protocol being used.
▼ Documentation incudes specific results and recommendations.

Chapter 21

Otoacoustic Emissions

Martin S. Robinette and Theodore J. Glattke

The discovery of otoacoustic emissions (OAEs) by David Kemp in 1977 set the stage for dramatic changes in our understanding of how the auditory system is able to respond to the vanishingly small energy levels that are required to reach the threshold of perception of humans. Kemp's (1978) report of stimulated or evoked otoacoustic emissions (EOAEs) and later description of spontaneous otoacoustic emissions (SOAEs) (Kemp, 1979) provided important evidence that fueled the development of modern auditory theory. Contemporary theory is an amalgamation of elements proposed by von Helmholtz more than 100 years ago; von Bekesy, approximately 70 years ago; and Gold, approximately 50 years ago. Von Helmholtz's (1863) observations called for the existence of precise resonators that are tuned to individual frequencies. The resonators were thought by Helmholtz to respond to the motion of the basilar membrane and to vibrate in and of themselves. Von Bekesy's (1928) report of a traveling wave disturbance that progressed along the cochlea's basilar membrane from base to apex had a profound effect on auditory theory. von Bekesy was critical of von Helmholtz's theory because he believed that the resonators that were proposed by von Helmholtz could not be tuned with sufficient precision to

explain precipitous high-frequency hearing loss that had been reported clinically. It is ironic that the lack of precision in the traveling wave formed the basis for a major criticism of von Bekesy's theory of cochlear analysis. Gold (1948) examined the theories of von Helmholtz, the data of von Bekesy, and the data on auditory perception that had accumulated and concluded that the mechanisms proposed by von Helmholtz and the mechanical activity recorded by von Bekesy were both important components of the response of the inner ear to sound. In addition, he argued that some form of positive feedback, or amplification, must be in place to allow humans to respond to low energy levels and do so with great sensitivity to small changes in stimulus frequency. Gold recognized that the positive feedback mechanism might reveal itself through episodes of oscillation like the audible tonal feedback associated with hearing aids and public address systems. He also considered that it should be possible to detect the presence of the amplifier mechanism through detection of the oscillation.

Today, the feedback predicted by Gold is commonly recorded as SOAEs. The mechanism of emission production is not known. However, the discovery of outer hair cell motility (Brownell, 1983) coupled with recordings of enhanced basilar membrane vibration in response to low-intensity stimulation (Johnstone et al, 1986, 1993; Ruggero & Rich, 1991) has led to a consensus that the outer hair cells supply the driving force for the emissions and the "cochlear amplifier" described by Davis (1983). Today, the traveling wave is thought to be the basis for the spatial representation and temporal dispersion of the inner ear's response to sound, and micromechanical activity originating in the outer hair cells is thought to provide the threshold sensitivity and tuning that characterizes normal-hearing (Dallos, 1992). Hearing loss of cochlear origin in the mild to moderate range now is thought to be due to the loss of a biomechanical amplifier system rather than the reduction in sensitivity of sensory cells. Because OAEs are intimately related to the operation of the outer hair cells and because those cells are critical components in the normal cochlear response to sound, it follows that OAE properties are sensitive to the presence of hearing loss caused by hair cell abnormalities.

The emissions are low-intensity sounds that may be detected in the external earcanal by a microphone. They offer a record of the pattern of ossicle and tympanic membrane motion in response to motion that originates within the cochlea. The motion is transduced to acoustic energy by the action of the ossicles and tympanic membrane on the air in the

Audiology: Diagnosis. Edited by Roeser, Valente, and Hosford-Dunn. Thieme Medical Publishers, Inc., New York © 2000

middle and external ear cavities. In this sense the middle ear apparatus functions like a loudspeaker diaphragm system. If the middle ear system is compromised, it is likely that the acoustic energy produced by that ear will also be compromised. In addition, the action of the middle ear muscles can be expected to influence the characteristics of OAEs (e.g., Margolis & Trine, 1997). Finally, outer hair cells receive a rich efferent innervation from the central nervous system (CNS) (e.g., Warr, 1992) and the interaction of OAEs with external stimulation reflects the influence of the CNS on the operation of the cochlear biomechanical system.

MEASUREMENT OF OTOACOUSTIC EMISSIONS

As Probst (1990) stated, any sound that is produced by the cochlea and detected in the earcanal is an otoacoustic emission. The various types of OAEs share several common features.

1. They are low-intensity sounds, ranging from the noise floor of the instrumentation (approximately −20 dB sound pressure level [SPL]) to a maximum between 20- and 30-dB SPL. The amplitude of an EOAE is related to the stimulus amplitude in a complex manner. Early investigations (e.g., Wilson, 1980) demonstrated that EOAEs obtained in response to near-threshold click stimuli contained more energy than was present in the stimulus. EOAEs reach saturation for stimuli in the mid-intensity range. A click stimulus at peak amplitude of 80 dB SPL will produce an emission with amplitude that is approximately 60- to 70-dB below the stimulus amplitude. Similar results occur for continuous tonal stimuli presented at moderate intensities.

2. The temporal and spectral characteristics of the emission will reflect the region of the cochlea that produces it. In a healthy ear an EOAE will mirror the stimulus: click stimuli will produce emissions with complex waveforms and spectra that extend over a broad frequency range; tone bursts elicit brief tonal emissions; and continuous tones produce continuous emissions at frequencies predicted by the frequency of the tonal stimuli.

3. Emissions can be suppressed or reduced in amplitude by presentation of ipsilateral or contralateral stimuli.

4. Emission properties are altered in the presence of slight hearing loss (Harris & Probst, 1991) and the probability of detecting emissions in the frequency region where hearing loss exceeds 30 dB HL is low (Harris & Probst, 1997).

5. Emissions are extracted from the background noise in the external earcanal by sampling the sound in the earcanal to develop an average time waveform or a spectral analysis or a combination of temporal and spectral averaging techniques.

Otoacoustic emissions are classified after Probst (1990) according to their relationship with the stimuli used to produce them. As summarized in Table 21–1, there are two broad categories of emissions. Spontaneous emissions, or SOAEs, as their name implies, occur without intentional stimulation of the ear. When detected in the absence of any external stimulus, they are registered through the use of spectral analysis of the sound in the external earcanal. Figure 21–1 provides an illustration of the typical representation of an SOAE. SOAEs can be synchronized with an external stimulus and when recorded this way, they are designated as *synchronized spontaneous otoacoustic emissions* (SSOAEs) (Prieve & Falter, 1995). The synchronous behavior of the SSOAE allows it to be captured using time-averaged sampling to improve the signal to noise

TABLE 21–1   Types of OAEs

Type of Emission	Stimulus	Recording/Analysis Technique
Spontaneous (SOAE)	None	Signal from microphone is submitted to high-resolution spectral analysis Spectral averaging usually used to reduce noise artifacts.
Synchronized spontaneous (SSOAE)	Click at 70 dB pSPL	Signal from microphone is submitted to time averaging over an 82 ms period. This is followed by a spectral analysis of the average waveform. A synchronized response detected in the time period between 60- and 80-ms after stimulus presentation is considered to be an SSOAE.
Transient evoked (TEOAE)	Click at 80 dB pSPL	Signal from microphone is submitted to time averaging. Average response waveform in buffer "A" is compared with average response waveform in buffer "B." Correlation between waveforms is expressed as response reproducibility. Response amplitude is based on a comparison of the cross power spectrum of the "A" and "B" buffer contents with a waveform computed as the difference between "A" and "B."
Stimulus frequency (SFOAE)	Swept sinusoid (low SPL)	SPL of signal in earcanal is monitored as stimulus at constant SPL is swept through the frequency region of interest. Changes in SPL are reflections of the combination of incident energy and emission produced by the cochlea.
Distortion product (DPOAE)	Paired sinusoids (no standard SPL)	Signal from microphone is submitted to time averaging. Spectral analysis is obtained for average waveform. Energy at the appropriate frequency is considered to be the DPOAE. Energy at other frequencies is "noise."

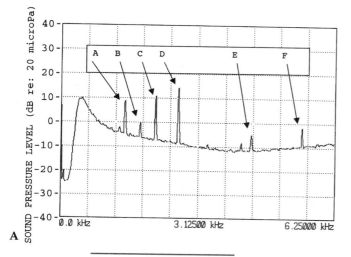

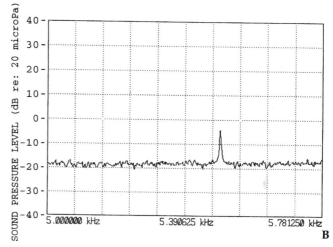

Figure 21–1 **(A)** Multiple SOAEs recorded from a subject with normal auditory thresholds. Frequency and SPL values of the SOAEs are as follows: A, 1437 Hz, 7 dB; B, 1796 Hz, −1 dB; C, 2156 Hz, 10 dB; D, 2671 Hz, 14 dB; E, 4328 Hz, −6 dB; F, 5480 Hz, −3 dB. **(B)** Single SOAE recorded with increased resolution. The example illustrated here is SOAE "F" from panel **A**. The frequency is 5480 Hz and the SPL now reads −5 dB. Note that the noise floor is now approximately −18 dB, but in panel A the noise floor is approximately −10 dB. The drop in noise floor (and improvement in the difference between the emission and the noise floor) is due to the increased resolution of the spectral analyzer. Total frequency span in panel A is 6250 Hz. In panel **B**, the total span is 578 Hz.

ratio of the recording. Pacheco (1997) recently replicated earlier findings of Wable and Collet (1994) by analyzing SOAE and SSOAE records obtained in a large population of normal listeners. She determined that the two recording techniques identify the same emissions and that the SSOAE method represents the emission and noise floor more favorably because of the time-averaging process. As reviewed by Bright (1997), SOAEs occur more frequently in women than in men and more often in the right ear than in the left. SOAEs are stable over long periods of time, but they are not used in clinical screening programs because they may be absent in nearly 50% of ears with normal pure tone thresholds.

EOAEs occur either during long-term stimulation or after a brief stimulus. Responses to brief stimuli are known as transient evoked otoacoustic emissions (TEOAEs). Although important exceptions exist (Gorga et al, 1993; Prieve, et al, 1993), most of the data regarding TEOAEs have been obtained through the use of hardware and software supplied by Otodynamics, Ltd, and known as ILO-88. The typical TEOAE stimulus is a brief, broad-spectrum click, but tone bursts also may be used to elicit the response (e.g., Xu et al, 1994). The response follows the stimulus with a latency that is determined by cochlear traveling wave dynamics. Responses that contain high-frequency components appear with a short latency, and responses with mid-frequency and low-frequency components appear after a latency of 8- to 10-ms. This response property makes separation of the stimulus and response records relatively easy through the use of techniques that are identical to those used in recording the short-latency auditory-evoked potentials. Approximately 2000 stimuli are presented to improve the signal-to-noise ratio of the response

record. The repeated sampling procedure is identical to that used for the purpose of obtaining auditory brain stem and other auditory-evoked potentials. The typical clinical recording involves stimulation at a level of 80 dB peak-equivalent SPL (e.g., Glattke, 1983), and response amplitudes are typically at levels approximately 60- to 70-dB below the level of the stimulus.

Stimulus-frequency otoacoustic emissions (SFOAE) occur during stimulation of the ear with tonal stimuli. They appear at the frequency of the external stimulus and, as a consequence, it is difficult to separate the response and the stimulus (Kemp & Chum, 1980). SFOAEs result from energy leaking back into the earcanal from the cochlear amplifier and their amplitudes increase as the stimulus intensity decreases. However, because of the difficulty associated with recording them, they have not been used in clinical investigations.

Distortion product otoacoustic emissions (DPOAE) also occur simultaneously with the stimulus. Unlike SFOAEs, they are relatively easy to detect because they occur at frequencies that are different than the stimulus frequencies. DPOAEs represent distortions of the stimulus, hence their name. DPOAEs are recorded clinically in response to the presentation of a pair of primary tones, called F_1 and F_2. The DPOAEs appear at several frequencies when the two primary tones are applied to the ear. The most robust is located at a frequency equal to $(2F_1 - F_2)$. In a practical situation the DPOAE frequency is found to be as far below F_1 as F_2 is above F_1. The DPOAE response appears at a level that is approximately 50 to 60 dB below the level of the primary stimulus, and it occurs only when the primary stimuli are located in a region of the cochlea that responds normally.

In summary, OAEs are small signals that depend on the integrity of the entire auditory periphery, including the external and middle ear apparatus, and the cochlea and its interactions with the CNS. No responsible author has suggested that OAEs can be used to estimate the amount of hearing loss with great precision, but it is clear that clinical recordings of OAEs are important elements in the audiologist's toolbox. They are finding widespread application in several areas, including the following:

1. Screening for hearing loss in the newborn and pediatric population

2. Augmenting behavioral test results in difficult-to-test patients

3. Developing a true differential diagnosis in terms of separating hearing loss into "sensory" and "neural" components

4. Identifying individuals with subtle abnormalities of CNS function

NORMATIVE DATA AND CLINICAL INTERPRETATION

Transient Evoked Otoacoustic Emissions

TEOAEs can be recorded from nearly all persons with normal pure tone thresholds and normal middle ear function. An example of the display associated with the ILO88 system is provided in Figure 21–2. The data display contains information about the stimulus, recording situation, and properties of the response. The key elements of the display are as follows:

1. **Stimulus:** The panel labeled stimulus includes an illustration of the stimulus waveform that was sampled before the onset of data collection. The display spans 5 ms. The

amplitude scale is indicated in Pascals (Pa). A value of 0.3 Pa is equivalent to 83.5 dB SPL.

2. **Patient/software:** The center panels identify the version of the software used to display the data and information about the patient, ear tested, and stimulus mode. The designation MX NONLIN CLICKN indicates that the ILO 88 default nonlinear stimulus mode was used to obtain the data. Responses are gathered for sets of four stimuli. Three are presented in one phase at the indicated amplitude and the fourth is presented in the opposite phase at a level that is three times greater than each of the three previous stimuli. The sum of the responses to the four stimuli consists of waveforms that follow the stimulus precisely (linear components) and components that do not change in a simple fashion with stimulus intensity or phase (nonlinear components). Kemp et al (1986) estimated that the linear stimulus artifacts and response components could be reduced by 40 dB, whereas the desired nonlinear portion of the emission would be reduced by only 6 dB with this stimulus method. In the default setting, the ILO 88 software stores the average response to one-half of the stimuli in a memory buffer identified as "A." The response for other stimuli is stored in a buffer identified as "B." The sampling process continues until responses from 260 sets of stimuli have been stored in each of the two memory areas. Therefore the A and B waveforms each represent the mean of responses to 260 × 4 transients or 1040 stimuli, and the total number of stimuli used in the default condition is 2080.

3. **Response waveform:** The display illustrates the time-averaged waveforms sampled for a 20.48 ms period after the onset of the transient stimulus. Tracings are plotted for the "A" and "B" memory locations, and each tracing consists of 512 data points. Each data point corresponds to a time period of 40 μs. The first 2.5 ms, or 63 data points, have been eliminated to reduce the contribution of a stimulus

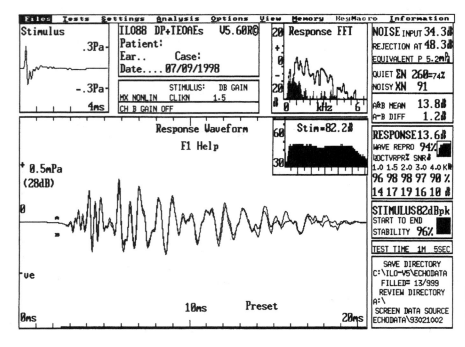

Figure 21–2 Example of TEOAE obtained from a cooperative child. See text for explanation of data display.

artifact to the average response waveform. The sensitivity of the vertical scale in the response waveform panel is 55 dB greater than the scale used to represent the click stimulus in the upper left-hand panel.

4. **Response FFT:** This display provides illustrations of the fast Fourier transforms (FFT) that are based on the A and B waveforms. The resolution of the FFT analysis is approximately 49 Hz per line. The open histogram reflects the spectrum of the response that is common to the A and B tracings. The cross-hatched display represents the spectrum of the difference between the A and B waveforms or the noise that remains in the average waveform. The horizontal scale extends from 0 to 6000 Hz. The vertical scale extends from less than -20 dB SPL to approximately $+20$ dB SPL.

5. **Stim:** This display provides a tabular representation of the peak equivalent SPL of the stimulus at the onset of the sampling. The spectrum of the stimulus is illustrated by the solid histogram. The horizontal scale of the stimulus spectrum is identical to the horizontal scale for the response FFT. The vertical scale extends from 30 dB SPL to greater than 60 dB SPL. For a typical transient stimulus with a peak level of 80 dB SPL, the spectrum level (or level per cycle) will be 40- to 45-dB SPL.

PITFALL

If the noise floor of your OAE recording is constant across frequency, the probe is not fitted properly in the earcanal.

---

6. **Noise:** The tabular value of the noise is the average SPL detected by the microphone during the samples that were not rejected by the software.

7. **Rejection at ___ dB:** The software permits the examiner to select a rejection threshold to reduce unwanted noise. The default rejection threshold is 47 dB SPL and the range available to the examiner extends from 24- to 55-dB SPL. The rejection level can be adjusted continuously throughout the sampling period, and the tabular value is the threshold selected by the examiner at the end of the sampling. The rejection threshold value also is shown in milliPascals.

8. **Quiet ΣN:** This entry is the number of responses accepted for the A and the B waveforms. The percentage of all samples accepted for the average waveform also is listed in tabular form.

9. **Noisy XN:** This entry is a tally of the number of response sets that were rejected during the sampling procedure.

10. **A & B Mean:** This is the sound pressure level of the average of the A and B waveforms. In this instance, the value is 13.8 dB.

11. **A-B Diff:** This is the average difference between the A and B waveforms and is the level of energy represented by the cross-hatched area of the "Response FFT" window. It is computed by taking the difference between the A and B waveforms on a point-by-point basis, less 3 dB. In this case, the A-B value is 12.6 dB less than the average power of the A and B waveforms.

12. **Response:** This value is the overall level of the correlated portions of the A and B response waveforms and is obtained from the FFT displayed in the Response FFT window.

13. **Wave Repro:** This is known as "whole-wave reproducibility." The entry is actually the value of the cross correlation between the A and B waveforms expressed as a percentage. The correlation is recomputed after every 20 stimulus sets, and the value of the correlation is represented in the small histogram to the right of the percent value. The result in this case is 94%, reflecting a near-perfect correlation, which is compatible with the small A-B Diff value.

14. **Band Repro % SNR dB:** The reproducibility and signal-to-noise ratio values are listed below column headings of 1.0 through 4.0 kHz. To obtain these results, the A and B waveforms are filtered into bandwidths of approximately 1000 Hz centered at the indicated frequencies. The correlations are recomputed, and the difference between the powers computed for the FFTs represented by the open and cross-hatched histograms in the "Response FFT" window are represented as the signal-to-noise ratio at each frequency.

15. **Stimulus ___ dB pk:** The stimulus intensity is measured after every 16 stimulus sets. The tabular value listed at this location is the result of the final computation. The final result may be different than the value obtained at the outset of the sampling procedure. The initial value is tabulated in the portion of the display containing the stimulus spectrum (see No. 5).

16. **Stability ___ %:** This entry and the accompanying histogram reflect changes that occur in the stimulus intensity. The single % entry expresses that greatest difference detected between the first and any subsequent stimulus throughout the sampling period as a % rather than dB value (1 dB is approximately 10%). The small histogram to the right of the entry chronicles the history of the stimulus intensity measurements.

17. **Test time:** This entry records the duration of the test.

CHARACTERISTICS OF TRANSIENT EVOKED OTOACOUSTIC EMISSIONS ELICITED WITH DEFAULT STIMULI

Clinical appraisal of electrophysiological responses, such as the auditory brain stem response (ABR) or electrocochleographic (ECoG) recordings obtained from the eighth cranial nerve, rely on estimates of response *threshold, latency, and amplitude*, to estimate the integrity of the auditory system. At the outset of studies of emissions, Kemp (1978) observed the highly nonlinear nature of the response, and he and his coworkers have reported that the minimum intensity at which a TEOAE can be detected rarely corresponds with perceptual threshold (e.g., Kemp et al, 1990). Kemp warns that the apparent "threshold" of the response is critically dependent on the noise in the recording situation and the status of the ear under test. For example, although a newborn may have robust emissions, physiological noise produced by the neonate may preclude detection of the emissions at levels corresponding to the infant's auditory threshold. An ear with strong emission responses may reveal little attenuation of the response with significant reductions of the stimulus intensity, as little as 0.1 dB per 1 dB change (Kemp et al, 1990). Thus it is impossible to estimate the threshold of hearing from the apparent threshold of the emission response or extrapolate from detected responses to presumed threshold on the basis of amplitude measurements. Kemp (1978), Prieve et al (1993), Grandori and Ravazzani (1993), Stover and Norton (1993), Prieve and Falter (1995) and Prieve et al (1997) are among the investigators who have examined the complex interaction between click stimulus intensity and response characteristics, including threshold. As Kemp et al (1990) suggested, we are far from having a standard against which response threshold, latency, and growth characteristics can be evaluated in a clinical setting. In this sense the TEOAEs share difficulties encountered in the interpretation of cochlear microphonic (CM) potentials, which, like the emissions, are intimately related to the status of the hair cells in the cochlea (e.g., Glattke, 1983).

The most common clinical application of TEOAEs involves click stimuli presented at moderate intensities, 80 dB peak equivalent SPL or about 45 dB greater than perceptual threshold. The default stimulus used by the ILO 88 equipment was selected to screen for hearing loss: if no response can be obtained, then it is possible that a hearing loss is present. In the most general sense the *spectrum* of a TEOAE elicited from a healthy ear reflects the spectrum of the stimulus. TEOAEs obtained in response to click stimuli are expected to have broad response spectra. The amplitudes of TEOAEs vary directly with the amplitudes of the stimuli, but the relationships between stimulus and response are complicated by the fact that TEOAEs result from highly nonlinear phenomena. From the outset, reports of properties of TEOAEs elicited from normal ears have emphasized the idiosyncratic nature of the responses. Unfortunately, few studies have provided tabular summaries of the data provided by the ILO 88 software or grouped data in terms of subject characteristics such as age, gender, and right/left differences. The data that are summarized in the sections that follow were obtained using ILO 88 default stimulus conditions: (a) 80 μs transients; (b) nominal stimulus level of 80- to 83-dB peak equivalent SPL; and (c) nonlinear mode, unless stated otherwise.

Although a number of studies have described the properties of OAEs in healthy infants and children, there are few large-scale studies of emission characteristics in children whose audiometric status has been documented by behavioral tests (e.g., Glattke et al, 1995). One report of the results of a newborn screening program in which control for sensitivity and specificity of the screening procedure was evaluated has appeared in the literature (Lutman et al, 1997). The salient property of TEOAEs obtained from healthy newborns is a robust response amplitude. Kok et al (1993) reported that the median response amplitude for infants is approximately 20 dB SPL, and the response reproducibility is directly related to response amplitude. As Prieve et al (1997) reviewed, the largest changes in TEOAE amplitude appear to occur between birth and 4 years of age. The average amplitude of the response to default stimuli (80 dB) declines from 20 dB to approximately 15 dB for preschool children and to 10 dB for adults.

Glattke and Robinette (1997) and Prieve and Falter (1995) have reported that TEOAE amplitude does not decrease with age when the responses obtained from older adults are compared with those obtained from young adults, so long as adequate control is provided for normal-hearing thresholds. Glattke and Robinette (1997) observed a continuing attenua-

tion of response with age if "normal" thresholds were defined as 25 dB HL or better. If the "normal" criterion was adjusted to 15 dB HL or better, then no age correction was needed. Prieve and Falter (1995) noted that the presence of SOAEs was associated with a robust TEOAE, regardless of age of the subject.

Other measures of TEOAEs proposed for clinical measurements include *response reproducibility* and *signal-to-noise ratio* as a function of frequency. A reproducibility score of 50% or greater signals the presence of an emission in the frequency region of interest (Kemp et al, 1990). The signal-to-noise ratio computed by the ILO software is based on a comparison of the power of the reproducible portion of the A and B response waveforms with the power in a waveform that is computed as the difference between the A and B memories. A reproducibility score of 50% or greater usually is associated with a signal-to-noise ratio of 3 dB or more, but the relationship between the reproducibility and signal-to-noise measures is complex.

DISTORTION PRODUCT OTOACOUSTIC EMISSIONS

DPOAEs are attractive as clinical tools because the frequency at which the response occurs is predicted exactly by the frequencies of the primary tones. The relationship among the primary stimuli and the frequency at which the distortion product is located helps to reduce the ambiguity in determining whether or not a response is present. A typical DPOAE display is illustrated in Figure 21–3. Primary tone frequency is plotted on the horizontal axis. Said another way, the abscissa is a representation of the region of the cochlea stimulated by the primary tones. The display may be arranged in terms of the value of F_2, or F_1, or some intermediate frequency. The ordinate of the illustration depicts SPL.

The manufacturers of DPOAE systems use a number of algorithms to create stimuli and sample the sound present in the earcanal during stimulation. In general terms DPOAE data are obtained by presenting the primary tones through independent transducers to reduce the possibility of the creation of distortion caused by the instrumentation. The waveform of the sound in the earcanal is submitted to time-averaging procedures that are synchronized to the stimuli. This has the effect of reducing background noise. The averaged waveform is submitted to a spectral analysis to determine the SPL at the DPOAE frequency and the background noise at frequencies near the DPOAE.

Regardless of the sampling and analysis methods, the display typically represents the magnitude of the DPOAE and the noise present in the earcanal in the frequency region of the DPOAE. Responses obtained from ears with normal audiometric thresholds are influenced by: (1) stimulus amplitude (designated as L for level); (2) relative amplitude of F_1 (L_1) and F_2 (L_2); and (3) ratio F_2 and F_1 frequencies.

The optimal intensities for stimuli to elicit DPOAEs from ears with normal audiometric thresholds are between 50- and 70-dB SPL, with L_2 approximately 10- or 15-dB below L_1 (Prieve et al, 1997). The optimal ratio of F_2/F_1 is approximately 1.2:1, which places the DPOAE at a point that is one-half octave below F_2 (Lonsbury-Martin et al, 1997). Under stimulus conditions such as these, the DPOAE response appears at a level of about 10 dB SPL in children and adults (Pafitis et al,

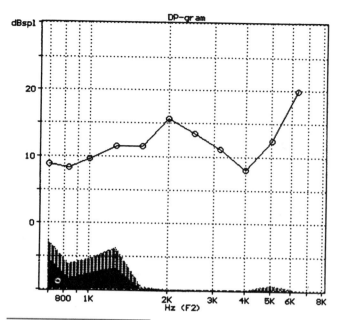

Figure 21–3 DPOAE amplitude as a function of F_2 frequency recorded from a cooperative child with normal auditory thresholds.

1994) and at approximately 15 dB SPL in infants (Prieve et al, 1997). As illustrated in the example in Figure 21–3, the typical response pattern reveals a slight reduction in DPOAE amplitude when the primary tones are in the mid-frequency (2 to 5kHz) region. This finding has been replicated in virtually all studies that have presented group data from ears with normal audiometric thresholds (Lonsbury-Martin et al, 1997). As is the case with TEOAEs, an individual's DPOAE response is idiosyncratic, and, consequently, clinical measurements have no universally accepted norms. For example, some protocols require that the response be at least 10 dB above the noise floor to be considered valid. Others require a response-to-noise ratio of 3- or 1-dB. In the example illustrated in Figure 21–3, the DPOAE amplitude is more than 10 dB above the noise floor for every data point.

Gorga et al (1993) and Prieve et al (1997) have provided data that are important to the development of response norms. The relationship between the stimulus and response amplitudes may signal the presence of cochlear abnormalities (e.g., Harris & Probst, 1997). DPOAE response latency measures may provide important information about the status of the ear under test (Lonsbury-Martin et al, 1997), but no large-scale studies of response latency properties in normal and disordered populations have been completed.

CLINICAL CONCEPTS

TEOAE or DPOAE responses are indices of the same cochlear phenomenon (the electromotile activity of outer hair cells in response to acoustic stimuli). The choice between TEOAE and DPOAE instrumentation may be influenced by the frequency range of interest. In terms of separating patients with normal-hearing sensitivity (20 dB or better) from those with mild or

greater hearing loss, TEOAEs are more sensitive at 1000 Hz, TEOAEs and DPOAEs are essentially equivalent for 2000 and 3000 Hz, and DPOAEs are more sensitive from 4000 through 6000 Hz (Gorga et al, 1993; Gorga et al, 1997; Prieve et al, 1993).

The preferred EOAE stimulus levels that optimize the separation between patients with normal versus impaired cochlear function are 80- to 82-dB pSPL for click stimuli used for TEOAE measures and pure tone stimulus levels of L_1 and L_2 at 65- and 55-dB SPL, respectively, for DPOAE measures. Under these conditions, the tests are effective in separating patients with pure tone hearing sensitivity of 20- to 25-dB HL or better from patients with hearing losses of 35 dB HL or poorer (Gaskill & Brown, 1990; Gorga et al, 1993; Gorga et al, 1997; Prieve et al, 1993; Probst & Harris, 1993; Robinette, 1992a; Stover et al, 1996; Whitehead et al, 1995a).

Figures 21–4 and 21–5 illustrate the probability of obtaining EOAEs as a function of hearing loss of cochlear origin in dB HL compiled by Harris and Probst (1997). For example, segment A of Figure 21–4 indicates a 99% probability of measurable TEOAEs for patients with hearing sensitivity of 20 dB or better. Harris and Probst summarized these data from eight reports in the literature. Segment C reflects the absence of TEOAEs for sensorineural hearing loss (SNHL) of 40 dB HL or more compiled from 13 reports in the literature. The HL in segment B represents a "zone of uncertainty" that extends from approximately 25- to 35-dB HL. In this range TEOAEs

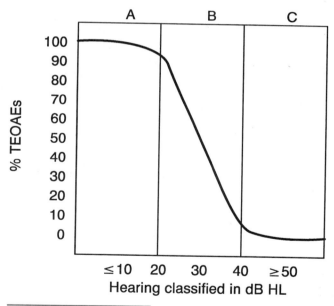

Figure 21–4 Schematic representation of the average pure tone threshold results associated with percentage of TEOAEs present. *Segment A,* overall hearing is better than 20 dB HL and TEOAEs are present in 99% of ears. *Segment C,* sensorineural hearing loss greater than 40 dB HL with no complicating etiological factors: TEOAEs are always absent. *Segment B,* a "zone of uncertainty" that extends from approximately 25- to 35-dB HL. In this range, TEOAEs may be present but are generally reduced in amplitude and in frequency content compared with findings from ears with thresholds falling within segment A. (Adapted from Harris & Probst [1997], with permission.)

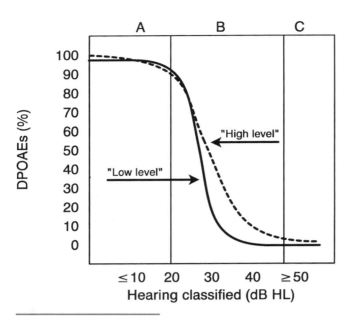

Figure 21–5 Schematic representation of the association between DPOAE presence and average pure tone threshold levels. The two curves represent probabilities of obtaining a response from either low-level (*solid line*) or high-level (*dashed line*) stimulation. When hearing is better than 25 dB HL, DPOAEs are routinely present for both high-level and low-level stimulation for most audiometric frequencies from 1-6 kHz, as represented in segment A. Depending on the stimulus parameters, it is possible to generate distortion even when hearing loss exceeds 50 dB HL, as represented in segment C. When low levels of stimulation are used, DPOAEs are not present above hearing levels of approximately 40 dB HL which is similar to TEOAEs as illustrated in Figure 21–4. The zone of uncertainty represented in segment B is wider than that identified for TEOAEs as illustrated in Figure 21–4. (Adapted from Harris & Probst [1997], with permission.)

may or may not be measurable. Figure 21–5 illustrates the A, B, C segments by hearing loss for DPOAEs from review of eight reports in the literature (Harris and Probst, 1997). The two curves represent probabilities of obtaining a response for either low-level (generally, 65 dB SPL or lower) or high-level (generally, 70- to 75-dB SPL) stimulation. DPOAEs are routinely present for both low-level and high-level stimulation when hearing is better than 25 dB HL (segment A). For low-level stimulation the curve is similar to that in Figure 21–4 for TEOAEs, but for high-level stimulation, DPOAEs on occasion may be measured with hearing loss as great as 40- to 50-dB HL. Consequently, the zone of uncertainty (segment B) is increased by about 10 dB. This uncertainty can make interpretation of DPOAEs measures more difficult, especially as a screening test for the identification of hearing loss. It is suggested that initial DPOAE measures be completed with low-level stimulation. If DPOAEs are absent for low-level stimulation but present for high-level stimulation, an interpretation of mild cochlear hearing loss is defensible. However, as illustrated in Figure 21–5, for hearing loss greater than 30 dB HL, even with high-level stimulation, the probability of a measurable DPOAE response is less than 50%.

However, it is not appropriate to estimate pure tone hearing sensitivity (audiometric thresholds) from EOAE data. EOAEs show evidence of normal to near-normal middle ear and cochlear function but do not reflect hearing thresholds. Although trends from group data suggest that EOAE amplitudes are inversely related to audiometric thresholds within the normal range (Gaskill & Brown, 1993; Gorga et al, 1993; LePage & Murray, 1993), the between-subject variability of EOAE amplitudes is about 25 dB.

Figures 21–6 and 21–7 illustrate the within-subject and between-subject variability of EOAE amplitudes across frequency for TEOAE and DPOAE measures, respectively. Figure 21–6 represents TEOAE data from 30 adults between the ages of 20 and 60 years with pure tone sensitivity of 20 dB HL or better for the frequency range of 500 through 6000 Hz (Mayo Clinic Rochester, 1997). The QuickScreen* and low-frequency filter options were used. Across-subject amplitudes for the half-octaves from 1000 through 4000 Hz ranged

from 3 dB to 37 dB above the noise floor for the 10th to 95th percentiles. It was not uncommon for subjects with thresholds ≤10 dB HL to have amplitudes below the 50th percentile and subjects with thresholds ≥15 dB HL to have TEOAE amplitudes above the 50th percentile.

Within-subject variability is very small. The shaded area around the 50th percentile represents the test-retest variability (95% confidence interval) of ± 3 dB per half-octave band reported by Marshall and Heller (1996). Figure 21–7 summarizes the amplitude range and test-retest variability from DPOAE data (Gorga et al, 1996). Between-subject amplitudes for DPOAEs for the half-octaves from 1000 through 8000 Hz ranged from 2- to 34-dB above the noise floor from the 10th to the 95th percentiles. Test-retest variability reported by Franklin et al (1992) is shown in the gray area surrounding the 50th percentile. They reported variability to be lowest between 3000 and 6000 Hz. The test-retest 95% confidence interval was ± 3 dB for 3000 through 6000 Hz, ± 4 dB at 2000 and 8000 Hz, and ± 5 dB at 1000 Hz. The clinical implications of the

---

*See Appendix for a description and example of the QuickScreen recording option.

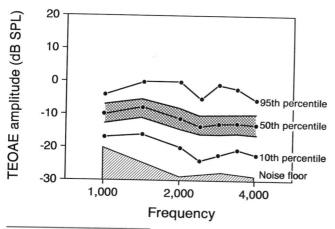

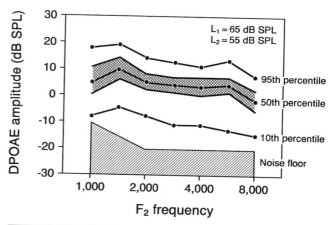

Figure 21–6 Comparison of the 10th, 50th, and 95th percentiles of the amplitude spectra of TEOAEs from 30 ears of adult subjects (age range, 20 through 60 years) with pure tone hearing sensitivity ≤20 dB HL for the frequency range of 500-6000 Hz *(dark circles connected by solid lines lines)*. Measures were made with the ILO88 instrument (Otodynamics Ltd.) with an 80 dB peak SPL click stimulus. QuickScreen stimulus was used, which presents the clicks at 80/s and displays the time-averaged response waveform from 2.5 to 12.5 ms after the stimulus. The low cut filter was also used, which reduces interference caused by noise by adding response attenuation below 1000 Hz. The use of QuickScreen and the low cut filter resulted in a reduction of the amplitude of the TEOAE response and an increase in the reproducibility percent and the signal-to-noise ratio in dB. The noise floor is displayed by the shaded area at the bottom of the figure. The shaded area around the 50th percentile of the spectra represents the small test-retest variability of TEOAE amplitudes reported by Marshall and Heller (1996).

Figure 21–7 Comparison of the 10th, 50th, and 95th percentiles of the amplitude of DPOAEs from 103 subjects (age range, 7 through 86 years) with pure tone hearing sensitivity ≤20 dB HL for the frequency range of 500-8000 Hz *(dark circles connected by solid lines)*. Measurements were made with a custom-designed system (Neely & Liu, 1993), in which response and noise were measured at the same frequency ($2f_1$-f_2) and in which a stopping rule was used (Gorga et al, 1996). The ratio of primary frequencies (f_2/f_1) was 1.2 and primary frequency levels were 65 dB SPL (f_1) and 55 dB SPL (f_2). The noise floor is displayed by the shaded area at the bottom of the figure. The shaded area around the 50th percentile of amplitude represents the small test-retest variability of DPOAE amplitude reported by Franklin et al (1992). (Adapted from Gorga et al, [1996], with permission.)

data represented in Figures 21–6 and 21–7 are that one should not predict pure tone thresholds from EOAE amplitude data, but after establishment of a threshold baseline, EOAE amplitude changes of 4 dB or more provide evidence of changes in cochlear and/or middle ear function.

HIGH-FREQUENCY COCHLEAR HEARING LOSS

A high correlation has been observed between the frequencies of pure tone hearing loss and frequency region of decreased or absent EOAEs (Bonfils & Uziel, 1989; Harris, 1990; Harris & Probst, 1991; Johnsen et al, 1993; Kemp et al, 1986; Lind & Randa, 1989; Probst et al, 1987; Robinette, 1990). Studies of the

relationship between DPOAE amplitude and temporary threshold shift (TTS) reveal that, for both animal and human models, the DPOAE amplitude decrease is frequency specific. The greatest reduction in amplitude occurred approximately half an octave above the frequency of the fatiguing stimuli (Engdahl & Kemp, 1996; Martin et al, 1987). This reduction in response is similar to that demonstrated by psychoacoustic measurements in humans that also reveal the greatest TTS at one-half octave above the frequency of the fatiguing stimulus (Davis et al, 1950). Figure 21–8 provides an example of TEOAE frequency specificity for high frequency hearing loss (Robinette, 1990). The composite audiogram in Figure 21–8A represents the mean thresholds (circles) and composite range (shaded area) for 35 ears of adults with normal-hearing sensitivity through 3000 Hz and pure tone thresholds >25 dB HL for frequencies >3000 Hz. The composite audiogram in Figure 21–8B incorporates the same data for 76 ears with normal sensitivity through 2000 Hz and hearing loss for frequencies >2000 Hz.

The left audiogram ordinate is dB HL; the right ordinate indicates the percentage of patients with the indicated hearing loss who reveal emissions. The square shows the percent of ears for which TEOAEs were present for each frequency band at center frequencies of 1, 1.5, 2, 2.5, 3, 3.5 and 4 kHz. As illustrated on the audiogram (Fig. 21–8A) TEOAEs were present for 33 (94%) of the 35 ears. TEOAEs were present for all 33 ears at 1000 and 1500 Hz, decreasing to 45% at the highest frequency within the normal range (3000 Hz) and fewer TEOAEs at the frequencies with hearing loss. In Figure 21–8B

PEARL

EOAE amplitude change of 4 dB or more provides evidence of changes in cochlear and/or middle ear function.

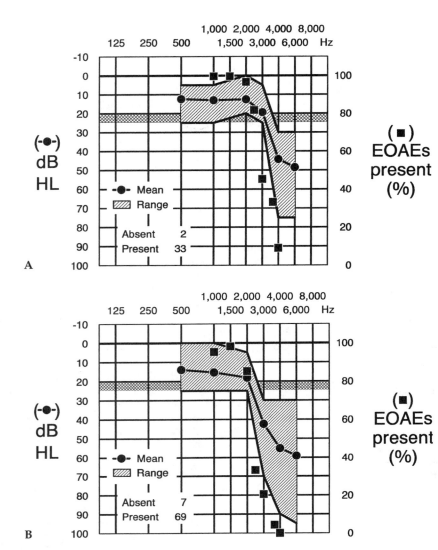

(■)
EOAEs
present
(%)

(■)
EOAEs
present
(%)

Figure 21–8   Examples of TEOAE frequency specificity obtained from patients with high-frequency sensorineural hearing loss. **(A)** Shaded area of audiogram represents the composite pure tone thresholds of 35 ears of adult patients with pure tone thresholds ≤25 dB HL for the frequencies of 500, 1000, 2000, and 3000 Hz, and pure tone thresholds ≥30 dB HL for the frequencies of 4000 and 6000 Hz. Mean thresholds are represented by solid circles. The left ordinate is dB HL for interpretation of audiometric data. The right ordinate represents percent of TEOAEs measured; 0% is at the bottom of the right ordinate, and 100% is near the top of the right ordinate. The solid squares represent the percent of TEOAEs present for each frequency band (1, 1.5, 2, 2.5, 3, 3.5, and 4 kHz) for the 35 patient ears tested. **(B)** Audiogram represents the same audiometric and TEOAE data for 76 ears of patients with pure tone thresholds ≤25 dB HL for the frequencies of 500, 1000, and 2000 Hz and pure tone thresholds ≥30 dB for the frequencies of 3000, 4000, and 6000 Hz. Measures were made with the IL088 instrument (Otodynamics Ltd.) at the default settings as shown in Figure 21–2.

it is shown that TEOAEs were present for 69 (91%) of the 76 ears. TEOAEs were generally present for frequencies with thresholds of ≤25 dB HL (i.e., 97%, 98%, and 85% for 1000, 1500, and 2000 Hz, respectively) and absent for frequencies with hearing loss (i.e., 33%, 21%, 4%, and 0% for 2500, 3000, 3500, and 4000 Hz, respectively). Good frequency specificity of TEOAEs is demonstrated by hearing loss because TEOAEs tend to be present for frequencies corresponding to thresholds within the normal range and absent for frequencies with hearing losses of ≥30 dB HL.

Figure 21–8 also demonstrates that, when hearing loss is present at some frequencies, the probability of obtaining a measurable TEOAE at any frequency is decreased. No TEOAEs were detected for 6 and 9% of the ears represented by the composite audiograms (Figures 21–8A,B). Robinette (1990) also found that the percent of absent TEOAEs increased to 20% for a group of 45 patients with hearing loss above 1000 Hz.

Monitoring Cochlear Status

The measurement of EOAEs may be more sensitive than behavioral audiometry to decreases in cochlear function. Data

displayed in Figure 21–8 are in agreement with other observations that EOAEs often tend to decrease about a half-octave below the knee of the high-frequency hearing loss (Avan et al, 1995; Haran et al, 1993; Harris, 1990, LePage & Murray, 1993). This observation is supported in animal studies regarding the relationship of the outer hair cell (OHC) population and behavioral thresholds (Altschuler et al, 1992; Avan et al, 1995). Figure 21–9 illustrates the behavioral threshold shift for a guinea pig (closed circles) following introduction of kanamycin ototoxicity versus remaining OHC and inner hair cell (IHC) populations (LePage & Murray, 1993). Pure tone behavioral thresholds remained unchanged from 125 through 8000 Hz. However, OHC populations across the same frequency range were decreased for OHC rows 1, 2, and 3. Behavioral thresholds did not decline until OHCs were decreased more than 50%. Figure 21–10 provides an example of DPOAEs and audiometric threshold measures before and after cisplatin treatment resulting in a high-frequency sensorineural hearing loss. Figure 21–10A shows the pretreatment audiogram for a female age 4 diagnosed with an ovarian carcinoma (James-Trychel, Personal communication, Arnold Palmer Hospital for Children and Women, Orlando, FL, 1997). Audiometric

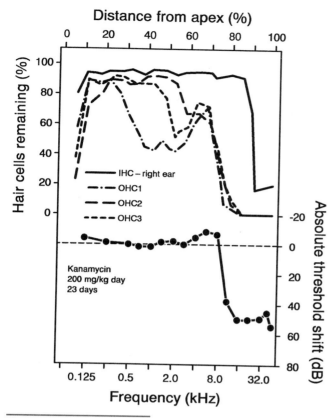

Figure 21–9 Comparison of the percentage loss of OHCs in a guinea pig, obtained postmortem, with the guinea pig's behavioral threshold after kanamycin-induced loss of OHCs. This evidence suggests that extensive damage is necessary to the OHCs before a behavioral hearing loss is evident. (Adapted from Altschuler et al [1992], with permission.)

thresholds were within normal limits (250 to −8000 Hz), and DPOAEs were present for F2 from 1000 to 6000 Hz. After cisplatin treatment, a moderate to severe sensorineural hearing loss developed above 3000 Hz (Figure 21–10B). Posttreatment DPOAEs decreased significantly before 3000 Hz. For this patient, EOAEs appear to be more sensitive to changes in cochlear function than the pure tone audiogram.

DIFFERENTIAL DIAGNOSIS

The diagnostic implications of OAEs are of considerable interest. Classically, audiological tests separate hearing loss into two categories, conductive and sensorineural. EOAEs provide a unique, objective measure of preneural cochlear function and therefore assist in the discrimination between sensory and neural auditory dysfunction. Most congenital and acquired sensory pathological conditions result in OHC dysfunction, which will affect EOAE test results. However, sensory pathological conditions caused by IHC dysfunction will not be reflected in EOAE measures.

For patients with moderate to profound hearing loss, the presence of EOAEs supports the diagnosis of retrocochlear hearing loss. Reports in the literature generally are focused on four patient groups: (a) those with *acoustic neuromas* (Bon-

fils & Uziel, 1988; Cane et al, 1994; Durrant et al, 1993; Prasher et al, 1995; Robinette et al, 1992; Robinette & Durrant, 1997; Telischi et al, 1995); (b) those with *idiopathic sudden hearing loss* (Cevette et al, 1995; Nakamura et al, 1997; Robinette & Facer, 1991; Sakashita et al, 1991; Truy et al, 1993); (c) those with *auditory neuropathy* (Hood et al, 1994; Starr et al, 1996; Stein et al, 1996; Widen et al, 1995; Wright & Dyck, 1995); and (d) those with *pseudohypacusis* (Durrant et al, 1997; Kvaerner

> ### PITFALL
> The recording of OAEs provides us with an opportunity to examine the function of the OHCs, but we lack a similar tool to study the status of IHCs.

et al, 1996; Musiek et al, 1995; Robinette, 1992a). In addition, a number of case studies have been published to highlight the contribution of EOAEs to the evaluation of retrocochlear hearing disorders (Cevette & Bielek, 1995; Doyle et al, 1996; Gravel & Stapells, 1993; Jerger et al, 1992; Katona et al, 1993; Konradsson, 1996; Laccourreye et al, 1996; Lutman et al, 1989; Monroe et al, 1996; Prieve et al, 1991; Robinette, 1992a,b; Welzl-Muller et al, 1993).

Acoustic Neuroma

For patients with acoustic neuromas, EOAEs have been used as a diagnostic indicator for intraoperative monitoring and to provide preoperative and postoperative information on cochlear reserve. The diagnositc value of EOAEs in identification of acoustic neuromas is limited. From a review of seven reports, Robinette and Durrant (1997) found that only 20% of 316 patients with surgically confirmed eighth nerve tumors had mild or greater hearing loss with EOAEs present to support the diagnosis of retrocochlear hearing loss. This lack of diagnostic precision may be attributed to cochlear hearing losses that frequently accompany eighth-nerve tumors. The cochlear loss is thought to be due to the restriction of the blood supply to the cochlea related to tumor growth (Levine et al, 1984).

Intraoperative monitoring of cochlear function by EOAEs during acoustic tumor removal has been demonstrated and found to provide earlier evidence of cochlear compromise than ABR monitoring (Cane et al, 1992; Telischi et al, 1995).

The measurement of EOAEs preoperatively and postoperatively, in conjunction with other tests, is helping to define the site of surgical insult when hearing is decreased or not preserved (Robinette et al, 1992; Robinette & Durrant, 1997). From a group of 11 patients with hearing preservation after acoustic neuroma removal, about half of the patients had poorer hearing postoperatively. Neural function was improved postoperatively for most patients (as measured by ABR), whereas cochlear function was decreased for most patients postoperatively (as measured by EOAEs) (Robinette & Durrant, 1997). These data suggest that neural function is often improved when the auditory nerve is preserved with tumor pressure removed, but subsequent hearing loss may be related more to cochlear damage from vascular compromise during surgery. Therefore even though EOAEs may

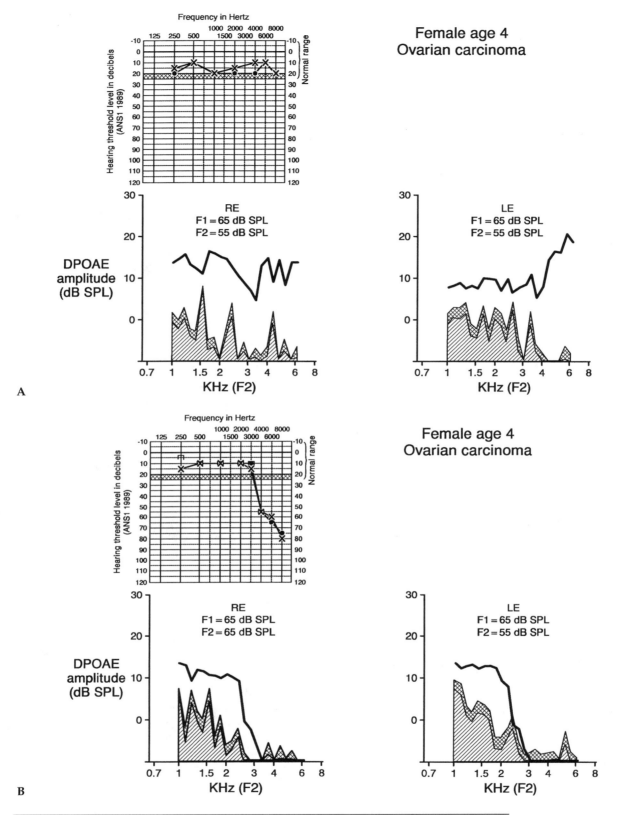

Figure 21–10 Audiometric thresholds and DPOAE amplitudes for a patient diagnosed with ovarian carcinoma. **(A)** Normal-hearing and normal DPOAE amplitudes for a before cisplatin treatment hearing evaluation. **(B)** Hearing evaluation results at 5 months after cisplatin treatment. Audiogram shows normal-hearing from 250 through 3000 Hz with a moderate-to-severe sensorineural hearing loss for 4000, 6000, and 8000 Hz. The DPOAE results show robust emissions from 1000 through 2500 Hz and significant decline in amplitude for higher frequencies. DPOAE measures were made with an ILO92 instrument (Otodynamics Ltd.). The ratio of primary frequencies (f_2/f_1) was 1.2 and primary frequency levels were 65 dB SPL (f_1) and 55 dB (f_2). The dark shading represents the mean noise floor + 1 standard deviation and the light shading represents the mean noise floor + 2 standard deviations.

have a limited role in the diagnosis of acoustic neuromas, they do have promise as a measure of preoperative, perioperative, and postoperative cochlear function.

Sudden Hearing Loss

Some patients with idiopathic sudden hearing loss (ISHL) have EOAEs despite significant hearing loss. Sakashita et al (1991) reported on two groups of patients with moderate-to-severe sensorineural hearing loss. About 50% of the group with ISHL had measurable EOAEs, whereas none of the group with long-standing hearing loss had EOAEs. They concluded that for many patients in the ISHL group, the inner-ear injury was not to the OHCs but to other cochlear structures. Of course, sudden hearing loss may also involve the eighth nerve or central auditory tracts. Figure 21–11 is an illustration of the audiometric and EOAE findings for a 30-year-old man with sudden left ear hearing loss (Robinette & Facer, 1991). The patient reported a history of multiple sclerosis. The initial clinical impression was that the sudden loss could be due to one of the following: multiple sclerosis; a cochlear dysfunction, such as a perilymph fistula; or a space-occupying retrocochlear lesion. Because sudden, profound unilateral hearing loss is not normally associated with multiple sclerosis (Durlovic et al, 1994), it seemed the least likely cause. Negative findings for the pure tone Stenger test ruled out pseudohypoacusis, and negative computed tomography results ruled out a space-occupying lesion. The findings of

normal TEOAEs for this patient in the ear with the profound hearing loss ruled out a perilymph fistula or other cochlear causes. On this basis the hearing loss was diagnosed as being due to an exacerbation of multiple sclerosis. The patient was treated with a short course of steroids and 2 weeks later experienced complete recovery of hearing in his left ear. Before EOAE testing ruling out cochlear hearing loss, surgical management for a perilymph fistula was being considered. For this patient, EOAE measurements influenced diagnosis and medical management.

Auditory Neuropathy

As mentioned previously, OAEs can be suppressed by ipsilateral or contralateral sound stimulation. Ipsilateral suppression studies have demonstrated the precision of tuning in the auditory periphery and probable contributions of the uncrossed olivocochlear efferent neural supply to the cochlea (e.g., Harris & Glattke, 1992; Tavartkiladze et al, 1997). In addition, a number of investigations have demonstrated that contralateral stimuli of low or moderate intensity are effective in reducing the amplitude of OAEs, although the question of tuning of the contralateral effect remains controversial. The primary effect of contralateral stimulation with broadband noise is a slight reduction in the amplitude of the emission (Collet et al, 1990, 1992).

Auditory neuropathy is a relatively new term used to categorize patients with a triad of symptoms: (1) mild to

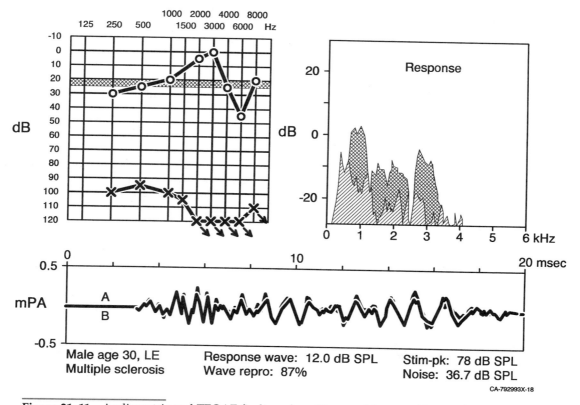

Figure 21–11 Audiometric and TEOAE findings for a 30-year-old man with a profound left ear hearing loss associated with multiple sclerosis. (Adapted from Robinette & Facer [1991], with permission.)

profound behavioral hearing loss on the basis of audiometric thresholds; (2) normal cochlear OHC function as evidenced by the presence of EOAEs and/or CMs; and (3) abnormal auditory pathway function as shown by absent or abnormal auditory brain stem evoked potentials, elevated or absent acoustic reflex thresholds, and absent contralateral supression of TEOAEs (Sininger et al, 1995; Starr et al, 1996). Before the use of EOAEs as an objective clinical measure of cochlear function leading to the identification of auditory neuropathy, patients with absent auditory-evoked potentials and mild-to-moderate hearing loss were considered a curious paradox (Davis & Hirsh, 1979; Hildesheimer et al, 1985; Kraus et al, 1984; Lenhardt, 1981; Worthington & Peters, 1980). Figures 21–12 and 21–13 provide examples obtained from a sister and brother with symptoms consistent with auditory neuropathy. A 15-month-old female patient with delayed speech development was seen for an audiological evaluation. Pure tone visual response audiometry (VRA) testing showed a profound sensorineural hearing loss with normal tympanometry and absent acoustic reflexes (Fig. 21–12A). Four-channel ABR recordings to 85 dB nHL rarefaction clicks were also abnormal, with only a reproducible wave I for the right ear (Fig. 21–12B). The measurement of robust normal EOAEs (Fig. 21–12C) were unexpected and altered clinical management considerations. Birth history and developmental milestones were unremarkable. Both a genetic workup and temporal bone imaging were negative. The patient's 4-month-old brother also was evaluated with similar results. Figure 21–13 shows normal TEOAEs (Fig. 21–13A) and abnormal ABR recordings (Fig. 21–13B) at 4 months of age. Figure 21–13C shows the profound sensorineural hearing loss obtained by VRA testing at age 6 months. Four additional cases of infants with normal EOAEs and abnormal ABRs are presented by Stein et al (1996). Although cases of auditory neuropathy are relatively uncommon, they highlight the value of EOAEs in clinical assessment. Generally EOAEs support behavioral test results in documenting the presence or absence of pediatric sensorineural hearing loss.

Pseudohypacusis

The audiology literature is replete with descriptions of methods for identification of pseudohypacusis. The Stenger test is the procedure of choice in detecting unilateral pseudohypacusis (Robinette & Gaeth, 1972). Cases of bilateral pseudohypacusis are more difficult to document by objective procedures, with auditory-evoked potential testing being the most reliable (Sanders & Lazenby, 1983). However, even evoked potentials may be misleading under some conditions (Glattke, 1983). EOAEs have been found to be a quick and reliable screening test of both unilateral and bilateral pseudohypacusis (Durrant et al, 1997; Kvaerner et al, 1996; Musiek et al, 1995; Robinette, 1992a). Figure 21–14A shows the initial audiometric thresholds obtained from a 35-year-old woman. She spoke Arabic and explained through an interpreter that she had progressive bilateral hearing loss. Speech audiometry was not attempted. Tympanometry, acoustic reflex thresholds, and decay were within normal limits. Pure tone test results were judged reliable with no indication of possible pseudohypacusis with the exception of her appearing to understand the speech of the interpreter better than one might expect with a severe sensorineural hearing loss. Figure 21–14B reveals normal TEOAE responses bilaterally that are consistent with normal to near-normal cochlear function. ABR waveforms and latencies were within normal limits for 85 dB nHL rarefaction click stimuli, ruling out eighth nerve involvement. Threshold ABR testing revealed repeatable wave V at stimulus levels of 20 dB nHL bilaterally, supporting the impression of pseudohypacusis. The patient's audiometric pure tone thresholds improved about 20 dB bilaterally, after reinstruction of response criteria and procedures.

Cochlear Implant Candidate

Several patients under consideration for cochlear implantation demonstrate measurable EOAEs despite profound sensorineural hearing loss (Mayo Clinic Rochester, 1997). One such patient has been previously reported (Robinette, 1992b). Figure 21–15 illustrates the EOAE and CM findings of a second patient. The 60-year-old man was seen for consideration of a cochlear implant (CI) 10 months after a sudden profound bilateral hearing loss. At the time of CI consideration, he had no measurable hearing audiometrically, tympanometry was normal, and acoustic reflexes were absent. He had a long history of progressive sensorineural hearing loss and had worn binaural hearing aids for 3 years before the sudden loss. After his sudden hearing loss, he was treated with a course of steroids without improvement. Magnetic resonance and computed tomography imaging were negative, and he was referred for consideration of a CI. During the CI evaluation, DPOAEs were measured in his right ear from 1000 through 2500 Hz (Fig. 21–15A). The presence of cochlear function was verified by the identification of bilateral CMs by comparison of ABR waveforms from rarefaction versus. condensation click stimuli. Specifically, Figure 21–15B illustrates a 180-degree phase shift between rarefaction and condensation click elicited waveforms during the first 2 ms of the response. The initial stimuli was presented at 100 dB nHL. As the stimulus levels were reduced to 80 dB nHL, microphonics remained at the same latency while the amplitudes decreased. These data were interpreted to suggest significant cochlear function with a retrocochlear component to the hearing loss and consequently a favorable prognosis from a CI was questioned. From such clinical experiences, it seems reasonable to recommend EOAE and CM assessment as part of pre-CI evaluations.

PEARL

EOAE testing is recommended as part of pediatric auditory evaluations of patients with normal middle ear function when history and/or behavioral tests suggest hearing loss.

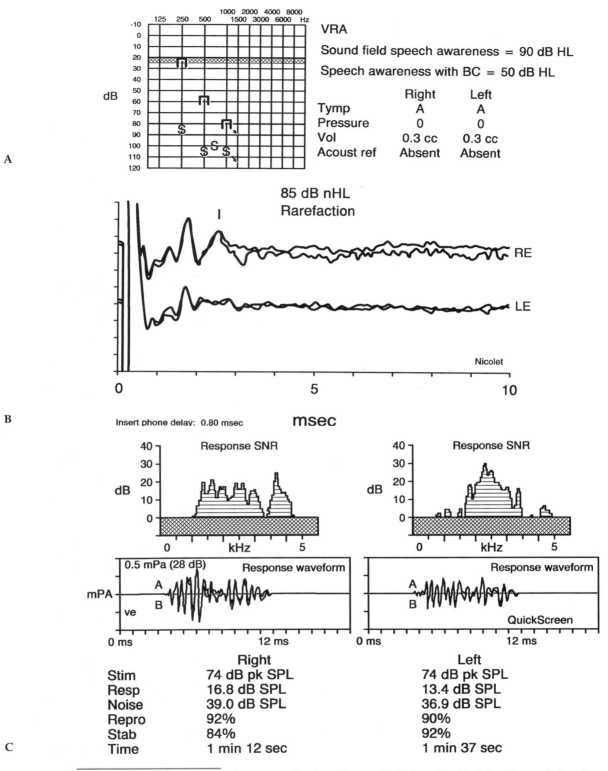

Figure 21–12 Audiologic evaluation results for a 15-month-old female with delayed speech development. **(A)** Profound hearing loss obtained from visual response audiometry and acoustic immittance findings. **(B)** Abnormal ABR tracings. Stimuli were rarefaction clicks at a level of 85 dB nHL at a rate of 11.1/s. Only wave I for the right ear was judged to be present. The large positive deflection preceding wave I was judged to be wave I prime. **(C)** Normal TEOAE response measured with QuickScreen. The box labeled *Response* shows the spectrum of the TEOAE above the subtracted noise floor. Below is the replicated response waveform displayed in the time domain from 2.5 ms to 12.5 ms after each stimulus pulse. (Adapted from Robinette & Durrant [1997], with permission.)

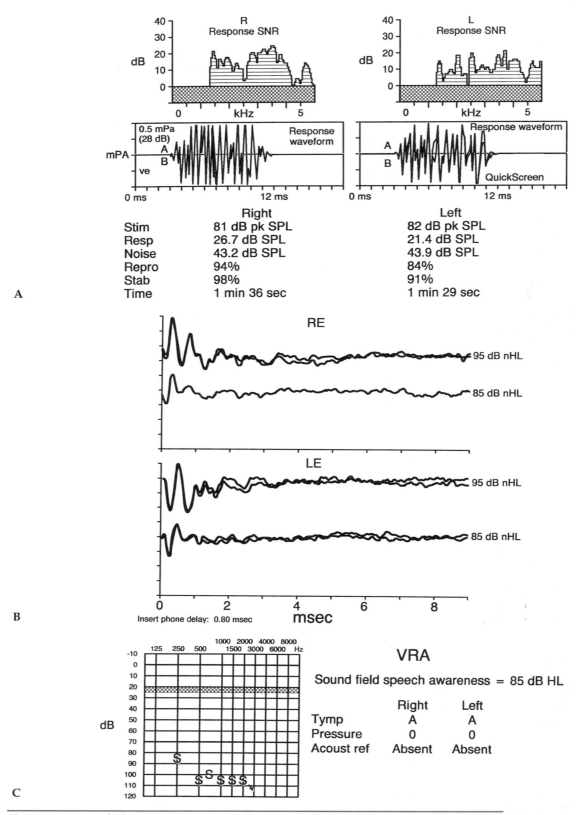

Figure 21–13 Audiologic evaluation results for a 4-month-old male, the sibling of the female patient presented in Figure 21-12. **(A)** Normal TEOAE response measured with QuickScreen. The box labeled *Response* shows the spectrum of the TEOAE above the subtracted noise floor. Below is the replicated response waveform displayed in the time domain from 2.5 ms to 12.5 ms after each stimulus pulse. **(B)** Abnormal ABR tracings. Stimuli were rarefaction clicks at levels of 95- and 85-dB nHL at a rate of 11.1/s. No response waves were judged to be present. **(C)** Profound hearing loss obtained from visual response audiometry, when the child was later tested at the age of 6 months.

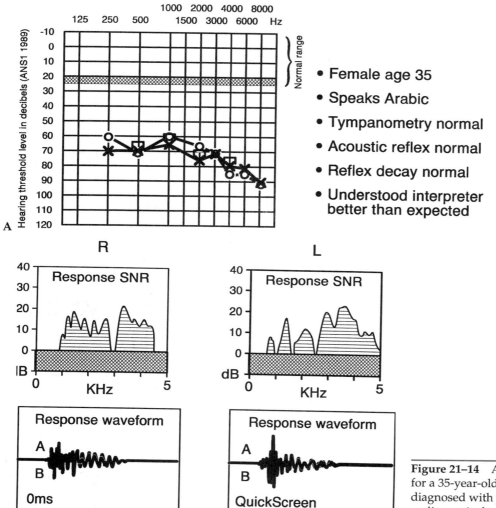

- Female age 35
- Speaks Arabic
- Tympanometry normal
- Acoustic reflex normal
- Reflex decay normal
- Understood interpreter better than expected

A

B

ABR thresholds 20 dB bilaterally
ABR: Neurodiagnostics WNL
Tympanometry WNL
Acoustic reflex thresholds and decay WNL

Figure 21–14 Audiometric and EOAE findings for a 35-year-old non-English-speaking woman diagnosed with pseudohypacusis. **(A)** Initial audiometric thresholds consistent with a severe bilateral sensorineural hearing loss. **(B)** Normal TEOAE (QuickScreen) responses bilaterally, consistent with normal to near-normal cochlear function. Subsequent threshold search ABR test results were within normal limits.

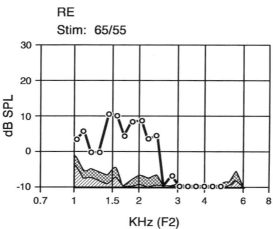

- NR audiometrically: Progressive then sudden HL
- Speech awareness 105 R, 110 L
- Tympanometry WNL
- Acoustic reflex absent
- No benefit from amplification

A

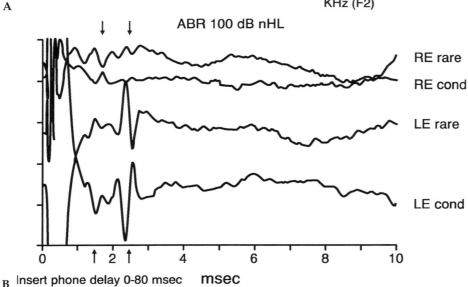

B Insert phone delay 0-80 msec   msec

Figure 21–15 DPOAE and CM findings for a 60-year-old man recorded as part of an evaluation for CI candidacy. **(A)** Normal DPOAE amplitudes from 1000 through 2500 Hz and absent DPOAEs from 3000 through 6000 Hz, measured from the patient's right ear. Primary stimulus frequency levels were 65 dB SPL (f_1) and 55 dB SPL (f_2). **(B)** shows the presence of CMs for both ears. The arrows indicate the location of phase reversals between responses to rarefaction and condensation clicks in the first 2 ms of the ABR response. Click stimuli was 100 dB nHL.

CONCLUSIONS

The discovery of otoacoustic emissions by David Kemp in 1978 has led to dramatic changes in our understanding of the physiology of auditory perception of exquisitely soft sounds by humans. In the clinical setting the methods of assessing evoked emissions by both TEOAEs and DPOAEs provide the opportunity to assess sensory function and, specifically, to document normal to near-normal cochlear function. An additional value is that the clinical measurement is objective, efficient, and noninvasive, which is very appealing in screening the hearing of newborns and other populations unable to provide reliable behavioral responses. The disadvantage, however, is that the absence of EOAEs does not reflect the actual magnitude of the hearing loss (i.e., mild, moderate, severe, or profound) or the site of the disorder leading to the loss. Even with this limitation, the examples provided in this chapter demonstrate the value of EOAEs as a part of the diagnostic test battery. Researchers and clinicians have much to learn about this new clinical tool as applications continue to open our professional eyes.

Appendix
TEOAE QuickScreen Option

In the ILO88 default program, time-averaged waveforms are sampled for 20.5 ms after the onset of the transient stimulus. The length of this time frame allows transient responses as low as 500 Hz to be recorded (Kemp et al, 1990). In 1992 the QuickScreen mode was introduced to improve the efficiency of TEOAEs in newborn screening (Kemp & Ryan, 1993). The QuickScreen option samples response waveforms for 12.5 ms, long enough to capture TEOAE data for 1000 Hz while reducing contamination by low-frequency physiological and ambient noise. Specifically, abbreviation of the time window reduces the contribution of low-frequency energy to the OAE, hence both noise and signal in the low-frequency region have relatively smaller contributions to the final result. Studies on adult patients and newborns show that reduced response window duration decreases TEOAE amplitudes for low frequencies while decreasing noise at all frequencies and increasing the signal-to-noise ratio (SNR) of TEOAEs, resulting in increased measurement efficiency (Hills, 1995; Whitehead et al, 1995).

Displayed in Figure 21A-1 are comparisons between TEOAE data collected with the default program and Quick-Screen. Data are from a 23-year-old woman with normal-hearing. The tests were conducted in a room without sound-reducing treatment. The TEOAE probe was inserted into the subject's right ear and removed after the test series. Figure 21A-1A shows responses from the default program and Figure 21A-1B from the QuickScreen program. The following differences in overall response may be noted from the QuickScreen results: Noise level reduced by 7.5 dB from 34.3 dB SPL to 26.8 dB SPL; response amplitude reduced by 2.5 dB from 9.7 dB SPL to 7.2 dB SPL; wave repro % increased by 8% from 88 to 96%. Improvements in band repro % and SNR are more difficult to assess from this figure because of the difference in displayed frequency bands for the two programs. However, the trend for higher band repro % and SNR with QuickScreen is apparent. A direct comparison may be made by reconfiguring each screen display to provide an analysis in one-half octave bands (strike key "H") (Table 21A-1).

As shown in Table 21A-1, band frequency reproducibility and SNR improved for each band with QuickScreen. The increase in SNR was quite dramatic, ranging from 5- to 9-dB (mean increase, 6.8 dB).

TABLE 21A-1   Comparison between the two programs in one-half octave bands

Frequency Band Hz	Default Repro %	Default SNR	Quickscreen Repro %	Quickscreen SNR
1000	00	−1	69	4
1500	78	6	96	15
2000	96	14	98	19
3000	97	16	99	23
4000	97	16	99	24

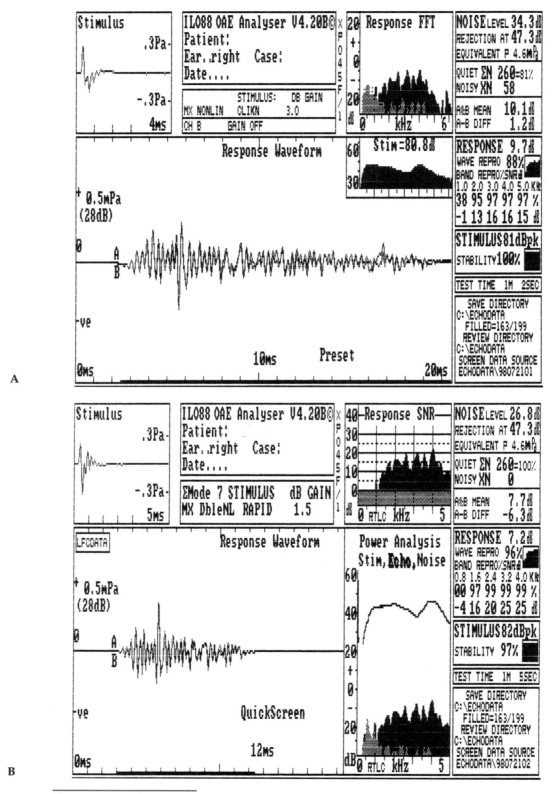

A

B

Figure 21A-1 Comparisons between TEOAE data collected with a 20.5 ms time-window after the onset of the transient stimulus **(A)** and data collected by QuickScreen with a 12.5 ms time-window after stimulus onset **(B)**. Subject was a 23-year-old woman with normal-hearing.

REFERENCES

ALTSCHULER, R.A., YEHOASH, R., PROSEN, C.A., DOLAN, D.F. & MOODY, D.B. (1992). Acoustic stimulation and overstimulation in the cochlea: A comparison between basal and apical turns of the cochlea. In: A.L. Dancer, D. Henderson, R.J. Salvi, & R.P. Hamernik (Eds.), *Noise-induced hearing loss* (pp. 60–72). St. Louis: Mosby–Year Book.

AVAN, P., BONFILS, P., LOTH, D., ELBEZ, M., & ERMINY, M. (1995). Transient-evoked otoacoustic emissions and high-frequency acoustic trauma in the guinea pig. *Journal of the Acoustical Society of America, 97*(5),3012–3020.

VON BEKESY, G. (1928). Zur Theorie des Horens: Die Schwingungsform der Basilarmembran. *Physik, Zeits, 29,*793–810. Translated by E.G. Wever (1960): Vibratory Pattern of the Basilar Membrane. In *Experiments in hearing* (pp. 404–429). New York: McGraw Hill.

BONFILS, P., & UZIEL, A. (1988). Evoked otoacoustic emissions in patients with acoustic neuromas. *American Journal of Otology, 9,*412–417.

BONFILS, P., & UZIEL, A. (1989). Clinical applications of evoked acoustic emissions: Results in normally hearing and hearing-impaired subjects. *Annals of Otology, Rhinology, and Laryngology, 98,*326–331.

BRIGHT, K. (1997). Spontaneous otoacoustic emissions. In: M.S. Robinette & T.J. Glattke (Eds.), *Otoacoustic emissions: Clinical applications* (pp. 46–62). New York: Thieme Medical Publishers, Inc.

BROWNELL, W.E. (1983). Observations on a motile response in isolated outer hair cells. In R.W. Webster, & L.Em. Aitken (Eds.). *Mechanisms of hearing* (pp. 5–10). Clayton, Australia: Monash University Press.

CANE, M.A., LUTMAN, M.E., & O'DONOGHUE, G.M. (1994). Transiently evoked otoacoustic emissions in patients with cerebellopontine angle tumors. *American Journal of Otology, 15,*207–216.

CANE, M.A., O'DONOGHUE, G.M., & LUTMAN, M.E. (1992). The feasibility of using evoked otoacoustic emissions to monitor cochlear function during acoustic neuroma surgery. *Scandinavian Audiology, 21,*173–176.

CEVETTE, M.J., & BIELEK, D. (1995). Transient evoked and distortion product otoacoustic emissions in traumatic brain injury. *Journal of the American Academy of Audiology, 6,*225–229.

CEVETTE, M.J., ROBINETTE, M.S., CARTER, J., & KNOPS, J.L. (1995). Otoacoustic emissions in sudden unilateral hearing loss associated with multiple sclerosis. *Journal of the American Academy of Audiology, 6,*197–202.

COLLET, L., KEMP, D.T., VEUILLET, E., DUCLAUX, R., MOULIN, A., & MORGON, A. (1990). Effect of contralateral auditory stimuli on active cochlear micro-mechanical properties in human subjects. *Hearing Research, 43,*251–262.

COLLET, L., VEUILLET, E., BENE, J., & MORGON, A. (1992). Effects of contralateral white noise on click-evoked emissions in normal and sensorineural ears: Towards an exploration of the medial olivocochlear system. *Audiology, 31,*1–17.

DALLOS, P. (1992). The active cochlea. *The Journal of Neuroscience, 12,*4575–4585.

DAVIS, H. (1983). An active process in cochlear mechanics. *Hearing Research, 9,*79–90.

DAVIS, H., & HIRSH, S.K. (1979). A slow brain stem response for low-frequency audiometry. *Audiology, 18,*445–61.

DAVIS, H., MORGAN, C.T., HAWKINS, J.E. GALAMBOS, R. & SMITH, F.K. (1950). Temporary deafness following exposure to loud tones and noise. *Acta-Otolaryngologica* (Suppl.), *88,*1–57.

DOYLE, K.J., FOWLER, C., & STARR, A. (1996). Audiologic findings in unilateral deafness resulting from contralateral pontine infarct. *Otolaryngology–Head and Neck Surgery, 114,*482–486.

DURLOVIC, B., RIBARIC-JANKES, K., KOSTIC, V., & STERNIC, N. (1994). Multiple sclerosis as the cause of sudden "pontine" deafness. *Audiology, 33,*195–201.

DURRANT, J.D., KAMERER, D.B., & CHIN, D. (1993). Combined OAE and ABR studies in acoustic tumor patients. In: D. Hochmann (Ed.), *EcoG, OAE and intraoperative monitoring* (pp. 231–239). Amsterdam: Kugler.

DURRANT, J.D., KESTERSON, R.K., & KAMERER, D.B. (1997). Evaluation of the nonorganic hearing loss suspect. *American Journal of Otology, 18,*361–367.

ENGDAHL, B., & KEMP, D.T. (1996). The effect of noise exposure on the details of distortion product otoacoustic emissions in humans. *Journal of the Acoustical Society of America, 99* (3),1573–1587.

FRANKLIN, D.J., McCoy, M.J., MARTIN, G., & LONSBURY-MARTIN, B.L. (1992). Test/retest reliability of distortion-product and transiently evoked otoacoustic emissions, *Ear and Hearing, 13*(6),417–429.

GASKILL, S.A., & BROWN, A.M. (1990). The behavior of the acoustic distortion product, 2f1-f2, from the human ear and its relation to auditory sensitivity. *Journal of the Acoustical Society of America, 88,*821–839.

GASKILL, S.A., & BROWN, A.M. (1993). Comparing the level of the acoustic distortion product, 2f1-f2 with behavioral threshold audiograms from normal-hearing and hearing-impaired ears. *British Journal of Audiology, 27,*397–407.

GLATTKE, T.J. (1983). *Short latency auditory evoked potentials.* Baltimore: University Park Press.

GLATTKE, T.J., PAFITIS, I., CUMMISKEY, C., AND HERER, G. (1995). Identification of hearing loss in children and young adults using measures of transient otoacoustic emission reproducibility. *American Journal of Audiology, 4,*71–86.

GLATTKE, T.J. & ROBINETTE, M.S. (1997). Transient evoked otoacoustic emissions. In: M.S. Robinette, & T.J. Glattke (Eds.), *Otoacoustic emissions: Clinical applications* (pp. 63–82). New York: Thieme Medical Publishers, Inc.

GOLD, T. (1948). Hearing II: The physical basis of the action of the cochlea. *Proceedings of the Royal Society of London. Series B: Biological Sciences, 135,*492–498.

GORGA, M.P., NEELY, S.T., BERGMAN, B.M., BEAUCHAINE, K.L., KAMINSKI, J.R., PETERS, J., SCHULTE, L., & JESTEADT, W. (1993). A comparision of transient evoked and distortion product otoacoustic emissions in normal-hearing and hearing-impaired subjects. *Journal of the Acoustical Society of America, 94,*2639–2648.

GORGA, M.P., NEELY, S.T., OHLRICH, B., HOOVER, B., REDNER, J., & PETERS, J. (1997). *Ear and Hearing, 18,*440–455.

GORGA, M.P., STELMACHOWICZ, P.G., BARLOW, S.M., AND BROOKHOUSER, P.E. (1995). Case of recurrent, reversible, sudden sensorineural hearing loss in a child. *Journal of the American Academy of Audiology, 6,*163–172.

GORGA, M.P., STOVER, L., NEELY, S.T., & MONTOYA, D. (1996). The use of cumulative distributions to determine critical values and levels of confidence for clinical distortion product otoacoustic emission measurements. *Journal of the Acoustical Society of America, 100*(2)968–997.

GRANDORI, F., & RAVAZZANI, P. (1993). Non-linearities of click-evoked otoacoustic emissions and the derived non-linear response. *British Journal of Audiology, 27,*97–102.

GRAVEL, J.S., & STAPELLS, D.R. (1993). Behavioral electrophysiologic, and otoacoustic measures from a child with auditory processing dysfunction: Case report. *Journal of the American Academy of Audiology, 4,*441–419.

HARAN, I.R., ATTIAS, J. & FURST, M. (1993). Characteristics of click-evoked otoacoustic emissions in ears with normal-hearing and with noise-induced hearing loss. *British Journal of Audiology, 27,*387–395.

HARRIS, F.P. (1990). Distortion-product otoacoustic emissions in humans with high-frequency sensorineural hearing loss. *Journal of Speech and Hearing Research, 33,*594–600.

HARRIS, F.P., & GLATTKE, T.J. (1992). The use of suppression to determine the characteristics of otoacoustic emissions. *Seminars in Hearing, 13,*67–80.

HARRIS, F., & PROBST, R. (1991). Reporting click-evoked and distortion-product otoacoustic emission results with respect to the pure tone audiogram. *Ear and Hearing 12,*399–405.

HARRIS, F. & PROBST, R. (1997). Otoacoustic emissions and audiometric outcomes. In: M.S. Robinette, & T.J. Glattke (Eds.), *Otoacoustic emissions: Clinical applications* (pp. 151–180). New York: Thieme Medical Publishers, Inc.

VON HELMHOLTZ, H.L.F. (1863). *Die Lehre von den Tonempfindungen als physiologische Grundlage fur die Theorie der Musik.* Brunswick: Vieweg-Verlag.

HILDESHEIMER, M., MUCHNIK, C., & RUBINSTEIN, M. (1985). Problems in interpretation of brain stem-evoked response audiometry results. *Audiology, 24,*374–79.

HILLS, D.A. (1995). *The effect of reducing analysis time on TEOAE reproducibility.* Unpublished MS Thesis. University of Arizona.

HOOD, L.J., BERLIN, C.I., & ALLEN, P. (1994). Cortical deafness: a longitudinal study. *Journal of the American Academy of Audiology, 5,*330–42.

JAMES-TRYCHEL, M. (1997). Personal Communication. Arnold Palmer Hospital for Children & Women, Orlando, FL.

JERGER, J., ALI, A., FONG, K., & TSENG, E. (1992). Otoacoustic emissions, audiometric sensitivity loss, and speech understanding: A case study. *Journal of the American Academy of Audiology, 3,*283–286.

JOHNSEN, J., PARBO, J. & ELBERLING, C. (1993). Evoked acoustic emissions from the human ear VI. Findings in cochlear hearing impairment. *Scandinavian Audiology, 22,*87–95.

JOHNSTONE, B., PATUZZI, R., & YATES, G.K. (1986). Basilar membrane measurements and the traveling wave. *Hearing Research, 22,*147–153.

KATONA, G., BUKI, B., FARKAS, Z., PYTEL, J., SIMON-NAGY, E., & HIRSCHBERG, J. (1993). Transitory evoked otoacoustic emission (TEOAE) in a child with profound hearing loss. *International Journal of Pediatric Otorhinolaryngology, 26,*263–267.

KEMP, D.T. (1978). Stimulated acoustic emissions from within the human auditory system. *Journal of the Acoustical Society of America, 64,*1386–1391.

KEMP, D.T. (1979). Evidence of mechanical nonlinearity and frequency selective wave amplification in the cochlea. *Archives of Otorhinolaryngology, 224,*37–46.

KEMP, D.T., BRAY, P., ALEXANDER, L., & BROWN, A.M. (1986). Acoustic emission cochleography—practical aspects. *Scandinavian Audiology, 9*(Suppl.), 71–95.

KEMP, D.T., & CHUM, R.A. (1980). Properties of the generator of stimulated acoustic emissions. *Hearing Research, 2,*312–232.

KEMP, D.T., RYAN, S., & BRAY, P. (1990). A guide to the effective use of otoacoustic emissions. *Ear and Hearing, 11,* 93–105.

KOK, M.R., VAN ZANTEN, G.A., BROCAAR, M.P., & WALLENBURG, H.C.S. (1993). Click-evoked otoacoustic emissions in 1036 ears of healthy newborns. *Audiology, 32,*213–223.

KONRADSSON, K.S. (1996). Bilaterally preserved otoacoustic emissions in four children with profound idiopathic unilateral sensorineural hearing loss. *Audiology, 35,*217–227.

KRAUS, N., OZDAMAR, V., STEIN, L., & REED, N. (1984). Absent auditory brain stem response: Peripheral hearing loss or brain stem dysfunction? *Laryngoscope, 94,*400–06.

KVAERNER, K.J., ENGDAHL, B., AURSNES, J., ARNESEN, A.R., & MAIR, I.W.S. (1996). Transient evoked otoacoustic emissions—helpful tool in the detection of pseudohypacusis. *Scandinavian Audiology, 25,*173–177.

LACCOURREYE, L., FRANCOIS, M., HUY, E.T.B., & NARCY, P. (1996). Bilateral evoked otoacoustic emissions in a child with bilateral profound hearing loss. *Annals of Otology, Rhinology, and Laryngology, 105,*286–288.

LENHARDT, M.L. (1981). Childhood central auditory processing disorder with brain stem evoked response verification. *Archives of Otolaryngology, 107,*623–25.

LEPAGE, E.L., & MURRAY, N.M. (1993) Click-evoked otoacoustic emissions: Comparing emission strengths with pure tone audiometric thresholds. *Australian Journal of Audiology, 15*(1)9–22.

LEVINE, R.A., OJEMANN, R.G., MONTGOMERY, W.W., & McGAFFIGAN, P.M. (1984). Monitoring auditory evoked potentials during acoustic neuroma surgery: Insights into the mechanism of the hearing loss. *Annals of Otology, Rhinolology, and Laryngology, 93,*116–123.

LIND, O., & RANDA, J. (1989). Evoked acoustic emissions in high-frequency vs. low/medium-frequency hearing loss. *Scandinavian Audiology, 18,*21–25.

LONSBURY-MARTIN, B.L., MARTIN, G.K., AND WHITEHEAD, M.L. (1997). Distortion product otoacoustic emissions. In: M.S. Robinette, & T.J. Glattke (Eds.), *Otoacoustic emissions: Clinical applications* (pp. 83–109). New York: Thieme Medical Publishers, Inc.

LUTMAN, M.E., DAVIS, A.C., FORTNUM, H.M., & WOOD, S. (1997). Field sensitivity of targeted neonatal hearing screening by transient evoked otoacoustic emissions. *Ear and Hearing, 18,*265–276.

LUTMAN, M.E., MASON, S.M., SHEPPARD, S., & GIBBIN, K.P. (1989). Differential diagnostic potential of otoacoustic emissions: A case study. *Audiology, 28,*205–210.

MARGOLIS, R.H. & TRINE, M.B. (1997). Influence of middle-ear disease on otoacoustic emissions. In: M.S. Robinette & T.J. Glattke (Eds.), *Otoacoustic emissions: Clinical applications* (pp. 130–150). New York: Thieme Medical Publishers, Inc.

Marshall, L., & Heller, L.M. (1996). Reliability of transient-evoked otoacoustic emissions. *Ear and Hearing, 17,* 237–254.

Martin, G.K., Lonsbury-Martin, B.L., Probst, R., Scheinin, S.A., & Coates, A.C. (1987). Acoustic distortion products in rabbit ear canal. II: Sites or origin revealed by suppression contours and pure tone exposures. *Hearing Research, 28,*191–208.

Mayo Clinic Rochester. (1997). Audiology Section, Rochester, MN: Unpublished data.

Monroe, J.A.B., Krauth, L., Arenberg, I.K., Prenger, E., & Philpot, P. (1996). Normal evoked otoacoustic emissions with a profound hearing loss due to a juvenile pilocytic astrocytoma. *American Journal of Otology, 17,*639–642.

Musiek, F.E., Bornstein, S.P., & Rintelmann, W.F. (1995). Transient evoked otoacoustic emissions and pseudohypacusis. *Journal of the American Academy of Audiology, 6,*293–301.

Nakamura, M., Yamasoba, T., & Kaga, K. (1997). Changes in otoacoustic emissions in patients with idiopathic sudden deafness. *Audiology, 36,*121–135.

Neely, S, & Liu, Z. (1993). *EMAV: Otoacoustic emission averager* (Tech. Memo No. 17). Boys Town National Research Hospital, Omaha, NE.

Pacheco, M. (1997). *A comparison of SOAEs and SSOAEs.* Unpublished Senior Honor's Thesis, University of Arizona.

Pafitis, I., Cummiskey, C., Herer, G., & Glattke, T.J. (1994). Detection of hearing loss using otoacoustic emissions. *Proceedings of Internoise 94* (pp. 763–768). Osaka: Institute of Noise Control Engineering/Japan & Acoustical Society of Japan.

Prasher, D.K., Tun, T., Brooks, G.B., & Luxon, L.M. (1995). Mechanisms of hearing loss in acoustic neuroma: An otoacoustic emission study. *Acta Otolaryngologica,115,*375–381.

Prieve, B.A. & Falter, S.R. (1995). COAEs and SSOAEs in adults with increased age. *Ear and Hearing, 16,*521–528.

Prieve, B.A., Fitzgerald, T.S., & Schulte, L.E. (1997). Basic characteristics of click-evoked otoacoustic emissions in infants and children. *Journal of the Acoustical Society of America, 102,*2860–2870.

Prieve, B.A., Gorga, M.P., & Neely, S.T. (1991). Otoacoustic emissions in an adult with severe hearing loss. *Journal of Speech and Hearing Research, 34,*379–385.

Prieve, B.A., Gorga, M.P., Schmidt, A., Neely, S., Peters, J., Schulte, L., & Jesteadt, W. (1993). Analysis of transient-evoked otoacoustic emissions in normal-hearing and hearing-impaired ears. *Journal of the Acoustical Society of America, 93,*3308–3319.

Probst, R. (1990). Otoacoustic emissions: An overview. *Advances in Otorhinolaryngology, 44,*1–91.

Probst, R., & Harris, F.P. (1993). Transiently evoked and distortion-product otoacoustic emissions: comparison of results from normally hearing and hearing-impaired human ears. *Archives of Otolaryngology—Head and Neck Surgery, 119,* 858–860.

Probst, R., Lonsbury-Martin, B.L., & Coats, A. (1987). Otoacoustic emissions in ears with hearing loss. *American Journal of Otolaryngology, 8,*73–81.

Robinette, M.S. (1990). *Frequency specificity of click evoked otoacoustic emissions for sensorineural hearing loss.* American Speech-Language-Hearing Association, Seattle, WA, November 18.

Robinette, M.S. (1992a). Clinical observations with transient evoked otoacoustic emissions with adults, *Seminars in Hearing, 13,*23–36.

Robinette, M.S. (1992b) Otoacoustic emissions in cochlear vs retrocochlear auditory dysfunction. *The Hearing Journal, 45,*32–34.

Robinette, M.S., Bauch, C.B., Olsen, W.O., Harner, S.G., & Beatty, C.W. (1992). Use of TEOAE, ABR, and acoustic reflex measures to assess auditory function in patients with acoustic neuroma. *American Journal of Audiology, 1,* 66–72.

Robinette, M.S., & Durrant, J.D. (1997) Contributions of evoked otoacoustic emissions in differential diagnosis of retrocochlear disorders. In: M.S. Robinette & T.J. Glattke (Eds.), *Otoacoustic emissions: Clinical applications* (pp. 205–232). New York: Thieme Medical Publishers, Inc.

Robinette, M.S., & Facer, G.W. (1991). Evoked otoacoustic emissions in differential diagnosis: A case report. *Otolaryngology–Head and Neck Surgery, 105,*120–123.

Robinette, M.S., & Gaeth, J.H. (1972). Diplacusis and the Stenger Test. *Journal of Auditory Research, 12,* 91–100.

Ruggero, M. & Rich, N.C. (1991). Application of a commercially manufactured Doppler shift laser velocimeter to the measurement of basilar membrane vibration. *Hearing Research, 51,*215–230.

Sakashita, T., Minowa, W., Hachikawa, K., Kubo, T., & Nakai, Y. (1991). Evoked otoacoustic emissions from ears with idiopathic sudden deafness. *Acta Oto-Laryngologica, 486* (Suppl.),66–72.

Sanders, J.W., & Lazenby, P.B. (1983). Auditory brain stem response measurement in the assessment of pseudohypacusis. *American Journal of Otology, 4,*292–299.

Sininger, Y.S., Hood, L.J., Starr, A., Berlin, C.I., & Picton, T.W. (1995). Hearing loss due to auditory neuropathy. *Audiology Today, 7,*(2)10–13.

Starr, A., Picton, T.W., Sininger, Y., Hood, L.J., & Berlin, C.I. (1996). Auditory neuropathy. *Brain, 119,*741–753.

Stein, L., Tremblay, K., Pasternak, J., Banerjee, S., Lindemann, K., & Kraus, N. (1996). Brain stem abnormalities in neonates with normal otoacoustic emissions. *Seminars in Hearing, 17*(2)197–213.

Stover, L., Gorga, M.P., Neely, S.T., & Montoya, D. (1996). Towards optimizing the clinical utility of distortion product otoacoustic emission measurements, *Journal of the Acoustical Society of America, 100,*956–967.

Stover, L., & Norton, S.J. (1993). The effects of aging on otoacoustic emissions. *Journal of the Acoustical Society of America, 94,*2670–2681.

Tavartkiladze, G.A., Fronlenkov, G.I., Krglov, A.V., & Artamasov, S.V. (1997). Ipsilateral suppression of transient evoked otoacoustic emissions. In: M.S. Robinette, & T.J. Glattke (Eds.), *Otoacoustic emissions: Clinical applications* (pp. 110–129). New York: Thieme Medical Publishers Inc.

Telischi, F.F., Roth, J., Lonsbury-Martin, B.L., & Balkany, T.J. (1995). Patterns of evoked otoacoustic emissions associated with acoustic neuroma. *Laryngoscope, 105,*675–682.

Telischi, F.F., Widick, M.P., Lonsbury-Martin, B.L., & McCoy, M.J. (1995). Monitoring cochlear function intraoperatively using distortion product otoacoustic emissions. *American Journal of Otology, 16,*597–608.

TRUY, E., VEUILLET, E., COLLET, L., & MORGON, A. (1993). Characteristics of transient otoacoustic emissions in patients with sudden idiopathic hearing loss. *British Journal of Audiology, 27,*379–385.

WABLE, J., & COLLET, L. (1994). Can synchronized otoacoustic emissions really be attributed to SOAEs? *Hearing Research, 80,*141–145.

WARR, W.B. (1992). Organization of olivocochlear efferent systems in mammals. In: D.B. Webster, A.N. Popper, & R.R. Fay (Eds.), *The mammalian auditory pathway: Neuroanatomy.* (Vol 1.) (pp. 410–488). New York: Springer-Verlag.

WELZL-MULLER K, STEPHAN, K., & STADLMANN, A. (1993). Click-evoked otoacoustic emissions in a child with unilateral deafness. *European Archives of Otorhinolaryngology, 250,* 366–368.

WHITEHEAD, M.L., JIMENEZ, A., STAGNER, B.B., McCOY, M.J., LONSBURY-MARTIN, B.L., & MARTIN, G.K. (1995a). Time-windowing of click-evoked otoacoustic emissions to increase signal-to-noise ratio. *Ear and Hearing, 16,*599–611.

WHITEHEAD, M.L., McCOY, M.J., LONSBURY-MARTIN, B.L., & MARTIN, G.K. (1995b). Dependence of distortion product otoacoustic emissions on primary levels in normal and impaired ears. I. Effects of decreasing L2 below L1. *Journal of the Acoustical Society of America, 97,*2346–2358.

WIDEN, J.E., FERRARO, J.A., & TROUBA, S.E. (1995). Progressive neural hearing impairment: Case report. *Journal of the American Academy of Audiology, 6,*217–224.

WILSON, J.P. (1980). Evidence for a cochlear origin for acoustic re-emissions, threshold fine-structure and tonal tinnitus. *Hearing Research, 2,*233–252.

WORTHINGTON, D.W., & PETERS, J.F. (1980). Quantifiable hearing and no ABR: Paradox or error? *Ear and Hearing, 1,*281–85.

WRIGHT, A., & DYCK, P.J. (1995). Hereditary sensory neuropathy with sensorineural deafness and early-onset dementia. *Neurology, 45,*560–562.

XU, L., PROBST, R., HARRIS, F.P., & ROEDE, J. (1994). Peripheral analysis of frequency in human ears revealed by tone burst evoked otoacoustic emissions. *Hearing Research, 74,*173–180.

## Chapter 22

Neonatal Hearing Screening: Follow-Up and Diagnosis

Joy O'Neal, Terese Finitzo, and Thomas A. Littman

Outline

In the United States, 4 million babies are born each year. Until 1998, fewer than 20% of the nation's births were screened for hearing loss as newborns (NIDCD Working Group, March 1998). In 1998, 20 states had a mandate for detection of hearing loss in newborns. Ten states had passed legislation supporting universal detection before hospital discharge, including the state of California with one eighth of the nation's births. The nine other states with legislation before the end of 1998 were Colorado, Connecticut, Hawaii, Massachusetts, Mississippi, Rhode Island, Utah, Virginia, and West Virginia. Large states like Texas and Florida have major initiatives in progress. In the coming decade, newborns will be screened routinely during their birth admission.

One only has to examine the early hearing detection and intervention (EHDI) programs from Rhode Island, Colorado, New York, and Texas to understand why EHDI is becoming the standard of care. In general, these states and others such as Hawaii, Wyoming, and Florida are identifying between two and four of every 1000 infants with neonatal hearing loss. These identification rates suggest that 8000 to 16,000 newborns a year have hearing loss. Fifty percent of these infants manifest no known risk factors for hearing loss. Such numbers challenge the common assumption that hearing loss is a low-incidence disorder. Texas Department of Health data (1996) show that of 100,000 babies screened for metabolic disorders, 4 are identified with sickle cell disease, 3 with phenylketonuria, 28 with hypothyroid disease, 2 with galactosemia, and 2 with adrenal hyperplasia, for a total of 82 infants. In this same population, between 220 and 314 infants have hearing loss (Finitzo et al, 1998). The prevalence of hearing loss is more than twice that of the other screenable newborn disorders combined (Finitzo et al, 1998).

Data show that an infant with a significant hearing impairment who receives intervention by 6 months of age will perform significantly better in language development than the infant who is identified after 6 months of age (Yoshinago-Itano et al, 1998). Although the average age of identification in the United States is being reduced with EHDI programs, until very recently, it has been 2½ years of age (Harrison & Roush, 1996; Stein, 1995b). Children with mild-to-moderate losses are often not identified until school age. A child identified at 2½ years of age will not have the same language developmental outcome as the infant identified before 6 months of age.

Audiologists must tackle the multifaceted task of implementing and managing EHDI programs if an impact is to be

Audiology: Diagnosis. Edited by Roeser, Valente, and Hosford-Dunn. Thieme Medical Publishers, Inc., New York © 2000

made on the age of identification and intervention for the infant with hearing loss. Establishing and maintaining an EHDI program require more than just screening a baby during the birth admission. It may be the most consequential role of audiologists (Stein, 1995a).

COMPONENTS OF EHDI

This chapter will examine the three components and the process involved in setting up programs to screen all newborns before discharge. In addition, a protocol for the diagnostic evaluation of newborns and infants is provided. Neonatal hearing screening has been evolving for the past three decades; historical information can be found in Jacobson (1994) and Hall (1992).

The EHDI process consists of three components: the birth admission screen, follow-up and diagnostic evaluation, and intervention. All three components of an EHDI program have to be in place and the links between each component must be robust for a program to benefit the infant. Many protocols are effective in screening an infant. The only caveat is that no rationale exists for screening for hearing loss in the neonatal period without effective follow-up, diagnosis, and intervention in place.

The Birth Admission Screen

The first component, the *birth admission hearing screen,* is defined as the testing performed on newborns after their birth and before discharge. Typically, this requires that a normal newborn be screened within 24 hours and certainly within 48 hours of birth. The birth admission screen uses a physiological measure of auditory function, either auditory brain stem responses (ABRs) or otoacoustic emissions (OAE). Whichever measure is used, the interpretation should be automated to eliminate errors and minimize delays in reporting screening information. Other chapters in this volume can be referenced for information on technologies, including Chapters 19 and 21 on the auditory brain stem response and otoacoustic emissions.

The Follow-Up Screen

The second component of an EHDI program is the *follow-up.* The follow-up may consist of a rescreen using the same screening protocol as the birth admission screen. The follow-up screen is on an outpatient basis, often in the birthing hospital when the baby is between 1 and 3 weeks of age. A rescreen keeps family costs low. If an infant fails the rescreen, an infant audiological diagnostic assessment is recommended and performed by an audiologist to identify the severity and type (conductive, sensorineural, or mixed) of hearing loss and to

begin the intervention process. The goal is to begin this diagnostic process between 1 and 3 months of age. Specific details on the infant diagnostic assessment conclude this chapter.

Intervention Services

The third component of an effective EHDI program encompasses all *intervention* services. Early childhood intervention (ECI) from Part C of the Individuals with Disabilities Education Act is contacted when an infant is not cleared at follow-up. The habilitative services are provided to ensure that an infant who has a significant hearing loss will develop language normally. The goal is to begin the intervention services before the baby is 6 months of age.

BUILDING THE CASE FOR EHDI

The following describes how the audiologist can build the case for an EHDI program to hospital and physician staff. Armed with information on state, local, federal, and professional standards; the incidence of hearing loss; and the effects of early identification, the audiologist will be able to make a strong case for support.

Standards

Standards can be examined as state and local standards, federal standards, and professional standards. Standard of care is what reasonably prudent practitioners do (Tharpe & Clayton-Wright, 1997). Standard of care is also defined by each state's statutory regulation.

State Governmental and Local Standards

State regulations and mandates are changing rapidly. A careful reader will check the most recent publications on state requirements. Community and state standards are important in defining standard of care, although increasingly there is reference to a single national standard, particularly in professional and governmental pronouncements on EHDI programs.

Since the early 1990s, EHDI has been supported from national block grants in state agencies. Some states use funding from the Individuals with Disabilities Education Act, Part C (formerly Part H) to fund universal newborn hearing screening. Others use Title V funding and grants from the

Bureau of Maternal and Child Health (MCHB). The U.S. Public Health Service funded a multistate effort that established the Marion Downs National Center for Infant Hearing in 1996, named in honor of this pioneer in pediatric audiology. Seventeen states agreed voluntarily to support the implementation of universal newborn hearing screening. The participating states were Alabama, Arizona, Arkansas, Colorado, Hawaii, Kansas, Louisiana, Massachusetts, Michigan, Minnesota, New Mexico, Oklahoma, Rhode Island, Tennessee, Texas, Virginia, and Wyoming. Their goal was to screen 85% of the births in these states by the year 2000. Diagnosis of hearing loss would be complete by 4 months of age, and appropriate intervention would be initiated by 6 months of age.

A further impetus to establishing a state standard was introduced in mid-1998 by MCHB. MCHB requires states to report the number of newborns screened at birth for hearing in their annual requests for the Title V Block Grant funding.

Federal Governmental Standards

Federal governmental positions include *Healthy People 2000* and the more recent *Healthy People 2010* currently in preparation. *Healthy People 2000*: Objective 17.16 states "Reduce the average age at which children with significant hearing impairment are identified to no more than 12 months." (*Healthy People 2000*, 1990). In that document, the baseline for identification was estimated as 24 to 30 months in 1988 in the United States. Other reports give an average age of identification between 12 and 25 months (Harrison & Roush, 1996; Parving, 1993). In *Healthy People 2010*, the focus remains on hearing, but the goals are more ambitious. *Healthy People 2010* has proposed setting the following objectives for EHDI:

- Increase to 100% the proportion of newborns served by state-sponsored EHDI programs.
- Access to screening by 1 month: 100%
- Follow-up diagnostic tests by 3 months: 100%
- Access to intervention for infants who are deaf/hard of hearing by 6 months: 100%

In 1993 and again in 1997, a National Institutes of Health (NIH) panel stated that newborns should be screened for hearing loss before hospital discharge (National Institutes of Health, 1993). The NIH panel convened in 1997 as an ongoing working group to address technology, outcomes, and research needed if EHDI is to succeed. The Centers for Disease Control and Prevention (CDC) and MCHB have also taken a major governmental role in advocating EHDI, focusing on interest in data reporting. CDC sponsored a series of workshops and telephone conferences throughout 1998 on important issues related to EHDI programs. In conjunction with Directors of Speech and Hearing Programs in State Health and Welfare Agencies (DSHPSHWA), they facilitated a dialogue on national database issues in newborn hearing screening.

Professional Standards

EHDI as standard of care is bolstered by the Joint Committee on Infant Hearing (JCIH) (ASHA, 1994). The JCIH has become an important unifying voice among professional organizations on the topic of early hearing detection. The committee, formed more than 30 years ago, published its first position statement in 1970, identifying a list of known conditions that placed an infant at risk for hearing loss. This list became known as the High-Risk Register. Identifying factors included a family history of childhood hearing loss, craniofacial defects, hyperbilirubinemia, low birth weight, and rubella or other viral infections known to cause hearing loss. At that time, the JCIH encouraged further research to determine methods for screening newborns. This document was important because the authors were representatives from the professional groups that worked with newborns, infants, and hearing.

The original group of JCIH organizations has evolved and changed. JCIH is composed of representatives from the American Academy of Audiology, American Speech-Language-Hearing Association, American Academy of Otolaryngology–Head and Neck Surgery, American Academy of Pediatrics, Councils for the Education of the Deaf, and the Directors of Speech and Hearing Programs in State Health and Welfare Agencies.

The JCIH position statements have reflected both the expert opinions of the committee and research in the field since 1970. The 1994 position statement was written in 1992, achieved consensus by member organizations in 1993, and was published in 1994. The statement:

- Endorses the goal of universal detection of infants with hearing loss
- Encourages continuing research and development to improve techniques for detection of and intervention for hearing loss as early as possible
- Maintains a role for the high-risk factors (hereafter termed indicators) described in the 1990 position statement and modifies the list of indicators associated with sensorineural and/or conductive hearing loss in newborns and infants
- Identifies indicators associated with late-onset hearing loss and recommends procedures to monitor infants with these indicators
- Recognizes the adverse effects of fluctuating conductive hearing loss from persistent or recurrent otitis media with effusion (OME) and recommends monitoring infants with OME for hearing loss
- Endorses provision of intervention services in accordance with Part H of the Individuals with Disabilities Education Act (IDEA)
- Identifies additional considerations necessary to enhance early identification of infants with hearing loss. (ASHA, 1994).

The JCIH 2000 position statement moved EHDI further into the mainstream, focusing on the infrastructure necessary for high-quality programs and emphasizing the need to educate parents to allow them to make knowledgeable choices for their children. Although JCIH endorsed universal detection as a goal for the nation, JCIH 2000 advocated strongly that the time had passed for discussion.

PEARL

Universal detection of neonatal hearing loss is the standard that the nation's hospitals should follow.

Many professional organizations have followed the JCIH's lead and published their own statements endorsing universal newborn hearing screening. An American Academy of Audiology Task Force prepared a report in 1994 that addressed the importance of early identification of hearing loss in infants and children and supported the idea that the hearing of every infant should be screened at birth, before hospital discharge (AAA, 1994). The DSHPSHWA, a group supported by the national MCHB, wrote a position statement on universal hearing detection in 1996. The statement endorsed universal newborn and infant hearing detection as described by the JCIH 1994 position statement. Similarly, in early 1999, the Academy of Pediatrics published its own strong position statement, coming on board to support EHDI. This document provided pediatricians and family practitioners with the information they needed to support EHDI (American Academy of Pediatrics, 1999).

The Incidence of Hearing Loss in Newborns

Screening at-risk infants identifies about 50% of the babies with congenital hearing loss. In addition, one half of the moderate-to-profound sensorineural hearing loss present at birth or in early childhood is the result of genetic factors (Rose et al, 1977).

Because many states have become involved in screening the hearing of all newborns, incidence information can be based on universal screening rather than at-risk screening. In Texas an incidence rate of 3 infants identified per 1000 screened has been reported (Finitzo, et al, 1998). Because most hospitals in the Texas project had fewer Medicaid births than present overall in the state, the interactions of incidence with demographics and income or socioeconomic status are still unknown. One could hypothesize that the real numbers of infants with hearing loss will increase in certain regions of the country because of the effects of poverty and poorer public health access.

The Effect of Early Identification of Hearing Loss on Development

Yoshinaga-Itano and colleagues (1998) followed a cohort of 72 children identified by 6 months of age compared with 78 identified after the age of 6 months. All hearing-impaired children received intervention within 2 months of diagnosis. For children with normal cognitive abilities, language was significantly better at all test ages regardless of communication modes, degree of hearing loss, or socioeconomic status. It was independent of gender, ethnicity, and the presence of additional disabilities. They reported that children identified between birth and 6 months of age have significantly higher developmental functioning in General Development, Expressive Language, Comprehension-Conceptual, Personal-Social, Communicative Gestures, Receptive Vocabulary, Expressive Vocabulary, Number of Consonants and Number of Vowels. Those children who had normal cognitive symbolic play skills and mild-to-severe hearing loss had median expressive vocabulary skills comparable to the median level for children with normal-hearing at 31 to 36 months of age. At 40 months of age, even profoundly hearing-impaired children identified at birth were not functioning significantly below their typically developing peers (Yoshinaga-Itano et al, 1998).

These data suggest that there is a window of opportunity for these young infants.

The Challenges in Screening All Babies at Birth

States face multiple challenges in expanding neonatal programs for the detection of hearing loss: crowded urban and sparsely populated rural areas; immigrant populations with diverse cultures, languages, and limited financial resources; urban and public hospitals with annual birth rates exceeding 12,000; and communities with rural hospitals that need funds and expertise to screen fewer than 50 births per year. Every state department of health faces such challenges. They must be surmounted if effective programs are to be implemented across the nation.

Quality of services is another enormous challenge. How does a healthcare system screen all babies before discharge when discharge may be as early as 12 to 18 hours after birth? All babies who do not pass the birth screen, must be rescreened within 14 days. Of the approximately 3.5% of babies who are referred for additional hearing testing after the birth screen, only 70% return for the follow-up testing (Finitzo et al, 1998). New paradigms must be created to ensure that infants will be connected to needed services "one baby at a time." Audiologists must be stewards of hearing healthcare for newborns (Finitzo, 1995).

Program reimbursement is another serious challenge. Before 1999, most agencies and insurance companies that paid for testing for hearing loss did so only for the at-risk population and not for well-babies. With government and state standards, individual states like Rhode Island have required insurers to reimburse for well-baby as well as at-risk infants. The actual cost to screen a baby is approximately $20 and $25 per baby; however, other state legislatures are concerned with total cost (Carpenter et al, 1996). It would cost $120 million to screen 4 million annual births if hospitals were reimbursed at a rate of $30 per baby. Although the cost of the service is borne by healthcare, savings accrue over the long-term in education and rehabilitative services. This is the cogent argument for early hearing programs but requires that decisions be made by the groups that are charged with managing both the nation's healthcare and education costs.

ESSENTIAL ELEMENTS OF A SUCCESSFUL EHDI PROGRAM

Three elements are essential if an EHDI program is to succeed. They are:

- A cascading sponsorship of support
- Audiologic involvement
- Effective data and information management (Finitzo, 1998)

Cascading Sponsorship of Support

Any successful newborn screening program must build the case for EHDI and gain the support of the people in the organization who will be needed to sustain a program, from administrators and physicians to nursing leadership. Audiologists must assume the leadership when it comes to building and maintaining an EHDI program.

> **PEARL**
>
> EHDI programs are new programs, providing us the opportunity to create service from the ground up.

Creating a new program is very rewarding, but newborn hearing screening is being promoted to the healthcare system when it is overwhelmed with demands. One way to overcome this is to be armed with information. Current re-engineering literature states that change efforts (and EHDI is change) must present a clear business case for change and address the human impact of change on the system if efforts are to succeed (Block, 1993).

THE BUSINESS CASE FOR EHDI

To present a clear business case for implementing programs, we must move beyond the argument that EHDI is the right thing to do for our children. Hospital administrators understand that there are many right things to do in healthcare today, but they often make hard choices and choose one program over many others. Without a simple mechanism for covering screening cost, an advocate must first capitalize on support from other sources. The Department of Health is the audiologist's primary supporter, often supporting EHDI through grants or contracts. The Department of Health can send letters to hospital chief executives that advocate implementation of newborn hearing screening.

Second, addressing how EHDI is standard of care helps administrators understand the need to change. Standard of care information has been discussed already as has the information on state regulations and mandates. The hospital's chief financial officer, risk managers, and quality assurance personnel will be interested in standard of care issues because they face risk and liability daily. Liability for a hospital can be prevented through an effective EHDI program. A poor program can increase liability (Tharpe & Clayton-Wright, 1997). A hospital can implement a good program and prevent the liability of failing to identify a hearing-impaired infant or can take the risk that they will not be sued.

EHDI programs can be a marketing and public relations tool to demonstrate quality care in maternal and neonatal services at each hospital by holding press conferences, having parties on program birthdays, and bringing in Department of Health staff to applaud the hospital for its efforts.

THE HUMAN SIDE OF EHDI

Once the business case for change has been addressed, the human issues cannot be overlooked. Change efforts fail in organizations because the human side of change is not sufficiently addressed. Each program must have strong sponsors. It should begin with senior administration, include physician leadership, and move to deliver the message throughout the hospital.

Administration

> **PITFALL**
>
> An uninformed supervisor who does not understand its value can cut a program without adequate administrative support.

The authorizing sponsor of a program must be identified. Often the hospital administrator will commission and own the program. The authorizing sponsor has a significant role, especially at budget time when an uninformed administrator who does not understand its value can cut a program without adequate support. Programs have been lost when hospital management changed and program directors failed to attend to the new leaders quickly enough to convince them of the value of the newborn screening. Program directors should meet with the authorizing sponsor on a yearly basis to summarize program outcomes. Authorizing sponsors may not attend other meetings where program statistics are reviewed.

Nursing

> **SPECIAL CONSIDERATION**
>
> Develop a shared commitment with the nursery leadership team.

Each program director should identify a reinforcing sponsor who is available to ensure that the program happens in the nursery. Nurse clinicians will partner with the audiologist if they understand what benefit hearing screening has for their babies. The first task is to communicate a compelling rationale for the universal detection of hearing loss in newborns. Here again is a role for the JCIH position statements, *Healthy People 2000*, and the NIH 1993 and 1997 statements. A parent of a young child with a hearing loss is an excellent resource. Parents who talk about their feelings surrounding the identification of hearing loss in their infant or young child can have a powerful impact on administrators who are unsure of the importance of universal screening.

It is necessary to identify who is available to screen the newborns on a daily basis. The screeners in the nursery can be EEG technicians, nurses, licensed vocational nurses, respiratory therapists, unit aides, or audiologists, but a limited number should be responsible for screening in a nursery. A maximum of six screeners is recommended, even in a hospital of 5000 births per year. Education and training are critical, but in most cases a director will be cross-training individuals who have other responsibilities.

> **SPECIAL CONSIDERATION**
>
> Keep in mind that one definition of cross-training is to take a competent individual and make him or her feel incompetent, so one must have patience when training staff.

The staff who must implement any new program feel the impact of the changes it brings more than anyone else in the organization. The program alters the day-to-day work routine. It is helpful to explore "WIFM" (what's in it for me) from the perspective of the staff. It could be a raise for taking on this new responsibility, new job skills or expanded opportunity. Letters should be written to supervisors, staff efforts should be supported, and staff should be assisted as they come up for a yearly review. Behavior needs to be reinforced. Yearly conferences should be sponsored and screeners from the hospitals should be invited to attend at no charge. One or two screeners will usually come forth to own the program.

Physicians/Pediatricians

> ### PEARL
>
> Physicians can be program champions. They may no longer have sufficient power to implement programs in every hospital, but their support is crucial to keep programs operating. Physicians are quality and data driven.

Physicians, like nurses, have a clinical perspective and will want different information than hospital administrators. Pediatricians need to review the rationale for EHDI and may ask, "why screen for hearing loss?" Pediatricians need to have data on age of identification of hearing loss in the nation and in the state and need to be provided the information from Yoshinaga-Itano et al (1998). Data on outcomes from New York, Texas, or Rhode Island, that document that a good program screens 97 to 98% of the babies before discharge should be provided. Physicians ask about pass rates, the fail rate, the follow-up, and the identification rate. Each program should select a data management procedure that will yield these numbers and performance measures for each screener. The hospital should research and choose what meets program needs.

Pediatricians may be concerned about false negative and false positive identification. Audiologists should have that information from the equipment manufacturer used because every test generates some false positive and false negative results.

Audiologist Involvement

The audiologist's role in universal newborn hearing is multidimensional. Audiologists should screen babies on a daily basis if it is a cost-effective and acceptable solution for the hospital. The audiologist can serve as the reinforcing sponsor in some hospitals. Screening by audiologists is no more expensive than screening with neonatal nurse practitioners (NNP), as long as time to complete the follow-up rescreening and the infant diagnostic assessments is available. In some hospitals NNPs, who are often in the nursery with other responsibilities that do not require full time effort, are conducting screening. The hospital's perspective is that NNPs can add screening without adding cost to the hospital.

THE ENVIRONMENTAL ASSESSMENT

Before implementing an EHDI program, the audiologist should conduct an *environmental assessment* to evaluate a hospital's readiness for this new service. The environmental assessment summarizes conversations with administration and physician leadership regarding program implementation and addresses technology selection, cost, personnel, supervision, follow-up, and quality assurance for the hospital. The technology decision depends on hospital needs. OAE and ABR are both acceptable as long as the screening technology provides an automated pass/refer option. With automated interpretation, outcomes are available at the completion of the test. This eliminates the need for nonaudiological personnel to make the decision, even with established guidelines. Equipment manufacturers and some information management companies provide automated interpretive routines or algorithms, and handheld units will soon be commonplace. Automation offers the advantage of providing uniform screening procedures and substantially reducing the potential risks of errors.

A cost analysis of different program options for technology, for personnel, for supervision, for information management, for ongoing audiological support, and for follow-up is extremely helpful. It should include a charge for audiologists as the service coordinators. This could be a flat fee or variable fee structure agreed on by the hospital and audiologist. As EHDI becomes a national effort, service coordination will ensure a robust link to follow-up. The cost analysis should include all costs of staff employed to screen, including fringe benefits, test time, and time to prepare documentation. If the screener is a multitask worker, the portion of time and, hence, salary needed for screening must still be considered. The cost of information management should also be included. A program should factor in supply costs as well.

The environmental assessment must also include an examination of the noise levels and reverberation in the proposed spaces for screening. Hard-walled surfaces are highly reverberant, rendering spaces composed of only hard surfaces as potentially too noisy for acceptable screening protocol. The environmental assessment can be a written document providing the hospital with appropriate and useful information regarding EHDI.

PREIMPLEMENTATION PLANNING

Before screening begins, decisions on the protocols for the birth admission screen, the protocols for the follow-up and the infant audiological assessment, and the protocol for referral to intervention services must be in place. These are the three basic components of EHDI programs. The links between these components must be strong or babies will be lost to follow-up. At this stage in planning, the hospital will have selected who will screen the infant and will understand that staff must be available 7 days a week. The audiologist should establish a day-to-day protocol for the screener in the nursery. Under almost no circumstance should a baby be discharged without screening. For details on protocols, refer to Finitzo et al (1998).

PARENT COMMUNICATION

Communication regarding hearing screening and its benefits should begin before the birth of a baby. Inservice training to prenatal nurse educators can lead to better informed parents. Obstetricians, pediatricians, and the counselors in the high schools can also be provided information packets. Parents must also have the option to elect not to screen their baby. This requires that information be available to parents to read during a preadmission visit. If a mother elects not to screen her baby, a release must be signed stating that she understands the consequences of missing a congenital hearing loss. A note of the parental decision in the information management system allows the program director to differentiate babies missed at birth admission from those not available because of parental or physician decision. Such differentiation allows the hospital to know which infants need to be contacted for follow-up.

Results of screening should be communicated to parents before discharge. A nurse, an audiologist, a physician, or a well-trained technician often communicates these results. This decision is hospital dependent. Ideally, hearing screening can be addressed by the discharge planning nurse with the family. Regardless of who communicates the information, the audiologist should write out sample scenarios and observe to see that the process is effective. Parents should also receive the information in writing. If a follow-up appointment is necessary, it should be scheduled before families leave the nursery. A telephone number of an expert should be provided in case of additional questions. This ability to provide an immediate answer to a family is another reason that automated interpretations are essential.

PHYSICIAN COMMUNICATION

Physicians must have easy access to hearing screening results. The issue of liability is of concern for them and for the audiologist. Some pediatricians may elect to receive information only on babies who need follow-up because the primary reason for the information is to ensure that the baby is connected to service. A concern with this approach is that if a baby fails a screen and the letter is lost in the mail, a physician or parent may assume erroneously that no news is good news. Consequently, effective management software should be able to print a summary listing for each pediatrician over different periods. Figure 22–1 represents one type of physician report; babies who are lost to follow-up are listed. Other paradigms, including Internet access, should be explored to provide results to physicians.

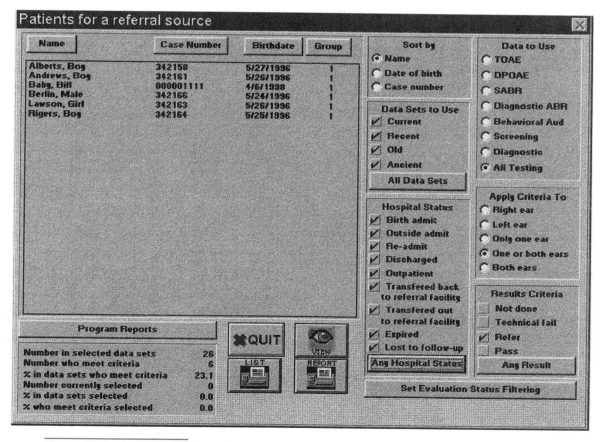

Figure 22–1 An example of an information management system providing data on babies who need follow-up services from one "pediatrician." (Courtesy of OZ Corporation, Dallas, Texas.)

EFFECTIVE INFORMATION MANAGEMENT, QUALITY INDICATORS, AND BENCHMARKS

In a survey on EHDI programs, Diefendorf and Finitzo (1997) noted that information management systems were considered in programs implemented before 1995 less than 50% of the time. As audiologists have learned more about this field, information management and quality monitoring are now well accepted. The selection of an information system should be based on specific needs of each program. The system should answer four questions:

- What is happening to each individual baby?
- How are screeners performing?
- Who are the babies who need . . . something?
- How is the program performing?

If the information management system assists with these questions, it will accomplish the most important goal, that of caring for the baby. In such a "babycentric"approach the needs of the baby are at the center of a system and the needs of the screener, the audiologist, the hospital, the state, and even the nation can be met (Pool, 1996). Quality indicators should be built into the information system as much as possible to minimize reliance on manual data entry and facilitate answering the preceding questions.

Quality indicators should be determined jointly with the hospital and physician leaders to avoid future misunderstandings. Indicators should be those items that make a difference to the hospital budget, the staff, or the family. The quality indicators used in many EHDI programs around the nation are related to important components of the process. The available infants, the birth admission screening rate, the follow-up rescreen, the diagnostic assessment, the number who receive intervention services, and the number identified with hearing loss are monitored. It is encouraged that sites add risk indicators for progressive loss. Missed and lost babies and parent refusal rates are tracked.

A birth screening performance index (BSPI) is a common denominator some programs use to cut across technology differences (Finitzo et al, 1998). The BSPI is obtained by multiplying the percent of newborns receiving a birth admission screen with the percent of newborns passing a birth admission screen. The BSPI is a single number that communicates the effectiveness of the hospital's screening program. Screening all babies and passing most of them before discharge reduces costs because fewer families need contact to return for follow-up. It also reduces parental anxiety that may result in some families with high failure rates at this stage.

> ### PITFALL
>
> **Whatever the dimensions of quality used by the screening program, it should not be assumed that the definitions are congruent with those used in the hospital.**

To be successful, an EHDI program must not only screen the infants it must also be capable of an effective follow-up process.

> ### PEARL
>
> **The four reasons for rescreening are :**
> - **the baby was missed at the birth admission;**
> - **the baby failed the birth admission screen;**
> - **the baby has a risk indicator for a delayed or progressive loss;**
> - **the birth admission screen was incomplete.**

Follow-up can take place in the birth hospital for parent convenience or at a regional or local audiology center. Some babies should not be followed because of a medical contraindication or parent or physician refusal. As more hospitals seek reimbursement for the hearing screening, some parents may refuse either the birth admission screen or the follow-up rescreen. A program director should track the families who elect not to have their infant screened. If refusal rate increases in a hospital screening program, the program director should examine how parents are being counseled about the program, including what they are told about the risks of not screening their infant. Well-counseled families seldom refuse the screening.

Prospective quality monitoring is essential in all programs and for all aspects of the program. Accountability does end with the hospital screening. Equal attention should be paid to follow-up. Ensuring that infants receive effective early intervention services in a timely manner is paramount. Wheeler and Chambers (1993) note that no program is ever static. A program director must understand when change in the status of a program requires intervention. Audiologists should review statistical process control theory to understand how to monitor programs successfully. The audiologist can make changes in a program before problems affect it.

> ### PEARL
>
> **Outcome measures are a vital part of a program. They are essential as the allocation of funds becomes more in demand.**

AUDIOLOGICAL EVALUATION OF INFANTS WHO FAIL NEONATAL HEARING SCREENING TESTS

A protocol for the diagnostic evaluation of hearing in infants who fail newborn screening should provide a battery of tests designed to achieve the following two purposes:

- To facilitate the prompt and accurate diagnosis of hearing loss
- To permit intervention, including fitting of hearing aids, before 6 months of age

Various components of a protocol may be adapted to fit the needs and resources of different settings. A shorter section will outline the protocol itself. The following discussion will assume that the child has failed a two-step screening process; that is, screening on birth admission and a second screening at follow-up or, in some cases, before discharge.

DIAGNOSTIC PHILOSOPHY

Overview

After a child fails newborn hearing screening, a sequence of events must occur quickly and smoothly, to meet our goal of effective intervention by 6 months of age. Minimally, these events include a diagnostic audiological evaluation, ECI referral, otologic referral/treatment, hearing aid evaluation and fitting, and initiation of habilitative and support programs. Because of the time constraints involved in getting through all stages of the intervention process, the diagnostic evaluation must rely heavily on electrophysiological measures.

The Auditory Brain Stem Response

The ABR is the cornerstone of the diagnostic process for newborns and infants. The click-evoked ABR is particularly useful for assessment of the auditory nervous system. For evaluation of auditory sensitivity, ABR thresholds evoked by frequency-specific stimuli correlate closely ($r > 0.93$) with behavioral thresholds in infants and children (Stapells et al, 1995). However, when behavioral thresholds are estimated from the click-evoked ABR alone, substantial errors can be made (Gravel, 1989; Oates & Stapells, 1998; Picton & Durieux-Smith, 1988; Picton et al, 1979).

PITFALL

The click-evoked ABR is inadequate for inferring hearing loss configuration and fitting hearing aids.

The example in Figure 22–2 illustrates the limitations of the click-evoked ABR in determining the configuration of a hearing loss. In Figure 22–2A, normal click ABR thresholds are seen bilaterally, with thresholds of 10- and 20-dB nHL for the right and left ears, respectively. However, a high-frequency cochlear loss is suggested by the distortion product otoacoustic emissions (DPOAEs) in the lower panel of Figure 22–2A. Frequency-specific ABR, using unmasked Blackman-gated tone bursts indicates a high-frequency loss bilaterally as shown in the top of Figure 22–2B. The sensorineural loss was subsequently confirmed by use of visual reinforcement audiometry and insert earphones as shown in the lower panel of Figure 22–2B.

As the foregoing paragraph suggests, the click-evoked ABR threshold is of dubious value when fitting hearing aids. Reasonable correlation between click thresholds and behavioral thresholds in the 2000 to 4000 Hz range have been reported for group data (Coats & Martin, 1977; Jerger & Mauldin, 1978; Van der Drift, 1989). However, when individual data are

considered, a given click-evoked ABR threshold can correspond to behavioral thresholds that range over 20- to 80-dB (Stapells et al, 1994). See also Chapter 19 in this volume. The usefulness of the click-evoked ABR threshold is perhaps best put in perspective by considering it the electrophysiological equivalent of the speech awareness threshold as suggested by Oates and Stapells (1998).

Frequency-Specific ABR

Because of the limitations of the click-evoked ABR, inclusion of frequency-specific stimuli is essential in evaluating infants who fail newborn screening. Although a number of options are available, the current methods of choice are either tone bursts presented in notched noise (Stapells et al, 1995) or unmasked tone bursts generated with a nonlinear gating function such as the Blackman window (Gorga & Thornton, 1989). Notched noise stimulus generators are not widely available yet but should be an option for clinical ABR equipment in the near future.

The morphology of the ABR waveform evoked by tone bursts is different from that evoked by clicks, particularly for lower frequencies. As shown in Figure 22–3, the 500 Hz response has a broad, rounded peak, with wave V frequently occurring as a "shoulder" rather than a well-defined peak. Note that latency at threshold is roughly 4 to 8 ms longer than what is expected for click stimuli. Therefore a longer analysis window of approximately 20 ms is needed. As with click stimuli, threshold responses must be replicated.

PEARL

It may be necessary to make several attempts at replicating a tone burst response at or near threshold.

The tone burst ABR is more variable than the click-evoked response. Three, four, or more attempts at replication may be needed before a threshold is confirmed.

Bone Conduction ABR

Stimulation through bone conduction is a key component of the ABR battery because it permits differential diagnosis of type of hearing loss (Stapells & Ruben, 1989). Furthermore, the bone-conducted ABR can be reliably recorded from neonates and infants (Hooks & Weber, 1984; Yang et al, 1987). For infants with aural atresia, bone conduction ABR measurement accurately reflects cochlear reserve (Gravel et al, 1989), and can overcome potential masking dilemmas which plague behavioral tests (Jahrsdoerfer et al, 1985). Given the limitations of immittance audiometry in this population, the bone conduction ABR may provide the clearest indicator of middle ear dysfunction.

Temporal rather than forehead placement of the vibrator is recommended (Yang et al, 1987). Placement of the vibrator in different regions of the temporal area results in significantly

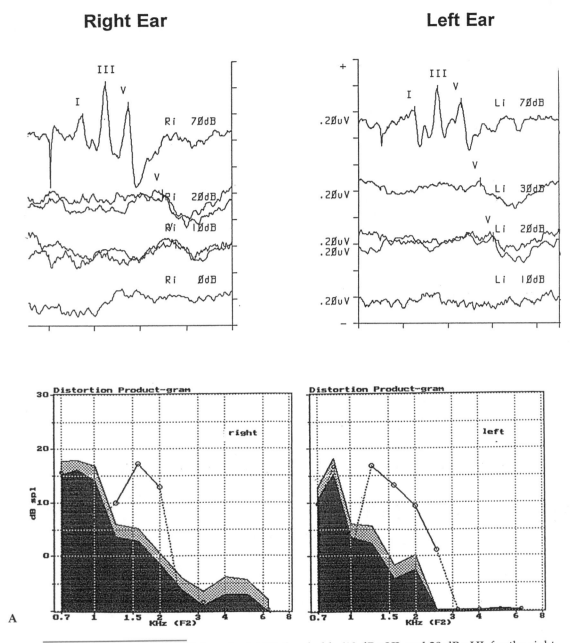

Right Ear

Left Ear

Figure 22–2   (A) Normal click-evoked ABR thresholds (10 dB nHL and 20 dB nHL for the right and left ear, respectively) for a 3-month-old male (*top*). Despite the normal click ABR, DPOAEs suggest high-frequency cochlear damage bilaterally (*bottom*).

different wave V latencies (Stuart et al, 1990). Therefore consistent placement during testing is important in reducing variability. Use of alternating polarity will minimize stimulus artifact.

Maintaining proper position and pressure on the bone conduction vibrator can be difficult with small children. The traditional metal headband is often too large, may slip, and can be disturbed when the child turns his or her head. In addition, pressure from the headband may wake a lightly sleeping child. Use of a cloth headband may have similar shortcomings.

PEARL

During ABR testing, the bone conduction vibrator may be handheld against the head, without any form of headband.

Proper technique is critical when holding the bone conduction vibrator against the head. Pressure must be applied

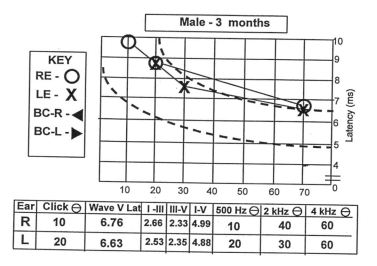

Ear	Click ⊖	Wave V Lat	I-III	III-V	I-V	500 Hz ⊖	2 kHz ⊖	4 kHz ⊖
R	10	6.76	2.66	2.33	4.99	10	40	60
L	20	6.63	2.53	2.35	4.88	20	30	60

Figure 22–2 (**B**) Latency-intensity function (*top*) for patient described in **A**. ABR thresholds for clicks are 10- and 20-dB nHL for the right and left ear, respectively. Thresholds for 500 Hz tone bursts are 10- and 20-dB nHL for the right and left ear, respectively. Thresholds for 2000 Hz tone bursts are 40- and 30-dB nHL for the right and left ear, respectively. Thresholds for 4000 Hz tone bursts are 60 dB nHL bilaterally. Behavioral responses (*bottom*) obtained at 7 months of age using visual reinforcement audiometry and insert earphones confirm the high-frequency loss suggested by the tone burst ABR.

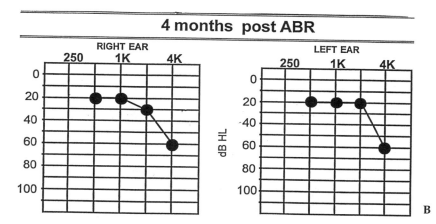

B

using one finger. When the vibrator is held between the thumb and two fingers, output is damped (see Bachmann & Hall, 1998, Fig. 22–4) and test accuracy will suffer. The vibrator must be held against the mastoid with sufficient pressure to just begin to move the child's head. Practice with the handheld technique is recommended before incorporating it into a clinical protocol. By comparing bone conduction responses obtained by using a metal headband with those obtained by using the handheld procedure, consistent positioning and pressure of the vibrator can be learned. When the bone vibrator is positioned and held properly, results similar to those in Figure 22–4 can be obtained routinely.

Amplifier Filter Settings

Because the ABR contains information in the 50 to 1000 Hz range (Domico & Kavanagh, 1986; Elberling, 1979), it is important that amplifier filters be set wide enough to include these frequencies. A high-pass filter setting of 30 to 50 Hz combined with a low-pass filter of 1500 to 3000 Hz is generally appropriate. (The reader is referred to Hall [1992] and Schwartz et al [1994] for comprehensive reviews of the topic.)

When noise interferes with the ABR recording, clinicians may be tempted to "close" the biological filters, often raising the high-pass filter to 100 Hz or higher. This will indeed

PITFALL

Narrowing the filter bandpass beyond 30 to 1500 Hz restricting the bandpass range) will reduce the amount of ABR information collected, especially near threshold.

reduce the noise but at the cost of reducing the ABR as well. Rather than change filter settings, it is preferable that the noise be eliminated at its source. Reducing electrical interference in the ABR recording environment will help considerably. In a hospital setting staff from the biomedical engineering department are often helpful in this endeavor. In other settings the ABR equipment representatives can be asked to make a site visit and help with electrical noise reduction. Repositioning the patient, using sedation, and careful routing of cables may also help.

A noncephalic inverting electrode can increase the amplitude of wave V by as much as 50% and can improve wave V detection at threshold (King & Sininger, 1992; Sininger & Don, 1989). Figure 22–5 demonstrates the increase in wave V amplitude at 70 dB nHL using the noncephalic (labeled "Nape"

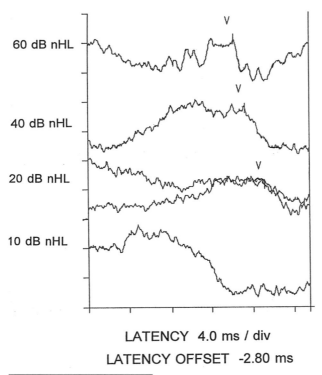

LATENCY 4.0 ms / div

LATENCY OFFSET -2.80 ms

Figure 22–3 ABR evoked by a 500 Hz Blackman-gated tone burst. Wave V latency at threshold (20 dB nHL) is 14.6 ms. The responses were recorded from a 2-month-old female.

PEARL

Wave V detection can be facilitated by using a noncephalic inverting (reference) electrode.

---

here) electrode. In Figure 22–6, the noncephalic (Nape) electrode yields a click ABR threshold that is 30 dB better than for the ipsilateral inverting electrode placed on the earlobe. The noncephalic reference can improve wave V detection for bone conduction and tone burst testing as well.

Acoustic Immittance Audiometry

The acoustic immittance battery is an important component in the infant audiological evaluation. However, test protocol and interpretation of results may not be as straightforward as with older children. For example, when low-frequency probe tones (226 Hz) and standard tympanometry are used, both notched and normal tympanograms were obtained in as many as 60% of infants with confirmed middle ear effusion (Marchant et al, 1986; Paradise et al, 1976). In contrast, Groothuis et al (1978, 1979) reported similar findings in less than 10% of infants studied.

In an attempt to improve test accuracy with young infants, tympanometry using probe tones greater than 220/226 Hz,

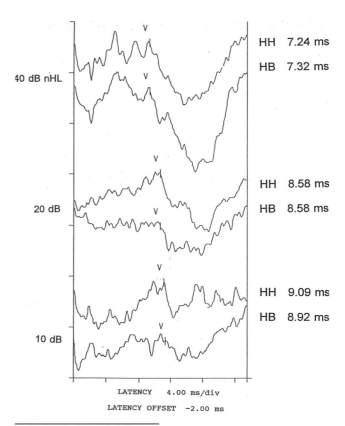

Figure 22–4 Comparison of click-evoked bone conduction responses obtained using the handheld (*HH*) technique versus the standard metal headband (*HB*). Note that wave V latencies and amplitudes are comparable, and, in some cases, the HH response has a clearer structure. The responses were recorded from a 4-month-old male.

has been advocated (Marchant et al, 1986). Multifrequency tympanometry indeed seems to reduce both false negative and false positive results in children less than 2 months old. However, it also appears that tympanogram configuration can be quite idiosyncratic in infants up to 4 months old (Holte et al, 1991). That is, tympanogram patterns to high-frequency probe tones do not follow established patterns.

In addition to higher frequency probe tones, multicomponent tympanometry, which analyzes immittance in terms of admittance, susceptance, and conductance, has been evaluated in infants, with the hope of improving test accuracy. Again, the pattern of results tends to be more variable than what is seen with older children and adults (Himelfarb et al, 1978; Holte et al, 1991).

Because of the dearth of normative data regarding multifrequency/multicomponent tympanometry in young infants, it is difficult to make an unequivocal recommendation for a specific protocol for clinical practice. However, what is clear, is that identification of middle ear disorders in infants improves when acoustic reflex measurement is included in the battery (Freyss et al, 1980; Schwartz & Schwartz, 1978, 1980). Test performance is further enhanced when reflexes are monitored using a higher frequency probe tone, such as 660 Hz or 800 Hz (McMillan et al, 1985; Sprague et al, 1985).

COMPARISON OF REFERENCE ELECTRODE SITES
Click ABR

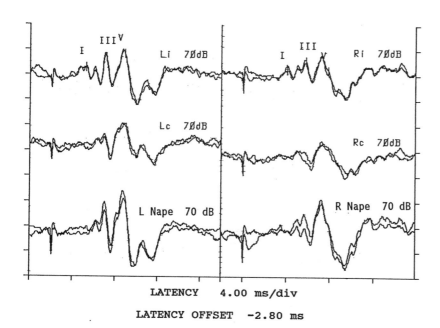

LATENCY   4.00 ms/div

LATENCY OFFSET   -2.80 ms

Figure 22–5 Click-evoked ABR at 70 dB nHL, obtained from a 3-month-old male. Inverting electrodes are the ipsilateral earlobe (*top*), contralateral earlobe (*middle*), and noncephalic (C_7), labeled Nape (*bottom*). Note that the amplitude of wave V, particularly the downslope, is substantially larger for the noncephalic reference.

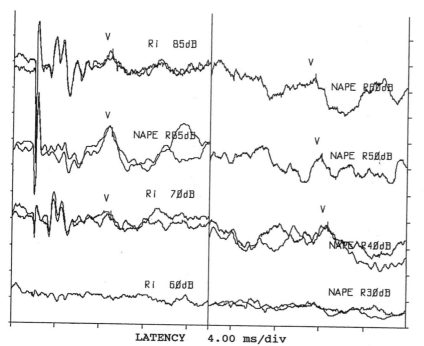

LATENCY   4.00 ms/div

Figure 22–6 Comparison of click-evoked ABR thresholds for inverting electrodes at ipsilateral earlobe and noncephalic locations. Note that the noncephalic recording (*Nape*) yielded a threshold, which was 30 dB better than for the ipsilateral recording. Responses were obtained from a 6-week-old male with a confirmed mild-to-moderate sensorineural hearing loss as a result of bacterial meningitis.

Either ipsilateral or contralateral acoustic reflexes appear to be effective with young infants.

We recommend that tympanometry and acoustic reflexes be evaluated in every infant seen in the diagnostic clinic. When test results are unclear or seem inconsistent with other test findings, referral to an experienced pediatric otologist is recommended.

Finally, because of the dependence of normal OAEs on good middle ear function, it might be argued that the finding of normal OAEs obviates the need for tympanometry in that ear. However, this possibility requires further exploration before it can be recommended as a standard of care.

Otoacoustic Emissions

Although they assess different aspects of the auditory system, OAEs provide an important cross-check for behavioral and ABR findings in young children. As shown in Figure

Right Ear

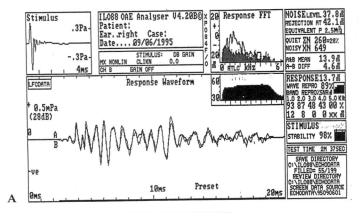

Left Ear

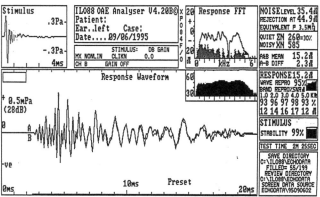

Figure 22–7 **(A)** DPOAEs of a 6-month-old female (*top*), suggesting cochlear damage at and above 2000 Hz for the right ear and cochlear damage at 6000 Hz for the left ear. In the lower panel, TEOAEs reflect a similar pattern, although the emission for the right ear in the 2000 Hz band appears to be somewhat stronger than the DPOAE at that frequency.

22–2A, DPOAEs suggested areas of cochlear damage despite a normal click-evoked ABR. Furthermore, in Figure 22–2B, DPOAEs confirmed or served as a cross-check for the high-frequency hearing loss suggested by the tone burst ABR.

Normal and hearing-impaired newborns and infants can be effectively differentiated using either transient-evoked otoacoustic emissions (TEOAEs) (Bonfils et al, 1988; Glattke, 1995; Norton, 1994) or DPOAEs (Lafreniere et al, 1991). Figure 22–7A demonstrates that both DPOAEs and TEOAEs are sensitive to mild-to-moderate sensorineural loss, depicted in the ABR latency-intensity function of Figure 22–7B.

Although both TEOAEs and DPOAEs provide frequency-specific information, DPOAEs perform somewhat better at higher frequencies (Gorga et al, 1993). DPOAEs might therefore be the tool of choice when factors such as ototoxicity or extracorporeal membrane oxygenation treatment put the child at risk for hearing loss onset at high frequencies.

OAEs also have an important role in the hearing aid fitting process. Sininger et al (1995), Berlin et al (1996), and Starr et al (1996) have described a series of adults and older children who demonstrate normal OAEs, along with a variety of other abnormal findings, including absent or abnormal ABRs,

mild-to-moderate elevation of behavioral thresholds, absent acoustic reflexes, and abnormally depressed word recognition abilities. This constellation of disorders has been described as "auditory neuropathy." Both Berlin et al and Sininger et al advise that hearing aids are not helpful for such patients because cochlear outer hair cells, and presumably cochlear mechanics, are normal.

A profile similar to auditory neuropathy may be seen in young children. For example, Lafreniere et al (1991) and Stein et al (1996) described newborns at risk for hearing loss caused by hyperbilirubinemia. These children exhibited abnormal ABRs but normal DPOAEs and/or TEOAEs. Like the adults described in the preceding paragraph, the abnormal ABR and normal OAEs suggest normal cochlear outer hair cell function, and hearing aids are presumably inappropriate for these newborns.

By extension, the data in the preceding two paragraphs caution against fitting hearing aids on any newborn or infant who demonstrates normal OAEs and an abnormal ABR. These children must be followed closely and monitored by both behavioral and electrophysiological means. Referrals to appropriate parent-infant programs are essential to arrange habilitation, including stimulation programs. Use of low-gain

Figure 22–7 **(B)** The latency-intensity function for the patient presented in **A**, where the mild-to-moderate sensorineural loss for the right ear is apparent (see Fig. 22–2B for interpretation of latency-intensity function). The left ear thresholds were within normal limits through 4000 Hz consistent with the OAE findings. The left ear 8000 Hz ABR threshold was 60 dB nHL (not shown), also consistent with the apparent high-frequency drop in the OAEs.

Ear	Click ⊖	Wave V Lat	I-III	III-V	I-V	500 Hz ⊖	2 kHz ⊖	4 kHz ⊖
R	30	6.79	2.24	2.12	4.36	10	30	50
L	10	6.31	2.50	2.19	4.69	10	20	20

assistive listening devices (ALDs) may prove helpful, but efficacy reports are not yet in the literature.

It is important to remember that an abnormal ABR and normal OAEs may reflect delayed neuromaturation in young infants. Neurological referral, serial ABR testing, behavioral testing, and a complete developmental assessment will help resolve the issue. Such children should not languish without intervention. Referral to local ECI programs and stimulation using low-gain ALDs are suggested as alternatives to traditional amplification until the relative sensory and neural components of the disorder are documented.

A great deal of additional research is needed to better understand this population. What is clear, however, is that the presence of normal OAEs is a signal to the audiologist that the child does not have a classic cochlear hearing loss. Options other than traditional amplification should be explored to deal with what may be a neural or "central" disorder. In such cases, increased emphasis should be placed on behavioral testing because it provides the most valid estimate of the child's functional hearing.

Behavioral Audiometry

Diagnostic audiometry with young infants is an ongoing process. The initial steps rely on electrophysiological techniques, but behavioral evaluation of aided and unaided performance should be attempted as soon as possible. Visual reinforcement audiometry can be effectively used with infants as young as 5 months old (Wilson & Thompson, 1984). Insert earphones can also be used with these children to obtain reliable, ear-specific threshold data (Gravel, 1994).

Hearing Aid Fitting

The initial hearing aid fitting can proceed after a single, carefully performed ABR test session. Unless the ABR data are flawed, withholding hearing aids while confirming and reconfirming ABR results is not necessary. Tone burst threshold data can be entered into any fitting strategy or program in the same manner that behavioral thresholds would be used. However,

because the ABR thresholds are generally more variable than behavioral thresholds, a hearing aid with flexible output characteristics is needed. In addition, the fitting must account for the acoustics of a newborn's ear. A fitting method such as the desired sensation level (Seewald, 1994) is an approach that seems well suited to infants. The hearing aid fitting should not proceed until OAE testing has been completed.

Follow-Up Testing

Within 3 to 6 months of the initial diagnostic ABR, it should be possible to confirm electrophysiological thresholds by means of behavioral means. If this cannot be done, a repeat ABR is justified to monitor stability of the loss. In cases with an increased likelihood of progressive hearing loss (meningitis, congenital cytomegalovirus [CMV] infection), repeat ABR testing every 3 months may be justified until ear-specific behavioral testing is possible.

Asymptomatic congenital CMV may account for as much as 40% of the sensorineural hearing losses in well babies (Littman et al, 1996). This virus is termed *asymptomatic* because no overt signs of abnormality are present other than the positive CMV titer. However, approximately 3600 to 6000 newborns with asymptomatic CMV have sensorineural hearing loss develop each year (Demmler, 1991). Within this group of hearing-impaired children, progressive hearing loss has been reported in 67% (Williamson et al, 1992) to 100 % (Littman et al, 1996) of the cases. It is therefore recommended that newborns with sensorineural loss of unknown cause be tested for CMV within 3 weeks of birth. If asymptomatic CMV is confirmed, follow-up testing every 3 months is indicated, at least until the child reaches school age.

DIAGNOSTIC EVALUATION PROTOCOL

High-Intensity ABR

The diagnostic evaluation begins with an otoscopic examination. A click-evoked ABR is then performed at a moderately high intensity level (70- to 80-dB nHL) to permit examination of waveform morphology and absolute and interpeak latencies in each ear. Use of age-specific and gender-specific norms is essential.

Threshold ABR for Click-Evoked Stimuli

A click-evoked threshold search is conducted for each ear by means of air conduction. Dropping in 30 dB steps, the response is monitored until wave V disappears. Stimulus intensity is then increased in 10 dB steps, until a replicable wave V is recorded. Threshold is defined as the lowest intensity at which a repeatable wave V is recorded.

To reduce test time without sacrificing important information, a possible "shortcut" protocol includes testing at 70- and 20-dB nHL only, if the latency values at 70 dB are normal. If a replicable wave V is seen at 20 dB nHL and if all latency values are age-appropriate, the click ABR may be considered normal. The reader is referred to Bachmann and Hall (1998) for a review of other options that may help reduce test time.

Bone Conduction Click ABR

If the click-evoked air conduction threshold is abnormal, a threshold search using click-evoked bone conduction stimuli is indicated. Tonal stimuli may also be presented by means of bone conduction (Nousak & Stapells, 1992).

Otoacoustic Emissions

If the click-evoked ABR yields normal latency and threshold values, OAEs should be assessed next. If normal OAEs are obtained, testing can be halted, and it can be inferred that sensitivity is normal at all frequencies for which a normal emission was noted. This approach requires that the ABR earphones be removed and the OAE probe inserted in the ear. Although these manipulations may rouse a few children, the time saved in avoiding the frequency-specific ABR testing justifies the risk. If OAEs are abnormal, frequency-specific ABR

testing is indicated. Similarly, frequency-specific ABR evaluation is indicated whenever the click-evoked ABR is abnormal.

Frequency-Specific ABR

If either the click-evoked ABR or OAEs are abnormal, ABR using air-conducted, frequency-specific stimuli is necessary. For hearing aid fitting, stimuli at 500, 2000, and 4000 Hz are most useful. Other frequencies may be evaluated as time permits. When a reason to suspect early onset of a loss at higher frequencies exists, it may be helpful to include 8000 Hz as well.

Acoustic Immittance Battery

Tympanometry and acoustic reflex testing should always be included. Use of a high-frequency probe tone is recommended for reflex measurement. Until the child is 4 to 7 months old, results must be interpreted with caution when they are inconsistent with other data. Referral to a pediatric otologist is recommended whenever results are questionable.

CONCLUSIONS

For decades, pediatric audiologists have championed the importance of early detection and been frustrated by the lack of response from medical colleagues. In the late 1990s outcome measures have become available to support early detection. Effective programs can be implemented. The roadmaps in this chapter and given by others should be followed (Joint Committee, 1994; Spivak, 1998). Establishing a newborn hearing detection program requires expertise and knowledge on the part of the pediatric audiologist. The audiologist's role is multifaceted. In some hospitals it may be one of expert or consultant. Audiologist's role is substantial in follow-up and diagnostic assessments. Only through diligence on the part of the pediatric audiologist will babies be detected in the nursery and connected to effective habilitation and intervention services.

REFERENCES

AMERICAN ACADEMY OF PEDIATRICS (TASK FORCE ON NEWBORN AND INFANT HEARING). (1999). Newborn and infant hearing loss: Detection and intervention. *Pediatrics, 103;* 527–530.

AMERICAN SPEECH-LANGUAGE & HEARING ASSOCIATION. (1994). Joint Committee on Infant Hearing 1994 Position Statement. *ASHA, 36;*38–41.

BACHMANN, K.R., & HALL, J.W. (1998). Pediatric auditory brain stem response assessment: The cross-check principle twenty years later. *Seminars in Hearing, 10;*1,41–60.

BERLIN, C.I., HOOD, L.J., HURLEY, A., & WEN, H. (1996). Hearing aids: Only for hearing-impaired patients with abnormal

otoacoustic emissions. In: C.I. Berlin (Ed.), *Hair cells and hearing aids* (pp. 99–111). San Diego, CA: Singular.

BLOCK, P. (1993). *Stewardship: Choosing service over self-interest.* San Francisco, CA: Berrrett- Koehler.

BONFILS, P., UZIEL, A., & PUJOL, R. (1988). Evoked oto-acoustic emissions from adults and infants: Clinical applications. *Acta Otolaryngologica, 105;*445–449.

CARPENTER, C., BENDER, A.D., NASH, D.B., & CORNMAN, J.C. (1996). Must we choose between quality and cost containment? *Quality in Health Care, 5;*223–229.

COATS, A.C., & MARTIN, J.L. (1977). Human auditory nerve action potentials and brain stem evoked responses. Effects of audiogram shape and lesion location. *Archives of Otolaryngology, 103;*605–622.

DEMMLER, G. (1991). Infectious diseases society of America and Centers for Disease Control. Summary of a workshop on surveillance for congenital cytomegalovirus disease. *Reviews of Infectious Diseases 13;*315–329.

DIEFENDORF, A., & FINITZO, T. (1997). The state of the information: A report to the Joint Committee on Infant Hearing *American Journal of Audiology, 6;*91–94.

DOMICO, W., & KAVANAGH, K. (1986). Analog and zero-phase shift digital filtering of the auditory brain stem response waveform. *Ear and Hearing, 7;*377–382.

DOWNS, P.P., & STERRITT, G.M. (1967). A guide to newborn and infant hearing screening programs. *Archives of Otolaryngology, 85,*37–44.

EARLY IDENTIFICATION OF HEARING IMPAIRMENT IN INFANTS AND YOUNG CHILDREN. (1993). *National Institutes of Health Consensus Statement* (11).

ELBERLING, K. (1979). Auditory electrophysiology: Spectral analysis of cochlear and brain stem evoked potentials. *Scandinavian Audiology, 8;*57–64.

FINITZO, T. (1995) Stewardship in universal infant hearing detection. *Audiology Today, 7;*25.

FINITZO, T. (1998). *The sounds of Texas project: Principles from the 1994 Joint Committee on Infant Hearing Position Statement.* Presentation to the European Union, May 1998, Milan, Italy.

FINITZO, T., ALBRIGHT, K., & O'NEAL, J. (1998). The newborn with hearing loss: Detection in the nursery. *Pediatrics, 102;*1452–1460.

FREYSS, G., NARCY, P., & MANAC'H, Y. (1980). Acoustic reflex as a predictor of middle ear effusion. *Annals of Otology, Rhinology and Laryngology, 89*(suppl. 68);196–199.

GLATTKE, T.J., PAFITIS, I.A., CUMMISKEY, C., & HERER, G.R. (1995). Identification of hearing loss in children using measures of transient otoacoustic emission reproducibility. *American Journal of Audiology 4;*71–86.

GORGA, M.P., NEELY, S.T., BERGMAN, B.M. BEAUCHAINE, K.L., KAMINSKI, J.R., PETERS, J., SCHULTE, L., & JESTEADT ,W. (1993). A comparison of transient-evoked and distortion product emissions in normal-hearing and hearing-impaired subjects. *Journal of the Acoustical Society of America, 94;*2639–2648.

GORGA, M.P., & THORNTON, A.R. (1989). The choice of stimuli for ABR measurements. *Ear and Hearing, 10;*217–230.

GRAVEL, J.A. (1989). Behavioral assessment of auditory function. *Seminars in Hearing, 10;*216–228.

GRAVEL, J.A. (1994). Auditory assessment of infants. *Seminars in Hearing, 15;*100–113.

GRAVEL, J.A., KURTZBERG, D., STAPELLS, D.R., VAUGHAN, H.G., & WALLACE, I.F. (1989). Case studies. *Seminars in Hearing, 10;*272–287.

GROOTHUIS, J.R., ALTEMEIER, W.A., WRIGHT, P.F., & SELL, S.H. (1978). The evolution and resolution of otitis media in infants: tympanometric findings. In: E.R. Harford, F.H. Bess, C.D. Bluestone, & J.O. Klein. (Eds.), *Impedance screening for middle ear disease in children* (pp. 105–109). New York: Grune and Stratton.

GROOTHUIS, J.R., SELL, S.H., & WRIGHT, P.F. (1979). Otitis media in infancy: Tympanometric findings. *Pediatrics, 63;*435–442.

HALL, J. (1992). *Handbook auditory evoked responses* (pp. 177–220). Boston: Allyn & Bacon.

HARRISON, M. & ROUSH, J. (1996). Age of suspicion, identification and intervention for infants and young children with hearing loss: A national study. *Ear and Hearing, 17,*55–62.

HIMELFARB, M.Z., POPELKA, G.R., & SHANON, E. (1978). Tympanometry in normal neonates. *Journal of Speech and Hearing Research, 22;*179–191.

HOLTE, L., MARGOLIS, R.H., & CAVENAUGH, R.M. (1991). Developmental changes in multifrequency tympanograms. *Audiology, 30;*1–24.

HOOKS, R., & WEBER, B. (1984). Auditory brain stem responses of premature infants to bone-conducted stimuli: A feasibility study. *Ear and Hearing 5;*42–46.

JACOBSON, J.T. (1994). *Principles and applications in auditory evoked potentials.* Boston: Allyn & Bacon.

JAHRSDOERFER, R.A., YEAKLEY, J.W., HALL, J.W., ROBBINS, K.T., & GRAY, L.C. (1985). High-resolution CT scanning and auditory brain stem response in congenital aural atresia: Patient selection and surgical correlation. *Otolaryngology – Head and Neck Surgery, 83;*292–298.

JERGER J, & MAULDIN L. (1978). Prediction of sensorineural hearing level from the brain stem evoked response. *Archives of Otolaryngology, 104;*456–461.

KING, A.J., & SININGER, Y.S. (1992). Electrode configuration for auditory brain stem response audiometry. *American Journal of Audiology, 1;*63–67.

LAFRENIERE, D., SMURZYNSKI, J., JUNG, M., LEONARD, G., & KIM, D.O. (1991). Otoacoustic emissions in full-term newborns at risk for hearing loss. *Laryngoscope, 103;*1334–1341.

LITTMAN, T., DEMMLER, G., WILLIAMS, S., ISTAS, A., & GRIESSER, C. (1996). Congenital asymptomatic cytomegalovirus infection and hearing loss. *Abstracts Association of Research Otolaryngology, 19;*40.

MARCHANT, C., McMILLAN, P., SHURIN, P., JOHNSON, C., TURCZYK, V., FEINSTEN, J., & PANEK, D. (1986). Objective diagnosis of otitis media in early infancy by tympanometry and ipsilateral acoustic reflex thresholds. *Journal of Pediatrics, 109;*590–595.

McMILLAN, P., BENNETT, M., MARCHANT, C., & SHURIN, P. (1985). Ipsilateral and contralateral acoustic reflexes in neonates. *Ear and Hearing, 6;*320–324.

NATIONAL INSTITUTE ON DEAFNESS AND OTHER COMMUNICATION DISORDERS. (1997). Working group on early identification of hearing impairment on acceptable protocols for use in state-wide universal newborn hearing programs. Chevy Chase, MD: September 4–5.

NORTON, S.J. (1994). The emerging role of evoked otoacoustic emissions in neonatal hearing screening. *American Journal of Otolaryngology, 15;* Supplement 1,4–12.

NOUSAK, J.M.K., & STAPELLS, D.R. (1992). Frequency specificity of the auditory brain stem response to bone-conducted tones in infants and adults. *Ear and Hearing, 13;*87–95.

OATES, P., & STAPELLS, D.R. (1998). Auditory brain stem response estimates of the pure tone audiogram: Current status. *Seminars in Hearing, 10;*1,61–85.

PARADISE, J., SMITH, C., & BLUESTONE, C. (1976). Tympanometric detection of middle ear effusion in infants and young children. *Pediatrics, 587;*198–210.

PARVING, A. (1993). Congenital hearing disability: Epidemiology and identification: A comparison between two health authority districts. *International Journal of Pediatric Otolaryngology, 27,*29–46.

PICTON, T.W., & DURIEUX-SMITH, A. (1988). Auditory evoked potentials in the assessment of hearing. *Neurologic Clinics, 6;*791–808.

PICTON, T.W., OUELLETTE, J., HAMEL, G., & SMITH, A.D. (1979). Brain stem evoked potentials to tonepips in notched noise. *Journal of Otolaryngology, 8;*289–314.

POOL, K.D. (1996). Infant hearing detection programs: Accountability and information management. *Seminars in Hearing, 17;*139–151.

SCHWARTZ, D.M., MORRIS, D.M., & JACOBSON, J.T. (1994). The normal auditory brain stem response and its variants. In: J.T. Jacobson (Ed.), *Principles and applications in auditory evoked potentials* (pp. 123–153). Boston: Allyn & Bacon.

SCHWARTZ, D.M., & SCHWARTZ, R.H. (1978). A comparison of tympanometry and acoustic reflex measurements for detecting middle ear effusion in infants below seven months of age. In: E.R. Harford, F.H. Bess, C.D. Bluestone, & J.O. Klein (Eds.), *Impedance screening for middle ear disease in children* (pp. 91–96). New York: Grune and Stratton.

SCHWARTZ, D.M., & SCHWARTZ, R.H. (1980). Tympanometric findings in young infants with middle ear effusion: Some further observations. *International Journal of Pediatric Otolaryngology, 2;*67–72.

SEEWALD, R.C. (1994). Fitting children with the DSL method. *Hearing Journal, 47;*10,48–51.

SININGER, Y.S., & DON, M. (1989). Effects of click rate and electrode orientation on threshold of the auditory brain stem response. *Journal of Speech and Hearing Reseach, 32;*880–886.

SININGER, Y.S., HOOD, L.J., STARR, A., BERLIN, C.I., & PICTON, T.W. (1995) Hearing loss due to auditory neuropathy. *Audioloty Today, 7;*11–13.

SPIVAK, L. (1998). *Universal newborn hearing screening.* New York: Thieme Medical Publishers, Inc.

SPRAGUE, B., WILEY, T., & GOLDSTEIN, R. (1985). Tympanometric and acoustic-reflex studies in neonates. *Journal of Speech and Hearing Research 28;*265–272.

STAPELLS, D.R., GRAVEL, J.S., & MARTIN, B.A. (1995). Thresholds of auditory brain stem responses to tones in notched noise from infants and young children with normal-hearing or sensorineural hearing loss. *Ear and Hearing, 16;* 361–371.

STAPELLS, D.R., & RUBEN, R.J. (1989). Auditory brainstem responses to bone-conducted tones in infants. *Annals of Otology, Rhinology and Laryngology, 98;*941–949.

STAPELLS, D.R., PICTON, T.W., & DURIEUX-SMITH, A. (1994). Electrophysiologic measures of frequency-specific auditory function. In: J.T. Jacobson (Ed.), *Principles and applications in auditory evoked potentials* (pp. 251–283). Boston: Allyn & Bacon.

STARR, A., PICTON, T.W., SININGER, Y., HOOD, L.F., & BERLIN, C.I. (1996). Auditory neuropathy. *Brain, 119;*741–753.

STEIN, L. (1995a). The volunteer audiologist. *Audiology Today, 7;*17.

STEIN, L. (1995b). On the real age of identification of congenital hearing loss. *Audiology Today, 17;*10–11.

STEIN, L., TREMBLAY, K., PASTERNAK, J., BANERJEE, S., LINDEMANN, K., & KRAUS, N. (1996). Brain stem abnormalities in neonates with normal otoacoustic emissions. *Seminars in Hearing, 17;*197–213.

STUART, A., YANG, E.Y., & STENSTROM, R. (1990). Effect of temporal area bone vibrator placement of auditory brain stem response in newborn infants. *Ear and Hearing, 11;*363–369.

TEXAS DEPARTMENT OF HEALTH, 1996 State Health Data, Austin, Texas.

THARPE, A.M., & CLAYTON-WRIGHT, E.W. (1997). Newborn hearing screening: Issues in legal liability and quality assurance. *American Journal of Audiology,* July.

U.S. DEPARTMENT OF HEALTH AND HUMAN SERVICES. (1990). *Healthy People 2000. Public Service.* DHHS Publication No. 91-50213. Washington, D.C.: U.S. Government Printing Office.

VAN DER DRIFT, J., VAN ZANTEN, G., & BROCAAR, M. (1989). Brain stem electric response audiometry: Estimation of the amount of conductive hearing loss with and without use of the response threshold. *Audiology, 28;*181–193.

WHEELER, D.J., & CHAMBERS, D.S. (1993). *Understanding statistical process control.* Knoxville, TN: SPC Press, Inc.

WILLIAMSON, W.D., DEMMLER, G.J., PERCY, A.K., & CATLIN, F.I. (1992). Progressive hearing loss in infants with asymptomatic congenital cytomegalovirus infection. *Pediatrics, 90;*862–866.

WILSON, W.R., & THOMPSON, G. (1984). Behavioral audiometry. In: J. Jerger (Ed.), *Pediatric audiology* (pp. 1–44). San Diego: College-Hill.

YANG, E., RUPERT, A., & MOUSHEGIAN, G. (1987). A developmental study of bone conduction auditory brain stem response in infants. *Ear and Hearing, 8;*244–251.

YOSHINAGA-ITANO, C., SEDLEY, A., COULTER, D., & MEHL, A. (1998). Language of early- and later-identified children with hearing loss. *Pediatrics, 102;*1161–1171.

Chapter 23

Intraoperative Neurophysiological Monitoring

Aage R. Moller

Outline

Operations that involve the nervous system always involve risks of death and neurological deficits. Such risks can never be eliminated because not all factors that are involved can be controlled, and the possibility always exists that mistakes may be done or that unforeseen circumstances can cause injuries or death. If it is physically possible to make a mistake, it will be made eventually, but the likelihood that a mistake occurs can be reduced. It is the goal of procedures in the operating room to make the likelihood for mistakes as small as possible. Intraoperative neurophysiological monitoring (IOM) is one of many means that can reduce the likelihood of mistakes that can lead to injury and permanent postoperative deficits, but it cannot eliminate surgically induced deficits.

IOM is based on the assumption that recordable neuroelectric potentials change while the injury is still reversible and before the severity of the injury has reached the level where permanent deficits result. Besides reducing the risk of permanent deficits, IOM may also give the surgeon an

Audiology: Diagnosis. Edited by Roeser, Valente, and Hosford-Dunn. Thieme Medical Publishers, Inc., New York © 2000

increased feeling of security and can often help the surgeon in identifying neural structures that are not directly visible. In some operations these electrophysiological methods can help the surgeon achieve the therapeutic goal of an operation.

IOM uses recordings of neuroelectric potentials, such as sensory evoked potentials and electromyographic (EMG) potentials, to detect changes in the function of specific systems. Far field sensory evoked potentials and near field potentials recorded directly from nerves, nuclei, and muscles are now commonly monitored in the operating room. Electrical stimulation of neural structures in the operative field is used for identifying specific nerves. EMG activity elicited by surgical manipulations of motor nerves is used as an indicator of activation of motor nerves and to detect injuries to motor nerves.

HISTORICAL BACKGROUND

It was not until the beginning of the 1970s that IOM came into general use, first for monitoring the integrity of the spinal cord in operations for scoliosis (Brown & Nash, 1979) and later for monitoring the auditory nerve and cranial motor nerves. But it was perhaps preservation of the facial nerve in operations for acoustic tumors that first demonstrated the benefits from the use of electrophysiological methods in the operating room. Electrophysiological methods made it possible to find the facial nerve during operations to remove acoustic tumors and test its function. Being able to find the facial nerve is naturally a prerequisite for being able to preserve its function. Krauze (1912) is reported to have used electrical stimulation of the facial nerve before the turn of the century for finding the facial nerve in the operative field during removal of acoustic tumors. Only a few reports on the use of facial nerve monitoring appeared during the next 50 years (Hilger, 1964; Jako, 1965), and monitoring of facial function in operations for acoustic tumors did not gain common use in operations of acoustic tumors until the end of the 1970s (Babin et al, 1982; Delgado et al, 1979; Harner et al, 1988; Kartush & Bouchard, 1992; Moller & Jannetta, 1984; Prass et al, 1987; Sugita & Kobayashi, 1982).

Monitoring of the function of the auditory nerve in microvascular decompression operations for hemifacial spasm and for face pain was described in the 1980s (Fischer, 1989; Friedman et al, 1985; Grundy, 1983; Linden et al, 1988; Radtke et al, 1989; Raudzens, 1982); and gained general use during the following decade. During the 1990s, the use of electrophysiological methods for preserving neural function increased rapidly and the methods are now in general use in many other kinds of operations (Moller, 1995).

Besides the facial nerve and the auditory-vestibular nerve, which are at risk in operations in the cerebellopontine angle (CPA), several cranial nerves are at risk of being injured in operations to remove large tumors of the brain that are located near the base of the skull (skull base tumors). When operations were developed to treat skull base tumors other than acoustic tumors (Sekhar & Moller, 1986, Sekhar & Schramm, 1987), IOM helped to reduce the risks of neurological deficits. These major operations involve high risk of permanent neurological deficit from surgical injuries to many different kinds of neural tissue. The development of the surgical technique used in these operations also benefited from the use of the electrophysiological methods used for IOM because these techniques can identify specific neural structures. That was important because the normal anatomy was often distorted by such tumors.

WHAT CAN BE MONITORED?

Neural conduction in nerves and fiber tracts in the brain and synaptic transmission in nuclei can be monitored intraoperatively by recording sensory evoked potentials or by recording evoked responses directly from exposed neural tissue. Nerve conduction in peripheral nerves can be monitored by electrically stimulating a nerve and recording compound action potentials (CAP) from the nerve. The function of motor nerves can be monitored by recording EMG potentials from the muscles they innervate.

PRINCIPLES OF INTRAOPERATIVE MONITORING

The use of intraoperative monitoring as a means to decrease the risk of postoperative neurological deficits is based on the assumption that surgical manipulations cause measurable changes in neural conduction in nerves and fiber tracts before permanent injuries to the nerve fibers occur. In a similar way it is assumed that synaptic transmission becomes impaired and even ceases to occur before permanent injury to the nerve cells in question occurs. To reduce the risk of permanent injury, it is therefore important that changes in neural function are detected as soon as possible after the injury has occurred and before they reach a level where the injury leads to a permanent neurological deficit. In addition, it must be possible to reverse the surgical manipulation that has caused the injury. The surgeon must know not only that a change in function has occurred but also which neural structures are affected and what surgical manipulations caused the injury to occur. That emphasizes the importance of informing the surgeon as soon as possible after a change in function has occurred. The recording techniques used in the operating room must be chosen with this in mind. It is naturally important that the recorded neuroelectric potentials reflect the function of the structures that are at risk.

Most of the electrophysiological methods used in IOM are similar to those used for diagnostic purposes. However, the fact that the records obtained in the operating room must be interpreted as soon as they are available requires that the person who performs the IOM be capable to immediately interpret the recordings that are obtained. It is also important that the surgeon can identify which step in the operation caused the change in function.

USE OF SENSORY EVOKED POTENTIALS IN INTRAOPERATIVE MONITORING

Sensory evoked potentials such as the brain stem auditory evoked potentials (BAEP) and somatosensory evoked potentials (SSEP) are far field potentials that are recorded from electrodes placed on the scalp. The amplitude of such potentials is small, and much smaller than the EEG activity picked up by the same electrodes. To make far field sensory evoked potentials interpretable, the responses to many stimuli must be added. That takes time and thus means a delay in interpretation. Such delay may not be of any great importance when evoked potentials are used in the clinic, but it is a serious obstacle to their use in the operating room for monitoring. A long delay between an injury and its detection may cause the injury to become permanent before it can be reversed. A long delay also makes it difficult to identify which surgical manipulation caused the injury when the time between the occurrence of an injury and its detection is long.

Several factors affect the time it takes to obtain an interpretable record. The following list summarizes the factors that are important for obtaining a clean interpretable record in as short a time as possible:

1. Decrease the electrical interference that reaches the recording electrodes.
2. Use optimal stimulus repetition rate.
3. Use optimal stimulus strength.
4. Use optimal filtering of the recorded potentials.
5. Use optimal placement of recording electrodes.
6. Use quality control that does not require replicating records.

Optimizing stimulation to increase the amplitude of the potentials, selection of optimal recording parameters, and reduction of electrical interference are all factors that can shorten the time it takes to obtain an interpretable record.

Electrical interference in the operating room is often great because of all the electronic equipment used, but interference from biological potentials (such as ongoing brain activity, EEG potentials, and EMG potentials generated by muscles) may also be noticeable. Methods for reducing the electrical interference from other equipment are described elsewhere (Moller, 1995) and will not be repeated here. The interference from muscles is not a problem when the patient is paralyzed, but muscle relaxants cannot be used in operations where EMG potentials are recorded.

Optimal filtering of the recorded evoked potentials can shorten the time it takes to obtain an interpretable result because it reduces the number of responses that must be collected (Doyle & Hyde, 1981; Moller, 1988a, 1995; Sgro et al, 1989). Interpretation of evoked potentials does not require that all the information contained in evoked potentials is preserved. When unnecessary parts of the recorded potentials are eliminated by filtering, the number of responses that need to be collected is reduced because more noise is eliminated by aggressive filtering. Modern digital filters offer much more flexibility than electronic filters, and it is possible to enhance certain portions of a record that are important for interpretation. Figure 23–1 illustrates what can be accomplished by optimal filtering. A clean record allows computer programs to identify the peaks and automatically print out their latencies in BAEPs as shown in Figure 23–1.

Under the best circumstances, it takes at least 20 seconds to obtain an interpretable BAEP record in an individual with normal-hearing, provided that the electrical interference is reduced to negligible values and optimal stimulus parameters are used together with aggressive (digital) filtering of the recorded responses. In patients with hearing loss the time can be several times longer and electrical interference can make it necessary to average many more responses, which can further prolong the time it takes to obtain an interpretable record.

Replication of records is the common method for quality control of evoked potentials in the clinic. However, if that method is used in the operating room, it will increase the time it takes to detect changes in function because two interpretable records must be obtained. Better ways of quality control that do not require replication of records have been devised (Hoke et al, 1984; Schimmel, 1967), and such methods are suitable for use in the operating room. These matters are discussed in detail elsewhere (Moller, 1995).

Stimulation

The optimal stimulation for recording of the BAEP in the operating room is clicks presented at a rate of 30 to 40 pulses/s (pps) and with an intensity of 100- to 105-dB peak equivalent sound pressure level (PeSPL), corresponding to 65 dB hearing level (HL) when presented at a rate of 20 pps. The most suitable earphones are insert earphone (such as the tubephone) or the miniature stereo earphones used in connection with Walkman tape players (Radio Shack) that have been used for more than 15 years (Moller, 1995). Either rarefaction or condensation clicks should be used. It is not recommended that clicks with alternating polarity be used because the response to these two kinds of clicks is different, particularly in individuals with hearing loss.

PITFALL

The use of clicks with alternating polarity may result in adding responses that have different waveforms, which decreases the amplitude of the response and may make individual peaks become broader than the peaks elicited by either rarefaction or condensation clicks.

Recording Electrodes

Needle electrodes are more suitable for recordings of BAEP in the operating room than the conventional surface electrodes, such as the common gold cup electrodes. It is common to use a subdermal needle electrode such as the Grass Instrument Co. type E2. These are equipped with a lead to connect to the electrode box of the amplifier. The electrodes should be inserted after the patient is anesthetized and secured by adhesive tape of good quality. Adhesive tape that can "breathe" such as the Blenderm adhesive tape manufactured by the Minnesota Mining Corporation should be used. If recording is done in only one channel, recording electrodes should be placed at the vertex and the ipsilateral earlobe. It is advantageous to use two channels of recordings. One channel should be connected to electrodes placed on the earlobes and the other channel should record from the vertex and upper neck.

Amplifiers and Filters

The amplification should be set at 50,000×. Use of higher amplification may prolong stimulus artifacts and other interference signals because of overloading the amplifier. If only electronic filters are used, a setting of 150 to 1500 Hz is suitable. If digital filters are used, the electronic filters in the

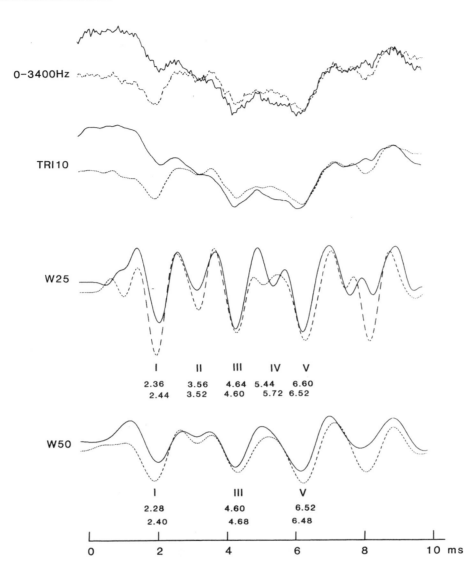

Figure 23–1   Effects on the waveform of the BAEP of different types of digital filters. The upper tracing was filtered with electronic filters only; the second tracing from top *(TRI10)* shows the same recordings after low-pass filtering with a digital filter that had a triangular weighing function with a base length of 0.4 ms. The two lower tracings show the effects of filtering of the same record with two different digital band-pass filters *(W25* and *W50)* that had W-shaped weighing functions (similar to a truncated sin(x)/x function) with the base length being 1 and 2 ms, respectively. The numbers on the two bottom curves are the latency values obtained using computer programs that automatically identified peaks of the BAEP and printed their latencies. The two tracings *(solid and dashed)* show replications. (From Moller [1988b], with permission.)

amplifiers should be set at 10 to 3000 Hz, and the digital filters should be set to enhance the peaks of the BAEP (Moller, 1988a, 1995).

Interpretation of the BAEP

The BAEP is characterized by a series of peaks and valleys. Interpretation of abnormalities in the BAEP has mainly concerned the vertex positive peaks that are traditionally labeled by Roman numerals. The two earliest peaks (I and II) are generated by the distal and the proximal portion of the auditory nerve, respectively. The auditory nerve is about 2.5 cm long (Lang, 1985), and the conduction velocity of the auditory nerve is approximately 20 m/s. This explains the interval of 1 to 1.2 ms between peak I and II. When the BAEP is used to detect changes in the neural conduction of the auditory nerve in operations involving the CPA, peak I is not likely to change, but peak II and all following peaks will be affected. It is mainly the latencies of the peaks that have been used as indicators of injuries. Because the changes in the latency of earlier peaks are imposed on later peaks, it is most convenient to use the latency of peak V or peak III as an indicator of

changes in the conduction time in the auditory nerve, especially because the large amplitudes of peak III and peak V make them easy to identify and their latencies can be accurately determined. The amplitude of these peaks is also affected by injuries to the auditory nerve, but the large variability of their amplitudes has detracted from using changes in amplitude as indicators of trauma. However, recent studies have shown that the change in amplitude may be valuable for detecting changes in neural conduction of the auditory nerve (Hatayama & Moller, 1998).

MONITORING BRAIN STEM STRUCTURES BY RECORDING BRAIN STEM AUDITORY EVOKED POTENTIALS

Surgical manipulations of the brain stem may occur in operations of larger tumors of the CPA such as large acoustic tumors. Such manipulations have traditionally been detected by observing changes in cardiovascular parameters such as heart rate and blood pressure. However, the systems that control the heart are under the influence of feedback systems that tend to keep conditions stable. Therefore blood pressure and heart rate may not change noticeably until rather large surgical manipulations have been made. Monitoring of the BAEP elicited by stimulation of the ear contralateral to the operated side can give earlier warnings about manipulations of the brain stem than observations of cardiac parameters (Angelo & Moller, 1996).

When BAEP is used to monitor neural conduction in the auditory nerve in the CPA, all peaks except peak I are expected to change when the neural conduction in the auditory nerve is affected and at risk of being surgically injured. The question is more complex when recording of BAEP is used to monitor specific structures of the brain stem. For that use, it is important to know what anatomical structures generate the different components of the BAEP.

As mentioned previously, the earliest two vertex positive peaks of the BAEP (peak I and II) are generated by the auditory nerve. These are the only components of the BAEP that have single generators. The subsequent peaks have contributions from more than one structure. Peak III and the following trough (negative peak) are generated mostly by the cochlear nucleus. Less is known about the generators of peak IV, but evidence has been presented that its generators are located close to the midline (Moller et al, 1995), probably the superior olivary complex. The sharp tip of peak V is generated mainly by the lateral lemniscus, probably where it terminates in the inferior colliculus. The slow negative wave that follows peak V (SN_{10}, Davis & Hirsch, 1979) is probably generated by dendrites in the inferior colliculus. The subsequent peaks of the BAEP (VI and VII) may be generated by cells in the inferior colliculus and the brachium of the inferior colliculus and perhaps neurons in the medial geniculate body.

PEARL

The fact that peaks I and II are generated by the auditory nerve shows that a nerve in the auditory nervous system can generate stationary peaks in recordings made at a long distance from the auditory nerve (far fields). It may also be assumed that fiber tracts of the ascending auditory pathway can generate stationary peaks in the BAEP. It is less certain, however, that cells in nuclei can generate noticeable far field potentials, but it has been convincingly demonstrated that the inferior colliculus can generate slow far field potentials (i.e., a broad peak in the BAEP). This component is known as the SN_{10} for slow negative at 10 ms. (For further details about the neural generators of the BAEP, see Moller, 1994.)

RECORDINGS DIRECTLY FROM THE AUDITORY NERVOUS SYSTEM

To provide the surgeon with timely information about injuries to the auditory nerve it is important to obtain an interpretable record in as short a time as possible. Even when all efforts are made to optimize recordings of BAEP and under the best circumstances, it takes at least 20 seconds to obtain an interpretable BAEP record in an individual with normal-hearing. In patients with hearing loss it may take several times longer. The problems obtaining an interpretable record in a short time can be overcome by recording evoked potentials directly from exposed portions of the nervous system because the amplitude of such near field evoked potentials is much larger than that of the BAEP. In fact, the amplitude of the evoked potentials recorded directly from the auditory nerve and the cochlear nucleus is large enough to be interpreted directly or after only a few responses have been added together (Moller & Jannetta, 1983a). Changes can therefore be detected almost immediately when they occur, which makes it possible to provide the surgeon with nearly instantaneous information about the function of the auditory nerve. Recordings of the CAP from the intracranial portion of the auditory nerve is now in routine use (Colletti et al, 1994; Linden et al, 1988; Silverstein et al, 1984) in operations for acoustic tumors and operations in the CPA (Moller, 1995; Moller & Jannetta, 1983a). Evoked potentials recorded from the cochlear nucleus (Moller & Jannetta, 1984, Moller et al, 1994a) are also used in operations in which the auditory nerve is at risk of being injured such as microvascular decompression operations of cranial nerves.

Recording Electrodes

Recordings of evoked potentials from the intracranial portion of the exposed eighth cranial nerve for monitoring purposes use a monopolar recording electrode (Moller & Jannetta, 1981, 1983b) that is placed directly on the exposed intracranial portion of the eighth nerve. The recording electrode should be placed as close to the brain stem as possible because it must be located proximally to the parts of the auditory nerve that are at risk of being injured (Fig. 23–2). The electrode wire should be tucked under the sutures that hold the dura open to minimize the risk that surgical manipulations dislocate the recording electrode.

A suitable monopolar recording electrode can be made from a multistrand Teflon insulated silver wire (Medwire Corp, Type Ag 7/40 T) with a small cotton wick sutured to its uninsulated tip, which is bent over, using a 5-0 silk suture (Fig. 23–2B). The purpose of the cotton wick is to reduce the risk of injury to the auditory nerve and to obtain more stable recordings than can be obtained by using a metal electrode in direct contact with the auditory nerve. It is naturally imperative that the cotton is sutured well to the wire so that it is not lost inside the brain. If that is a concern, cotton can be replaced by shredded Teflon felt that does not cause inflammatory reactions if accidentally left in the brain. It is important that the wire is flexible so that it does not injure the nerve on which it is placed and yet stiff enough that it will remain in position.

Amplifiers

The electrode wire is connected to the electrode box of the amplifier through an electrically shielded cable. The recording electrode should be connected to the inverting input so

---

PEARL

Bipolar recording electrodes are often used when recording from neural tissue for research purposes because such electrodes are more spatially selective (i.e., record from more specific neural structures). Bipolar recording electrodes have been used in recordings from the auditory nerve for research purposes (Moller et al, 1994a) and for finding the cleavage plane between the vestibular nerve and the auditory nerve (Moller et al, 1994a; Rosenberg et al, 1993). However, little reason exists to use bipolar electrodes for monitoring neural conduction in the auditory nerve because other neural structures that might contribute to the response are located anatomically far from the auditory nerve, and their contributions to the recordings from the auditory nerve using a monopolar electrode are small. It is more difficult to place a bipolar recording electrode on the exposed eighth cranial nerve.

---

that a negative potential results in an upward deflection. The other (reference) input to the amplifier should be connected to a needle electrode placed in the wound. The shielded cable should be anchored at the drape with a towel clip so that accidental pulling of that cable will not dislocate the electrode. The filters should be set at 30 to 3000 Hz, and no digital filtering is required.

Stimuli

The same stimuli as used for monitoring BAEP are suitable for eliciting direct recorded evoked potentials from the auditory nerve.

Responses

A typical CAP recorded from the exposed auditory nerve in response to click stimulation CAP is shown in Figure 23–3, together with the simultaneously recorded BAEP. The CAP has a triphasic waveform, typical for the response recorded with a monopolar electrode from a long nerve in which a brief depolarization travels past the recording electrode. The initial positive deflection is generated when the region of depolarization approaches the recording electrode and the main negative peak occurs when the depolarization passes under the recording electrode. The positive deflection that follows is generated when the depolarization moves away from the location of the recording electrode (Moller, 1995). The latency of the large negative peak of the CAP is approximately the same as peak II of the BAEP (Fig. 23–3). The latency of the CAP increases with decreasing stimulus intensity and the amplitude decreases (Fig. 23–4).

Interpretation

The waveform of the CAP is closely related to the discharge pattern of auditory nerve fibers (Goldstein, 1960) and thus provides more direct information about abnormalities in the discharge pattern of auditory nerve fibers than the BAEP.

When a monopolar recording electrode is placed on the eighth nerve close to the brain stem, passively conducted potentials from the cochlear nucleus may contribute to the

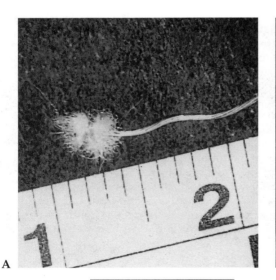
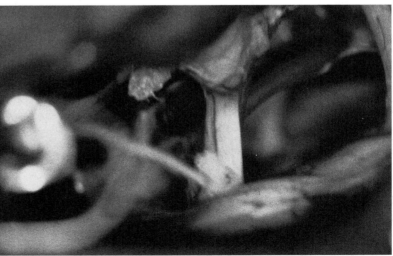

A   B

Figure 23–2   **(A)** Wick electrode used for intracranial recordings. The small divisions on the scale are millimeters. **(B)** Placement of a wick recording electrode on CN VIII for an operation to relieve hemifacial spasm. (From Moller [1988b], with permission.)

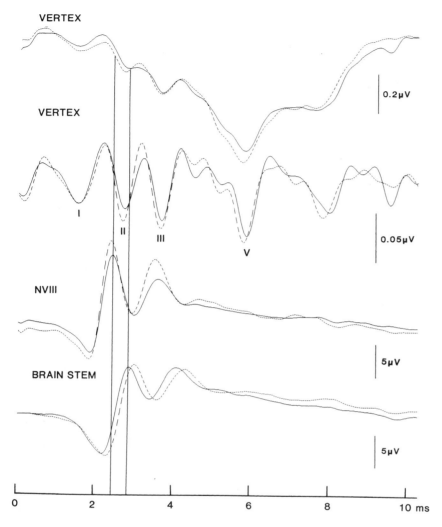

Figure 23–3 Comparison of the BAEP recorded from electrodes placed on the vertex without digital filtering (*upper tracings*) and with digital filtering (*second tracings*). Vertex positivity is a downward deflection. CAP recorded from the exposed eighth nerve (CNVIII) at two different locations, near the porus acousticus and near the brain stem. *Solid lines,* responses to rarefaction clicks; *dashed lines,* responses to condensation clicks (105 dB PeSPL). The results were obtained in a patient with normal-hearing undergoing a microvascular decompression operation.

recorded potentials, but these potentials will have longer latencies than those caused by propagated neural activity in the auditory nerve. Comparison between bipolar and monopolar recordings from the exposed eighth cranial nerve have confirmed that the CAP recorded by a monopolar electrode for the most part reflects propagated neural activity in the auditory nerve. The slow deflection seen to occur at latencies longer than that of the initial triphasic waveform probably has noticeable contributions from the cochlear nucleus. These components are more prominent in the responses to low-intensity clicks, and they are probably generated by dendrites of cochlear nucleus cells and conducted passively to the recording site on the eighth nerve from the cochlear nucleus (Fig. 23–4).

The waveform of the CAP recorded from the auditory nerve in patients with hearing loss depends on the degree of hearing loss and the nature of the pathological condition that causes the hearing loss (Fig. 23–5). The waveform of the CAP in response to condensation and rarefaction clicks is similar in patients with normal-hearing but is often very different in patients with hearing loss. The amplitude of the responses to clicks of opposite polarity may differ considerably. In some individuals the CAP in response to clicks exhibits several

waves (damped oscillations) that may last more than 10 ms (Fig. 23–5) (Moller et al, 1991). The waveform of such prolonged oscillations reverses with reversing click polarity, suggesting that these waves are the result of abnormal motion of the basilar membrane and not a sign of abnormal neural conduction in the auditory nerve.

When the polarity of a click stimulus is reversed, the initial deflection of the basilar membrane is reversed and its subsequent oscillations will be of the opposite direction (shifted 180 degrees). Thus, when the polarity of recorded potentials reverses when the stimuli are changed from condensation to rarefaction clicks, it means that the recorded potentials are depending on the direction of the deflection of the basilar membrane. Cochlear microphonic potentials have that property, but the recordings made from the intracranial portion of the auditory nerve contain negligible amounts of cochlear microphonics because of the long distance to the cochlea from the recording site. Nerve action potentials in auditory nerve fibers are initiated mainly when the basilar membrane is deflected in one direction and therefore potentials that are related to the discharges in the auditory nerve, such the CAP recorded from the intracranial portion of the auditory nerve, will also be related to the deflection of the basilar membrane.

NVIII DISTAL

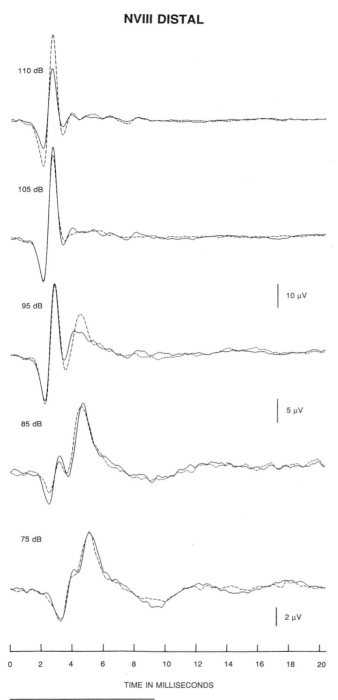

Figure 23–4 CAPs recorded from the intracranial portion of the eighth cranial nerve in a patient with normal-hearing undergoing a microvascular decompression operation for trigeminal neuralgia. The stimuli were rarefaction clicks (*solid lines*) and condensation clicks (*dashed lines*). The stimulus intensity is given by legend numbers, in dB PeSPL. (From Moller & and Jho [1991], with permission.)

Such potentials are the sum of the neural activity in many nerve fibers. Therefore large CAPs are associated with simultaneous discharges in many nerve fibers. The normal traveling wave motion of the basilar membrane does not generate such synchronous activity, and only the initial deflection of the basilar membrane generates synchronized neural activity. That is the reason the normal CAP is a single peak (N_1).

PEARL

Only when large parts of the basilar membrane vibrate in phase can prolonged oscillations occur. A standing wave motion, caused by reflections from a certain point on the basilar membrane, is a plausible explanation for these prolonged oscillations.

CHANGES IN THE COMPOUND ACTION POTENTIALS FROM INJURY TO THE AUDITORY NERVE

Injury from surgical manipulations of the eighth nerve that cause changes in the neural conduction result in different kinds of changes in the CAP when recorded from a location that is central to the location of the injury. A slight injury such as may occur from a slight stretching of the auditory nerve causes a slowing of neural conduction (decrease in conduction velocity), causing the latency of the CAP to increase (Fig. 23–6). The auditory nerve is particularly sensitive to injury from stretching where it passes through the area cribrosa (a thin bone with many perforations through which the fibers of the auditory nerve pass). Even slight stretching may cause slight bleeding in the nerve in that region (Sekiya & Moller, 1987). More severe stretching also causes broadening of the negative peak of the CAP and decreased amplitude because the increase in conduction time is different for different nerve fibers. More severe injuries may cause some nerve fibers to cease conducting nerve impulses, which results in an increase in the amplitude of the initial positive deflection and a decrease in the amplitude of the negative peak (Fig. 23–7). (Notice the difference in the response to condensation and rarefaction clicks, which is typical in patients with hearing loss.) If all fibers cease to conduct nerve impulses at a location that is distal to the location of the recording electrode, the CAP will become reduced to a single positive deflection. This is what is known as a "cut end" potential that can be recorded from a nerve that has been cut or crushed (Moller, 1995).

Severe injury to the auditory nerve that causes arrest of propagation of neural activity (Fig. 23–7) can be caused by heat that may be transferred from electrocoagulation of a vein close to the auditory nerve. Bipolar radio frequency coagulation that is now the standard form of electrocoagulation used in the brain only leak a very small amount of radio frequency current compared with monopolar electrocoagulation previously used. However, bipolar electrocoagulation does use

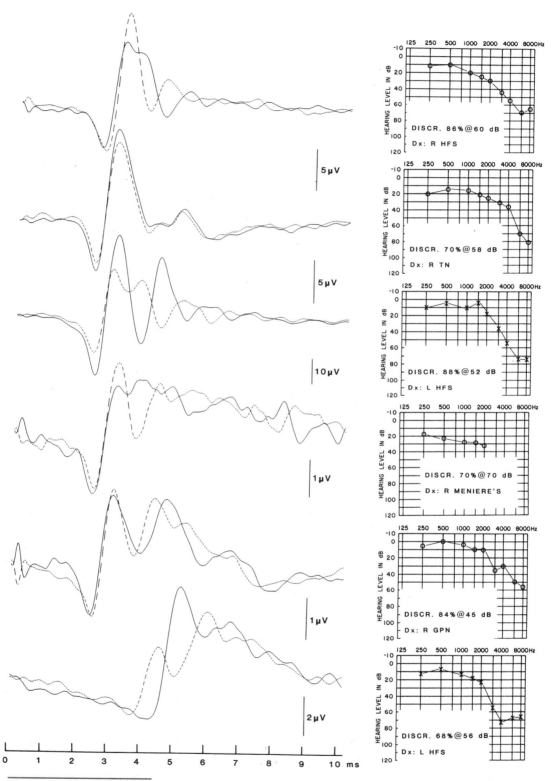

Figure 23–5 Examples of recordings from the exposed intracranial portion of the eighth cranial nerve in patients with different degrees of hearing loss. The recordings were obtained in during microvascular decompression operations before the eighth cranial nerve was manipulated. The diagnosis is given below the pure tone audiograms. (From Moller et al [1991], with permission.)

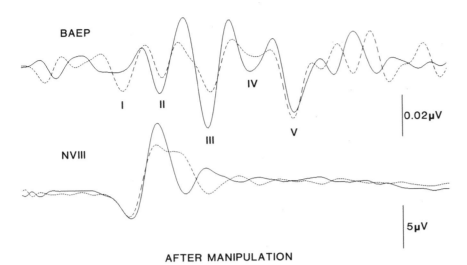

BEFORE MANIPULATION

BAEP

I II III IV V

0.02µV

NVIII

5µV

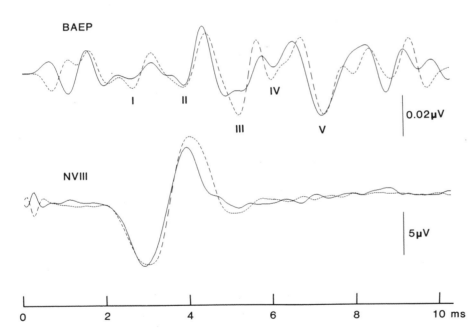

AFTER MANIPULATION

BAEP

I II III IV V

0.02µV

NVIII

5µV

0   2   4   6   8   10 ms

Figure 23–6 Comparison between the BAEP and the CAP recorded from the exposed eighth nerve before (*top tracing*) and after (*bottom tracings*) the eighth nerve was stretched to show the effect of slight injury to the auditory nerve and to the BAEP. Top recordings were obtained in the beginning of the operation and the bottom recordings were obtained after surgical manipulations of the eighth nerve. (From Moller [1995], with permission.)

heat to coagulate tissue and heat may be transferred to neural tissue and cause irreversible damage. The transfer of heat can be reduced by placing heat-insulating material between the nerve and the site of coagulation, or by using the coagulator at the lowest possible setting and by coagulating in several short spurts instead of one long burn.

The vestibular nerve cannot be monitored as readily as the auditory nerve, but protecting the auditory nerve from injury can also help to protect the vestibular nerve from injuries because these two nerves are close to each other. Manipulations that affect the auditory nerve will most likely also affect neural conduction in the vestibular nerve. The postoperative consequences of injuries to the vestibular nerve are not as obvious as those that follow from injuries to the auditory nerve; however, many people with surgically induced hearing loss also experience vestibular symptoms (Sekiya et al, 1991).

DIRECT RECORDED POTENTIALS FROM THE COCHLEAR NUCLEUS

When recording directly from the auditory nerve during operations for acoustic tumors, it may be difficult to keep the recording electrode in its correct position during tumor removal because of its proximity to the tumor. A better solution to direct recording is to place the recording electrode on (or close to) the surface of the cochlear nucleus (Moller & Jannetta, 1983a; Moller et al, 1994b). The surface of the cochlear nucleus is the floor of the lateral recess of the fourth ventricle, and a recording electrode placed in the lateral recess of the fourth ventricle will record evoked potentials from the cochlear nucleus (Moller & Jannetta, 1983a). The electrode can be placed so that it is not dislocated by surgical manipulations in

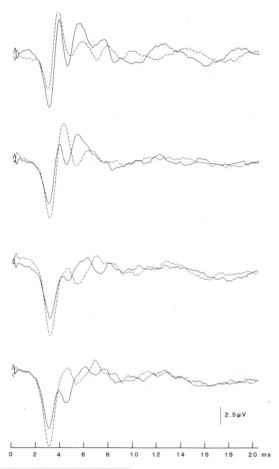

2.5 μV

0 2 4 6 8 10 12 14 16 18 20 ms

Figure 23–7 The effect of heating from electrocoagulation on the CAP recorded from the exposed intracranial portion of the eighth nerve in an individual with preoperative hearing loss. The top recording was obtained before coagulation, and the recordings below were obtained with short time intervals during electrocoagulation of a vein close to the eighth nerve. *Solid lines,* responses to rarefaction clicks; *dashed lines,* responses to condensation clicks. (From Moller [1988b], with permission.)

removing a tumor from the eighth nerve. This is the main advantage of recording from the cochlear nucleus over recording from the exposed auditory nerve.

Recording Electrodes

The same wick electrode as described earlier for recording from the exposed auditory nerve is also suitable for recordings from the cochlear nucleus. The lateral recess can be reached through the foramen of Luschka, which is located dorsal to the entrance of the ninth and tenth cranial nerves (Kuroki & Moller, 1995, Moller et al, 1994b) (Fig. 23–8). Often, a small tuft of choroid plexus can be seen to protrude from that opening, but that may be shrunk by electrocoagulation to make room for the recording electrode. In fact, suitable recordings can be obtained by placing the recording electrode on the brain stem dorsal to the entrance of the ninth and tenth cranial nerves.

When the electrode wire is placed along the caudal wall of the wound and tucked under the dura sutures, it is far away from the area of operation, and it is not at risk of being dislocated or caught by the drill used to drill the wall of the porus acousticus (Fig. 23–8).

PITFALL

Because the electrode may be placed inside the lateral recess of the fourth ventricle, it is even more critical that the cotton wick does not become dislocated or the wire break so that the wick is left inside the brain where recovering it is difficult.

Responses

The recorded potentials from the cochlear nucleus have nearly the same amplitude as those recorded from the exposed auditory nerve (Fig. 23–9). The response to transient sounds consists of an initial positive-negative deflection that signals the arrival of a volley of nerve impulses from the auditory nerve followed by a slow negative deflection that represents electrical activity in the cochlear nucleus. Recordings from the cochlear nucleus reflect injuries to the auditory nerve in a similar way as those recorded from the proximal portion of the auditory nerve. The initial positive-negative deflection is probably a better indicator of injury to the auditory nerve than the slow potential that follows.

USE OF ELECTROCOCHLEOGRAPHY TO MONITOR AUDITORY FUNCTION

As a means of obtaining auditory evoked potentials of larger amplitude than the BAEP, some investigators have used recordings of electrocochleographic (ECoG) potentials for monitoring purposes (Levine et al, 1984; Sabin et al, 1987). However, ECoG potentials only reflect the neural activity in the most distal portion of the auditory nerve. The intracranial portion of the auditory nerve can therefore be injured without any noticeable change in the ECoG.

PITFALL

Only if the blood supply to the cochlea is compromised will the ECoG potentials change noticeably. That means recording of ECoG potentials is not suitable for monitoring neural conduction in the auditory nerve in operations where the intracranial portion of the auditory nerve is at risk.

MONITORING CRANIAL MOTOR NERVES

Cranial motor nerves are at risk in operations of tumors located at the base of the skull. (We have 12 cranial nerves; some are sensory nerves, some are motor nerves, and some

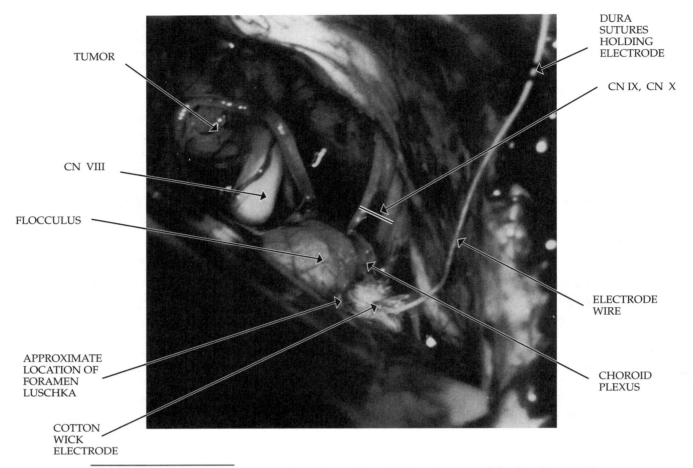

TUMOR

CN VIII

FLOCCULUS

APPROXIMATE
LOCATION OF
FORAMEN
LUSCHKA

COTTON
WICK
ELECTRODE

DURA
SUTURES
HOLDING
ELECTRODE

CN IX, CN X

ELECTRODE
WIRE

CHOROID
PLEXUS

Figure 23–8 Placement of the recording electrode in the lateral recess of the fourth ventricle. (From Moller et al [1994b], with permission.)

are part of the autonomic nervous system–see Fig. 23–10 and Table 23–1.) The most common skull base tumor is the acoustic tumor, and operations to remove acoustic tumors place the auditory and the facial nerves at risk. The auditory nerve is naturally at risk because it is directly involved in the tumor, and many patients with acoustic tumors already have hearing loss. Preservation of hearing is feasible in operations for small acoustic tumors if the patient has good hearing before the operation. In addition to the need for efforts to decrease the risk of hearing loss from surgically induced injuries to the auditory nerve, it is perhaps even more important to reduce the risks of injuries to the facial nerve causing facial weakness, synkinesis, or facial palsy. The facial nerve runs close to the auditory-vestibular nerve and it is therefore at eminent risk of being injured during removal of acoustic tumors. Impairment or loss of facial function has severe consequences and affects the entire life of a person.

Less than 20 years ago, facial nerve function was rarely preserved in operations for acoustic tumors. Now, facial function can be preserved in most operations for acoustic tumors. Several factors have contributed to the improvement in preservation of the facial nerve. Many tumors that are surgically removed are smaller now than they were some years ago because they are often detected early as a result of better diagnostic methods. The introduction of better operating equipment and refinement of surgical technique have also

contributed to a higher success rate in preserving function of these two nerves.

The introduction of IOM has also contributed to reduce the risks of impairment of facial function in operations for acoustic tumors. IOM of the facial nerve is now in common use in operations for acoustic tumors and its use has been supported by an official statement from the National Institutes of Health (1991), which stated, "There is a consensus that intraoperative real-time monitoring improves the surgical management of vestibular schwanoma, including the preservation of facial nerve function, and possibly improves hearing preservation by use of intraoperative auditory brainstem response monitoring. New approaches to monitoring acoustic nerve function may provide more rapid feedback to the surgeon, thus enhancing their usefulness. Intraoperative monitoring of cranial nerves V, VI, IX, X and XI also has been described, but the full benefits of this monitoring remains to be determined."

Removal of other skull base tumors such as those invading the cavernous sinus may place several cranial nerves in jeopardy, particularly those that innervate the extraocular muscles (i.e., the third, fourth, and sixth cranial nerves). Loss of the function of the third cranial nerve makes the eye essentially useless because that nerve, in addition to controlling three of the five extraocular muscles, controls accommodation and the size of the pupil. Impairment of the function of the other two nerves, the fourth (trochlearis) and the sixth (abducens) cranial

IPSILATERAL

VERTEX - NECK

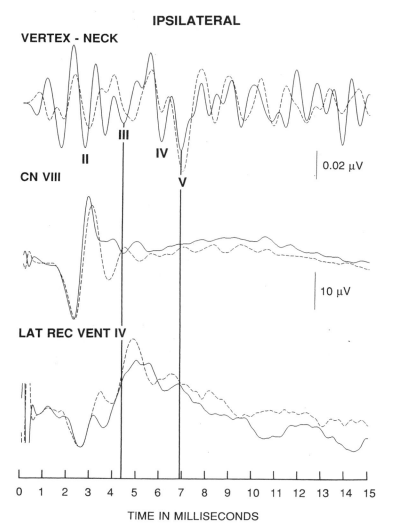

II   III   IV   V

CN VIII

0.02 µV

10 µV

LAT REC VENT IV

0   1   2   3   4   5   6   7   8   9   10   11   12   13   14   15

TIME IN MILLISECONDS

Figure 23–9 Comparison of the BAEP (*upper tracings:* digitally filtered as in Fig. 23–1, W25) together with the responses recorded from the exposed eighth nerve (*middle tracings*) and the responses recorded from an electrode placed in the lateral recess of the fourth ventricle (*lower tracings*), as shown in Figure 23–8. *Solid lines,* responses to rarefaction clicks; *dashed lines,* responses to condensation clicks. All recordings were obtained at about the same time during an operation to relieve hemifacial spasm. (From Moller et al [1994a], with permission.)

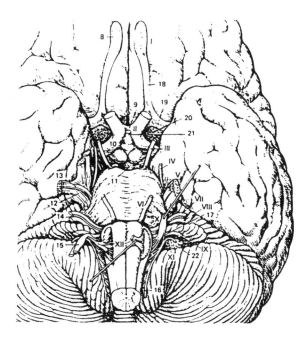

Figure 23–10 We have 12 pairs of cranial nerves; some are sensory nerves, some are motor nerves, and some are part of the autonomic nervous system. Diagram shows the anatomical location of the cranial nerves. (From Roeser [1996], with permission.)

557

TABLE 23–1   List of the main functions of cranial nerves

Number	Name	Type	Function	Description
I.	Olfactory	Sensory	Smell	
II.	Optic	Sensory	Vision	
III.	Oculomotor	Motor	Eye movements	Innervates all extraocular muscles, except the superior oblique and lateral rectus muscles; innervates the striated muscle of the eyelid
			Autonomic	Mediates pupillary constriction and accommodation for near vision
IV.	Trochlearis	Motor	Eye movements	Innervates superior oblique muscle
V.	Trigeminal	Sensory		Mediates cutaneous and proprioceptive sensations from skin, muscles, and joints in the face and mouth, including the teeth, and from the anterior two-thirds of the tongue
		Motor		Innervates muscles of mastication
VI.	Abducens	Motor	Eye movements	Innervates the lateral rectus muscle
VII.	Facial	Motor		Innervates muscles of facial expression
		Autonomic		Lacrimal and salivary glands
		Sensory		Mediates taste and possible sensation from part of the face (behind the ear)
	Nervous intermedius			Pain around the ear; possibly taste
VIII.	Vestibulocochlear	Sensory	Hearing	Equilibrium, postural reflexes, orientation of the head in space
IX.	Glossopharyngeal	Sensory	Taste	
		Sensory	Swallowing	Mediates visceral sensation from palate and posterior third of the tongue. Innervates the carotid body; innervates taste buds in the posterior third of tongue.
		Motor		Muscles in posterior throat (stylopharyngeal muscle)
		Autonomic		Parotid gland
X.	Vagus	Sensory		Mediates visceral sensation from the pharynx, larynx, thorax, and abdomen; innervates the skin in the earcanal and taste buds in the epiglottis
		Autonomic		Contains autonomic fibers that innervate smooth muscle in heart, blood vessels, trachea, bronchi, esophagus, stomach, and intestine
		Motor		Innervates striated muscles in the soft palate, pharynx, and larynx
XI.	Spinal accessory	Motor		Innervates the trapezius and sternocleidomastoid muscles
XII.	Hypoglossal	Motor		Innervates intrinsic muscles of the tongue

From Moller, A.R. (1995). *Intraoperative neurophysiologic monitoring.* Luxembourg: Harvard Academic Publishers.

nerves, causes noticeable disturbances. Loss of the fifth (trigeminal) cranial nerve is perhaps less debilitating, but loss of sensation in the face (the sensory portion of the nerve) and function of mastication (the motor portion of the nerve) may imply a considerable inconvenience.

Skull base tumors that extend caudally on the clivus (the downward sloping surface of the base of the skull to the foramen magnum) may be close to the lower cranial nerves, which therefore may become at risk of being injured during removal of such tumors. Although loss of the ninth cranial nerve on one side will affect swallowing, loss of that nerve bilaterally is life threatening because of its role in controlling blood pressure. The most noticeable deficits from loss of the function of the tenth cranial (vagus) nerve on one side is probably disturbance of closure of the vocal cords and impairment of speech. Bilateral loss of function of the vagus nerve is life threatening. Loss of function of the twelfth cranial nerve on one side paralyzes one side of the tongue and affects swallowing, and bilateral loss of the twelfth nerve may be life threatening.

In general, monitoring the function of motor nerves involves the use of a handheld electrical stimulating probe to find the anatomical location of the respective nerve while observing contractions of muscles innervated by the motor nerve in question. Injured motor nerves are likely to have spontaneous activity that can also be monitored by recording EMG potentials from the muscles innervated by the respective motor nerve. Mechanical manipulations of a nerve can cause neural activity that may persist after the manipulation has been stopped. Examination of the pattern of the spontaneous activity provides important information about the degree of injury to the nerve. Injured nerves are more likely to respond to mechanical stimulation than uninjured nerves, and the sensitivity to mechanical stimulation can therefore provide information about how much a nerve is injured. A motor nerve may have been injured before the start of the operation because of a tumor or other disease process, and it may be useful to have preoperative tests of the function of the motor nerves that are to be monitored during an operation.

MONITORING THE FACIAL NERVE IN OPERATIONS FOR ACOUSTIC TUMORS

Intraoperative monitoring of the facial nerve has been the model for monitoring other cranial motor nerves. The methods used for stimulation have been little changed during the past century, but the methods for detecting when the facial muscles contracted have been different. Earlier, the patient's face was observed by the surgeon or by an assistant. This was replaced by the use of electronic sensors introduced by Sugita and Kobayashi (1982) and further developed by other investigators (Silverstein et al, 1984). Later the use of recordings of EMG potentials has become the method of choice for detecting contraction of facial muscles (Moller & Jannetta, 1984; Prass et al 1987), and it is used in a variety of commercially available equipment.

Stimulation

A handheld electrical stimulating electrode that delivers short (0.1 ms) electrical impulses is used to probe the operative field. A return electrode is placed in the wound. Electrical stimulation of a nerve can either be constant current or constant voltage or a mixture of these two. Constant current means that the stimulator delivers an electrical current that is independent of the resistance of the tissue that is being stimulated. An electrode connected to a constant voltage stimulator applies a constant voltage to the tissue with which the stimulating electrode is in contact. That means that the electrical current that flows through the tissue that is being stimulated depends on the electrical resistance of the tissue. It is preferrable to use constant (or semiconstant) voltage rather than constant current because constant voltage stimulation will deliver a stimulus to the facial nerve that depends less on how wet the operative field is, whereas the current delivered to a nerve with constant current stimulation will vary with the electrical conductivity of the surrounding media that will shunt current away from the facial nerve to a degree that depends on how wet the operative field is. (Moller, 1995; Moller & Jannetta, 1984; Yingling, 1994).

Recording of EMG Potentials

As for recording, the BAEP needle electrodes are preferred to surface electrodes because they provide a stable recording condition over a longer period (Moller, 1995). Some investigators have advocated recording from muscles of the upper face and the lower face separately by use of two amplifiers. One amplifier is connected to electrodes placed in the forehead and the orbicularis oculi (the muscle around the eye), and the other amplifier is connected to electrodes placed in the orbicularis oris (the muscle around the mouth) and in the nasal fold. Because the objective is not to differentiate between contractions of muscles of the upper face and the lower face, others use recording of EMG potentials in only one channel with electrodes placed in the upper and the lower face (Fig. 23–11). Such recordings will reveal contractions of most muscles of the face, including the masseter and temporal muscles. These muscles are innervated by the motor portion of the trigeminal nerve, and stimulation of that nerve will therefore result in EMG activity that might be misinterpreted as resulting from stimulation of the facial nerve. However, the EMG response from the facial nerve can easily be distinguished from that of the trigeminal nerve because of the much longer latency of the response from facial muscles compared with those innervated by the trigeminal nerve (6.5 to 8 ms, vs. 1.5 to 2 ms) (Fig. 23–12). A second amplifier may become more useful when connected to electrodes placed in the masseter muscle (Fig. 23–11) to record from muscles innervated by the (motor) trigeminal nerve. This makes it easier to differentiate between the responses from muscles innervated by the facial and the trigeminal nerves including activity elicited by mechanical stimulation of the respective nerves and activity caused by injuries to these nerves.

It is now common to make the EMG potentials audible through a loudspeaker (Moller & Jannetta, 1984; Prass et al, 1987) so that the surgeon can hear when electrical stimulations cause a contraction of facial muscles. The output of mechanotransducers contains mostly low frequencies and is therefore not suitable to be presented through a loudspeaker. Instead, it has been used to trigger a tone that then signals muscle contraction. A similar method is available in commercial equipment used for recording EMG potentials. The EMG signal contains valuable information that is lost if it is used to trigger a tone.

PEARL

One reason to use mechanotransducers is to avoid the stimulus artifact from reaching the amplifier in EMG recordings. When the recorded EMG potentials are made audible, such stimulus artifacts will be disturbing and may mask the sound of the EMG potentials. The stimulus artifact can, however, be easily prevented from reaching the audio amplifier by a suitable gating circuit (Moller & Jannetta, 1984).

PRACTICAL ASPECTS OF MONITORING THE FACIAL NERVE IN OPERATIONS FOR ACOUSTIC TUMORS

Monitoring of the facial nerve in operations for acoustic tumors has three parts: finding areas of the tumor where no part of the facial nerve is present, identifying the location of the facial nerve, and detecting when the facial nerve has been injured.

Finding Areas of a Tumor Where No Part of the Facial Nerve Is Present

When operating on large acoustic tumors, the earliest use of facial nerve monitoring is to identify regions of the tumor where *no* parts of the facial nerve are present. That is done by probing the regions of the tumor before it is being removed while observing facial muscle contractions. This form of monitoring allows the surgeon to remove large volumes of the tumor without risk of injuring the facial nerve, and it shortens the operation. It also gives the surgeon an increased feeling of security in addition to decreasing the risk of permanent postoperative impairment of facial function.

At this point in a surgical procedure, preservation of the facial nerve depends on absence of a response. This places a greater demand on the settings of the stimulus intensity and the reliability of electrodes and electronic equipment because the absence of a response can also be caused by malfunction of equipment, including recording and stimulating electrodes and by the use of too low a stimulus intensity. The stimulus strength must be sufficient to activate the facial nerve at a small distance so that probing extends a few millimeters from the stimulating electrode. The stimulus strength should not be so strong that it activates the facial nerve at too large a distance because that would result in a response from large parts of the tumor. The greatest risk is to have too low a stimulus strength because that might lead to the conclusion that a certain amount of a tumor tissue could be safely removed when in fact it might contain parts of the facial nerve that then would be destroyed when the tumor tissue is removed.

Equipment failure or misplacement of recording electrodes that prevent recording of facial muscle contractions would give the surgeon the impression that no facial nerve was present in the tumor volume probed when in actuality the nerve was present. Extracting a portion of the tumor that contains parts of the facial nerve would cause severe injury to the facial nerve. To reduce that risk, the recording and stimulation system must be tested meticulously before its use. The best way of testing the facial nerve monitoring equipment is to stimulate the facial nerve before tumor removal begins. This can be done in operations for small tumors, but it is usually not possible in operations for large tumors in which other methods must be used. Observation of the stimulus artifact in the EMG recording displayed on an oscilloscope is a useful indicator that the stimulator delivers a stimulus current and that the EMG amplifier is working, but it does not guarantee that the stimulation is sufficient to elicit a facial muscle contraction, nor does it guarantee that the amplifiers of the EMG potentials work correctly. One common cause of failure is that the return electrode for the stimulator, usually a needle placed in the wound, becomes dislocated. That would affect, but not necessarily abolish, the stimulus artifact.

Another serious risk of a malfunction is that the patient has inadvertently been paralyzed, a situation that would not be revealed by observing the stimulus artifact. The best way to reduce that risk for the team that is performing the intraoperative monitoring is to keep in close contact with the anesthesia team. This would allow the monitoring team to know whether changes are made in administering anesthesia such as adding neuromuscular blocking agents.

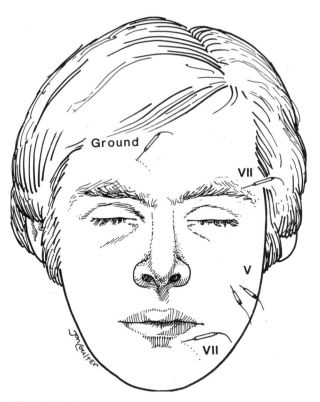

Figure 23–11 Placement of recording electrodes for recording EMG from face muscles (*VII*). Also shown is how recording can be done from the masseter muscle (*V*). (From Moller [1995], with permission.)

Identifying the Location of the Facial Nerve

When the bulk of a large tumor has been removed, the task of facial nerve monitoring is to help find the facial nerve so that the surgeon knows where it is located at all times. Finding the anatomical location of the facial nerve can be done by probing the surgical field with the handheld electrical stimulator. If moving the stimulating electrode results in an increase in the amplitude of the recorded EMG response, the facial nerve is located in the direction the electrode was moved. If moving the electrode results in a smaller response, the electrode was moved away from the nerve. The use of this method requires frequent adjustments of the stimulus strength to keep the response below its maximal amplitude. The use of this method also requires close collaboration between the person who does the monitoring and the surgeon.

The facial nerve is often divided in several parts, and it should therefore not be assumed that the entire facial nerve has been found when a response to electrical stimulation has been obtained. The entire operative field must therefore be explored with the facial nerve stimulator.

Continuous Monitoring of Facial Muscle Activity

Monitoring of the function of the facial nerve can be a great help in reducing the risk of injury to the facial nerve. Removing parts of a tumor that adhere to the facial nerve is a challenge, and safe removal of such tumor tissue is facilitated by listening to the EMG activity elicited by surgical manipulations of the facial nerve or activity elicited by injury to the facial nerve. Such activity may have several different forms, and the nature of the sound generated by the EMG activity provides information about the risks of postoperative impairments of facial function. The activity that causes the least concern is the EMG activity that is a direct response to touching the nerve with a surgical instrument and that stops immediately when the manipulation stops. The activity that continues after the manipulation is stopped may suggest a greater risk of permanent impairment of facial function. The risk of permanent impairment increases with the

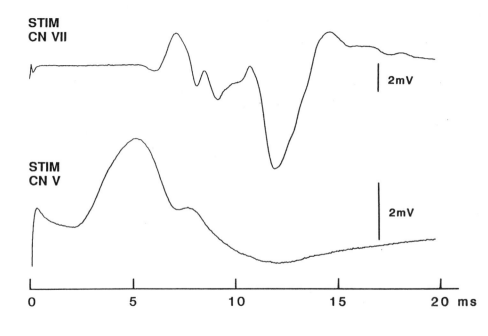

Figure 23–12 EMG potentials recorded from electrodes placed on the face, as shown in Figure 23–11, when the intracranial portion of the facial nerve was stimulated electrically (*upper tracing*) and when the motor portion (of CN V) was stimulated (*lower tracing*). (From Moller [1995], with permission.)

length of time that such activity lasts and by the number of times during the operation that surgical manipulations of the facial nerve have caused such activity. This means that surgically induced muscle activity should be avoided as much as possible. That can best be achieved by making the EMG activity audible so that the surgeon can hear the activity and moderate the manipulations accordingly (Moller & Jannetta, 1984; Prass et al, 1987). It is also important that the EMG activity of all facial muscles are represented so that manipulations of all parts of the facial nerve are monitored.

Another critical part of operations for acoustic tumors occurs when a tumor is to be removed from the facial nerve or its vicinity along its course inside the internal auditory meatus (IAC). Drilling of the bone of the IAC generates heat than can injure the facial nerve. Monitoring EMG activity from facial muscles can detect such injuries, and the surgeon should be encouraged to make pauses in manipulations or drilling that elicit such activity. Use of irrigation to cool the bone may help reduce the risk from drilling.

OTHER CRANIAL NERVES MAY BE AT RISK

Large acoustic tumors may extend rostrally to the fifth cranial nerve. Electrically stimulating the fifth nerve elicits contractions of the temporal muscle and the masseter muscle because

PEARL

The most critical part of operations for large acoustic tumors regarding preservation of the facial nerve occurs when tumor tissue is removed from near the facial nerve where it emerges from the internal auditory meatus and turns downward. That part of the facial nerve is often severely injured by the tumor, and it is often spread out to form a thin sheath of nerve tissue that has the consistency of wet tissue paper. It is therefore extremely fragile and even the slightest manipulation can destroy the nerve. Continuous monitoring of facial muscle EMG through a loudspeaker can facilitate safe removal of tumor tissue from such an injured facial nerve without causing further injury to the nerve.

PITFALL

Probing the surgical field with a surgical instrument to find the location of the facial nerve should never be used as a substitute for probing the surgical field with a handheld electrical stimulation electrode. The reason that surgical manipulations of the facial nerve often elicit facial muscle activity is most likely that the nerve is injured. A normal nerve has a low degree of sensitivity to mechanical manipulations.

they are innervated by the (motor portions of) trigeminal nerve. EMG electrodes placed on the scalp may pick up activity from these muscles. As mentioned previously, the responses from these two nerves can be distinguished on the basis of the latency of the EMG response. This requires that responses be displayed on an oscilloscope. It is even better to record from the masseter muscle with a separate recording channel (Fig. 23–11). If two recording channels for EMG potentials are available, one channel may be used to record EMG potentials from the masseter muscles (Fig. 23–12), which makes it possible to distinguish between the EMG activity elicited by mechanical stimulation of these two nerves.

OTHER SKULL BASE TUMORS

Although acoustic tumors are the most common neoplasm in the CPA, a variety of tumors may occur near the base of the skull. These tumors are often benign, and they may grow to large sizes before they give noticeable symptoms. At that stage, such tumors may affect several cranial nerves, and they may extend inside the cavernous sinus. Surgical removal of such tumors can place several cranial nerves at risk of being injured or destroyed. The nerves of the extraocular muscles are often displaced, and it may be difficult to find these nerves by visual inspection of the surgical field. Intraoperative monitoring using a handheld electrical stimulating electrode in connection with recording of EMG potentials from the extraocular muscles is often the only way to find these nerves.

Loss of function of the extraocular muscles can have severe consequences. Thus loss of function of the oculomotor nerve (third cranial nerve) renders the eye essentially useless because that nerve not only innervates three of the five extraocular muscles, it also controls accommodation and the size of the pupil. Loss of function of the lateral rectus muscle, innervated by the sixth cranial (abducens nerve) nerve makes it impossible to move the eye laterally from the midline. Loss of function of the fourth cranial nerve that innervates the superior oblique muscle has the least severe consequences but makes it difficult to look down. Tumors (chordomas) found adjacent to the base of the skull (clivus) may involve lower cranial nerves such as the hypoglossal (twelfth cranial) nerve, the loss of which may have severe and even life-threatening consequences. Loss of the fifth cranial nerve results in numbness in the face and degeneration of mastication muscles.

MONITORING THE NERVES OF THE EXTRAOCULAR MUSCLES

The principles of monitoring these cranial motor nerves intraoperatively are similar to that of monitoring the facial nerve as described above.

Recording Electrodes

EMG potentials from the extraocular muscles can be recorded by placing needle electrodes through the skin (percutaneously) into these muscles or their close vicinity (Fig. 23–13) (Moller, 1995; Moller, 1987; Sekhar & Moller, 1986). Only one electrode is placed in each muscle, and the reference elec-

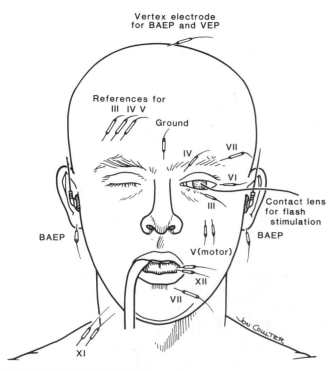

Figure 23–13 Electrode placements for recording EMG potentials from the extraocular muscles (*III, IV, VI*), the masseter muscle (*V motor*), the facial muscles (*VII*), shoulder muscles (*XI*) and the tongue (*XII*). Electrode placement for recording BAEP and a contact lens for delivering visual stimuli for recording visual evoked potentials are also shown. (From Moller [1990], with permission.)

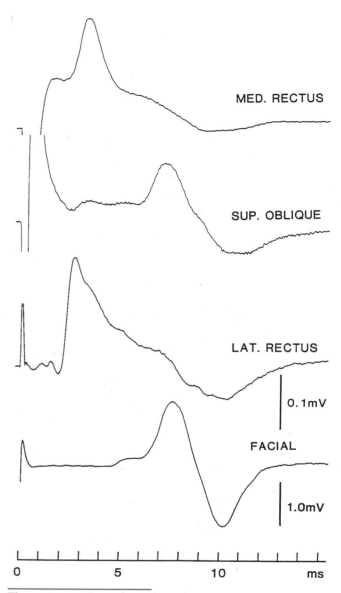

Figure 23–14 Recordings from the extraocular muscles and from facial muscles with electrodes placed as shown in Figure 23–13. The muscle contractions were elicited by electrical stimulation of the respective motor nerves intracranially. (From Moller [1987], with permission.)

trodes for all the recording electrodes should be placed on the forehead on the opposite side to avoid the interference from facial muscle contractions on the operated side. This technique has a low risk, provided that it is done by a person who is trained in the procedure and well acquainted with the anatomy. It should only be done after the patient is anesthetized, and the electrodes should be carefully removed before the patient wakes up. Such recordings yield EMG potentials of sufficient amplitude to make them visible and interpretable without averaging (Fig. 23–14). EMG potentials can also be recorded from the extraocular muscles using noninvasive recording electrodes in the form of small wire rings placed under the eyelids (Sekiya et al, 1992).

Amplifiers

One amplifier and display is required for each muscle from which EMG recordings are to be made. In most skull base operations it is also justified to record from muscles innervated by several motor nerves, a technique that may require six to eight recording channels with oscilloscopic displays. The option to mix all channels for making the EMG potentials audible or to listen to a selected channel should be available. Filter settings should be 30 to 3000 Hz.

Stimulation

The use of a handheld electrical stimulating electrode is recommended as described previously. The same principles as described for monitoring the facial nerve can be used for finding areas of a tumor where none of these other nerves are present. Identification of the location of these nerves and monitoring the neural conduction in individual nerves can be done by using the same methods as described earlier for the facial nerve. The EMG activity elicited by mechanical stimulation of the facial nerve or elicited by injury to the nerve can be monitored in the same way as described previously for the facial nerve.

MONITORING LOWER CRANIAL MOTOR NERVES

Lower cranial nerves (CN IX, CN X, CN XI, and CN XII) may be at risk in operations for large tumors at the base of the skull and in large acoustic tumors that extend caudally. Several of these nerves are mixed nerves, and it is the motor portion that is monitored. It is assumed that preserving the motor portions also preserves the sensory portions of these nerves. In general, the same principles can be used for preserving these nerves as described for preservation of the function of the facial nerve.

The motor portion of the glossopharyngeal (ninth cranial) nerve can be monitored by recording EMG potentials from muscles in the posterior palate (Lanser et al, 1992; Moller, 1995; Yingling, 1994). This nerve should be stimulated cautiously because of its possible effect on circulation (blood pressure) and the heart. When stimulating that nerve, the anesthesia team should be informed and encouraged to watch the patient's blood pressure and heart rate.

The motor portion of the vagal nerve (CN X) can be monitored by recording EMG potentials from laryngeal muscles (Lanser et al, 1992; Stechison, 1995; Yingling, 1994). The recording electrodes may be inserted in the vocal folds under laryngoscopic guidance or percutaneously or by use of a tracheal tube with conductive rings that act as recording electrodes. The vagal nerve should be stimulated with caution, and it is particularly important that a high rate of stimulation be avoided. Use of stimulus rates of 5 pps or less seems safe, but the anesthesia team must be informed when electrical stimulation is to be done.

The spinal accessory nerve (eleventh cranial nerve) can be monitored by placing EMG recording electrodes in muscles innervated by that nerve, such as the shoulder muscles (Fig. 23–13).

The hypoglossal (twelfth cranial) nerve is very small and difficult to find by visual observation, but it is easily located by probing the surgical field with a handheld electrical stimulating electrode. Its motor portion can be monitored by placing EMG recording electrodes in the lateral side of the tongue (Lanser et al, 1992; Moller, 1987, 1995; Sekhar & Yingling, 1994) (Fig. 25–13).

MONITORING THE SENSORY PORTION OF THE TRIGEMINAL NERVE

PITFALL

Monitoring the sensory portion of the trigeminal nerve is not widely performed, and evoked potentials recorded from electrodes placed on the scalp are affected by common anesthetics, which, together with uncertainties regarding the neural generators of these potentials, has prevented the general use of trigeminal evoked potentials in intraoperative monitoring.

OPTIC NERVE

Intraoperative monitoring of the optic nerve has gained some use. Visual evoked potentials recorded from electrodes placed on the scalp have been the most common method for such monitoring, but evoked potentials have also been recorded directly from the exposed optic nerve and optic tract (Moller, 1987). However, several technical factors have made it difficult to use visual evoked potentials in intraoperative monitoring. Clinical studies have shown that the optimal stimulus for eliciting visual evoked potentials for detecting pathological conditions of the optic nerve is a reversing pattern of a checkerboard (Chiappa, 1983). Because that requires that a pattern can be focused on the retina, that kind of stimulus cannot be used in an anesthetized patient, and the only stimuli that can be used in anesthetized individuals are light flashes. It has been shown that changes in the visual evoked potentials elicited by light flash are not generally good indicators of intraoperative injuries to the optic nerve and optic tract (Cedzich et al, 1988) in agreement with clinical experience (Chiappa, 1983). More recently, it has been indicated that visual evoked potentials evoked by high-intensity light flashes are better indicators of pathological conditions than evoked potentials elicited by conventional flashes generated by light-emitting diodes (Pratt et al, 1994). Therefore it may be recommended that monitoring of the optic nerve be performed using high-intensity light flashes.

MONITORING THE PERIPHERAL PORTION OF THE FACIAL NERVE

Monitoring of the peripheral portion of the facial nerve can be done by the use of similar methods as described for monitoring the intracranial portion of the facial nerve in operations of the skull base. Such monitoring is of value in several kinds of operations of the face such as operations of the parotid gland and in reconstructive and cosmetic operations of the face. Usually only one branch of the facial nerve is affected, and EMG potentials should be recorded from muscles innervated by that branch. The wound can be probed by an electrical stimulating electrode in the same way as described for removal of acoustic tumors. The latencies of the responses are shorter than those elicited by stimulation of the intracranial portion of the facial nerve, which must be taken into account when setting the duration of the suppression of the stimulus artifact.

INTRAOPERATIVE RECORDINGS THAT CAN AID THE SURGEON IN CARRYING OUT THE OPERATION

In a few operations, intraoperative neurophysiological recordings can help the surgeon carry out the operation so that the therapeutic goal is achieved. One example of that are recordings of the abnormal muscle response in patients who are treated for hemifacial spasm using the microvascular decompression technique (Haines & Torres, 1991; Moller & Jannetta, 1987). Another example is the use of recordings from the eighth nerve to help find the cleavage plane between the auditory nerve and the vestibular nerve in operations where the vestibular nerve is to be cut to treat vestibular disorders caused by hyperactivity of the vestibular organ (Rosenberg et al, 1993). Operations aimed at specific neural tissue that may not be identified visually in the surgical field may benefit from electrophysiologic recordings to identify such tissue. Considerable individual variations in anatomy are easily overlooked and may lead to mistakes. The risk of these errors may be reduced by use of electrophysiological methods as an aid in identification.

VESTIBULAR NERVE SECTION

Vestibular nerve section is one example of an operation where electrophysiological identification may help to perform a selective section of the vestibular nerve without injuring the auditory nerve (Rosenberg et al, 1993). The superior vestibular nerve and the auditory nerve have a slight difference in grayness, but it may be difficult to distinguish between these two parts of the eighth cranial nerve from visual inspection. Recording of auditory evoked potentials with a bipolar recording electrode can help in identifying the demarcation line between these two nerves (Moller et al, 1994a; Rosenberg et al, 1993) (Fig. 23–15). The evoked potentials change as the recording electrode is moved around the circumference of the intracranial portion of the eighth nerve, and the best separation between recordings from the these two nerves is achieved when a low stimulus sound intensity is used (Rosenberg et al, 1993).

HEMIFACIAL SPASM

Hemifacial spasm (HFS) is characterized by involuntary contractions of muscles in one side of the face. It can be cured by moving a blood vessel off the intracranial portion of the facial nerve, an operation known as microvascular decompression (MVD). The operation has a success rate of about 80% (Barker et al, 1995; Moller, 1991), and the reason for failure is almost always inability to identify the blood vessel that is the cause of the spasm. Monitoring the abnormal muscle response can help identify the vessel that causes the disorder. It can ensure that the therapeutic goal of the operation has been reached before the operation is ended. The abnormal muscle response (Esslen, 1957) is specific for patients with HFS and can be demonstrated by electrically stimulating one branch of the face while recording the EMG response from a muscle innervated by another branch (Fig. 23–16, Moller & Jannetta, 1987). It can be recorded during surgical anesthesia, provided that muscle relaxants are not used. This response disappears totally when the blood vessel that is related to the spasm is moved off the facial nerve. The success rate of these operations increased considerably after the recording method was introduced as routine monitoring during MVD operations for HFS (Haines & Torres, 1991; Moller & Jannetta, 1987). Introduction of these electrophysiological techniques has nearly eliminated the need for re-operations. In addition to increasing the success rate, such monitoring also gives the surgeon an increased feeling of

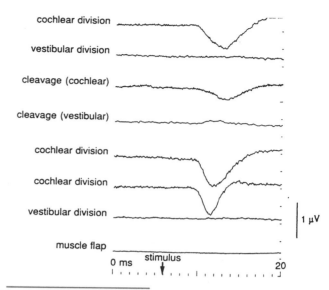

Figure 23–15 Bipolar recordings of auditory evoked potentials from the intracranial portion of the eighth cranial nerve. The stimuli were clicks at 25 dB above threshold for the BAEP. (From Rosenberg et al [1993], with permission.)

security. It has often shortened the operating time because it makes it unnecessary to look for other vessels when the one that caused this abnormal muscle response to disappear has been found.

RISKS AND PROBABILITIES

Intraoperative monitoring should not be regarded as a method for providing warnings of imminent disasters but instead as a source of information that can help the surgeon carry out the operation in the safest possible way and reduce the likelihood of emergency situations. To fulfill that goal, it is important that the person who is responsible for the monitoring is knowledgeable about the physiology of the systems that are monitored and understands what signs indicate change in neural function. The person who conducts the monitoring must also have good knowledge about the operation and be present in the operating room at all times when risk of injury to neural tissue exists. It is also essential that frequent contact with the surgeon and the anesthesia team be maintained. The latter is especially important in monitoring motor nerves. Not only surgical manipulations cause change in the potentials that are monitored, and the person who is responsible for monitoring must be able to discriminate significant changes from insignificant changes.

PRACTICAL ASPECTS OF PERFORMING ELECTROPHYSIOLOGICAL RECORDINGS IN THE OPERATING ROOM

Monitoring must be well planned so that all necessary equipment is available immediately, and contingency plans must be in place for covering equipment failure and other unforeseen events.

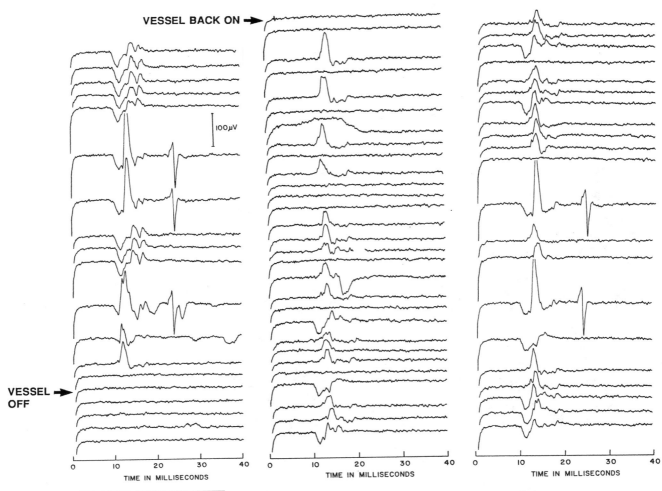

VESSEL BACK ON →

100 μV

VESSEL → OFF

TIME IN MILLISECONDS

TIME IN MILLISECONDS

TIME IN MILLISECONDS

Figure 23–16 Recordings of the abnormal muscle response from the mentalis muscle in response to electrical stimulation of the peripheral portion of the zygomatic branch of the facial nerve presented at a rate of 10 pps obtained in a patient undergoing a microvascular decompression operation for hemifacial spasm. The top part of the left column shows consecutive EMG recordings before the offending blood vessel was lifted off the facial nerve. At the arrow, the vessel was lifted off the nerve, and it fell back on the nerve as marked at the top of the middle column. (From Moller & Jannetta [1985], with permission.)

Clinical use of electrophysiological tests such as evoked potentials customarily involves comparison of the obtained results with a standard that is the average of results obtained in many individuals without (known) pathological conditions. Intraoperative recordings instead compare the obtained responses with the patient's own preoperative test results. That provides a higher sensitivity, which means that smaller changes in the recorded potentials can be used as signs of injuries than would be the case if the results were compared with a laboratory standard. The baseline recording of evoked potentials such as the BAEP is preferably obtained after the patient is anesthetized but before the operation is started.

Although recording evoked potentials and EMG potentials in the clinic and the operating room is similar in many ways, they are also different in many ways. One important difference is that the recordings in the operating room must

be interpreted immediately. Another difference is that it is the deviation from individual patient's own recordings that are important in the operating room and not deviations from a standard. To do recordings in unconscious individuals is naturally different from clinical tests of awake patients.

It has often been claimed that the large amount of electrical equipment in the operating room produces so much electrical interference that it is difficult (or impossible) to record small electrical potentials such as the BAEP. However, it is possible to reduce the effect of such interference to a degree that makes it possible to obtain high-quality evoked potentials, even when the amplitude is small as with the BAEP. The technique for reducing the electrical interference in the operating room has been described in detail elsewhere (see, e.g., Moller, 1995).

Electrodes placed on the head are usually out of reach after the patient has been draped and therefore must be secured to reduce the risk that they will come off. Having extra electrodes placed can be valuable in ensuring that monitoring does not need to be aborted because an electrode fails. Needle electrodes usually provide a stable recording condition over many hours, whereas surface electrodes may be dislocated or change recording conditions over time. Needle electrodes, however, involve a small risk of causing burns where they are inserted. This may occur when electrocautery is used. It is mainly electrocautery equipment of old types that have such a risk. It may also occur if the return electrode of the electrocautery is faulty in one way or another. It is extremely rare when modern equipment is used (see Moller, 1995).

EFFECT OF ANESTHESIA

Anesthesia does not affect the auditory evoked potentials discussed in this chapter, but a common component of anesthesia, namely muscle relaxation, makes it impossible to record EMG potentials from muscles. That means that the anesthesia regimen must often be altered when muscle contractions are recorded. The patient's temperature may fall during long operations and that may affect auditory evoked potentials slightly. When monitoring depends on recording of muscle contractions with EMG recordings or other methods, arrangements must be made with the anesthesiologist before the operation, preferentially the previous day to ensure that the patient will not be paralyzed. Equipment for stimulating the facial nerve should be in place and tested before the operation begins.

WHEN ARE PREOPERATIVE AND POSTOPERATIVE TESTS IMPORTANT?

The patients who are to be monitored in an operation should have preoperative tests of the systems that are to be monitored. If it is not possible to obtain a response before the operation, it is unlikely that it would be possible in the operating room and it would be wasted effort to try. Failure to obtain a response in the operating room could be a result of equipment failure and that should be remedied. Alternately, it could be a preoperative pathological conditions that prevented successful recording. For similar reasons, it is important to test motor systems that are to be monitored preoperatively. The preoperative evoked potential recordings may be used as baseline for the intraoperative recordings, but it is better to obtain a baseline recording after the patient is anesthetized but before the operation begins. Having adequate preoperative hearing tests is important for interpretation of intraoperative tests. It is also important to have preoperative tests for detecting any postoperative deficits or worsening of preoperative deficits. For that, it is also necessary to repeat the preoperative tests after the operation.

RISK INVOLVED IN INTRAOPERATIVE MONITORING

Intraoperative monitoring that is intended to reduce risk can itself be a risk, much like medication intended to be beneficial to health may have side effects that can cause pathological conditions. Inadvertently stimulating nervous tissue with too high electrical current is one mistake that may occur. It can be avoided if the stimulating equipment is not able to deliver currents that pose risks. It can be reduced, but not eliminated, by adequate training of the people who operate the equipment. Another, more complex risk is to monitor the wrong system and by that not detect changes from surgical manipulations. An example is placing the EMG recording electrodes on the wrong side of the face in an operation for an acoustic tumor or applying the sound stimulation to the ear opposite to the side where an operation involves the auditory nerve.

WHAT SHOULD BE REPORTED TO THE SURGEON?

It has been suggested that the surgeons should only be informed when the changes in the recorded potentials indicate a high likelihood for permanent neurological deficits if the manipulation that caused the changes was not reversed. However, it is our experience that it is preferable to inform the surgeon immediately when a change has occurred that was larger than the normal small variations that occur without any known cause (Moller, 1995). That makes it easy for the surgeon to identify the cause of the change and it gives the surgeon several options. One option is to do nothing and wait to see whether the changes increase. If the surgeon knows what caused the change, the manipulation may be reversed at any time. Another option is to immediately reverse the manipulation, and that has the advantage that the surgeon does not need to be concerned about the problem in the future. If the surgeon is not informed until the change has reached a dangerous level, his or her options become limited. If attempts to reverse the injury are unsuccessful, the results may be that the patient will get a permanent postoperative neurological deficit. It may not be known what has caused the change because of the time that has elapsed between the occurrence of the change in function and the time the surgeon was informed. Surgeons who choose to reverse an injury immediately after it has been discovered have far fewer incidents of permanent neurological deficits than surgeons who choose the "wait and see" option.

WHICH OPERATIONS TO MONITOR?

Intraoperative monitoring that is aimed at reducing the risk of surgically induced injuries to neural tissue should be considered whenever neural tissue is being surgically manipulated. Because the risk involved in different operations varies and the reduction of the risks of postoperative permanent deficits that can be achieved by IOM varies between different kinds of operations, it has been thought to be unnecessary to monitor some operations. The risks and the benefits of IOM also vary between surgeons with different degrees of training and experience. The selection of operations for monitoring must therefore rely on the availability of resources, the risk without monitoring, and the reduction in risks that can be achieved with monitoring. Most risk calculations, however, show that IOM is economically sound because of large costs involved in caring for people with neurological deficits. IOM can also act as a teaching aid in that electrophysiological recordings can point to which manipulations may cause injuries and therefore which manipulations should be avoided. From a human perspective, the advantages of IOM are even greater and may serve as an example of a situation in which suffering can be reduced by a small economic sacrifice.

WHICH SURGEONS MAY BENEFIT FROM MONITORING?

Intraoperative monitoring is likely to benefit surgeons in different ways, depending on the experience of doing a particular operation. Also, surgeons with different levels of experience may benefit from different aspects of intraoperative monitoring. Monitoring the facial nerve in operations for acoustic tumors may serve as an example. An extremely experienced surgeon may feel more comfortable having IOM available to help confirm anatomy, even if it may provide only a modest reduction of facial nerve injuries. The slightly less experienced surgeon may have a greater reduction in facial nerve injuries and will be able to carry out the operation considerably faster with IOM than without IOM. The moderately experienced surgeon will always benefit from confirmation of the anatomical location of the facial nerve and will benefit from knowing when surgical manipulations cause injuries. IOM will usually help any surgeon to do the operation much faster and is likely to help improve surgical skills, regardless of experience.

PEARL

Many highly experienced surgeons who can operate with a high degree of safety with few complications will not operate without the aid of IOM because they believe that IOM reduces the risks of complications and because it gives them a feeling of safety so that they can operate with greater ease.

HOW TO DETERMINE THE BENEFITS OF INTRAOPERATIVE MONITORING

For several reasons, it has been difficult to do controlled studies of the benefits of IOM. Ethical reasons and the surgeons' reluctance to deprive their patients from the benefit of intraoperative monitoring have made it difficult to do studies of the benefits from IOM using randomly selected patients for monitoring. Studies based on comparisons between the rate of complications before and after introduction of monitoring have been published (Moller & Moller, 1989, Radtke et al, 1989), but such studies have been criticized because it has been claimed that other improvements in the operations could have accounted for the lower rate of complications. The fact that different surgeons achieve different degrees of reduction of complications, depending on their experience, is also a factor that adds to the difficulty in determining what operations would benefit from intraoperative monitoring. This is one reason why intraoperative monitoring has been officially regarded as beneficial in relatively few operations, but regarded as indispensable by many individual surgeons performing a variety of the operations. IOM for preservation of facial function during operations for acoustic tumors is an exception because it has received official recommendation (Consensus Statement by the National Institutes of Health, 1991).

CONCLUSIONS

IOM is foremost an aid that can help to reduce the risk of permanent neurological injuries, but surgeons also benefit in other ways from the use of intraoperative electrophysiological recordings. Thus IOM often helps the surgeon to perform better, and the use of IOM can reduce operating time in some operations. It is also important for developing better operating techniques, and IOM is an important teaching aid for surgical residents. In some operations IOM may directly help the surgeon achieve the therapeutic goals of the operation. These benefits are difficult to evaluate quantitatively but they should nevertheless not be ignored when the value of IOM is assessed.

REFERENCES

ANGELO, R., & MOLLER, AR. (1996). Contralateral evoked brain stem auditory potentials as an indicator of intraoperative brain stem manipulation in cerebellopontine angle tumors. *Neurology Research, 18*;528–540.

BABIN, R.W., JAI, H.R., & McCABE, B.F. (1982). Bipolar localization of the facial nerve in the internal auditory canal. In: M.D. Graham, & W.F. House (Eds.). *Disorders of the facial nerve: Anatomy, diagnosis, and management* (pp. 3–5). New York: Raven Press.

BARKER, F.G., JANNETTA, P.J., BISSONETTE, D.J., SHIELDS, P.T., & LARKINS, M.V. (1995). Microvascular decompression for hemifacial spasm. *Journal of Neurosurgery, 82*;201–210.

BROWN, R.H., & NASH, JR., C.L. (1979). Current status of spinal cord monitoring. *Spine, 4*;466–478.

CEDZICH, C., SCHRAMM, J., MENGEDOHT, C.F., & FAHLBUSCH, R. (1988). Factors that limit the use of flash visual evoked potentials for surgical monitoring. *Electroencepholography and Clinical Neurophysiology, 71*;142–145.

CHIAPPA, K.H. (1983). Evoked potentials in clinical medicine. In: A.B. Baker, & L.H. Baker (Eds.). *Clinical neurology* (Vol. 1.) (pp. 1–55). Philadelphia, PA: JB Lippincott.

COLLETTI, V., BRICOLO, A., FIORINO, F.G., & BRUNI, L. (1994). Changes in directly recorded cochlear nerve compound action potentials during acoustic tumor surgery. *Skull Base Surgery, 4*;1–9.

DAVIS, H. & HIRSH, S.K. (1979). A slow brain stem response for low-frequency audiometry. *Audiology, 18*;445–461.

DELGADO, T.E., BUCHHEIT, W.A., ROSENHOLTZ, H.R., & CHRISSIAN, S. (1979). Intraoperative monitoring of facial muscle evoked responses obtained by intracranial stimulation of the facial nerve: A more accurate technique for facial nerve dissection. *Journal of Neurosurgery, 4;*418–421.

DOYLE, D.J., & HYDE, M.L. (1981). Analogue and digital filtering of auditory brain stem responses. *Scandinavian Audiology. (Stockholm),* 10;81–89.

ESSLEN, E. (1957). Der spasmus facialis—eine Parabioseerscheinung. *Dtsch Z Nervenh,* 176;149–l72.

FISCHER, C. (1989). Brain stem auditory evoked potential (BAEP) monitoring in posterior fossa surgery. In: J.E. Desmedt (Ed.). *Neuromonitoring in surgery* (pp. 191–218). Amsterdam: Elsevier Science Publishers.

FRIEDMAN, W.A., KAPLAN, B.J., GRAVENSTEIN, D., & RHOTON, A.L. (1985). Intraoperative brain stem auditory evoked potentials during posterior fossa microvascular decompression. *Journal of Neurosurgery,* 62;552–557.

GOLDSTEIN, M.H., JR. (1960). A statistical model for interpreting neuroelectric responses. *Information and Control,* 3;1–17.

GRUNDY, B.L. (1983). Intraoperative monitoring of sensory evoked potentials. *Anesthesiology,* 58;72–87.

HAINES, S.J., & TORRES, F. (1991). Intraoperative monitoring of the facial nerve during decompressive surgery for hemifacial spasm. *Journal of Neurosurgery,* 74;254–257.

HARNER, S.G., DAUBE, J.R., BEATTY, C.W., & EBERSOLD, M.J. (1988). Intraoperative monitoring of the facial nerve. *Laryngoscope,* 98;209–212.

HATAYAMA, T. & MOLLER, A.R. (1998). Correlation between latency and amplitude of peak in the BAEP: Intraoperative recordings in microvascular decompression operations. *Acta Neurochirugica. (Wien),* 140;681–687.

HILGER, J. (1964). Facial nerve stimulator. *Transactions of the American Academy of Ophthalmology and Otolaryngology,* 68;74–76.

HOKE, M., ROSS, B., WICKESBERG, R., & LUETKENHOENER, B. (1984). Weighted averaging—Theory and application to electrical response audiometry. *Electroencephalography and Clinical Neurophysiology,* 57;484–489.

JAKO, G. (1965). Facial nerve monitor. *Transactions of the American Academy of Ophthalmology and Otolaryngology,* 69;340–342.

KALMANCHEY, R., AVILA, A., & SYMON, L. (1986). The use of brain stem auditory evoked potentials during posterior fossa surgery as a monitor of brain stem function. *Acta Neurochirurgica (Wien),* 82;128–136.

KARTUSH, J.M., & BOUCHARD, K.R. (1992). Intraoperative facial nerve monitoring. Otology, neurotology, and skull base surgery. In: J.M. Kartush, & K.R. Bouchard (Eds.). *Neuromonitoring in otology and head and neck surgery* (pp. 99–120). New York: Raven Press.

KRAUZE, F. (1912). *Surgery of the brain and spinal cord* (First English Edition) (pp. 738–743). Rebman Company.

KUROKI, A., & MOLLER, A.R. (1995). Microsurgical anatomy around the foramen of Luschka with reference to intraoperative recording of auditory evoked potentials from the cochlear nuclei. *Journal of Neurosurgery,* 82;933–939.

LANG, J. (1985). Anatomy of the brain stem and lower cranial nerves, vessels, and surrounding structures. *American Journal of Otology,* (suppl. November); 1–19.

LANSER, M.J., JACKLER, R.K., & YINGLING, C.D. (1992). Regional monitoring of lower (ninth through twelfth) cranial nerves.

In: J.M. Kartush, & K.R. Bouchard (Eds.). *Neuromonitoring in otology and head and neck surgery* (pp. 131–150). New York: Raven Press.

LEONETTI, J.P., BRACKMANN, D.E., PRASS, R.L. (1992). Improved preservation of facial nerve function in the infratemporal approach to the skull base. *Otolaryngology–Head and Neck Surgery,* 101;74–78.

LEVINE, R.A., OJEMANN, R.G., MONTGOMERY, W.W., & McGAFFIGAN, P.M. (1984). Monitoring auditory evoked potentials during acoustic neuroma surgery. Insights into the mechanism of the hearing loss. *Annals of Otology, Rhinology and Laryngology,* 93;116–123.

LINDEN, R.D., TATOR, C.H., BENEDICT, C., CHARLES, D., MRAZ, V., & BELL, I. (1988). Electrophysiological monitoring during acoustic neuroma and other posterior fossa surgery. *Le Journal Canadien des Sciences Neurologiques,* 15;73–81.

MOLLER, A.R. (1987). Electrophysiological monitoring of cranial nerves in operations in the skull base. In: L.N. Sekhar, & V.L. Schramm, Jr. (Eds.).*Tumors of the cranial base: Diagnosis and treatment* (pp.123–132). Mt. Kisco, NY: Futura Publishing Co.

MOLLER, A.R. (1988a). Use of zero-phase digital filters to enhance brain stem auditory evoked potentials (BAEPs). *Electroencephalography and Clinical Neurophysiology,* 71;226–232.

MOLLER, A.R. (1988b). *Evoked potentials in intraoperative monitoring.* Baltimore, MD: Williams & Wilkins

MOLLER, A.R. (1990). Intraoperative monitoring of evoked potentials: An update. In: R.H. Wilkins, & S.S. Rengachary (Eds.). *Neurosurgery update I. Diagnosis, operative technique, and neuro-oncology* (pp. 169–176). New York: McGraw-Hill Inc.

MOLLER, A.R. (1991). The cranial nerve vascular compression syndrome: I. A review of treatment. *Acta Neurochirurgica. (Wien),* 113;18–23.

MOLLER, A.R. (1994). Neural generators of auditory evoked potentials. In: J.T. Jacobson (Ed.). *Principles and applications in auditory evoked potentials* (pp. 23–46). Boston, MA: Allyn & Bacon.

MOLLER, A.R. (1995). *Intraoperative neurophysiologic monitoring.* (pp. 1–343) Luxembourg: Harwood Academic Publishers.

MOLLER, A.R., COLLETTI, V., & FIORINO, F. (1994a). Click evoked responses from the exposed intracranial portion of the eighth nerve during vestibular nerve section: Bipolar and monopolar recordings. *Electroencephalography and Clinical Neurophysiology,* 92;17–29.

MOLLER, A.R., & JANNETTA, P.J. (1981). Compound action potentials recorded intracranially from the auditory nerve in man. *Experimental Neurology,* 74;862–874.

MOLLER, A.R., & JANNETTA, P.J. (1983a). Monitoring auditory functions during cranial nerve microvascular decompression operations by direct recording from the eighth nerve. *Journal of Neurosurgery,* 59;493–499.

MOLLER, A.R., & JANNETTA, P.J. (1983b). Auditory evoked potentials recorded from the cochlear nucleus and its vicinity in man. *Journal of Neurosurgery,* 59;1013–1018.

MOLLER, A.R, & JANNETTA, P.J. (1984). Preservation of facial function during removal of acoustic neuromas: Use of monopolar constant-voltage stimulation and EMG. *Journal of Neurosurgery,* 61;757–760.

MOLLER, A.R., & JANNETTA, P.J. (1985). Microvascular decompression in hemifacial spasm: Intraoperative electrophysiological observations. *Neurosurgery,* 16;612–618.

Moller, A.R, & Jannetta P.J. (1987). Monitoring facial EMG responses during microvascular decompression operations for hemifacial spasm. *Journal of Neurosurgery, 66;*681–685.

Moller, A.R. & Jho, H.D. (1991). Effect of high-frequency hearing loss on compound action potentials recorded from the intracranial portion of the human eighth nerve. *Hearing Research, 55;*9–23.

Moller, A.R, Jho, H.D., & Jannetta, P.J. (1994b). Preservation of hearing in operations on acoustic tumors: An alternative to recording BAEP. *Neurosurgery, 34;*688–693.

Moller, A.R., Jho, H.D., Yokota, M., & Jannetta, P.J. (1995). Contribution from crossed and uncrossed brain stem structures to the brain stem auditory evoked potentials (BAEP): A study in human. *Laryngoscope, 105;*596–605.

Moller, A.R, & Moller, M.B. (1989). Does intraoperative monitoring of auditory evoked potentials reduce incidence of hearing loss as a complication of microvascular decompression of cranial nerves? *Neurosurgery,24;*257–263.

Moller, A.R., Moller, M.B., Jannetta, P.J., & Jho, H.D. (1991). Auditory nerve compound action potentials and brain stem auditory evoked potentials in patients with various degrees of hearing loss. *Annals of Otology, Rhinology, and Laryngology, 100;*488–495.

National Institutes of Health (NIH) Consensus Development Conference (held December 11-13, 1991). (1991). *Consensus Statement, 9*(4);1–24.

Prass, R.L., Kinney, S.E., Hardy, R.W., Hahn, J.F., & Lueders, H. (1987). Acoustic (loudspeaker) facial EMG monitoring: Part II. Use of evoked EMG activity during acoustic neuroma resection. *Otolaryngology–Head and Neck Surgery, 97;*541–551.

Pratt, H., Martin, W.H., Bleich, N., Zaaroor, M., & Schacham, S.E. (1994). A high-intensity, goggle-mounted flash stimulator for short-latency visual evoked potentials. *Electroencephalography and Clinical Neurophysiology, 92;*469–472.

Radtke, R.A., Erwin, W., & Wilkins, R.H. (1989). Intraoperative brain stem auditory evoked potentials: Significant decrease in post-operative morbidity. *Neurology, 39;*187–191.

Raudzens, P.A. (1982). Intraoperative monitoring of evoked potentials. *Annals of the New York Academy of Science, 388;*308–326.

Rosenberg, S.I., Martin, W.H., Pratt, H., Schwegler, J.W., & Silverstein, H. (1993). Bipolar cochlear nerve recording technique: A preliminary report. *American Journal of Otology, 14;*362–368.

Sabin, H.I., Bentivoglio, P., Symon, L., Cheesman, A.D., Prasher, D., & Momma, F. (1987). Intraoperative electrocochleography to monitor cochlear potentials during acoustic neuroma excision. *Acta Neurochirurgica (Wien), 85;*110–116.

Schimmel, H. (1967). The $(+/-)$ reference: Accuracy of estimated mean components in average response studies. *Science, 157;*92–94.

Sekhar, L.N., & Moller, A.R. (1986). Operative management of tumors involving the cavernous sinus. *Journal of Neurosurgery, 64;*879–889.

Sekhar, L.N., Schramm, Jr., V.L. (1987). (Eds.) *Tumors of the cranial base: Diagnosis and treatment.* Mt. Kisco, NY: Futura Publishing Co., Inc.

Sekiya, T., Hatayama, T., Iwabuchi, T., & Maeda, S., (1992). A ring electrode to record extraocular muscle activities during skull base surgery. *Acta Neurochirurgica. (Wien), 117;*66–69.

Sekiya, T., Iwabuchi, T., Hatayama, T., & Shinozaki, N. (1991). Vestibular nerve injury as a complication of microvascular decompression. *Neurosurgery, 29;*773–775.

Sekiya, T., & Moller, A.R. (1987). Cochlear nerve injuries caused by cerebellopontine angle manipulations. An electrophysiological and morphological study in dogs. *Journal of Neurosurgery, 67;*244–249.

Sgro, J.A.S., Emerson, R.G., & Pedley, T.A. (1989). Methods for steadily updating the averaged responses during neuromonitoring. In: J.E. Desmedt (Ed.). *Neuromonitoring in surgery* (pp. 49–60). Amsterdam: Elsevier Science Publishers.

Silverstein, H., Norrell, H., Hyman, S. (1984). Simultaneous use of CO_2 laser with continuous monitoring of eighth cranial nerve action potential during acoustic neuroma surgery. *Otolaryngology–Head and Neck Surgery, 92;*80–84.

Stechison, M.T. (1993). The trigeminal evoked potential: Part II. Intraoperative recording of short-latency responses. *Neurosurgery, 33;*639–644.

Sugita, K., & Kobayashi, S. (1982). Technical and instrumental improvements in the surgical treatment of acoustic neurinomas. *Journal of Neurosurgery, 57;*747–752.

Yingling, C.D. (1994). Intraoperative monitoring in skull base surgery. In: R.K. Jackler, & D.E. Brackmann (Eds.). *Neurotology* (pp. 967–1002). St. Louis, MO: Mosby–Year Book.

## Chapter 24

Assessment of Vestibular Function

M. Wende Yellin

Dizziness and vertigo are subjective sensations that afflict an estimated 5 million individuals a year (National Ambulatory Medical Care Survey, 1991). Symptoms may be mild, lasting only a few minutes, to quite severe, resulting in total incapacity. In addition to dizziness, individuals may experience headaches and muscle aches; motion sickness, nausea and vomiting; and fatigue and loss of stamina. Balance disturbance in the form of dizziness, vertigo, or disequilibrium affects people of all ages and walks of life. It is predicted that as the population of the United States ages, the number of individuals seeking medical attention for dizziness will dramatically increase.

Evaluation of patients reporting vertigo and dizziness is complicated and complex. To maintain balance, information from the visual, somatosensory, and vestibular systems must be acquired and integrated. A disorder in any one of these systems may induce dizziness, vertigo, or disequilibrium, but compensatory contributions from the unaffected systems often obscure the true site of the lesion. The challenge faced in evaluating vestibular function lies in differentiating input received from each system and determining the area of dysfunction.

Audiologists working in medical settings are assuming a major role in evaluating balance disturbance because many patients have both auditory and vestibular problems. In fact, a thorough evaluation of the patient with dizziness should include assessments of both auditory and balance function to provide a comprehensive analysis of the patient's condition (Rubin, 1990; Yellin and Mainord, 1996). This responsibility often lies with the audiologist because of the link between the auditory and vestibular systems and the audiologist's expertise in these areas. The American Academy of Audiology (AAA) and American Speech-Language and Hearing Association (ASHA) have recognized vestibular assessment within the audiologist's scope of practice (AAA, 1997; ASHA, 1996).

This chapter will provide a comprehensive overview of procedures involved in the clinical assessment of vestibular function. The purpose is to familiarize audiologists with tests available to assess the balance system and to describe practical aspects of integrating these tests into the clinical workup of the patient with dizziness. The anatomy and physiology of the vestibular system and evaluation of the auditory system through electrocochleography (ECoG) and auditory brain stem response (ABR) audiometry are discussed in other chapters within this volume (see Chapters 4, 18, and 19). This chapter will discuss the evaluation of balance dysfunction by reviewing patient case history and preparation for assessment, describing evaluation procedures and the physiological processes assessed, and reviewing the interpretation of test results.

PATIENT HISTORY

The causes of dizziness, vertigo, and balance disorder are numerous and considerable (Brown, 1990; Dickins & Graham, 1986; Ojala & Palo, 1991). The pathological conditions associated with balance disturbance are as follows:

Head trauma or neck injury
Central nervous system (CNS) disorders, such as multiple sclerosis (MS) or seizure disorder
Embolism, aneurysm, tumor, or transient ischemic attack (TIA)
Metabolic disorders such as diabetes, hypoglycemia, and thyroid disease
Ocular problems, such as glaucoma, refractive errors, and ocular muscular imbalance

Audiology: Diagnosis. Edited by Roeser, Valente, and Hosford-Dunn. Thieme Medical Publishers, Inc., New York © 2000

Proprioceptive or musculoskeletal system disorder, including Paget's disease, and spinal degeneration with cervical arthritis

Vestibular dysfunction caused by Meniere's disease, perilymph fistula, vestibular neuronitis, benign paroxysmal positional vertigo, and labyrinthitis

Cerebellopontine angle (CPA) tumor

Cerebral hypoxia, arteriosclerosis and hypertensive cardiovascular disease, and postural hypotension

Symptoms may develop after injury or trauma to the head or neck. CNS disorders, such as MS or seizure disorder may cause dizziness. Embolism, aneurysm, tumor, or TIA often present with symptoms of balance disturbance. Dizziness can be induced by metabolic disorders such as diabetes, hypoglycemia, and thyroid disease. Ocular problems, such as glaucoma, refractive errors, and ocular muscular imbalance, and disorders of the proprioceptive or musculoskeletal system, including Paget's disease and spinal degeneration with cervical arthritis, can cause dizziness. Vestibular dysfunction caused by Meniere's disease, perilymph fistula, vestibular neuronitis, benign paroxysmal positional vertigo, and labyrinthitis may induce balance disturbance. The presence of a CPA tumor must be considered. In older patients dizziness can be related to cerebral hypoxia, arteriosclerosis and hypertensive cardiovascular disease, and postural hypotension. Because of the numerous possibilities, the evaluation should begin with a complete medical history to explore the presence of these precipitating disorders or illnesses.

After obtaining the medical history, it is important to define the symptoms comprehensively. Areas explored should include onset of symptoms, characteristics of symptoms at onset, the progression of symptoms over time, current symptoms, the nature and duration of typical spells, and past or current medications and treatment strategies (Shepard & Telian, 1994). Generally, dizziness refers to one's perception of the body in space, but it is important to encourage the patient to provide a more precise description. The patient may include terms such as giddiness, wooziness, faintness, light-headedness, or vertigo, and although dizziness may include the sensation of vertigo, vertigo itself refers to the sensation or hallucination of movement. A patient who reports that the environment is spinning is experiencing objective vertigo, whereas the patient who feels a spinning sensation is experiencing subjective vertigo. The patient may report disequilibrium and describe symptoms of stumbling or falling, clumsiness, swaying, or instability. Defining the patient's symptoms provides a better understanding of the total disability.

The impact of the symptoms on the patient's daily activities is another area to be discussed with the patient. Transitory symptoms may be a mere annoyance to one person but debilitating to another. To evaluate the functional, physical, and emotional effects of balance disturbance on the patient, the Dizziness Handicap Inventory (DHI) was developed (Jacobson & Newman, 1990; Jacobson et al, 1991). The DHI consists of 25 items requiring a "yes," "no," or "sometimes" response (see Appendix). Responses provide insight into the patient's perception of the balance disturbance and its effect on the quality of the patient's life.

Once the patient's symptoms have been clarified and their impact determined, a patient profile develops and differential diagnosis begins (Baloh, 1995). In general, dizziness accompanied by light-headedness or floating indicates a nonvestibular balance disorder. Symptoms tend to be continuous and constant, can be precipitated by stress, and exacerbate in specific situations. Episodic vertigo or spinning is usually consistent with a vestibular site of the disorder. Accompanying the vertigo are sensations of drunkenness or motion sickness and feelings of falling to one side or tilting. Severe vertigo associated with hearing loss, tinnitus, nausea, and vomiting is usually of peripheral origin, whereas vertigo with neurological symptoms of diplopia, dysarthria, numbness, or weakness is of central origin. Once symptoms are categorized, formal assessment begins.

PRETEST PREPARATION

For convenience to the patient and consistency of results, all balance function tests should be scheduled during a single block of time. Patients undergoing the complete battery should report to their appointment prepared for 3 to 4 hours of testing. Information regarding test procedures and patient preparation should be provided at least 1 week before the scheduled appointment and should include the following pre-evaluation patient information:

Information regarding test procedures
  Name of the test.
  Purpose of the test.
  Brief description of test procedures.
  Expectations of the patient.
  Length of time for test battery.
Patient responsibilities
  Wear loose and comfortable clothing.
    Women should wear pants instead of dresses or skirts.
  No make-up and no oil to skin the day of the test.
  Little or nothing to eat for the 4 hours before testing.
    If a morning appointment, skip breakfast or toast and juice.
    If an afternoon appointment, early breakfast and skip lunch or only a clear broth or dry sandwich allowed.
    No consumption of caffeine drinks, such as coffee or cola beverage, the day of the test.
  No use of tobacco the day of the test.
  Medications
    Medications taken for heart problems, high blood pressure, diabetes, seizure prevention, or other medical conditions should not be interrupted.
    Tranquilizers, sedatives, vestibular suppressants, and alcohol must be discontinued for at least 48 hours before testing.

To ease anxiety, the patient should receive information about the tests ordered. This information should include the name of the test, the purpose of the test, a brief description of test procedures, and expectations of the patient. When the patient understands the nature of the tests and the variety of procedures that are included, concern over 4 hours of testing can be reduced.

Instructions should be provided regarding test day protocol. The patient should be told to wear loose and comfortable clothing. It is preferable that women wear pants instead of dresses or skirts. Women also should not wear make-up, and both men and women should not apply oil to their skin the day of the test. Because some of the tests may cause dizziness and/or nausea, the patient should have little or nothing to eat for the 4 hours before testing. If a morning appointment is scheduled, it is preferable for the patient to skip breakfast; if some nourishment is necessary, only toast and juice should be allowed. If an afternoon appointment is scheduled, it is preferable for the patient to eat breakfast early in the morning and skip lunch; if some nourishment is required, only a clear broth or dry sandwich should be allowed. The patient should not consume any caffeine drinks, such as coffee or cola beverage, or use tobacco the day of the test because caffeine and tobacco may affect test results.

It is critical and mandatory that instructions be provided to the patient concerning the use of medications before testing. Medications taken for heart problems, high blood pressure, diabetes, seizure prevention, or other medical conditions should not be interrupted. Tranquilizers, sedatives, vestibular suppressants, and alcohol must be discontinued for at least 48 hours before testing (Cass & Furman, 1993; Goebel et al, 1995). The presence of these medications in the patient's system can inaccurately indicate brain stem–cerebellar dysfunction, CNS dysfunction, or vestibular system dysfunction. If discontinuing these medications incapacitates the patient to the point that testing cannot be performed, the patient should be allowed to take the medications, but use of the medications should be included in the report, and results should be cautiously reviewed and interpreted, indicating the possible influence of the medications on all findings.

ELECTRONYSTAGMOGRAPHY

One of the oldest tests developed to evaluate vestibular function is electronystagmography (ENG). ENG is based on electro-oculography, a technique that objectively records eye movements by measuring the corneoretinal potential (Coats, 1975). ENG can provide important information often missed in more recently developed imaging and electrophysiological procedures and therefore continues to be an essential part of the diagnostic battery of inner ear function.

Because of the complex organization of the vestibulo-ocular system, innervation of the semicircular canal receptors influences eye motion on the horizontal plane. When the head is rotated, movement of the endolymph causes the normal individual to produce compensatory eye movements away from the fluid motion. The eyes will move slowly until they reach maximum deviation and then return quickly back into position because of CNS correction before repeating the compensatory motion. This activity generated by the vestibulo-ocular reflex (VOR) is identified as nystagmus.

Nystagmus has a saw-tooth appearance. The slow phase is induced by inner ear fluid movements that produce eye motion; the fast phase reflects the CNS correction. Nystagmus is identified by the direction of the fast phase of the eye movement, being left beating or right beating on the horizontal plane and up beating or down beating on the vertical plane (Fig. 24–1). The intensity of nystagmus is determined by measuring the angle of the slow phase of the nystagmoid movement, known as the slow phase velocity (SPV). SPV is reported in degrees of rotation per second.

To perform the test, electrodes are placed near the outer canthi of each eye to record horizontal movements and above and below one eye to measure vertical movements

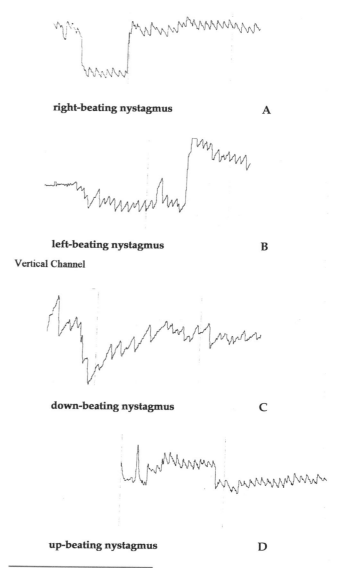

right-beating nystagmus **A**

left-beating nystagmus **B**

Vertical Channel

down-beating nystagmus **C**

up-beating nystagmus **D**

Figure 24–1 Examples of **(A)** right-beating nystagmus; **(B)** left-beating nystagmus; **(C)** up-beating nystagmus; and **(D)** down-beating nystagmus.

(Fig. 24–2). The individual undergoes various forms of stimulation, and the ocular response is recorded by means of the corneoretinal potential and sent to equipment for analysis. Traditionally, recordings were made using a strip chart, and the clinician would subjectively evaluate the accuracy of the responses and measure and calculate the SPV of nystagmus. More recently, computer programs have been developed that present the stimuli, filter and amplify the recordings, and analyze the response. With computer technology, more precise interpretation can be achieved.

SPECIAL CONSIDERATION

If a patient is blind in one eye or if the clinician notes disconjugate eye movements, electrodes should be coupled only around the better eye.

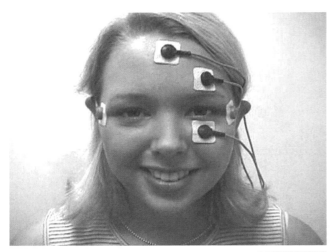

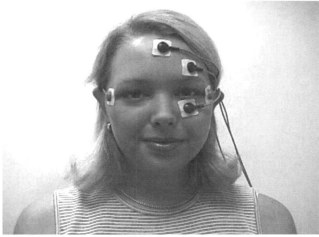

Figure 24–2 Electrode placement for ENG testing.

The ENG evaluation consists of a battery of subtests that includes measurements of spontaneous nystagmus, the saccade test, gaze test, sinusoidal tracking test, optokinetic test, Dix-Hallpike positional test, positional tests, bithermal caloric test, and assessment of the ability to suppress nystagmus by fixation (Brookler, 1991; Coats, 1975; Resnick & Brewer, 1983; Stockwell, 1983; Teter, 1983; Therapeutics and Technology Assessment Subcommittee, 1996). The ENG test battery and an overview explanation of ENG results is described in the following and listed in Table 24–1.

Spontaneous Nystagmus

Spontaneous nystagmus is involuntary, unprovoked, repetitive eye movement that can appear in any direction or be rotary. It is present in all head positions when the eyes are closed or opened. It is measured early in the ENG evaluation because the presence of spontaneous nystagmus can influence the interpretation of all subsequent test results (Teter, 1983).

To perform this procedure, the patient is seated upright with the back supported. Eyes are closed. Ocular movements are recorded continuously for approximately 30 seconds while the patient performs a concentration task to prevent suppression of the response.

The presence of spontaneous nystagmus is a nonlocalizing finding but indicates the presence of a pathological condition within the vestibular system (Brandt, 1993; Stockwell, 1983). In acute stages of peripheral vestibular disease, spontaneous horizontal nystagmus appears toward the unaffected ear. In later stages it may reverse itself or diminish. If spontaneous nystagmus is maintained when the eyes are open, or if direction-changing spontaneous nystagmus is observed, it is indicative of a CNS disorder.

Saccade Test

The saccade test evaluates the eyes' ability to rapidly shift the point of visual fixation. The saccade movement is the most rapid movement the oculomotor system is capable of performing (Evans & Melancon, 1989). This test requires the patient to fixate at a point for several seconds, then rapidly switch to a new point and fixate for several seconds without any head movement. This test is often performed as the ENG test equipment is calibrated.

To perform the test, the patient is seated upright with the back supported facing the stimulus bar. The patient is asked to follow a target that randomly moves back and forth in an arc ranging from 5 to 30 degrees. Testing is performed with the stimulus bar in the horizontal position to measure horizontal saccadic movements. The bar is then turned 90 degrees so that vertical saccadic eye movements can be evaluated. Testing proceeds for approximately 60 seconds in each direction or until eye movements have been measured at several points on the stimulus bar.

TABLE 24–1   ENG test battery and description of findings

Test	Abnormality	Interpretation
Saccadic eye movement	Ocular dysmetria, characterized by overshoot, undershoot, glissades, pulsions occurring over 50% of the time in the recording.	CNS pathological condition, involving the cerebral cortex, brain stem, or cerebellum.
Gaze test	Persistent nystagmus recorded for ocular displacements of 30 degrees or less.	CNS pathological condition, indicating brain stem or cerebellar disturbance.
Sinusoidal tracking test	Breakup of smooth pursuit.	Cerebellar dysfunction and inner ear, eye, and neurological disorder, and systemic conditions affecting the CNS.
Optokinetic test	Asymmetry in amplitude of response.	CNS pathological condition.
Spontaneous nystagmus test	Involuntary, unprovoked, repetitive eye movement that can appear in any direction.	Nonlocalizing finding but indicates the presence of pathological condition within the vestibular system.
Dix-Hallpike positional test	Sudden onset of nystagmus approximately 10 seconds after positioning that intensifies 20–30 seconds after positioning, then diminishes. Fatigued response when repeated.	Peripheral site of disorder consistent with benign paroxysmal positional vertigo.
Positional nystagmus test	Involuntary, unprovoked, repetitive eye movement that can appear in any direction.	Nonlocalizing, consistent with lesions in either the peripheral or central vestibular pathway, or both.
Bithermal caloric tests	UW: SPV differs by 20–30% or more between ears DP: Nystagmus in one direction is more intense than responses in the other direction. If no UW, a difference of 20% or more between right-beating and left-beating nystagmus is significant; if UW is present, a difference of 30% or more right-beating and left-beating nystagmus is significant. BW: SPV on each side is less than approximately 12 degrees/s.	UW: Peripheral (nerve and/or end organ) vestibular site of lesion. DP: Nonlocalizing finding, suggesting either a peripheral or central vestibular abnormality. BW: Either CNS disorder or peripheral vestibular abnormality.
Ability to suppress nystagmus by fixation	Inability of CNS to attenuate caloric nystagmus when the eyes are opened.	Brain stem and/or cerebellar disease.

Eye motion is evaluated for latency, velocity, and accuracy of the response (Honrubia, 1995). Normal tracings are rectangular in shape and occur within a specified latency. In pathological cases, the patient is unable to accurately follow the target. The four most common patterns of saccadic inaccuracy are undershoot dysmetria, overshoot dysmetria, glissades, and pulsions (Hain, 1993). Although these patterns are sometimes observed transiently in normal patients, they are considered abnormal if they occur more than 50% of the time in the recording. The presence of ocular dysmetria indicates a CNS pathological condition involving the cerebral cortex, brain stem, or cerebellum (Konrad, 1991; Sataloff & Hughes, 1988).

Gaze Test

The gaze test looks for nystagmus when the head is stable and upright and the eyes are in a fixed position.

To perform the test, the patient is seated upright with the back supported facing the stimulus bar. Five separate, 30-second recordings are made as the patient fixates at a target placed at 0 degrees azimuth, displaced 30 degrees to the right of the center spot, 30 degrees to the left of the center spot, 30 degrees above the center spot, and 30 degrees below the center spot.

PEARL

Eye blinks may appear as right-beating or left-beating nystagmus in the horizontal channel. If horizontal nystagmus is observed, check the vertical channel response for the presence of sharp, eye-blink movements.

Any persistent nystagmus recorded for ocular displacements of 30 degrees or less is considered abnormal. The presence of gaze nystagmus is consistent with a CNS pathological condition, indicating brain stem or cerebellar disturbance (Coats, 1975; Sataloff & Hughes, 1988).

Sinusoidal Tracking Test

The sinusoidal tracking test examines the ocular smooth pursuit system.

To perform the test, the patient is seated upright with the back supported facing the stimulus bar. The patient is instructed to fixate on a target moving in a sinusoidal pattern that extends 20 degrees to the right and left from center. The head must remain stable. The target movement progresses from low frequency (slow moving) to high frequency (fast moving). If an automated light bar is not available, gross assessment may be obtained by having the patient watch the movement of a pendulum. To make a pendulum, a small weight may be suspended from a pencil.

Normal responses from the sinusoidal tracking test are characterized by smooth, sinusoidal movements whose amplitudes correspond to the motion of the target. The most common abnormality observed is breakup of smooth pursuit, which suggests cerebellar dysfunction. Abnormal patterns have also been associated with diseases of the inner ear, eyes, neurological disorders, and systemic conditions affecting the CNS (Evans & Melancon, 1989; Hain, 1993). However, results from this test must be interpreted with caution because performance is strongly affected by attention.

Optokinetic Test

The optokinetic (OPK) test measures nystagmus elicited by repetitive movement of stimuli across the visual field. The test has been compared with "watching cars on a moving train" because the stimuli are constantly moving lights or stripes. Although the test is intended to test OPK nystagmus, it is actually considered a fast pursuit ocular task because the entire visual field is usually not filled in the ENG setting.

To perform the test, the patient is seated upright with the back supported facing the stimulus bar. Specific instructions depend on the stimulus being used. If a stimulus bar with moving lights is incorporated, the patient is instructed to watch the lights as they move across the center of the stimulus bar. If a stimulus drum, consisting of alternating black and white stripes, is used, the patient is instructed to watch either the black stripes or white stripes as they appear in the visual field. It is critical to remind the patient not to fixate but to watch the series of moving stimuli.

Stimuli are presented horizontally, moving from right to left for approximately 20 seconds, then left to right for 20 seconds. Stimuli are next presented vertically, moving from bottom to top for approximately 20 seconds, then top to down for approximately 20 seconds. The stimuli are presented at a fast speed (40 degrees/s), and a slow speed (20 degrees/s). Be aware that responses from vertical upward movements may be contaminated by eye blinks.

Results of the OPK test are analyzed for symmetry in each direction of pursuit. If asymmetry is observed, responses are considered abnormal and indicative of a CNS pathological condition (Teter, 1983).

Dix-Hallpike Positional Test

The Dix-Hallpike positional test is designed to elicit nystagmus caused by benign paroxysmal positioning vertigo (BPPV). BPPV is caused by dislodged otoconia settling in the posterior semicircular canal, generating a gravity-dependent cupula deflection (cupulolithiasis). Symptoms of BPPV include brief attacks of vertigo precipitated by rapid head extension and tilt toward the affected ear, like rolling from side to side in bed.

Patient cooperation is essential for accurate test performance. The patient should be instructed to lie down quickly in the supine position and to remain in that position for at least 1 minute. The patient should be told that the maneuver may induce intermittent dizziness and that it is important to report the onset of dizziness and its resolution to the clinician. As a check on patient reporting, the clinician should ask if the patient is "dizzy" during testing.

> ### PITFALL
>
> **The patient must be screened for a history of neck or back injury or impairment before performing the Dix-Hallpike maneuver and positional tests. If the patient reports any such problems, perform these tests only after obtaining medical clearance.**

To perform the Dix-Hallpike maneuver, the patient is seated upright and unsupported with the head turned. At the count of 3, the clinician quickly repositions the patient to the supine position with the head turned and extended off the end of the table. This position is maintained for a minimum of 60 seconds, with the patient's eyes opened and fixed. The clinician observes the eyes as ocular recordings are made.

A classical, positive Dix-Hallpike test is characterized by the sudden onset of nystagmus approximately 10 seconds after the head is positioned that intensifies to maximum severity approximately 20 to 30 seconds after positioning and then diminishes and resolves approximately 40 to 60 seconds after positioning. Linear-rotary nystagmus that the patient is unable to fixate will be observed by the clinician (Katsarkas, 1987). The patient will also report a burst of severe vertigo and nausea (Brandt, 1993). Once the first set of symptoms resolve, the patient remains in position because another attack may occur and resolve. When the patient returns to the seated position, nystagmus may reappear but in the opposite direction. If the response just described is obtained, the maneuver is repeated in the same direction with the same results, albeit with reduced intensity.

The Dix-Hallpike maneuver is performed with the head turned to the right then to the left. It must be completed before positional testing is performed because positional testing may diminish or obliterate the response. Spontaneous nystagmus must be assessed before the maneuver so the presence of spontaneous nystagmus is not interpreted as a positive, non-classical result.

Positional Nystagmus Test

Positional testing is performed to determine the effect of head and body movement on spontaneous nystagmus or to elicit nystagmus in response to stationary head and body positions.

Testing is performed after the Dix-Hallpike maneuver. The patient is instructed to turn into a position and remain in that position with the eyes closed for approximately 30 seconds. While in position, the patient performs concentration tasks to prevent suppression. Positions commonly used include head hanging, supine, head right and head left in supine position, and right lateral and left lateral (completely on side).

After spontaneous nystagmus is ruled out, the presence of positional nystagmus is nonlocalizing, consistent with lesions in either the peripheral or central vestibular pathway or both (Evans and Melancon, 1989; Stockwell, 1983). In general, horizontal positional nystagmus caused by peripheral lesions has a latency of 2 to 10 seconds, is maintained for 10 to 20 seconds, and fatigues with repetition, whereas that of central origin has no latency, lasts 30 seconds or longer, is not fatiguable, and may be direction changing (Parker, 1993). The presence of up-beating or down-beating vertical positional nystagmus is usually indicative of midbrain, brain stem, or cerebellar lesions (Kanaya et al, 1994; Parker, 1993).

Bithermal Caloric Tests

Bithermal caloric testing is often considered the most important part of the ENG battery because it specifically isolates and evaluates the ability of each horizontal semicircular canal to respond to a stimulus. Irrigating the external auditory canal (EAC) warms or cools the skin of the EAC and tympanic membrane, transmitting a temperature change to the endolymph in the horizontal semicircular canal (Jacobson & Newman, 1993). This temperature change causes induction currents in the horizontal semicircular canals, simulating endolymphatic fluid movements like those that occur during head rotation. Warm stimulation causes ampullopetal (toward the ampulla) movement of the horizontal canal cupula, and cool stimulation causes ampullofugal (away from the ampulla) movement of cupula. In response to this movement hair cell activity in the crista increases and generates nystagmus. The expected physiological responses to thermal stimulation are left-beating nystagmus to right cool stimulation, right-beating nystagmus to left cool stimulation, left-beating nystagmus to left warm stimulation, and right-beating nystagmus to right warm stimulation. By stimulating each external auditory canal with a warm stimulus and a cool stimulus, the physiological integrity of the left and right horizontal semicircular canals can be evaluated separately and compared.

Before testing begins, instructions should be given to prepare the patient for the test. Start off by explaining that this part of the ENG isolates the contributions of each inner ear system to balance function. Each system will be presented a

---

> **PEARL**
>
> To help remember the expected direction of nystagmus induced by caloric stimulation, the acronym, COWS, is used, meaning cold (stimulation)—opposite (direction nystagmus); warm (stimulation)—same (direction nystagmus).

cool stimulus followed by a warm stimulus to change the temperature of the inner ear fluids. Responses will be measured and compared to determine whether each system is responding and whether the contribution from each system is "equal." Explain that each system will be measured separately, starting with cool to the right ear, then to the left ear, then warm to the left ear and finally to the right ear. Breaks of 5 to 10 minutes will be taken between each stimulation. The patient will need to stay relaxed throughout testing with the eyes closed performing concentration tasks until told to open the eyes and fixate on a point. It is important to warn the patient that caloric stimulation may induce vertigo and/or nausea that will diminish as the inner ear fluids return to normal so that if symptoms occur the patient will not be alarmed. Once any questions are answered that the patient may have, testing begins.

Three types of irrigators have been developed for caloric stimulation. The water irrigator consists of two "baths" containing warm and cool water, temperature-sensing devices, thermostats to heat the water, a switch that gates water flow controlled by a foot pedal, a switch that controls the volume of water flow, and a delivery system that presents the water in the EAC. The main disadvantages of water irrigation include the inconvenience of purging the system before each caloric stimulation to ensure correct water temperature, the need to recover water flowing out of the EAC, the possibility of water contamination, and the potential for electrical shock. To address these concerns, the closed-loop water irrigation system was developed. The closed-loop system also consists of two "baths" with thermostats; however, water flows through a thin-walled silicone balloon that is placed in the EAC to induce the temperature change. The problems associated with water flow are therefore avoided. The third type of irrigation system is the air caloric irrigator. The air irrigator consists of an air flow regulator, a heater, a thermostat, and a hose or speculum through which air is delivered to the EAC. The advantages of air stimulation are the ability to visualize the tympanic membrane during stimulation and convenience.

The patient is placed in a supine position, eyes closed, with the head lifted and resting at a 30-degree angle. Recordings begin as the temperature-controlled stimulus is presented to the ear for approximately 30 seconds. During stimulation, the patient performs a concentration task. Once stimulation ends, the patient maintains his or her position with the eyes closed and continues performing the concentration task for approximately 30 more seconds. Finally, the clinician asks the patient to open his or her eyes and fixate on a point for 10 to 15 seconds. Once fixation is obtained, testing is completed, recording stops, and the patient may relax until the next stimulation.

PITFALL

The EAC and tympanic membrane must be examined for abnormalities before caloric stimulation. If the patient has a perforation of the tympanic membrane, air calorics must be used to prevent water from entering the middle ear space. Caution must be taken, however, because warm air can cool fluid moistening the canal of a draining ear, resulting in a cool stimulation and the presence of nystagmus that is opposite from that which is expected.

Each EAC is stimulated twice, once using a stimulus 7° C greater than (44° C) and once at 7° C (30° C) less than normal body temperature. A 5 to 10 minute rest is taken between each stimulation to allow the inner ear system to return to a neutral condition.

The SPV of the induced nystagmus is the most useful variable for quantifying the caloric response. For each caloric stimulation, the SPV is quantified by averaging 10 consecutive beats of nystagmus at the peak of the caloric response. Right ear responses are compared with left ear responses to determine unilateral weakness (UW) or canal paresis, and right-beating nystagmus is compared with left-beating nystagmus to determine directional preponderance (DP) (Coats, 1975).

Results from the caloric test can identify several abnormalities (Evans & Melancon, 1989; Jacobson et al, 1993). A UW is present when the SPV differs by 20 to 30% or more between ears and suggests a peripheral (nerve and/or end organ) vestibular site of the lesion (Fig. 24–3). A DP is identified when responses in one direction of nystagmus are more intense than responses in the other direction. If no UW is present, a difference of 20% or more between right-beating and left-beating nystagmus is considered significant; if a UW is present, a difference of 30% or more between right-beating and left-beating nystagmus is considered significant. The presence of a DP is a nonlocalizing finding, suggesting either a peripheral or central vestibular abnormality. Fixation suppression (FS) evaluates the ability of the CNS to control vestibular nuclei and attenuate caloric nystagmus when the eyes are opened. Failure of fixation suppression suggests brain stem and/or cerebellar disease. A bilateral weakness (BW) is demonstrated when the SPV induced from caloric irrigations on each side is less than approximately 12 degrees/s. BW can be caused by both CNS disorders and peripheral vestibular abnormalities. The presence of a BW therefore must be interpreted with information from other diagnostic procedures.

Advantages and Disadvantages of Electronystagmography

ENG offers several advantages over other measures of balance function. First, because nystagmus is the only physical sign uniquely linked to the vestibular system, ENG is a crucial tool in evaluating the vestibular system. Second, ENG recordings can be made with the eyes closed as well as open, which becomes critical when it is realized that pathologically significant nystagmus is completely suppressed by visual fixation and cannot be seen by any examiner with the patient's eyes open. Third, ENG is capable of detecting subtle abnormalities of both volitional and reflex eye movement controlled at the brain stem and higher levels that cannot be detected by any other techniques. Thus ENG may provide the only substantial and documentable evidence of brain stem dysfunction. Fourth, ENG is the only clinical test that can unequivocally isolate one labyrinth from its contralateral partner. Finally, ENG provides a permanent, objective record that can be reviewed after it was made and compared with new tracings to establish a serial record of the evolution of dysfunction or to document improvement.

PITFALL

Although ENG testing is able to identify the site of the lesion, the sensitivity is low and rarely is it possible to identify the site of the lesion from test results.

Despite these advantages, the test has some drawbacks. The caloric part of ENG testing does not use a true physiological stimulus because caloric irrigation is not a natural occurrence. The caloric stimulus is also subject to a variety of variables that are not under the examiner's control. Such variables include the shape and size of the individual patient's external auditory canal, the thickness and position of the tympanic membrane, the size of the tympanic cavity, and the thickness of bone and pneumatization of the patient's middle ear and mastoid. To minimize the effects of such variables, test protocol demands that the examiner efficiently prepares the skin to ensure good contact between the electrodes and skin, recalibrates equipment before every examination, and removes cerumen that might compromise caloric stimulation. The most effective ENG clinician must be firm and thorough but treat the patient tactfully and compassionately to gain confidence and cooperation. Only with the patient's full cooperation can accurate and consistent results be obtained.

SINUSOIDAL HARMONIC ACCELERATION

Sinusoidal harmonic acceleration (SHA) testing assesses balance function by measuring eye movements (nystagmus) induced in response to back-and-forth sinusoidal movement of a motorized chair. Barany (1907) first demonstrated the presence of nystagmus after rapidly turning a patient from side-to-side, but research was limited because of difficulties controlling chair acceleration and deceleration and the inability to effectively measure eye movements.

The development of torque-driven motors to control chair rotation and computer software to record nystagmus led to renewed interest in rotational testing. Because SHA testing simulates natural environmental motion to evaluate vestibular function, it has become an integral part of the standard balance function protocol.

When the head is rotated on the vertical axis, the horizontal semicircular canals on each side of the head are simultaneously stimulated (Jacobson & Newman, 1991). This activity is complementary but proportional. Head movements to the

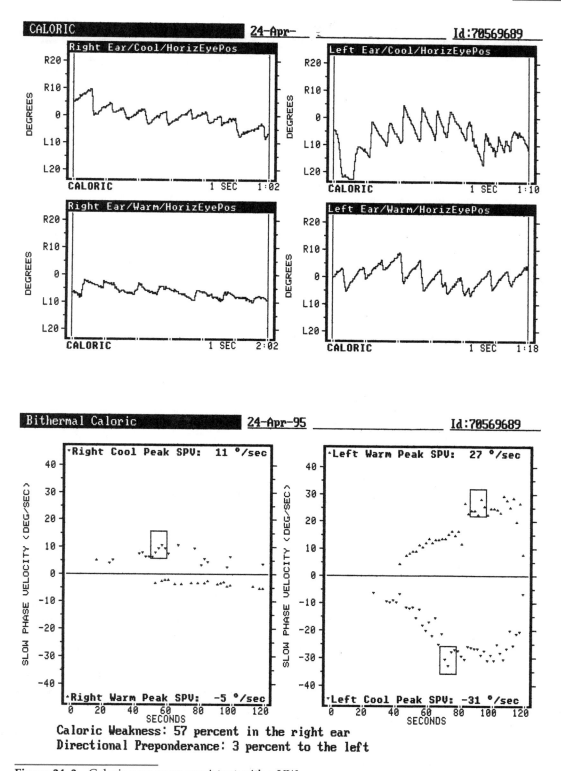

Figure 24–3 Caloric responses consistent with a UW.

right increase neural discharge from the right labyrinth and decrease neural discharge from the left labyrinth, whereas head movement to the left increases left labyrinth neural activity and decreases right labyrinth neural activity. These changes in discharge rate induce nystagmus. By measuring the VOR response, information can be obtained concerning the activity and interactions of the right and left vestibular systems.

The SHA software includes several subtests and the rotational test battery (Jacobson & Newman, 1991) is as follows:

Saccadic eye movement test*
Smooth pursuit*
Optokinetic nystagmus
Gaze nystagmus*
Spontaneous nystagmus
Rotational testing
Fixation of nystagmus during rotational testing

Subtests include measurements of spontaneous nystagmus, the saccade test, gaze test, sinusoidal tracking test, and the OPK test. Although these tests may be excluded if ENG testing is being performed, it is necessary to repeat the spontaneous nystagmus test, and it is beneficial to perform the OPK test. The spontaneous nystagmus test allows the clinician to calculate the influence of spontaneous nystagmus on SHA results. OPK testing in SHA conditions provides a true measure of OPK nystagmus that is not achieved with ENG parameters because the entire visual field can be stimulated with rotating stripes, and the patient's ability to stabilize the condition can be assessed.

To perform the SHA test, the patient is seated in a computer-driven chair located in a concentric booth that is lightproofed and completely darkened to prevent visual input. A seatbelt is worn for safety. With the aid of a sculpted cushion and head band, the patient's head is fixed and tilted at a 30-degree angle to provide maximum stimulation of the horizontal semicircular canals. Electrodes are placed close to the outer canthi of the eyes to record compensatory eye movements elicited in response to the chair's rotation. A ground electrode is placed in the middle of the forehead. To maintain contact with the patient, an infrared camera is focused on the patient's face, and a two-way voice communication system is set up between patient and tester.

Instructions to the patient should include the following: The SHA test is an attempt to simulate everyday head motion in a controlled manner. The chair will be rotated at several different speeds, with short rest periods between each rotational speed. The first rotation will be very slow, turning the chair 360 degrees in both directions. The speed of rotation will be progressively faster until the final rotation, which results in a back and forth, sinusoidal motion. The patient should be told to relax in the chair and keep his or her eyes open while the test is being performed and to participate in concentration tasks. It is essential that the clinician watch the patient through the infrared monitor and be diligent performing the alerting tasks to ensure that the nystagmoid response is not suppressed. The clinician should also tell the patient when rotation has stopped because there may be a lag between cessation of movement and perception of cessation of movement by the patient.

A minimum of five test frequencies is incorporated into SHA testing to evaluate vestibular output over a wide operating range. Testing at only one frequency would be equated to performing a hearing test at only one frequency to assess hearing sensitivity. Frequencies commonly used include 0.01 Hz, 0.02 Hz, 0.04 Hz, 0.08 Hz, 0.16 Hz, 0.32 Hz, and 0.64 Hz (Hamid et al, 1986; Hirsch, 1986; Jacobson & Newman, 1991).

---

*Not necessary to repeat if performed during ENG test.

PEARL

To successfully perform SHA testing, concentration tasks that keep the patient thinking and talking for several minutes must be used to prevent suppression of the response. Distractions that have been successful include asking what the patient would do with a million dollars; how to bake a cake; stories about children or grandchildren, hobbies, favorite vacations, and so forth.

At 0.01 Hz, 1/100 of a cycle is completed in 1 second, taking 100 seconds to complete 1 cycle; at 0.16 Hz, 16/100 of a cycle is completed in 1 second, taking 6.25 seconds to complete 1 sinusoidal cycle. For each frequency, the chair reaches a maximum velocity of 50 degrees/s, whereas the rate of acceleration depends on the frequency of rotation (Wolfe et al, 1978).

After stimulation at the five frequencies indicated, fixation support (FS) to rotational testing is evaluated. The chair is again rotated at the two highest frequencies of rotation, first at 0.32 Hz, then 0.64 Hz, and the patient is instructed to fixate on a light located at eye level directly in the forward visual field. During this part of the testing, no alerting tasks are performed so the patient can concentrate on suppressing the nystagmoid response.

Rotation on a vertical axis generates compensatory eye movements in the direction opposite rotation; saccadic eye movement brings the eyes back into the central position. These nystagmoid movements are recorded, then analyzed using fast Fourier transform (FFT) to remove the fast phase component of the movement. The SPV of the eyes can then be compared with the velocity of the head movement controlled by the rotating chair. The parameters used to analyze the nystagmoid movements include phase, gain, and symmetry (Fig. 24–4) (Cyr et al, 1989; Hamid et al, 1986; Hirsch, 1986; Li et al, 1991; Wall, 1990). In general, low-frequency rotations reveal abnormal phase and gain responses, whereas high-frequency rotations demonstrate asymmetries (Stockwell & Bojrab, 1993).

Phase analysis measures the temporal relationship between the initiation of changes in head (chair) movement velocity to changes in eye movement velocity. As chair movement is initiated, eye movement is elicited after a known latency that depends on the frequency of the rotation. Although the induced eye movement is opposite in direction to the movement of the head (chair), responses are inverted so latencies can be compared.

Phase abnormalities represent differences in how long after the start of the stimulus (change in head movement) the compensatory eye movement occurs. When eye movement velocity occurs later in time with respect to head (chair) movement, phase lag occurs. When eye movement occurs earlier in time to head (chair) movement, phase lead occurs. Most peripheral vestibular disorders have been associated with phase abnormalities, characterized by pronounced phase differences at low frequencies that improve to near normal phase values at high frequencies (Hamid et al, 1986; Hirsch, 1986; Li et al, 1991). The phase pattern often remains abnormal for years despite successful physiological adaptation and compensation,

ROTATIONAL CHAIR SUMMARY

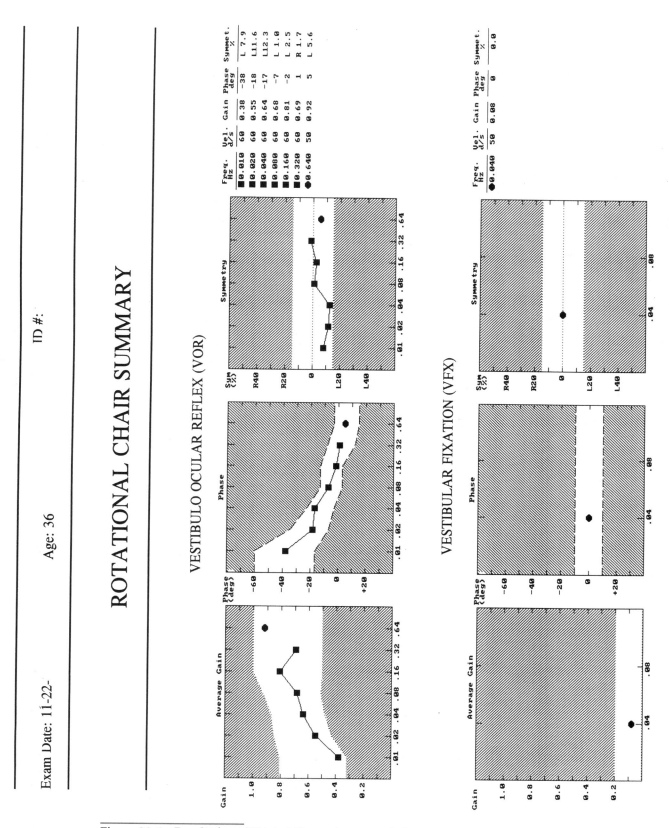

Figure 24–4 Results from SHA test illustrating normal phase, gain, and symmetry.

making phase evaluation beneficial when assessing chronic vestibular disorder (Jacobson & Newman, 1991; Parker, 1993). When phase abnormality is the same over all measured frequencies or shows increased abnormality as rotation frequency increases, CNS dysfunction should be suspected (Gresty et al, 1977).

Symmetry evaluates and compares clockwise and counterclockwise eye displacements or nystagmus. When the head (chair) is rotated in the clockwise direction, counterclockwise eye movements are induced, whereas head (chair) rotation in the counterclockwise direction induces clockwise eye movements. Symmetry is determined by comparing the peak SPV generated by right movement to the peak SPV generated by left movement and calculating the percentage difference or DP (Hirsch, 1986).

Before interpreting symmetry, the influence of underlying spontaneous nystagmus must be examined. If a patient has a 10-degree right-beating spontaneous nystagmus, responses to left rotations, which elicit right-beating nystagmus, will be enhanced 10 degrees/s, whereas responses to right rotations, which elicit left-beating nystagmus, will be reduced 10 degrees/s. It will appear to the clinician that the individual's eyes "prefer" to beat to the right, and a right DP is present. However, this bias is not due to rotational stimulation. The clinician must calculate the influence of spontaneous nystagmus on the response and, once the influence of spontaneous nystagmus has been ruled out or clarified, symmetry results can be interpreted.

In the early stages of acute, peripheral lesions, significant asymmetry will be observed but will not necessarily indicate the side of disorder because both systems are stimulated simultaneously. Studies have shown that active Meniere's disease may cause increased response toward the diseased ear, whereas responses after labyrinthectomy or removal of acoustic neuroma will show increased responses toward the normal ear (Hirsch, 1986; Parker, 1993). Therefore early on, only if phase lag is observed in conjunction with an asymmetry can the side of vestibular loss be deduced (Hamid, 1991). In later stages of peripheral vestibular disorder, asymmetry disappears as compensation takes place, whereas phase lag remains, limiting the usefulness of symmetry results when evaluating patients with chronic vestibular dysfunction. However, patients with central lesions demonstrate persistent low-level asymmetry that is associated with minimal changes in symptoms (Hamid et al, 1986).

Gain measures the amplitude of eye movements induced in response to head movement and depends on the velocity of rotation (Hirsch, 1986). When head (chair) velocity is low, compensatory eye movements are small because the stimulus is not strong enough to elicit a strong eye response. As head (chair) velocity increases, eye velocity increases, and at high velocities, eye movement velocity approaches chair velocity. For example, if the amount of eye movement induced by a given degree of rotation (in degrees per second) were exactly the same as the magnitude of the chair rotation (also in degrees per second), the gain would be 1; if the induced eye movements were half as large, the gain would be 0.5; and if the induced eye movement were twice as large, the gain would be 2. It is not surprising that the amplitude of gain depends on the velocity of rotation. Very slow rotational movements induce relatively small eye movements, with a typical gain of 0.5 for 0.01 Hz stimuli. As rotation speed increases, eye movement similarly increases but at a faster rate, so that at a rotational speed of 0.16 Hz, normal gains are in the 0.7 range.

Gain results must be considered before interpreting any SHA results. When gain is low, the vestibular system has not been stimulated sufficiently to provide meaningful data. Therefore phase and symmetry calculations cannot be interpreted. Low gains are usually a consequence of bilateral chronic vestibular weakness. In fact, patients with bilateral vestibular paresis who demonstrate no measurable response to bithermal caloric stimulation may actually respond to higher frequency rotations, providing evidence of remaining vestibular function (Furman & Kamerer, 1989; Parker, 1993). However, low gains occasionally occur in response to acute unilateral labyrinthine lesions when the cerebellum deliberately suppresses output from all vestibular nuclei to minimize symptoms of rotation, nausea, and vomiting (Hirsch, 1986; Jacobson & Newman, 1991). In such cases obvious signs of acute vestibular pathological conditions will generally be present, especially spontaneous nystagmus. Individuals with CNS injury occasionally show increased gain because of the absence of descending inhibition (Baloh et al, 1981). Such increased gain is similar to other varieties of "release" pathological neurological symptoms. However, it is essential to interpret gain with caution because it is highly variable and is significantly influenced by the alertness of the patient (Möller et al, 1990).

FS must be considered separately from all other SHA results. In normal individuals, staring at a fixed point during rotation results in suppression of the nystagmoid response. Gain scores will be low or at least 50% less than the gain observed at the corresponding rotational frequency speed. Inability to suppress nystagmus while fixating during rotational testing is consistent with CNS pathological conditions (Baloh & Furman, 1989).

Advantages and Disadvantages of SHA Testing

SHA testing has several advantages over the more traditional tests of vestibular function such as ENG (Hirsch, 1986; Parker, 1993). First, because the stimulus that initiates the VOR is mechanically generated by the chair in which the patient sits, the stimulus can be precisely and accurately controlled and modified. The clinician does not need to be concerned about adequate transfer of thermal energy through skin tissue and bone as in bithermal calorics to adequately stimulate each inner ear system. Second, the stimulus used in SHA is physiological, simulating the sort of rotational movement one might encounter in everyday life. The semicircular canals are therefore stimulated in a more natural way. Third, compensation and adaptation (or its lack) can be confirmed by monitoring changes in symmetry. Fourth, SHA testing may be performed immediately after ear surgery because direct stimulation of the earcanal is not necessary. Fifth, SHA testing can be performed when the patient is taking vestibular suppressant drugs because the VOR is not affected by such medications and phase relationships will not be altered. Finally, SHA testing is more comfortable and acceptable to the patient because it does not induce the nausea and vertigo of caloric stimulation.

SHA testing, though, has two distinct disadvantages. First, both labyrinths are tested simultaneously during sinusoidal testing, preventing ear-specific information and making it more difficult to obtain unequivocal side of lesion data. Second, the test requires the installation of expensive, fixed equipment, resulting in limited clinical application.

DYNAMIC PLATFORM POSTUROGRAPHY

Dynamic platform posturography (DPP) is a systematic test of balance function that assesses the patient's ability to use sensory input to coordinate the motor responses necessary to maintain balance (Nashner & Peters, 1990). Although other tests of balance function concentrate on evaluating the integrity of the vestibular system by assessing peripheral and central components of the vestibulo-ocular system, DPP assesses the individual's ability to use information from the vestibular, somatosensory, and visual sensory systems, both singularly and together, to coordinate motor responses to maintain center of gravity (COG) and balance (Nashner, 1971; Nashner et al, 1982).

To stand in an upright position, body mass must be centered over a base formed by the feet (Nashner, 1971). The COG can sway within certain limits of stability over this base with no adverse consequences, but if these limits are exceeded, a step or stumble must re-establish this base of support so the individual does not fall. Movement of the COG around a fixed point is termed sway, and sway can be measured in both the anteroposterior and lateral planes. During DPP, the patient is placed in a variety of circumstances that compromise the COG. Use of sensory input is necessary to coordinate motor responses to compensate for this disruption. Sensory input is provided by the visual, vestibular, and somatosensory systems and is constantly updated and integrated so that the motor system can make appropriate musculoskeletal adjustments to maintain the COG. By evaluating both the sensory and motor components of balance, DPP not only assesses vestibular function but also isolates compensatory interactions of the visual and proprioceptive systems used to maintain balance.

To understand DPP, the contributions of each sensory system to balance function must be understood (Nashner & McCollum, 1985; Nashner et al, 1982). Visual input orients the eyes and head and is derived from sway-dependent motions of the head relative to the visual surround. Somatosensory input orients body parts and is derived from the forces and motions exerted by the feet on the support surface. Vestibular input measures gravitational, linear, and angular accelerations of the head in relation to inertial space and is derived from head motions related to active or passive body sway in reference to gravity. When the visual field is stable and the support surface is fixed, vision and somatosensation dominate balance control because they are sensitive to subtle changes in body position. Specifically, the somatosensory system is sensitive to rapid changes, whereas the visual system is sensitive to slower changes in body orientation.

Inaccurate sensory information provides conflicting input to the brain that must be compensated for. Sensory breakdown can occur when objects in the visual field are moving, when the eyes are closed and visual information is absent, or

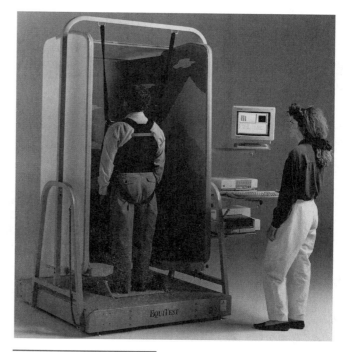

Figure 24–5 Photograph of dynamic platform posturography. (Figure courtesy of NeuroCom International, Inc., Clackamas, OR.)

when the support surface is compliant or moving. When visual and somatosensory information is conflicting or insufficient, the vestibular system resolves the situation and sends accurate information to the brain (Black & Nashner, 1984). If an abnormality or lesion occurs in any of the sensory systems, this coordination of compensating activity will be affected, resulting in disequilibrium and balance disorder.

DPP hardware consists of a dual support forceplate surface and visual surround coupled to a computer software program (Fig. 24–5) (Hunter & Balzer, 1991; Nashner, 1993). The forceplate is a flat, rigid surface supported on three or more points by independent force-measuring devices or sensors. Sensors located under the toes and heels of each foot transduce vertical forces into voltage changes and calculate the position of the COG over time. Sensors between the center plate and lower plate measure horizontal forces and the accelerations of the body COG in the anteroposterior and lateral directions. By knowing the height and weight of the patient, computer analysis derives the COG sway angle over time from vertical movements and horizontal shear forces exerted by the patient's feet and compares these movements to a computer model of body dynamics. It also analyzes the latency, strength, and pattern of patient response to brief movements (translations) of varying size and direction of the support surface.

To perform DPP, the patient must be able to stand erect and unassisted with eyes open for periods of at least 1 minute. During testing, the clinician should watch for signs of fatigue and give breaks if necessary. Shoes must be removed, although socks or stockings may be worn. The patient should be told that balance will be assessed while standing on a movement-sensitive platform. At times, the platform and visual surround will move in response to patient movements, whereas at other times, platform movement will cause the patient to move. The battery of tests begins with easy tasks that become progressively more difficult. A description of each subtest and instructions to the patient will be provided before each trial.

PEARL

If a patient is unable to stand unassisted, testing may be carried out with the patient using a walker, cane, or other mobility device. However, the device must be placed on the forceplate to be a part of forceplate movement.

For safety, the patient wears a parachute type harness connected to an overhead bar. The harness should be adjusted so that patient's weight is transferred through the patient's lower trunk rather than the upper trunk and shoulders. The straps connecting the harness to the overhead bar must allow for complete freedom of motion within the limits of normal stability. If the overhead straps are too tight, they may hold the patient up when extreme sway or even a fall would have occurred. They may also interfere with the patient's movement strategy.

PEARL

It is convenient to have surgical scrubs available for female patients who wear a dress or skirt.

Once instructions have been given and the harness adjusted, the patient's feet must be positioned on the forceplate. To ensure proper alignment, the medial maleolus of the ankle joint (the bone protruding from the ankle on the inside of the foot) should be centered directly over a marking stripe that transects the two footplates. To ensure this alignment, the clinician's hand may be vertically positioned from the bone to the stripe. Once the patient is in place, testing begins.

PITFALL

If the patient moves during the test, the clinician must re-establish the patient's foot position over the marking stripe.

The DPP test battery is divided into two parts (Hunter & Balzer, 1991; Nashner, 1993). The sensory organization test (SOT) assesses the patient's ability to integrate correct sensory information while ignoring inaccurate sensory cues. These findings isolate the site of breakdown and contribute to overall diagnosis of the disorder. The motor control test (MCT) measures the patient's ability to adapt to increasing anterior and posterior rocking and body sway. These results objectively demonstrate the degree of disability experienced by the patient.

Sensory Organization Test

The SOT assesses the patient's stability under six conditions of increasing difficulty (Fig. 24–6). Conditions 1 and 2 are essentially Romberg tests. In condition 1 the patient stands on the forceplate with eyes open, whereas in condition 2 the eyes are closed, preventing the reception of visual input. In condition 3 the eyes are open and the forceplate is stable, but the visual surround moves, providing inaccurate visual input. In condition 4 the eyes are open and the visual surround is stationary, but the support surface moves, providing inaccurate proprioceptive input. In condition 5 the eyes are closed while the forceplate moves. The patient is deprived of visual information and somatosensory input is inaccurate so the patient is completely dependent on vestibular information. In condition 6 the eyes are open, but both the visual surround and the forceplate move, providing inaccurate visual and somatosensory information and forcing the patient to, again, rely on vestibular information to maintain balance. The patient is assessed in each condition with three separate 20-second trials.

The patient's ability to maintain equilibrium, the COG, and strategies used to maintain equilibrium are recorded and analyzed (Fig. 24–7). Equilibrium scores are compared with age-matched normal controls and are provided for each test condition. They are expressed as percent of stability, ranging from 0%, representing a fall, to 100%, representing no sway and good stability. Sensory analysis scores assess the use of sensory input over the six test conditions. This analysis also compares the patient's response to age-matched normal controls and is expressed as percent of stability, ranging from 0 to 100%. "Somatosensory" assesses the patient's ability to use input from the somatosensory system by comparing responses in conditions 2 and 1. A low score indicates that the patient makes poor use of somatosensory reference. "Visual" assesses the patient's ability to use input from the visual system, comparing responses of conditions 4 and 1. Low scores indicate that the patient makes poor use of visual reference. "Vestibular" assesses the patient's ability to use vestibular input, comparing conditions 5 and 1. Low scores indicate that the patient makes poor use of vestibular cues or that vestibular cues are unavailable. "Preference to visual input" assesses the degree to which the patient relies on visual information to maintain balance, comparing conditions 2 and 5 with conditions 3 and 6. Low scores indicate that the patient relies on visual cues even when they are incorrect. COG is a scatterplot of the patient's COG position at the start of each trial, indicating the patient's ability to align himself or herself before each trial. Strategy analysis differentiates the use of ankle versus hip movement to maintain equilibrium. Well-functioning, normal individuals move their COG around their ankles in response to impending disequilibrium, whereas individuals with balance dysfunction often incorporate a maladaptive, counterproductive hip strategy. These analyses not only assess the patient's use of sensory input but

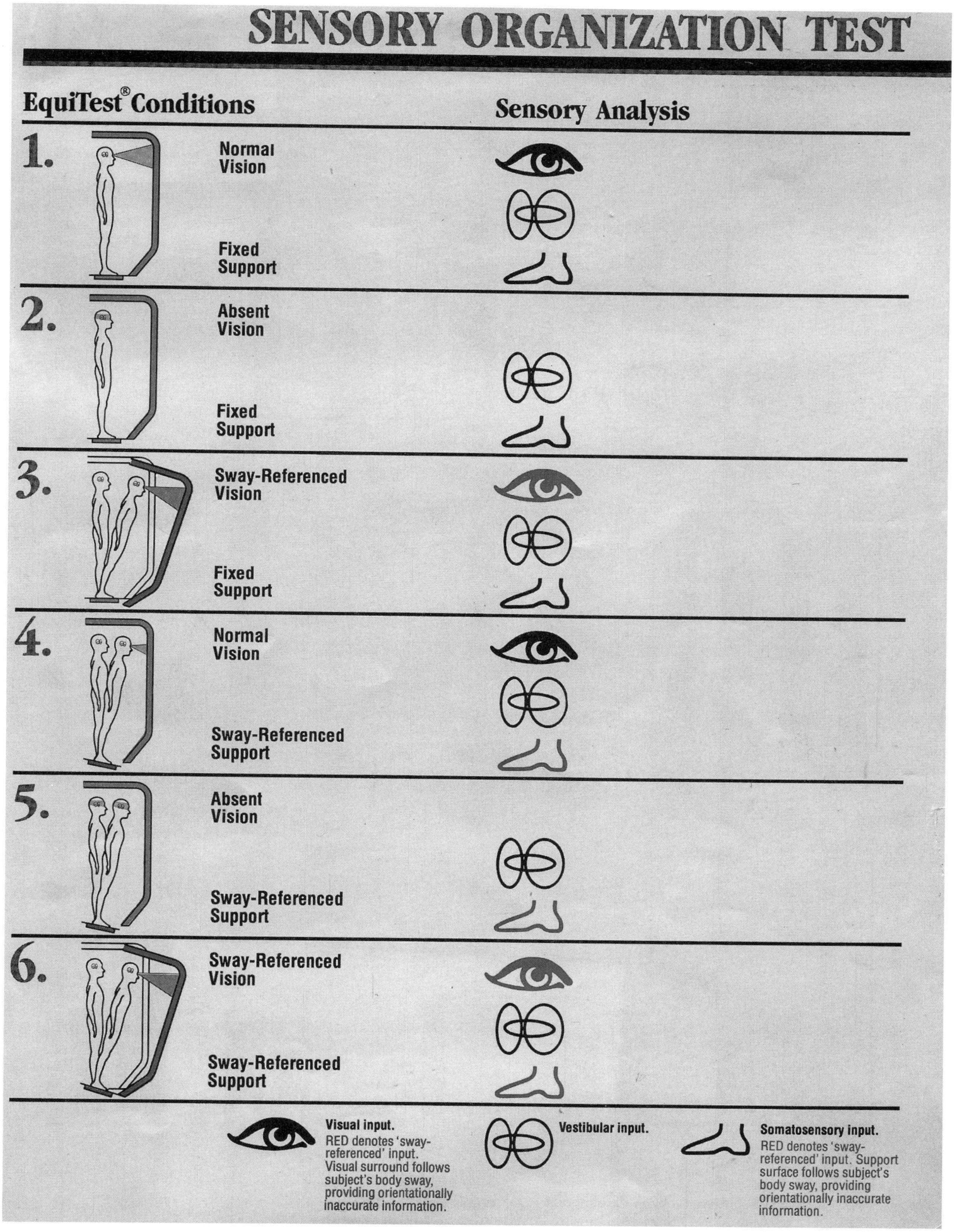

SENSORY ORGANIZATION TEST

EquiTest® Conditions

Sensory Analysis

1. Normal Vision

Fixed Support

2. Absent Vision

Fixed Support

3. Sway-Referenced Vision

Fixed Support

4. Normal Vision

Sway-Referenced Support

5. Absent Vision

Sway-Referenced Support

6. Sway-Referenced Vision

Sway-Referenced Support

Visual input. RED denotes 'sway-referenced' input. Visual surround follows subject's body sway, providing orientationally inaccurate information.

Vestibular input.

Somatosensory input. RED denotes 'sway-referenced' input. Support surface follows subject's body sway, providing orientationally inaccurate information.

Figure 24–6   Six conditions of the SOT.

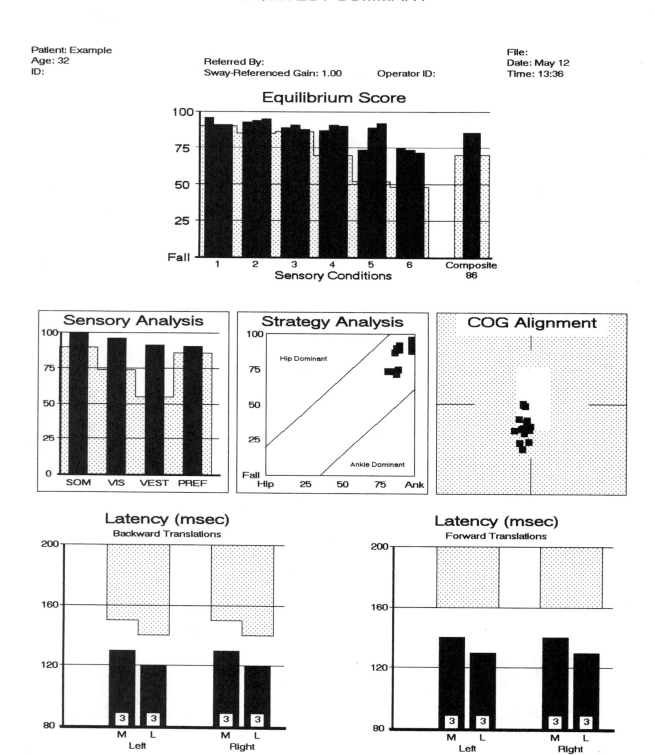

Figure 24–7 Normal results from the SOT.

also have strong implications for patient prognosis and rehabilitation recommendations.

Motor Control Test

The MCT assesses the patient's responses to jerky movements, or perturbations, of the forceplate. Two types of perturbations are used. In the first part of the test, random small, medium, and large forward and backward translations in the horizontal direction are presented. The size of the translation is based on the patient's height. The patient's ability to adapt to these sudden, quick movements is measured. In the second part of the test the patient's ability to adapt when the support surface is disrupted at an angle, forcing the toes up or down, is measured. Each translation stimulus consists of three presentations, and results are averaged to characterize the response.

Computer analysis measures four aspects of the patient's response and compares the results to age-matched normal control subjects (Fig. 24–8). Weight symmetry assesses the distribution of weight during the active response incorporated to maintain balance. In normal individuals, each leg uses equal amounts of strength in the process of balance recovery. Dynamic strength assesses the amplitude or strength of corrective movements for each leg. Responses are judged in reference to the size of the stimulus and the symmetry of leg movements. Latency assesses the time of onset between platform movement and the first corrective muscle contractions for each leg. Adaptation assesses the patient's ability to decrease response latency when platform elevations are predictable and expected. Responses to forward and backward translations are analyzed separately because the pathways responsible for postural responses are separate and may be affected differently by a disease process. Responses of the left and right legs are analyzed separately because the pathways mediating responses on the two sides can be affected separately by disease processes.

Abnormalities in MCT results can be due to a variety of problems and can contribute to the diagnosis of balance dysfunction (Hunter & Balzer, 1991; Nashner & Peters, 1990). Before analyzing results for evidence of automatic postural response abnormalities, the influence of orthopedic and/or musculoskeletal problems such as peripheral muscle atrophy and unilateral hip disease must be ruled out because these disorders produce abnormal response patterns. In general, prolonged latencies for either leg to forward or backward translations is indicative of a pathological condition within the long-loop automatic response pathways and demonstrate extravestibular CNS lesions (Nashner et al, 1983; Voorhees, 1989). Abnormally large strength differences between the two legs indicates long-loop automatic response abnormality (Nashner et al, 1983). Patients with CNS abnormalities caused by MS or spinocerebellar degeneration exhibit characteristic MCT abnormality patterns (Williams et al, 1997).

Responses from the MCT also describe the patient's ability to perform and adapt in a complex environment and provide insight into a patient's ability to perform daily balance tasks (Horak et al, 1988). Amplitude scaling scores indicate whether the patient's responses to external perturbations are too strong or too weak. Overreactions are characterized by extreme sway to maintain balance, whereas underreactions disrupt

the patient's ability to return to a balanced position. Adaptation indicates a patient's ability to adjust to uneven or compliant walking surfaces. Low scores suggest that the patient is unable to suppress the influence of disruptive stimuli to maintain balance. This information can be used in the development of rehabilitation programs and to monitor progress during rehabilitation efforts.

Interpretation of DPP Results

Interpretation of DPP results is based on response patterns of the SOT and MCT. Decreased performance on conditions 5 and 6, condition 5 only, and condition 6 only of the SOT suggests peripheral vestibular deficits, because visual and somatosensory input is inaccurate and the patient is depending on correct vestibular information to maintain balance (Black et al, 1983; Bowman & Mangham, 1989; Dickins et al, 1992; Keim et al, 1990). Decreased performance on several conditions simultaneously indicates multisensory abnormalities and can be interpreted in several ways (Nashner & Peters, 1990). If scores in conditions 4, 5, and 6 are abnormal, the patient is dependent on somatosensory information; if scores in conditions 2, 3, 5, and 6 are abnormal, the patient is dependent on visual information. The inability to effectively use two of the three available senses to maintain balance is indicative of vestibular and extravestibular central disorders (Keim et al, 1990). Patients with benign paroxysmal positional nystagmus (BPPN) demonstrate normal performance on conditions 2 and 5 and reduced performance on conditions 3 and 6, indicating that inaccurate visual input disrupts the use of somatosensory and vestibular information (Black & Nashner, 1984). If scores in conditions 2, 3, 4, 5, and 6 are abnormal, the patient is dependent on a combination of visual and somatosensory inputs, another indication of vestibular and extravestibular central pathological conditions (Nashner & Peters, 1990). When scores on conditions 4, 5, and 6 are equal to or better than scores on conditions 1, 2, and 3, results are physiologically inconsistent and suggest either patient anxiety or exaggeration of disability (Nashner & Peters, 1990). Prolonged latencies and/or strength asymmetries for either leg in either direction of the MCT indicate a pathological condition within the long-loop automatic response pathways and suggest extravestibular CNS lesions (Ackermann et al, 1986; Nashner et al, 1983; Voorhees, 1989).

Advantages and Disadvantages

Results from DPP provide unique information that can be reviewed with other tests of balance function to determine the site of balance disorder (DiFabio, 1995; Nashner & Peters, 1990). In general, if vestibular function tests indicate normal peripheral input and DPP indicates balance abnormality, a central pathological condition localized to central vestibular and/or extravestibular pathways and to the long-loop motor pathways of the brain stem, spinal cord, and peripheral nerves is suspected. When tests of vestibular function are abnormal, indicating peripheral vestibular disorder, and DPP is normal, it is assumed that the patient has adapted to and compensated for the peripheral lesion. Abnormal vestibular function tests and abnormal DPP are indicative of a central and/or peripheral pathological condition.

MOTOR CONTROL TEST

Patient: Example
Age: 32
ID:

Referred By:
Sway-Referenced Gain: 1.00

Operator ID:

File:
Date: May 12
Time: 13:36

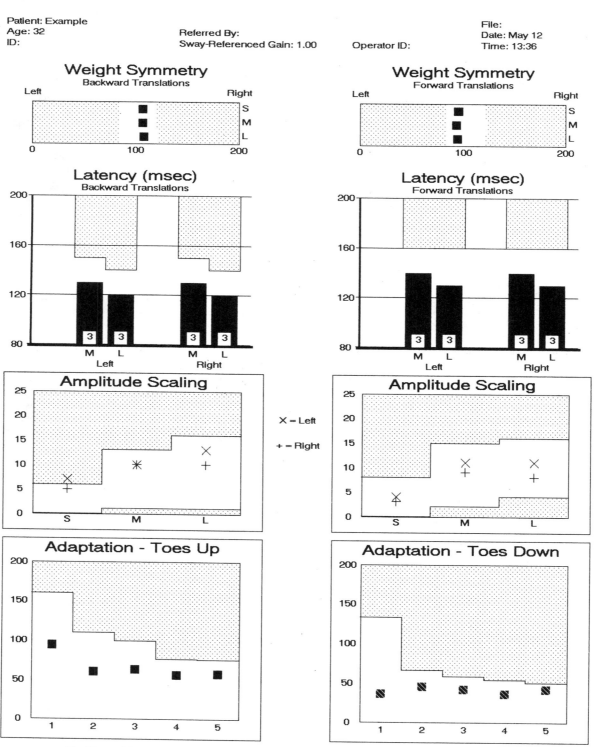

EquiTest ® Version 4.04 Copyright © 1992 NeuroCom ® International Inc. - All Rights Reserved
TEST NOTES: NeuroCom Data Range: 20 - 59; Data from version 4.04

Figure 24–8 Normal results from the MCT.

DPP results also assess the patient's risk for falling and guide balance rehabilitation efforts. Patients who perform poorly on DPP are at greater risk for falling than patients who perform normally. Specific pattern abnormalities in the SOT and MCT correlate closely with risk for falling. When DPP shows the patient is using maximal strategies to compensate for perturbations to his balance system, vestibular rehabilitation therapy can be tailored to teach the patient more adaptive techniques. For example, individuals using a maladaptive hip strategy can be redirected toward the more appropriate and helpful ankle strategy. Individuals overly dependent on vision can be given tasks to enhance their ability to use vestibular and proprioceptive information.

CONCLUSIONS

Balance is an extremely complex process that involves reception of input from the vestibular, somatosensory, and visual systems, processing and integration of this sensory input, and coordination of motoric responses to maintain balance. No single procedure can identify the site of the lesion and assess the impact of balance disturbance on a patient's quality of life. Therefore a test battery approach has been developed.

The battery described in this chapter evaluates components involved in balance separately and together to determine where in the system breakdown occurs and balance is disrupted. Once the battery of tests is completed, a patient profile begins to emerge. The profile can be used to confirm diagnosis or to recommend further assessment with imaging techniques. The profile can also be used to determine whether medical or surgical intervention is necessary or if rehabilitation efforts provide the optimum alternative.

For patients with auditory and vestibular problems, a test battery approach is necessary to ensure quality patient care. Audiologists have been on the forefront with electrophysiological assessment of the auditory system. With the expanded scope of practice, audiologists in medical settings must incorporate vestibular tests into their diagnostic protocols.

Appendix
The Dizziness Handicap Inventory
(Reprinted with permission)

Instructions: The purpose of this scale is to identify difficulties that you may be experiencing because of your dizziness or unsteadiness. Please answer "yes," "no," or "sometimes" to each question. *Answer each question as it pertains to your dizziness or unsteadiness problem only.*

P1.	Does looking up increase your problem?

E2.	Because of your problem do you feel frustrated?

F3.	Because of your problem do you restrict your travel for business or recreation?

P4.	Does walking down the aisle of a supermarket increase your problem?

F5.	Because of your problems do you have difficulty getting into or out of bed?

F6.	Does your problem significantly restrict your participation in social activities such as going out to dinner, movies, dancing, or parties?

F7.	Because of your problem do you have difficulty reading?

P8.	Does performing more ambitious activities like sports, dancing, and household chores such as sweeping or putting dishes away increase your problem?

E9.	Because of your problems are you afraid to leave your home without having someone accompany you?

E10.	Because of your problem have you been embarrassed in front of others?

P11.	Do quick movements of your head increase your problem?

F12.	Because of your problem do you avoid heights?

P13.	Does turning over in bed increase your problem?

F14.	Because of your problem is it difficult for you to do strenuous housework or yardwork?

E15.	Because of your problem are you afraid people may think you are intoxicated?

F16.	Because of your problem is it difficult for you to go for a walk by yourself?

P17.	Does walking down a sidewalk increase your problem?

E18.	Because of your problem is it difficult for you to concentrate?

F19.	Because of your problem is it difficult for you to walk around your house in the dark?

E20.	Because of your problem are you afraid to stay home alone?

E21.	Because of your problem do you feel handicapped?

E22.	Has your problem placed stress on your relationships with members of your family or friends?

E23.	Because of your problem are you depressed?

F24.	Does your problem interfere with your job or household responsibilities?

P25.	Does bending over increase your problem?

A "yes" response is scored 4 points. A "sometimes" response is scored 2 points. A "no" response is scored 0 points.
"F" represents an item contained on the functional subscale, "E" represents an item contained on the emotional subscale, and "P" represents an item contained on the physical subscale.

REFERENCES

ACKERMANN, H., DIENER, H.C., & DICHGANS, J. (1986). Mechanically evoked cerebral potentials and long-latency muscle responses in the evaluation of afferent and efferent long-loop pathways in humans. *Neuroscience Letters, 66*; 233–238.

AMERICAN ACADEMY OF AUDIOLOGY (1997). Audiology: scope of practice. *Audiology Today, 9*;12–13.

AMERICAN SPEECH-LANGUAGE-HEARING ASSOCIATION (1996). Scope of practice in audiology. *ASHA, 38*(Suppl. 16);12–15.

BALOH, R.W. (1995). Approach to the evaluation of the dizzy patient. *Otolaryngology–Head and Neck Surgery, 112*;3–7.

BALOH, R.W., & FURMAN, J.M.R. (1989). Modern vestibular function testing. *Western Journal of Medicine, 150*;59–67.

BALOH, R.W., YEE, R.E., KIMM, J., & HONRUBIA, V. (1981). The vestibulo-ocular reflex in patients with lesions of the vestibulocerebellum. *Experimental Neurology, 12*;141–152.

BARANY, R. (1907). *Physiologie und pathologie des bogengangapparates biem menschen.* Vienna: Franz Deuticke.

BLACK, F.O., & NASHNER, L.M. (1984). Postural disturbance in patients with benign paroxysmal positional nystagmus. *Annals of Otology, Rhinology and Laryngology, 93*;595–599.

BLACK, F.O., WALL, C., & NASHNER, L.M. (1983). Effect of visual and support surface references upon postural control in vestibular deficit subjects. *Acta Otolaryngologica, 95*;199–210.

BOWMAN, C.A., & MANGHAM, C.A. (1989). Clinical use of moving platform posturography. *Seminars in Hearing, 10*;161–171.

BRANDT, T. (1993). Background, technique, interpretation, and usefulness of positional and positioning testing. In: G.P. Jacobson, C.P. Newman, & J.M. Kartush (Eds.). *Handbook of balance function testing.* (pp. 123–155). St. Louis, MO: Mosby–Year Book.

BROOKLER, K.H. (1991). Standardization of electronystagmography. *American Journal of Otology, 12*;480–483.

BROWN, J.J. (1990). A systematic approach to the dizzy patient. *Neurology Clinics, 8*;209–224.

CASS, S.P., & FURMAN, J.M.R. (1993). Medications and their effects on vestibular function testing. *ENG Report.* Chicago: ICS Medical Corporation.

COATS, A.C. (1975). Electronystagmography. In: *Physiological measures of the audio-vestibular system* (pp. 37–83). New York: Academic Press.

CYR, D.G., MÖLLER, C.G., & MOORE, G.F. (1989). Clinical experience with the low-frequency rotary chair. *Seminars in Hearing, 10*;172–190.

CYR, D.G., MÖLLER, C., NASHNER, L., SHEPARD, N., & STOCKWELL, C. (1987). *State of the art methods for vestibular/ocular motor assessment.* Instructional course presented at the Annual Convention of the American Speech-Language-Hearing Association, New Orleans, LA.

DICKINS, J.R.E., CYR, D.G., GRAHAM, S.S., WINSTON, M.E., & SANFORD, M. (1992). Clinical significance of type 5 patterns in platform posturography. *Otolaryngology–Head and Neck Surgery, 107*;1–6.

DICKINS, J.R.E., & GRAHAM, S.S. (1986). Evaluation of the dizzy patient. *Ear and Hearing, 7*:133–137.

DIFABIO, R.P. (1995). Sensitivity and specificity of platform posturography for identifying patients with vestibular dysfunction. *Physical Therapy, 75*;290–305.

EVANS, K.M., & MELANCON, B.B. (1989). Back to basics: A discussion of technique and equipment. *Seminars in Hearing, 10*;123–140.

FURMAN, J.M., & KAMERER, D.B. (1989). Rotational responses in patients with bilateral caloric reduction. *Acta Otolaryngologica, 108*;355–361.

GOEBEL, J.A., DUNHAM, D.N., ROHRBAUGH, J.W., FISCHEL, D., & STEWART, P.A. (1995). Dose-related effects of alcohol on dynamic posturography and oculomotor measures. *Acta Otolaryngologica Supplement, 520*;212–215.

GRESTY, M.A., HESS, K., & LEECH, J. (1977). Disorders of the vestibulo-ocular reflex producing oscillopsia and mechanisms of compensating for loss of labyrinthine function. *Brain, 100*;693–716.

HAIN, T.C. (1993). Interpretation and usefulness of ocular motility testing. In: G.P. Jacobson, C.P. Newman, & J.M. Kartush (Eds.). *Handbook of balance function testing* (pp. 101–122). St. Louis, MO: Mosby–Year Book.

HAMID, M.A. (1991). Determining side of vestibular dysfunction with rotatory chair testing. *Otolaryngology–Head and Neck Surgery, 105*;40–43.

HAMID, M.A., HUGHES, G.B., KINNEY, S.E., & HANSON, M.R. (1986). Results of sinusoidal harmonic acceleration test in one thousand patients: preliminary report. *Otolaryngology–Head and Neck Surgery, 94*;1–5.

HIRSCH, B.E. (1986). Computed sinusoidal harmonic acceleration. *Ear and Hearing, 7*;198–203.

HONRUBIA, V. (1995). Contemporary vestibular function testing: Accomplishments and future perspectives. *Otolaryngology–Head and Neck Surgery, 112*;64–77.

HORAK, F.B., SHUMWAY-COOK, A., CROWE, T.K., & BLACK, F.O. (1988). Vestibular function and motor proficiency of children with impaired hearing, or with learning disability and motor impairments. *Developmental Medicine and Child Neurology, 30*;64–79.

HUNTER, L.L., & BALZER, G.K. (1991). Overview and introduction to dynamic platform posturography. *Seminars in Hearing, 12*;226–247.

JACOBSON G.P., & NEWMAN C.W. (1990). The development of the dizziness handicap inventory. *Archives in Otolaryngology Head Neck Surgery, 116*;424–427.

JACOBSON, G.P., & NEWMAN, C.W. (1991). Rotational testing. *Seminars in Hearing, 12*;199–225.

JACOBSON, G.P., & NEWMAN, C.W. (1993). Background and technique of caloric testing. In: G.P. Jacobson, C.P. Newman, & J.M. Kartush (Eds.). *Handbook of balance function testing.* (pp. 156–192). St. Louis, MO: Mosby–Year Book.

JACOBSON, G.P., NEWMAN, C.W., HUNTER, L., & BALZER, G.K. (1991). Balance function test correlates of the dizziness handicap inventory. *Journal of the American Academy of Audiology, 2*;253–260.

JACOBSON, G.P., NEWMAN, C.W., & PETERSON, E.L. (1993). Interpretation and usefulness of caloric testing. In: G.P. Jacobson, C.W. Newman, & J.M. Kartush (Eds.). *Handbook of balance function testing* (pp. 193–233). St. Louis, MO: Mosby–Year Book.

KANAYA, T., NONAKA, S., KAMITO, M., UNNO, T., SAKO, K., & TAKEI, H. (1994). Primary position upbeat nystagmus localizing value. *Otolaryngology-Rhinology-Laryngology, 56*;236–238.

KATSARKAS, A. (1987). Nystagmus of paroxysmal positional vertigo: Some new insights. *Annals of Otology, Rhinology, and Laryngology, 96*;305–308.

KEIM, R.J., DICKINS, J.R.E., & NASHNER, L.M. (1990). *Computerized dynamic posturography: Fundamentals and clinical applications.* Instructional course presented at the Annual Convention of the American Academy of Otolaryngology–Head and Neck Surgery, San Diego, CA.

KONRAD, H.R. (1991). Clinical application of saccade-reflex testing in man. *Laryngoscope, 101*;1293–1302.

LI, C.W., HOOPER, R.E., & COUSINS, V.C. (1991). Sinusoidal harmonic acceleration testing in normal humans. *Laryngoscope, 101*;192–196.

MÖLLER, C., ÖDKVIST, L., WHITE, V., & CYR, D. (1990). The plasticity of compensatory eye movements in rotary tests. *Acta Otolaryngologica, 109*;15–24.

NASHNER, L.M. (1971). A model describing vestibular detection of body sway motion. *Acta Otolaryngologica, 72*;429–426.

NASHNER, L.M. (1993). Computerized dynamic posturography. In: G.P. Jacobson, C.P. Newman, & J.M. Kartush (Eds.). *Handbook of balance function testing* (pp. 280–307). St. Louis, MO: Mosby–Year Book.

NASHNER, L.M., BLACK, F.O., & WALL III, C. (1982). Adaptation to altered support and visual conditions during stance: Patients with vestibular deficits. *Journal of Neuroscience, 2*;536–544.

NASHNER, L.M., & McCOLLUM, G. (1985). The organization of human postural movements: A formal basis and experimental synthesis. *Behavioral Brain Science, 8*;135–172.

NASHNER, L.M., & PETERS, J.F. (1990). Dynamic posturography in the diagnosis and management of dizziness and balance disorders. *Neurologic Clinics, 8*;331–350.

NASHNER, L.M., SHUMWAY-COOK, A., & MARIN, O. (1983). Stance posture control in selected groups of children with cerebral palsy: Deficits in sensory organization and muscular coordination. *Experimental Brain Research, 197*;393–409.

OJALA, M., & PALO, J. (1991). The aetiology of dizziness and how to examine a dizzy patient. *Annals of Medicine, 23*;225–30.

PARKER, S.W. (1993). Vestibular evaluation—electronystagmography, rotational testing, and posturography. *Clinics in Electroencephalography, 24*;151–158.

RESNICK, D.M., & BREWER, C.C. (1983). The electronystagmography test battery: Hit or myth? *Seminars in Hearing, 4*;23–32.

RUBIN, W. (1990). How do we use state of the art vestibular testing to diagnose and treat the dizzy patient? *Neurology Clinics, 8*;225–234.

SATALOFF, R.T., & HUGHES, M.E. (1988). How I do it: An easy guide to electronystagmography interpretations. *American Journal of Otology, 9*;144–151.

SHEPARD, N.T., & TELIAN, S.A. (1994). Evaluation of balance system function. In: J. Katz (Ed.). *Handbook of clinical audiology* (4th Ed.) (pp. 424–447). Baltimore, MD: Williams & Wilkins.

STOCKWELL, C.W. (1983). *ENG workbook.* Baltimore: University Park Press.

STOCKWELL, C.W., & BOJRAB, D.I. (1993). Background and technique of rotational testing. In: G.P. Jacobson, C.P. Newman, & J.M. Kartush (Eds.). *Handbook of balance function testing* (pp. 237–258). St. Louis, MO: Mosby–Year Book.

TETER, D.L. (1983). The electronystagmography test battery and interpretation. *Seminars in Hearing, 4*;11–21.

THERAPEUTICS AND TECHNOLOGY SUBCOMMITTEE; AMERICAN ACADEMY OF NEUROLOGY. (1996). Assessment: Electronystagmography. *Neurology, 46*;1763–1766.

VOORHEES, R.L. (1989). The role of dynamic posturography as a screening test in neurotologic diagnosis. *Laryngoscope, 99*;995–1001.

WALL, C. (1990). The sinusoidal harmonic acceleration rotary chair test: Theoretical and clinical basis. *Neurology Clinics, 8*;269–285.

WILLIAMS, N.P., ROLAND, P.S., & YELLIN, W. (1997). Vestibular evaluation in patients with early multiple sclerosis. *The American Journal of Otology, 18*;93–100.

WOLFE, J.W., ENGELKEN, E.J., OLSON, J.E., & KOS, C.M. (1978). Vestibular responses to bithermal caloric and harmonic acceleration. *Annals of Otology, Rhinology, and Laryngology, 87*;861–867.

YELLIN, M.W., & MAINORD, J.C. (1996). *Evaluation of the dizzy patient: The package.* Instructional course presented at the Annual Convention of the American Academy of Audiology, Salt Lake City, UT.

## Chapter 25

Genetic Intervention and Hearing Loss

Bronya J. B. Keats

Approximately 1 in 1000 children is born with profound hearing impairment, and at least 70% have no associated anomalies (Gorlin et al, 1995). Analysis of data collected by Gallaudet University in the 1969-1970 Annual Survey of Hearing-Impaired-Children and Youth estimated that 50.7% of cases are attributable to genetic causes (Nance et al, 1977), whereas analysis of the survey data collected two decades later (1988 to 1989) estimated a genetic cause in 62.8% of cases (Marazita et al, 1993). A major reason for the increase in the proportion of profound hearing impairment caused by genetic factors is the reduction in environmental causes (such as rubella). However, an underlying genetic predisposition is likely to be a factor even when an environmental insult is known to have contributed to the cause of the hearing loss.

Adult-onset hearing loss is also a significant health problem, with 14% of individuals between the ages of 45 and 64 and 30% of those older than 65 having hearing problems (Hotchkiss, 1989). Sill et al (1994) collected extensive population data in an attempt to delineate the causes of later-onset hearing loss. The data strongly suggested a genetic cause in a large percentage of the participants, but a precise estimate could not be determined.

PEARL

A genetic cause must be considered for all patients with hearing impairment, and consultation with a clinical geneticist is recommended as standard practice for audiologists.

Documentation of awareness that inheritance is important in hearing impairment can be traced back to the sixteenth century. According to Goldstein (1933), the earliest known author to have recognized that some forms of deafness may be hereditary was Johannes Schenck (1531–1598) who noted a family in which several children were born deaf. Stephens (1985) includes a pedigree drawing of a sixteenth century family of the Spanish aristocracy in which members in three generations were documented as deaf. In 1621 the papal physician Paolus Zacchias (1584–1659) recommended that the deaf abstain from marriage because of evidence that their children will also be deaf (Cranefield & Federn, 1970), indicating his conviction that heredity is important in deafness. Reardon (1990) ascribes to Sir William Wilde (1815–1876) the demonstration of autosomal dominant and recessive inheritance of deafness, the relevance of consanguinity, and the awareness of an excess of males among the congenitally deaf. These findings were confirmed by Hartmann (1881), who carried out his studies in schools for the deaf in Germany.

More recently, Konigsmark (1969), Konigsmark and Gorlin (1976), and Fraser (1976) provided comprehensive reviews of hereditary hearing impairment and associated clinical abnormalities, emphasizing the extensive clinical and genetic variability. This heterogeneity is underscored by Gorlin et al (1995) who list 427 forms of hereditary hearing impairment. Several studies attempted to estimate the number of genes for deafness in various populations (Brownstein et al, 1991; Chung & Brown, 1970; Chung et al, 1959; Costeff & Dar, 1980; Sank, 1963; Stevenson & Cheeseman, 1956), with the results ranging from less than 10 to several thousand. As far as pattern of inheritance is concerned, general agreement exists that approximately 77% is autosomal recessive, 22% is autosomal

593

dominant, and the remainder is X-linked and mitochondrial (Gorlin et al, 1995). Fraser (1976) pointed out that inheritance pattern is useful but not sufficient for categorizing type of hearing impairment and he predicted that "within the foreseeable future it will be possible to define each type of genetically determined deafness by other criteria, such as can be employed at present, for example, for defining galactosemia and phenylketonuria, on biochemical grounds as two specific forms of mental subnormality." Twenty years later this prediction is becoming a reality.

PEARL

Genetic research on hearing impairment is leading to the development of new clinical diagnostic and therapeutic technologies.

The purpose of this chapter is to review the present genetic knowledge of hearing impairment and to discuss the potential for the development of gene-based approaches to treatment. The major goals of ongoing genetic research are to provide a complete battery of molecular diagnostic tests that will pinpoint the defective gene and to develop effective therapies on the basis of this underlying cause that will complement the present approaches to management of symptoms.

THE HUMAN GENOME

The human genome consists of 24 different types of chromosomes designated 1 to 22 (autosomes), X and Y (sex chromosomes). An offspring inherits one set of chromosomes from each parent, providing a total of 46 chromosomes (22 autosomal pairs plus XX or XY) in the nucleus of a cell. If both parents transmit an X chromosome, the offspring is female (XX); if the father transmits a Y chromosome, the offspring is male (XY). Each of these chromosomes consists of a single molecule of deoxyribonucleic acid (DNA), which has a double helical structure. DNA is composed of a sugar-phosphate backbone and four bases, adenine (A), guanine (G), thymine (T), and cytosine (C). The double helix is formed through the pairing of A with T, and C with G, and the bases are held together by hydrogen bonds. Thus, knowing the sequence of bases on one DNA strand automatically gives the sequence on the other strand. This precise pairing means that DNA can replicate by separation of the two strands followed by each strand serving as a template for a new complementary strand.

The set of 24 chromosomes has 3 billion base pairs, of which 5 to 10% make up the estimated 80,000 to 120,000 human genes. Genes consist of both coding sequences (exons) and intervening sequences (introns), and it is the exons that encode the amino acid sequence of the protein product. The connecting link between the gene (DNA) and the protein is messenger ribonucleic acid (mRNA). The sequence of bases in the exons is called the complementary DNA (cDNA) sequence because it can be synthesized with the mRNA as a template. There are 20 different amino acids, and each set of three bases in the mRNA constitutes a codon, which specifies either a particular amino acid or a stop signal. Thus the amino acid sequence of a protein can be deduced from the cDNA (or mRNA) sequence.

One goal of genetic research is to localize, identify, and establish the base sequence of all genes. Genetic linkage analyses of families in which some members have an inherited disorder provide the chromosomal location of the defective gene. The transmission from parents to offspring of genetic markers (usually short fragments of DNA) that are found to be close to the defective gene can then be analyzed to provide precise risks and diagnoses for relatives of affected individuals. When the gene is identified and mutations are detected, diagnostic tests that examine the DNA within the gene itself are applicable to all individuals. The techniques that are used to localize and identify the gene causing a disorder in family members are described later in this chapter.

PHENOTYPE AND GENOTYPE

The findings that result from a clinical examination are an individual's phenotype. They may include biochemical, physiological, and morphological characteristics. This phenotype can result from genetic factors, environmental factors, or a combination of both. The genetic factors are the individual's genotype. An individual has pairs of chromosomes and therefore pairs of genes and pairs of genetic markers. The different forms of genes and genetic markers are called alleles; thus an individual has two alleles for each gene and genetic marker and the pair of alleles is the genotype. If the two alleles are the same, the individual is homozygous; if they are different, the individual is heterozygous. A disease gene may be considered to have two alleles, one of which is normal (N) and the other is abnormal (D). Thus the individual's genotype can be NN, ND, or DD. A genetic marker often has many alternate forms, usually given arbitrary designations such as a, b, c, d, . . . or 1, 2, 3, 4, . . ., and consequently many different possible genotypes exist. An individual's genotype at a single gene is often the cause of a phenotype such as hearing impairment. In other cases the phenotype may be the result of an individual's genotype at several different genes, and environmental factors may play a role.

Syndromic versus Nonsyndromic Hearing Loss

Hearing impairment may be only one feature of the phenotype, in which case the disorder is known as a syndrome; if no associated clinical anomalies are apparent, the hearing impairment is called nonsyndromic. In their comprehensive monograph, Gorlin et al (1995) describe 30 syndromes in which hearing loss is associated with abnormalities of the external ear, 40 with the eye, 87 with the musculoskeletal system, 23 with the kidney, 56 with the skin, 63 with the central nervous system, 51 with endocrine and metabolic conditions, 12 with chromosomal anomalies, 8 with oral and dental problems, and 35 with miscellaneous disorders, and 22 forms of nonsyndromic hearing impairment. Examples of these syndromes include Treacher Collins syndrome, branchio-otorenal (BOR) syndrome, Usher's syndrome, Norrie's disease, Stickler syndrome, Alport's syndrome, neurofibromatosis type 2, Pendred's syndrome, Waardenburg's syndrome, and

Jervell and Lange-Nielsen syndrome. The underlying cause of all of these syndromes is a mutation in a single gene. However, the gene may be different from one patient to another (e.g., at least nine different genes cause Usher's syndrome), and the phenotypic expression of defects in the same gene may be variable among affected individuals (e.g., Waardenburg's syndrome). The clinical features and gene defects in each of these syndromes are discussed in this chapter.

PATTERNS OF INHERITANCE

Autosomal Dominant Inheritance

The pattern of inheritance is probably autosomal dominant if individuals in each generation are affected, and males and females are equally likely to be affected. Affected individuals usually have one normal and one abnormal copy of the gene for the disorder and each offspring of an affected individual has a 50% chance of inheriting the abnormal allele. If all individuals who inherit an abnormal allele exhibit features of the disease, the penetrance is complete. With some disorders individuals who must have the abnormal allele (because, for example, they have an affected parent and an affected child) show no phenotypic signs. In this case penetrance is incomplete, perhaps because of the effect of other genetic factors or possibly environmental factors. Penetrance is defined as the probability of expressing the phenotype given the presence of a particular genotype. For example, for a dominant disorder, if 70% of individuals who have the abnormal allele show features of the disorder, then the penetrance value is 0.7. Figure 25–1 shows examples of pedigree structures that might be observed for dominant disorders with complete (Fig. 25–1A) and incomplete (Fig. 25–1B)

penetrance. Penetrance may also be age dependent, such as with adult-onset hearing loss. In this case the probability that a person who has the abnormal allele will have hearing loss increases with age. Thus penetrance may be close to 0 at 10 years of age, 0.3 at 20 years of age, 0.7 at 30 years of age, and 1.0 at 50 years of age.

PITFALL

The degree of penetrance needs to be taken into account when providing information on recurrence risks to individuals who have relatives with an autosomal dominant disease. Also, remember that the phenotype of an individual with features of the disease but a negative family history may be due to a new mutation, meaning that the individual has a 50% chance of transmitting the gene to an offspring.

With many disorders, the penetrance may be complete, but the phenotype may vary among affected individuals. This variable expression suggests that additional genes or environmental factors are contributing to the phenotype. Thus knowing the genotype may not be adequate for predicting the phenotypic expression.

Treacher Collins syndrome, BOR syndrome, Stickler syndrome, neurofibromatosis type 2, and Waardenburg's syndrome are examples of syndromes that show an autosomal dominant pattern of inheritance. In addition, nonsyndromic hearing impairment and auditory neuropathy may show dominant inheritance.

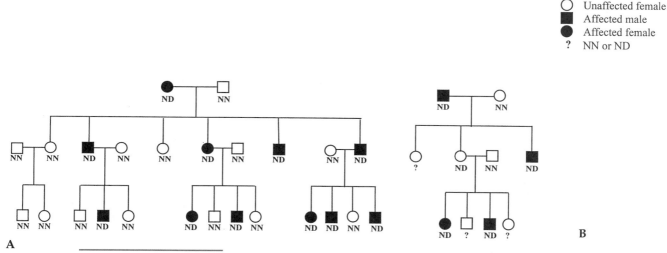

☐ Unaffected male
○ Unaffected female
■ Affected male
● Affected female
? NN or ND

Figure 25–1 Autosomal dominant patterns of inheritance with **(A)** complete penetrance, and **(B)** incomplete penetrance. The genotypes (NN, ND, DD) are shown below each individual. Those who are affected have one normal (N) allele and one abnormal (D) allele, and the probability that a child inherits the D allele is 50%. If penetrance is complete, every individual with the ND genotype is affected. However, if penetrance is incomplete, the genotype of unaffected individuals cannot always be determined with certainty; they may be NN or ND. (Spouses of ND individuals are unaffected and assumed to be NN.)

Treacher Collins Syndrome

The characteristic findings in patients with Treacher Collins syndrome are malformed pinnae, external canals, and middle ear structures; conductive hearing loss; coloboma of the lower eyelid; downslanting palpebral fissures; depressed cheekbones; and a receding chin. The face is narrow, making the nose appear large, but this perception is a result of the other facial abnormalities. Extra ear tags and blind fistulas are found anywhere from behind the ear lobes to the mouth. At least 55% of individuals with this syndrome have bilateral conductive hearing loss because of the deformities of the middle ear structures and external canals (Gorlin et al, 1995). Treacher Collins syndrome is autosomal dominant with variable expression within and between families. However, studies of family members indicate that all individuals who have the defective gene show some of the features of the disease, meaning that penetrance is complete.

Branchio-Oto-Renal Syndrome

The features of BOR syndrome are a branchial cleft, fistulas, or cysts; malformed pinnae; preauricular pits; hearing loss; and renal anomalies. Approximately 75% of affected individuals have hearing loss that is conductive in about 30% of cases, sensorineural in 20%, and mixed in 50%. Age of onset varies from early childhood to young adulthood, and the hearing loss is usually not progressive. The mode of inheritance is dominant with close to complete penetrance, but the expression of the phenotype is quite variable with some patients having only branchial features and others having only otologic features. Also, families have been described in which some affected members have conductive hearing loss, others have sensorineural loss, yet others have a mixed loss, and the type of loss may even be different in the two ears (Gorlin et al, 1995).

Stickler Syndrome

Characteristic features of Stickler (STL) syndrome include a flat midface, cleft palate, severe myopia with retinal detachment and cataracts, hearing loss, joint hypermobility, mild spondyloepiphyseal dysplasia, and mitral valve prolapse. Progressive sensorineural high-frequency hearing loss is found in about 80% of cases, and conductive hearing loss has been reported in some patients (Gorlin et al, 1995). The phenotypic expression of this syndrome is highly variable both within and between families, but penetrance is close to complete.

Neurofibromatosis Type 2

This autosomal dominant disorder is characterized by bilateral vestibular schwannomas (acoustic neuromas) of the eighth cranial nerve, with usual age of onset between 15 and 30 years. Progressive unilateral or bilateral sensorineural hearing loss in the second or third decade is often the presenting symptom, and the loss is usually profound within 5 to 10 years. Also, vestibular function is abnormal and decreasing vision is common. The incidence is about 1 in 40,000 and penetrance is estimated to be 95% after age 30. Neurofibromatosis type 2 (NF2) is clinically and genetically distinct from neurofibromatosis type 1 (NF1). Almost all patients with NF1 have several café-au-lait spots and Lisch nodules of the iris, findings that are much less frequent in NF2 patients. In addition, vestibular schwannomas are found in only 2 to 4% of NF1 cases and they are almost never bilateral (Gorlin et al, 1995).

Waardenburg's Syndrome

The most common features of Waardenburg's syndrome type I (WS1) are widely spaced medial canthi (dystopia canthorum), synophrys (joined eyebrows), and a broad nasal root. Heterochromia irides and a white forelock are seen in about 30% of patients. Two clinical types have been described; the major phenotypic characteristic differentiating WS2 from WS1 is the lack of dystopia canthorum in WS2. The frequency of sensorineural hearing impairment is about 20% in WS1 and 50% in WS2. The degree of impairment varies from minimal to severe and may be unilateral or bilateral (Gorlin et al, 1995). Waardenburg's syndrome is autosomal dominant, and most individuals with a defective gene show some signs of the disease. However, occasionally individuals who must have the gene are unaffected; thus penetrance is less than 100%, and a child who has no features of the disease may still have inherited a defective gene from an affected parent. DNA analysis is necessary to determine whether the child has inherited the parent's gene for Waardenburg's syndrome.

Autosomal Dominant Nonsyndromic Hearing Impairment

As discussed later in this chapter, a large number of genes cause nonsyndromic hearing impairment. Genes for autosomal dominant nonsyndromic hearing impairment are designated as DFNA* (* = 1,2,3,. . .). Autosomal dominant forms of sensorineural hearing impairment without associated anomalies are usually progressive. The frequencies at which the loss is first noticed tend to be consistent, and the progression pattern is similar among members of the same family. Although age of onset may vary from one family member to another, it is usually after the first decade. An exception is the hearing loss in members of the family described by Chaib et al (1994), in whom the onset was before 4 years of age and was severe to profound across all frequencies.

Autosomal Dominant Auditory Neuropathy

The auditory neuropathies are a clinically and genetically heterogeneous set of hearing disorders in which neural function is impaired but the outer hair cells of the cochlea appear to function normally. Patients have abnormal auditory brain stem responses, but otoacoustic emissions and cochlear microphonics are present, which means that the deficit is probably of neural origin and that the outer hair cells and endocochlear potential are not affected (Berlin et al, 1998; Starr et al, 1996). Some families show an autosomal dominant pattern of inheritance, and affected members of these families usually have a peripheral neuropathy resembling Charcot-Marie-Tooth disease. The hearing problems tend to begin with difficulty understanding what is being said when there is background noise and may progress to severe hearing loss.

Autosomal Recessive Inheritance

The mode of inheritance of a disorder is autosomal recessive if the abnormal phenotype is expressed only in individuals who have two copies of the defective gene. If both parents are carriers of the same abnormal (D) allele (that is, both have the genotype ND), their child may inherit two copies of the D allele, one from each parent. In this situation the child has the disorder, but neither of the parents is affected. Assuming complete penetrance, the probability that a child of carrier parents will be affected is one quarter; the probability that an unaffected sibling is a carrier is two-thirds (Fig. 25–2). If a hearing-impaired child of normal hearing parents has an affected sibling or the parents are related, then the cause is most likely to be a defective gene with the mode of inheritance being autosomal recessive. Alternately, if family history is negative and a known environmental insult such as an infectious agent or a drug is present, the presence of a defective gene is less likely. However, the possibility of recessive inheritance must always be considered. Note that a positive family history is not expected with a recessive disorder because the abnormal allele may be passed on from one (unaffected) carrier to the next for many generations before a couple, who by chance both carry the same abnormal allele, has an affected child. Usher's syndrome, Pendred's syndrome, and Jervell and Lange-Nielsen syndrome are examples of disorders that show an autosomal recessive pattern of inheritance. At least 19 different genetic forms of autosomal recessive nonsyndromic hearing impairment exist and most are congenital and profound. In addition, auditory neuropathy is often found in siblings whose parents are both unaffected. This finding is consistent with the existence of autosomal recessive forms of auditory neuropathy.

SPECIAL CONSIDERATION

Recessive inheritance probably explains most cases of profound sensorineural hearing loss when family history is negative and no known environmental factor could be responsible.

Usher's Syndrome

Usher's syndrome is made up of a group of clinically and genetically heterogeneous disorders characterized by sensorineural hearing impairment and pigmentary retinopathy.

Clinically, three types of Usher's syndrome have been described. Patients with Usher's syndrome type I have severe-to-profound congenital hearing impairment, vestibular dysfunction, and retinal degeneration beginning in childhood, whereas those with type II have moderate-to-severe hearing impairment, normal vestibular function, and later onset of retinal degeneration (Smith et al, 1994). The hearing loss in Usher's syndrome type III is progressive and age of onset of retinal degeneration is variable (Davenport & Omenn, 1977). Among profoundly hearing-impaired infants, approximately 3 to 6% are likely to have Usher's syndrome. Night blindness is often the first symptom of the retinal degeneration.

Pendred's Syndrome

The combination of goiter (thyroid enlargement) and severe-to-profound congenital sensorineural hearing impairment is known as Pendred's syndrome. It is estimated to account for between 4.3 and 7.5% of all cases of congenital deafness (Fraser, 1976). Associated characteristics include a Mondini-type developmental defect of the cochlea and autosomal recessive inheritance. The goiter is usually detected before puberty and it remains small in most patients. A thyroidectomy followed by thyroid therapy may be performed but the goiter tends to recur.

Jervell and Lange-Nielsen Syndrome

Congenital profound sensorineural hearing loss and an electrocardiogram that has a prolonged Q–T interval characterize this syndrome. Fainting spells of variable frequency and severity begin by the age of 3, and, if untreated, cardiac dysrhythmia leads to sudden death by the age of 15 in more than 70% of patients. The percentage of profoundly hearing-impaired individuals with Jervell and Lange-Nielsen syndrome (JLNS) may be as high as 1% (Gorlin et al, 1995). Thus an electrocardiogram (ELG) is warranted in all congenitally deaf children to rule out this syndrome.

Autosomal Recessive Nonsyndromic Hearing Impairment

The different genetic forms of autosomal recessive nonsyndromic hearing impairment are assigned a DFNB* symbol (* = 1,2,3,. . .). Severe-to-profound hearing impairment with onset before 12 months of age is a characteristic finding in most of those affected. An exception to preverbal onset is a

Parents		**ND**	**X**	**ND**	

↓

Possible Genotypes	**NN**	**ND**	**DN**	**DD**
Probability	¼	¼	¼	¼

Figure 25–2 Autosomal recessive inheritance. Both parents have the ND genotype; that is, they are unaffected but are carriers of the abnormal (D) allele. Each parent transmits either an N or a D to a child. Thus four outcomes are possible, but two are the same (ND = DN), so the probability of an affected (DD) child is one-fourth and the probability of a carrier child is one-half. However, three of the four possible outcomes give an unaffected child (NN, ND, DN), and of these three outcomes, two are carriers. Thus the probability that an unaffected offspring is a carrier is two-thirds.

large consanguineous kindred from Pakistan in which affected individuals had normal hearing until about 10 years of age but the loss was profound within 4 to 5 years (Veske et al, 1996). Finding the genes involved usually requires the analysis of several families, in which there are at least two hearing-impaired siblings. Because the same gene may not be responsible for the hearing impairment in two different families, a set of families from an isolated or endogamous (marrying within the ethnic group) population is likely to be much more informative than a random set of families with various ethnic backgrounds. Thus many of the studies that have been successful have worked with families from countries such as Pakistan, India, Tunisia, Bali, Lebanon, Palestine, Israel, and Syria. In some of these studies the affected siblings are the offspring of consanguineous matings such as first cousin marriages. When the parents are closely related, the affected offspring are likely to be identically homozygous for genetic markers in the vicinity of the gene. This identity facilitates finding the gene.

Autosomal Recessive Auditory Neuropathy

Infants with autosomal recessive forms of auditory neuropathy often have profound hearing impairment. However, although their auditory brain stem responses and middle ear muscle reflexes are absent, they have robust otoacoustic emissions (Berlin et al, 1998; Starr et al, 1996). Longitudinal studies of some children suggest that, in the absence of middle ear effusion or other middle ear disorders, the otoacoustic emissions can be lost as they get older. Thus a subset of individuals with recessive nonsyndromic hearing impairment may have originally had an auditory neuropathy. An alternative presentation is an audiogram showing a mild-to-moderate hearing impairment but poor speech discrimination and great difficulty hearing in noise. Associated peripheral neuropathy is usually not found with autosomal recessive auditory neuropathy. An exception is a gypsy family in which the affected members have hereditary sensory motor neuropathy and neural deafness (Kalaydjieva et al, 1996, 1998).

X-Linked Inheritance

Males have both an X and Y chromosome; females have two X chromosomes. Thus a necessary condition for X-linked inheritance is no father-to-son transmission because a son must receive his X chromosome from his mother. If a disorder has an X-linked dominant pattern of inheritance with complete penetrance, all daughters of affected fathers are affected and each child of an affected mother has a 50% chance of being affected. In the case of an X-linked recessive trait, most affected individuals are male because they have only one X chromosome. Females have two X chromosomes and may be carriers but are unlikely to be affected. Sons of a carrier mother each have a 50% chance of inheriting the abnormal allele, whereas daughters have a 50% chance of being carriers. Of course, if the father is affected and the mother is a carrier, then the daughters must receive an abnormal allele from their father and, therefore, have a 50% chance of inheriting two abnormal alleles and being affected. Figure 25–3 shows examples of pedigree structures that may be found with X-linked dominant (Fig. 25–3A) and X-linked recessive (Fig. 25–3B) inheritance. The possibility that a new mutation may be

responsible for the disorder in an affected son needs to be considered when no other family members are affected. Alport's syndrome and Norrie's disease are examples of X-linked disorders, and nonsyndromic X-linked forms of hearing impairment have also been described.

SPECIAL CONSIDERATION

Several families have been described showing X-linked patterns of inheritance in which all affected members have hearing impairment and some also have other anomalies. In general, the phenotype is specific to a single family such as the one described by Priest et al (1995) in which affected males have axonal motor-sensory neuropathy with deafness and mental retardation. Finding more families with similar phenotypes will facilitate the identification of the defective gene.

Alport's Syndrome

The bilateral sensorineural hearing loss in Alport's syndrome is progressive and is associated with nephritis. Patients show ultrastructural abnormalities in basic membranes because of defective type IV collagen. Males who have the abnormal allele on their X chromosome are affected. In addition, the mode of inheritance is X-linked dominant meaning that females with one abnormal and one normal copy of the gene have symptoms of the disease, but they are generally less severely affected and have later ages of onset than males. Renal failure leads to death between the ages of 20 and 40 in 50 to 75% of men and 10 to 35% of women. Hearing loss generally begins in the first or second decades and is found in 55% of men and 40% of women (Gorlin et al, 1995). The loss in women is usually mild and has a later age of onset than in men. Although the X-linked form of Alport's syndrome is the most common, both autosomal dominant and autosomal recessive forms of Alport's syndrome are known to occur.

Norrie's Disease

The major characteristic of Norrie's disease is congenital blindness caused by retinal dysplasia, which is associated with sensory hearing loss and severe mental retardation in about 35% of cases. The hearing loss is progressive and usually begins after 10 years of age. It originates in the cochlea and does not appear to involve the brain stem. The mode of inheritance is X-linked recessive (Gorlin et al, 1995).

X-Linked Nonsyndromic Hearing Impairment

As mentioned earlier in the chapter, nineteenth century authors had noted that more males than females were hearing-impaired. This observation suggests that some types of hearing impairment are X-linked recessive. Many families in which the nonsyndromic hearing impairment shows an X-linked recessive pattern of inheritance have now been reported. They differ in type, severity, and age of onset, but affected members are usually males and no father-to-son transmission exists. One X-linked recessive form of severe

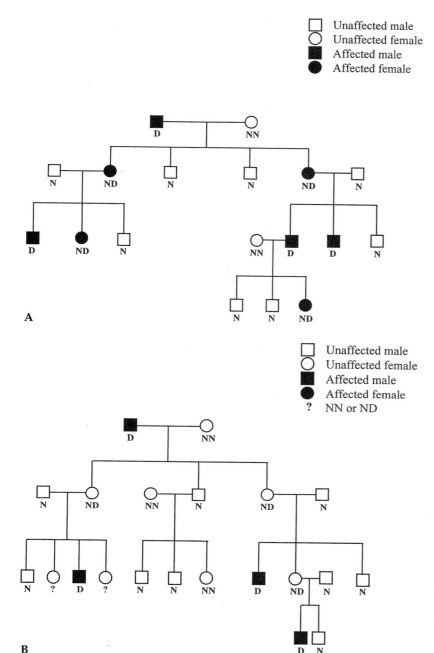

Figure 25–3 **(A)** X-linked dominant inheritance and **(B)** X-linked recessive inheritance. Genotypes are shown below each individual. Females (XX) have two alleles (NN, ND, DD), but males (XY) have only one (N or D). A male who inherits D is affected. With dominant inheritance, ND females are affected, whereas with recessive inheritance they are carriers. In **(B)** the ? means that the genotype of these two females cannot be determined from the pedigree structure; they may be NN or ND.

mixed hearing impairment is associated with a developmental, bony abnormality of the cochlea that can be seen on a CT scan and fixation of the stapedial footplate (Cremers & Huygen, 1983). If a stapedectomy is attempted, a perilymphatic gusher occurs.

Mitochondrial Inheritance

Mitochondria are small organelles that are located within the cytoplasm of a cell; they are independent of the nucleus and have their own DNA (mtDNA). A process called oxidative phosphorylation takes place in the mitochondria and is responsible for energy (adenosine triphosphate) production in the cell. Each mitochondrion has multiple copies of mtDNA,

and each cell contains several hundred mitochondria, and thus many copies of mtDNA. The mutation rate is 10 times higher in mtDNA than in nuclear DNA and cells may contain both mutant copies and normal copies, a condition known as heteroplasmy. If the normal copies can successfully provide the energy requirements of the cell, normal function will be retained. However, different cell types have differing energy requirements. The organs with the most demand for energy are the skeletal muscle, heart, and brain. Thus the typical symptoms found in mitochondrial disorders are muscle weakness, nervous system disorders, visual problems, hearing loss, and dementia.

The mtDNA molecule is circular and consists of about 16,000 base pairs. Mitochondria are maternally inherited, so

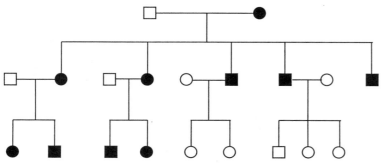

Figure 25–4 Mitochondrial pattern of inheritance. All offspring of affected females are affected, but no offspring of affected males are affected.

the expected family history for a mitochondrial disorder is that all children of an affected mother are affected and children of an affected father are never affected. However, because of heteroplasmy, the mother and siblings of an affected individual may show only minor symptoms or none at all. Figure 25–4 shows a pedigree structure that might be found for a disorder caused by (a) mtDNA mutation.

Sensorineural hearing loss is often one of the characteristic findings in mitochondrial disorders such as (MELAS) (mitochondrial encephalomyopathy, lactic acidosis, strokelike episodes, and sensorineural hearing loss) and (MERRF) (mitochondrial encephalomyopathy, myoclonus epilepsy, ragged-red fibers and sensorineural hearing loss) (Fischel-Ghodsian, 1998). In some families showing a mitochondrial inheritance pattern, sensorineural hearing loss is the only finding. Prezant et al (1993) reported evidence for maternal inheritance in aminoglycoside-induced hearing loss. In this case both a defective mitochondrial gene and an environmental insult were found to be necessary to cause hearing impairment.

METHODS FOR IDENTIFYING HEARING LOSS GENES

Linkage Analysis

The process by which genes for hereditary disorders are localized and identified is called positional cloning. The first step is a linkage study to find a genetic marker that is close to the disease gene. DNA is extracted from blood samples drawn from both affected and unaffected family members and marker types are obtained for each individual using the polymerase chain reaction (PCR). The genome contains thousands of these markers, which usually consist of a string of short repeats (e.g., CACACACACA. . .) that vary in length among individuals. These markers have unique chromosomal locations and thus serve as landmarks on the chromosomes. Markers are amplified by PCR using an individual's DNA sample, and the marker sizes are determined by electrophoresis. Because chromosomes come in pairs, an individual may have two

DNA fragments (alleles) of the same size or two different sizes for each marker. Figure 25–5 shows the results for a family in which three of the children have Usher's syndrome type IC (USH1C). The genetic marker is on chromosome 11 and is designated as D11S921. It has three alleles (*a, b, c*), and the three affected children all have two copies of the *a* allele (genotype *aa*), one inherited from each parent, whereas the unaffected children have the genotypes *bc* and *ab*. This type of association between a marker allele and presence of the disorder within a family suggests that the genetic marker may be close to the gene for the disorder. In fact, linkage analyses of more families showed the same pattern confirming that the USH1C gene is likely to be very close to D11S921. A linkage study may require typing hundreds of genetic markers before the disease gene is localized, but once this step is accomplished, research to identify candidate genes in the region begins. As well as providing the approximate location of a disease gene, linkage analysis permits more precise genetic counseling. For example, the marker genotype results shown in Figure 25–5 indicate that individual 6 probably has two normal copies of the USH1C gene, whereas individual 7 is likely to be a carrier of the defective allele. (That is, she has one normal copy and one abnormal copy of the USH1C gene.)

If age of onset is variable among family members, then linkage analysis must allow for age-dependent penetrances. Children may be unaffected because they are too young to have developed symptoms, not because they do not have the abnormal allele. Thus ignoring age and coding them as unaffected in the analysis would give misleading results and delay finding the location of the gene.

For recessive hearing impairment, affected individuals who are related are likely to have the same homozygous genotype. Thus the search for the location of the gene may be accelerated by screening pooled DNA samples from these individuals and selecting markers for which they are all homozygous for the same allele (Sheffield et al, 1994). If pooling is feasible, the number of samples that needs to be typed can be reduced dramatically. This approach has successfully located several of the genes for hearing impairment.

PITFALL

Affected individuals in unrelated families are not expected to have the same genotypes at markers that are close to the disease gene. Thus pooling samples from affected individuals in different families is not likely to be helpful. In addition, the same gene may not necessarily be responsible for the phenotype in each family.

Heterogeneity

Results from linkage studies of several families may be pooled to increase the probability that the correct location has been found for the disease gene. This convenience may also be a complication if the disease is caused by different genes in some of the families.

PITFALL

Many different genes and genotypes may lead to the same clinical phenotype; conversely, the same genotype may result in variable phenotypes. This genetic heterogeneity often precludes accurate diagnosis.

Studying endogamous populations or large pedigrees minimizes heterogeneity but does not necessarily eliminate it. A phenotype such as nonsyndromic hearing impairment is caused by many different genes and the cause may not be the same even for affected members of the same family. In some cases auditory testing may detect phenotype differences among members of the same kindred. Such findings may be the result of etiological differences and provide critical information for

genetic studies. For example, in the family studied by Vahava et al (1998) auditory testing showed that the hearing impairment in one member was different from that in the other members. Knowing that this individual was a phenocopy (same clinical phenotype but different cause) facilitated the linkage analysis.

Many sophisticated auditory tests can now be done that complement the standard pure tone audiogram and provide a much more comprehensive and accurate assessment of the hearing impairment. New techniques can distinguish between hair cell (sensory) deafness and neural deafness (Berlin et al, 1998; Starr et al, 1996) and between deafness caused by brain malfunction in contrast to cochlear malfunction. The same pure tone audiogram might be observed in one patient with a genetically based loss of outer hair cells and another with normal outer hair cells but damaged nerve fibers. However, cause and genotypes are probably quite different and classifying both patients according to their pure tone audiograms alone would not be adequate for genetic analysis. A more precise categorization of the hearing loss can be made by testing otoacoustic emissions that allow cochlear function to be assessed somewhat independently of neural function. Recent studies suggest that they may be helpful in discriminating between those who carry certain mutations that cause recessive nonsyndromic sensorineural hearing impairment and those who do not (Morell et al, 1998). In addition, by performing tests for both auditory brain stem response and otoacoustic emissions, a patient with sensorineural hearing impairment can be distinguished from one with an auditory neuropathy.

Physical Mapping, cDNA Libraries, and Candidate Genes

The development of high-resolution genetic and physical maps, together with the construction of genomic and cDNA libraries, and the availability of sequence databases for many

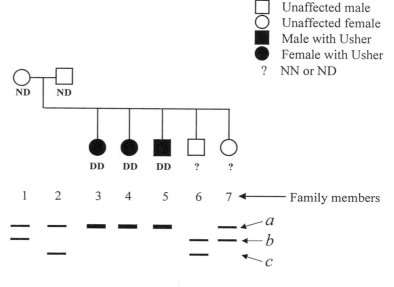

Figure 25–5 Genotypes for the genetic marker D11S921 in members of a family in which three of the offspring have Usher's syndrome type IC. The family members are labeled 1 through 7; the parents are 1 (mother) and 2 (father); the affected children are 3, 4, 5; and the unaffected children are 6 and 7. The genotypes for USH1C (NN, ND, DD) are shown below each individual. The D11S921 genotypes *(aa, ab, ac, bb, bc, cc)* for each family member are given beneath the representation of the DNA fragments visualized after electrophoresis. The three affected individuals have two copies of the *a* allele, whereas the other family members have two different alleles.

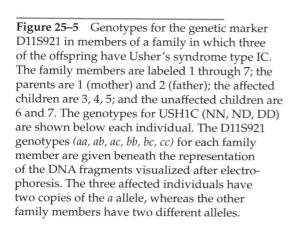

species provide the tools for finding genes once they have been localized by linkage analysis. Figure 25–6 provides a schematic illustration of the series of steps that lead from approximate location to gene identification. The map of markers used for linkage analysis is called the genetic map. The physical map consists of overlapping fragments of DNA that are relatively easy to manipulate. DNA fragments are inserted into specialized vectors (carriers of DNA material) such as yeast artificial chromosomes (YACs) and bacterial artificial chromosomes (BACs). YACs may hold more than a million base pairs of human DNA, whereas the size of the human DNA contained in BACs is usually about 200,000 base pairs. YAC and BAC genomic libraries are commercially available for gene identification studies. These libraries may be screened to find those clones that contain the genetic markers known from linkage analysis to be close to the disease gene. Another type of library, a cDNA library, has been constructed for many different tissues; these libraries are likely to contain cDNA sequence of most of the genes that are expressed in the tissue, although the sequence may not be complete. A human fetal cochlear cDNA library (Robertson et al, 1994) has been valuable in the identification of several of the hearing impairment genes.

If the location of a gene can be narrowed to a single BAC, determining the sequence of base pairs becomes feasible. This sequence can be searched using computer programs to find subsets of sequence that are likely to be exons and therefore part of a gene. Once potential exons are identified, their sequence is used to obtain a full-length cDNA usually with the help of a cDNA library. The final step is to compare the normal sequence of each candidate gene with the sequence in patients. If a mutation is found in the gene in affected individuals but not in those who are unaffected, the search for the gene responsible for the hearing impairment may be over. However, DNA sequence varies from one individual to another, so a sequence difference may not necessarily make the gene defective. Some mutations, though, such as a deletion or insertion of several bases, or a point mutation (single base change) that gives rise to a codon that does not correspond to an amino acid (e.g., a stop codon), are likely to be causal.

Transgenic and Knockout Mice

Finding a mutation that probably makes a gene defective is a critical step, but it does not prove that the defect actually

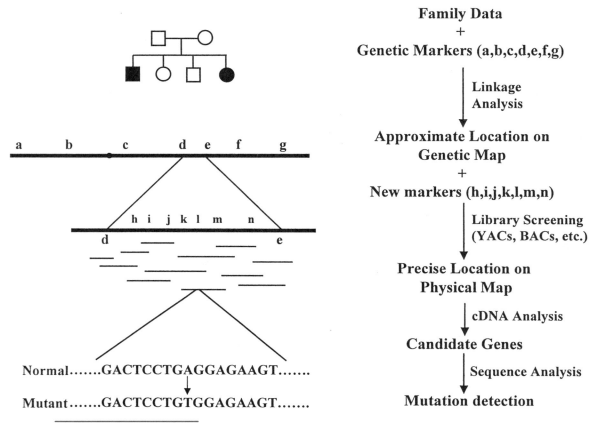

Figure 25–6 The steps involved in the positional cloning approach to identifying a gene.

causes the hearing impairment. However, if a transgenic or knockout mouse is hearing-impaired, the argument that the defect causes the abnormal phenotype is convincing. To obtain a transgenic mouse, copies of the gene are injected into mouse oocytes just after fertilization. The otocytes are then implanted into a foster mother whose uterus has been prepared for pregnancy by treatment with hormones. The transgene may incorporate anywhere in the genome and usually several copies (sometimes as many as 200 copies) are found at a single location. In general, between 10 and 30% of the progeny are found to have the injected gene in their germline DNA and can therefore pass it on to their offspring, thus allowing the development of a colony of transgenic mice.

The construction of a knockout mouse is a much more controlled and precise experiment than generating a transgenic mouse. The first step is to replace the normal copy of the gene with a copy containing the mutation of interest. This procedure is carried out in embryonic stem (ES) cells derived from mouse blastocysts (an early stage of embryonic development) and grown in tissue culture. The mutant gene may insert anywhere in the genome, but only those cells in which the normal copy is replaced by the mutant copy are selected for the next step. The selected ES cells are then injected into a recipient blastocyst, which is implanted into a foster mother. The resulting offspring will be chimeric, meaning that some of their cells are derived from the ES cell line and some are from the recipient blastocyst. Mating experiments may then be set up to determine whether the ES cells have contributed to the germline and to generate a colony of knockout mice. Knockout mice provide excellent animal models for studying the effect of gene mutations that are associated with human disorders.

Gene Therapy

Gene therapy is the term used to describe a method of treatment of a human disorder in which a gene is transferred into the cells of the particular organ that is affected. A normal copy of the gene that is defective in the patient is packaged into a vector and introduced to the cells. Note that the gene is not incorporated into the germline cells. The purpose of gene therapy is to treat the patient, not to change the genetic material that is passed on to the next generation. Many research studies are in progress to determine effective vectors and suitable approaches for delivering genetic material to specific tissues. Certain classes of viruses may be used as vectors, and ongoing investigations are exploring their potential in gene therapy. Nonviral strategies such as coating the gene in a lipid layer are also being developed.

Although still in its infancy, gene therapy holds great promise for future treatment of genetic disorders, including hearing impairment. More than 100 gene therapy protocols have been approved, most of them being for the treatment of cancer patients. However, a few protocols have been approved for monogenic disorders such as cystic fibrosis. Within the next 10 years medical treatment based on gene therapy is likely to become available for many disorders.

LOCALIZED AND IDENTIFIED GENES FOR HEARING IMPAIRMENT

Figure 25–7 shows the chromosomal locations of genes for hearing impairment (Van Camp & Smith, 1998). Those for which the defective gene has been identified are denoted by an asterisk and the proteins encoded by these genes are listed beneath the chromosome.

PEARL

Many regions of the mouse genome are similar (homologous) to the human genome, and some of the human genes for hearing impairment have been identified because mutations in the homologous mouse genes had been shown to cause deafness in mice.

Mouse mutants for which the genes are known to be, or are likely to be, the same as those in humans are also shown in Figure 25–7.

Syndromes

As might be anticipated, mapping and identification of genes for several syndromic forms of hearing impairment preceded nonsyndromic forms. However, as will become clear, the distinction between syndromic and nonsyndromic and also between dominant and recessive is blurred at the level of the gene. These words describe the phenotype and the pattern of inheritance, not the defective gene. The same gene may cause syndromic hearing loss in one case and nonsyndromic hearing loss in another case. Similarly, a dominant pattern of inheritance may be seen in one family and a recessive pattern in another, but the defective gene may be the same in both. For example, the unconventional myosin VIIa (MYO7A) was shown to be the Usher's syndrome type IB gene (Weil et al, 1995) before mutations in that gene were also found to cause a recessive nonsyndromic hearing loss, DFNB2 (Liu et al, 1997a; Weil et al, 1997), and a dominant nonsyndromic hearing loss, DFNA11 (Liu et al, 1997b). Similarly, mutations in the gene (PDS) for Pendred's syndrome, in which congenital sensorineural hearing impairment is combined with thyroid goiter, also appear to be associated with nonsyndromic hearing impairment (Everett et al, 1997; Li et al, 1998). In addition, mutations in the connexin 26 gene (GJB2) were shown to cause recessive nonsyndromic hearing impairment (DFNB1) (Kelsell et al, 1997), and Denoyelle et al (1998) recently reported a family with dominant deafness in which a mutation in GJB2 is most likely to be responsible.

Syndromic hearing impairment tends to be less genetically heterogeneous than nonsyndromic hearing impairment, although the number of genes that have so far been mapped for Usher's syndrome type I (USH1*) is six, and analyses of some families suggest that there are more. It is of interest to note that USH1C (Smith et al, 1992) maps to the same location as DFNB18 (Jain et al, 1998) on the short arm of chromosome 11, and USH1D (Wayne et al, 1996) and DFNB12 (Chaib et al,

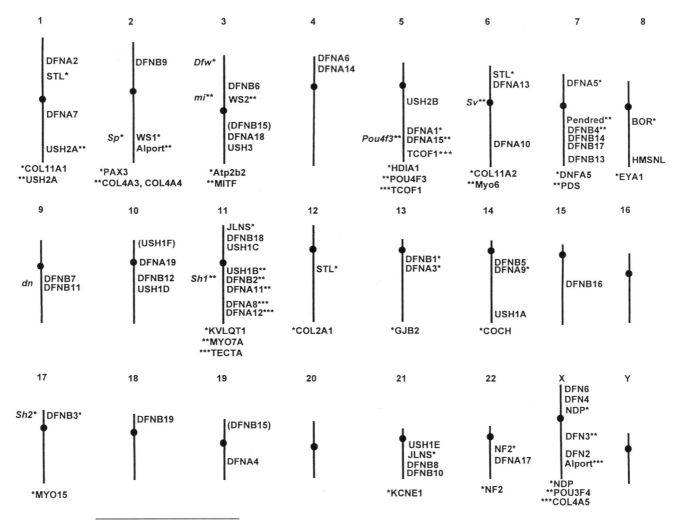

Figure 25–7 Chromosomal locations of genes for hearing impairment. Those genes that have been identified are denoted by asterisks, and the encoded protein is shown below the chromosome. Mouse genes that are known to be, or likely to be, homologous are shown to the left and human genes to the right. DFNB15 is in parentheses because it is equally likely to be on chromosomes 3 and 19 (Chen et al, 1997), and USH1F is in parentheses because its precise location on chromosome 10 is unknown. This figure was constructed from the Hereditary Hearing Loss Homepage. (From Van Camp & Smith [1998], with permission.)

1996) are both in the same region of the long arm of chromosome 10. Thus more examples of different mutations in the same gene causing both syndromic and nonsyndromic hearing impairment are likely to be found.

Treacher Collins Syndrome

Linkage studies showed that the Treacher Collins gene is on the long arm of chromosome 5 (Jabs et al, 1991; Dixon et al, 1991). Positional cloning led to the isolation of a novel gene (TCOF1) of unknown function in which different mutations were found in affected members of five unrelated families (Treacher Collins Syndrome Collaborative Group, 1996). All these mutations were predicted to result in premature termination of the gene product and none were found in control samples, providing evidence that TCOF1 is the Treacher Collins gene. The clinical phenotype of Treacher Collins syndrome

suggests that the gene plays a fundamental role in early embryonic development, particularly in the development of the craniofacial complex. Wise et al (1997) showed that the gene shares motifs with nucleolar trafficking proteins in other species and postulated that Treacher Collins syndrome results from defects in a nucleolar trafficking protein that is critical for normal human craniofacial development.

Branchio-Oto-Renal Syndrome

Kumar et al (1992) mapped the BOR gene to the long arm of chromosome 8 by linkage analysis. Abdelhak et al (1997) identified the defective gene (EYA1) as the human homologue of the *Drosophila* "eyes absent" gene. The expression pattern of the mouse EYA1 homologue suggested that the gene may have a role in the development of all components of the inner ear. As was found for the TCOF1 gene, mutations in the EYA1 gene tend to be family specific with unrelated affected individuals having different mutations.

Stickler Syndrome

Francomano et al (1987) demonstrated linkage between the disease gene and the procollagen 2 gene (COL2A1) on chromosome 12 in several families, and Williams et al (1996) demonstrated the presence of a mutation in the COL2A1 gene in affected members of the kindred originally described by Stickler et al (1965). Subsequent mutational analyses of the COL2A1 gene in affected individuals have revealed the presence of many different mutations, which lead to a truncated procollagen 2 alpha chain with no carboxy terminus (Brown et al, 1995). However, defects in COL2A1 do not explain all cases of Stickler syndrome because approximately 50% of families with affected individuals do not show linkage to COL2A1. Brunner et al (1994) described a large Dutch kindred in which they localized the gene causing Stickler syndrome to the short arm of chromosome 6. The gene encoding the alpha$_2$-subunit of type XI collagen (COL11A2) had been assigned to the candidate region of chromosome 6, and Vikkula et al (1995) found a nonsense mutation (base change resulting in a stop codon) in the COL11A2 gene in affected members of the Dutch kindred. A four-generation family studied by Richards et al (1996) did not show linkage to either COL2A1 or COL11A2; instead, additional analyses demonstrated linkage to the COL11A1 gene region on chromosome 1 and a mutation was found in this gene in affected members of the family. Type II and type XI collagen copolymerize within collagen fibrils (Mendler et al, 1989) and are necessary for skeletal development.

Neurofibromatosis Type 2

The NF2 gene was mapped to chromosome 22 (Rouleau et al, 1990; Seizinger et al, 1986) and identified by Trofatter et al (1993). Rouleau et al (1993) showed that both copies of the NF2 gene are inactivated in vestibular schwannomas (Rouleau et al, 1993). The mode of inheritance of NF2 is dominant with one abnormal allele being inherited. But a spontaneous mutation must occur in the other NF2 allele in a cell for a tumor to form. This process of tumor formation was originally proposed by Knudson (1971) for retinoblastomas. Many different mutations have been reported in the NF2 gene, and each one tends to be unique to a patient or family. However, point mutations leading to stop codons that terminate protein synthesis prematurely have been found in a number of patients and may be a basis for screening to provide presymptomatic diagnosis (Sainz et al, 1995). Mutations in the NF2 gene also are often present in sporadic vestibular schwannomas (Lekanne Deprez et al, 1994) and other human tumor types (Bianchi et al, 1994).

Waardenburg's Syndrome

Genetic linkage analysis of DNA samples from affected individuals and their family members allowed the assignment of the gene for Waardenburg's syndrome type 1 to chromosome 2 and suggested that it may be homologous to the mouse *Splotch (Sp)* mutation (Farrer et al, 1992), which was known to

be caused by mutations in *pax-3*, a paired box gene (Epstein et al, 1991; Goulding et al, 1991). These types of genes encode DNA binding proteins that are important in development (Gruss & Walther, 1992). Studies by Baldwin et al (1992) and Tassabehji et al (1992) of the human homologue, PAX3, demonstrated mutations in patients with Waardenburg's syndrome type 1. Different mutations in PAX3 are usually found in unrelated affected individuals, and affected members of the same family often show considerable variation in expression of the phenotype. Thus predicting phenotype on the basis of the mutation is not feasible at present, although Pandya et al (1996) suggest that ultimately it may be possible.

A gene for Waardenburg's syndrome type 2 was mapped to chromosome 3 (Hughes et al, 1994) and shown to be the human homologue of the mouse *microphthalmia* mutant (Tassabehji et al, 1994). Mutations in this gene (MITF), which encodes a transcription factor, explain about 20% of cases of Waardenburg's syndrome type 2, whereas most cases of Waardenburg's syndrome type 1 are caused by mutations in PAX3. Many different mutations have been documented in both PAX3 and MITF (Tassabehji et al, 1995). Thus different genotypes lead to the same clinical phenotype. Conversely, the variation in phenotypic expression among affected individuals within a family demonstrates that the same genotype can result in different clinical phenotypes.

Usher's Syndrome

The mode of inheritance for all types of Usher's syndrome is autosomal recessive, and linkage studies of affected families have led to the localization of nine different genes. Six Usher-type I genes have been mapped to chromosomes 14q (USH1A) (Kaplan et al, 1992), 11q (USH1B) (Kimberling et al, 1992), 11p (USH1C) (Smith et al, 1992), 10q (USH1D) (Wayne et al, 1996), 21q (USH1E) (Chaib et al, 1997), and 10 (USH1F) (Wayne et al, 1997). An Usher type II gene (USH2A) was assigned to chromosome 1q (Kimberling et al, 1990, Lewis et al, 1990), and a second (USH2B) to chromosome 5q (Pieke Dahl et al, 1998). Sankila et al (1995) localized a gene for Usher's syndrome type III (USH3) to chromosome 3q.

The USH1B gene on 11q has been shown to encode the protein, myosin VIIa (Weil et al, 1995). This finding provides the basis for a molecular diagnostic test to search for mutations in this gene in individuals who may have Usher type I or who may be carriers. However, it needs to be emphasized that this is just one of several genes that causes Usher's syndrome. Before mutational analysis is performed, genetic marker testing of affected individuals and their family members is necessary to determine the location of the defective gene. If the results indicate that the gene on 11q is responsible, searching for a mutation in the myosin VIIa gene would be meaningful. Eudy et al (1998) showed that the USH2A gene on 1q encodes a novel protein, which resembles an extracellular matrix protein or a cell adhesion molecule. Three different mutations were found, with one of them appearing to be relatively frequent in affected individuals of northern European ancestry. Mutations in USH2A probably explain most cases of Usher type II, but at least one other gene (USH2B) is associated with this phenotype.

Sometimes ancestry may suggest the likely gene. For example, Usher's syndrome type I gene (USH1C) on 11p has been found only in the Acadian population, and genetic marker studies are consistent with a single mutation being responsible for all cases of Acadian Usher's syndrome type I (Keats et al, 1994). Thus, for profoundly hearing-impaired infants of Acadian ancestry, genetic marker analyses may allow differentiation between nonsyndromic hereditary hearing impairment and Usher's syndrome type I.

Pendred's Syndrome

Linkage analysis of families, in which some members have this syndrome, localized the defective gene to the long arm of chromosome 7 (Coyle et al, 1996; Sheffield et al, 1996). Positional cloning of the critical region led to the identification of a gene (PDS) that encodes a highly conserved (meaning that it is found in many different species) but unknown protein (Everett et al, 1997). Mutational analyses of affected members in three families were carried out, and a different mutation was found in each family. A fourth mutation appears to cause nonsyndromic hearing impairment in a family reported by Li et al (1998).

Jervell and Lange-Nielsen Syndrome

Neyroud et al (1997) showed that mutations in the KVLQT1 gene cause the recessive Jervell and Lange-Nielsen syndrome. Mutations in this gene also cause the Ward-Romano syndrome, a dominant disorder in which affected individuals have a prolonged Q-T interval in their ECG but are not hearing-impaired. Thus parents of children with Jervell and Lange-Nielsen syndrome may have Ward-Romano syndrome. Tyson et al (1997) found that most of the families they studied showed linkage to markers in the region on chromosome 11 containing the KVLQT1 gene; however, linkage to KVLQT1 was excluded for a small consanguineous British family. The affected children in this family were found to be homozygous for markers on chromosome 21 flanking the KCNE1 gene, suggesting that mutations in this gene may be responsible for the phenotype. Both KCNE1 and KVLQT1 encode proteins that form the delayed rectifier potassium channel, which is necessary for endolymph homeostasis within the inner ear.

Alport's Syndrome

Most cases of Alport's syndrome are caused by mutations in the gene (COL4A5) for the alpha$_5$-subunit of type IV collagen (Barker et al, 1990). This gene is on the long arm of the X chromosome, and female carriers usually show some signs of the disease, although not as severe as males. A large number of COL4A5 mutations causing Alport's syndrome have been reported, and many more are likely to be found. The gene consists of 51 exons making the search for mutations a time-consuming process. In addition, some families with Alport's syndrome show an autosomal recessive pattern of inheritance and mutations in the genes for the alpha$_3$- and alpha$_4$-subunits of collagen type IV on the long arm of chromosome 2 have been found in affected individuals (Mochizuki et al, 1994).

Norrie's Disease

The gene for Norrie's disease was assigned to the short arm of the X chromosome by linkage analysis, and Berger et al (1992) and Chen et al (1992) isolated a novel candidate gene (NDP) from the critical region. The proportion of cases of Norrie's disease caused by new mutations is relatively high (as is often found for X-linked disorders), and diagnosis on the basis of clinical findings is often difficult. However, the coding sequence of NDP is small, making the process of detecting mutations for Norrie's disease much less time consuming than for most of the other hearing impairment disorders. Chen et al (1993) showed that NDP consists of three exons, and they proposed that the protein product may be involved in regulation of neural cell differentiation and proliferation. Sequence pattern searches and three-dimensional modeling by Meitinger et al (1993) indicated that Norrie's disease protein has a tertiary structure similar to that of transforming growth factor beta.

MELAS and MERRF

MELAS syndrome can be caused by several different mtDNA mutations in transfer RNA (tRNA) genes, which are essential for protein synthesis. The mitochondrial genome contains 22 tRNA genes, and most of the mutations causing MELAS syndrome are in one of these genes. A specific mutation associated with MERRF in a mtDNA tRNA gene was first demonstrated by Shoffner et al (1990). This mutation accounts for 80 to 90% of MERRF cases (Shoffner & Wallace, 1992). Although the genetic defect is transmitted through the maternal lineage in both of these syndromes, the clinical phenotype varies greatly within a pedigree, consistent with a heteroplasmic population of mtDNAs, some of which are normal and others mutant.

Auditory Neuropathies

Many families with auditory neuropathy have been identified, but the location of the gene has been determined in only one. The difficulties with finding these genes are the small sizes of the families and the high level of heterogeneity, with many different genes resulting in similar phenotypes. In addition, in some children diagnosed with an auditory neuropathy, otoacoustic emissions disappear as they get older. Thus diagnosing the disorder in older children may be problematic. The gene (HMSNL) that has been localized is on the long arm of chromosome 8, and the study was done in a large gypsy kindred (Kalaydjieva et al, 1996). The disorder is recessive in this kindred, but because of the isolated and endogamous nature of the gypsy population, 14 affected individuals spanning four generations participated in the study. Otoacoustic emissions were not obtained on these patients. However, Butinar et al (1999) performed extensive auditory testing on members of another gypsy family with a similar phenotype and showing linkage to the same region of chromosome 8. The affected members in this family had abnormal auditory brain stem responses but robust otoacoustical emissions, indicating an auditory neuropathy.

Nonsyndromic Hearing Impairment

As might be expected, the first hearing impairment gene mapped was in families showing X-linked inheritance (Brunner et al, 1988; Wallis et al, 1988). This mixed (conductive and sensorineural) hearing impairment (DFN3) is associated with perilymphatic gushers if stapedectomy is done. The gene was localized to the long arm of the X chromosome, and analyses of DNA from patients showed that mutations in the POU3F4 gene, a member of the POU family of transcription factors that are expressed in early development, cause this hearing impairment (de Kok et al, 1995). Three other nonsyndromic hearing impairment genes have been localized on the X chromosome, but they have not yet been identified.

PITFALL

Rule out a defect in POU3F4 before performing stapedectomy.

The number of genes for hearing impairment that have been mapped increases from one month to the next. As of November 1998, the Hereditary Hearing Loss Homepage (Van Camp & Smith, 1998) listed the autosomal locations of 19 genes for dominant (DFNA*) and 19 for recessive (DFNB*) nonsyndromic sensorineural hearing impairment. Several of these autosomal genes have been identified: DFNA1, DFNA8 (also DFNA12), DFNA15, DFNB1 (also DFNA3), DFNB2 (also DFNA11), DFNB3, and DFNB4 encode the highly conserved diaphanous (HDIA1) (Lynch et al, 1997), alpha tectorin (TECTA) (Verhoeven et al, 1998), the transcription factor, POU4F3 (Vahava et al, 1998), the gap junction protein, connexin 26 (GJB2) (Kelsell et al, 1997), the unconventional myosin VIIA (MYO7A) (Liu et al, 1997a,b; Weil et al, 1995, 1997), another unconventional myosin (MYO15) (Wang et al, 1998), and the protein that is defective in Pendred's syndrome (Li et al, 1998), respectively. DFNA5 and DFNA9 have also been identified, but the function of their protein products is unknown (Robertson et al, 1998; Van Laer et al, 1998). The protein encoded by DFNA9 is called COCH because the gene was isolated from the human fetal cochlear cDNA library (Robertson et al, 1994) before it was shown to be DFNA9. All of these advances in our knowledge of the major role played by genes in the cause of hearing impairment have occurred over the past 6 years.

Mutations in GJB2 may account for more than 50% of cases of nonsyndromic recessive sensorineural hearing impairment (Gasparini et al, 1997). In addition, the same GJB2 mutation is found in a large percentage of these individuals (Denoyelle et al, 1997; Zelante et al, 1997). This mutation is referred to as either 30delG or 35delG because it is a one base pair deletion occurring in a string of six guanines, which begin at position 30 in the coding sequence. Interestingly, a different mutation (167delT) in the GJB2 gene probably accounts for most cases of nonsyndromic recessive deafness in the Ashkenazi Jewish population (Morell et al, 1998).

As discussed in the section on syndromes, hearing impairment is often one of the components of the phenotype in mitochondrial myopathies that are caused by specific mtDNA mutations (Fischel-Ghodsian, 1998). However, in some families hearing impairment may be the only anomaly. An mtDNA mutation (A1555G) in the 12S ribosomal RNA (rRNA) gene was found to be the cause of hearing impairment in a family showing a maternal pattern of inheritance.

This same mutation is associated with heightened sensitivity to hearing loss after aminoglycoside antibiotic treatment (Prezant et al, 1993). Estimates of the frequency of this mutation suggest that screening of hearing-impaired individuals may be beneficial in some populations (Estivill et al, 1998).

Another form of hearing loss that may be associated with mtDNA mutations is presbycusis. Fischel-Ghodsian et al (1997) found a significant increase in mtDNA mutations in the temporal bones of patients with presbycusis, and evidence is mounting that the accumulation of mtDNA mutations may be relevant to many aspects of the aging process (Nagley et al, 1993).

SPECIAL CONSIDERATION

Consider testing individuals for the presence of the A1555G rRNA mutation before administering aminoglycoside antibiotic treatment.

Mouse Models

Because of the high degree of similarity (homology) of genes in humans and mice, studies of mouse mutants have made many valuable contributions to human disease gene identification (Meisler, 1996), and hearing impairment is no exception (Brown and Steel, 1994). An example was the identification of PAX3 as the gene for Waardenburg's syndrome type 1 after the detection of *pax-3* mutations in the *splotch* mouse, as discussed earlier in the chapter. Major advantages of using the mouse for finding disease genes are the ability to set up specific matings and the relative ease of obtaining large numbers of informative progeny for linkage analysis to localize the gene. A relevant example is human USH1B and the mouse deafness mutant *shaker-1 (sh1)*, which were hypothesized to be caused by mutations in homologous genes because they had been mapped by linkage to a conserved region on human chromosome 11q13 and mouse chromosome 7. This hypothesis was proven to be correct when Gibson et al (1995) showed that the *sh1* gene encoded myosin VIIa, and Weil et al (1995) quickly found mutations in the human MYO7A gene in Usher type IB patients. Similarly, the mouse mutant *shaker-2 (sh2)* and DFNB3 are both caused by mutations in another unconventional myosin (MYO15), and complementary work in mice and humans led to this finding (Probst et al, 1998; Wang et al, 1998).

The POU4F3 gene became a candidate for the dominant hearing impairment in the DFNA15 family when it was mapped to a region of the long arm of chromosome 5 that was likely to share homology with the region on mouse chromosome 18 containing the *Pou4f3* (also known as Brn3c and Brn-3.1) gene (Vahava et al, 1998). Targeted deletion of both alleles of *Pou4f3* had been shown to cause deafness in mice (Erkman et al, 1996; Xiang et al, 1997). Although the critical region on chromosome 5 was too large to begin a physical mapping approach to finding the gene, the hunch that POU4F3 may be the defective gene proved to be true.

No human genes have yet been mapped to the homologous region of mouse chromosome 9 to which the *Snell's waltzer (sv)* gene was mapped and shown to encode an unconventional myosin heavy chain, myosin VI (Avraham et al, 1995). This mouse is deaf and shows the typical circling and head-tossing behavior of mice with inner ear defects, and hearing-impaired patients with defects in this gene on human chromosome 6 will probably be found. Similarly, Street et al (1998) showed that the *Deafwaddler (Dfw)* gene on mouse chromosome 6 encodes a plasma membrane Ca^{2+}-ATPase type 2 pump *(Atp2b2)* that may be necessary for sensory transduction in stereocilia of hair cells and neurotransmitter release from the basolateral membrane. Although no patients have yet been identified with mutations in the human homologue of this gene that is on the short arm of chromosome 3, it is a likely candidate for a phenotype with both deafness and vestibular dysfunction.

Another probable homologue of a human gene for hearing impairment is the *deafness (dn)* gene on mouse chromosome 19 (Keats et al, 1995). This region shares homology with human chromosome 9q13-q21 to which both DFNB7 and DFNB11 have been mapped (Jain et al, 1995; Scott et al, 1996).

MOLECULAR GENETIC DIAGNOSTIC TESTS FOR HEARING LOSS

In theory, once a disease gene is identified, diagnostic tests can be developed to detect mutations in individuals who may have the disease. Offering such diagnostic tests can be beneficial if one or two mutations are responsible for most cases of hearing impairment caused by that gene. An example is the GJB2 gene.

PEARL

Diagnostic testing for GJB2 mutations may provide the cause for a large percentage of congenitally deaf infants.

For many genes, however, unrelated affected individuals are likely to have different mutations, making detection a time-consuming and expensive task especially if the gene is large. Moreover, finding a sequence difference does not necessarily mean that the responsible mutation has been found; sequence variation among individuals is common and very few of the variants are associated with a disorder. Thus setting up diagnostic tests that are commercially available may not be economically feasible. On the other hand, once a mutation is identified in one family member, related individuals can be tested for this mutation. This can be beneficial for (1) presymptomatic diagnosis in later age of onset hearing impairment; (2) detecting the presence of the defective gene when penetrance is not complete, meaning that unaffected individuals may have the gene; and (3) identifying carriers of the gene when the inheritance pattern is recessive.

GENETIC COUNSELING

Genetic counseling attempts to answer questions concerning cause (e.g., Why is our child hearing-impaired?) and risk (e.g., What is the chance that we will have a hearing-impaired

CONTROVERSIAL POINT

Should molecular diagnostic testing be offered routinely if the result will not provide an alternative approach to treatment and management of the disorder? What are the psychological effects of presymptomatic genetic testing? Should parents be able to have their children tested for the presence of a disease gene for which the age of onset of symptoms is after they reach adulthood? What is the obligation to other family members if a defective gene is detected? Remember, genes are transmitted from one generation to the next, and the results for one individual are pertinent to many relatives.

child?). These questions may come from the parents of a child with hearing impairment, from a hearing-impaired individual who wants to have a child, or from a person who has hearing-impaired relatives. As well as answering these questions, the genetic counselor can provide information concerning the availability of genetic diagnostic testing. The first step in the counseling session is to assess the results of audiological testing, physical examination, and any other medical findings of the patient and obtain a complete family history. The audiological tests and physical examination may provide insight into the cause of the hearing impairment. In particular, abnormal physical findings such as ear pits or tags, hyperpigmentation or depigmentation, or goiter may aid in making a diagnosis. Similarly, evidence of retinal degeneration or an abnormal electrocardiogram or CT scan would suggest specific disorders. The family history provides information for estimating the risk of having a hearing-impaired child. The genetic counselor will ask questions concerning the hearing and general health of all known relatives going back as many generations as possible and construct a family tree. Information concerning parental consanguinity is particularly pertinent and needs to be provided. The complete medical and family history will then be used to answer the questions of the consultant.

A critical part of genetic counseling is making sure that the patient understands the information being conveyed. It is essential that no communication barriers are present, and genetic counseling of hearing-impaired individuals must be done in an appropriate manner using visual material and/or a sign language interpreter.

Marriages between two deaf individuals are relatively common. The offspring of two deaf parents are likely to be hearing because the cause of the deafness is probably different in the parents. Even if both parents have recessive deafness, the chance that the same gene is defective in both of them is not high. Thus the offspring will probably be carriers of two different genes for deafness, but they will have normal hearing. An outcome of the identification of many of the genes for deafness is that tests will become available that determine which gene is causing an individual's deafness. If spouses with recessive deafness find out that they have the same defective gene, they will know that all of their children will be hearing-impaired.

FUTURE OF GENETIC INTERVENTION IN HEARING LOSS

Routine molecular diagnostic testing for many of the genes causing hearing impairment is likely to be available within the next few years, but the development of effective therapies based on gene identification is still in its infancy. However, promising new advances through research are arising at a rapid rate and the potential for developing molecular intervention strategies as a treatment and perhaps cure is encouraging. A prerequisite, though, is understanding the normal function of proteins encoded by hearing impairment genes, such as unconventional myosins (MYO7A, MYO15, myo6), in the inner ear. The stereocilia of the hair cells in the cochlea consist of an actin core and a myosin outer cover, and without them normal hearing cannot take place. The bending of the stereocilia in response to sound is critical for the activation of the afferent auditory pathway. Scanning electron microscopy shows that stereocilia are malformed when the MYO7A, MYO15, and myo6 genes are defective, suggesting that these myosins are needed to maintain the structure of the stereocilia (Steel & Brown, 1998). Thus effective molecular therapies will require finding alternate ways to ensure correct formation of the stereocilia, and the intervention may be necessary very early in development.

The prospect for molecular therapies in the near future is probably more promising for later age of onset hearing loss than for congenital deafness. If symptoms do not appear until adulthood, then decline in other cellular processes together with accumulation of environmental insults are likely to be playing a role in the onset of the hearing loss. Thus interventions aimed at protecting the cells from age-related damage may be effective.

CONCLUSIONS

Comprehensive medical histories for all family members are important for determining the cause of a disorder, especially if genetic factors are likely to play a role. Family history may demonstrate a clear pattern of inheritance on which recurrence risk calculations can be based and the information provided to family members. These calculations become more definitive when the location of the gene causing the disorder is known. Laboratory testing of genetic markers that are very close to the gene can be done to determine which alleles are transmitted from parents to offspring, and this information can be used to predict with high probability (usually greater than 98%) whether a family member has the defective gene. Identification of the gene allows direct mutational analysis to be performed on an individual's DNA without the need for DNA samples from other family members.

Genetic studies of many disorders over the past few years, including those in which hearing impairment is a characteristic finding, have led to the localization and identification of a large number of causative genes. The goal of such research is to provide the knowledge necessary for precise prenatal and postnatal diagnostic testing and for developing more effective therapies for genetic disorders. In addition, this research is demonstrating the vast amount of variation at both the phenotypic and genotypic levels. Individuals with identical genotypes have varying clinical phenotypes, whereas the same clinical phenotype may result from different genotypes and, in fact, from defects in different genes.

As described in this chapter, defects in many different genes cause hearing impairment, and the cause may be different even among family members. Conversely, both syndromic and nonsyndromic hearing impairment may be caused by mutations within the same gene. Also, different mutations within the same gene may cause dominant and recessive forms of hearing impairment. These findings drive home the point that the adjectives, dominant and recessive, describe the relationship between a specific phenotype and genotype, not the gene itself. In contrast, different mutations within the same gene and different genes may give the same clinical phenotype as is found for recessive nonsyndromic hearing impairment. Thus the problem of useful categorization on the basis of the clinical phenotype and mode of inheritance has been clarified substantially by the localization and, in some cases, identification of the gene.

Identification of genes for hearing impairment provides an important step toward understanding the molecular mechanism of hearing. In some cases a single gene defect may be the major contributor to the hearing impairment, in others it may be an environmental insult. But they are just the initiating factors; they set in motion a cascade of cellular events that inhibit the ability of the cell to function correctly. In many cases the relationship between the initiating factor (the gene mutation) and the abnormal phenotype (hearing impairment) is not obvious. Research is providing insight into the function of the proteins encoded by these genes, and as a consequence, understanding of the auditory system is advanced. The goal, which is to characterize all the genetic and nongenetic factors that play a role in hearing impairment and to determine the interactions among them is within reach. Effective molecular intervention therapies for some forms of hearing impairment may be achievable in the near future.

REFERENCES

ABDELHAK, S., KALATZIS, V., HEILIG, R., COMPAIN, S., SAMSON, D., VINCENT, C., WEIL, D., CRUAUD, C., SAHLY, I., LEIBOVICI, M., BITNER-GLINDZICZ, M., FRANCIS, M., LACOMBE, D., VIGNERON, J., CHARACHON, R., BOVEN, K., BEDBEDER, P., VAN REGEMORTER, N., WEISSENBACH, J., & PETIT, C. (1997). A human homologue of the drosophila eyes absent gene underlies branchio-oto-renal (BOR) syndrome and identifies a novel gene family. *Nature Genetics, 15*;157–164.

AVRAHAM, K.B., HASSON, T., STEEL, K.P., KINGSLEY, D.M., RUSSELL, L.B., MOOSEKER, M.S., COPELAND, N.G., & JENKINS, N.A. (1995). The mouse *Snell's waltzer* deafness gene encodes an unconventional myosin required for structural integrity of inner ear hair cells. *Nature Genetics, 11*;369–375.

BALDWIN, C.T., HOTH, C.F., AMOS, J.A., DA-SILVA, E.O., & MILUNSKY, A. (1992). An exonic mutation in the HuP2 paired domain gene causes Waardenburg's syndrome. *Nature, 355*;637–638.

BARKER, D.F., HOSTIKKA, S.L., ZHOU, J., CHOW, L.T., OLIPHANT, A.R., GERKEN, S.C., GREGORY, M.C., SKOLNICK, M.H., ATKIN, C.L., & TRYGGVASON, K. (1990). Identification of mutations in the COL4A5 collagen gene in Alport syndrome. *Science, 248*;1224–1226.

BERGER, W., MEINDL, A., VAN DE POL, T.J.R., CREMERS, F.P.M., ROPERS, H.H., DOERNER, C., MONACO, A., BERGEN, A.A.B., LEBO, R., WARBURG, M., ZERGOLLERN, L., LORENZ, B., GAL, A., BLEEKER-WAGEMAKERS, E.M., & MEITINGER, T. (1992). Isolation of a candidate gene for Norrie disease by positional cloning. *Nature Genetics, 1*;199–203.

BERLIN, C.I., BORDELON, J., ST. JOHN, P., WILENSKY, D., HURLEY, A., KLUKA, E., HOOD, L.J. (1998). Reversing click polarity may uncover auditory neuropathy in infants. *Ear and Hearing, 19*;37–47.

BIANCHI, A.B., HARA, T., RAMESH, V., GAO, J., KLEIN-SZANTO, A.J.P., MORIN, F., MENON, A.G., TROFATTER, J.A., GUSELLA, J.F., SEIZINGER, B.R., & KLEY, N. (1994). Mutations in transcript isoforms of the neurofibromatosis 2 gene in multiple human tumour types. *Nature Genetics, 6*;185–192.

BROWN, D.M., VANDENBURGH, K., KIMURA, A.E., WEINGEIST, T.A., SHEFFIELD, V.C., & STONE, E.M. (1995). Novel frameshift mutations in the procollagen 2 gene (COL2A1) associated with Stickler syndrome (hereditary arthro-ophthalmopathy). *Human Molecular Genetics, 4*;141–142.

BROWN, S.D.M., & STEEL, K.P. (1994). Genetic deafness—Progress with mouse models. *Human Molecular Genetics, 3*;1453–1456.

BROWNSTEIN, Z., FRIEDLANDER, Y., PERITZ, E., & COHEN, T. (1991). Estimated number of loci for autosomal recessive severe nerve deafness within the Israeli Jewish population, with implications for genetic counseling. *American Journal of Medical Genetics, 41*;306–312.

BRUNNER, H., BENNEKOM, C., LAMBERMON, E., OEI, L., CREMERS, C., WIERINGA, B., & ROPERS, H. (1988). The gene for X-linked progressive deafness with perilymphatic gusher during surgery (DFN3) is linked to PGK. *Human Genetics, 80*;337–340.

BRUNNER, H.G., VAN BEERSUM, S.E.C., WARMAN, M.L., OLSEN, B.R., ROPERS, H.H., & MARIMAN, E.C.M. (1994). A Stickler syndrome gene is linked to chromosome 6 near the COL11A2 gene. *Human Molecular Genetics, 3*;1561–1564.

BUTINAR, D., ZIDAR, J., LEONARDIS, L., POPOVIC, M., KALAYDJIEVA, L., ANGELICHIVA, D., SININGER, Y., KEATS, B., & STARR, A. (1999). Hereditary auditory, vestibular, motor, and sensory neuropathy in a Slovenia Roma (Gypsy) kindred. *Annals of Neurology*; in press.

CHAIB, H., KAPLAN, J., GERBER, S., VINCENT, C., AYADI, H., SLIM, R., MUNNICH, A., WEISSENBACH, J., & PETIT, C. (1997). A newly identified locus for Usher syndrome, USH1E, maps to chromosome 21q21. *Human Molecular Genetics, 6*;27–31.

CHAIB, H., LINA-GRANADE, G., GUILFORD, P., PLAUCHU, H., LEVILLIERS, J., MORGON, A., & PETIT, C. (1994). A gene responsible for a dominant form of neurosensory non-syndromic deafness maps to the NSRD1 recessive deafness gene interval. *Human Molecular Genetics, 3*;2219–2222.

CHAIB, H., PLACE, C., SALEM, N., DODE, C., CHARDENOUX, S., WEISSENBACH, J., EL ZIR, E., LOISELET, J., & PETIT, C. (1996). Mapping of DFNB12, a gene for a non-syndromal autosomal recessive deafness, to chromosome 10q21-22. *Human Molecular Genetics, 5*;1061–1064.

CHEN, A., WAYNE, S., BELL, A., RAMESH, A., SRISAILAPATHY, C.R.S., SCOTT, D.A., SHEFFIELD, V.C., VAN HAUWE, P., ZBAR, R.I.S., ASHLEY, J., LOVETT, M., VAN CAMP, G., & SMITH, R.J.H. (1997). New gene for autosomal recessive non-syndromic hearing loss maps to either chromosome 3q or 19p. *American Journal of Medical Genetics, 71*;467–471.

CHEN, Z.Y., BATTINELLI, E.M., HENDRIKS, R.W., POWELL, J.F., MIDDLETON-PRICE, H., SIMS, K.B., BREAKEFIELD, X.O., & CRAIG, I.W. (1993). Norrie disease gene: characterization of deletions and possible function. *Genomics, 16*;533–535.

CHEN, Z.Y., HENDRIKS, R.W., JOBLING, M.A., POWELL, J.F., BREAKEFIELD, X.O., SIMS, K.B., & CRAIG, I.W. (1992). Isolation and characterization of a candidate gene for Norrie disease. *Nature Genetics, 1*;204–208.

CHUNG, C.S., & BROWN, K.S. (1970). Family studies of early childhood deafness ascertained through the Clarke School for the Deaf. *American Journal of Human Genetics, 22*;630–644.

CHUNG, C.S., ROBISON, O.W., & MORTON, N.E. (1959). A note on deaf mutism. *Annals of Human Genetics, 23*;357–366.

COSTEFF, H., & DAR, H. (1980). Consanguinity analysis of congenital deafness in Northern Israel. *American Journal of Human Genetics, 32*;64–68.

COYLE, B., COFFEY, R., ARMOUR, J.A.L., GAUSDEN, E., HOCHBERG, Z., GROSSMAN, A., BRITTON, K., PEMBREY, M., REARDON, W., & TREMBATH, R. (1996). Pendred syndrome (goitre and sensorineural hearing loss) maps to chromosome 7 in the region containing the nonsyndromic deafness gene DNFB4. *Nature Genetics, 12*;421–423.

CRANEFIELD, P.F., & FEDERN, W. (1970). Paulus Zacchias on mental deficiency and on deafness. *Bulletin of the New York Academy of Medicine, 46*;3–21.

CREMERS, C.W.R.J., & HUYGEN, P.L.M. (1983). Clinical features of female heterozygotes in the X-linked mixed deafness syndrome (with perilymphatic gusher during stapes surgery). *International Journal of Pediatric Otorhinolaryngology, 6*;179–185.

DAVENPORT, S.L.H., & OMENN, G.S. (1977). *The heterogeneity of Usher syndrome* [abstract 215]. Publication 426. (pp. 87–88).

Amsterdam: Excerpta Medica Foundation, International Congress Series.

DE KOK, Y.J., VAN DER MAAREL, S.M., BITNER-GLINDZICZ, M., HUBER, I., MONACO, A.P., MALCOLM, S., PEMBREY, M.E., ROPERS, H.H., & CREMERS, F.P. (1995). Association between X-linked mixed deafness and mutations in the POU domain gene POU3F4. *Science, 267*;685–688.

DENOYELLE, F., LINA-GRANADE, G., PLAUCHU, H., BRUZZONE, R., CHAIB, H., LEVI-ACOBAS, F., WEIL, D., & PETIT, C. (1998). Connexin 26 gene linked to a dominant deafness. *Nature, 393*;319–320.

DENOYELLE, F., WEIL, D., MAW, M.A., WILCOX, S.A., LENCH, N.J., ALLEN-POWELL, N.R., OSBORN, A.H., DAHL, H.M., MIDDLETON, A., HOUSEMAN, M.J., DODE, C., MARLIN, S., BOULILA-ELGAIED, A., GRATI, M., AYADI, H., BENARAB, S., BITOUN, P., LINA-GRANADE, G., GODET, J., MUSTAPHA, M., LOISELET, J., EL-ZIR, E., AUBOIS, A., JOANNARD, A., LEVILLIERS, J., GARABEDIAN, E., MUELLER, R.F., MCKINLAY GARDNER, R.J., & PETIT, C. (1997). Prelingual deafness: High prevalence of a 30delG mutation in the connexin 26 gene. *Human Molecular Genetics, 6*;2173–2177.

DIXON, M.J., READ, A.P., DONNAI, D., COLLEY, A., DIXON, J., & WILLIAMSON, R. (1991). The gene for Treacher Collins syndrome maps to the long arm of chromosome 5. *American Journal of Human Genetics, 49*;17–22.

EPSTEIN, D., VEKEMANS, M., & GROS, P. (1991). Splotch (Sp2H), a mutation affecting development of the mouse neural tube, shows a deletion within the paired homeodomain of Pax-3. *Cell, 67*;767–774.

ERKMAN, L., MCEVILLY, R.J., LUO, L., RYAN, A.K., HOOSHMAND, F., O'CONNELL, S.M., KEITHLEY, E.M., RAPAPORT, D.H., RYAN, A.F., & ROSENFELD, M.G. (1996). Role of transcription factors Brn-3.1 and Brn-3.2 in auditory and visual system development. *Nature, 381*;603–606.

ESTIVILL, X., GOVEA, N., BARCELO, A., PERELLO, E., BADENAS, C., ROMERO, E., MORAL, L., SCOZZARI, R., D'URBANO, L., ZEVIANI, M., & TORRONI, A. (1998). Familial progressive sensorineural deafness is mainly due to the mtDNA A1555G mutation and is enhanced by treatment with aminoglycosides. *American Journal of Human Genetics, 62*;27–35.

EUDY, J.D., WESTON, M.D., YAO, S., HOOVER, D.M., REHM, H.L., MA-EDMONDS, M., YAN, D., AHMAD, I., CHENG, J.J., AYUSO, C., CREMERS, C., DAVENPORT, S., MOLLER, C., TALMADGE, C.B., BEISEL, K.W., TAMAYO, M., MORTON, C.C., SWAROOP, A., KIMBERLING, W.J., & SUMEGI, J. (1998). Mutation of a gene encoding a protein with extracellular matrix motifs in Usher syndrome type IIa. *Science, 280*; 1753–1757.

EVERETT, L.A., GLASER, B., BECK, J.C., IDOL, J.R., BUCHS, A., HEYMAN, M., ADAWI, F., HAZANI, E., NASSIR, E., BAXEVANIS, A.D., SHEFFIELD, V.C., & GREEN, E.D.H. (1997). Pendred syndrome is caused by mutations in a putative sulphate transporter gene (PDS). *Nature Genetics, 17*;411–422.

FARRER, L.A., GRUNDFAST, K.M., AMOS, J., ARNOS, K.S., ASHER, J.H., BEIGHTON, P., DIEHL, S.R., FEX, J., FOY, C., FRIEDMAN, T.B., GREENBERG, J., HOTH, C., MARAZITA, M., MILUNSKY, A., MORELL, R., NANCE, W., NEWTON, V., RAMESAR, R., WILCOX, E.R., WINSHIP, I., & READ, A.P. (1992). Waardenburg syndrome (WS) type I is caused by defects at multiple loci, one of which is near ALPP on chromosome 2: First report of the WS consortium. *American Journal of Human Genetics, 50*;902–913.

FISCHEL-GHODSIAN, N. (1998). Mitochondrial mutations and hearing loss: Paradigm for mitochondrial genetics. *American Journal of Human Genetics, 62*;15–19.

FISCHEL-GHODSIAN, N., BYKHOVSKAYA, Y., TAYLOR, K., KAHEN, T., CANTOR, R., EHRENMAN, K., SMITH, R., & KEITHLEY, E. (1997). Temporal bone analysis of patients with presbycusis reveals high-frequency of mitochondrial mutations. *Hearing Research, 110*;147–154.

FRANCOMANO, C.A., LIBERFARB, R.M., HIROSE, T., MAUMENEE, I.H., STREETEN, E.A., MEYERS, D.A., & PYERITZ, R.E. (1987). The Stickler syndrome: Evidence for close linkage to the structural gene for type II collagen. *Genomics, 1*;293–296.

FRASER, G.R. (1976). *The causes of profound deafness in childhood.* Baltimore, MD: The Johns Hopkins University Press.

GASPARINI, P., ESTIVILL, X., VOLPINI, V., TOTARO, A., CASTELLVI-BEL, S., GOVEA, N., MILA, M., DELLA MONICA, M., VENTRUTO, V., DE BENEDETTO, M., STANZIALE, P., ZELANTE, L., MANSFIELD, E.S., SANDKUIJL, L., SURREY, S., & FORTINA, P. (1997). Linkage of DFNB1 to non-syndromic neurosensory autosomal-recessive deafness in Mediterranean families. *European Journal of Human Genetics, 5*;83–88.

GIBSON, F., WALSH, J., MBURU, P., VARELA, A., BROWN, K.A., ANTONIO, M., BEISEL, K.W., STEEL, K.P., & BROWN, S.D.M. (1995). A type VII myosin encoded by the mouse deafness gene Shaker-1. *Nature, 374*;62–64.

GOLDSTEIN, M.A. (1933). *Problems of the deaf.* St. Louis, MO: The Laryngoscope Press.

GORLIN, R.J., TORIELLO, H.V., & COHEN, M.M. (1995). *Hereditary hearing loss and its syndromes.* Oxford: Oxford University Press.

GOULDING, M.D., CHALEPAKIS, G., DEUTSCH, U., ERSELIUS, J.R., & GRUSS, P. (1991). Pax-3, a novel murine DNA-binding protein expressed during early neurogenesis. *EMBO Journal, 10*;1135–1147.

GRUSS, P., & WALTHER, C. (1992). Pax in development. *Cell, 69*;719–722.

HARTMANN, A. (1881). *Deafmutism and the education of deaf mutes by lipreading and articulation.* Translated by J.P. Cassels. London: Balliere, Tindall and Cox.

HOTCHKISS, D. (1989). *Demographic aspects of hearing impairment: Questions and answers* (2nd ed.). Center for Assessment and Demographic Studies, Gallaudet University.

HUGHES, A., NEWTON, V.E., LIU, X.Z., & READ, A.P. (1994). A gene for Waardenburg syndrome type 2 maps close to the human homologue of the *Microphthalmia* gene at chromosome 3p12-p14.1. *Nature Genetics, 7*;509–512.

JABS, E.W., LI, X., COSS, C.A., TAYLOR, E.W., MEYERS, D.A., & WEBER, J.L. (1991). Mapping the Treacher Collins syndrome locus to 5q31.3-q33.3. *Genomics 11*;193–198.

JAIN, P.K., FUKUSHIMA, K., DESHMUKH, D., ARABANDI, R., THOMAS, E., KUMAR, S., LALWANI, A.K., PLOPLIS, B., SKARKA, H., SRISAILAPATHY, C.R.S., WAYNE, S., ZBAR, R.I.S., VERMA, I.C., SMITH, R.J.H., & WILCOX, E.R. (1995). A human recessive neurosensory nonsyndromic hearing impairment locus is a potential homologue of the murine deafness (dn) locus. *Human Molecular Genetics, 4*;391–394.

JAIN, P.K., LALWANI, A.K., LI, X.C., SINGLETON, T.L., SMITH, T.N., CHEN, A., DESHMUKH, D., VERMA, I.C., SMITH, R.J.H., & WILCOX, E.R. (1998). A gene for recessive nonsyndromic sensorineural deafness (DFNB18) maps to the chromosomal region 11p14-p15.1 containing the Usher syndrome type 1C gene. *Genomics, 50*;290–292.

KALAYDJIEVA, L., HALLMAYER, J., CHANDLER, D., SAVOV, A., NIKO-LOVA, A., ANGELICHEVA, D., KING, R.H.H., ISHPEKOVA, B., HONEYMAN, K., CALAFELL, F., SHMAROV, A., PETROVA, J., TURNEV, I., HRISTOVA, A., MOSKOV, M., STANCHEVA, S., PETKOVA, I., BITTLES, A.H., GEORGIEVA, V., MIDDLETON, L., & THOMAS, P.K. (1996). Gene mapping in gypsies identifies a novel demyelinating neuropathy on chromosome 8q24. *Nature Genetics, 14*;214–217.

KALAYDJIEVA, L., NIKOLOVA, A., TURNEV, I., PETROVA, J., HRIS-TOVA, A., ISHPEKOVA, B., PETKOVA, I., SHMAROV, A., STANCHEVA, S., MIDDLETON, L., MERLINI, L., TROGU, A., MUD-DLE, J.R., KING, R.H.M., & THOMAS, P.K. (1998). Hereditary motor and sensory neuropathy-Lom, a novel demyelinat-ing neuropathy associated with deafness in gypsies: Clin-ical, electrophysiological and nerve biopsy findings. *Brain, 121*;399–408.

KAPLAN, J., GERBER, S., BONNEAU, D., ROZET, J., DELRIEU, O., BRI-ARD, M., DOLLFUS, H., GHAZI, I., DUFIER, J., FREZAL, J., & MUNNICH, A. (1992). A gene for Usher syndrome type I (USH1) maps to chromosome 14q. *Genomics, 14*;979–988.

KEATS, B.J.B., NOURI, N., HUANG, J.M., MONEY, M., WEBSTER, D.B., & BERLIN, C.I. (1995). The deafness locus (dn) maps to mouse chromosome 19. *Mammalian Genome, 6*;8–10.

KEATS, B.J.B., NOURI, N., PELIAS, M.Z., DEININGER, P.L., & LITT, M. (1994). Tightly linked flanking microsatellite markers for the Usher syndrome type I locus on the short arm of chro-mosome 11. *American Journal of Human Genetics, 54*;681–686.

KELSELL, D.P., DUNLOP, J., STEVENS, H.P., LENCH, N.J., LIANG, J.N., PARRY, G., MUELLER, R.F., & LEIGH, I.M. (1997). Con-nexin 26 mutations in hereditary non-syndromic sen-sorineural deafness. *Nature, 387*;80–83.

KIMBERLING, W.J., MÖLLER, C.G., DAVENPORT, S., PRILUCK, I.A., BEIGHTON, P.H., GREENBERG, J., REARDON, W., WESTON, M.D., KENYON, J.B., GRUNKMEYER, J.A., PIEKE DAHL, S., OVERBECK, L.D., BLACKWOOD, D.J., BROWER, A.M., HOOVER, D.M., ROWLAND, P., & SMITH, R.J.H. (1992). Linkage of Usher syndrome type I gene (USH1B) to the long arm of chromo-some 11. *Genomics, 14*:988–994.

KIMBERLING, W.J., WESTON, M.D., MÖLLER, C.G., DAVENPORT, S.L.H., SHUGART, Y.Y., PRILUCK, I.A., MARTINI, A., & SMITH, R.J.H. (1990). Localization of Usher syndrome type II to chromosome 1q. *Genomics, 7*;245–249.

KNUDSON, A.G. (1971). Mutation and cancer: Statistical study of retinoblastoma. *Proceedings of the National Academy of Sciences, USA, 68*;820–823.

KONIGSMARK, B.W. (1969). Hereditary deafness in man. *New England Journal of Medicine, 281*;713–720,774–778,827–832.

KONIGSMARK, B.W., & GORLIN, R.J. (1976). *Genetic and metabolic deafness.* Philadelphia, PA: W.B. Saunders.

KUMAR, S., KIMBERLING, W.J., KENYON, J.B., SMITH, R.J.H., MAR-RES, E.H.M.A., & CREMERS, C.W.R.J. (1992). Autosomal dominant branchio-oto-renal syndrome—Localization of a disease gene to chromosome 8q by linkage in a Dutch family. *Human Molecular Genetics, 1*;491–495.

LEKANNE DEPREZ, R.H., BIANCHI, A.B., GROEN, N.A., SEIZINGER, B.R., HAGEMEIJER, A., VAN DRUNEN, E., BOOTSMA, D., KOPER, J.W., AVEZAAT, C.J.J., KLEY, N., & ZWARTHOFF, E.C. (1994). Frequent NF2 gene transcript mutations in sporadic menin-giomas and vestibular schwannomas. *American Journal of Human Genetics, 54*;1022–1029.

LEWIS, R.A., OTTERUD, B., STAUFFER, D., LALOUEL, J.M., & LEP-PERT, M. (1990). Mapping recessive ophthalmic diseases:

Linkage of the locus for Usher syndrome type II to a DNA marker on chromosome 1q. *Genomics, 7*;250–256.

LI, X.C., EVERETT, L.A., LALWANI, A.K., DESMUKH, D., FRIEDMAN, T.B., GREEN, E.D., & WILCOX, E.R. (1998). A mutation in PDS causes non-syndromic recessive deafness. *Nature Genetics, 18*;215–217.

LIU, X.Z., WALSH, J., MBURU, P., KENDRICK-JONES, J., COPE, M.J.T.V., STEEL, K.P., & BROWN, S.D.M. (1997a). Mutations in the myosin VIIA gene cause non-syndromic recessive deafness. *Nature Genetics, 16*;188–190.

LIU, X.Z., WALSH, J., TAMAGAWA, Y., KITAMURA, K., NISHIZAWA, M., STEEL, K., & BROWN, S. (1997b). Autosomal dominant non-syndromic deafness (DFNA11) caused by a mutation in the myosin VIIA gene. *Nature Genetics, 17*;268–269.

LYNCH, E.D., LEE, M.K., MORROW, J.E., WELCSH, P.L., LEON, P.E., & KING, M.C. (1997). Non-syndromic deafness DFNA1 associated with mutation of the human homolog HDIA1 of the *Drosophila* diaphanous gene. *Science, 278*;1315–1318.

MARAZITA, M.L., PLOUGHMAN, L.M., RAWLINGS, B., REMINGTON, E., ARNOS, K.S., & NANCE, W.E. (1993). Genetic epidemio-logical studies of early-onset deafness in the U.S. school-age population. *American Journal of Medical Genetics, 46*;486–491.

MEISLER, M.H. (1996). The role of the laboratory mouse in the Human Genome Project. *American Journal of Human Genet-ics, 59*;764–771.

MEITINGER, T., MEINDL, A., BORK, P., ROST, B., SANDER, C., HAASEMANN, M., & MURKEN, J. (1993). Molecular model-ing of the Norrie disease protein predicts a cystine knot growth factor tertiary structure. *Nature Genetics, 5*;376–380.

MENDLER, M., EICH-BENDER, S.G., VAUGHAN, L., WINTERHAL-TER, K.H., & BRUCKNER, P. (1989). Cartilage contains mixed fibrils of collagen types II, IX, and XI. *Journal of Cellular Biology, 108*;191–197.

MOCHIZUKI, T., LEMMINK, H.H., MARIYAMA, M., ANTIGNAC, C., GUBLER, M.C., PIRSON, Y., VERELLEN-DUMOULIN, C., CHAN, B., SCHRODER, C.H., SMEETS, H.J., & REEDERS, S.T. (1994). Identification of mutations in the alpha 3(IV) and alpha 4(IV) collagen genes in autosomal recessive Alport syn-drome. *Nature Genetics, 8*;77–81.

MORELL, R., KIM, J.J., HOOD, L.J., GOFORTH, L., FRIDERICI, K., FISHER, R., VAN CAMP, G., BERLIN, C.I., ODDOUX, C., OSTRER, H., KEATS, B.J.B., & FRIEDMAN, T.B. (1998). Mutations in the connexin 26 gene (GJB2) among Ashkenazi Jews with non-syndromic recessive deafness. *New England Journal of Med-icine, 339*;1500–1505.

NAGLEY, P., ZHANG, C., MARTINUS, R.D., VAILLANT, F., & LINNANE, A.W. (1993). Mitochondrial DNA mutations and human aging: molecular biology, bioenergetics, and redox therapy. In: S. DiMauro, & D.C. Wallace (Eds.). *Mitochondrial DNA in human pathology* (pp. 137–157). New York: Raven Press.

NANCE, W.E., ROSE, S.P., CONNEALLY, P.M., & MILLER, J. (1977). Opportunities for genetic counseling through institutional ascertainment of affected probands. In: H.A. Lubs, & F. de la Cruz (Eds.). *Genetic counseling* (pp. 307–331). New York: Raven Press.

NEYROUD, N., TESSON, F., DENJOY, I., LEIBOVICI, M., DONGER, C., BARHANIN, J., FAURE, S., GARY, F., COUMEL, P., PETIT, C., SCHWARTZ, K., & GUICHENEY, P. (1997). A novel mutation in the potassium channel gene KVLQT1 causes the Jervell and Lange-Nielsen cardioauditory syndrome. *Nature Genetics, 15*;186–189.

PANDYA, A., XIA, X.J., LANDA, B.L., ARNOS, K.S., ISRAEL, J., LLOYD, J., JAMES, A.L., DIEHL, S.R., BLANTON, S.H., & NANCE, W.E. (1996). Phenotypic variation in Waardenburg syndrome: Mutational heterogeneity, modifier genes or polygenic background? *Human Molecular Genetics, 5;*497–502.

PIEKE DAHL, S., KELLY, P.M., ASTUTO, L.M., WESTON, M.D., KENYON, J.B., & KIMBERLING, W.J. (1998). *Localization of USH2B to 5q14.3-q21.3.* Abstract presented at the Molecular Biology of Hearing and Deafness meeting, Bethesda, October 8-11, 1998.

PREZANT, T.R., AGAPIAN, J.V., BOHLMAN, M.C., BU, X., OZTAS, S., QIU, W.Q., ARNOS, K.S., CORTOPASSI, G.A., JABER, L., ROTTER, J.I., SHOHAT, M., & FISCHEL-GHODSIAN, N. (1993). Mitochondrial ribosomal RNA mutation associated with both antibiotic-induced and non-syndromic deafness. *Nature Genetics, 4;*289–294.

PRIEST, J.M., FISCHBECK, K.H., NOURI, N., & KEATS, B.J.B. (1995). A locus for axonal motor-sensory neuropathy with deafness and mental retardation maps to Xq26-q27. *Genomics, 29;*409–412.

PROBST, F.J., FRIDELL, R.A., RAPHAEL, Y., SAUNDERS, T.L., WANG, A., LIANG, Y., MORELL, R.J., TOUCHMAN, J.W., LYONS, R.H., NOBEN-TRAUTH, K., FRIEDMAN, T.B., & CAMPER, S.A. (1998). Correction of deafness in shaker-2 mice by an unconventional myosin in a BAC transgene. *Science, 280;*1444–1447.

REARDON, W. (1990). Sex linked deafness: Wilde revisited. *Journal of Medical Genetics, 27;*376–379.

RICHARDS, A.J., YATES, J.R.W., WILLIAMS, R., PAYNE, S.J., POPE, F.M., SCOTT, J.D., & SNEAD, M.P. (1996). A family with Stickler syndrome type 2 has a mutation in the COL11A1 gene resulting in the substitution of glycine 97 by valine in alpha-1(XI) collagen. *Human Molecular Genetics, 5;*1339–1343.

ROBERTSON, N.G., KHETARPAL, U., GUTIERREZ-ESPELATA, G.A., BIEBER, F.R., & MORTON, C.C. (1994). Isolation of novel and known genes from a human fetal cochlear cDNA library using subtractive hybridization and differential display. *Genomics, 23;*42–50.

ROBERTSON, N.G., LU, L., HELLER, S., MERCHANT, S.N., EAVEY, R.D., MCKENNA, M., NADOL, J.B., MIYAMOTO, R.T., LINTHICUM, F.H., LUBIANCA NETO, J.F., HUDSPETH, A.J., SEIDMAN, C.E., MORTON, C.C., & SEIDMAN, J.G. (1998). Mutations in a novel cochlear gene cause DFNA9, a human nonsyndromic deafness with vestibular dysfunction. *Nature Genetics, 20;*229–303.

ROULEAU, G.A., MEREL, P., LUTCHMAN, M., SANSON, M., ZUCMAN, J., MARINEAU, C., HOANG-XUAN, K., DEMCZUK, S., DESMAZE, C., PLOUGASTEL, B., PULST, S.M., LENOIR, G., BIJLSMA, E., FASHOLD, R., DUMANSKI, J., DE JONG, P., PARRY, D., ELDRIDGE, R., AURIAS, A., DELATTRE, O., & THOMAS, G. (1993). Alterations in a new gene encoding a putative membrane-organizing protein causes neurofibromatosis type 2. *Nature, 363;*515–521.

ROULEAU, G.A., SEIZINGER, B.R., WERTELECKI, W., HAINES, J.L., SUPERNEAU, D.W., MARTUZA, R.L., & GUSELLA, J.F. (1990). Flanking markers bracket the neurofibromatosis type 2 (NF2) gene on chromosome 22. *American Journal of Human Genetics, 46;*323–328.

SAINZ, J., FIGUEROA, K., BASER, M.E., MAUTNER, V.F., & PULST, S.M. (1995). High frequency of nonsense mutations in the NF2 gene caused by C to T transitions in five CGA codons. *Human Molecular Genetics, 4;*137–139.

SANK, D. (1963). Genetic aspects of early total deafness. In: J.D. Rainer, K.Z. Altshuler, & F.J. Kallman (Eds.). *Family and mental health problems in a deaf population* (pp. 28–81). New York: New York State Psychiatric Institute.

SANKILA, E.M., PAKARINEN, L., KÄÄRIÄINEN, H., AITTOMÄKI, K., KARJALAINEN, S., SISTONEN, P., & DE LA CHAPELLE, A. (1995). Assignment of an Usher syndrome type III (USH3) gene to chromosome 3q. *Human Molecular Genetics, 4;*93–98.

SCOTT, D.A., CARMI, R., ELBEDOUR, K., YOSEFSBERG, S., STONE, E.M., & SHEFFIELD, V.C. (1996). An autosomal recessive nonsyndromic-hearing-loss locus identified by DNA pooling using two inbred Bedouin kindreds. *American Journal of Human Genetics, 59;*385–391.

SEIZINGER, B.R., MARTUZA, R.L., & GUSELLA, J.F. (1986). Loss of genes on chromosome 22 in tumorigenesis of human acoustic neuroma. *Nature, 322;*644–647.

SHEFFIELD, V.C., CARMI, R., KWITEK-BLACK, A., ROKHLINA, T., NISHIMURA, D., DUYK, G.M., ELBEDOUR, K., SUNDEN, S.L., & STONE, E.M. (1994). Identification of a Bardet-Biedl syndrome locus on chromosome 3 and evaluation of an efficient approach to homozygosity mapping. *Human Molecular Genetics, 3;*1331–1335.

SHEFFIELD, V.C., KRAIEM, Z., BECK, J.C., NISHIMURA, D., STONE, E.M., SALAMEH, M., SADEH, O., & GLASER, B. (1996). Pendred syndrome maps to chromosome 7q21-34 and is caused by an intrinsic defect in thyroid iodine organification. *Nature Genetics, 12;*424–426.

SHOFFNER, J.M., LOTT, M.T., LEZZA, A.M.S., SEIBEL, P., BALLINGER, S.W., & WALLACE, D.C. (1990). Myoclonic epilepsy and ragged-red fiber disease (MERRF) is associated with a mitochondrial DNA tRNA-lys mutation. *Cell, 61;*931–937.

SHOFFNER, J.M., & WALLACE, D.C. (1992). Mitochondrial genetics: principles and practice [editorial]. *American Journal of Human Genetics, 51;*1179–1186.

SILL, A.M., STICK, M.J., PRENGER, V.L., PHILLIPS, S.L., BOUGHMAN, J.A., & ARNOS, K.S. (1994). Genetic epidemiologic study of hearing loss in an adult population. *American Journal of Medical Genetics (Neuropsychiatric Genetics), 54;*149–153.

SMITH, R.J.H., BERLIN, C.I., HEJTMANCIK, J.F., KEATS, B.J.B., KIMBERLING, W.J., LEWIS, R.A., MÖLLER, C.G., PELIAS, M.Z., & TRANEBJÆRG, L. (1994). Clinical diagnosis of the Usher syndromes. *American Journal of Medical Genetics, 50;*32–38.

SMITH, R.J.H., LEE, E.C., KIMBERLING, W.J., DAIGER, S.P., PELIAS, M.Z., KEATS, B.J.B., JAY, M., BIRD, A., REARDON, W., GUEST, M., AYYAGARI, R., & HEJTMANCIK, J.F. (1992). Localization of two genes for Usher syndrome type 1 to chromosome 11. *Genomics, 14;*995–1002.

STARR, A., PICTON, T.W., SININGER, Y.V., HOOD, L.J., & BERLIN, C.I. (1996). Auditory neuropathy. *Brain, 119;*741–753.

STEEL, K.P., & BROWN, S.D.M. (1998). More deafness genes. *Science, 280;*1403.

STEPHENS, S.D.G. (1985). Genetic hearing loss: A historical overview. *Advances in Audiology, 3;*3–17.

STEVENSON, A.C., & CHEESEMAN, E.A. (1956). Hereditary deaf mutism, with particular reference to Northern Ireland. *Annals of Human Genetics, 20;*177–207.

STICKLER, G.B., BELAU, P.G., FARRELL, F.J., JONES, J.D., PUGH, D.G., STEINBERG, A.G., & WARD, L.E. (1965). Hereditary progressive arthro-ophthalmopathy. *Mayo Clinic Proceedings, 40;*433–455.

STREET, V.A., MCKEE-JOHNSON, J.W., FONSECA, R.C., TEMPEL, B.L., & NOBEN-TRAUTH, K. (1998). Mutations in a plasma membrane Ca^{2+}-ATPase gene cause deafness in deafwaddler mice. *Nature Genetics, 19;*390–394.

TASSABEHJI, M., NEWTON, V.E., LIU, X.Z., BRADY, A., DONNAI, D., KRAJEWSKA-WALASEK, M., MURDAY, V., NORMAN, A., OBERSZTYN, E., REARDON, W., RICE, J.C., TREMBATH, R., WIEACKER, P., WHITEFORD, M., WINTER, R., & READ, A.P. (1995). The mutational spectrum in Waardenburg syndrome. *Human Molecular Genetics,* 4;2131–2137.

TASSABEHJI, M., NEWTON, V.E., & READ, A.P. (1994). Waardenburg syndrome type 2 caused by mutations in the human microphthalmia (MITF) gene. *Nature Genetics,* 8;251–255.

TASSABEHJI, M., READ, A.P., NEWTON, V.E., HARRIS, R., BALLING, R., GRUSS, P., & STRACHAN, T. (1992). Waardenburg syndrome patients have mutations in the human homologue of the Pax-3 paired box gene. *Nature,* 355;635–636.

TREACHER COLLINS SYNDROME COLLABORATIVE GROUP. (1996). Positional cloning of a gene involved in the pathogenesis of Treacher Collins syndrome. *Nature Genetics,* 12; 130–136.

TROFATTER, J.A., MACCOLLIN, M.M., RUTTER, J.L., MURRELL, J.R., DUYAO, M.P., PARRY, D.M., ELDRIDGE, R., KLEY, N., MENON, A.G., PULASKI, K., HAASE, V.H., AMBROSE, C.M., MUNROE, D., BOVE, C., HAINES, J.L., MARTUZA, R.L., MACDONALD, M.E., SEIZINGER, B.R., SHORT, M.P., BUCKLER, A.J., & GUSELLA, J.F. (1993). A novel moesin-, ezrin-, radixin-like gene is a candidate for the neurofibromatosis 2 tumour suppressor. *Cell,* 72;791–800.

TYSON, J., TRANEBJAERG, L., BELLMAN, S., WREN, C., TAYLOR, J.F., BATHEN, J., ASLAKSEN, B., SORLAND, S.J., LUND, O., MALCOLM, S., PEMBREY, M., BHATTACHARYA, S., & BITNER-GLINDZICZ, M. (1997). IsK and KvLQT1: Mutation in either of the two subunits of the slow component of the delayed rectifier potassium channel can cause Jervell and Lange-Nielsen syndrome. *Human Molecular Genetics,* 12;2179–2185.

VAHAVA, O., MORELL, R., LYNCH, E.D., WEISS, S., KAGAN, M.E., AHITUV, N., MORROW, J.E., LEE, M.K., SKVORAK, A.B., MORTON, C.C., BLUMENFELD, A., FRYDMAN, M., FRIEDMAN, T.B., KING, M., & AVRAHAM, K.B. (1998). Mutation in transcription factor POU4F3 associated with inherited progressive hearing loss in humans. *Science,* 279;1950–1954.

VAN CAMP, G., SMITH, R.J.H. (1998). *Hereditary hearing loss homepage.* World Wide Web URL: *http://dnalab-www.uia.ac.be/dnalab/hhh.*

VAN LAER, L., HUIZING, E.H., VERSTREKEN, M., VAN ZUIJLEN, D., WAUTERS, J.G., BOSSUYT, P.J., VAN DE HEYNING, P., MCGUIRT, W.T., SMITH, R.J.H., WILLEMS, P.J., LEGAN, P.K., RICHARDSON, G.P., & VAN CAMP, G. (1998). Nonsyndromic hearing impairment is associated with a mutation in DFNA5. *Nature Genetics,* 20;194–197.

VERHOEVEN, K., VAN LAER, L., KIRSCHHOFER, K., LEGAN, P.K., HUGHES, D.C., SCHATTEMAN, I., VERSTREKEN, M., VAN HAUWE, P., COUCKE, P., CHEN, A., SMITH, R.J.H., SOMERS, T., OFFECIERS, F.E., VAN DE HEYNING, P., RICHARDSON, G.P., WACHTLER, F., KIMBERLING, W.J., WILLEMS, P.J., GOVAERTS, P.J., & VAN CAMP, G. (1998). Mutations in the human alpha-tectorin gene cause autosomal dominant non-syndromic hearing impairment. *Nature Genetics,* 19;60–62.

VESKE, A., OEHLMANN, R., YOUNUS, F., MOHYUDDIN, A., MULLER-MYHSOK, B., QASIM MEHDI, S., & GAL, A. (1996). Autosomal recessive non-syndromic deafness locus (DFNB8) maps on chromosome 21q22 in large consanguineous kindred from Pakistan. *Human Molecular Genetics,* 5;165–168.

VIKKULA, M., MARIMAN, E.C.M., LUI, V.C.H., ZHIDKOVA, N.I., TILLER, G.E., GOLDRING, M.B., VAN BEERSUM, S.E.C., DE WAAL MALEFIJT, M.C., VAN DEN HOOGEN, F.H.J., ROPERS, H.H., MAYNE, R., CHEAH, K.S.E., OLSEN, B.R., WARMAN, M.L., & BRUNNER, H.G. (1995). Autosomal dominant and recessive osteochondrodysplasias associated with the COL11A2 locus. *Cell,* 80;431–437.

WALLIS, C., BALLO, R., WALLIS, G., BEIGHTON, P., & GOLDBLATT, J. (1988). X-linked mixed deafness with stapes fixation in a Mauritian kindred: linkage to Xq probe pDP34. *Genomics,* 3;299–301.

WANG, A., LIANG, Y., FRIDELL, R.A., PROBST, F.J., WILCOX, E.R., TOUCHMAN, J.W., MORTON, C.C., MORELL, R.J., NOBEN-TRAUTH, K., CAMPER, S.A., & FRIEDMAN, T.B. (1998). Association of unconventional myosin MYO15 mutations with human nonsyndromic deafness DFNB3. *Science,* 280; 1447–1451.

WAYNE, S., DER KALOUSTIAN, V.M., SCHLOSS, M., POLOMENO, R., SCOTT, D.A., HEJTMANCIK, J.F., SHEFFIELD, V.C., & SMITH, R.J.H. (1996). Localization of the Usher syndrome type ID gene (USH1D) to chromosome 10. *Human Molecular Genetics,* 5;1689–1692.

WAYNE, S., LOWRY, R.B., MCLEOD, D.R., KNAUS, R., FARR, C., & SMITH, R.J.H. (1997). Localization of the Usher syndrome type IF (Ush1F) to chromosome 10 [abstract]. *American Journal of Human Genetics,* 61;A300.

WEIL, D., BLANCHARD, S., KAPLAN, J., GUILFORD, P., GIBSON, F., WALSH, J., MBURU, P., VARELA, A., LEVILLIERS, J., WESTON, M.D., KELLEY, P.M., KIMBERLING, W.J., WAGENAAR, M., LEVI-ACOBAS, F., LARGET-PIET, D., MUNNICH, A., STEEL, K.P., BROWN, S.D.M., & PETIT, C. (1995). Defective myosin VIIA gene responsible for Usher syndrome type 1B. *Nature,* 374;60–61.

WEIL, D., KUSSEL, P., BLANCHARD, S., LEVY, G., LEVI-ACOBAS, F., DRIRA, M., AYADI, H., & PETIT, C. (1997). The autosomal recessive isolated deafness, DFNB2, and the Usher 1B syndrome are allelic defects of the myosin VIIA gene. *Nature Genetics,* 16;191–193.

WILLIAMS, C.J., GANGULY, A., CONSIDINE, E., MCCARRON, S., PROCKOP, D.J., WALSH-VOCKLEY, C., & MICHELS, V.V. (1996). A(-2)-to-G transition at the 3-prime acceptor splice site of IVS17 characterizes the COL2A1 gene mutation in the original Stickler syndrome kindred. *American Journal of Medical Genetics,* 63;461–467.

WISE, C.A., CHIANG, L.C., PAZNEKAS, W.A., SHARMA, M., MUSY, M.M., ASHLEY, J.A., LOVETT, M., & JABS, E.W. (1997). TCOF1 gene encodes a putative nucleolar phosphoprotein that exhibits mutations in Treacher Collins syndrome throughout its coding region. *Proceedings of the National Academy of Science,* 94;3110–3115.

XIANG, M., GAN, L., LI, D., CHEN, Z.Y., ZHOU, L., O'MALLEY, B.W., KLEIN, W., & NATHANS, J. (1997). Essential role of POU-domain factor Brn-3c in auditory and vestibular hair cell development. *Proceedings of the National Academy of Science,* 94;9445–9450.

ZELANTE, L., GASPARINI, P., ESTIVILL, X., MELCHIONDA, S., D'AGRUMA, L., GOVEA, N., MILA, M., DELLA MONICA, M., LUTFI, J., SHOHAT, M., MANSFIELD, E., DELGROSSO, K., RAPPAPORT, E., SURREY, S., & FORTINA, P. (1997). Connexin26 mutations associated with the most common form of non-syndromic neurosensory autosomal recessive deafness (DFNB1) in Mediterraneans. *Human Molecular Genetics,* 6;1605–1609.

## Chapter 26

The Future of Diagnostic Audiology

James F. Jerger, Alison M. Grimes, Gary P. Jacobson, Kathryn A. Albright, and Deborah Moncrieff

In this chapter five noted audiologists provide their insights into the future of diagnostic audiology. All agree that the role of diagnostic audiology is changing rapidly and will continue to change with the almost daily modifications that are occurring in healthcare. Because each contributor represents his or her view of the future of the profession, it is not surprising that opinions vary, sometimes diverge, and are contradictory at times. However, interleaved throughout the presentations is the undeniable fact that audiology as a profession has matured to a level that it is recognized nationally as a vital part of the healthcare arena.

Appropriately, Dr. James F. Jerger, the individual who has developed most of the diagnostic audiological tests over the past several decades, and a highly respected visionary of the profession, begins with the role of diagnostic audiology in medical diagnosis. Jerger's "no holds barred" look at the future of medical tests in audiology may be alarming in parts for some. However, a continuing refrain runs throughout his presentation: that newer, more sophisticated and sensitive technology will improve reliability of diagnostic results and eventually replace older technology.

Other audiologists also provide their views by examining specific areas in which they have cultivated professional expertise. Comments are provided in the following areas by well-recognized audiologists:

- Diagnostic audiology in private practice (Alison M. Grimes)
- Intraoperative neurophysiological monitoring (Gary P. Jacobson)
- Audiologists' role in universal newborn hearing screenings (Kathryn A. Albright)
- Diagnosing central auditory disorders (Deborah Moncrieff)

As one author, Dr. Gary Jacobson, muses, "It is difficult to make predictions about anything in an age when the impact of technologic innovations affects us so profoundly and constantly." Only time will be the judge of the accuracy of these wise panelists.

AUDIOLOGIC TESTS IN MEDICAL DIAGNOSIS

James F. Jerger

When thinking about future trends in diagnostic audiology, it is important to distinguish between the two different arenas in which audiologists perform diagnostic tests: as consultants in diagnoses and as managers of nonmedical interventions. One arena is related to medical, especially otological, diagnosis. The audiologist supplies intended information to help the medical practitioner diagnose the basis of the hearing complaint. A common example is differentiating cochlear from auditory nerve site as an aid to the diagnosis of acoustic tumors or other neoplastic lesions of the cerebellopontine angle. When functioning in this mode, audiologists provide a clinical laboratory service. They are supplying the results of an evaluation ordered by another individual to be used for the purpose of medical diagnosis; in this setting the audiologist is not the gatekeeper.

In the second arena the audiologist carries out diagnostic procedures to understand fully the nature of the auditory disorder. Such understanding helps the audiologist to devise optimal intervention strategies. A common example is the differentiation between peripheral and central auditory deficits in children whose academic difficulties appear to be related to listening problems.

Audiology: Diagnosis. Edited by Roeser, Valente, and Hosford-Dunn. Thieme Medical Publishers, Inc., New York © 2000

Audiologists typically find themselves immersed in the first arena when working with or for otolaryngologists, neurologists, and neurosurgeons. This is a perfectly valid audiological activity as long as the audiologist understands that the activity is a laboratory (or consultative) service to another profession. In this respect the audiologist functions in very much the same way that radiologists, or pathologists, for example, provide a service for other professionals. However, the second arena, the evaluation of hearing function to design and execute suitable nonmedical intervention strategies, is the core of audiology. It is the "raison d'être" of the audiologist, an important part of the foundation of the profession.

This said, the following sections will consider future trends separately in each of these two arenas.

With the advent and continuing improvement of methods for brain and temporal bone imaging, much of differential audiological testing has been rendered obsolete. In the 1950s and 1960s tests such as the Short Increment Sensitivity Index (SISI), the alternate binaural loudness balance test (ABLB), and Bekesy-type tracings were helpful in differentiating cochlear from eighth nerve sites (see Chapter 1). In the 1970s and 1980s they were largely replaced by the acoustic reflex, the performance versus intensity (PI) function for speech, and the auditory brain stem response (ABR) tests. With this new battery accuracy was improved substantially. But, by the 1990s otologists concerned with the diagnosis of neoplasms, such as acoustic tumors, had largely taken the position that imaging had become the "gold standard" and should be ordered for anyone with progressive unilateral or asymmetrical sensorineural hearing losses (Naessens et al, 1996; Ruckenstein et al, 1996; Wilson et al, 1997). Thus the concept of specialized behavioral tests to delineate site of lesion (or disorder) has become less and less viable. To be sure, imaging facilities are not yet universally available. A continuing role exists for auditory tests in geographical regions where imaging is still available only at considerable distance. But the trend is inexorably toward wider availability of imaging facilities. However, imaging everyone with unilateral or asymmetrical hearing loss to uncover the relatively rare acoustic tumor may not be the most cost-effective way to deliver healthcare. Perhaps imaging need only be performed on those patients who fail an ABR. But as the cost of imaging decreases because of technological improvements and increased volume, this argument becomes less persuasive.

In this same medical arena, as discussed later in this chapter by Dr. Gary Jacobson, some audiologists are participating in the intraoperative monitoring of surgical procedures by means of evoked potentials, sometimes auditory but usually somatosensory. Here, also, the audiologist functions as a provider of clinical services to someone else. And here, too, the future is uncertain, principally because other professionals may claim territorial rights. When such an activity becomes

financially rewarding, electroencephalographers and other medical technicians are likely to raise interested eyebrows. Whether persons who follow the course of an operation by means of somatosensory evoked potentials are in any way practicing audiology is also open to question.

It is reasonable to ask to what extent tests of middle ear function, immittance audiometry, and indirectly otoacoustic emissions can assist in the medical diagnosis of middle ear disease. As pointed out in Chapter 17, multifrequency tympanometry, for example, is a powerful technique for evaluating the status of the tympanic membrane and the middle ear mechanism. But otologists, pediatricians, other medical specialists and audiologists concerned with the daily evaluation of middle ear disorder have, by and large, shown little interest in the finer nuances of middle ear measurement. As imaging techniques of the temporal bone improve further, this situation is not likely to change. Visualization of the tympanic membrane and of the middle ear structures, either by imaging or by direct observation, are preferred. To be sure, pediatricians rely more and more on tympanograms to evaluate otitis media, but few audiologists are employed in carrying out this testing.

Diagnostic Audiology and Audiological Intervention

It is clear that significant growth will occur in the use of diagnostic audiological tests in the following three distinct patient populations:

1. Newborns
2. Children with suspected auditory processing disorders
3. Elderly persons

Newborns

Screening the hearing of every newborn is rapidly becoming a reality in state after state (Downs, 1990; Johnson et al, 1993; Mehl & Thompson, 1998). As of this writing, 20 states have mandated universal screening programs. Many more states are in the process of developing such mandates. In this arena the audiologist will bear heavy responsibility for designing and implementing appropriate screening protocols. Central to such activities will be the use of otoacoustic emissions (OAEs) (Bonfils et al, 1988; Martin et al, 1990) as the first stage in the screening process. Whether the transient or the distortion-product approach is best remains to be determined. But it seems certain that some form of evoked OAE will be the first stage of a two-stage screen (Anon, 1993). All children failing the OAE screen will be screened by ABR. Only those babies who fail the second-stage (ABR) screen will be referred for follow-up evaluation. This is a future trend that will pay rich dividends in early identification and intervention.

As a result of mandated screening, an ever-growing need for the thorough diagnostic evaluation of babies who fail the two-stage screen may be anticipated. Such testing, both unaided and aided, must necessarily rely heavily on the early auditory evoked potentials, in particular the ABR and the auditory steady-state response (Picton et al, 1998). For this reason heightened interest in methods for improving the frequency specificity of such measures will undoubtedly occur. Another important trend will be the greater application of the bone-conducted ABR as a means of avoiding the problems created by the high prevalence of outer earcanal and middle-ear problems in the newborn population.

Children With Suspected Auditory Processing Disorder

Children suspected of central auditory processing disorder (CAPD) are a potentially large pool of individuals in need of more sophisticated audiological evaluation (Bellis, 1996; Keith, 1977). Test instruments in use at present are largely scaled-down versions of behavioral testing techniques designed many years ago for the evaluation of adults with suspected central auditory disorders. The major problem with such behavioral tests is that they are not necessarily specific to auditory processing disorder. Behavioral tests of CAPD typically require the child to listen to a speech target presented through earphones or loudspeaker, then make an appropriate motor response. Performance below an established norm for absolute scores is taken as evidence of CAPD. But a child's absolute scores on such behavioral tests may fall below the norm for many reasons other than CAPD. A host of extraauditory disorders (e.g., attention deficit hyperactivity disorder, language disorder, emotional disorder, intellectual challenge) can result in poor performance on listening tests and in the misdiagnosis of CAPD. The long-term consequence of such overdiagnosis is not likely to be helpful to the profession.

An urgent need exists for more effective behavioral tests designed specifically for this population. The result will be that the tests will be designed in such a way that they rely less heavily on comparisons of absolute performance with norms. Instead they will emphasize using each child as his or her own control by comparing (1) performance on equivalent tests presented both in the auditory and visual modes, (2) performance across the range of listening levels, and (3) interaural asymmetries in performance.

Future trends in testing for CAPD, however, are likely to be in the expanded use of electrophysiological measures of auditory processing (Baran et al, 1988; Kileny & Berry, 1983). We have only begun to exploit the possibilities inherent in all the auditory evoked potentials, both exogenous and endogenous. Exogenous potentials include the ABR, the middle latency response (MLR), and, to some extent, the N1 and P2 waves of the late vertex response (LVR). Endogenous potentials include the event-related potentials (ERPs), chief among which are the P300, the N400, and the mismatched negativity (MMN) response.

Seldom is the ABR abnormal in these children, but it must be obtained to rule out speech processing problems at the brain stem level. In the future its use will grow as a part of the comprehensive evaluation of such children. The MLR, on the other hand, is less likely to enjoy increased use. Its clinical

value in this population remains to be demonstrated in convincing fashion. However, the LVR will, in all probability, realize expanded use as an essential component of comprehensive assessment. In the past its application was largely limited to simple pure tone stimuli, but with advances in instrumentation the capability of measuring LVRs to various dimensions of speech signals is anticipated.

The most significant future trend in this population, however, likely will be in the area of the ERPs. They will be used to probe the actual processing of contrasting speech features (Kraus et al, 1993), of syntactic and semantic processing of speech (Herning et al, 1987), and of interhemispheric processing asymmetries.

A growing body of evidence shows that language-impaired children are deficient in the temporal resolution of short events (Wright et al, 1997) and that such deficits may respond to systematic training (Merzenich et al, 1996). If it is shown that children with CAPD are also deficient in this dimension of auditory function, we may anticipate a considerable future interest, both in testing for temporal resolution deficits and in intervening with training stratagems.

Elderly Persons

Senior citizens will continue to constitute the bulk of users of hearing aids and other amplification systems. Hopefully, their problems will be better understood. We can expect to see more concern for the central processing component of auditory deficits (Divenyi & Haupt, 1997; Gatehouse, 1991; McCandless & Parkin, 1979), and the implications of that component for successful intervention (Chmiel & Jerger, 1996; Fire et al, 1991). It is becoming increasingly clear that not all elderly persons will automatically benefit from a binaural fitting. Some may actually do better with a monaural hearing aid. Still others may be better served by an assistive listening device (ALD) than by any arrangement of aids. For these reasons, we can expect to see more concern for realistic outcome measures, procedures that evaluate how well the elderly person is able to function in the sound field with various amplification arrangements including unaided, monaural-aided, binaural-aided, and ALD-aided alternatives (e.g., Jerger & Jordan, 1992; Newman et al, 1991).

Auditory deprivation (Silman et al, 1992) is a recently described phenomenon. It can best be described as a progressive loss in speech understanding resulting from prolonged lack of auditory stimulation. In particular, persons who have worn a monaural aid for a period of time show poorer speech understanding ability in the unaided than in the aided ear. The recent interest in this phenomenon will undoubtedly translate into more follow-up investigation for the success of a particular fitting after 4 to 6 weeks of use. An important role exists here for the many excellent scales and questionnaires that have been developed to assess benefit from amplification (e.g., Cox & Alexander, 1995). Another probable consequence of the work in deprivation in elderly persons will be renewed dedication to early intervention with amplification for both ears to prevent the development of the kinds of functional asymmetries that can interfere with the subsequent successful use of binaural amplification (Jerger et al, 1993).

Studies of asymmetries in the interhemispheric transfer of auditory information (Jerger et al, 1995) suggest that a test of dichotic listening should be included in every assessment of an elderly person, especially in the eighth decade (80 to 89 years). Such testing will prove valuable in assessing the central processing component of the auditory deficit (Jerger et al, 1990; Musiek & Pinheiro, 1985). Results will impact not only the prognosis for successful binaural amplification but also the issue of whether any amplification should be recommended.

In general, less interest will be present in the peripheral component of the auditory disorder and more interest in the total functional deficit. As a result, we can expect to see a declining interest in the aided audiograms of elderly persons and more concern for the overall communication disorder. More efficacious intervention will come from a better understanding of the complexity of senescent changes in auditory function.

Auditory evoked potentials will prove useful in differentiating peripheral from central deficits in elderly persons. The same principles described for children with suspected CAPD also apply to elderly persons. The ABR is likely to be affected only by the high-frequency peripheral component, but the later potentials, especially the ERPs, will be increasingly useful for studying the auditory processing capabilities of elderly persons.

CONCLUSIONS

Evaluation of auditory function as an aid to medical diagnosis is likely to undergo considerable attenuation as the technology of brain and temporal bone imaging becomes more widespread and less expensive. But the role of auditory tests as an aid to audiological intervention has a bright future. Three populations are particularly relevant: newborns, children with suspected CAPD, and elderly persons. Mandated universal hearing screening of the newborn will sharply increase the use of OAEs and ABR as two-stage screening devices and the use of conventional ABR in the subsequent follow-up examination of those who fail the two-stage screen. A considerable thrust to improve behavioral evaluation of children suspected of CAPD will occur along with further exploitation of auditory evoked potentials, especially ERPs, to achieve more accurate identification. A greater concern for the complexities of age-related auditory deficits and a focus on realistic outcome measures to assess the success of audiological intervention is anticipated in the elderly population.

DIAGNOSTIC AUDIOLOGY IN PRIVATE PRACTICE

Alison M. Grimes

New opportunities and challenges face the profession of audiology. Some, for better or for worse, are of the profession's own making, whereas others have resulted from factors seemingly beyond our control. As never before, it is imperative that audiologists be "on the same page" about factors that can and will critically impact the ability to practice and the ability to be compensated commensurate with the level of training, skills, and expertise that audiologists have.

The practice of diagnostic audiology, arguably the "bread and butter" of the private practice audiologist of yesterday, has experienced significant, and primarily negative, change in the recent past as a consequence of the following several factors:

- A belief that diagnostic audiology equates to a pure tone audiogram, which can be adequately performed by someone other than an audiologist. The common practice of having a nurse perform a pure tone audiogram on a patient in the primary care physician's (PCP) office is the most obvious example. In addition, the frequent use of tympanometry in the pediatrician's office and, indeed, the ability for a consumer to purchase a rudimentary tympanometric device from local retail stores decrease the likelihood that audiologists will be routinely authorized for or reimbursed for acoustic immittance measurements.

- Consumers' confusions regarding what constitutes a "hearing test," where it should be obtained, and who should perform it. With hearing aid salespeople and indeed some audiologists, advertising "free hearing tests" ("for the purpose of fitting and selling a hearing aid" in small print), consumers are uncertain as to the value and resultant expense of an audiologist's examination as opposed to a "free test."

- Physicians increasingly turn to computed tomography (CT) or magnetic resonance imaging (MRI) scans in cases of suspected eighth nerve lesions as opposed to a referral to the audiologist for an ABR evaluation or other "special tests."

- Although two common procedural terminology (CPT) codes for OAE testing exist, many third-party payers are either unaware of these codes or unwilling to pay for a procedure with which they are not familiar.

- Automated equipment, such as automated ABR screeners and handheld OAE devices, make testing by the nonaudiologist more likely.

- Managed care in general has very effectively reduced the number of CPT codes that are authorized for evaluations and the frequency of evaluations permitted.

This last item may single-handedly be most responsible for the significant reduction in diagnostic audiological activities. As is the case with all areas of healthcare, managed care has had a critical impact on audiology. Although its effects have been felt more in some geographical regions than in others, its implications are nationwide. Third-party payers, including Medicare, which is often viewed as a standard for other reimbursement protocols, are unwilling to pay for services deemed duplicative, unnecessary, or available at a lower cost from another provider.

Audiologists bear some of the responsibility for this decline in third-party payers' willingness to reimburse for diagnostic evaluations. In managed care arrangements, audiologists or audiology groups vie for the privilege of providing services to a group of beneficiaries. One of many factors that a managed care organization considers when choosing a provider is what the cost will be to the health plan to contract with that provider. Naturally, the lower the cost, the more desirable the provider is to the health plan. Unfortunately, some audiologists have taken this situation to the extreme by offering diagnostic services to healthcare plans at no charge. In exchange, the healthcare plan refers their insureds to the same audiology providers for hearing aids, which are paid for by the patient, not the health plan.

> ## CONTROVERSIAL POINT
>
> **Some audiologists offer diagnostic services to healthcare plans at no cost in exchange for referrals for hearing aids. This policy gives the impression to referral sources that diagnostic audiology has limited or no value.**

In so doing, the managed care plan may come to believe that the diagnostic audiological evaluation has no value; if it were a thing of value, why would it be given away? And unfortunately, what one managed care plan may arrange with a provider may be imitated by other managed care plans. Negotiations between audiology and managed care plans must lead to a contractual agreement to supply services at a discounted rate in return for referrals, while recognizing the value of the services offered (i.e., fair and reasonable reimbursement for services).

For these reasons, diagnostic audiology as it has been historically taught and practiced will be a shrinking piece of audiology practice in most settings. Indeed, many private practice audiologists already have seen their proportion of revenue shift markedly from the diagnostic income to the income generated from hearing aid sales. It is imperative that training programs continue to provide a thorough grounding in routine and advanced diagnostic procedures, including their anatomical, physiological, and psychoacoustic underpinnings and their interpretation and implications. However, the role of rehabilitation, which was the genesis of the audiology profession and likely will play the major role in its future, cannot be understated.

The future for audiology and audiologists is bright, however, in selected areas of diagnostic assessments. Chief among these is the area of pediatric evaluation, in which audiologists are in the strongest position to be diagnosticians. Assessment of hearing in newborns, infants, and children is a challenge to audiologists and is certainly beyond the reach of nonaudiologists such as nurses or technicians.

With the increasing emergence of universal newborn hearing screening programs, the audiologist has a critical role to play in the diagnosis of hearing impairment: not in the screening itself, which will certainly be performed by hospital personnel, but in the follow-up evaluations of babies who fail their newborn screens. Combining the techniques of objective and behavioral diagnostic test batteries, skilled pediatric audiologists are in a unique position as the sole professional able to appropriately assess young children.

Diagnosis of central auditory processing has been an area to which both audiologists and speech-language pathologists have laid claim, yet it remains an area fraught with questions. Because the diagnosis of CAPD has no "gold standard," persistent, and justified, concerns exist regarding the reliability and particularly the validity of behavioral tests. Although speech-language pathologists and audiologists alike have generally relied on behavioral, language-based measures of central auditory function, with the advent of electrophysiological tests such as MMN, it is possible that audiologists may one day be in the position to assess central function by means of objective tests of auditory perception. Whether such measures would ever become routine clinical procedures, however, is open to question because of the equipment requirements.

Assessment of balance disorders is an area that historically has been in the purview of audiologists, both because balance is an important aspect of the auditory system and because no other professional group has laid claim to the lengthy testing and interpretation involved in electronystagmography evaluations. As balance system function assessment becomes more sophisticated with tools such as dynamic platform posturography (see Chapter 24) and rotary chair testing, it is likely that audiologists can continue to be at the forefront of the diagnosis and research associated with disorders of balance and vestibular function.

Diagnosis of hearing loss as it is related to communication impairment is an important way in which the audiologist's evaluation is superior to the hearing test performed by the nurse in the primary care physician's office. With 85% or more of adult hearing impairment a result of nonmedically treatable conditions (i.e., presbyacusis/noise exposure), the audiologist who can not only diagnose the hearing impairment but also relate the hearing loss to the patient's communication difficulty provides a much greater value. Diagnosis of hearing loss, coupled with subsequent assessment of communication impairment and rehabilitation planning are the services that the adult with acquired hearing loss requires, and it is only the audiologist who is in a position to provide such comprehensive services to the patient.

CONCLUSIONS

In summary, although some of the traditional diagnostic procedures that audiologists have performed for many years may be threatened by issues of reimbursement and competition from nonaudiologists, no professional is better skilled and more knowledgeable than the audiologist to diagnose and provide nonmedical treatment for hearing loss. This is especially true in the areas of pediatric diagnostic evaluation and in the diagnosis of communication impairment for both children and adults as a result of hearing loss. It is imperative that audiologists lay strong claim to these activities, not only in the diagnostic activity itself but also in the research that provides the foundation for the procedures and assessments that are used. Finally, the importance of audiologists advocating for the profession, including reimbursement, licensure, and educational issues, cannot be overstated.

INTRAOPERATIVE NEUROPHYSIOLOGICAL MONITORING

Gary P. Jacobson

Neurophysiological monitoring during surgical procedures began in the late 1970s with the pioneering work of Drs. Clyde Nash and Richard Brown (Nash et al, 1977). These forward-thinking clinical scientists applied basic neurophysiological principles and clinical evoked potential recording techniques to the preservation of spinal cord function during orthopedic procedures. By recording somatosensory evoked potentials intraoperatively from patients undergoing procedures designed to correct scoliotic spinal deformities, it was possible to predict when patients were in the process of developing permanent motor system deficits. In so doing, clinical scientists gained a modality by which spinal cord function could be preserved.

Since that time, clinicians from a myriad of training backgrounds have become involved in this subspecialty of clinical neurophysiology. These backgrounds have included neurology and neurosurgery, anesthesiology, neurophysiology, and audiology. In addition, textbooks that provide comprehensive accounts of the area of neurophysiological monitoring have been published (e.g., Nuwer, 1986). Also, a professional society was conceived called the American Society of Neurophysiological Monitoring (ASNM) that has been in existence since 1990 and whose leadership has included such presidents as Drs. Jack Kartush and Aage R. Moller.

PEARL

The American Society of Neurophysiological Monitoring as been in existence for about 10 years to promote and support the use of monitoring during surgical procedures.

Audiologists' involvement started early because they often possessed the first instrumentation (i.e., evoked potential systems) that could be used to record neurophysiological responses in the operating rooms. The cadre of audiologists and auditory scientists who opened the door for future audiologists in neurophysiological monitoring (NPM) include Aage R. Moller, Daniel Schwartz, Paul R. Kileny, H.B. Calder, and J. Michael Dennis. Soon, audiologists who had interests and expertise only in clinical electrical recordings from the auditory system became engaged in aggressive self-study to make it possible for them to record and interpret data from other sensory (e.g., somesthetic, visual) and motor systems. Accordingly, those individuals whose initial intent was to restrict focus on preservation of the auditory system were soon involved in monitoring activities designed to preserve function of the entire nervous system.

During the interval when rapid growth in the understanding of techniques and limitations of NPM was occurring, questions arose regarding the sensitivity of the ABR for the identification of eighth nerve tumors. In fact, with the advent of gadolinium-enhanced MRI the sensitivity of the ABR for the detection of small vestibular schwannoma (i.e., tumors <1 cm) reportedly decreased from better than 95% to as poor as 40 to 83% (Chandrasekhar et al, 1995; Gordon & Cohen, 1995; Ruckenstein et al, 1996). Clinicians argued that the ABR had limited usefulness if it could not identify, with precision, small tumors that had the best likelihood of being removed without significant loss of functional hearing. Accordingly, many audiologists who witnessed a decrease in referrals for neurodiagnostic ABRs saw an increase in referrals for NPM to help preserve useful hearing during removal of vestibular schwannoma. Thus it is likely that, in the future, electrophysiological activities that will receive widespread use in audiology may be limited to balance function testing (i.e., electronystagmography, rotary chair testing, and dynamic computerized posturography), infant hearing screening (i.e., use of both ABR and otoacoustic emissions techniques), and intraoperative NPM. It is difficult to make predictions about anything in an age when the impact of technical innovations affects us so profoundly and constantly in our business and personal lives. However, it is likely that intraoperative monitoring will assume great importance for those who are interested in developing a career path in clinical neurophysiology.

NPM monitoring has been included in the scope of practice statements of both the American Speech-Language-Hearing Association (ASHA) and the American Academy of Audiology (AAA).* Indeed, many audiologists have incorporated intraoperative NPM of both motor (e.g., seventh nerve) and sensory (e.g., eighth nerve) cranial nerve monitoring into their clinical practices. However, audiologists cannot bill and collect from Medicare for NPM as independent practitioners. In fact, as of this date, the HealthCare Financing Administration (HCFA) has proposed that only a physician may interpret neurophysiological recordings. Furthermore, the physician (i.e., physician other than the surgeon) must be present for the entire procedure.

The problem stems, in part, from the realization that audiologists have, at present, no mechanism by which they can demonstrate entry level competence in the area of NPM. In comparison, physicians (e.g., neurologists) have three mechanisms by which they can become board certified in activities associated with clinical neurophysiology. The American Board of Medical Specialties (ABMS) has sanctioned these board examinations. Two of these boards, the American Board of Clinical Neurophysiology and the American Board of Electrodiagnostic Medicine are affiliated with professional medical societies (i.e., the American Electroencephalography Society and the American Association of Electrodiagnostic Medicine, respectively). The third board examination is administered by the American Board of Psychiatry and Neurology with Added Qualifications in Clinical Neurophysiology, which is not associated with any professional medical association. At this writing (winter 1999), audiologists have no mechanism by which to become board certified in NPM. The ASNM and the legally separate entity, the American

---

*It is important to be clear about the term *scope of practice*. Scope of practice means that a particular activity may be performed by a professional. That an activity falls within the scope of practice of a profession does not infer that every practitioner in that specialty possesses the knowledge and skills to perform that activity, nor does it imply that that profession has sole ownership of that activity.

Board of Neurophysiological Monitoring (ABNM), have announced an intent to offer a two-part examination to practitioners (i.e., including medical doctors and nonmedical doctors) holding, at a minimum, the master's degree. Part I is a written examination that was administered on October 16 and 17, 1999. Part II will be an oral examination. Applicants will have a 3-year period to pass Part II; during this time they will be designated as "board eligible." When applicants pass Part II, they will become "board certified" and receive a certificate as a "Diplomate of the American Board of Neurophysiological Monitoring." In time, it is hoped that this credential will gain credibility in such a manner that diplomates will be able to act as autonomous providers of NPM services.

It is of marginal significance that audiologists also may take an examination offered by the American Board of Registration of Electroencephalographic and Evoked Potential Technologists, Inc. (i.e., ABRET) offered by the American Society of Electroneurodiagnostic Technologists (ASET). Passing the written examinations results in Certification in Neurophysiological Intraoperative Monitoring (CNIM). However, the code of ethics of ASET does not permit interpretation of the data collected, thus greatly limiting the usefulness of the credential for audiologists who work in the operating room independently. Accordingly, it is hoped that, as the twenty first century nears, audiologists will have greater opportunities to demonstrate expertise and proficiency in intraoperative NPM in such a way as to be credentialed to perform, and be reimbursed for, these services. However, to demonstrate proficiency in NPM, the onus has been placed on audiologists to improve the knowledge base in those areas not commonly required or taught in graduate school curricula.

In this regard, for the past 20 years tremendous growth has occurred in the activities that constitute the field of NPM. Intraoperative NPM now encompasses identification of cell structures in, and proximal to, the globus pallidus, intraoperative and extraoperative identification of eloquent cerebral cortex, measurement of cerebral blood flow, cranial nerve monitoring, sensory and motor spinal cord pathway monitoring, nerve root identification, and peripheral nerve monitoring. This list is not inclusive.

Surgeries for which intraoperative NPM has demonstrated efficacy include carotid endarterectomy; epilepsy; neurovascular decompression of cranial nerves V, VII, and VIII; removal of cerebral and brain stem tumors; correction of arteriovenous malformations of the cerebral cortex and brain stem; aneurysm removal; correction of scoliosis and kyphoscoliosis; removal of intramedullary and extramedullary spinal cord tumors and correction or removal of spinal cord arteriovenous malformations; correction of tethered cord; rhizotomy surgery for pediatric patients with cerebral palsy; peripheral nerve repair in the presence of trauma or tumor; and repair of vertebral and pelvic fractures. Yet, this list is not inclusive. New areas where intraoperative NPM may have application include surgery for prostate cancer where bladder and sexual function might be at risk.

Devices that practitioners must be familiar with range from the transcranial Doppler ultrasonogram, magnetic brain stimulators, electrode fabrication, and sophisticated digital evoked potential and electroencephalographic recording systems. Practitioners are expected to understand normal anatomy and physiology of the entire neuraxis, the actions and effects of anesthetic agents on nervous system function, electrophysiological instrumentation, data processing, and technical aspects of physiological monitoring. Further, they are expected to understand methods to record and interpret digitally processed EEG, and evoked responses generated by all sensory and motor systems. Finally, clinicians must understand the surgical procedures that put various sensory and motor structures at risk.

SPECIAL CONSIDERATION

Because few universities teach NPM, audiologists who desire to work in this area need to be trained in apprenticeships.

None of this is taught well, or at all, at either the master's or doctoral level in most universities. Accordingly, NPM skills will eventually need to be learned in apprenticeship settings and through independent study. After being involved in the field of NPM for 15 years, it has become clear that the operating room is the last place where the incompetent belong. An incompetent monitorist complicates surgeries at best, and, at worst, can put a patient's nervous system and life in jeopardy. A competent monitorist may play an integral role in the delivery of healthcare to a patient, have a direct effect on that patient's quality of life, and may earn a good living in the process. Thus it is likely that, in the future, audiologists who intend to become engaged in NPM will seek out graduate school coursework to include intensive study in the basic sciences. It might be possible for future monitorists to obtain practical experience through paid internships. That is, throughout the United States a number of Centers have been willing, for a fee, to accept qualified interns who wished to learn the practice of NPM.

CONCLUSIONS

As a new millennium approaches, audiologists with an interest and demonstrated expertise in NPM will hopefully continue to effect positive changes in the outcomes of surgeries as independent providers.

AUDIOLOGISTS' ROLE IN UNIVERSAL NEWBORN HEARING SCREENING

Kathryn A. Albright

Establishing early hearing detection and intervention (EHDI) programs has been one of the focused objectives of audiology for more than 40 years. The road traveled from the early 1960s by Dr. Marion Downs to the programs in place today is remarkable. However, many challenges are ahead for audiologists. To date (early 1999) only 20 states have legislation mandating universal newborn hearing screening. In fact, audiologists are often faced with significant resistance when attempting to implement universal newborn hearing screening (UNHS) programs without a legislative initiative. Coupled with a lack of understanding for the importance of early identification, there continues to be only minimum financial reimbursement for many aspects of the EHDI process. Three significant challenges for the continuing evolution of successful UNHS programs in the future will revolve around (1) appropriate screening measures that provide beneficial service for newborns and their families, (2) understanding technology, and (3) providing relevant outcomes measures.

To identify hearing loss in a newborn baby adequately from a procedural and cost perspective, the method must be quick, effective, accurate, and inexpensive. It has taken almost 40 years to overcome the challenges of development and refinement of techniques to detect hearing loss in newborns and infants. With the advent of microchip technology, ABR and OAE equipment has became portable and automated, further reducing many of the challenges of interpretation and manageability. Advances in technology for universal neonatal hearing screening now make it possible to carry out effective programs.

Outcome measures evaluate the results of a process or technique. In newborn hearing screening, they answer the question, "Does early identification of hearing loss benefit the baby?" Evidence is strong that such early identification is of great benefit to the baby, refuting previous criticisms that early identification of hearing loss is not efficacious (Allen, 1986; Yoshinaga-Itano et al, 1998). A challenge for the future is to educate those who are not yet aware of or who do not understand the possible implications.

Role Redefinition

As long-time advocates for universal newborn hearing screening, audiologists are uniquely qualified to play a key role in EHDI programs. They have the clinical training, expertise in the diagnosis and management of hearing impairment, and have or know of the resources needed to assist families once hearing loss is identified in infants.

Historically, audiologists functioned as screeners in many programs because audiological expertise was needed to operate the equipment and interpret the data. Today, automated ABR and OAE screening formats do not require that audiologists act as screening personnel. In fact, in all of the position and consensus statements concerning early identification of hearing loss, audiologists are clearly designated as diagnostic clinical service providers and as program supervisors rather than as screening staff. Although some audiologists continue to function as primary screeners, others are acting in a supervisory capacity in the screening arena and are providing clinical services either for rescreening or for the diagnostic audiological evaluation.

In the future it is expected that continuing technological advancement will further remove audiologists from being front-line screeners and into supervisory roles. One potential repercussion created by the role change from screener to supervisor is that as other trained professionals and technicians perform screenings, the audiologist will become unfamiliar with and removed from the day-to-day screening program. A possible result is for the audiologist to becoming "out of touch" with the technology, screening staff, and the families whose babies are being screened. As is true for all professionals in supervisory roles, audiologists in neonatal screening programs will need to take measures not to lose contact with the day-to-day operations of their programs.

SPECIAL CONSIDERATION

Although audiologists have the training and skills, in the future they typically will not perform the day-to-day activities of the screening program. Rather, they will act in a supervisory capacity.

As part of their expanding supervisory role in the future, audiologists will have to address quality assurance issues such as screener competence, program outcome measures, and cost containment. At the same time, communicating and maintaining visibility in the nursery environment will be necessary. This will allow both screening and nursing staff to recognize the audiologist's contribution to a successful program. Physicians and nurses seek to ensure that patients are well cared for. Once it is understood that screening for hearing loss is more than simply the procedure that takes place in the hospital, the audiologist's supervision and program management skills will be recognized and valued. However, the acknowledgment of value will not be recognized unless the audiologist establishes a presence in the day-to-day program operation.

Financial Obstacles

Today, and probably even more in the future, financial reimbursement will be the most difficult obstacle for any facility to overcome to implement hearing screening programs. Many significant changes in the healthcare arena over the past decade have created a paradigm of creating services that will meet most needs at the lowest cost. Little incentive exists to add new programs, especially those that do not break even or generate significant income. Despite all the evidence that newborn hearing screening is "the right thing to do," administrators must decide which "right thing " is most important and yet economically viable. Audiologists in the future will find an increasing need to have business skills to negotiate managed care contracts successfully and partner with insurance companies to provide services that are considered valuable and reimbursable. Likewise, designing effective and cost-efficient hearing screening programs that meet the requirements of current and future healthcare paradigms will continue to be a necessity.

Relationship with other Professionals

Not surprisingly, the nursing profession has turned an interested eye to newborn hearing screening. After all, nurses have been in neonatal nurseries since their early inception and are familiar with a variety of screening tools. When nurses act as the primary screener, audiologists will need to ensure that the program design includes more than just the birth-screening component—that appropriate referral and follow-up take place with those who are identified with hearing loss. The need to market and educate other medical practitioners with hospital administrators to the services and roles that audiologists play in UNHS will be greater. Equipped with the JCIH (1995) and

NIH (1993) statements that support a supervisory function in these programs, audiologists are in a position to assist hospitals that do not have these components in place.

Legislation and Consensus Statements

Many exciting developments have taken place for EHDI programs in recent times. Consensus statements (American Academy of Audiology, 1988; American Academy of Pediatrics, 1995, 1998; NIH, 1993) supporting universal screening of all newborns with a screening technology are now available, making many goals attainable. Indeed, research has confirmed that early identification is beneficial to both infant and family. Nevertheless, obstacles still impede screening all infants for hearing loss born in this nation. Such obstacles will drive audiologists in the future to seek creative solutions and develop new partnerships outside the profession to overcome those remaining problems.

To make universal newborn hearing screening a reality for all babies born in this nation in the future, legislation requiring and funding universal newborn hearing screening must be drafted and passed. While leaving room for "creative local solutions," the language of the legislation must clearly spell out the appropriate components of good screening programs and they must clearly define the role of audiologists as program supervisors and diagnostic service providers. Twenty states currently have legislation for universal newborn screening, and 20 more have legislation pending. The burden to build relationships with local, state, and national legislators must be shouldered by audiologists to secure a defined position in the newborn hearing screening arena.

CONCLUSIONS

Audiologists have long advocated early detection of hearing loss, and in recent times effective technology has been made available to provide effective programs. These advances have allowed the audiologist, who was initially functioning as a bedside screener, to focus more on the clinically challenging components of the EHDI process, namely the diagnostic and intervention components. The future role of the audiologist will depend on what current audiologists do and whether programs managed by audiologists are demonstrated to be superior to others. The future of audiology will be secured in the newborn hearing screening arena if the following critical components are achieved and maintained: (1) audiologists are able to secure positions as supervisors and diagnostic service providers; (2) links are forged with the legislative community to write mandates that require audiology input; (3) critics are educated regarding the life-changing benefit provided to the early identified child; and (4) insurance and healthcare providers are convinced that audiologists' services of are valuable enough to reimburse. Audiologists should act now to secure a defined role in neonatal hearing screening by training audiology students to understand the importance of their role in neonatal screening and by clarifying all the objectives and guidelines for competent audiological services needed in the care of newborns.

CENTRAL AUDITORY PROCESSING DISORDERS

Deborah Moncrieff

It is well established that the standard audiogram fails to reflect the entire audiological diagnosis for patients routinely seen in a clinical setting. As an example, some patients complain of difficulties with speech intelligibility or hearing in the presence of background noise, yet they have normal audiometric results. In the past these patients have been labeled as having obscure auditory dysfunction (OAD) (Saunders & Haggard, 1989). The term *OAD* itself addresses the inability of the diagnsotic procedures used in standard audiological practice to identify the nature of this type of hearing disorder successfully. In other cases dispensing audiologists have been confronted with adults who receive successful amplification from hearing aids but who continue to experience significant problems understanding speech. Similarly, children who demonstrate disorders of phonology, language, or reading are often referred to the audiologist to rule out hearing loss and are found to have normal auditory sensitivity. All three of these types of patients, the OAD adult, the amplified adult with speech perception problems, and a number of the children with language or reading disorders, are likely to share common traits among a variety of auditory processing measures.

Even though many of the tests have been available for many years, most audiologists do not routinely perform the diagnostic tests that identify specific components of the disorders experienced by these patients. As a result, little is being done to address the problems caused by their auditory processing disorder, generically referred to as disorders of central auditory processing. As many authors have previously stated throughout this book, there appears to be a rich future in diagnostic audiology in the development and application of procedures to assess central auditory processing.

ASHA (1996) defined central auditory processes as those responsible for sound localization and lateralization, auditory discrimination, auditory pattern recognition, the temporal aspects of audition (temporal resolution, temporal masking, temporal integration, and temporal ordering), auditory performance with competing acoustic signals, and auditory performance with degraded acoustic signals. To assess an individual thought to have a CAPD properly, a battery of assessments to address each of these processes individually must be used. As detailed in Chapter 15 of this volume, diagnostic tests of central auditory processing must begin with carefully designed questionnaires that include the patient's case history and the observations and comments from significant individuals in the patient's daily life. The questionnaires should then be used to determine which specific assessments would best target the problems the patient is having and define the battery that the audiologist will use.

Many of the CAPD test batteries recommended for diagnostic purposes were developed or extensively evaluated by audiologists or researchers trained in auditory processes. Several have been used on patients with known lesions of the central auditory system to validate the test's sensitivity in identifying disorders related to those regions of the brain. Some of these tests can be used to reasonably evaluate children older than 8, and some screening measures are helpful with children as young as 3 years old. An important goal for future research is to develop assessment tools for a comprehensive evaluation of both children and adults and, most especially, for the evaluation of children less than the age of 8. Too many children are identified only after they have begun to fall behind in elementary school, even though parents and preschool teachers may have suspected a central auditory processing problem at a much younger age.

Electrophysiology has been used to characterize normal development in the central auditory system and could ultimately be used to help identify children at risk for language and reading disorders. Much of the evoked potential research has focused on normal and abnormal responses to very short duration pure tone stimuli, but recent studies have used synthesized and natural speech to examine central auditory responses to more complex stimuli. These procedures can measure the preattentive responses centered around N100 (i.e., MMN) and other evoked responses, which can occur as a positivity centered at 100, 200, or 800 ms after stimulus presentation or as a negativity occurring at 200 to 400 ms after stimulus presentation. Results have demonstrated that changes in latency and amplitude occur in several of the waveforms from birth to adolescence (Eggermont et al, 1997; Kraus et al, 1993; Sharma et al, 1997; Shibasaki & Miyazaki, 1992; Tonnquist-Uhlen, 1996a). It is expected that future studies in this area will be fruitful in identifying children and adults whose auditory responses reflect either maturational delays or disorders in processing.

Parallel work on analyzing the processing skills of children with cochlear implants (Deggouj & Gersdorff, 1998; Eggermont et al, 1997; Kileny et al, 1997) and on the language acquisition skills of infants and very young children (Mills & Neville, 1997; Molfese & Molfese, 1985; 1997) also promise to contribute significant electrophysiological evidence that will help the audiologist understand how speech is processed into language through the central auditory system. As more of these electrophysiological measures are characterized and normalized on populations across the developmental range, they should become part of the standard clinical practice, just as the ABR is now considered part of routine audiological evaluation. Abnormalities in electrophysiological results will be able to provide powerful confirmation of behavioral measures within a comprehensive CAPD evaluation. With their training in the application and interpretation of auditory electrophysiological measures, audiologists are the professionals best prepared to perform these types of evaluations.

Topographic brain mapping techniques are making it possible to examine not only the latency and amplitude of late cortical responses but also to graphically display the region of the brain in which maximal activation is distributed (Tonnquist-Uhlen, 1996b). Latency measures of the P100 have been used to assess central auditory maturation in cochlear implant patients (Eggermont et al, 1997), and P300 measures have been used to reflect behavioral changes after treatment in children with CAPD (Jirsa, 1992). Once the latencies and

regional distributions of normal evoked potentials to pure tone and speech stimuli are reliably established across the span of normal development, it will be possible to use electrophysiological measures to better determine the nature of an auditory processing disorder. In adults who have difficulties listening in the presence of background noise or who demonstrate poor speech intelligibility, electrophysiology and topographic brain mapping will provide important evidence that a CAPD is present and will help to identify the region of the brain that is involved (Jerger et al, 1995). It will be well within the scope of practice for the audiologist to provide the assessment and interpretation of electrophysiological results to direct remediation and to provide outcome measures after rehabilitation.

Another potentially powerful tool for diagnostic assessment of central auditory processing is fMRI (see Chapter 7). Availability and expense may limit fMRI use in some areas, but where it is available, it promises to provide important information on brain regions that respond differently during speech processing tasks in individuals with suspected auditory processing disorders. Although fMRI research is the newest area examining these questions, it is rapidly detailing which regions of the brain are involved in processing complex auditory stimuli. To date, most fMRI studies have examined activation levels in the auditory cortex after speech input to determine hemispheric lateralization for language and measure degree of activation (Binder et al, 1996). However, recent fMRI studies are beginning to explore subcortical regions of activation after auditory stimuli (Guimaraes et al, 1998). Together with other imaging techniques such as PET and SPECT, fMRI will not only yield important information about which regions of the brain are predominantly activated by specific central auditory processes but will also help to characterize the levels of activation and function the activation represents. In this way, differences in activation after input to one ear or the other can be identified, and difficulties with processing particular types of language-based stimuli can be analyzed. It would not be surprising if fMRI eventually becomes a standard tool for differential diagnosis of CAPD in adults and children.

Once an individual is identified as having a CAPD, providing remediation information and strategies is vital. A number of techniques are available that are currently being used to assist in remediation of CAPD, especially for children diagnosed with phonological processing problems or reading disorders. Many of these techniques have yielded successful outcomes for a number of patients, but few studies by researchers in auditory science have confirmed the benefits by taking preintervention and postintervention measures of auditory processing skills in these children (Jirsa, 1992). Confirmation of the remedial benefits of these techniques will provide powerful evidence that a particular intervention can be successfully used with patients whose CAPD fits particular profiles. More studies in this important area of research are needed and are likely to be conducted in facilities where electrophysiological and imaging techniques are readily available.

Future prospects for evaluating and treating CAPDs in both children and adults look promising. Emerging combinations of behavioral, electrophysiological, and imaging techniques will provide important information about how individuals process complex acoustic stimuli. Once norms are established and studies demonstrate differences in children and adults with central auditory processing difficulties, standard clinical practice can improve the specificity with which it can diagnose a person's CAPD. After specific disorders of central auditory processing are appropriately identified, remediation techniques can be developed and initiated for treatment. Throughout the course of treatment, outcome measures derived behaviorally, electrophysiologically, or through imaging methods will confirm which remediation procedures provide the best results with each specific procedure. All of these factors will ultimately make it possible for most audiologists to diagnose and treat persons with CAPD with confidence and efficiency.

CONCLUSIONS

A variety of behavioral, physiological and electrophysiological procedures sensitive to central auditory processes have been enumerated in many chapters throughout this book. As more audiology programs add CAPD assessment to the teaching curricula, emerging clinicians will be better equipped to include the battery in standard practice. With specific training in the neuroanatomy of the central auditory system, an understanding of the physiology involved in the processing of both simple and complex acoustic stimuli, and clinical skills in the application of behavioral and electrophysiological tests, audiologists are uniquely qualified to make diagnostic decisions when CAPD is involved.

REFERENCES

ALLEN, T.E. (1986). Patterns of academic achievement among hearing-impaired students: 1974 and 1983. In: A.N. Schildroth, & M.A. Karchmer (Eds.), *Deaf children in America* (pp. 161–206). Boston: College-Hill Press.

AMERICAN ACADEMY OF AUDIOLOGY. (1988). Position statement: Early identification of hearing loss in children. *Audiology Today, 1*;1–2.

AMERICAN ACADEMY OF PEDIATRICS. (1995). Joint Committee position statement: Infant Hearing 1994. *Pediatrics, 95*;1.

AMERICAN HOSPITAL ASSOCIATION. (1996). American Hospital Association Resource Center (E-mail inquiry and response).

AMERICAN SPEECH-LANGUAGE-HEARING ASSOCIATION. (1996). *Central auditory processing: Current status of research implications for clinical practice. Task force on central auditory processing consensus development.* Rockville, MD.

ANON. (1993). *Early identification of hearing impairment in infants and young children. Report of the National Institutes of Health Consensus Development Conference.* Bethesda, MD.

BARAN, J., LONG, R., MUSIEK, F., & OMMAYA, A. (1988). Topographic mapping of brain electrical activity in the assessment of central auditory nervous system pathology. *The American Journal of Otology, 9*(Supplement);72–6.

BELLIS, T.J. (1996). *Assessment and management of central auditory processing disorders in the educational setting.* San Diego, CA: Singular Publishing Group, Inc.

BINDER, J.R., FROST, J.A., HAMMEKE, T.A., RAO, S.M., & COX, R.W. (1996). Function of the left planum temporale in auditory and linguistic processing. *Brain, 119*;1239–1247.

BONFILS, P., UZIEL, A., & PUJOL, R. (1988). Screening for auditory dysfunction in infants by evoked otoacoustic emissions. *Archives of Otolaryngology–Head and Neck Surgery, 114*;887–890.

CHANDRASEKHAR, S.S., BRACKMANN, D.E., & DEVGAN, K.K. (1995). Utility of auditory brain stem audiometry in diagnosis of acoustic neuromas. *American Journal of Otology, 16*;63–67.

CHMIEL, R., & JERGER, J. (1996). Hearing aid use, central auditory disorder, and hearing handicap in elderly persons. *Journal of the American Academy of Audiology, 7*;190–202.

COX, R., & ALEXANDER, G. (1995). The abbreviated profile of hearing aid benefit. *Ear and Hearing, 16*;176–186.

DEGGOUJ, N., & GERSDORFF, M. (1998) Imaging and cochlear implant. *Acta Otorhinolaryngologica Belgium, 52*(2);133–143.

DIVENYI, P., & HAUPT, K. (1997). Audiological correlates of speech understanding deficits in elderly listeners with mild to moderate hearing loss III. Factor representation. *Ear and Hearing, 18*;189–201.

DOWNS, M. (1990). Twentieth century pediatric audiology: Prologue to the 21st. *Seminars in Hearing, 11*(4); 408–411.

EGGERMONT, J.J., PONTON, C.W., DON, M., WARING, M.D., & KWONG, B. (1997). Maturational delays in cortical evoked potentials in cochlear implant users. *Acta Otolaryngologica (Stockholm), 117*;161–163.

FIRE, K., LESNER, S., & NEWMAN, C. (1991). Hearing handicap as a function of central auditory abilities in the elderly. *American Journal of Otology, 12*;105–108.

GATEHOUSE, S. (1991). The contribution of central auditory factors to auditory disability. *Acta Otolaryngologica,* (Supplement)*476*;182–188.

GORDON, M.L., & COHEN, N.L. (1995). Efficacy of auditory brain stem response as a screening test for small acoustic neuromas. *American Journal of Otology, 16*;136–139.

GUIMARAES, A.R., MELCHER, J.R., TALAVAGE, T.M., BAKER, J.R., LEDDEN, P., ROSEN, B.R., KIANG, N. Y. S., FULLERTON, B.C., & WEISSKOFF, R.M. (1998). Imaging subcortical auditory activity in humans. *Human Brain Mapping, 6*;33–41.

HECOX, K., & GALAMBOS, R. (1974). Brainstem auditory evoked responses in human infants and adults. *Archives of Otolaryngology, 99*;30–33.

HERNING, R., JONES, R., & HUNT, J. (1987). Speech event related potentials reflect linguistic content and processing level. *Brain and Language, 30*;116–29.

JERGER, J., ALFORD, B., LEW, H., RIVERA, V., & CHMIEL, R. (1995). Dichotic listening, event-related potentials, and interhemispheric transfer in the elderly. *Ear and Hearing, 16*;482–498.

JERGER, J., STACH, B., JOHNSON, K., LOISELLE, L., & JERGER, S. (1990). Patterns of abnormality in dichotic listening. In: J. Jensen (Ed.), *Presbyacusis and other age related aspects.* Copenhagen: Stougaard Jensen.

JERGER, J., & JORDAN, C. (1992). Age increases asymmetry on a cued-listening task. *Ear and Hearing, 13*;272–277.

JERGER, J., SILMAN, S., LEW, H., & CHMIEL, R. (1993). Case studies in binaural interference: Converging evidence from behavioral and electrophysiologic measures. *Journal of the American Academy of Audiology, 4*;122–131.

JIRSA, R.E. (1992). The clinical utility of the P3 AERP in children with auditory processing disorders. *Journal of Speech and Hearing Research, 35*(4);903–912.

JOHNSON, M., MAXON, A., WHITE, K., & VOHR, B. (1993). Operating a hospital-based universal newborn hearing screening program using transient evoked otoacoustic emissions. *Seminars in Hearing, 14*(1);46–56.

KEITH, R. (1977). *Central auditory dysfunction.* New York: Grune & Stratton.

KILENY, P., & BERRY, D. (1983). Selective impairment of late vertex and middle latency auditory-evoked responses in multiply handicapped infants. In: G. Mencher, & S. Gerber (Eds.), *The multiply handicapped hearing-impaired child* (pp. 233–258). New York: Grune & Stratton.

KILENY, P.R., BOERST, A., & ZWOLAN, T. (1997) Cognitive evoked potentials to speech and tonal stimuli in children with implants. *Otolaryngology–Head and Neck Surgery, 117*(3Pt1); 161–169.

KRAUS, N., McGEE, T., CARRELL, T., SHARMA, A., MICCO, A., & NICOL, T. (1993). Speech-evoked cortical potentials in children. *Journal of the American Academy of Audiology, 4*(4); 238–248.

KRAUS, N., McGEE, T., CARRELL, T, SHARMA, A., & NICOL, T. (1995). Mismatch negativity to speech stimuli in school-age children. *EEG and Clinical Neurophysiology,* (Supplement) 44;211–217.

MARTIN, G., WHITEHEAD, M., & LONSBURY-MARTIN, B. (1990). Potential of evoked otoacoustic emissions for infant hearing screening. *Seminars in Hearing, 11*(2);186–203.

McCANDLESS, G., & PARKIN, J. (1979). Hearing aid performance relative to site of lesion. *Otolaryngology–Head and Neck Surgery, 87*;871–875.

MEHL, A., & THOMPSON, V. (1998). Newborn hearing screening:the great omission. *Pediatrics, 191*;1–6.

MERZENICH, M., JENKINS, W., JOHNSTON, P., SCHREINER, C., MILLER, S., & TALLAL, P. (1996). Temporal processing deficits of language-learning impaired children ameliorated by training. *Science, 271*,77–81.

MILLS, D.L., & NEVILLE, H.J. (1997). Electrophysiological studies of language and language impairment. *Seminars in Pediatric Neurology, 4*(2);125–134.

MOLFESE, D.L., & MOLFESE, V.J. (1985). Electrophysiological indices of auditory discrimination in newborn infants: The bases for predicting later language development? *Infant Behavior and Development, 8*;197–211.

MOLFESE, D.L. & MOLFESE, V.J. (1997). Discrimination of language skills at five years of age using event-related potentials recorded at birth. *Developmental Neuropsychology, 13*;135–156.

MUSIEK, F., & PINHEIRO, M. (1985). Dichotic speech tests in the detection of central auditory dysfunction. In M. Pinheiro & F. Musiek (Eds.). *Assessment of central auditory dysfunction; Foundations and clinical correlates* (pp. 201–219). Baltimore: Williams & Wilkins.

NAESSENS, B., GORDTS, F., CLEMENT, P., & BUISSERET, T. (1996). Reevaluation of the ABR in the diagnosis of CPA tumors in the MRI-era. *Acta Oto-Rhino-Laryngologica Belgica, 50;* 99–102.

NASH JR., C.L., LORIG, R.A., & SCHATZINGER, L.A., et al. (1977). Spinal cord monitoring during operative treatment of the spine. *Clinical Orthopedics and Related Research, 126*;100–105.

NATIONAL INSTITUTE OF HEALTH. (1993). Consensus statement. Identification of Hearing Impairment in Infants and Young Children, Bethesda, MD. *NIH, 11*;1–24.

NEWMAN, C., JACOBSON, G., HUG, G., WEINSTEIN, B., & MALINOFF, R. (1991). Practical method for quantifying hearing aid benefit in older adults. *Journal of the American Academy of Audiology, 2*;70–75.

NUWER, M.R. (1986). *Evoked potential monitoring in the operating room.* New York: Raven Press.

PICTON, T.W., DURIEUX-SMITH, A., CHAMPAGNE, S.C., WHITTINGHAM, J., MORAN, L.M., GIGUERE, C., & BEAUREGARD, Y. (1998). Objective evaluation of aided thresholds using the auditory steady-state responses. *Journal of the American Academy of Audiology, 9*;315–331.

RUCKENSTEIN, M., CUEVA, R., MORRISON, D., & PRESS, G. (1996). A prospective study of ABR and MRI in the screening for vestibular schwannomas. *American Journal of Otolaryngology, 17;* 317–320.

SAUNDERS, G.H., & HAGGARD, M.P. (1989). The clinical assessment of obscure auditory dysfunction - 1. Auditory and psychological factors. *Ear and Hearing, 10*(3);200–208.

SHARMA, A., KRAUS, N., McGEE, T.J., & NICOL, T.G. (1997). Developmental changes in P1 and N1 central auditory responses elicited by consonant-vowel syllables. *Electroencephalography and Clinical Neurophysiology, 104*(6);540–545.

SHIBASAKI, H., & MIYAZAKI, M. (1992). Event-related potential studies in infants and children. *Journal of Clinical Neurophysiology, 9*(3);408–418.

SILMAN, S., SILVERMAN, C.A., EMMER, M.B., & GELFAND, S.A. (1992). Adult onset auditory deprivation. *Journal of the American Academy of Audiology, 3*;390–396.

TONNQUIST-UHLEN, I. (1996a). Topography of auditory-evoked cortical potentials in children with severe language impairment. *Scandinavian Audiology Supplement, 44*;1–40.

TONNQUIST-UHLEN, I. (1996b). Topography of auditory-evoked long-latency potentials in children with severe language impairment: The P2 and N2 components. *Ear and Hearing, 17*(4);314–326.

WILSON, D., TALBOT, J., & MILLS, L. (1997). A critical appraisal of the role of ABR and MRI in AN diagnosis. *American Journal of Otology, 18*;673–681.

WRIGHT, B., LOMBARDINO, L., KING, W., PURANIK, C., LEONARD, C., & MERZENICH, M. (1997). Deficits in auditory temporal and spectral resolution in language-impaired children. *Nature, 387*,176–178.

YOSHINAGA-ITANO, C., SEDEY, A., COULTER, D., et al. (1998). Language of early- and later-identified children with hearing loss. *Pediatrics, 102*;1161–1171.

INDEX